THOMSON'S

SPECIAL VETERINARY PATHOLOGY

THOMSON'S SPECIAL VETERINARY PATHOLOGY

SECOND EDITION

William W. Carlton, D.V.M., Ph.D.

Diplomate, American College of Veterinary Pathologists
Leslie Morton Hutchings Distinguished Professor Emeritus
of Veterinary Pathology
Department of Veterinary Pathobiology
School of Veterinary Medicine
Purdue University
West Lafayette, Indiana

M. Donald McGavin, M.V.Sc., Ph.D., M.A.C.V.Sc.

Diplomate, American College of Veterinary Pathologists
Professor
Director of Necropsy Laboratories
Department of Pathology
College of Veterinary Medicine
University of Tennessee
Knoxville, Tennessee

with **828** *illustrations*

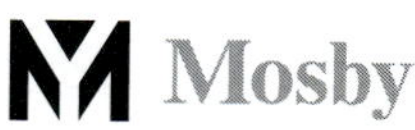

St. Louis Baltimore Boston Carlsbad Chicago Naples New York Philadelphia Portland
London Madrid Mexico City Singapore Sydney Tokyo Toronto Wiesbaden

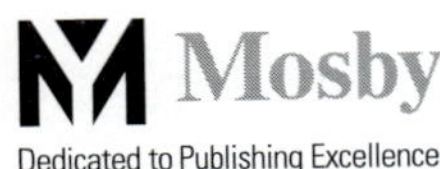

Dedicated to Publishing Excellence

A Times Mirror
Company

Publisher: Don Ladig
Editor: Linda L. Duncan
Developmental Editor: Jo Salway
Project Manager: Christopher J. Baumle
Production Editor: David Orzechowski
Editing and Production: University Graphics Production Services
Manufacturing Supervisor: Linda Ierardi
Designer: Sheilah Barrett

SECTION EDITION

Printed in the United States of America
Composition by University Graphics, Inc.
Printing/binding by Maple Vail—York

Mosby–Year Book, Inc.
11830 Westline Industrial Drive
St. Louis, Missouri 63146

International Standard Book Number 0-8016-7968-0

95 96 97 98 / 9 8 7 6 5 4 3 2 1

Contributors

Helen M. Acland, B.V.Sc.
Diplomate, American College of Veterinary Pathologists
Associate Professor of Pathology and Head, Laboratory of Large Animal Pathology
School of Veterinary Medicine
University of Pennsylvania
New Bolton Center
Kennett Square, Pennsylvania

Charles C. Capen, D.V.M., Ph.D.
Diplomate, American College of Veterinary Pathologists
Professor and Chairman
Department of Veterinary Biosciences
College of Veterinary Medicine;
Professor of Endocrinology
Department of Internal Medicine
College of Medicine
The Ohio State University
Columbus, Ohio

William W. Carlton, D.V.M., Ph.D.
Diplomate, American College of Veterinary Pathologists
Leslie Morton Hutchings Distinguished Professor Emeritus of Veterinary Pathology
Department of Veterinary Pathobiology
School of Veterinary Medicine
Purdue University
West Lafayette, Indiana

Anthony W. Confer, D.V.M., Ph.D.
Diplomate, American College of Veterinary Pathologists
Professor and Head
Department of Veterinary Pathology
College of Veterinary Medicine
Oklahoma State University
Stillwater, Oklahoma

John M. Cullen, V.M.D., Ph.D.
Diplomate, American College of Veterinary Pathologists
Professor
Department of Microbiology, Pathology, and Parasitology
School of Veterinary Medicine
North Carolina State University
Raleigh, North Carolina

Cecil E. Doige, D.V.M., Ph.D.†
Western College of Veterinary Medicine
University of Saskatchewan
Saskatoon, Saskatchewan

Richard R. Dubielzig, D.V.M.
Diplomate, American College of Veterinary Pathologists
Associate Professor
Department of Pathobiological Sciences
School of Veterinary Medicine
University of Wisconsin
Madison, Wisconsin

Victor J. Ferrans, M.D., Ph.D.
Diplomate, American College of Veterinary Pathologists
Chief, Ultrastructure Section
Pathology Branch
National Heart, Lung, and Blood Institute
National Institutes of Health
Bethesda, Maryland

Ann M. Hargis, D.V.M., M.S.
Diplomate, American College of Veterinary Pathologists
Director, DermatoDiagnostics
Edmonds, Washington;
Affiliate Associate Professor
Department of Comparative Medicine
School of Medicine
University of Washington
Seattle, Washington

Alfonso López, M.V.Z., M.Sc., Ph.D.
Associate Professor
Department of Pathology and Microbiology
Atlantic Veterinary College
University of Prince Edward Island
Charlottetown, Prince Edward Island
Canada

N. James MacLachlan, B.V.Sc., M.S., Ph.D.
Diplomate, American College of Veterinary Pathologists
Professor
Department of Veterinary Pathology, Microbiology, and Immunology
School of Veterinary Medicine
University of California
Davis, California

†Deceased.

M. Donald McGavin, M.V.Sc., Ph.D., M.A.C.V.Sc.
Diplomate, American College of Veterinary Pathologists
Professor
Director of Necropsy Laboratories
Department of Pathology
College of Veterinary Medicine
University of Tennessee
Knoxville, Tennessee

Roger J. Panciera, D.V.M., Ph.D.
Diplomate, American College of Veterinary Pathologists
Professor
Department of Veterinary Pathology
College of Veterinary Medicine
Oklahoma State University
Stillwater, Oklahoma

James A. Render, D.V.M., Ph.D.
Diplomate, American College of Veterinary Pathologists
Associate Professor
Department of Veterinary Pathology
College of Veterinary Medicine
Michigan State University
East Lansing, Michigan

Gene P. Searcy, D.V.M., Ph.D.
Diplomate, American College of Veterinary Pathologists
Professor
Department of Pathology
Western College of Veterinary Medicine
University of Saskatchewan
Saskatoon, Saskatchewan

Ralph W. Storts, D.V.M., Ph.D.
Diplomate, American College of Veterinary Pathologists
Professor
Department of Veterinary Pathology
College of Veterinary Medicine
Texas A & M University
College Station, Texas

Herbert J. Van Kruiningen, D.V.M., Ph.D., M.D.
Diplomate, American College of Veterinary Pathologists
Professor
Department of Pathobiology
University of Connecticut
Storrs, Connecticut

John F. Van Vleet, D.V.M., Ph.D.
Diplomate, American College of Veterinary Pathologists
Professor
Associate Dean of Academic Affairs
Department of Veterinary Pathobiology
School of Veterinary Medicine
Purdue University
West Lafayette, Indiana

Steven E. Weisbrode, V.M.D., Ph.D.
Diplomate, American College of Veterinary Pathologists
Professor
Department of Veterinary Biosciences
College of Veterinary Medicine
The Ohio State University
Columbus, Ohio

Preface

It is now 8 years since the first edition of *Special Veterinary Pathology* appeared. In this second edition, the editors and authors were committed to the goal of the first edition, which was "to provide the undergraduate veterinary student . . . with a textbook comprehensive enough to meet every need in veterinary pathology." Thus, the challenges to the authors have been to identify that information of primary importance and, because of space and cost limitations, to reduce or omit other material. An additional objective of the editors, authors, and publisher of this second edition was to produce a well-balanced book at a reasonable price. To achieve this end, some changes have been made. For a better balance in material, some chapters were shortened and others have been lengthened. Individual citations in the text were removed and the number of references reduced, but the core references and suggested reading lists have been retained.

In order to give the student a basic understanding of specific organ systems, all chapters now include a review of anatomy and a description of the response to injury of that system. Details of pathogenesis of individual diseases have been expanded also. Illustrations have been increased and the quality improved. Arrows, letters, and other indicators have been added to many illustrations, and most figure legends have been expanded. A standardized format has been used for the legends in an attempt to facilitate students' understanding of the lesions illustrated.

We have standardized nomenclatures using nomina anatomica veterinaria (NAV) for anatomic structures and the most current bacteriologic terminology. Older or previously used terms for bacteria have been included in parentheses where it was thought that this would be advantageous.

We considered changing the name of the book from *Special Veterinary Pathology* to Systemic Veterinary Pathology. The word "special" in the European sense of "systemic" is not always well understood. However, the decision, made with the concurrence of Ms. Linda Duncan, Executive Editor, of Mosby was to retain the name originally proposed by Dr. R. G. Thomson and also to incorporate his name into the title, in recognition of his contributions to veterinary pathology.

The editors have many people to thank for help and support. We are grateful to our respective departments for their support and especially to Mrs. Carolyn Arnold and Mrs. Paula Vitello of the office staff of the Department of Veterinary Pathobiology, Purdue University, for their help in producing the manuscripts and disks for the chapters and to Ms. Emily Swafford of the Department of Pathology, University of Tennessee, for her help in editing the photographs and legends.

We would like to extend our appreciation to Ms. Jo Salway, Associate Developmental Editor, and Ms. Linda Duncan, Executive Editor, of Mosby for smoothing the way and ensuring a quality production and also to our wives Jean and Beverley for their support and patience during the project.

We are well aware that some errors and inaccuracies may have found their way into the text. We hope that the users of the book will bring these to our attention so that we can make any needed corrections in the third edition.

WILLIAM W. CARLTON
M. DONALD McGAVIN

Dr. Cecil E. Doige
An Appreciation

Dr. Cecil E. Doige, who died in October 1992, was the author of the Skeletal System chapter in the first edition of *Special Veterinary Pathology*. A Gold Medal recipient upon graduation from the Ontario Veterinary College in 1959, Dr. Doige later obtained a Ph.D. in pathology at the Western College of Veterinary Medicine, University of Saskatchewan. During his subsequent career, he became known for his expertise in pathology of the skeletal system. He trained many graduate students, published numerous scientific papers, and received several teaching awards, including being named Master Teacher by the University of Saskatchewan. He served terms as Head of the Department of Veterinary Pathology and Associate Dean of Research at the Western College of Veterinary Medicine, University of Saskatchewan. In addition to his contributions to the teaching of Veterinary Pathology, Dr. Doige was respected as an unassuming, quiet, thoughtful man who was always a fair person and a gentleman.

Gene P. Searcy

Contents

THOMSON'S

SPECIAL VETERINARY PATHOLOGY

CHAPTER

1

Gastrointestinal System*

HERBERT J. VAN KRUININGEN

ANATOMIC FEATURES, DEFENSE MECHANISMS, AND RESPONSES TO INJURY

The alimentary tract is anatomically and functionally divided into segments: the oral cavity, esophagus, stomach, small intestine, large intestine, and rectum. The oral cavity is composed of such structures as skeletal musculature, teeth, tongue, salivary glands, and tonsils. The mucosal surface is lined by a thick, stratified squamous epithelium that provides surface integrity, even after rough boluses of ingested material scrape the surface. Saliva from the major and minor salivary glands provides lubrication for that surface, initiates the digestion process, and provides IgA that is helpful in containing the indigenous oral flora. The tonsils and scattered solitary lymphoid follicles act as sentinels in this system, sampling antigens and initiating immune responses as indicated. The oral cavity contains a microbial flora—composed of aerobic bacteria, anaerobic bacteria, spirochetes, and, sometimes, fungi—that fluctuate in number and kind in response to environmental factors such as carbohydrate or protein substrates, pH, oxygen tension, mucus, and antibodies. A lack of scabrous fibrous ingesta, poor hygiene, or immune compromise alters the ecologic balance and enhances the growth of some organisms, while suppressing the growth of others. Places of stagnation, such as gingival pockets or tonsilar crypts, provide special opportunities for bacterial growth.

The mucosal surface of the oral cavity may experience lacerations, contusions, erosions, ulcers, hyperplasia, and neoplasia; the lamina propria and submucosa are the sites of abscesses and granulomas; and the musculature is the site of parasitic myositis, deep bacterial infections, and a unique form of eosinophilic myositis in dogs. Mesenchymal neoplasms, such as fibrosarcomas and rhabdomyosarcomas, may occur in the lamina propria, submucosa, or muscle; the tonsils are sometimes the sites of squamous cell carcinoma or malignant lymphoma; and the major and minor salivary glands may have obstructed ducts, become inflamed, or develop neoplasms.

The pharynx is that place where involuntary muscles and peristalsis assume responsibility for the transport of ingesta. When a bolus is forwarded by the tongue to the pharynx, the upper esophageal sphincter relaxes, permitting material to enter the esophagus. Motility is the function of the esophagus, which serves solely as conduit from pharynx to stomach. The presence of a bolus in the upper esophagus initiates a peristaltic roll that transports materials distally. A coordinated reflex relaxation of the lower esophageal sphincter then allows entrance to the stomach. The cricopharyngeous muscle and striated muscle of the upper esophagus make up the upper esophageal sphincter.

The surface of the esophagus is a tough, white, stratified squamous epithelium similar to that of the oral cavity, and presumably for the same reason: to provide a cobblestone-type paving that will sustain surface integrity following the passage of feed boluses. The esophageal mucosa has pliability, providing a degree of expandability and flexibility with distention and contraction. Longitudinal folds running the length of the esophagus collapse the lumen in the resting state; the distal esophagus has transverse folds as well, that flatten out with distention or passage of feed.

The esophageal surface is lubricated by mucus produced in glands located in the lamina propria and submucosa. At the upper end of the esophagus, striated muscle is arranged in an inner and outer muscle coat; striated muscle arranged in an inner tight spiral layer and an outer loose spiral layer comprises the remainder of the esophagus in the dog. In the cat, opossum, nonhuman primates, and human beings, the distal two thirds of esophageal wall is composed of smooth muscle, an inner circular layer, and an outer longitudinal layer. The esophagus has a bacterial flora, but the

*With a section on Diseases of Teeth by R.R. Dubielzig, D.V.M., Department of Pathobiology, College of Veterinary Medicine, University of Wisconsin.

lack of a persistent substrate between meals and the strong emptying motility of this organ provide little opportunity for overgrowth. Salivary IgA, and some that undoubtedly is secreted with esophageal mucus, further protect the surface from bacterial colonization. Esophageal motility disorders allow stagnation of contents and alter that ecology, allowing a residue and development of significant numbers of bacteria.

The high-pressure zone, the lower esophageal sphincter (LES) at the distal end of the esophagus, protects the esophagus from the acidity of the gastric contents that might occur with regurgitation. When the sphincter is hypotonic, reflux is possible, and the stratified squamous epithelium undergoes inflammation, erosion, ulcerations, and, later, metaplasia to a gastric or intestinal epithelial type and transformation to neoplasia.

The esophageal mucosal surface experiences lacerations, contusions, erosions (often virus induced), ulceration, inflammations, hyperplasia, parakeratosis, and, uncommonly, neoplasia. The lamina propria and submucosa are sites for abscesses, phlegmon, or granulomas. The sphincters and body of the esophagus have a variety of motility disorders; some are congenital and some are acquired. Neoplasms may occur in the esophageal muscle coats.

The dog and cat have simple acid-pepsin–secreting stomachs comparable with those of human beings, whereas the pig and horse have a portion lined by stratified squamous epithelium; ruminants have a three-part forestomach (reticulum, rumen, omasum). The latter is more elaborately endowed with folds and subdivisions, a complex innervation and motility, and, most important, an extensive digestive, fermentative flora. The stratified squamous regions of the pig and horse have a unique peptic ulceration that may be comparable between the two, but not among other species. In the horse, this surface is the site for *Gastrophilus* parasitism.

The disorders of the ruminant stomach are disorders of its flora and its motility. Because of its fermentative functions, abrupt alterations in diet result in either paralysis of bacterial actions or an exuberant and unstable proliferation by one component or another. Often, alterations in one member of the flora lead to a chain of events that can produce rumen acidosis at one extreme and rumen bloat at the other. The competitive flora and a certain stability of substrate keep the rumen healthy. It is not clear to what extent IgA or other antibodies have any role in this complex milieu of carbohydrate and cellulose-rich ingesta, bacteria, fungi, and protozoa.

The stratified squamous mucosa of the reticulum, rumen, and omasum is subject to acute inflammation, often secondary to an acid pH of the contents and bacterial and mycotic overgrowth permitted by an abnormal milieu. The reticulum can trap foreign bodies as they exit the esophagus, and these are detrimental by irritation and penetration. The motility disorders of the forestomachs are poorly understood. Ruminants seldom have neoplasms of the forestomachs.

The acid-pepsin stomach of the simple-stomached animals and the abomasum of ruminants are similar in function and in their response to injury. In each, the proximal two thirds is composed of the fundus and body, the acid and pepsin secretory organ; and the distal third or antrum is lined by epithelium rich in gastrin-producing G cells and mucous glands. Simple stomachs have an indigenous flora, but it is of minor importance when compared with that of the ruminants. Motility under normal circumstances clears the mucosa of substrate. Foveolar mucus forms a protective blanket over the mucosa; IgA inhibits bacterial attachment; and the stomach is acid-washed several times daily. The stomach is protected from self-digestion during times of basal or maximal acid output by the gastric mucosal barrier, which includes a negative electric potential that prevents back diffusion of H^+ ions, cytoprotective prostaglandins, and foveolar and neck mucus secretions. Duodenal contents with bile reflux into the stomach only infrequently in normal animals; normal antral peristalsis (4.5 contractions per minute in the dog) and a normal pylorus prevent more frequent refluxes, which would damage the gastric mucosal barrier.

The mucosal surface of the simple stomach is thrown into convoluted folds called rugae, which are penetrated by the foveolae (numerous stellate-shaped crevices in the surface) through which gastric gland contents are delivered to the surface. The rugal pattern is sparse and longitudinally arrayed along the lesser curve of the stomach and sparse and spirally arranged in the antrum. The mucosa of the body and fundus is composed of parallel tubular glands containing mucous neck cells, parietal cells (secreting acid), chief cells (secreting pepsin), and enterochromaffin cells, while that of the antrum contains simple mucous-secreting glands. The submucosa of the antrum is rich in equidistantly spaced lymphoid follicles. Simple stomachs can be lacerated and contused by foreign bodies, develop ulcers from an imbalance of deleterious and protective factors, have acute and chronic inflammatory processes, and have acute and chronic motility disorders. Certain neoplasms, such as adenocarcinoma, malignant lymphoma, and leiomyoma, may also occur.

The small intestine is a variable-length muscular tube that begins at the pylorus and ends at the ileocolic or ileocecal valve. It takes origin from the stomach in the right cranial abdomen, proceeds caudally as the descending duodenum, then, after a variable length, cranially through 180 degrees around the root of the mesentery to enter the left side and become the jejunum. Both limbs of the duodenum are fixed in location by short mesenteries, as are the origin of the jejunum and the terminus of the ileum, the latter in the posterior right abdomen. In between, the loops of jejunum and ileum are convoluted on the margin of the mesentery. The anatomic distinction between the end of the jejunum and the beginning of the ileum is not clearly defined in most species. The ileum is less folded at the mesentery, a straighter portion of small bowel. The small intestine has inner circular and outer longitudinal smooth muscle coats, thicker in carnivores than in omnivores or herbivores, which provides progressive peristalsis that moves ingesta along the tube. The loops of small bowel are held more or less together within an omental sling.

The mucosa of the small intestine is specialized for absorption. The surface area is increased by mucosal folds, each of which is covered by hundreds of thousands of villi that extend into the lumen. The epithelium lining the villi is continuous with that of the crypts of Lieberkühn where cell replication takes place. New cells ascend from the crypts onto the margins of the villi, gradually differentiating into enterocytes, goblet cells, or enterochromaffin cells. As they ascend the villus, cells become mature, carry out their functions, reach senescence, and are desquamated into the lumen. The shapes and heights of villi vary with intestinal segments and among species. Duodenal villi are moderate in height, jejunal villi are the tallest, and ileal villi are short and plump. The height of the villi is often expressed as villus height: crypt depth ratio. In the dog or cat, jejunal villi maintain a ratio of 2:1; whereas in the pig, 5:1 is not extraordinary. These differences need to be considered before deciding that an animal has villous atrophy. Villous epithelial cells provide an exoskeleton for the villi; the greater the longevity of the surface cells, the taller the villi. Enterocyte longevity and, thus, villous height vary among species and with the composition of the intestinal flora. The villi of germ-free animals are almost twice as tall as those of conventional animals, and those of animals with bacterial overgrowth, akin to tropical sprue in human beings, are variably shortened.

The villus consists of a central lacteal (a lymph capillary that begins blindly near the villus tip), a connective tissue stroma, the lamina propria, smooth muscle, a resident cellular population, a capillary bed, and an epithelium. The resident cellular population is composed of lymphocytes, plasma cells, a few mast cells and histiocytes, and a variable population of eosinophils. The number of cells within villous cores increases with age, presumably in response to encounters with viral, bacterial, parasitic, and dietary antigens.

Scattered through the small intestine are numerous solitary submucosal lymphoid follicles and fewer aggregates of lymphoid follicles, called Peyer's patches. The latter are oval in some species and elongated strips in others and are located along the antimesenteric wall of the intestine. Grossly, Peyer's patches appear recessed because vestigial villi overlie the lymphoid tissue. (A mistake often committed at the necropsy is to incise the intestine along the antimesentric border, transecting Peyer's patches and preventing an evaluation of their undisturbed character.) Although originally described in the ileum, Peyer's patches are not restricted to this segment but are usually more numerous there.

Each aggregate is located in the submucosa and has a cone-shaped protuberance of lymphocytes extending through the muscularis mucosae into the mucosa between intestinal crypts. This portion, called the dome, is covered by a specialized epithelium of ''M'' cells, cells with the phagocytic capability to ''taste'' antigens at the intestinal surface and to convey them to macrophages (antigen-presenting cells) within the dome. M cell epithelium can be recognized because it lacks the goblet cells and microvillous border of adjacent epithelium and because it contains lymphocytes that have invaginated the basal borders of these cells to come into more intimate contact with the surface. M cells sometimes serve as portals of entry for disease-producing viruses and bacteria and have served to transport *Giardia.* Beneath the lymphoid follicles are lymph sinuses that communicate with mucosal and submucosal lymph vessels. Thus, the route for some microorganisms may extend from M cells, through the dome, and via lymph vessels to lymph nodes and, perhaps, beyond into the systemic circulation.

The luminal surface of the villous epithelium is protected by a glycocalyx and by secreted mucus and IgA. Pancreatic bicarbonate, released in response to consumption of feed, raises the pH of the gastric contents to make them alkaline and, thus, prevents acid damage. The small intestine has a bacterial flora, aerobic and anaerobic, with the numbers and kinds fewest proximally and increased aborally. In some animals, over 400 species of bacteria reside in the intestines, and all intestines have *Escherichia coli* and *Clostridium perfringens* as part of the flora. As in more proximal segments of the tract, constantly changing diet, competitiveness among organisms for ecologic niches, a mucous barrier, IgA, and progressive motility constitute defenses against bacterial overgrowth. In addition, Paneth cells present in the crypts in some species contribute to the control of the bacterial flora by the secretion of antibacterial substances called cryptdins. The crypts of Lieberkühn provide new cells each day sufficient to compensate for those lost through attrition and senility and those destroyed by the toxic by-products of the resident bacterial flora.

Shortly after death, these defenses are lost and bacterial toxin-induced autolysis rapidly damages the villi. If villous lesions are to be accurately defined, the intestines must be examined as soon as possible after death, and first in the necropsy. Sites to be sampled along the intestine should be promptly opened, carefully excised, labeled, and immediately placed in fixative. When a segment of intestine is deprived of its blood supply, the anaerobes shortly thereafter produce similar villous damage. In overeating disease or carbohydrate engorgement of ruminants, clostridial toxins efface villi much as autolysis does.

The intestinal mucosa suffers such injuries as acid burns;

lacerations and contusions from foreign bodies; idiopathic ulcers; diffuse villus necrosis induced by viruses, bacteria, or toxic chemicals; acute eosinophilic and chronic inflammation; villus atrophy; crypt and villus hyperplasia; and neoplasia. Parasites traumatize the epithelium, invade enterocytes, and move through the lamina propria, submucosa, or muscularis. Granulomatous diseases affect the connective tissue stroma, the lamina propria, and the submucosa. Vasculitis in these areas is rare, but lymph stasis, subsequent to lymphadenitis or neoplasia, is not uncommon. The intestine can have such lesions as intussusception, volvulus, and mesenteric ischemia. Muscle tunics are often thickened as a result of chronic inflammatory or neoplastic processes in the adjacent submucosa or serosa. Thickening also occurs proximal to obstructions, such as occurs from a poorly functioning ileocolic valve and constriction due to inflammatory or neoplastic diseases. Neoplasms of the mucosal epithelia are rare and include adenocarcinomas and carcinoids. Malignant lymphomas of the mucosa and submucosa are not uncommon; leiomyomas of the muscle coats are rare.

The ileum of the small intestine joins the cecum and colon, which are larger-diameter segments of the intestine. The large intestine reclaims water, electrolytes, and water-soluble vitamins and forms the feces. In animals with a large and functional cecum, cellulolytic digestion and bacterial and protozoal fermentation occur. Carnivores have a two-layered complete muscle wall in the colon, whereas omnivores and herbivores have sacculated large bowel segments. The sacculations are the result of semilunar contraction rings in the inner smooth muscle coat distributed along a modified outer longitudinal muscle coat organized as taenia extending the length of the segment. Species have varying diameters, varying zones of sacculation, and varying reflective and spiral arrangements of the colon on its mesentery. The dog and cat have the simplest and thickest colon and a vestigial cecum, whereas the pig, sheep, goat, and cow have a large cecum and a redundant centripetal and centrifugal spiral colon. The rectum presents as a straight terminal segment of the large intestine and is that portion contained within the pelvis.

The mucosa is similar throughout the cecum, colon, and rectum and is composed of parallel tubular glands of mucus-rich epithelial cells. Villi are lacking in the large intestine. Lamina propria is sparse between the colonic glands and contains scattered leukocytes, less numerous than those in the small intestine. Solitary lymphoid follicles and aggregates of follicles occur, but the latter are not called Peyer's patches, but rather lymphoid aggregates. They are often found in proximal colon, at the transition from the cecum to colon, and in the rectum, just cranial to the anus. In some of our species of domestic large animals, submucosal lymphoid follicles contain invaginated colonic crypt epithelium, with a zone of M cells. These have been called lymphoglandular complexes and may be functionally different from lymphoid follicles with classical domes.

The function of the cecum is to house an important bacterial and protozoal digestion process; the function of the colon is to retain and knead the small bowel effluent for the purpose of water and electrolyte reclamation. Colonic contractions are segmental and not progressive, except at several intervals through the day, when mass movements deliver material more distally. Mass movements often occur consequent to ingestion of a large meal, which triggers a gastrocolic reflex. Once fecal material has been forwarded to the rectum, this unit, unique in mucosal tactile sense, signals the urge for defecation.

Greater than 50% of the weight of feces is bacteria. Defense mechanisms in the large intestine are similar to those occurring in the small bowel. The large intestine requires fiber for proper stimulation of motility and for cellulolytic digestion and fermentation in omnivores and herbivores. The flora of the large intestine are more numerous than those of the small bowel and differ in kind as well. The ileocolic or ileocecal valve provides a barrier against appreciable reflux of colonic or cecal flora into the distal ileum.

The large bowel can suffer injuries similar to those of the small intestine, minus the various lesions of villi. These include lacerations and contusions from foreign bodies; necrosis induced by viruses, bacteria, and toxins (although most toxins have had their effect cranially in the tract and are absorbed or neutralized before reaching the large intestine); acute, chronic, eosinophilic, and granulomatous inflammations; hyperplasia; and neoplasia. The parasites of the large intestine are different from those of the small bowel. Surface neoplasms such as adenocarcinoma are more common, presumably in accord with the slower transit of ingested carcinogens. Malignant lymphoma sometimes originates in lymphoid aggregates of the large bowel. Motility disorders include intussusception, volvulus, functional obstipation, and aganglionic megacolon. Perforation of the rectum is sometimes a consequence of rough and unskilled rectal examination. During dystocia, laceration by a fetus may extend through the dorsal uterus into the ventral rectum.

The anus is composed of voluntary and involuntary muscular sphincters and a stratified squamous mucosa. The anus is always closed and without contents, except during defecation. Inflammations here are rare; contusions and lacerations occur in dystocia (rectal and anal tears in the equine) or the passing of foreign bodies that have made their way through the GI tract. Squamous cell carcinoma occurs rarely in the anal mucosa.

ORAL CAVITY

Obstructions and Functional Disorders

Salivary mucoceles

The salivary mucocele is a small or large, thin-walled, fluid-filled pseudocyst of the oral mucosa and is without an epithelial lining. Large mucoceles are rare and displace the tongue or cause obstruction in the oral cavity. Mucoceles of 1 cm or less probably go unrecognized but may be more numerous. Clinically, mucoceles cause salivation, displacement of the tongue, or difficulty in eating.

Salivary mucoceles are caused by trauma to the cheeks or to the undersurface of the tongue, as occurs when animals bite themselves during mastication or traumatize the mucosa during the chewing of rough boluses, foreign bodies, or bones. Saliva enters the interstices of the lamina propria or submucosa, thereby forming a mucocele.

The mucocele (a round, oval, or irregular lesion) is a translucent, saliva-filled bubble within the mucosa of the oral cavity and may measure 2 to 4 cm in diameter. Saliva within connective tissue stimulates a thin wall of granulation tissue, and, in some cases, the response is granulomatous. **Ranula** is a term used in some species to refer specifically to a mucocele of sublingual salivary gland origin.

Sialolithiasis

Sialolithiasis is a rare disorder of cattle, horses, dogs, nonhuman primates, and human beings. The hard sialolith may be a firm, palpable, submucosal mass along the course of the parotid duct or in the floor of the mouth. Affected animals salivate excessively, and dogs may traumatize the area in an attempt to deal with the discomfort resulting from distention and pressure within the occluded duct.

Sialoliths are chalky yellow or white calcium concretions that form in the ducts of either the parotid or the submandibular salivary glands and, in radiographs, often have concentric lamellae. The nidus is usually not identified, but could be bacteria, clumps of mucus, or desquamated epithelial cells. Sialoliths have high calcium phosphate content, a lesser proportion of calcium carbonate, other soluble salts, organic matter, and water. Some have reached almost 1 cm in length by 6 mm in diameter. Distention of salivary ducts proximal to the obstruction occurs secondarily.

Viral Stomatitides

Vesicular stomatitis

Stomatitis, characterized by vesicles and fluid-filled bullae of the oral mucosa, occurs in virus-induced diseases of large domestic animals. These diseases spread rapidly in epizootic proportions and have a major economic impact on the food industry. Four distinct diseases cause vesicular disease of the labia, buccal mucosa, and tongue; these are foot-and-mouth disease caused by a picornavirus, vesicular stomatitis caused by a rhabdovirus, swine vesicular disease caused by a picornavirus, and swine vesicular exanthema caused by a calicivirus. Clinically, these diseases are indistinguishable from one another; however, the viruses do have some species selectivity. Foot-and-mouth disease occurs in cloven-footed animals, which means that, under farm circumstances, the cow, sheep, goat, and pig are susceptible, but not the horse. Vesicular stomatitis may occur in the horse, cow, pig, and other large animal species, whereas swine vesicular disease and vesicular exanthema are limited to the pig. The four diseases are characterized by easy and rapid transmission, as the viruses are readily acquired from the fluid of the vesicles and from saliva and are carried from one premises to another. The incubation period is short, ranging from 2 to 4 days, and the diseases produced are all acute.

Clinical signs of vesicular stomatitis include aphthae (white spots in the mouth), vesicles, bullae, detached epithelium, raw ulcerated areas on the tongue and lips, salivation, lameness, fever, and anorexia. The diagnosis is made by gross and microscopic lesions, species affected, susceptibility of laboratory animal species to experimental inoculation, serology, and virus isolation.

The gross lesions begin as small, clear, fluid-filled vesicles of the lips, the buccal mucosa, and the surface and margins of the tongue. These enlarge and coalesce to create bullae, which subsequently ulcerate, creating irregular patches of red, denuded submucosa. The epithelium over large bullae may be readily pulled away by forceps or rubbed away with a gloved hand. Similar lesions occur in the nasal mucosa, particularly in swine, and in the esophagus and rumen. Some animals have conjunctivitis and vesicular dermatitis of the interdigital cleft, coronary band, teats, and vulva. Young animals with foot-and-mouth disease frequently have a viral myocarditis, characterized microscopically by Zenker's necrosis.

Microscopically, the lesions of these four diseases are very similar. Each begins as an intracellular edema, which results in ballooning degeneration of the cells of the stratum spinosum. These swollen cells have eosinophilic or clear, watery cytoplasm and pyknotic nuclei. Cell lysis and intercellular edema occur as well. The stratum granulosum, lucidum, and corneum above the virus-damaged zone serve as a roof for the vesicle, which contains variable amounts of blood and neutrophils. Vesicles coalesce, producing bulla (Fig. 1-1); ulceration occurs when the surface is abraded or eroded and is accompanied by a fibrinopurulent coating of the surface and granulation tissue at the base. The hydropic ballooning of epithelial cells of the stratum spinosum is characteristic. Viral inclusion bodies do not occur.

Ovine ecthyma

Contagious ovine ecthyma, ''sore mouth'' or ''orf,'' is a readily transmissible, but mild, poxvirus infection of sheep and goats. The disease occurs commonly in the United States when herds have not been vaccinated. Human beings are susceptible, and the disease is readily transmitted to the oral mucosa, conjunctiva, or hands.

The lesions of contagious ecthyma occur most often on the lips and are multiple (Fig. 1-2). Animals have similar lesions of the oral mucosae, and, in a few animals, the infection extends to include the mucosae of the esophagus and rumen. Ecthyma is frequently seen in young stock, and nursing by these animals may transmit the disease to the

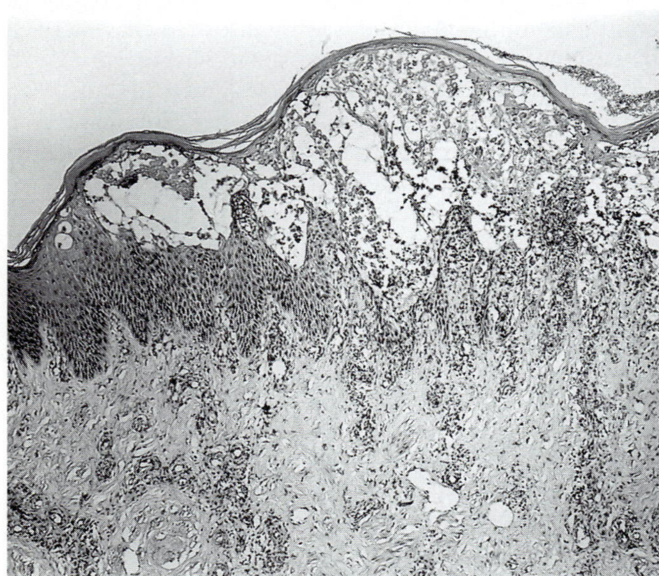

Fig. 1-1 Oral mucosa; cow. Foot and mouth disease. Vesicles are formed from multiple coalescing foci of hydropic degeneration, leading to multilocular intraepithelial bullae. Hematoxylin-eosin (H & E) stain. *Courtesy Dr. D. Gregg.*

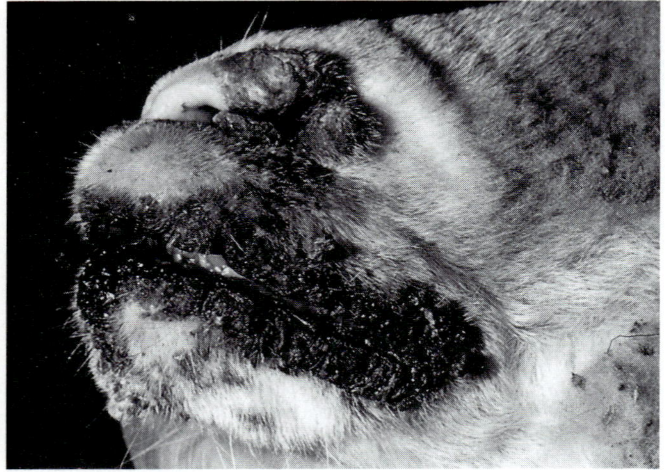

Fig. 1-2 Muzzle; lamb. Ovine contagious ecthyma. Lips and external nares are encrusted with coalesced, blackened sores. *Courtesy Dr. M.D. McGavin.*

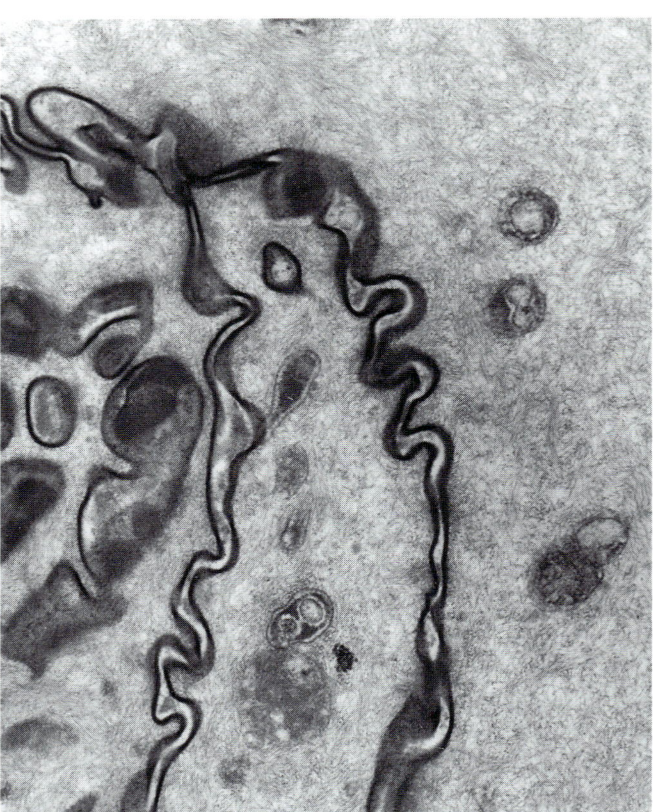

Fig. 1-3 Esophagus; cow. Bovine papular stomatitis. Virus particles approximately 200 nm in diameter are in epithelial cells.

teats, udder, or flank of the dams. The sores are round to irregular, firm, raised encrustations. They are usually dark red to violet, approximately 1 cm in diameter, and are well delineated from the adjacent healthy mucosa.

This disease is characterized by cytoplasmic ballooning (hydropic degeneration) accompanied by cytoplasmic eosinophilic inclusion bodies. Cell lysis and intercellular edema never reach the proportions that occur in the vesicular stomatitides, and fluid-filled bullae do not occur. In addition, the lesions are heavily infiltrated with inflammatory cells and have neovascularization and proliferation of basal cells so that the lesion has a cellular consistency. The ''sore'' is elevated above the surrounding mucosa, and superinfection of the surface by secondary bacteria, such as *Fusobacterium necrophorum,* causes a variable surface color and consistency. Such lesions are dry, dark-colored, and crusty. Leukocytosis and increased vascularity occur in the submucosa beneath.

Bovine papular stomatitis

This disease is caused by a virus related to that of contagious ovine ecthyma. It occurs in young stock, and the disease is milder than ovine ecthyma. The lesions either remain unrecognized or are found when the oral cavity is examined in an animal with excessive salivation or a fever of unknown origin. Several related viruses have been isolated from outbreaks of bovine papular stomatitis (Fig. 1-3).

The lesions are slightly raised papules several millimeters in diameter and macules up to a centimeter in size. The papules persist for several weeks before spontaneous re-

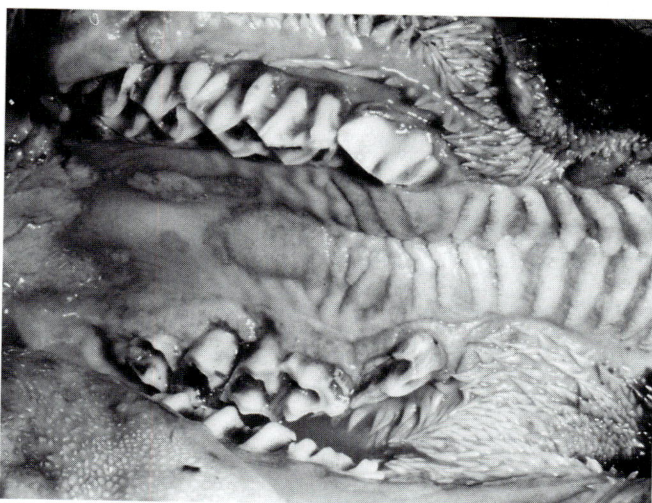

Fig. 1-4 Palate and tongue; cow. Bovine papular stomatitis. Multiple, oval, plaquelike, depressed macules with hyperemic margins occur in the soft palate and dorsum of the tongue. *Courtesy Dr. M.D. McGavin.*

covery occurs. The macules often have a pale center and a hyperemic rim demarcating the lesion from adjacent normal tissue. These lesions occur on the hard palate, lips, muzzle, and tongue (Fig. 1-4), and may extend into the esophagus (Fig. 1-5), reticulum, rumen, and omasum. The microscopic lesions are very similar to those of contagious ovine ecthyma and are characterized by ballooning degeneration of epithelial cells of the stratum spinosum and, in some infections, by intracytoplasmic inclusion bodies. The lesions seldom ulcerate or become superinfected.

Bacterial Stomatitides

Ulcerative gingivitis, oral necrobacillosis, and noma

Ulcerative gingivitis, also known as Vincent's disease and trench mouth, is a fusospirochetal disease that affects human beings, chimpanzees, and some other species of nonhuman primates. A similar gingivitis occurs rarely in puppies. The acute inflammation and necrosis characteristic of this infection induce painful gums, a fetid mouth odor, hemorrhages that occur with slight trauma, and increased salivation. The disease is caused by two anaerobes, *Borrelia vincentii,* a spirochete, and *Fusobacterium* sp, gram-negative fusiform bacilli. These organisms induce disease because of underlying nutritional deficiencies, debilitating conditions, or psychogenic factors.

The lesion is an acute, necrotizing inflammation of the gingiva. Punched-out, craterlike ulcers occur in the interdental gingiva and the gingival margin, and are sometimes covered by a gray pseudomembrane. In bacteriologic cultures and smears of the mouth, large numbers of spirochetes and fusiform bacteria can be demonstrated.

Oral necrobacillosis of calves (calf diphtheria) and young pigs is a disease caused by *F. necrophorum,* a part of the normal flora in many of these animals, and is endemic in the soil, in particular on farms where another *Fusobacterium* disorder, foot rot of cattle, is also prevalent. It is not clear if the *Fusobacterium* acts alone. Animals with oral necrobacillosis have swollen cheeks, anorexia, fever, and a characteristic fetid breath. The lesions are of greater severity than those of ulcerative gingivitis and are more localized, consisting of gray-to-tan foci of coagulation necrosis from 1 to several centimeters in diameter.

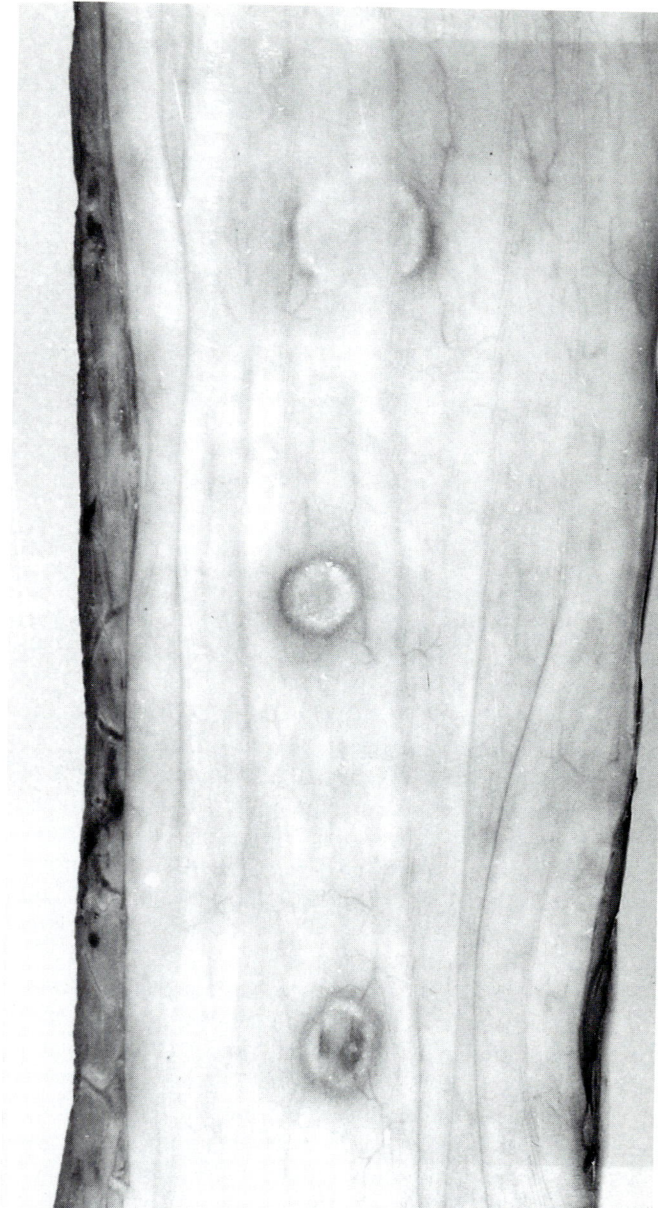

Fig. 1-5 Esophagus; cow. Bovine papular stomatitis. Slightly raised and depressed oval lesions with red margins are in the esophagus. *Courtesy Dr. R.G. Thomson.*

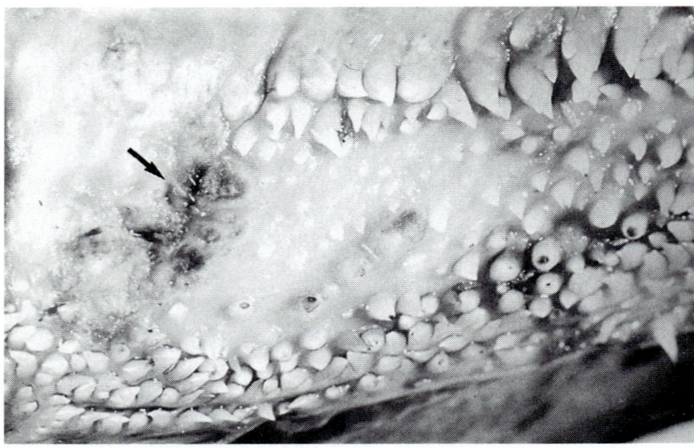

Fig. 1-6 Buccal mucosa; calf. Oral necrobacillosis. An irregular, blackened erosion *(arrow)* is in the buccal mucosa. *Courtesy Dr. R.G. Thomson.*

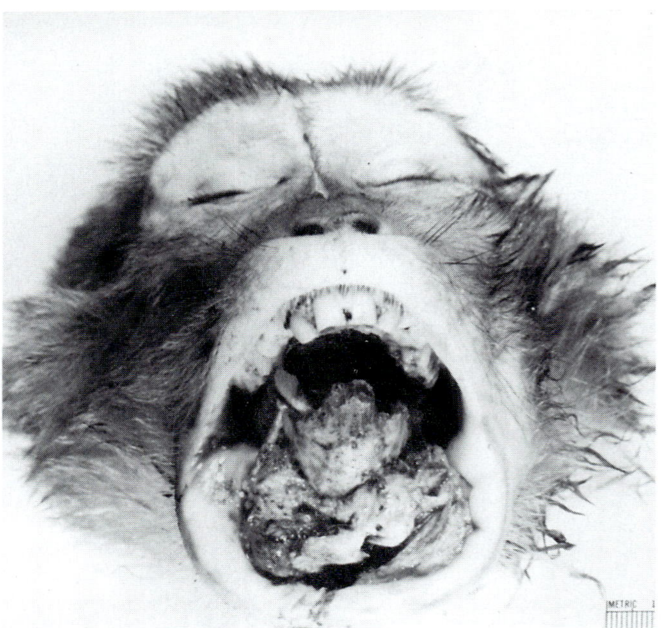

Fig. 1-7 Oral mucosa; rhesus monkey. Noma. The mouth contains a mass of necrotic and inflammatory tissue. There has been a loss of lower incisors. *Adams RJ, Bishop JL. Lab Anim Sci. 1980; 30:89.*

Affected animals usually have only one or two such foci, along the teeth, in the buccal mucosa of the cheeks (Fig. 1-6), or at the pharynx.

The lesion, grossly, consists of a raised core of tan-to-gray necrotic material, readily separated from the adjacent viable crater. Microscopically, the lesion is characterized by coagulation necrosis surrounded by a zone of granulation tissue and by hyperemia. The disease can be reproduced using pure cultures of *F. necrophorum,* a gram-negative anaerobe. This organism appears as long, thin filaments and sometimes as rods or cocci and is very difficult to demonstrate in tissue sections.

Noma, or cancrum oris, is an acute, gangrenous stomatitis that has been recognized in human beings, rhesus monkeys, cynomolgus monkeys, and dogs. This disease is caused by spirochetes and fusiforms, perhaps with participation by other organisms of the mouth. It is similar to necrobacillosis, except the lesions are more severe, progressing to gangrene, perforation of the cheeks, lysis of bone, and death (Fig. 1-7). Spirochetes may be demonstrated in the lesions with a Warthin-Starry stain.

Actinobacillosis

Infrequently, *Actinobacillus lignieresii* causes a deeply located infection and granulomatous inflammation of the oral tissues and the adjacent lymph nodes in cattle, small ruminants, and horses. This gram-negative bacillus, present in the environment, gains access to the submucosal tissues by erosions and penetration by the hulls and awns in feeds. Clinically, the animal cannot use its tongue, which may be enlarged and firm, so-called "wooden-tongue." Other clinical features include abnormal positioning of the tongue, salivation, difficulty in eating, or partial anorexia.

Grossly, the surface of the tongue is intact or may have small erosions or focal scars. The lesion, a circular or irregular, white, gray, or yellow-white firm granuloma up to 6 cm in size, displaces normal tissue. The cut surface contains small, 2 to 3 mm, irregular yellow granules, which have the appearance of and have been called "sulfur granules." The contents of the granulomas include the gram-negative rods, granulocytes, macrophages, and eosinophilic club-shaped structures. Regional lymph nodes have similar granulomas.

Microscopically, the granulomas have gram-negative bacilli at their centers, and the colonies are surrounded by a zone of palisaded, eosinophilic, club-shaped structures composed of immunoglobin products of host inflammatory cells. These rosettes are often surrounded by a collection of granulocytes, macrophages, epithelioid cells, and multinucleated Langhans-type giant cells. Within and surrounding this granulomatous collar are lymphocytes and plasma cells. Depending on the duration of the disease, fibrous tissue may surround and be incorporated into the granulomas. Regional lymph nodes may contain similar granulomas or have abscesses that drain to the surface.

Actinomycosis

Actinomycosis is a rare osteomyelitis of the jaw of cattle caused by *Actinomyces bovis,* an organism that appears as gram-positive rods or filaments. Clinical signs include progressive enlargement of one side of the mandible, anorexia, and progressive loss of weight.

The gross lesion is a gray or gray-white, firm and fibrotic, irregular, dense, nodular mass that may contain focal yellow "sulphur granules" similar to those described

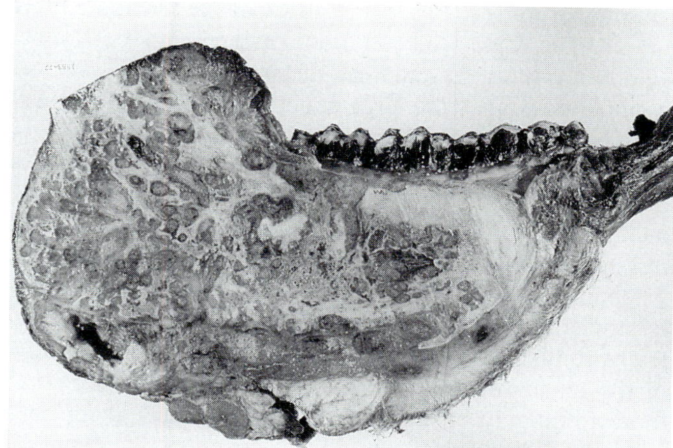

Fig. 1-8 Mandible; cow. Actinomycosis. The bone is greatly thickened and honeycombed by numerous granulomas. *Courtesy Dr. R.G. Thomson.*

in lesions of actinobacillosis. The granulomatous response in the mandible is accompanied by osteolysis, resulting in a honey-combed enlargement that has been called ''lumpy jaw'' (Fig. 1-8). Sinus tracts may drain to the exterior, and regional lymph nodes may contain granulomas or abscesses, as well as sinus tracts. Microscopically, the lesions of actinomycosis consist of aggregated or confluent granulomas of a cellular pattern similar to that of actinobacillosis. At the center of each granuloma, the gram-positive rods or filaments can be found.

Disorders of Undetermined Etiology

Oral eosinophilic granuloma

A focal granuloma or ulcer (''rodent ulcer'') of oral tissues has been described infrequently in young dogs and cats as oral eosinophilic granuloma. Lesions are similar in dogs and cats; occur on the tongue, lips, or palate; and appear etiologically related to similar lesions found interdigitally and in the skin of the trunk or flanks. The disease has been transmitted from one area of the skin to another on the same cat via autologous tissue. Oral eosinophilic granulomas have been identified in Siberian huskies, and most cases occur in animals under 3 years of age.

The cause of oral eosinophilic granuloma is not known; but the lesions are suggestive of an immune-mediated mechanism, and similar lesions can be induced in experimental animals by injection of immune complexes. Also, antiepithelial autoantibodies can be demonstrated in cats with eosinophilic granulomas. In both dogs and cats, a peripheral eosinophilia occurs in about half to two thirds of cases.

Gross lesions in the cat occur most frequently on the upper lips, particularly the commissure of the lips, but may also develop in the gums, palate, pharynx, tongue, or regional lymph nodes. In the Siberian husky, the ventral and lateral surfaces of the tongue and the palatine mucosa have been the sites of lesions (Fig. 1-9). The granuloma may occur as an ulcer with a firm, indurated base of 8 to 15 mm diameter and of irregular shape; alternatively, the mucosa may be intact and the lesion a firm, granulomatous plaque, which has an off-white or yellow-white cut surface. Microscopically, the base of the ulcer and the granulomatous plaque consist of multiple foci of inflammation similar to those seen in bacterial granulomas. The center of the lesion has necrotic collagen that appears as amorphous or granular eosinophilic material, with projections radiating into the surrounding inflammatory tissue. The latter is composed of eosinophils, mast cells, macrophages, epithelioid cells, and a few multinucleated giant cells. Perivascular aggregates of eosinophils and plasma cells have been described in these lesions in cats.

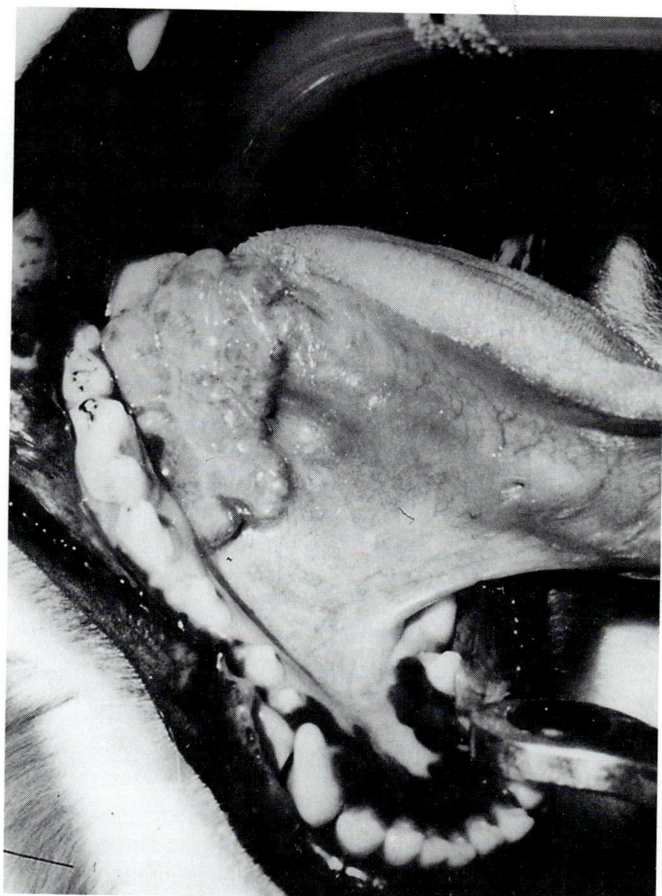

Fig. 1-9 Lingual mucosa; dog. Eosinophilic granuloma. An irregular, raised, firm mass protrudes from the lingual mucosa along the lateral margin of the tongue. *Potter, KA, Tucker RD, Carpenter JL, J Am Anim Hosp Assoc 1980; 6:595-600.*

Neoplasms

Oral papillomas

Papillomas occur in the oral tissues of young dogs, often puppies. The tumors are infectious in origin, are caused by

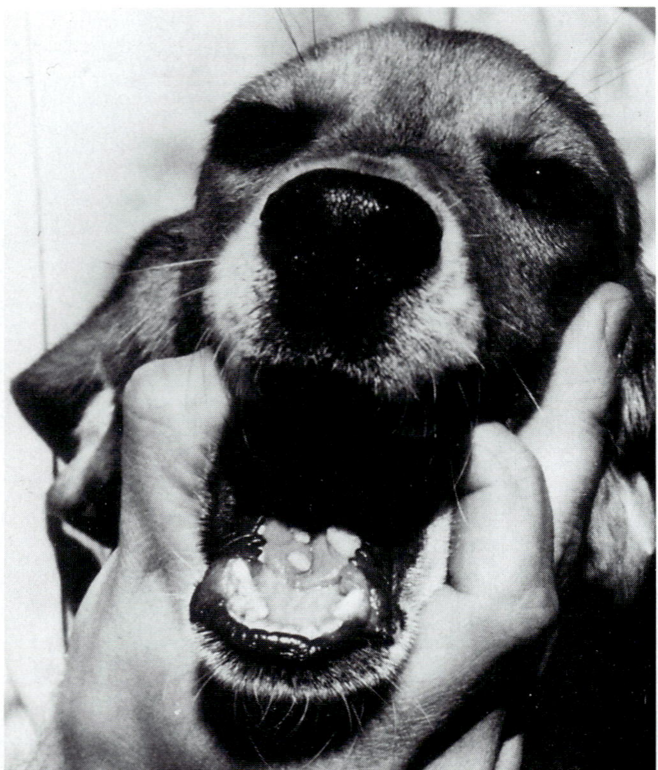

Fig. 1-10 Tongue and gingiva; dog. Oral papillomas. Multiple, raised, gray nodules protrude from the tip of the tongue and gingiva. *Sundberg JP Oncology 1987; 24:14.*

a papillomavirus, are transmissible and multiple, and occur in the buccal mucosa and on the tongue, palate, pharynx, and epiglottis (Fig. 1-10). Papillomas can be transmitted experimentally by exposing a scarified oral mucosa to cell cultures or cell-free material containing the virus. The incubation period is 30 to 33 days. Clinical disease is mild, and tumors persist for approximately 1.5 to 3 months, after which there is spontaneous remission and, finally, complete immunity.

Grossly, these multiple tumors appear white or gray, are flat or smooth early, and, later, are gray, raised, and pedunculated with a keratinized surface. Microscopically, papillomas consist of an acanthotic, hyperplastic, stratified squamous epithelium and a proliferated connective tissue stroma, creating folds and fronds. Cells of the stratum spinosum enlarge greatly and may have vesicular cytoplasm, so-called ballooning degeneration. At some stages, intranuclear inclusion bodies that contain virus particles are present.

Squamous cell carcinoma

Squamous cell carcinomas are relatively common in the oral mucosa of aged dogs and cats but occur less frequently in other species. The carcinoma may begin in the tongue, gingiva, or tonsils (Fig. 1-11); those of the tonsil are more frequent in dogs, whereas those of the tongue are more common in cats. Carcinomas of the oral mucosa are recognized when they are large enough to cause difficult eating and swallowing. The gingival neoplasms and those of the tongue may be seen by the owner, but carcinomas of the tonsil are unrecognized until clinical signs occur. These include attempts to regurgitate or cough out saliva and interference with respiration or swallowing.

About 5% to 10% of gingival squamous cell carcinomas metastasize to regional lymph nodes, and about 3% metastasize to distant sites, whereas squamous cell carcinomas of the tonsils metastasize to regional lymph nodes much more frequently, in up to 98% of cases, and about 63% metastasize to distant sites.

Squamous cell carcinomas, when small, appear as small granular lesions and, with increase in size, appear as beaded, cauliflower-like masses. In cats, squamous cell carcinoma of the tongue originates on the ventral-lateral surface adjacent to the reflection of the frenulum. Microscopically, irregular masses and cords of stratified squa-

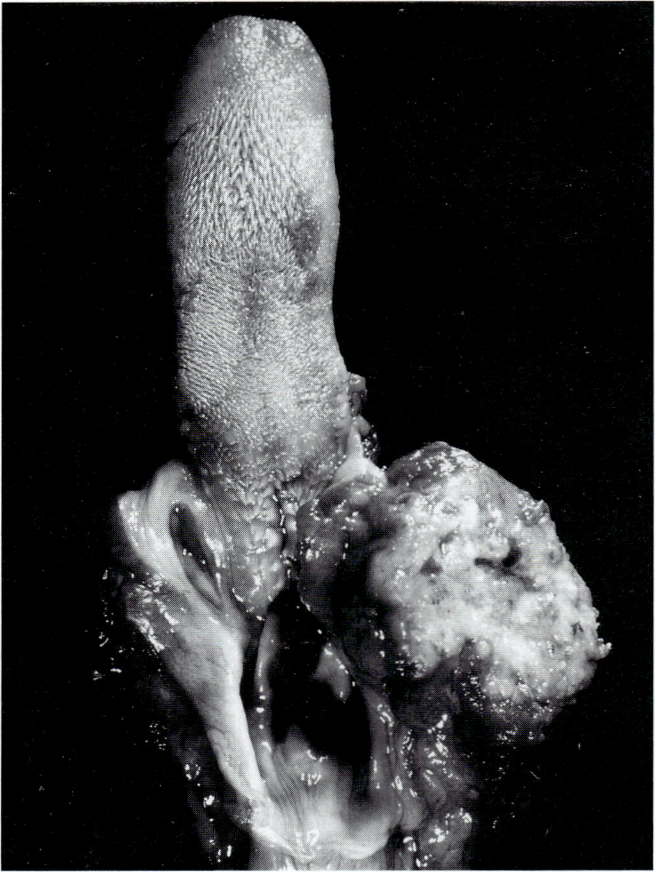

Fig. 1-11 Tonsil; cat. Squamous cell carcinoma. Regional tissues have been distorted and replaced by a large, cauliflower-like neoplasm. *Courtesy of Dr. R.W. Storts.*

mous epithelial cells invade the lamina propria and submucosa or even the muscle beneath, with the amount of keratin depending on the degree of maturation of the neoplastic cells. Well-differentiated neoplasms have numerous keratin pearls, but poorly differentiated neoplasms have only a few keratinized cells and numerous mitotic figures. A characteristic feature is the presence of intercellular bridges between adjacent epithelial cells. The amount of fibrous stroma varies considerably; some carcinomas have areas of necrosis as well.

Malignant melanoma

Melanomas are composed of melanocytes of neuroectodermal origin, normally located at the junction between the basal layer of the epithelium and the lamina propria beneath. The neoplasms commonly arise at this junctional location. Melanomas are usually solitary lesions occurring rather commonly in the pigmented portions of the mouths of dogs 7 to 14 years, but they may originate in the gums, buccal mucosa, palate, or lips.

The melanoma begins as a black macule and develops into a rapidly growing, firm mass. It may be dome-shaped and smooth or have an ulcerated, red, and bleeding surface. Depending on the amount of pigment present, the interior of the mass may be gray-white, dark brown, or black. Microscopically, the neoplasms consist of epithelioid or spindle-shaped melanocytes. Some neoplasms consist almost exclusively of epithelioid cells, whereas others are composed of spindle-shaped cells and resemble fibrosarcomas. Melanin content varies (Fig. 1-12), and some melanomas may be amelanotic. However, most amelanotic melanomas have a few clusters of cells containing melanin pigment. Nests of stellate or spindle-shaped malignant melanocytes commonly are found at the junction between the basal layer of epithelium and lamina propria in oral melanomas. Most oral melanomas are malignant and metastasize via lymph vessels to regional lymph nodes or by blood to the lungs.

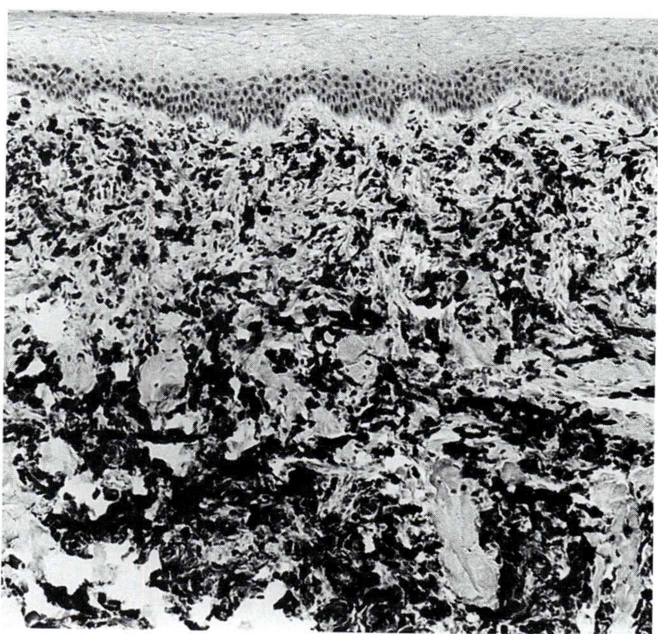

Fig. 1-12 Oral mucosa; dog. Malignant melanoma. Submucosa is markedly infiltrated with pigment-filled melanocytes. H & E stain.

DISEASES OF THE TEETH

Richard R. Dubielzig

Response of Dental Tissue to Disease

The proper function of dental tissue is to provide mechanical advantage for mastication. Dental function can be negatively affected by diseases that disrupt normal development and positioning of the teeth. Acquired disease can result in the loss of integrity of the dental tissue itself or result in the loss of rigid attachment of the teeth to the jaw bones. Neoplastic disease can affect dental function by compression and destruction of the structures of the oral cavity.

Dental Development and Morphology

Embryology

Tooth formation begins when ectodermally derived oral epithelium undergoes a proliferation and invasion of the adjacent mesenchyme of the jaws. The epithelial ingrowth thus formed is called the **dental lamina** (Fig. 1-13). Next, the dental lamina proliferates to form a cup-shaped epithelial structure. The mesenchyme adjacent to the concave surface of the epithelial cup is reorganized into a myxomatous mesenchyme that will become the dental pulp. The mesenchymal cells most closely associated with the concave surface of the epithelial cup elongate and differentiate to form odontoblasts. These cells are responsible for the production of the extracellular dentin matrix. The epithelial cells abutting the **odontoblasts** also undergo elongation and palisading and become the **ameloblasts.** The ameloblasts are responsible for the secretion of enamel matrix. In the

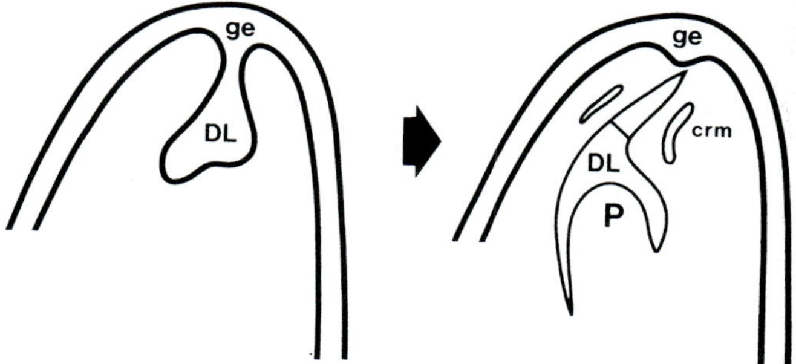

Fig. 1-13 Dental organogenesis begins with the downgrowth of the dental lamina *(DL)* from the gingival epithelium *(ge)*. Invagination to form an epithelial cup around dental pulp mesenchyme (*P*) follows. Epithelial cell rests can survive tooth formation to become the cell rests of Malassez *(crm).*

central portions of the epithelial cup, the epithelial cells separate slightly, accentuating the desmosomal attachments, and become known as **stellate reticulum.** The stellate reticulum then is invaded by blood vessels and fibroblasts from surrounding mesenchyme and eventually is replaced by mesenchyme. This leaves the ameloblastic cells supported by a vascularized epithelial layer known as the **condensed enamel organ.** The fully differentiated odontoblasts and the functional ameloblasts produce dentin matrix and enamel matrix (Fig. 1-14).

Dentin is a renewable collagenous matrix similar to acellular osteoid matrix. Dentin has tubules through which cellular processes from the odontoblasts penetrate into the dentin. Odontoblasts therefore maintain the dentin matrix throughout the life of the tooth.

Enamel matrix is deposited by individual ameloblasts in hexagonal rods and is approximately 98% mineral when fully mineralized. The mineralized enamel matrix is acellular and inert, and, once it becomes mineralized, the epithelial structures of the enamel organ (the ameloblasts and supporting condensed enamel organ) are unnecessary. Some of these cells continued to exist as small cell rests in the periodontal ligament or become incorporated in the superficial gingival epithelium. Proliferative, cystic, or neoplastic diseases of the dental arcade can originate from cell rests that form from the dental lamina or the enamel organ (the cell rests of Malassez). In simple-toothed animals, such as carnivores, the tooth root is not covered by enamel.

The root is anchored to the alveolar bone by fibrous strands that attach on a collagenous matrix known as **cementum.** In complex-toothed animals, such as domestic herbivores, enamel deposition continues far beyond eruption. In these animals, following mineralization of the enamel and atrophy of the ameloblastic epithelium, cementogenesis occurs immediately adjacent to the mineralized enamel matrix. In the central crown of large ruminant teeth, there is an enamel cup (infundibulum). Following eruption, the enamel cup becomes separated from its blood supply; therefore, cementogenesis within the infundibulum must occur prior to eruption. Incomplete infundibular cementogenesis can lead to infundibular impaction and inflammatory dental disease.

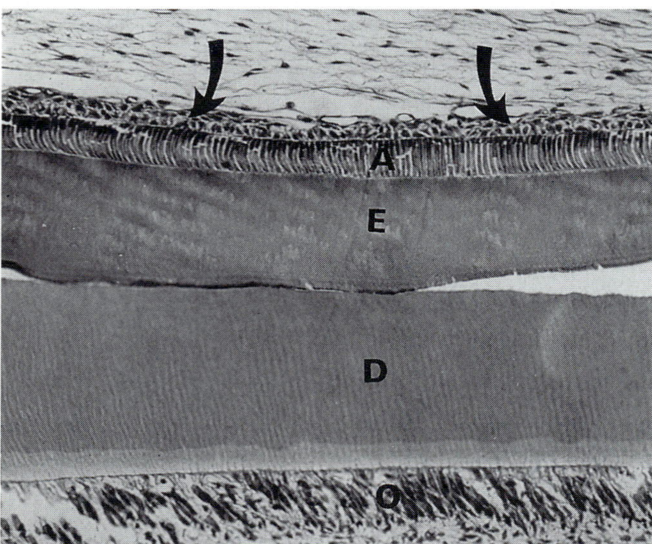

Fig. 1-14 The enamel organ showing condensed enamel organ *(arrows)*, ameloblasts (*A*), enamel matrix (*E*), dentin matrix (*D*), and odontoblasts (*O*).

Dental morphology

Domestic and laboratory animals have several different forms of teeth, which vary in form and function and include incisors, canines, premolars, and molars. Charts of dental formulas are available in standard anatomy texts. Generally, the teeth of domestic species can be divided into two forms most simply described as simple teeth and complex teeth.

Simple teeth. A diagrammatic representation of a simple tooth is shown in Fig. 1-15. The **crown** is the visible part

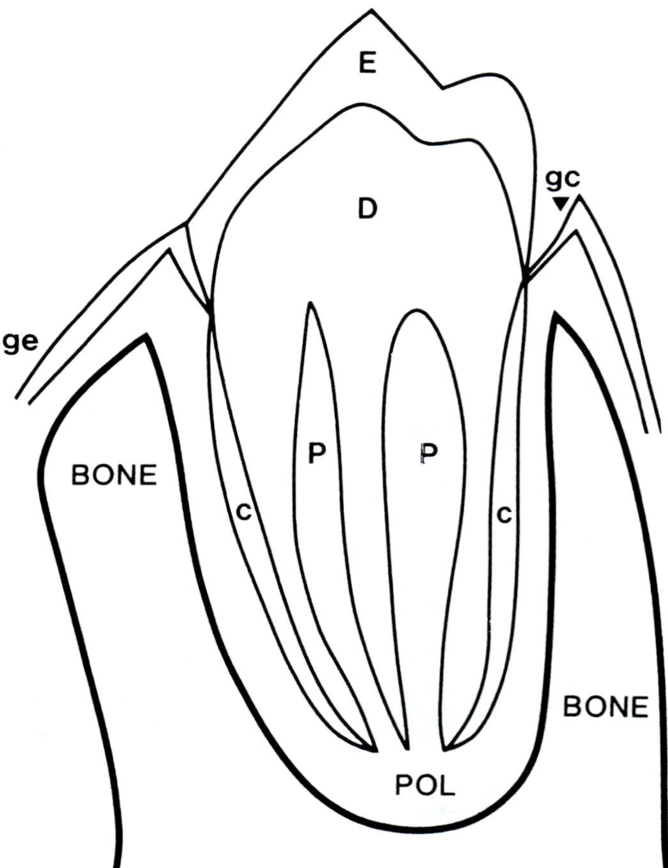

Fig. 1-15 Simple tooth diagram. Enamel (*E*), gingival crevice *(gc)*, periodontal ligament *(POL)*, cementum (*c*), dental pulp (*P*), and alveolar bone.

of the tooth, and in a simple tooth is that portion covered by an enamel cap. The **root,** made up of dentin covered by cementum and no enamel, is maintained rigidly within the alveolar socket by the firm, fibrous periodontal ligament. The **periodontal ligament** consists of fibrous tissue anchored firmly in both cementum and alveolar bone. The **alveolus** is the indentation of the jaw bone where the tooth root is inserted. The **dental pulp** is the highly vascular connective tissue that extends into the tooth root and nourishes the viable dentin. Odontoblasts produce and maintain the dentin and line the junction between the dental pulp and the dentin matrix. Nerve endings extend into the dentin.

Complex teeth. The large domestic herbivores have teeth modified for a rotating and grinding form of mastication. These teeth have a high, flat occlusal surface and undergo physiologic attrition; therefore, there is a need for continuous eruption. The distinction between the anatomic crown and root is less apparent than in simple teeth. As in the simple tooth, the viable dentin occurs closest to the dental pulp. Enamel is deposited flush against the dentin, not only on the crown but extending deep into the alveolar socket along the tooth root. Unlike in the simple tooth, cementum is adherent to the enamel layer so that dentin, enamel, and cementum make up the hard dental substance on both the crown and the root. Another feature of complex teeth is the infolding that occurs on the masticatory surface. A deep indentation lined by enamel and filled with cementum is referred to as the **infundibulum** (Fig. 1-16, *A*, and *B*).

Dental Anomalies

Anomalies of tooth positioning

Abnormal positioning of the teeth can be the result of jaw conformation or, more rarely, the result of spontaneous abnormal eruption patterns. In domestic herbivores, abnormal tooth positioning leads to uneven wear that has serious consequences.

Jaw conformation is an important contributory factor in

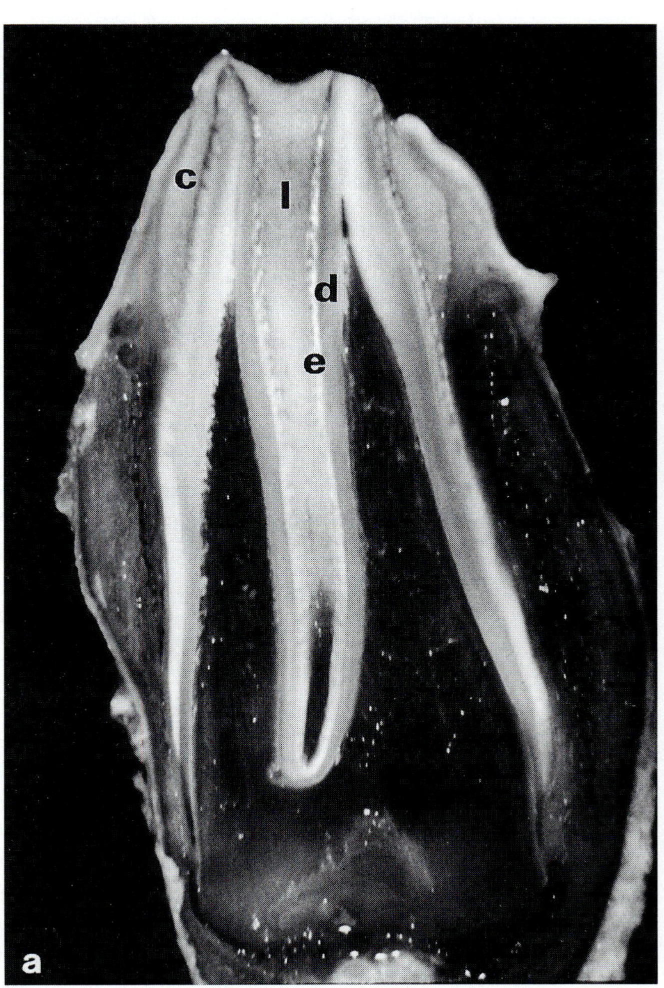

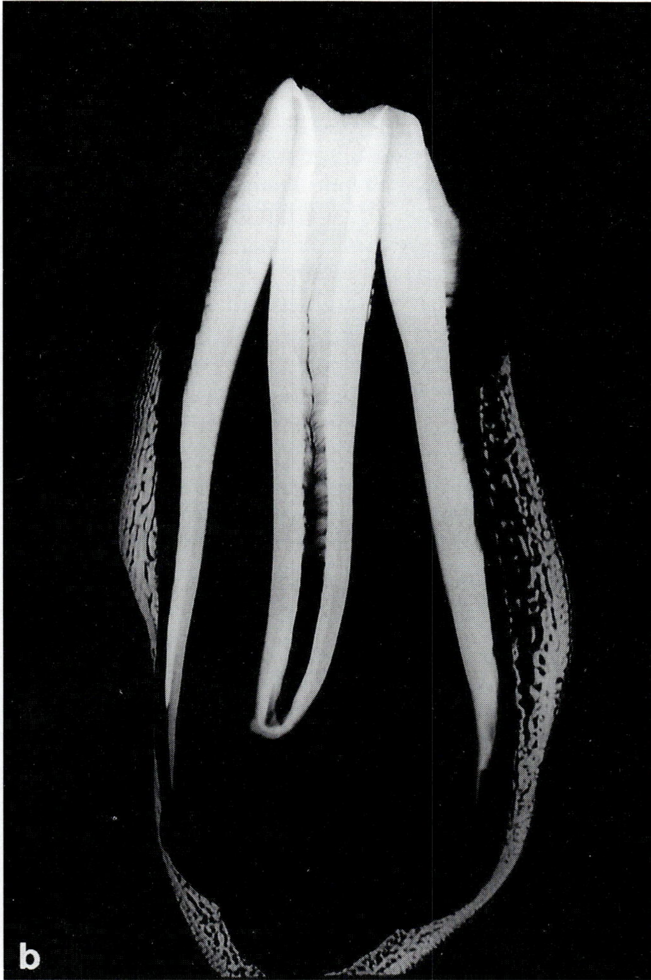

Fig. 1-16 **A,** Complex tooth (neonatal equine second premolar). Infundibulum (*I*), enamel (*e*), dentin (*d*), and cementum (*c*). **B,** Radiograph of same tooth. Horse.

dental occlusion abnormalities. The two forms of abnormal jaw conformation most commonly encountered are **brachygnathism,** in which the mandibular canine tooth is displaced caudally in relation to the maxillary canine (the maxilla is ''overshot'' rostrally), and **prognathism,** in which the mandibular canine tooth is abnormally positioned rostrally with regard to the maxillary canine tooth (the mandible is ''overshot'' rostrally). Problems of jaw conformation are most serious in herbivores and rodents because the resultant uneven tooth wear leads to abnormal dental attrition and eventually serious problems of mastication.

Anomalies of tooth development

Tooth agenesis is fairly common and of little clinical significance in animals with simple teeth. Supernumerary tooth development is a rare curiosity. Abnormalities of tooth development can result from either primary dysplasias of the enamel organ or secondary consequences of trauma, infection, toxicosis, or metabolic abnormalities affecting tooth development. Primary dysplasias of the enamel organ usually result in failure of tooth development or severe malocclusion.

Dentigerous cysts. These lesions are a result of abnormal tooth development giving rise to epithelial-lined, cystic structures in the bone or soft tissues of the jaw. This is a rare lesion, which can remain asymptomatic or lead to painful or destructive diseases of the jaw and occasionally can be the origin of neoplasms. Usually, the cysts are lined by stratified squamous epithelium and often become filled with keratin. Infrequently, fragments of poorly developed teeth form within dentigerous cysts. In horses, a dentigerous cyst can result in a painful fistulous lesion seen most often in the temporal region, rostral and ventral to the ear. Infrequently, dentigerous cysts develop in mature animals with normal dentition. In these cases, the cysts arise as a result of the proliferation of epithelial cell rests remaining from the enamel organ (the cell rests of Malassez).

Abnormal tooth development has been reported in horses with epitheliogenesis imperfecta. Affected teeth appeared normal clinically, but when carefully examined in radiographs the teeth had irregular dental margins and absence of normal enamel formation (Fig. 1-17).

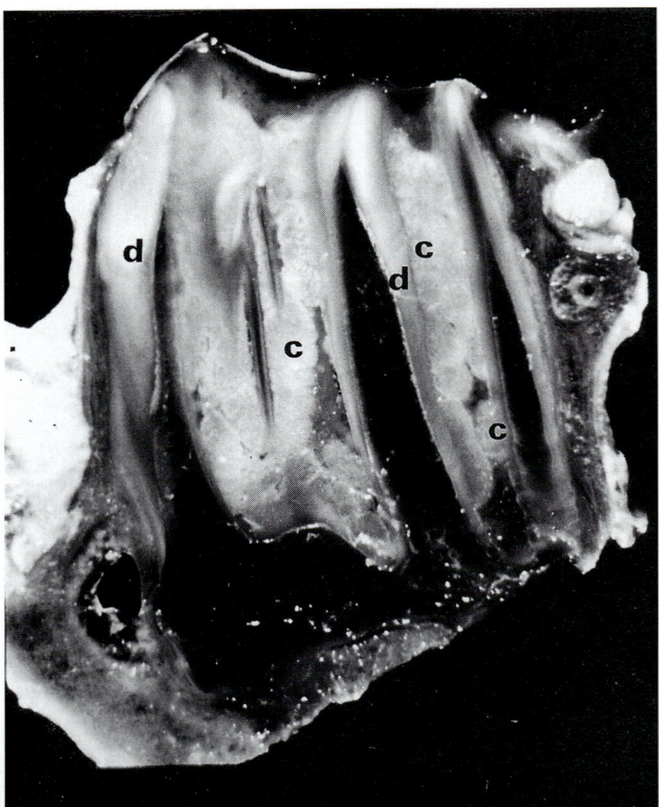

Fig. 1-17 Dysplastic tooth; foal. Epitheliogenesis imperfecta. Dentin (*d*) and cementum (*c*) are seen, but no enamel.

Segmental enamel hypoplasia occurs in the adult teeth of dogs infected with canine distemper virus during odontogenesis. The epithelium of the enamel organ during virus infection has typical viral infection lesions, including necrosis, disorganization, and lack of function in ameloblasts (Fig. 1-18, *A*, and *B*). After recovery from viral infection, the return of function and organization of the enamel organ is followed by reestablishment of normal enamel formation. Segmental enamel hypoplasia, corresponding to the zones of enamel formation during the time of distemper infection, is noted upon eruption of the permanent teeth.

Abnormal coloration of teeth can result from the incorporation of chemical agents, most typically tetracyclines, during mineralization. This frequently occurs with the use of pediatric medications during permanent tooth development. Incorporation of porphyrins into the dentin can cause pink discoloration of the teeth in animals with congenital porphyria. Accentuation of the discoloration of both tetracycline and porphyrin incorporation can be enhanced by ultraviolet light.

Excessive fluoride incorporation into the enamel and dentin occurs in fluoride toxicosis in cattle. Toxic dietary concentrations of fluorine during odontogenesis (from 6 to 36 months of age) can result in incorporation of the fluoride in the enamel and dentin of the permanent teeth leading to soft, chalky enamel. Yellow, dark-brown, or black discoloration of the enamel is common in fluorosis (Fig. 1-19, *A*, and *B*). Clinical disease results from rapid dental attrition and loss of dental function. Involvement of deciduous tooth has not been seen in experimentally induced fluorosis.

In a survey of dental disease in a fluoride-contaminated environment, several dental lesions were found that differ from those seen in experimentally affected cattle. The specific lesions reported in cattle exposed to industrial fluoride

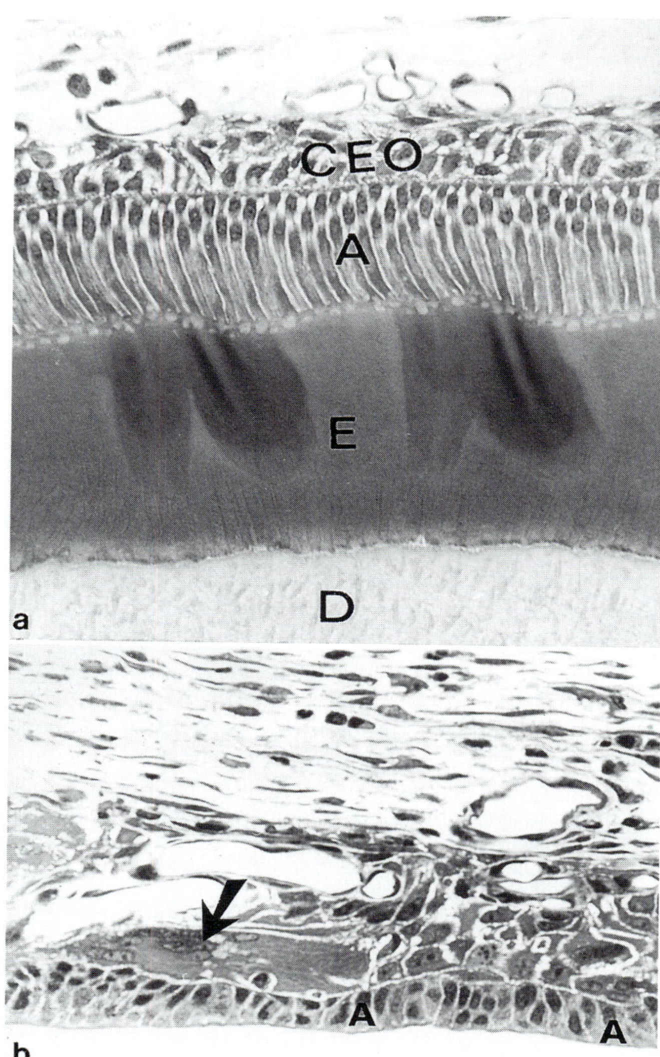

Fig. 1-18 **A,** Structures from enamel organ of control dog showing normal condensed enamel organ *(CEO),* ameloblasts (*A*), enamel matrix (*E*), and dentin (*D*). **B,** Enamel organ; dog. At 16 days after infection with distemper virus, there is shortening of the ameloblasts (*A*) and syncytial giant cells *(arrow)* are present.

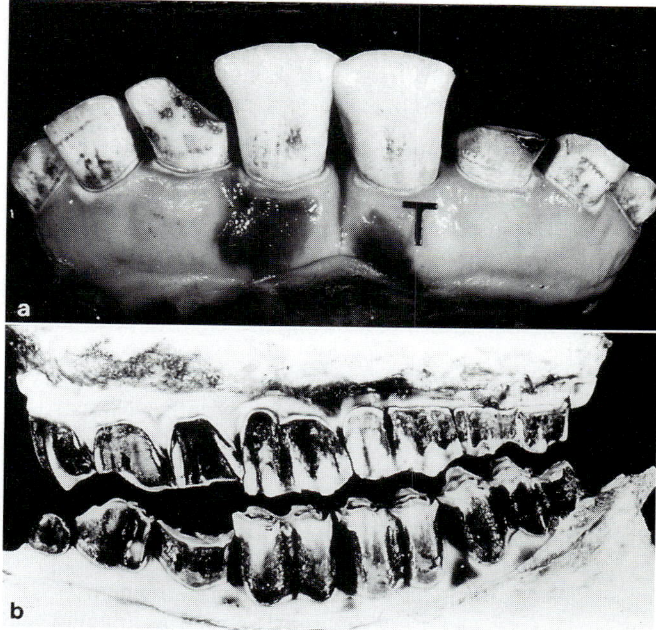

Fig. 1-19 **A,** Incisor tooth; cow. Cow was fed a nonconstant toxic fluoride diet. There is abnormal pigmentation and an unusual wear pattern. **B,** Molar and premolar tooth; cow. The abnormal wear pattern seen here can cause problems with mastication. *Courtesy J.W. Suttie.*

pollution were hypercementosis, delayed eruption, necrosis of alveolar bone, oblique eruption of permanent teeth, and rapid progression of dental lesions.

Abnormal tooth development or abnormal dental matrix formation is often attributed to dietary deficiencies or to nonspecific metabolic factors such as fever, infection, or exposure to toxins during odontogenesis. Abnormalities of this type can lead to rapid dental attrition or delayed dental eruption. In herbivores, delayed eruption of the permanent teeth can result in loss of masticatory function and inability to thrive on pasture.

Degenerative Dental Disease

Lesions caused by attrition and abnormal wear

Alterations in dental appearance and function can be caused by normal or abnormal wear as a result of grinding forces. Loss of dental function due to normal dental attrition is an age-limiting factor in domestic ruminants. Abnormal or irregular wear as a result of poor masticatory function or oral cavity conformation can lead to serious dental malformation in horses. Aggressive dental maintenance is necessary to control irregular wear. In simple-toothed animals, the enamel cap is not meant to be exposed to abnormally harsh grinding pressures. Habitual rock chewing or abnormal mastication can lead to erosion of the crown enamel and disfiguration of the tooth. Exposure of dentin or the pulp canal can lead to dental infection.

Feline external resorptive neck lesions

Cats with **external resorptive neck lesions** of their teeth can have clinical signs referable to pain during mastication. Failure to eat or abnormal masticatory movements may be noticed. Many cats have these tooth lesions and have no history of prior dental disease. The disease is characterized by odontoclastic resorption of dental tissues. The resorption can occur in the root, but, most commonly, resorption occurs in the neck area of the tooth. The resorptive cavity is subsequently lined completely or partially by either a cementum or osteoid ingrowth. The resorptive cavity can fill with a bacterial plaque that results in intense inflammation. However, it is unknown if the resorption is caused by inflammatory gum disease.

Inflammatory Dental Disease

Dental caries

These lesions are characterized by digestion of the inorganic matrix of enamel and dentin concurrent with demineralization resulting from the effects on the dental matrix of acids and enzymatic digestion from bacterial metabolic processes. Dental plaque is the accumulated, nonmineralized bacterial mass adherent to tooth surfaces because of the lack of regular cleaning either by masticatory movements or saliva flow or by prophylactic cleaning. If undisturbed, dental plaque can undergo calcification, with the calcium derived from saliva, to form dental calculus or dental tartar. Tartar does not contribute to destruction of the mineralized dental matrices; however, its presence signals an accumulation of plaque, which if left unchecked, can lead to perforation of the pulp canal and development of pulpitis. Pulpitis (inflammation of the dental pulp) causes pain and, eventually, periodontal abscesses. Dental caries are relatively uncommon in domestic animals.

Infundibular impaction

Impaction of the infundibulum is a cause of serious dental disease in ruminants, comparable in pathogenic mechanism to dental caries in simple-toothed animals. This disease has also been called infundibular necrosis and infundibular caries. The disease is important in both horses and cattle. Incomplete cementum formation in the infundibulum before adult tooth eruption likely predisposes to infundibular impaction. Feed material is ground into the infundibulum (Fig. 1-20), and resultant bacterial metabolic synthesis leads to acid formation, causing demineralization and enzymatic digestion of the organic matrix of enamel and dentin. As a result of matrix destruction, the pulp cavity is penetrated, resulting in pulpitis and periodontitis. Dental abscesses and formation of fistulous tracks lead to serious dental disease. The inflammatory cavities often continue to become impacted with feed, increasing the likelihood of lesion development.

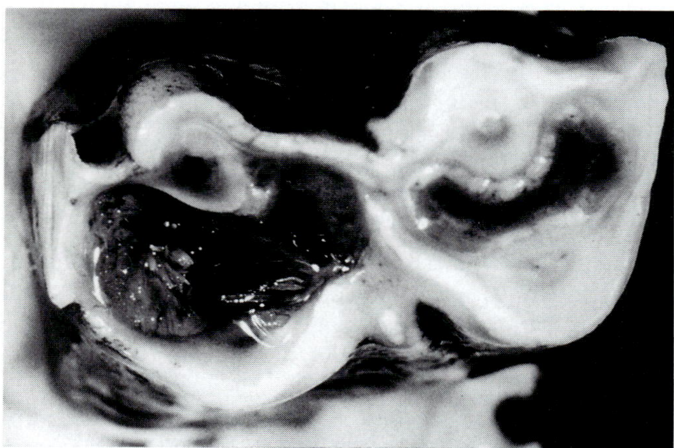

Fig. 1-20 Molar tooth; cow. The infundibulum is impacted with feed.

Periodontal disease

In addition to having a destructive effect on mineralized dental matrices, the accumulation of bacterial plaque has a destructive effect on the supporting soft tissues of the gingiva and periodontal ligament. Bacterial toxins and, possibly, the mechanical irritation of tartar lead to atrophy and inflammation of the gingival epithelium and supporting stroma. The initial site for destructive inflammation is in the gingival crevice, that portion of the gingival epithelium that folds inward adjacent to the crown and attaches at the cementum-enamel junction. Following atrophy and destruction of the gingival stroma adjacent to the gingival crevice, the attachment of the epithelium moves downward on the tooth. Eventually, attachment may occur on the root of the tooth, deep in the alveolar socket. As inflammation invades the connective tissues of the periodontal ligament, the suspensory apparatus is destroyed, and the tooth loosens. Additionally, alveolar osteomyelitis and pulpitis can result in abscesses, bacteremia, pain, reluctance to masticate, and a noxious odor to the breath. Periodontal disease is common in dogs and cats. Diets that fail to provide an opportunity for forceful grinding in mastication predispose to periodontal disease.

Dental Neoplasia

Epulides

These tumors are fairly common and are most frequently seen in dogs, but are also seen in cats. They occur in the gingiva near the tooth and usually appear as epithelium-covered, soft, nodular masses. These lesions have been subdivided into three categories based on morphology and biologic behavior. These subdivisions are fibromatous epulis, osseous epulis, and acanthomatous epulis. The common feature of all three forms is the presence of a stroma characterized by dense, fibrillar collagen; regularly spaced, stellate cells; and a regular, open, vascular pattern.

Fibromatous epulis is composed mainly of periodontal ligament stroma with occasional nests of collagenous matrix which may be bone, cementum, or dentin. Also present are long cordlike or ribbonlike, interbranching, epithelial fronds. When the bonelike matrix becomes a major component, the epulis is called an **osseous epulis.** Both fibromatous epulis and osseous epulis are considered benign overgrowths of periodontal ligament stroma and have been classified as hamartomas or benign tumors.

Acanthomatous epulis is distinguished by the presence of interconnecting broad sheets of acanthomatous epithelial cells. These cells are characterized by peripheral palisading and central, prominent, spinous processes. Keratinization does not occur in the epithelial sheets.

Acanthomatous epulis is differentiated from squamous cell carcinoma by such features as the lack of keratinization, the presence of the characteristic stroma, and the mineralized collagenous matrix in the acanthomatous epulis. Unlike fibromatous epulis and osseous epulis, the acanthomatous epulis infiltrates and destroys the periodontal apparatus, including the alveolar bone. Acanthomatous epulis is sensitive to radiation therapy, but recurrence has been observed following a long latent period. The recurrent lesion is usually a squamous cell carcinoma. However, fibrosarcoma and osteosarcoma have also been reported.

Editors' note: The classification of lesions of the gingiva of dogs referred to as the epulides is incomplete. The term epulis refers to any tumorous lesion of the gingiva, and, while clinically descriptive, it is a nonspecific term, and the real nature of these lesions must be determined by microscopic examination. Thus, in more recent studies, investigators have suggested that the canine epulides can be placed into the categories of focal fibrous hyperplasia (some fibromatous and ossifying epulides), peripheral odontogenic fibroma (some fibromatous epulides with fronds of odontogenic epithelium), and peripheral ameloblastoma (some acanthomatous epulides).

Neoplasms of the Enamel Organ

Neoplasms of the enamel organ are named according to the extent of differentiation and the extent of odontogenesis seen in the tumor. The enamel organ consists of all the various tissues responsible for odontogenesis, including the odontogenic epithelium, dental pulp, and odontoblasts. Odontogenic epithelium must be present in order to initiate the inductive events leading to dental pulp and odontoblast formation. For this reason, dental epithelium is present in all the common neoplasms arising from the enamel organ. Odontogenic tumors can arise from the original dental lamina or from epithelial cell rests of Malassez that remain in the periodontal ligament. Dental neoplasms can also arise from dental epithelium in the superficial gingiva, in either the gingival crest or the surface epithelium. Odontogenic neoplasms can also arise from the cystic remnants of dysplastic odontogenesis. Poorly differentiated, strictly epithelial neoplasms usually occur in mature animals, presumably from the cell rests of Malassez. More fully differentiated neoplasms, displaying inductive formation of dentin or well-differentiated enamel matrix, arise in young animals, probably from dysplastic remnants of the original dental lamina. Dental neoplasms can either arise deeply in the jaw or originate on the surface epithelium. They usually occur near the teeth.

Ameloblastoma

Ameloblastoma is the preferred generic name used for purely epithelial neoplasms of enamel organ origin. Although variations in the morphologic pattern of ameloblastoma occur within many species, not enough is known about the biologic significance of the morphologic variations to justify the use of more specialized nomenclature. Most is known about the morphologic and behavioral aspects of ameloblastoma in dogs. Ameloblastoma occurs anywhere in the dental arcade, usually in adult dogs. Neoplasms can be either superficial or deep and are usually locally invasive, resulting in lysis of alveolar bone. The histologic features characteristic of ameloblastoma in dogs include interbranching sheets of epithelial cells with palisading at the base and stellate, reticulum-like formation centrally; elongate, interbranching ribbons of epithelial cells; abrupt and intense keratinization, often with large, round, heavily keratinized cells; and the presence of extracellular hyalin bodies occurring between epithelial cells. These hyalin bodies often stain positive for amyloid. In addition, islands of mineralized, collagenous matrix of bone, cementum, or dentin can be found often intimately associated with the epithelium, suggesting an inductive effect. Ameloblastoma may be differentiated from acanthomatous epulis by the fact that the characteristic stroma is not found, keratinization does occur, and there is the unique finding of intercellular hyalin bodies. Ameloblastoma can be differentiated from squamous cell carcinoma by the nature and extent of the keratinization, the presence of intercellular hyalin bodies, and the formation of stellate, reticulum-like, epithelial sheets. Palisading of tall, columnar cells suggesting ameloblastic differentiation can occasionally be found.

Inductive fibroameloblastoma (ameloblastic fibroma)

Inductive fibroameloblastoma is a rare neoplasm of young cats. The neoplasm occurs in the cat approximately at the time of replacement of the deciduous teeth and may be either deep or superficial. Inductive fibroameloblastoma is characterized by interbranching epithelial fronds that tend to form cuplike clusters surrounding areas of mesenchyme having differentiation toward dental pulplike epithelium reminiscent of the cup state of odontogenesis (Fig. 1-21). These neoplasms have been removed successfully when bone infiltration has not occurred.

Ameloblastic odontoma (odontoameloblastoma)

Ameloblastic odontoma is a predominantly epithelial neoplasm with well-defined evidence of dental laminar origin, such as well-differentiated stellate reticulum or palisaded ameloblastic epithelium. For the neoplasm to be classified as ameloblastic odontoma, dentinlike matrix must be present. Usually, clusters within the neoplasm have well-differentiated, ameloblastic-type epithelium immediately adjacent to areas where dentin matrix is deposited (Fig. 1-22). Usually, areas of inductive dentin formation must be searched for. These neoplasms are rare and usually are seen in young animals. They have been re-

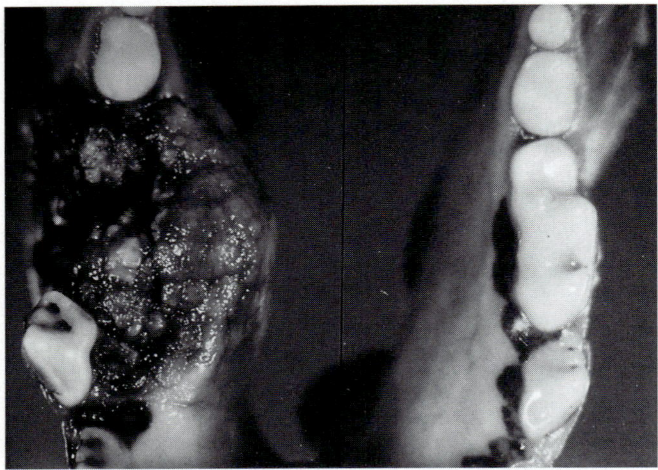

Fig. 1-21 Mandible; dog. Acanthomatous epulis.

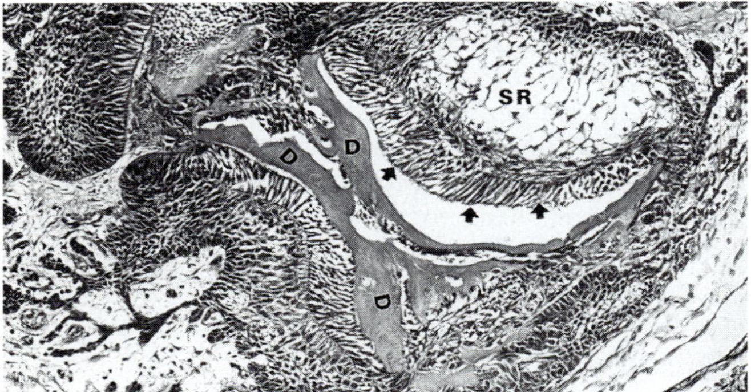

Fig. 1-22 Mandible; dog. Ameloblastic odontoma characterized by dentin matrix (*D*), ameloblastic epithelium *(arrows),* and stellate reticulum *(SR).*

ported in dogs, sheep, horses, cattle, nonhuman primates, and rats.

Ossifying (cementifying) fibroma

In this neoplasm, numerous small, round-to-ovoid islands of acellular mineralized material occur within an abundant, immature, highly cellular, fibrous connective tissue stroma composed of a population of tightly packed, interwoven, plump fibroblasts. The composition of the neoplasms varies from those that are predominantly fibroblastic to those that are composed predominantly of mineralized tissue.

Calcifying epithelial odontogenic tumor

This is a benign but locally invasive neoplasm composed of large, polyhedral epithelial cells that form sheets, islands, and strands within a fibrous stroma. Characteristic features are the presence of eosinophilic masses within the epithelial cells and concentrically laminated foci of calcification. The eosinophilic material stains as amyloid in some procedures and is considered a degradation product of lamina densa material.

Peripheral odontogenic fibroma

This neoplasm is characterized by abundant fibrous tissue containing a variety of osseous, osteoid, dentinoid, and cementoid-like materials. Strands, usually of two-cell thickness, and small clusters of odontogenic epithelium are present and are in close association with the foci of hard tissues. The epithelial cells are uniform and appear inactive. The fibrous connective tissue component varies in degree of cellularity but is typically arranged as cellular strands interwoven with less cellular areas.

Odontoma

Odontomas are hamartomas of enamel organ origin and contain fully differentiated dentin and enamel. Ameloblasts, odontoblasts, and dental pulp may also be present. Odontomas can be classified as **complex odontoma** if the dental substances are completely disorganized, having no resemblance to normal tooth formation, or as **compound odontoma** if the dental substances are arranged to form clusters of small toothlike structures known as denticles. Complex and compound odontomas are nearly always found in young animals, usually in dogs and horses.

ESOPHAGUS

Obstructions and Functional Disorders

Cricopharyngeal achalasia

This disorder of the upper esophageal sphincter is recognized infrequently in dogs, but occurs most often in terriers, cocker spaniels, and miniature poodles. After weaning and before 6 months of age, the disorder is characterized by dysphagia and regurgitation of ingested feed. After deglutition and failure of the sphincter to relax, short, sharp movements of the tongue, mandible, and neck are made in an attempt to dislodge the food bolus. Acquired cricopharyngeal achalasia occurs rarely in the dog. The etiology is unknown in both the congenital and acquired forms.

The lesion, a grossly discernible deformity of the cricopharyngeous muscle, has been variously described as hypertrophy, fibrosis, myositis, or atrophy. Few specimens have been available for microscopic study, as surgeons perform simple myotomy as a treatment for the disease rather than resection or biopsy.

Megaesophagus

Megaesophagus is an infrequent disorder of the dog, cat, and horse; it has been recognized in 28 purebred breeds of dogs and in mongrels as well. In the German shepherd dog and Great Dane, multiple cases among littermates suggest that the disorder is inherited. In the cat, a preponderance of cases has occurred in the Siamese breed, and some af-

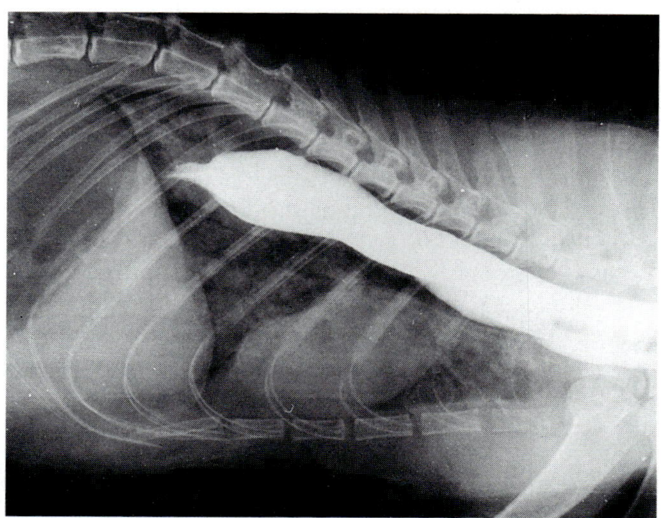

Fig. 1-23 Esophagus; cat. Megaesophagus. This lateral radiograph demonstrates a dilated esophagus, twice the diameter of normal. *Clifford DH, Soifer FK, Wilson CF, Waddel ED, Guilloud GL. J Am Vet Med Assoc 1971; 158:1558.*

fected cats have had pyloric stenosis as well. Congenital megaesophagus has been rarely recognized in young Thoroughbred colts. An acquired form is well recognized in old horses and in the dog. In each of the species affected, megaesophagus is indicated by regurgitation shortly after a meal, a distended cervical esophagus, fetid breath, and weight loss. Aspiration pneumonia occurs in some affected animals.

Dogs with megaesophagus have an absence of function of a portion of the upper and middle esophagus. However, the lower esophageal sphincter pressure is normal in both the congenital and acquired forms. Results of manometric and electromyographic studies of affected unanesthetized dogs indicate that sphincter relaxation occurs in response to swallowing less than 60% of the time. Megaesophagus has been attributed to a developmental immaturity of the vagus nervous supply, an immaturity that was demonstrated in a small proportion of normal dogs as well. Supranodosal vagotomy or electrolytic destruction of the nucleus ambiguous (the motor nucleus of the vagus) of the dog and cat produces megaesophagus without sphincter hypertonicity, which is similar to the naturally occurring disease. In some spontaneous cases, the nucleus ambiguous has much fewer neurons, but Siamese cats with congenital megaesophagus have normal numbers of myenteric ganglion cells and neurons in the dorsal motor nucleus of the vagus.

Grossly, megaesophagus is a prominently dilated, flaccid esophagus, two to three times normal diameter (Fig. 1-23), with the dilatation uniform in some animals, but quite eccentric in others. The dilated portions often contain a fetid fluid residue from previously consumed meals. The lower esophageal sphincter, a zone 1 to 2 cm in length, is unaffected. Microscopic examination and efforts to count myenteric ganglion cells are usually nondiagnostic. Vagus nerves may or may not contain lesions of a degenerative nature.

Injuries and Inflammation

Reflux esophagitis

This rare disorder of dogs and cats is caused by acid or acid and pepsin irritation of the stratified squamous epithelium of the distal esophagus. In the normal animal, reflux of acid and pepsin is prevented by a properly functioning cardia, but when this is hypotonic or for other reasons fails to perform its function adequately, as during anesthesia, acid and pepsin percolate into the distal esophagus, causing severe erosive esophagitis.

The lesions of reflux esophagitis may be focal ulceration or erosion with necrosis of the superficial epithelial layers, or, alternatively, the lesions may be inflammatory and hyperplastic. Chronic bathing of the lower esophagus with acid produces an acanthosis—a hyperplasia of the proliferating cells of the stratified squamous mucosa. The connective tissue ridges of the lamina propria beneath extend toward, and almost reach, the luminal surface. In chronic cases, the lamina propria and submucosa are extensively infiltrated with plasma cells and lymphocytes and are fibrotic due to chronic ulceration.

Chemical injury

Chemical burns of the esophagus from strong acids and alkalis are rare in animals, but were seen in the past in horses when harsh chemical agents were used as vermifuges. Clinically, affected animals have evidence of intense pain in the mouth and chest, are unable to swallow, and have tachycardia. Affected animals may retch, regurgitate, and bring up quantities of frothy mucus, blood, and devitalized esophageal tissue. This acute phase passes in 3 to 4 days and is followed by dysphagia secondary to stricture formation.

The lesions are coagulation necrosis with necrotic membrane, severe edema with blister formation, and diffuse erythema of the mucosae of the oral cavity, pharynx, and esophagus. Microscopically, coagulation necrosis extends through the epithelial layers, lamina propria, and submucosa and, in some cases, through the tunica muscularis.

Traumatic esophagitis and impaction

Traumatic esophagitis occurs with some frequency in dogs and horses, especially in puppies and young dogs, which have a propensity for chewing and swallowing foreign objects, such as safety pins, parts of toys, and sharp-edged bones. The splintered long bones of chicken legs and the sharp T bones of pork chops are particularly likely to cause damage to the esophagus. These foreign bodies may produce lacerations or become lodged. Horses have traumatic esophagitis secondary to "choke." Horses ''choke'' when esophageal motility is impaired, after consumption of dry feeds such as pelleted commercial rations or beet pulp, and after retention of improperly administered capsules or boluses. Cattle choke follows the ingestion of apples or similar fruits and vegetables, e.g., turnips. In cattle, complete obstruction interferes with eructation of rumen gases, rapidly resulting in a potentially fatal bloat. Choke on grain produces little damage to the esophageal mucosa, unless the condition goes unresolved for many days. On the other hand, obstruction of the esophagus by a mass, such as a bolus or apple, produces ischemic necrosis and ulceration, and more severe and extensive lesions occur when the obstructing mass contains irritating chemical ingredients, such as cathartics.

Clinical signs in animals that have esophageal injury or choke include an inability to swallow saliva and feed and peculiar movements with the head and neck, in an attempt to dislodge the choked material. In horses, and sometimes cattle, the material causing the choke may distend the esophagus to the extent that it can be seen and palpated.

The lesions in traumatic esophagitis vary with the cause and time. Small foreign bodies swallowed by dogs produce lacerations, foci of coagulation necrosis, ulceration, and granulocytic response. The diffuse choke that occurs in horses can be expected to cause pressure necrosis in the most compacted areas. Capsules and boluses in the equine esophagus produce focal severe coagulation necrosis involving the mucosa, lamina propria, and submucosa, and perforation may result. If the choke is relieved and perforation does not occur, fibrosis and stenosis are common secondary lesions.

Parasitic Esophagitis

Gongylonemiasis

This disease occurs in horses, cattle, sheep, goats, pigs, buffalo, wild boars, donkeys, deer, camels, zebra, rats, nonhuman primates, and human beings. The *Gongylonema* are long, thin, spiruroid nematodes up to 6 cm in length that inhabit the esophageal mucosa and are seen as accordion-pleated threads (Fig. 1-24). The parasites are essentially nonpathogenic and produce no local host response.

Spirocercosis

Spirocercosis caused by *Spirocerca lupi* is a parasitic granulomatous inflammation of the distal esophagus affecting carnivores in the southern United States and in tropical countries. The adult red spiruroid nematode, 30 to 80 mm in length, burrows into the mucosa of the distal esophagus, producing a cystic granuloma that communicates with the esophageal lumen by a fistula. Discharged embryonated ova pass through the fistulous opening into the lumen of the esophagus, down the GI tract, and into the feces of the host. The eggs are consumed by dung beetles, the intermediate host, and these in turn are consumed by reptiles, rodents, or chickens, which serve as paratenic hosts. The larvae encyst until the intermediate or paratenic host is consumed. Upon digestion in the carnivore, larvae penetrate the wall of the stomach, migrate in the adventitia of gastric arteries, and find their way to the proximal aorta, where they produce parasitic cysts, aneurysms, granulomas, and, sometimes, aortic rupture. After a time, the parasites leave the aorta and migrate in the interstitium or along small arteries to the distal esophagus. The lesions often produce no clinical illness or may be the cause of

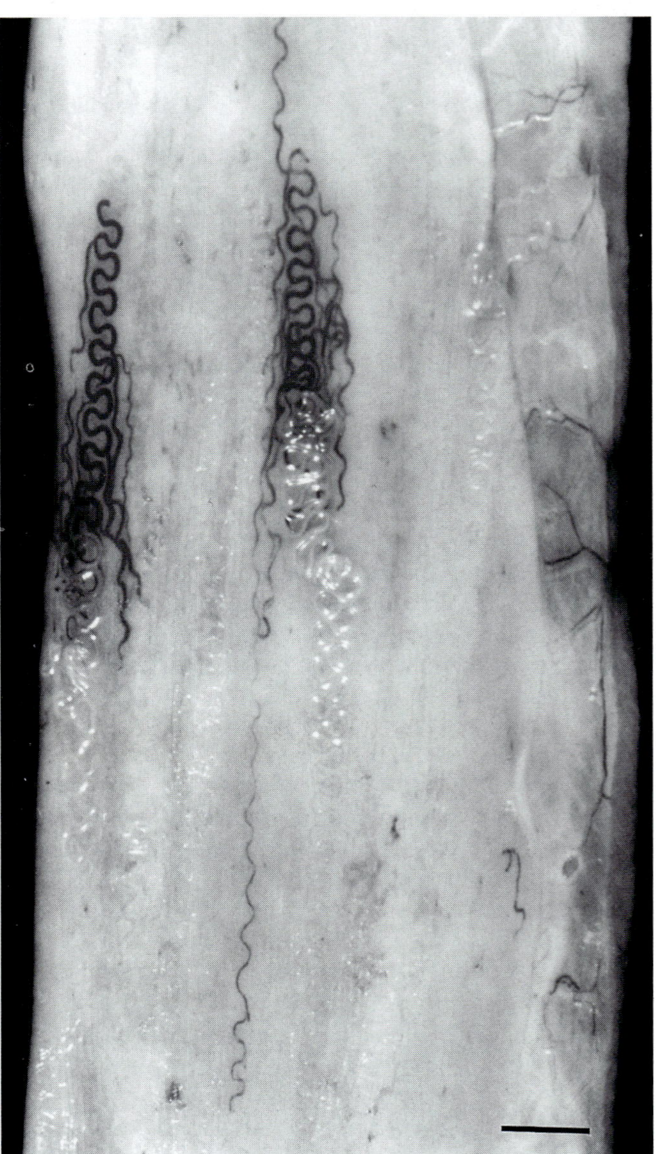

Fig. 1-24 Esophagus; deer. Gonglyonemiasis. The *Gonglyonema* are embedded within esophageal mucosa. Bar = 5 mm. *Courtesy Dr. M.D. McGavin.*

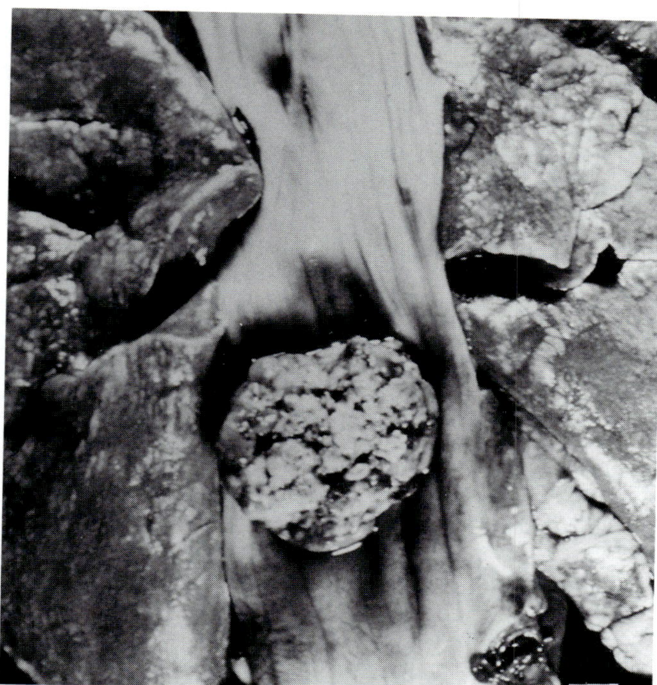

Fig. 1-25 Esophagus; dog. Spirocercosis. A 4-cm diameter granulomatous nodule protrudes into the lumen of the distal esophagus. Bar = 1 cm. *Courtesy the Department of Pathology and Parasitology, Auburn University.*

dysphagia, regurgitation, and dilatation of the esophagus proximal to the granulomatous segment.

Larval migration tracks contain necrotic tissue, hemorrhage, and eosinophils, but some tracks may be difficult to find when they are replaced by fibrous tissue. In the aorta, the lesions consist of mural granulomas and aneurysms; in the distal esophagus, a granulomatous, fibrous cystic nodule, varying from 1 to 10 cm in diameter, encases the parasites (Fig. 1-25). Within these nodules, *Spirocerca* females with flattened ovoid eggs are surrounded by a purulent exudate. Where the parasites have produced chronic granulomatous inflammation of a segment of the aorta, spondylitis deformans may occur in adjacent vertebral bodies. In dogs, chronic granulomatous disease of the distal esophagus rarely is the site for development of esophageal fibrosarcomas or osteosarcomas.

Mycotic Esophagitis

Candidiasis

Candidiasis, also known as ''thrush'' or moniliasis, is an infection of the stratified squamous epithelium of the esophagus, oral cavity, and crop, caused by the yeast, *Candida albicans,* a normal inhabitant of the upper GI tract. Candidiasis has been recognized in human beings, monkeys, chimpanzees, calves, goats, pigs, cetaceans, and birds. *Candida* becomes pathogenic when the resistance of the host has been lowered by systemic infection, leukopenia, severe neoplasia, immunosuppression, or chemotherapy. In calves, candidiasis results from reduction of competing bacterial flora when antibiotic therapy is prolonged. *Candida* can invade other parts of the GI tract but generally overgrows in parts with stratified squamous epithelium. Candidiasis of the esophagus of the dog and cat is uncommon.

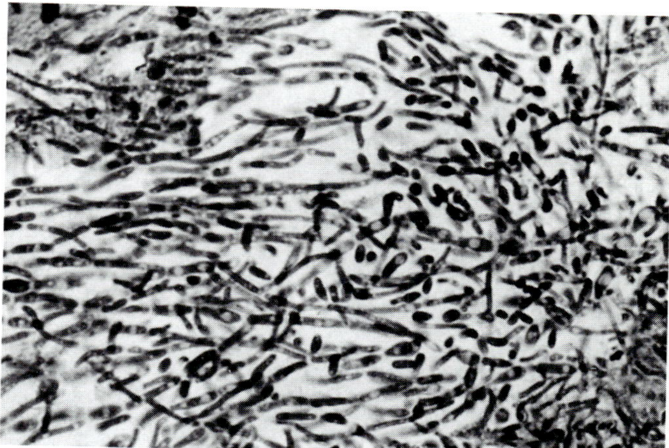

Fig. 1-26 Esophagus; calf. Candidiasis. Yeast and pseudohyphal forms of *Candida albicans* in a tangled mat on the surface of damaged epithelium. Grocott's methenamine-silver stain.

The lesions of candidiasis are white, raised, oval plaques (5 to 8 mm in diameter) on the epithelial surface. The coalesced lesions may comprise a pseudomembranous layer over red, raw areas of ulceration. In severe cases of candidiasis, the surface is encrusted by caseous material.

Microscopically, masses of the organisms, as yeast and pseudohyphal forms, make up the white-gray material on the surface (Fig. 1-26), which interdigitates with a parakeratotic stratified squamous epithelium.

Neoplasms

Squamous cell carcinoma

Neoplasms of the esophagus are rare in animals, but have been described in cats and horses and in cattle in Brazil and Great Britain, where consumption of bracken fern *(Pteris aquilina)* has been incriminated.

Clinically, esophageal carcinoma is accompanied by dysphagia, regurgitation, dilatation of esophagus proximal to the mass, weight loss, and a palpable cervical mass.

Squamous cell carcinomas are often not detected early because the neoplastic mass grows into the lumen. The surface is cauliflower-like and may be ulcerated. With time, the mass obstructs the esophagus and produces a stricture. Spread to contiguous tissue occurs readily, and the neoplasms metastasize to regional lymph nodes, liver, and lungs.

STOMACH

Obstructions and Functional Disorders

Acute gastric dilatation

Acute gastric dilatation occurs in all species of animals, but it is most frequent in cattle, horses, dogs, and nonhuman primates. The large, compartmentalized stomach of ruminants is specialized for digestion and fermentation; the latter creates a recurrent possibility for bloat (ruminant tympany). Three types of acute gastric dilatation are recognized: obstructive bloat, simple bloat, and frothy bloat. Obstructive bloat occurs when large fruits or vegetables cause obstruction of the esophagus. Simple bloat or frothy bloat occurs after the consumption of feeds rich in readily digestible carbohydrates and failure to eructate because of lack of scabrous material to stimulate the cardia, submersion of the cardia beneath fluid ingesta, and occlusion of the cardia by froth. Frothy bloat is characterized by entrapment of gas within the ingesta, and intubation fails to relieve the distention. Entrapment of gas occurs through increasing surface tension and stable foam formation. Decreased amounts of saliva and a pH below 6.0 favor foam stability.

Horses engorged on grain have acute gastric dilatation and, subsequently, gastric rupture. In Scotland, England, and Sweden, acute gastric dilatation occurs in horses on pasture as a part of a disease called "grass sickness." Grass sickness has been regarded as a separate disease entity by some, and, recently, serologic evidence has been provided for an association with *Clostridium perfringens* type A enterotoxin. However, certain features are consistent with acute gastric dilatation, including excessive salivation, dysphagia or inability to swallow, antiperistaltic contractions of the esophagus, gastric rupture, peritonitis, and death. Another cause of gastric rupture in the horse is reflux of intestinal contents, occurring with reverse peristalsis associated with small bowel obstruction.

Acute gastric dilatation constitutes a major cause of death in many large breeds of dogs and occurs after consumption of a large meal, suggesting that diet or engorgement is causative. Dogs fed a commercial dry product once daily develop larger stomachs that contain a greater feed residue hours after eating. Commercial dry dog food products that contain readily digestible and fermentable ingredients have been incriminated.

Acute gastric dilatation also occurs spontaneously in nonhuman primates. In captive monkeys, an increased frequency often occurs over a weekend when presumably there is a difference in the feeding pattern because of weekend caretakers. Evidence of the roles of *C. perfringens* and fermentable substrates comes from studies with monkeys and marmosets. *C. perfringens* was found in the gastric contents of 21 of 24 monkeys with acute gastric dilatation but in few samples (2 of 18) from normal monkeys. Twenty-nine cases of acute gastric dilatation occurred in marmosets over a 5-week period following therapy with gentamicin and Furoxone. *C. perfringens* type A was found in the gastric contents of all 25 animals that were necropsied.

In each of the species that experience this disease, the sudden gaseous distention of the stomach and an enigmatic failure to eructate result in abdominal distention, accompanied by compression of the lungs and occlusion of the posterior vena cava, resulting in hypovolemic shock. The dog, cat, pig, and human being often have concomitant gastric volvulus; dogs, horses, monkeys, and human beings have gastric rupture as a consequence, with resultant peritonitis.

Severe gaseous and fluid enlargement of the stomach causes the abdomen to be protuberant and tympanitic. With simple dilatation, the enlarged stomach assumes a longitudinal orientation within the abdomen, thereby displacing other viscera and causing collapse of the lungs and ileus of the small intestine (Figs. 1-27 and 1-28). From the se-

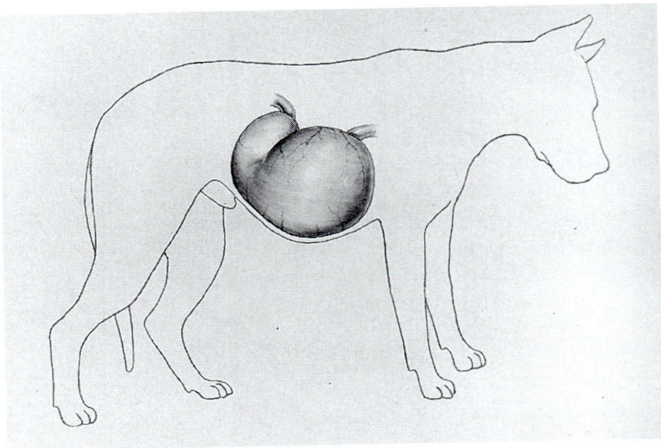

Fig. 1-27 Stomach; dog. Acute gastric dilatation. This diagram drawn from postmortem photographs illustrates the position of the distended stomach in the live animal. *Van Kruiningen HJ, Gregoire K, Meuten DJ. J Am Anim Hosp Assoc 1974; 10:306.*

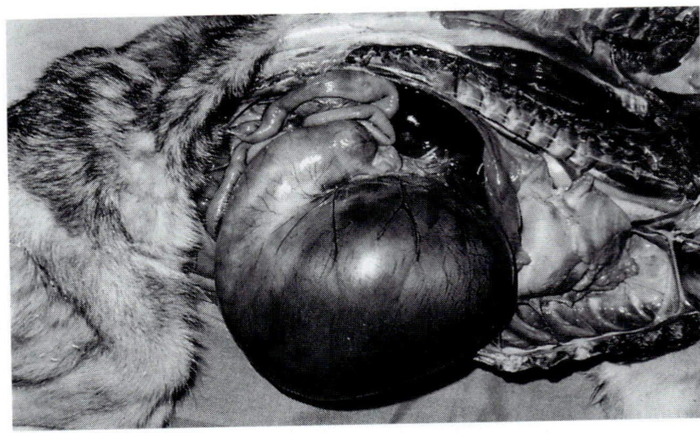

Fig. 1-28 Stomach; dog. Acute gastric dilatation. The stomach is distended by ingesta and gas and is red to violet. It has significantly displaced other abdominal viscera. Note the collapsed lung.

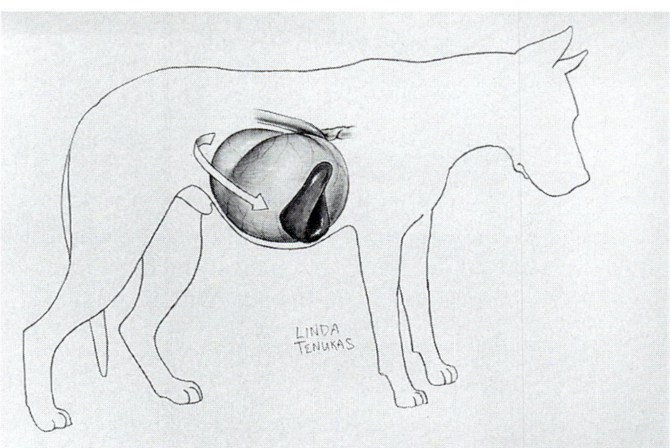

Fig. 1-29 Stomach; dog. Acute gastric dilatation. This diagram made from postmortem photographs illustrates the 360-degree rotation that occurs with volvulus. The spleen is folded and located in the right cranial abdomen up against the diaphragm. *Van Kruiningen HJ, Gregoire K, Meuten DJ. J Am Anim Hosp Assoc 1974; 10:306.*

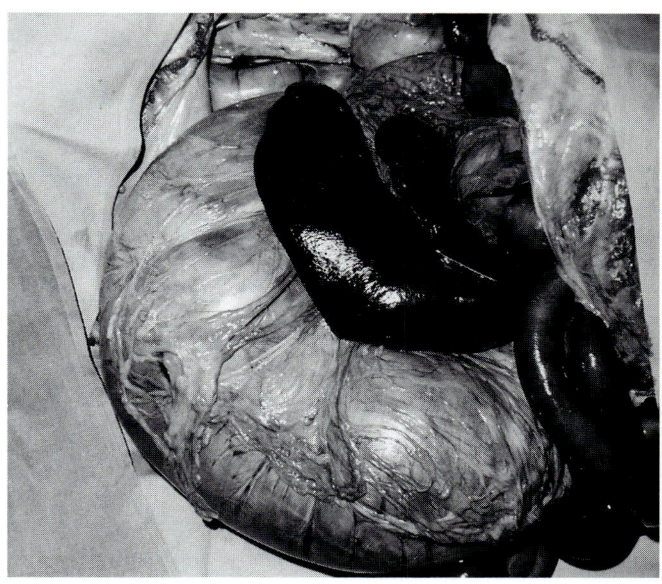

Fig. 1-30 Stomach; dog. Acute gastric dilatation with a 360-degree volvulus. The stomach is greatly enlarged and distended, and the spleen is folded in a V, located against the diaphragm adjacent to the last ribs on the right side of the abdomen. The intestines are dilated and congested.

rosal surface, the gastric wall has a dull blue to violet color; mucosal surface is maroon to red-black. Gastric contents are of thick-liquid consistency, containing partially digested feed. In animals with volvulus as well (an event that takes place during distention), the stomach is rotated on its mesenteric axis in a clockwise direction (as viewed ventrodorsally) (Fig. 1-29). The duodenum is entwined around the esophagus, and the spleen has been carried with the stomach from its location on the left side of the abdomen to a position caudodorsal to the stomach and thence to the right side. In most instances of volvulus, there is a 360 degree clockwise twist. The spleen does not follow the stomach for a full 360 degrees, but instead becomes trapped and folded in a V up against the right side of the diaphragm (Fig. 1-30). In fewer cases, the stomach twists from 180 to 270 degrees, and the displacement of the spleen is variable. The spleen is greatly enlarged and engorged with blood. Ileus is manifested by reddening and dilatation of the intestines.

Displaced abomasum

This disorder occurs infrequently in low-producing dairy cattle that are allowed to be outside much of the year and to consume normal quantities of roughage. On the other hand, displaced abomasum occurs with increased frequency in cows of high-producing herds that are intensively managed; that are fed greater amounts of succulent feeds, such as corn silage, and lesser amounts of dried, coarse roughages; and that have fewer days at pasture.

Clinical features of displaced abomasum include partial anorexia, weight loss, dehydration, scanty feces, and ketonuria. On auscultation, a characteristic high-pitched ping can be heard over the distended, displaced abomasum, whether it is on the left side or the right. Acute displacement of the abomasum to the right with volvulus is characterized by abomasal tympany and signs of abdominal pain such as grinding of the teeth, abnormal posture, repeated getting up and lying down, and kicking at the belly. Other clinical signs include anorexia, restlessness, rapid heart rate, modest grunting or groaning, lack of abdominal peristalsis, and scanty feces.

The abomasum is located on the ventral midline of the abdomen of the cow, sometimes slightly to the right of the midline. With atony, enlargment, and gaseous dilatation, the dilated abomasum can remain in its usual location, but usually it is displaced either to the left (80% to 90% of displacement cases in North America) or to the right. The left displaced abomasum occupies the anterior left quadrant of the abdomen of the cow, displaces the rumen medially, and is found in this location at the time of necropsy. When the abomasum is displaced to the right, it may continue to distend, curl dorsally, and then twist on its mesenteric axis, resulting in volvulus of the abomasum (Figs. 1-31 and 1-32). When in volvulus, the wall is dark red and blood-filled.

Chronic gastric dilatation

Chronic gastric dilatation is almost always a secondary event. In the dog, it is secondary to gastric ulcer, lymphoma of the gastric wall, uremia, pyloric stenosis, acute gastric dilatation, intervertebral disc disease, and vagotomy. In the horse, chronic gastric dilatation may occur as a conse-

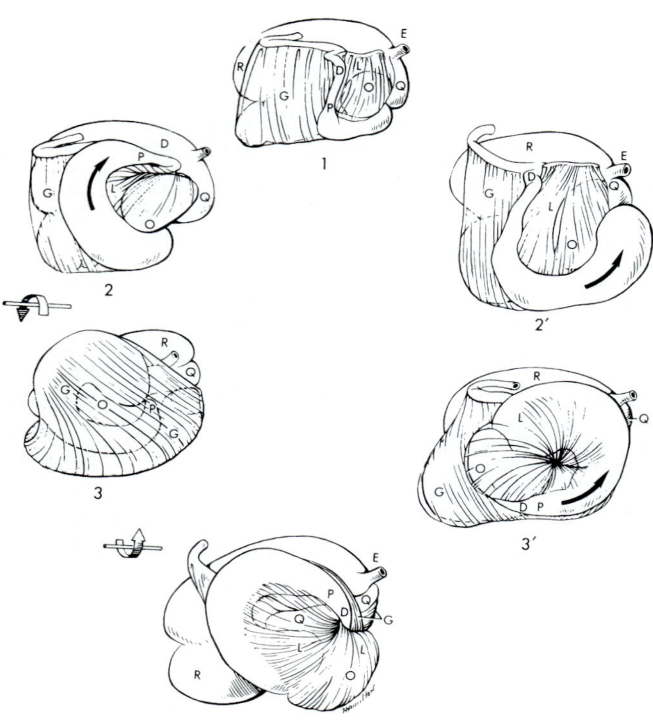

Fig. 1-31 Abomasum; cow. Displaced abomasum with volvulus. Diagrams to illustrate two possible modes of rotation of the omasum, abomasum, and cranial part of the duodenum in volvulus. *1,* normal relations; *2,* simple dilatation and displacement on the right; *3,* 180-degree volvulus around the longitudinal axis of the lesser omentum, counterclockwise as seen from the rear; *2′*, 90-degree rotation of the abomasum in a sagittal plane, counterclockwise as seen from the right; *3′*, 180-degree rotation of the abomasum and omasum around the transverse axis of the lesser omentum, drawing the duodenum cranially, medial to the omasum; *4,* 360-degree counterclockwise volvulus, final stage resulting from either mode of rotation. *D,* duodenum; *E,* esophagus; *G,* greater omentum; *L,* lesser omentum; *O,* omasum; *P,* pylorus; *Q,* reticulum; *R,* rumen. *Habel RE, Smith DF. J Am Vet Med Assoc 1981; 179:447-455.*

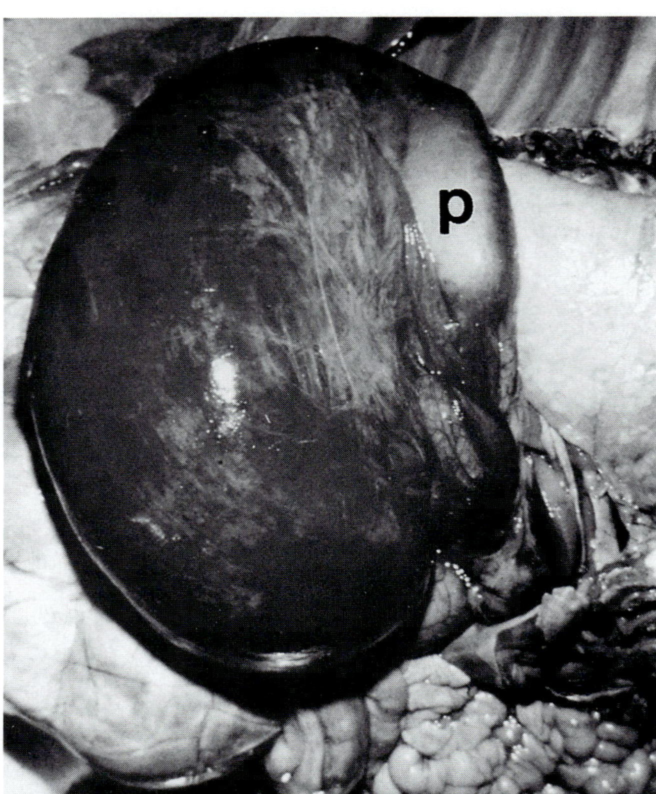

Fig. 1-32 Abomasum; cow. Right displaced abomasum with volvulus. The abomasum is enlarged and the wall is engorged with blood and edema. *P,* pylorus.

quence of the consumption of nonnutritious feed, but more frequently in horses that are "wind-suckers," those animals with the vice of cribbing and air-swallowing. In ruminants, chronic dilatation of the rumen occurs after engorgement, difficult parturition, transport fatigue, and metabolic disorders. Ruminants fed poorly nutritious feed such as straw, poor quality hay, and frozen silage develop chronic gastric dilatation. Chronic abomasal dilatation occurs in cows with abomasal ulcers, abomasal malignant lymphoma, and the disorder called "vagal indigestion." Vagal indigestion is considered a sequela to traumatic reticulitis, with the implication that inflammation and subsequent fibrosis of the diaphragm or of regional lymph nodes compromises vagal innervation. Selective vagotomy will produce chronic dilatation and atony of selected compartments of the ruminant stomach, but cattle with impacted abomasums do not have fibrosis of the diaphragm in the vicinity of the vagal nerves or degenerative changes within the vagal nerves.

Clinically, animals with chronic gastric dilatation have partial or complete anorexia, a lack of normal contraction sounds or peristaltic waves, greater than normal gaseous bubble, and, thus, noticeably distended abdomen. Chronic gastric dilatation contributes to a slowing of the entire GI system so that sounds and motility patterns of the small bowel are reduced and feces are scanty. Lesions in chronic gastric dilatation are few and consist of an enlarged stomach with an abnormal volume or character of feed residue. The dilated abomasum is enlarged and impacted with dry contents.

Engorgement toxemia

Engorgement toxemia, an acute atony of the rumen, occurs consequent to engorgement on carbohydrates and development of a lactic acidosis. Engorgement toxemia is seen more frequently in cattle than in other ruminants and usually occurs when animals accustomed to one level of dietary carbohydrates suddenly have access to a much greater amount or are inadvertently overfed.

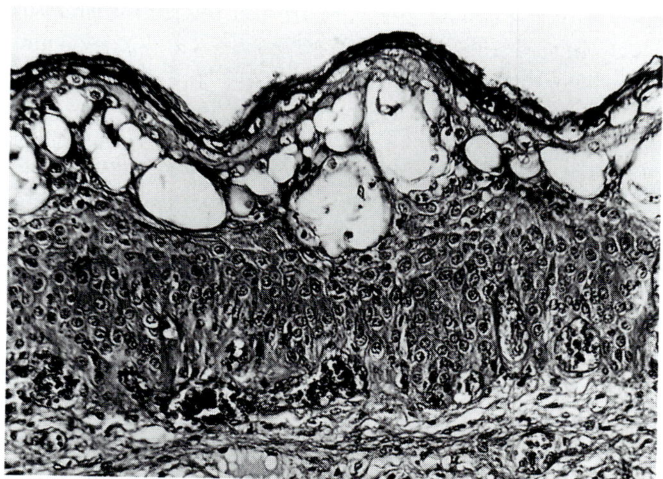

Fig. 1-33 Rumen; cow. Engorgement toxemia. Microvesicles, many of which contain granulocytes, occur in stratified squamous epithelium of rumen papillae. H & E stain.

When excessive quantities of readily digestible, fermentable carbohydrates are consumed, within several hours the rumen flora produce excessive quantities of volatile fatty acids, resulting in reduction in the rumen pH (the normal pH being 5.5 to 7.5). As the pH falls, protozoa and gram-negative bacteria are suppressed, and other bacteria, such as streptococci and lactobacilli, overgrow and produce excessive quantities of lactic acid. The excess of lactic and volatile fatty acids establishes a pH of 4.0 to 4.5 and a toxic acidosis. The increased content of fatty acids has an osmotic effect and attracts fluids from the systemic circulation into the rumen, resulting in dehydration, hypovolemia, acidosis, rumen atony, fluid distention of the rumen, and toxemia. Clinically, cattle with lactic acidosis have anorexia, cessation of milk flow, depression, rumen atony, splashy ruminal sounds on ballottment, cold extremities, and dilated, unresponsive pupils. In severe cases, there is prostration.

Cattle dying of engorgement toxemia have enlarged rumens containing excessive fluid contents and excessive carbohydrate-rich feeds, have a ruminal pH below 4.5, and are dehydrated. The lesions of lactic acidosis are granulocyte-containing microvesicles of the epithelium of the rumen papillae (Fig. 1-33). These lesions represent an avenue for invasion by fusobacteria *(Fusobacterium necrophorum)* and by fungi.

Pyloric stenosis

This lesion has been recognized in dogs, particularly the brachycephalic breeds and especially the boxer; in cats, particularly Siamese cats; and, sometimes, in association with megaesophagus, and in laboratory rabbits. Pyloric stenosis is familial in dogs, cats, and human beings.

The pyloric sphincter is composed of smooth muscle fibers of the inner muscle layer, and hyperplasia of this muscle coat may be due to prenatal, neonatal, or acquired hormonal or neurologic influences. Pentagastrin administration to pregnant bitches and newborn puppies has produced pyloric hypertrophy in a proportion of the puppies. Selective destruction of the myenteric plexuses of the canine pylorus failed to reproduce the lesion. Although most pyloric stenosis is recognized as congenital, with clinical signs occurring soon after the animal takes solid feed, an acquired pyloric stenosis occurring later in life is recognized also. When the disorder occurs in an older animal, it is usually regarded as secondary to pyloric ulceration, parasitic eosinophilic granuloma, focal inflammation, or fibrosis of the pyloric wall.

The stenotic pylorus interferes with gastric emptying, and this results in projectile vomiting shortly after a meal, enlargement of the stomach, retention of a gastric residue, and accentuated peristaltic waves that may be heard, seen, or felt coursing from left to right across the abdomen. The hypertrophied pylorus may be palpated in animals that have a thin abdominal wall.

The lesions of pyloric stenosis are grossly discernable enlargement and muscular hypertrophy, reduced lumen diameter, and accentuated mucosal folds. Microscopically, muscle hypertrophy is accompanied by variable submucosal edema, submucosal vascular ectasia, minimal leukocyte influx, and variable degeneration of myenteric ganglion cells.

Injuries and Inflammations

Gastric ulcers

Gastric ulcers occur infrequently in dogs, cats, and foals; and abomasal ulcers are seen in both young and adult cattle. In the dog, gastric ulcers have been seen with mastocytoma, thyroid neoplasia, hepatic cirrhosis, uremia, and the Zollinger-Ellison syndrome. Gastric ulcers also occur independent of other illnesses. In foals, gastric ulceration may be sporadic, affecting animals 1 to 6 months of age, or clusters of cases may be endemic to a farm or a particular management. About 1% of normal adult cattle have ulcers at the time of slaughter, whereas in feedlot cattle the prevalence is about 3.6%.

Ulcers may occur in the fundus, the body, and the antrum of the stomach; the proximal duodenum; and the esophagus. The distribution and microscopic features of the lesions are important in defining syndromes and relating ulcers to etiologic or predisposing events. Stress ulcers, gastric ulcers, duodenal ulcers, and ulcers of the forestomachs have been characterized.

Stress ulcers are multiple, shallow, well-demarcated, without fibrous base, 2 to 25 mm in size, and oval to stellate in shape. They occur most frequently in the fundus and body, and are found less frequently in the antrum and duodenum. Acid hypersecretion has been documented in some cases, but, in others, reduced perfusion of the gastric mucosa is significant. Gastric mucus, state of epithelial renewal, and prostaglandins are also etiologically important. Prostaglandin E_2 has a cytoprotective role, and other prostaglandins influence acid secretion.

Gastric ulcers in dogs are usually solitary, may be multiple (Fig. 1-34), and may occur with ulcers of the duodenum. Acid secretion is normal. The mechanism is a breakdown of the gastric mucosal barrier, permitting back diffusion of hydrogen ions. Bile reflux may alter the mucosal barrier, and the nonsteroidal antiinflammatory drugs—aspirin, phenylbutazone, and indomethacin—contribute to ulcer formation by interfering with local prostaglandin synthesis.

Duodenal ulcers occur idiopathically with gastric ulcers in the dog, and most are secondary to some significant disease in other organs. Dogs develop duodenal ulcers secondary to mastocytoma, uremia, cirrhosis, or neoplasms, especially those with metastases to multiple organs.

In young feedlot cattle, abomasal ulcers are often multiple, range from 2 to 4 cm in diameter, are more common during the first 45 days of winter-initiated fattening, and have perforations most frequently in the antrum. The majority of abomasal ulcers are located in the body of the abomasum, along the greater curvature, in the ventralmost portion of the organ, and vary from a few millimeters to 15 cm in size (Fig. 1-35). The ulcers are round to oval and often have their greatest dimension parallel to the long axis of the abomasum. Bleeding ulcers are found most frequently in cows less than 4 years of age; during the months of February, March, August, and September; during the postpartum month (75%); and in animals with such concurrent diseases as metritis, mastitis, or ketosis.

Gastric ulcers in foals occur most frequently in the stratified squamous portion of the stomach and may encompass 20% to 70% of this portion; perforation occurs most often at the margo plicatus. In a proportion of affected foals, both the stratified squamous portion and the gastric antrum have ulcers, and perforation sometimes occurs in the antrum. Ulcers of the antrum may occur as solitary lesions. Esophageal ulceration is common, perhaps occurring in as many as 80% of affected foals. In some foals, candidiasis has been found in the hyperkeratotic mucosa in the area of ulceration of the esophagus and squamous portion of the stomach. As in the pig, parakeratosis and hyperkeratosis appear to be early lesions in an injured squamous mucosa, with ulceration a secondary event and candidiasis an incidental superinfection. In adult horses, ulcers of the squamous portion of the stomach extend along the margo plicatus and are most severe in the region of the lesser curvature.

In the dog, gastric ulceration is manifested by vomiting,

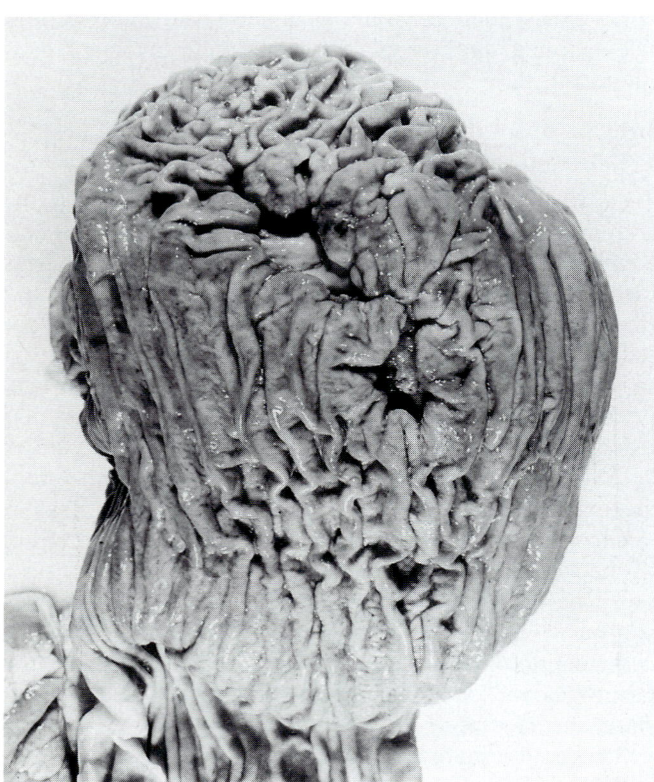

Fig. 1-34 Stomach; dog. Chronic gastric ulcers. Three stellate ulcers are in the body of this stomach, the upper two of which have perforated. Antrum is at the bottom. *Courtesy Dr. R.G. Thomson.*

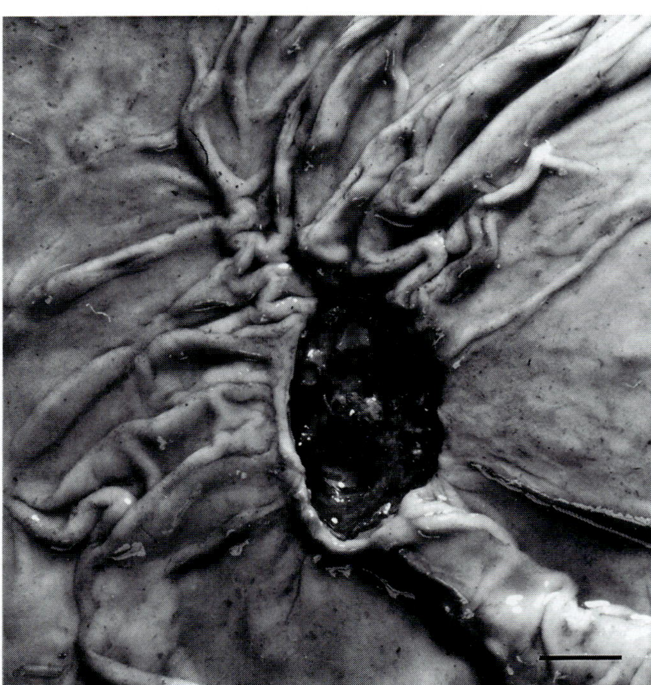

Fig. 1-35 Abomasum; cow. Abomasal ulcer. This solitary, 4-cm diameter ulcer penetrated the wall and the ensuing diffuse peritonitis resulted in death. Bar = 1 cm. *Courtesy Dr. M.D. McGavin.*

variable appetite, abdominal pain, anemia, and, occasionally, loss of weight. Foals with gastric ulcers have abdominal pain, bruxism, salivation, and gastric reflux and lie in dorsal recumbency. Cattle with abomasal ulcers have partial or complete anorexia, decreased milk production, palpable discomfort under the right xiphoid area, and melena. In any species, the vomiting of coffee grounds–like material (hematemesis) and/or melena are highly suggestive of gastric ulcer disease.

An **ulcer** is an excavation in the mucosa produced by coagulative necrosis that penetrates through to the muscularis mucosae. When focal coagulation necrosis produces excavation only partway through the depth of the mucosa, the lesion is termed **erosion.** Ulcers may be round, stellate, or linear. Acute stress ulcers are shallow, have soft hyperemic margins, and often occur in a diffusely congested mucosa. Ulcers that have been present for a time lack a hyperemic rim but have indurated margins and are deeper. The crater may be coated with a gray or tan, fibrinopurulent pseudomembrane. Microscopically, ulcers appear as an abruptly marginated focal excavation in the mucosa, with or without fibrinopurulent exudate above and granulation tissue beneath. Thrombosis of blood vessels beneath the crater occurs in some ulcers but is usually not regarded as a cause of the ulcer. Ulcers that penetrate through the submucosa into the tunica muscularis or to the subserosa are bordered by an acute inflammatory response.

Ulcers of the nonglandular stomach in swine are often subclinical, and the real incidence of this disease has perhaps been underestimated in the past. The incidence varies from 10% to 50% of slaughtered swine in various regions of the world.

The causes of these ulcers are multiple, with several dietary factors modifying the incidence. Corn is more ulcerogenic than wheat and oats; particle size of the feed appears important as the finer the feed, the greater the incidence of ulcers. Incidence of ulceration is greater with dry feeds than with wet feeds of similar products. Diets rich in unsaturated fatty acids appear more ulcerogenic than those rich in saturated fatty acids.

Pigs with mild to moderate ulceration may have no clinical signs of illness or may have reduced growth. When stressed, some seemingly healthy swine unexpectedly develop anorexia, weakness, and paleness of the nonpigmented portions of the skin and mucous membranes. The feces may be tarry and pasty, gradually becoming black and pelleted. Weakness is often severe. Death results from a severe loss of blood.

The ulcers are preceded by epithelial lesions characterized by hyperkeratotic and parakeratotic proliferation and degeneration, changes that cause a thickened, rough, and yellow-brown surface. The mucosa is irregularly thickened, the epithelial cells are swollen and vesicular, and edema and hemorrhage occur in the papillae of the lamina propria. Foci of intraepithelial necrosis occur and are infilitrated by granulocytes. Erosions soon follow, which progress to and though the muscularis mucosae, thereby establishing ulcers. In the acute stage, the ulcers are covered by a fibronecrotic membrane containing bacteria and fungal organisms; the underlying tissue is infiltrated with neutrophils. In later stages, connective tissue is increased at the base and at the edges of the ulcer. Grossly, the acute ulcer is covered with clotted blood, and the lumen of the stomach and intestines may be filled with unclotted blood. The chronic ulcer appears as a round, oval, or stellate crater, up to 8 to 10 cm in diameter, sometimes involving the entire stratified squamous gastric mucosa (Fig. 1-36). Thrombosed arteries and veins are often found in the granulation tissue and fibrous tissue adjacent to the ulcer. Some pigs have ulcers of the squamous portion of the stomach and smaller, more acute ulcers of the glandular gastric mucosa.

Gastritis

Acute erosive or **hemorrhagic gastritis** is poorly understood because cases are seldom studied either by biopsy or at necropsy. Gastritis is undoubtedly overdiagnosed clinically in animals that have vomiting as the presenting sign. Dogs with access to garbage have an increased incidence of gastritis. Cats are affected less frequently.

The earliest lesions of gastritis in animals spontaneously

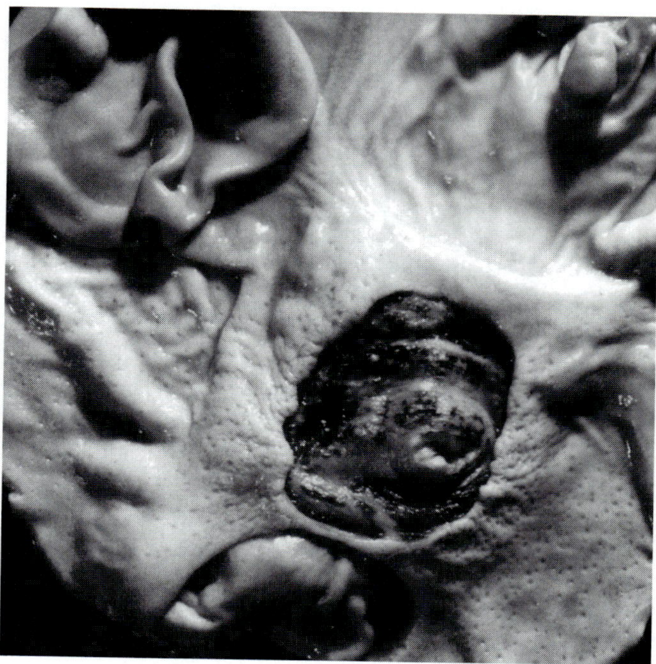

Fig. 1-36 Stomach; pig. Ulcer of the nonglandular stomach. This solitary chronic ulcer of the stratified squamous portion of the stomach surrounds the esophagus. Glandular portion of the stomach is toward the top. *Courtesy Dr. M.D. McGavin.*

affected or experimentally exposed to stress or infectious or chemical irritation of the stomach are characterized by congestion and focal hemorrhages in the gastric mucosa. These lesions are soon followed by degenerative changes in the surrounding epithelium, additional hemorrhages, edema, and erosion of the surface epithelium. Epithelial cell injury permits back-diffusion of hydrogen ions into the mucosa, leading to acid-pepsin digestion, which results in erosion and hemorrhages.

Clinically, acute erosive or hemorrhagic gastritis is characterized by epigastric discomfort, anorexia, nausea, and vomiting. In severe cases, the vomitus contains coffee grounds–like material or red blood. The more severe cases are characterized by repeated episodes of vomiting, either with an empty stomach or following the consumption of either feed or water.

The lesions of acute erosive or hemorrhagic gastritis may be localized or diffuse and consist of multiple mucosal hemorrhages, variable edema of the mucosa (Fig. 1-37), and oval, linear, or stellate surface erosions accompanied by extravasation of blood and plasma from damaged vessels into the lamina propria. The underlying gastric glands may be separated by edema and, in more severe cases, by edema and inflammatory cells.

Traumatic gastritis occurs in any species of animal but is seen with greatest incidence in dogs and cows. In dogs, traumatic gastritis is caused by swallowed bones, safety pins, toys, plastic balls, stockings, stones, and leather goods. Cattle consume wires, nails, electric fence clips, and screws as part of their dietary roughage.

These foreign bodies may remain in the stomach for a period of time before producing lesions and signs, or they may cause signs soon after ingestion. In dogs, some larger objects cause obstruction; leather goods, balls, and stockings act as ball valves and interfere with the function of the pylorus. Objects with jagged edges or sharp points cause damage by penetration.

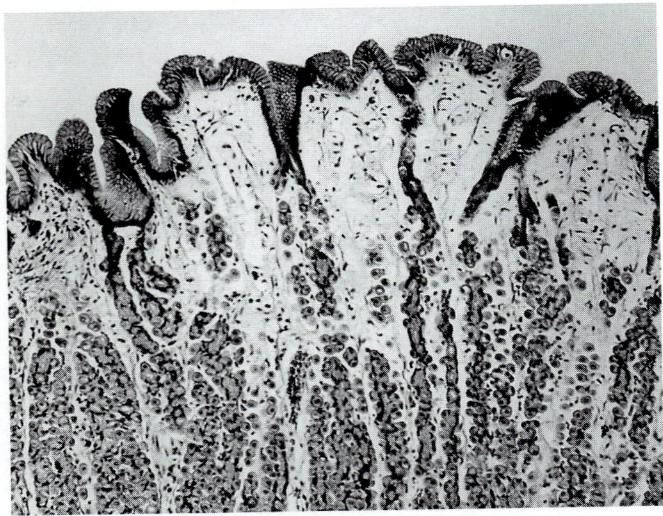

Fig. 1-37 Stomach; dog. Gastric mucosal edema. The surface is raised, and foveolae are separated by edema. Gastric glands are similarly separated in the neck region but appear normal at the base of the mucosa. H & E stain.

Clinically, animals with traumatic gastritis stop eating, become less active, and assume an abnormal stance. Cattle will have a pronounced arching of the back and audible groans on expiration. Small animals may vomit. Affected dairy cattle have an abrupt reduction in milk production and complete cessation of ruminal contractions. In any species, penetration of a foreign body may be accompanied by inflammation, a leukocytosis, and neutrophilia.

The lesions produced by foreign bodies include lacerations and contusions of the gastric mucosa, hemorrhages, and ulceration. With penetration, a localized, inflammatory response is initially characterized by granulocytes, and later development of an abscess or granuloma, scar tissue, and peritonitis. In cattle, traumatic gastritis is more often referred to as traumatic reticulitis and may result in traumatic pericarditis. The bacterial organisms in the stomach at the time of penetration determine, to great extent, the tissue response.

Chronic superficial gastritis probably occurs more frequently in animals than is diagnosed. The causes are not understood. Clinically, chronic superficial gastritis is characterized by episodes of inappetence, lethargy, and vomiting.

Chronic superficial gastritis is characterized by lymphocytic and plasma cell infiltration of the lamina propria adjacent to the gastric surface and about the gastric pits. A slight polymorphonuclear infiltrate is present in the epithelium. The surface mucous cells may be irregular or flattened and have decreased mucus in their apical cytoplasm. In the gastric antrum, hyperplasia of the submucosal lymphoid follicles produces a lesion designated follicular gastritis.

Chronic atrophic gastritis is not often described in veterinary medicine; diagnostic criteria include morphologic evidence of gastritis, atrophy of parietal and chief cells, and hypochlorhydria. In both dogs and nonhuman primates, atrophic gastritis can be produced by immunization with gastric antigens. These animals develop circulating antibodies to parietal cells and intrinsic factor.

The lesion of chronic atrophic gastritis is an infilitrate of lymphocytes, plasma cells, and a few eosinophils in the lamina propria of the stomach, about the gastric pits, and extending to the muscularis mucosae. The mucosa is variably thinned with partial or complete loss of gastric glands, and, when atrophic gastritis is severe, the residual glands may contain undifferentiated or pyloric-type cells. A lesion associated with chronic atrophic gastritis is a patchy or diffuse replacement of the gastric epithelium by an intestinal-type epithelium. This is referred to as **intes-**

tinal metaplasia and apparently results from an aberrant differentiation of the dividing cells in the depths of the gastric pits. The intestinal epithelium contains both goblet cells and absorptive cells that have microvilli and possess the enzymatic activity of intestinal epithelial cells.

Hypertrophic gastritis has been recognized in human beings, monkeys, horses, pigs, dogs, and mice. In monkeys, the condition occurs following the experimental dermal administration of shale oil and following consumption of polychlorinated biphenyls. It also occurs in monkeys infected with the gastric nematode, *Nochtia nochti*. In the horse, hypertrophic gastritis occurs in response to infection with *Habronema* sp and *Trichostrongylus axei*. The cause for the lesion in the canine is not known, but, experimentally, hyperplasia of the gastric mucosa has been produced by small bowel resection and by repeated injections of histamine, pilocarpine, or pentagastrin. Clinically, animals with hypertrophic gastritis have inappetence, weight loss, hypoalbuminemia, poor hair coat, upper abdominal tenderness, and, sometimes, vomiting.

The gastric lesions are enlarged, thickened, tortuous rugae, similar to cerebral convolutions (Fig. 1-38); the mucosa may be pink to red to violet; the sulci between folds are deep; and the mucosa is edematous and thickened. The mucosa may be diffusely thickened, or solitary plaques of hypertrophy may occur, particularly on the greater curvature. Microscopically, mucosa has pronounced hyperplasia (Fig. 1-39), and mucous cell metaplasia replaces parietal and chief cells. Cystic dilatation involves some of the gastric glands, and these dilated glands penetrate the muscularis mucosae, resulting in a lesion termed **gastritis cystica profunda.** Gastric glands contain polymorphonuclear leukocytes; the edematous lamina propria often contains an infiltrate of neutrophils, eosinophils, Russell bodies, lymphocytes, and plasma cells (Fig. 1-40); and the muscularis mucosae is fragmented and focally infiltrated with lymphocytes.

Eosinophilic gastritis probably occurs, but rarely, in most species of animals, but has been studied in dogs, cats, and human beings. In all three species, two forms of eosinophilic gastritis are recognized: a focal form caused by an eosinophil response to trapped nematode larvae and a diffuse form, believed allergic in nature, affecting a large portion of the stomach.

In the dog, focal eosinophilic gastritis occurs in response to the migration of larval *Toxocara canis.* Puppies obtain *T. canis* larvae through the milk of the bitch or from eating feed contaminated by the eggs or larvae, presumably from the feces of the bitch. These larvae may remain in the tissues for years, attracting eosinophils because of their waste products, saliva, and sheath. The lesion is a polypoid or nodular mass consisting of an embedded parasite surrounded by a collection of eosinophils and is often confined to the gastric antrum, where it may produce gastric outlet obstruction. A scirrhous eosinophilic gastritis occurs in

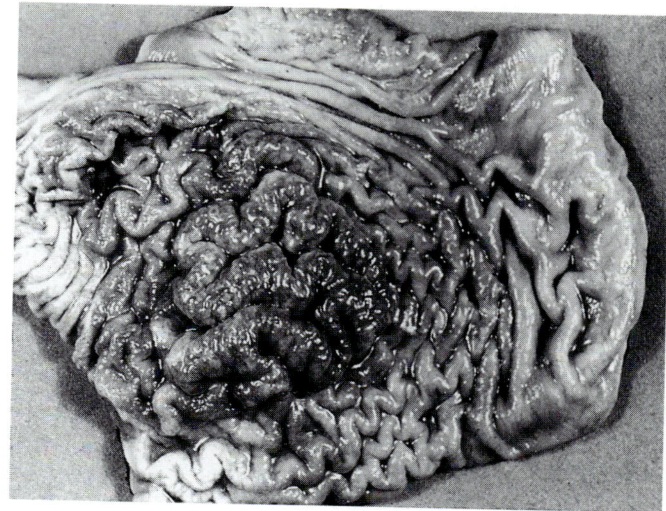

Fig. 1-38 Stomach; dog. Hypertrophic gastritis. A plaque of hyperplastic mucosa, composed of convoluted, reddened, and exaggerated rugae, occurs as a solitary mass several centimeters in diameter. *Van Kruiningen HJ. Vet Pathol 1977; 14:19-28.*

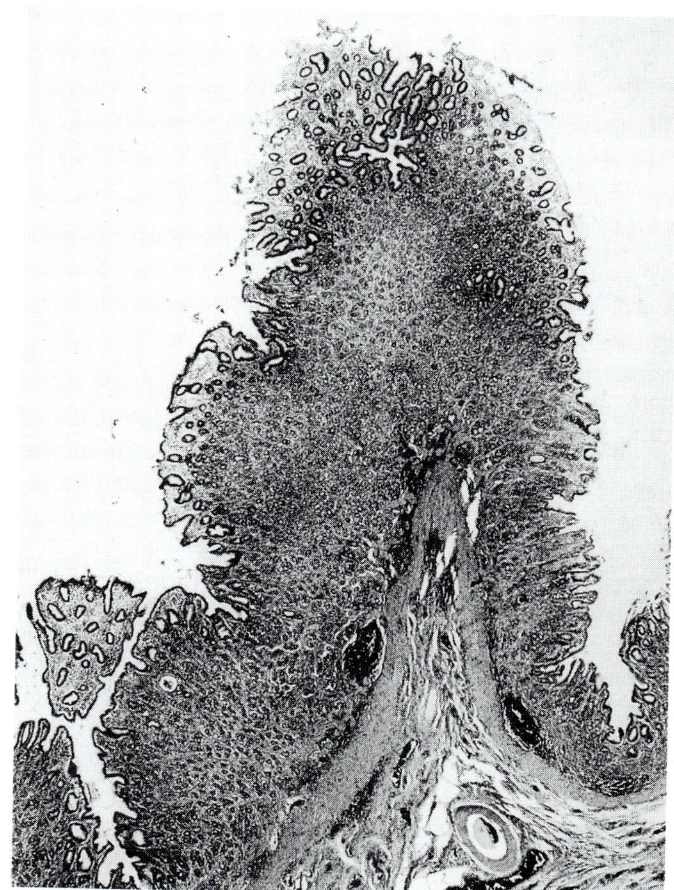

Fig. 1-39 Stomach; dog. Hypertrophic gastritis. Ruga. The mucosa is thickened irregularly. *Van Kruiningen HJ. Vet Pathol 1977; 14:19-28.*

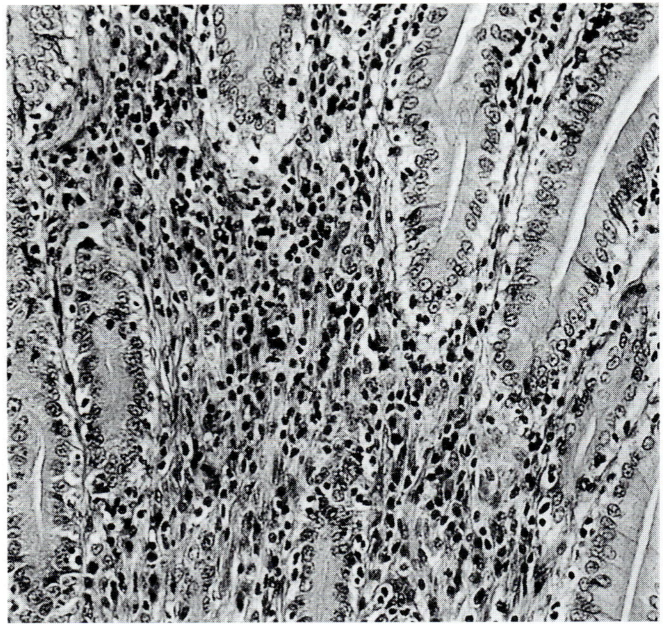

Fig. 1-40 Stomach; dog. Hypertrophic gastritis. Lamina propria is markedly infiltrated with lymphocytes and plasma cells. *Van Kruiningen HJ. Vet Pathol 1977; 14:19-28.*

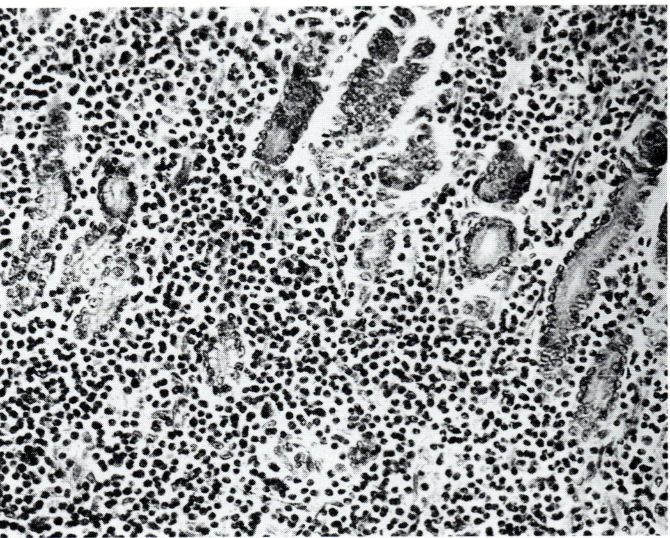

Fig. 1-41 Stomach; dog. Scirrhous eosinophilic gastritis. Gastric glands are separated by an infiltrate of eosinophils. H & E stain. *Hayden DW, Fleischmann RW. Vet Pathol 1977; 14:441-448.*

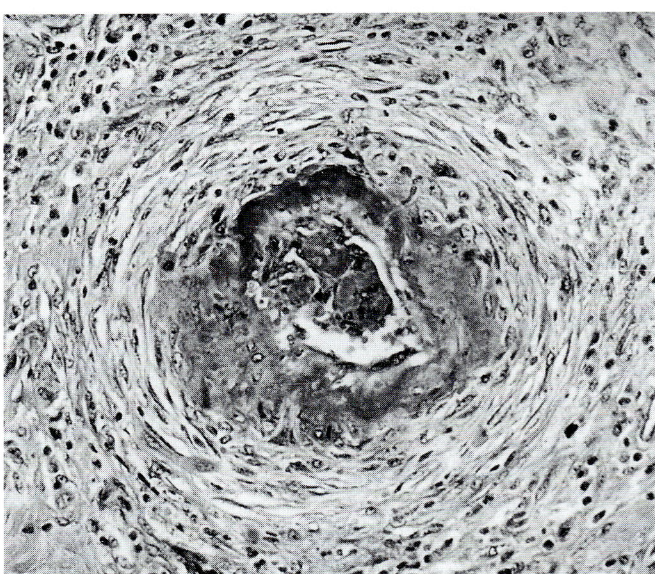

Fig. 1-42 Stomach; dog. Scirrhous eosinophilic gastritis. This submucosal artery has thrombosis, fibrinoid necrosis of the media, and adventitial cell proliferation. *Hayden DW, Fleischmann RW. Vet Pathol 1977; 14:441-448.*

dogs, and a similar disorder of the stomach and intestines affects cats. The cause is not known. Scirrhous eosinophilic gastritis is characterized by weight loss, lethargy, recurrent vomiting, sometimes a pendulous abdomen, and a thickened stomach. Affected animals have peripheral eosinophilia, as great as 30% in the dog.

The microscopic lesions are characterized by infiltrates of eosinophils in the mucosa, in the submucosa, extensively through the muscle layers of the stomach, and, sometimes, in segments of the small intestine and colon (Fig. 1-41). In the dog, some of the small- and medium-sized arterioles of the submucosa of the affected antrum have medial necrosis, adventitial proliferation, and eosinophilic perivasculitis (Fig. 1-42). The eosinophilic infiltrate may be followed by fibroplasia of the lamina propria, submucosa, and muscle layers (Fig. 1-43). Regional lymph nodes are enlarged and have eosinophilic infiltration, lymphoid hyperplasia, and fibrosis.

Parasitic gastritides. Haemonchosis, the most significant parasitic gastritis in animals, occurs in sheep, goats, and other ruminants. The cause, *Haemonchus contortus,* is a nematode parasite of 2.5 to 3 cm length, commonly called the ''barberpole worm.'' The common name is derived from the red and white striping in the females, resulting from a blood-engorged GI tract entwined with a white reproductive system. These parasites are acquired at pasture when the third-stage larvae are consumed with pasture grasses. The ingested larvae enter the abomasum, where they may reside within the gastric glands in a hypobiotic state, or they undergo development to adults and assume their location on the surface. Eggs of the nematode pass out in the feces, thereby completing the cycle. Haemonchosis is a serious problem when large numbers of larvae are ingested by lambs at pasture.

Sheep, goats, and cattle with mild haemonchosis have few clinical signs, except that they are unthrifty and fail to grow or make weight gains. Heavy infestations of the parasite result in hypoproteinemia and anemia with development of signs of ''bottle jaw,'' weakness or fatigue upon

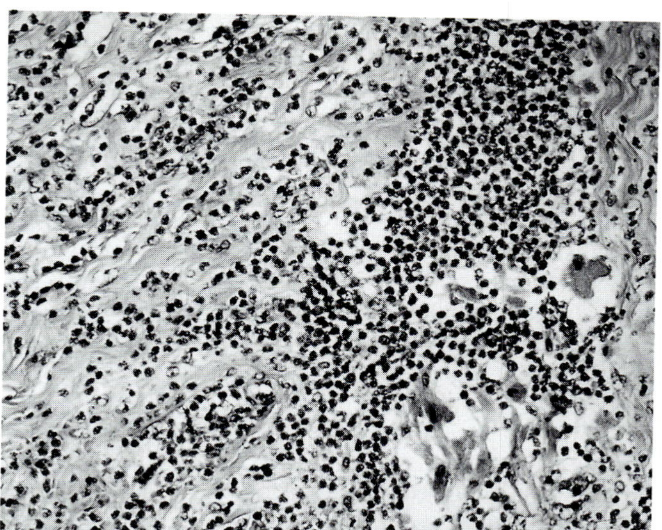

Fig. 1-43 Stomach; dog. Scirrhous eosinophilic gastritis. Eosinophils and fibrous tissue have replaced the gastric musculature. A few degenerate muscle fibers are present at right. *Hayden DW, Fleischmann RW. Vet Pathol 1977; 14:441-448.*

exertion, and diarrhea. At necropsy, parasitism is indicated by subcutaneous edema of the intermandibular space, pale conjunctiva and oral membranes, stunted growth, and liquid feces. The organs are pale, the blood is watery, and the abomasal contents are fluid and brown. The abomasal folds may have no lesions or have diffuse or patchy congestion and submucosal edema. Parasites are seen in the abomasal contents; they are seen best if the contents are emptied into a white pan. Handfuls of the parasite may be rolled from the abomasum in animals dying of haemonchosis.

Ostertagiasis causes significant disease in sheep, goats, and cattle. In sheep and goats, the most common species is *Ostertagia circumcincta,* and in cattle it is *O. ostertagi.* These nematode parasites are approximately 1.5 cm in length, they have a direct life cycle similar to that of *Haemonchus* sp, and reside as third-, fourth-, and fifth-stage larvae in the gastric glands of the abomasum. *Ostertagia* sp are often found in the company of other trichostrongyles that reside in the small intestine. This combined parasitism results in failure to make adequate weight gains, inappetence, lassitude, diarrhea, and, in later stages, hypoproteinemia and attendant ventral edema.

Ostertagia sp produce gastritis characterized by an infiltration of chronic inflammatory cells (lymphocytes and plasma cells), some eosinophils, an increase in globule leukocytes in the mucosa, a decrease in the number of parietal and chief cells, and a hyperplasia of mucous cells. The abomasal contents are fluid, brown-green, and fetid, as the ingesta is partially putrefied because of large populations of bacteria. Gross lesions in the abomasal mucosa are tiny pale nodules that may be few in number or so numerous as to become confluent, creating a cobblestone surface

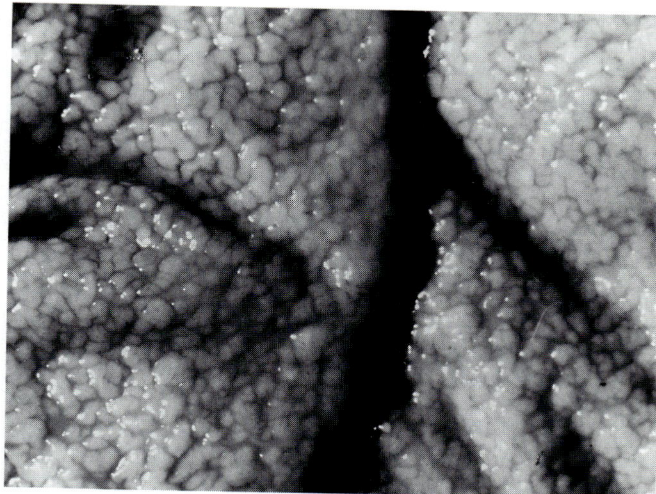

Fig. 1-44 Abomasum; cow. Ostertagiasis. The mucosa of the abomasal folds is studded with lymphoid nodules. *Courtesy Dr. M.D. McGavin.*

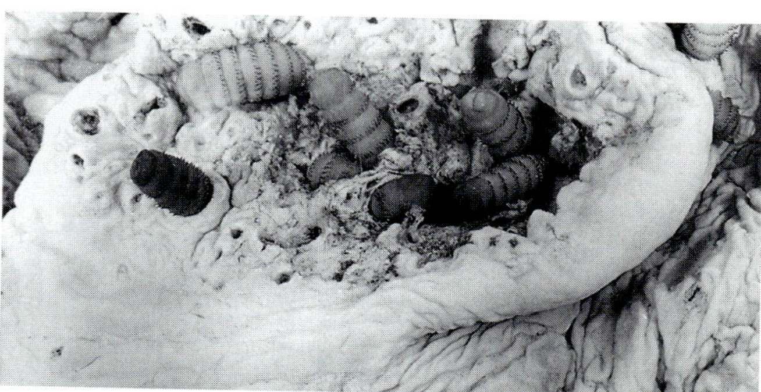

Fig. 1-45 Stomach; horse. Gastric bots. *Gastrophilus* larvae and the craters produced by them are present in the squamous portion of the stomach. *Thomson RG. General Veterinary Pathology. Philadelphia: Saunders, 1978:398.*

(Fig. 1-44). *Ostertagia* sp may be demonstrated at necropsy. The worms are brown, smaller than *H. contortus,* and more difficult to see without magnification. The parasites occur within the gastric glands and in areas of chronic inflammation.

Gastrophilus larvae **(gastric bots),** particularly those of *Gastrophilus nasalis* and *G. intestinalis,* are a common cause of parasitic gastritis in the horse. The bots are larvae of a fly that deposits its eggs on the forelegs and jaws of horses during spring and summer. The eggs—2 to 3 mm in length, oval, and white—are attached to hairs. Hatching occurs after the horse licks the eggs into the warm, moist environment of the oral cavity. The larvae migrate down the esophagus to the stomach and there develop into spiny, 2 cm long bots with anterior pinchers by which they attach to the gastric mucosa. *G. intestinalis* attaches to the stratified squamous portion of the stomach (Fig. 1-45), and *G. nasalis* attaches to the antral mucosa. After the parasites

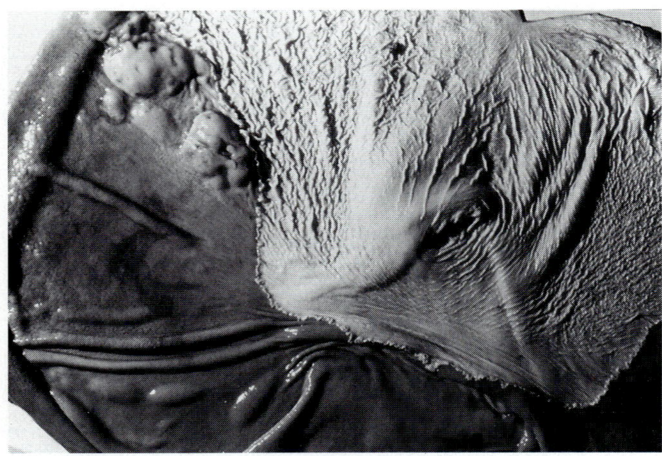

Fig. 1-46 Stomach; horse. Habronemiasis. Several raised parasitic nodules are present at the margo plicatus. *Courtesy Dr. M.D. McGavin.*

detach, they pass out in the feces, pupate, and develop into flies.

Grossly, the areas inhabited by the *Gastrophilus* larvae have multiple, 2 to 3 mm, craterous depressions, but there is little inflammation, usually no ulceration, hemorrhage, pseudomembranes, abscess formation, or other complications. Microscopically, the parasite causes little host response at points of pincher attachment. Bots are clinically silent, and no changes occur in leukocyte counts or concentrations of plasma proteins.

Habronemiasis, caused by the spirurid parasite *Draschia megastoma,* a worm 1 to 2 cm in length, infrequently results in parasitic gastritis in the horse. *Draschia* are acquired when the horse inadvertently eats the intermediate host, flies or larvae that have exited the fly via its proboscis. The larvae develop in the stomach and penetrate the glandular mucosa, usually near the margo plicatus, creating a granulomatous nodule with a cystic space. At necropsy, one or several nodules are found (Fig. 1-46). The adults in the cysts of the submucosal nodules release eggs through a fistulous pore. The eggs pass with the feces from the animal and are consumed by larvae of the fly that serves as the appropriate intermediate host.

Microscopically, granulomas of the submucosa bulge into the lumen, are covered by an intact mucosa, and have numerous eosinophils among the inflammatory cells. Rarely, the nodules undergo abscess formation or the parasite or inflammation extends through the serosa to cause peritonitis and death.

Ollulaniasis and **gnathostomiasis** of the cat rarely produce gastritis. *Ollulanus tricuspis,* a minute nematode approximately 0.8 mm long, is transmitted in the vomitus of an infected cat and, rarely, causes mild gastritis or, sometimes, chronic fibrosing gastritis, indicated by mucosal nodularity or gastric rugal hypertrophy. The other parasite, *Gnathostoma* sp, is a spirurid nematode with toothlike spines on the cephalic end that induces large, granulomatous masses.

Bacterial and mycotic gastritides. Acute phlegmonous gastritis occurs in the dog and represents infection of the gastric wall by bacteria. Infecting organisms may include streptococci, staphylococci, *Escherichia coli, Proteus vulgaris,* or *C. perfringens.* Clinically, phlegmonous gastritis is characterized by abrupt onset of midepigastric pain, nausea, and vomiting accompanied by fever, chills, and prostration. Death usually ensues from circulatory collapse. Purulent emesis, a rare occurrence, is specific for this entity, and emesis of a necrotic cast of the gastric wall is pathognomonic.

Grossly, the stomach is dilated with thickened walls, 1.5 cm in thickness, and deep red to purple, discolored mucosa. The submucosa is usually edematous and may ooze pus. Less often, emphysema of the submucosa results in bubbles of varying sizes in the thickened gastric wall and imparts a cobblestone texture to the mucosa. Emphysematous gastritis is due to gas-forming organisms such as *E. coli* or *C. perfringens* and sometimes occurs with acute gastric dilatation with volvulus. Microscopically, the mucosa and submucosa are thickened and distended by edema and a diffuse, granulocytic inflammatory infiltrate. The mucosa has hemorrhage, congestion, and coagulation necrosis. The causative bacteria usually can be seen enmeshed in a fibrinopurulent inflammation in the gastric wall.

Necrobacillary ruminitis occurs in cattle and, less frequently, in other ruminants. It occurs secondary to a mild ruminitis, which, in the calf, is caused by misfeeding of milk replacers and in the adult, by the consumption of excessive amounts of grain. Necrobacillary ruminitis occurs most frequently in feedlot cattle when animals are changed from a pasture-type feed to a diet rich in concentrates.

Necrobacillary ruminitis is caused by *Fusobacterium necrophorum,* a bacterium commonly found as a component of ruminal flora. The bacterium becomes pathogenic following ruminitis and an imbalance of the normal ruminal flora. In ruminal acidosis, vesicular degeneration of the surface stratified squamous epithelium is accompanied by granulocytic infiltrates into epithelium and into the vesicles. The lamina propria becomes engorged and infiltrated by granulocytes. If these changes are not reversed, *F. necrophorum* invades and causes other lesions. This form of ruminitis is characterized by inappetence, reduced milk production, decreased ruminal contractions, and diarrhea.

Necrobacillary ruminitis affects principally the ventral sac of the rumen and occasionally the pillars. Gross lesions are multiple, irregular dark patches from 3 to 15 inches in diameter. Within these patches, the ruminal papillae are swollen, dark red-black, slightly mushy, and matted together by inflammatory exudate. Microscopically, the affected areas have lesions of coagulation necrosis and a marked infiltration with neutrophils. The papillae are melded together by necrosis and a serofibrinous inflammatory response. If the disease is treated successfully, the necrotic patches of epithelium slough, creating an ulcer followed by epithelial regeneration. The regenerative epithelium is flat and white, without complete recovery of the specialized papillae, a small angular scar is formed. In necrobacillary omasitis, perforation of the leaves often occurs. *F. necrophorum* frequently translocates from the rumen or omasum to the liver, producing foci of coagulation necrosis and hepatic abscesses.

Mycotic gastritis (ruminitis) occurs secondary to indigestion, to improper feeding of young calves, or to rumen acidosis in adult cattle. In calves, the cause is *Candida albicans.* In adult cattle, fungi of the genera *Mucor, Rhizopus,* and *Absidia* are causes, and the disease is called **mucormycosis.** These fungi are opportunists and are pathogenic when the indigenous flora are altered or in the presence of antibiotics, inadequate gastric motility, and leukopenia. *C. albicans* appears to thrive on excessive keratin in the squamous mucosa. Although the *Candida* organisms are content to colonize the surface and produce necrosis of the surface epithelium, the fungi of mucormycosis extend into the mucosa and submucosa where they invade the walls of blood vessels, causing vasculitis and thrombosis, resulting in areas of coagulation necrosis. The fungi of mucormycosis may be translocated to the liver and produce foci of necrosis there as well.

Ruminal candidiasis is seldom diagnosed during life. Severe candidiasis is seen at necropsy of calves that have failed to respond to treatment for a concomitant disease. Mucormycosis of adult cattle is almost always fatal.

The lesions produced by *C. albicans* infection and invasion of the rumen are grossly and microscopically similar to those described for the esophagus. The ruminal lesion consists grossly of an accumulation of caseous, gray, necrotic, crumbly material covering focal areas or large patches of the rumen. Microscopically, these consist of necrotic squamous epithelium, hyperkeratotic material, and a mat of yeasts and pseudohyphae of *C. albicans.* The inflammatory response beneath this mat is slight and consists of neutrophils, lymphocytes, and histiocytes.

The lesions of mucormycosis resemble those of necrobacillary ruminitis, but are often more extensive, involving one half to two thirds of the rumen wall and large portions of the omasum (Figs. 1-47 and 1-48). Grossly, the affected areas of the mucosa are dark red to red-black with well-demarcated margins; they are firm, leathery, and thickened because of the congestion and hemorrhage within the damaged mucosa secondary to vascular thrombosis. The lesions of mucormycosis extend to the peritoneal surface. Microscopically, in areas of infarction of the mucosa, the ruminal papillae are melded together because of coagulation necrosis. Necrosis may extend deep into the submucosa with extensive hemorrhage, edema, vasculitis, and thrombosis of vessels. In sections stained with periodic acid–Schiff (PAS) or Grocott-Gomori methenamine-silver nitrate technique, fungi are readily apparent growing from the surface, through the necrotic mucosa and submucosa, and invading the vessels. Hyphae of fungi of mucormycosis are large, coarse, nonseptate, and branching.

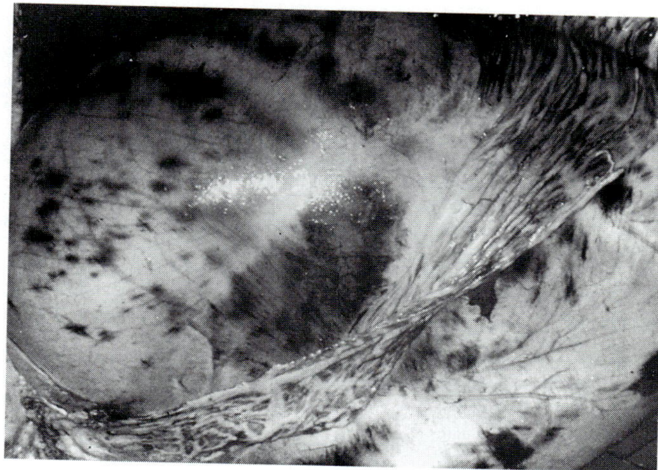

Fig. 1-47 Rumen, serosal surface; cow. Mycotic ruminitis. Circular black foci and larger aggregates of infarction are present in the gastric wall. *Courtesy Dr. M.D. McGavin.*

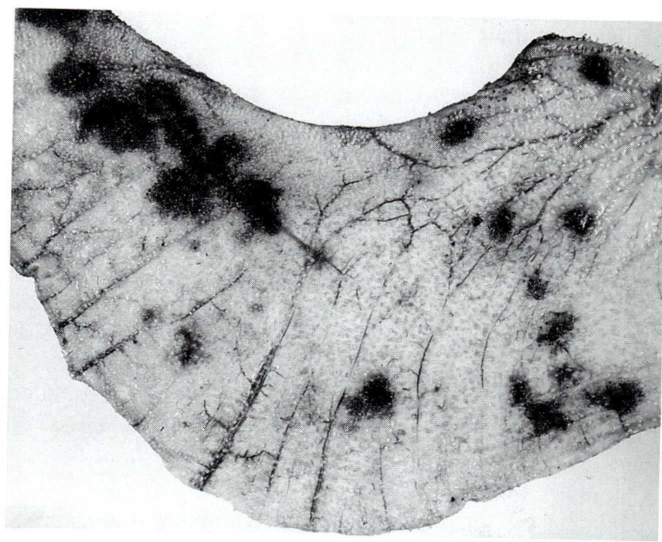

Fig. 1-48 Omasum; cow. Mycotic omasitis. Well-delineated black foci of infarction are scattered over the leaves of the omasum. *Courtesy Dr. R.G. Thompson.*

Granulomatous gastritis is caused by microorganisms that invade the deeper tissues of the gastric wall rather than just the mucosa. These include such organisms as *Mycobacterium tuberculosis* and *Histoplasma capsulatum.* Organisms gain access to the deeper tissues, i.e., the submucosa, the muscle layers, lymph vessels, subserosa, and adjacent lymph nodes, and cause a granulomatous inflammation. The wall of the stomach becomes increasingly thickened, and the stomach becomes less functional. Clinical features include postprandial epigastric pain, vomiting, weight loss, weakness, hematemesis, and gastric outlet obstruction.

Microscopically, the lamina propria and submucosa are infiltrated by chronic inflammatory cells; predominating are phagocytic cells of either the epithelioid or macrophage type, with a variable number of giant cells. Phagocytic cells occur in association with plasma cells, lymphocytes, fibroblasts, and variable numbers of neutrophils and eosinophils.

Gastric Neoplasms

Gastric adenocarcinoma

These are the most common neoplasms of the stomach of small animals and occur in horses and cattle as well. In the dog, gastric adenocarcinoma constitutes 1% to 2% of all malignant neoplasms and 47% to 72% of all gastric malignancies. These neoplasms are less common in cats. In the dog, adenocarcinomas occur in males more frequently than in females. Gastric neoplasms often go unrecognized until advanced because they either grow into the lumen or spread laterally within the wall. Clinical features include vomiting, anorexia, weight loss, and a palpable abdominal mass.

The gastric adenocarcinoma grossly may be fungating or ulcerating or may cause diffuse thickening of the wall (linitis plastica). Microscopically, gastric adenocarcinomas have been divided into two cellular types; about one third of canine gastric adenocarcinomas are composed of cells of intestinal type, and the neoplastic cells have a distinct glandular arrangement forming tubules or acini of well-differentiated epithelial cells with clear brush borders. These neoplasms have a mild to moderate desmoplastic reaction and a low mitotic index. The most common histologic type of gastric adenocarcinoma is the diffuse type; the neoplastic cells are of gastric type and are disseminated through the mucosa, submucosa, lymph vessels, and muscle layers as clusters and sheets of cells (without tubular or acinar arrangement).

The cells of the gastric adenocarcinoma may have little or no mucus content, or may have pseudopallisading of nuclei or nests of glands. Alternatively, the cells may have abundant mucus (signet-ring cells) and stain brightly with mucicarmine and PAS techniques. Those adenocarcinomas characterized by a great deal of extracellular mucus are termed **colloid carcinomas,** whereas those with marked concomitant desmoplasia are termed **scirrhous.** Gastric adenocarcinomas metastasize first to regional lymph nodes and then to liver, lungs, and adrenal glands.

Gastric malignant lymphoma

These neoplasms of the stomach occur with some frequency in dogs and human beings, and infiltrate the wall of the abomasum in cattle. Lymphosarcomas constitute from 12% to 15% of canine gastric neoplasms. Clinically, dogs with gastric lymphosarcoma have signs of abdominal pain, weight loss, vomiting, weakness, abdominal fullness, and eructation. In advanced cases, an epigastric mass may be palpable. With lymph node involvement, abdominal masses are multiple. Gastric lymphosarcoma may be accompanied by lymphosarcomatous infiltrates of other organs such as lymph nodes, liver, and spleen.

Lymphosarcomatous infiltration begins in the lamina propria, submucosa, or lymphoid follicles of the gastric wall. Lymphosarcomas are usually localized, the surface may ulcerate, or there may be diffuse infiltration of the lamina propria and submucosa, causing enlargement of gastric rugae similar to that seen in hypertrophic gastritis. Microscopically, neoplastic lymphocytes in a diffuse pattern distend and distort the lamina propria and submucosa. Neoplastic cells extend between the muscle fibers and sometimes to the serosa.

SMALL INTESTINE

Obstructions and Functional Disorders

Adynamic ileus

This disorder of the stomach and intestines is characterized by lack of normal tone and peristaltic movements. Once called paralytic ileus, the gut is not paralyzed, but rather adynamic because of sympathetic nerve inhibition. The stomach and intestines fail to respond to the presence of ingesta, cathartics, and enemas but can react to pharmacologic and electrical stimuli. Adynamic ileus represents a disease with a biochemical rather than a morphologic lesion.

Clinical signs of adynamic ileus are anorexia, abdominal distention, absence of bowel sounds, fluid- and gas-filled loops (detected by palpation or radiography), failure to pass flatus and feces, vomiting, and large volumes of fluid aspirated by nasogastric tube. Laboratory findings often associated with the disorder include hypochloremia, hyponatremia, hypokalemia, and eosinopenia (apparently related to adrenal cortical output).

Adynamic ileus occurs in all species of animals and is recognized in human beings, dogs, cats, cattle, and horses. Causes, in order of frequency, include manipulation of the stomach or intestines at surgery, other forms of abdominal surgery, peritonitis, severe painful stimuli elsewhere in the body, and states of abnormal metabolism, toxemia, and electrolyte imbalance, such as hypocalcemia, hypomagnesemia, hypokalemia, vitamin B deficiency, uremia, tetanus, diabetes, and lead poisoning. In the manipulation of abdominal viscera, afferent and efferent limbs of the neurologic reflex are conducted through splanchnic nerves. Because chloride, potassium, and calcium are essential for neuromuscular conductivity, electrolyte deficits have been regarded as at least contributory in many cases of ileus.

Foreign bodies

Foreign bodies occur in all species of animals, but with the greatest frequency in dogs and cats. Young dogs have a propensity to swallow objects such as soft rubber balls, rubber nipples, coins, aluminum foil, pieces of string, and socks. Although many such objects stop at the stomach, some pass beyond the pylorus and into the small intestine and produce obstruction. The cat is a more fastidious eater, but enjoys playing with and chewing at thread and yarns, sometimes with needles attached. Long-haired cats develop hair balls from grooming themselves.

Foreign bodies may produce transient clinical features, such as vomiting and diarrhea, and then be passed in feces without further incident, or they may become trapped in the small intestine, particularly at the ileocolic valve, where they produce complete or incomplete obstruction. The foreign body may be large enough so that it is arrested in the small intestine and produces ischemia by compression of blood vessels. Foreign bodies can precipitate exaggerated peristalsis and, thus, lead to intussusception. They may produce dilatation and a stagnant loop syndrome with bacterial overgrowth and, subsequently, damage to the villous surface proximal to the blockage.

Clinically, obstruction of the small intestine is characterized by vomiting. The time interval between the taking of a meal and the act of vomiting is roughly proportional to the distance from the mouth to the foreign body. There may be abdominal distention, anorexia, and a palpable abdominal mass. In the event of partial or transient obstructions, the animal may have signs of obstruction that are relieved by vomiting and diarrhea, only to recur later. Cats with lesions from linear foreign bodies, e.g., sewing thread lacerations, have clinical signs indicative of peritonitis, including fever, anorexia, elevated leukocyte counts, and signs of a painful abdomen.

The lesion produced is obstruction, segmental dilatation, collapse of intestines distal to the site, hyperemia and congestion at the site, and variable surface erosions, ulceration, or perforation. In the cat, long lengths of sewing thread sometimes extend through the length of the GI tract, very often with the craniad end around the base of the tongue. The result is a taut thread about which intestinal motility occurs, causing an accordion pleating, multiple lacerations of the intestine, and peritonitis at one or more points.

Intussusception

Intussusception is the invagination of one segment of intestine into another, and it occurs in all species. The telescoping of contiguous intestinal segments, one into another, takes place in the normal intestine; for intussusception to occur, peristalsis must be enhanced or exaggerated, and the telescoped segment must have a lesion upon which to stay fixed. In young animals, enlarged Peyer's patches, most often a consequence of viral infections, and foreign bodies frequently provide the nidus for fixation. In adult animals, polyps and neoplasms are very often the cause of intussusception (Fig. 1-49). For most animal cases, the cause is not established. In the dog, intussusception of the intestine has been related to or caused by the granulomas of visceral larva migrans and histoplasmosis, surgical exposure and manipulation of the small intestine, hypertrophied lymphoid nodules in salmon poisoning and *Yersinia pseudotuberculosis* infections, linear foreign bodies, and ascarids. Causes of intussusception in the cat include foreign bodies and adenocarcinomas of the intestine. In cattle, papillomas, abscesses, fibromas, and lipomas are causes; and, in the horse, ascarids, parasitic granulomas, verminous arteritis, and leiomyoma are identified as causes. Ileoileal, ileocecal, cecocecal, and cecocolic intussusceptions have been attributed to infestations with the horse tapeworm, *Anoplocephala perfoliata,* as the tapeworms can be demonstrated at the edge of the intussusceptum. Endoparasitism, malnutrition, protozoal infections, and the diarrheas that are often concomitant cause intussusception.

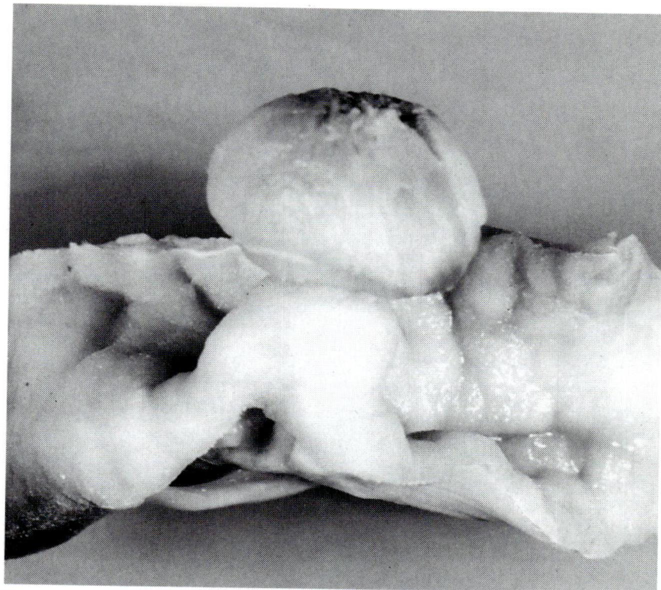

Fig. 1-49 Small intestine; dog. Intussusception. A 1-cm diameter polyp resulted in intussusception.

Most intussusceptions occur in the direction of peristalsis (direct); less often, they occur in the direction opposite to that of peristalsis (retrograde). Intussusceptions may be multiple; they may be compound, one intussusception becoming the nidus for another (Fig. 1-50); and they may be recurrent. Multiple intussusceptions sometimes occur agonally, apparently in response to hypoxia at the time of death, but these are readily distinguished from antemortem intussusceptions because of the lack of swelling, hyperemia, and congestion. After resection or at the time of necropsy, the intussusception should be carefully dissected in an attempt to define the cause.

Clinical features of intussusception are those of intestinal obstruction and include abdominal distention, dilated bowel loops, palpable abdominal mass, signs of abdominal pain, complete anorexia, and vomiting. After 24 hours, there may be melena, and then subsequently, a lack of feces.

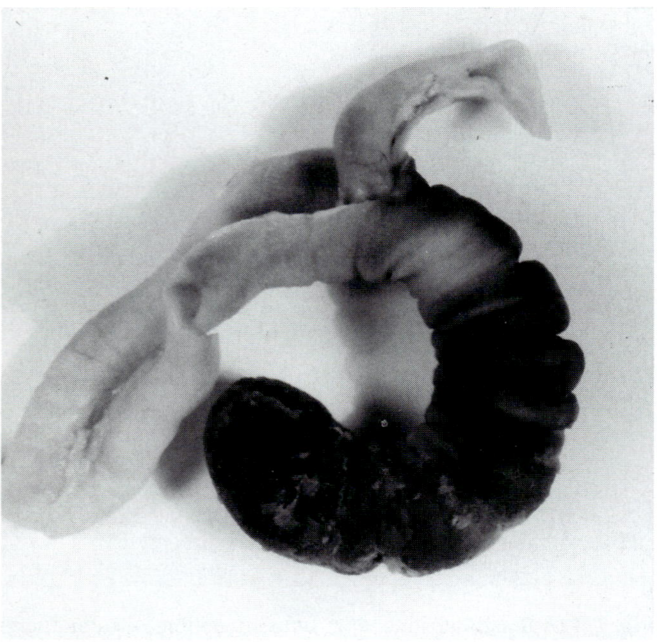

Fig. 1-50 Small intestine; young dog. Compound intussusception. This intussusception within an intussusception is black and coated with tags of fibrin.

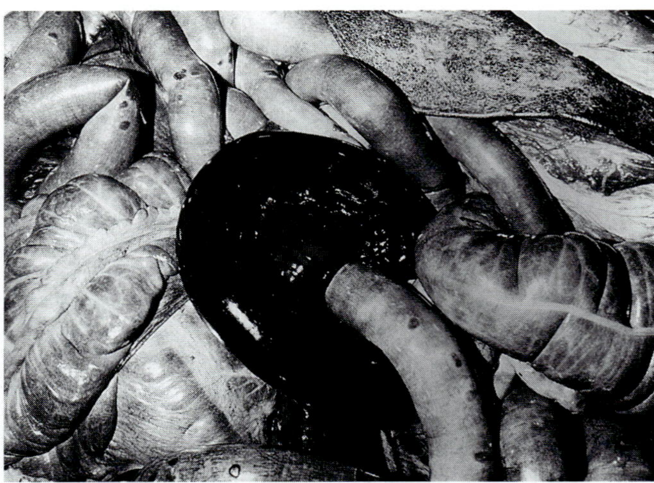

Fig. 1-51 Intestines; horse. Intestinal incarceration and volvulus. The affected segment is black and gas-filled, and the mesenteric vessels are distended. The dark nodules in the serosa of the nonincarcerated small intestine are strongyle-induced haemomelasma ilei. *Thomson RG. General Veterinary Pathology. Philadelphia: Saunders, 1978:103.*

The intussusception is an enlarged, thickened segment of intestine that may vary in length from several inches to a meter or more. It is grossly swollen, discolored, dark red or black because of congestion and hemorrhage and heavy because of the mass within. At one end of the intussusception, the invagination of the smaller segment is visible, and the mesentery of the intussuscepted portion is gathered up and engorged with blood and edema. Microscopically, after 24 hours, ischemic necrosis involves the mucosa of both segments, with congestion and edema of the submucosa, muscularis, and subserosa.

Intestinal volvulus

Volvulus is the pathologic twisting of a segment of intestine upon its mesenteric axis. This results in vascular strangulation, ischemia, and occlusion of the lumen of the intestine. It occurs in all species but has been recognized most often in horses, cattle, swine, dogs, and human beings.

In the horse, most cases of small bowel volvulus have occurred because of incarceration of a portion of the intestine through mesenteric rents and hernias (Fig. 1-51) or twisting around scars of fibrous umbilical remnants attached to Meckel's diverticulum. Small bowel volvulus has been seen in association with ileal infarction, severe ascarid infestations, equine viral arteritis, *Strongylus vulgaris*–induced thrombosis of the cranial mesenteric artery, and overeating on cracked corn. Dogs may suffer an acute volvulus of the entire small intestine; idiopathic canine small bowel volvulus may represent clostridial enterotoxemia. Canine volvulus has been attributed to the anthelminthic piperazine in combination with obstruction caused by ascarids and pebbles.

Horses and cattle with small bowel volvulus have a sudden onset of colic, complete anorexia, severe continuous pain, anxiety, delirium, and sweating. Animals make violent movements, bruising and abrading themselves; they tread, paw, and kick at the belly. Some roll, tremble, have a rising pulse and temperature, congested membranes, labored breathing, and an absence of peristalsis and feces. Tenesmus is a clinical sign of small bowel volvulus. Horses may attempt to vomit, and cattle may groan or bellow. Small animals haves signs of anorexia, abdominal distention, vomiting, prostration, evidence of acute abdomen, and death. Laboratory findings include leukocytosis and albuminuria. After the affected bowel has become necrotic, large animals become quiet and recumbent with a subnormal temperature that precedes death.

At necropsy, the volvulus is a small or large twisted segment of small intestine, sometimes including the cecum or proximal colon, which is considerably distended, ballooned with gas and fluid, and discolored dark red or black. The volvulus is often difficult to untangle; the twist may be 360 to 720 degrees, either clockwise or counterclockwise. In some animals, a neoplasm, foreign body, incarceration, or intussusception is coexistent. The entire wall of the affected segment is thickened by edema and severe congestion. The thin-walled veins of the mesentery are occluded first, while the nonoccluded arteries permit blood flow into the diseased segment. The mesentery is usually thickened, severely congested, and dark red. Lymph nodes adjacent to the intestine are congested and swollen. Microscopically, the affected intestine has lesions of necrosis, congestion, and hemorrhage. The flora entrapped in blood-filled anoxic loops produce toxins and gas, which cause distention of the part and necrosis of the mucosa. Gangrene, peritonitis, intestinal rupture, and death are the terminal events.

Intestinal lipofuscinosis

A brown discoloration of the small intestine occurs in the dog, "brown dog gut," and in human beings, "brown bowel syndrome." The brown, discolored small intestine occurs in conjunction with bile duct occlusion, pancreatic insufficiency, chronic enteritis, vitamin E deficiency, or excess dietary lipids. Brown pigmentation of smooth muscle is a well-known lesion of vitamin E deficiency in several species of laboratory animals; the canine and human intestinal pigmentation is also the result of vitamin E deficiency. The requirement for vitamin E is proportional to the concentration of polyunsaturated fatty acids in the diet. Intestinal lipofuscinosis probably does not cause clinical signs; however, the lesion has significance as an indicator of what has previously occurred in the patient.

The small intestine, from the serosal side, is brown. The color varies from tan to khaki in the mildly affected, to deep brown in the severely affected gut. In severely affected dogs, portions of the stomach, cecum, or colon are also pigmented. Microscopically, the brown color results from the accumulation perinuclearly of lipofuscin granules in the cytoplasm of the smooth muscle cells of the intestine (Figs. 1-52 and 1-53). These granules vary from basophilic to brown with hematoxylin-eosin (H & E) stain and are PAS and Sudan black B–positive. Older granules may be acid-fast when stained by the special acid-fast technique for lipofusion. Those granules that are acid-fast are referred to as **ceroid pigments.**

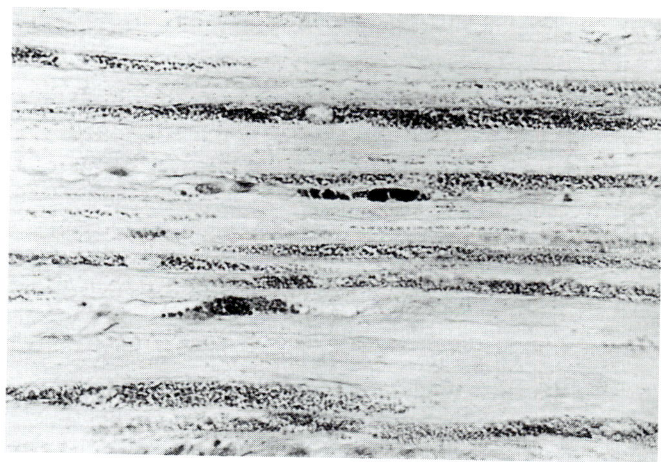

Fig. 1-52 Intestine; dog. Intestinal lipofuscinosis. Myocytes of the inner muscle layer contain numerous PAS-positive cytoplasmic granules. PAS reaction.

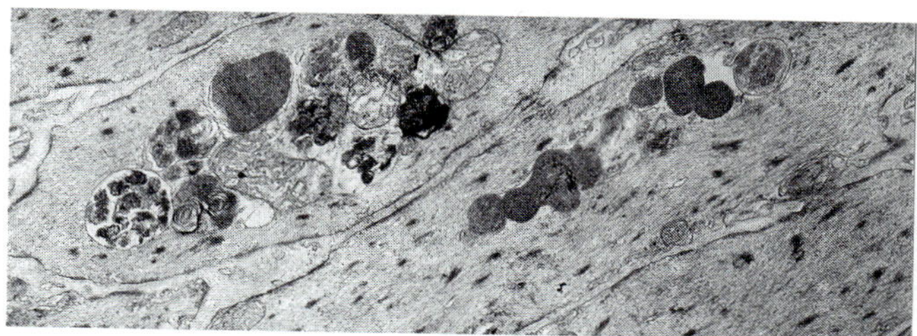

Fig. 1-53 Intestine; dog. Intestinal lipofuscinosis. In electron micrographs, the lipofuscin granules are electron-dense, round or irregular, lipid bodies approximately the size of mitochondria.

Intestinal muscular hypertrophy

Muscular hypertrophy occurs infrequently in several species of animals. In some horses, it is an idiopathic segmental disease affecting the ileum and progressing proximad to affect the jejunum and, subsequently, more anterior segments. In these cases, the lesion represents a work hypertrophy proximal to a damaged or stenotic ileocecal valve. In other horses, hypertrophy affects the duodenum and jejunum and is associated with diverticula. Muscular hypertrophy of the ileum in pigs occurs as a component of regional enteritis and as an independent disorder as well. Muscular hypertrophy associated with diverticulosis has been recorded in young Yorkshire pigs and in Romney Marsh and Hampshire sheep. Cats have a severe hypertrophy of the inner, circular muscle of the intestine, which appears to originate in the ileum and progress proximal. Segmental hypertrophy of muscularis of the antrum and variable segments of small intestine occurs in cats with hypereosinophilic syndrome, a disorder characterized by intramural eosinophil infiltrates. Muscular hypertrophy of the intestine and medial hyperplasia of pulmonary arteries occur in cats given large oral doses of *Toxocara cati* larvae. The exposed animals often had diarrhea and eosinophilic enteritis, and, later, had variable fibrosis of the lamina propria of the mucosa and hypertrophy of the inner muscle layer.

Clinically, horses with muscular hypertrophy of the intestine have intermittent or subacute colic, a variable appetite, exaggerated bowel sounds, and, finally, cachexia. In some species, diarrhea is a feature. Associated signs may include a "harsh" coat, "tucked-up" abdomen, depression, nasal discharge, and abnormal stance, with the hind limbs placed forward under the abdomen. An intestinal mass may be palpable, and, in small animals, vomiting may be a feature.

Injuries and Inflammations

Canine multifocal eosinophilic gastroenteritis

This is a disease of young dogs, usually less than 4 years of age, caused by migrating larvae of the canine ascarid, *Toxocara canis.* The disease often originates in kennels that have less than satisfactory hygiene and parasite control. As puppies, affected dogs were parasitized with ascarids, hookworms, and tapeworms, and received repeated treatments. Clinically, this disorder is characterized by chronic diarrhea, moderate weight loss, intermittent or persistent eosinophilia, and elevated serum beta-globulin concentrations. Serum albumin concentration is normal, and absorption tests and small bowel contrast radiographs usually are negative.

T. canis larvae enter by the oral route, invade the mucosa of the stomach and small intestine, and then become trapped and localized by the inflammatory response. Adult bitches often harbor significant larval parasite burdens in their tissues. Larvae migrate into the uterus and fetuses during late pregnancy. Shortly after birth, presumably in response to hormonal stimuli, larvae are directed to the mammary gland, where they are secreted in the milk of the bitch. Ascarid larvae also may be acquired from fecal contamination of the teats or the kennel environment. Larvae that are taken in by previously ascarid-free puppies usually transit the mucosa of the stomach and small intestine and travel via intestinal lymph vessels or the portal vein to the liver and then to the lungs. Here they develop into third-stage larvae, which are then coughed up and swallowed. In the GI tract, these larvae mature to adult roundworms. In the great majority of exposed dogs, ascarid larvae pass through tissues and complete the life cycle in several weeks, or the larvae are trapped and killed by granuloma formation, which results in necrosis of the parasite and calcification. Dogs that have developed multifocal eosinophilic gastroenteritis have *T. canis* larvae trapped in the gastrointestinal wall by an immune reaction. The incidence of this disease is low. In tissue sections of affected individuals, the entrapped larvae are surrounded by eosinophils, but still appear viable. Ascarid larvae, surrounded by aggregates of eosinophils, may remain trapped and viable in the wall of the stomach and small intestine for as long as 4 years. Waste products of the parasites are chemotactic for eosinophils. The multifocal aggregates of eosinophils occur along pathways traveled by ascarid larvae and are found in the mucosa and submucosa of the stomach and small intestine, in the mesenteric lymph nodes, in the connective tissue of the pancreas, in the portal areas of the liver, and in the kidneys and lungs.

Focal eosinophilic lesions that occur in this disease are 1 to 4 mm in diameter and may or may not be grossly visible (Fig. 1-54). In some dogs, as many as 40 to 80 white, firm nodules, the size of a pinhead, can be observed from the serosal side of the intestine. Few nodules occur in the wall of the stomach and in the colon. Regional lymph nodes may be slightly enlarged and variegated, or they may contain grossly visible, 4 to 5 mm diameter, white nodules (Fig. 1-55). Gross lesions may be seen in the renal cortex or as scattered foci throughout the pancreas, liver, and subpleurally. Microscopically, most of the lesions are composed of eosinophils, and some lesions have plasma cells and macrophages. Ascarid larvae can often be demonstrated in these aggregates (Fig. 1-56). Some of the lesions are granulomas. The larvae may be surrounded by an eosinophilic, amorphous, fringed material, which stains PAS-positive (the Hoeppli phenomenon). The multifocal nature and size of these lesions produce little deformity to the mucosal surface.

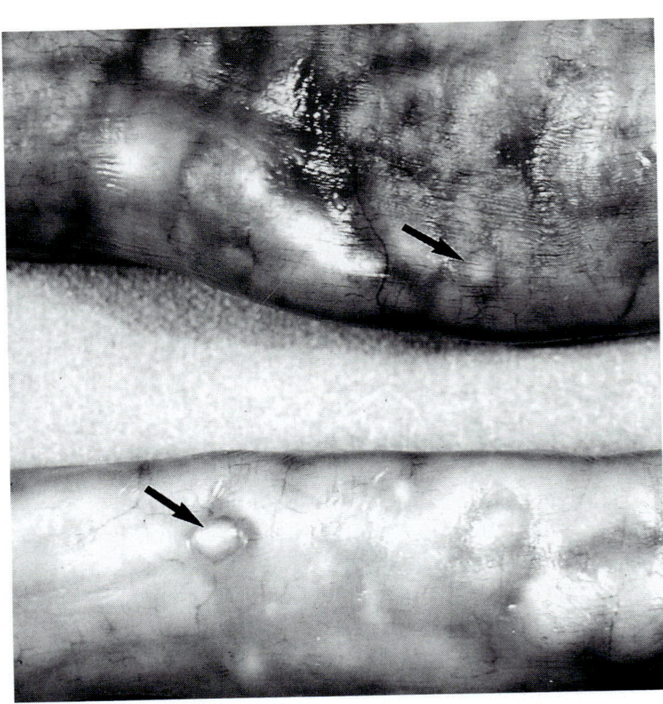

Fig. 1-54 Intestine; dog. Multifocal eosinophilic gastroenteritis. Multiple intramural eosinophilic nodules *(arrows)* are present throughout the jejunum in this dog with visceral larva migrans. *Courtesy Dr. D.W. Hayden.*

Diffuse eosinophilic gastroenteritis

This rather uncommon disease, recognized in dogs, cats, and human beings, may occur in other species as well. Allergy to some food ingredient is the cause in a proportion of human cases. Such is not true for other human and most canine and feline cases. Often the cause is not established.

Animals with diffuse eosinophilic gastroenteritis have diarrhea, signs of abdominal discomfort, weight loss, and eosinophilia. Some may vomit. When allergy is the cause, specific food intolerances may be recognized in the history.

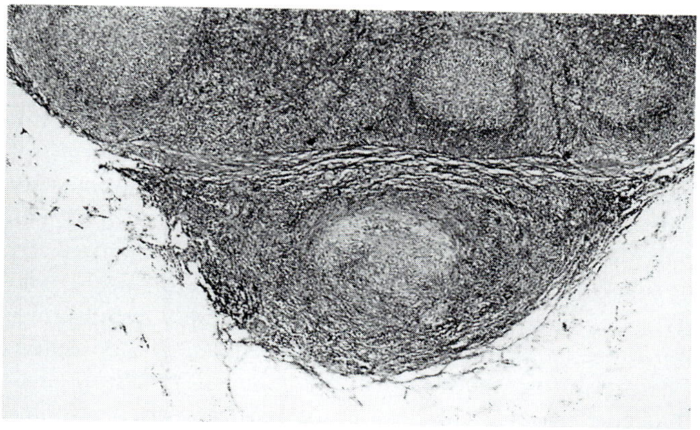

Fig. 1-55 Mesenteric lymph node; dog. Multifocal eosinophilic gastroenteritis. A capsular granuloma protrudes from lymph node of a dog with visceral larva migrans. *Hayden DW, Van Kruiningen HJ. J Am Vet Med Assoc 1973; 162:379-384.*

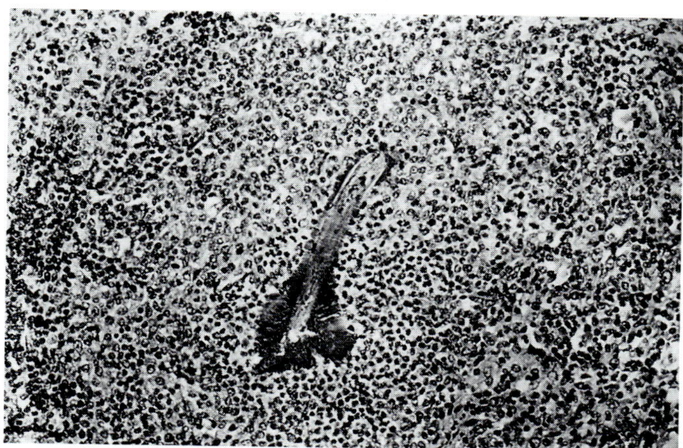

Fig. 1-56 Mesenteric lymph node; dog. Multifocal eosinophilic gastroenteritis. A nematode larva is located at the center of an eosinophilic granuloma. The larva is partially coated by fringed eosinophilic material (Hoeppli phenomenon). *Hayden DW, Van Kruiningen HJ. J Am Vet Med Assoc 1973; 162:379-384.*

Food items most often incriminated include milk protein, shellfish protein, soy protein, horse meat, chocolate, gluten, and egg protein.

In diffuse eosinophilic gastroenteritis, most of the lesions are in the mucosa and submucosa. Eosinophils occur diffusely in the lamina propria, just beneath the epithelium, surrounding the lacteals, and in a mantle beneath the crypts. Submucosal involvement is usually minimal, but, in some cases, the eosinophils extend not only into the submucosa but also into the muscle layers. The antrum of the stomach may have lesions, but it is unusual for the colon to be affected. Eosinophilic gastroenteritis does not produce gross distortions of the mucosa or changes in lumen diameter unless the muscle layers are involved. In such cases, there is segmental thickening of the intestine.

Canine lymphocytic-plasmacytic enteritis

German shepherd dogs and lesser numbers of other large, purebred dogs have a chronic enteritis characterized by a lymphocytic-plasmacytic infiltration of the small intestine. Clinically, this disease is characterized by chronic diarrhea, weight loss, hypoalbuminemia, and moderate malabsorption. The small intestine in contrast radiographs appears normal.

Lymphocytic-plasmacytic enteritis is a morphologic diagnosis for categorizing one group of chronic canine diarrheas. A cause has not been defined for this canine enteritis. The lesion may result from one agent, or, alternatively, it may represent a common response of the host to several inciting agents. Some affected animals have helminth and protozoan parasites, but the parasites appear not to be the cause of these lesions.

Lesions of lymphocytic-plasmacytic enteritis are not discernible grossly. Microscopically, significant infiltration with lymphocytes and plasma cells involves the lamina propria of the entire small intestine and, in some cases, of a portion of the stomach or colon. The number of inflammatory cells is excessive and well beyond proportions usually found in the villous core (Fig. 1-57). Villi may appear filled with lymphocytes and plasma cells. Often, plasma cells with Russell bodies (globules of immunoglobin) are found and are additional evidence of a pronounced immunologic response in the connective tissue of the intestine. In this disease, villi do not appear reduced in height, but do appear thickened and overly filled with mononuclear cells. The epithelium often is cuboidal rather than columnar. When intestinal lacteals are diffusely distended, protein loss occurs, and the animal may become hypoproteinemic and develop edema. Over time, the chronic inflammation results in adhesions of adjacent villi, fibrosis within the villous cores and among villi, and severe obliteration and distortion of mucosal lacteals.

Lymphocytic enteritis needs to be distinguished from the early stages of intestinal malignant lymphoma, in which the cellular infiltrate consists exclusively of neoplastic lymphocytes. In canine lymphocytic-plasmacytic enteritis, the solitary lymphoid follicles of the GI tract, Peyer's patches, and the regional lymph nodes may have reactive lymphoid hyperplasia.

Sprue

Sprue and tropical sprue are primary diseases of the villous epithelium of human beings, and counterparts of both diseases have been recognized in dogs. Sprue is synonymous with celiac disease and gluten enteropathy; the term **malabsorption syndrome** may be used to refer to sprue or it may have a more general connotation. Clinically, sprue is characterized by diarrhea, variable abdominal fullness, cramping, and chronic weight loss. The results of various tests include a flat oral glucose tolerance curve, a flat D-xylose curve, a flat vitamin A absorption curve, and ste-

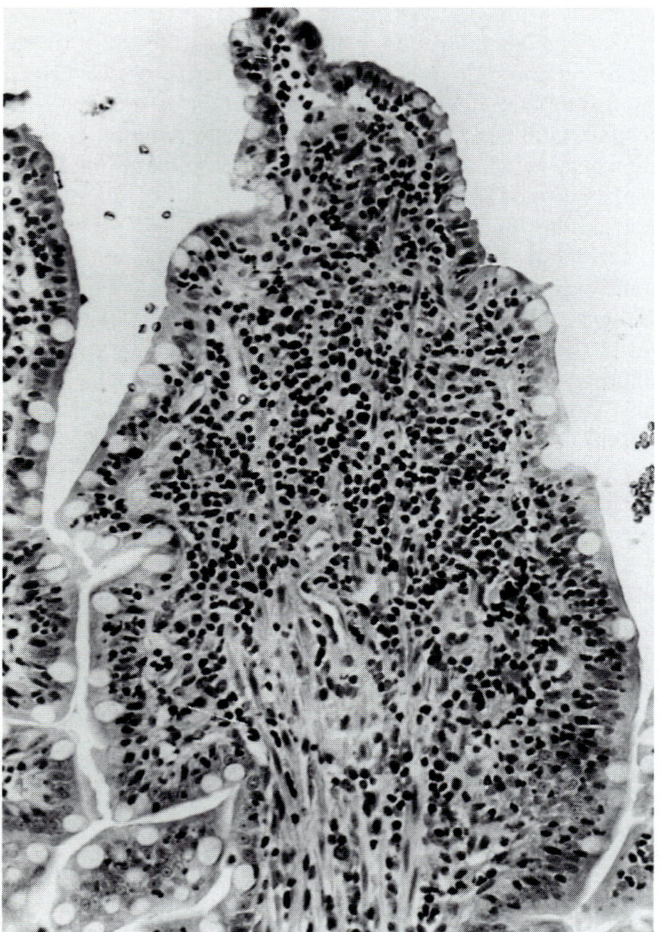

Fig. 1-57 Intestine; dog. Lymphocytic plasmacytic enteritis. The connective tissue core of the villus is infiltrated with lymphocytes and plasma cells. H & E stain.

atorrhea. Other findings may include vitamin deficiencies, anemia, or hypocalcemia.

Sprue or celiac disease is caused by an abnormal sensitivity of villous epithelial cells to gluten, the water-insoluble protein moiety of such cereal grains as wheat, barley, buckwheat, rye, and oats. Patients with gluten sensitivity have premature loss of absorptive villous epithelial cells. Instead of the cells surviving and performing their absorptive functions for 4 days, the cell cycle may be shortened to 1.5 days or less. The epithelium appears less differentiated, seems more cuboidal, and contains increased numbers of lymphocytes. In response to increased cellular loss along the periphery of the villi, epithelium of intestinal crypts becomes hyperplastic. Mitotic figures are increased, and the crypts increase in depth. The reduction in the number of villous epithelial cells and the increased number of crypt cells cause a change in the villus height: crypt depth ratio. Villi become shortened, crypts become lengthened, and the normal ratio of approximately 3:1 becomes reduced to 1:1. Simultaneously, the number of lymphocytes and plasma cells in the lamina propria is increased. Sequentially, the villi lose their scalloped appearance, become short and rigid, and contain excessive numbers of lymphocytes and plasma cells. Later, the villi appear thumb- or club-shaped and greatly reduced in height. In the most severe form of the disease, the mucosa becomes flat, with only nubbins of villi remaining over a zone of markedly hyperplastic crypts. These changes occur diffusely over large segments of the intestine and severely compromise the capacity of the animal to absorb nutrients. A gluten-free diet brings reversal of these changes. A wheat-sensitive enteropathy with lesions of partial villous atrophy, increased villous lymphocytes plasma cells, and intraepithelial lymphocytes, and biochemical abnormalities of the brush border has been described in Irish setter dogs.

In tropical sprue, similar morphologic changes occur, but are the result of bacterial colonization of the small intestine. Tropical sprue is endemic in some underdeveloped countries and often occurs in conjunction with parasitism or protein malnutrition. Toxic products from the offending bacterial flora appear to be deleterious to villous epithelial cells, and atrophy results. Bacterial overgrowth of the small intestine in a "naturally occurring enteropathy" has been reported in German shepherd dogs. These dogs have minimal microscopic lesions, but do have specific biochemical abnormalities of the jejunal mucosa. German shepherd dogs and Shetland sheepdogs have villous atrophy with increased villous lymphocytes, plasma cells, and intraepithelial lymphocytes, as well as reduced brush border enzymes. Affected dogs have reduced xylose absorption and low concentrations of serum and erythrocyte folate and vitamin B_{12}. These features resemble those of chronic tropical sprue disease of human beings.

Canine intestinal lymphangiectasia

This rare disorder is characterized by segmental or widespread dilatation of intestinal lacteals, stagnation of lymph, and enteric protein loss. In the canine, a **primary intestinal lymphangiectasia,** with no obstructive lesions of the intestinal lymph vessels or lymph nodes, has been described. **Secondary lymphangiectasia** occurs when granulomatous disease or neoplasia significantly distorts and obstructs mesenteric lymph nodes. Dilatation of intestinal lacteals with enteric protein loss occurs in some dogs with lymphocytic-plasmacytic enteritis.

An additional lymphangiectasia in the dog is associated with lipogranulomatous lymphangitis. Clinically, this disease is characterized by chronic diarrhea, weight loss, hypoalbuminemia, ascites, chylous ascites, and, less frequently, chylothorax or ventral edema. Some dogs with this disease recover in response to corticosteroids or medium-chain triglyceride diets. Grossly, the affected small intestine appears contracted and dull red, with prominent lymph vessels (Fig. 1-58). The mucosa of affected segments is

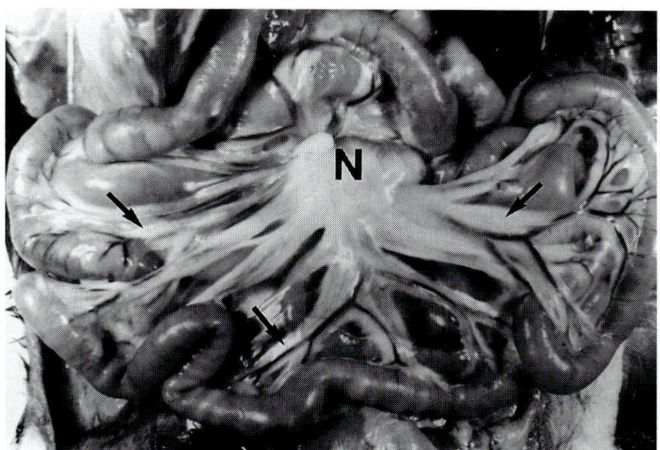

Fig. 1-58 Small intestine; dog. Lipogranulomatous lymphangitis. Lymph vessels in the mesentery are distended and milky white *(arrows)* as they course toward mesenteric lymph node (*N*). The intestine is eccentrically contracted and banded by rings of lighter coloring.

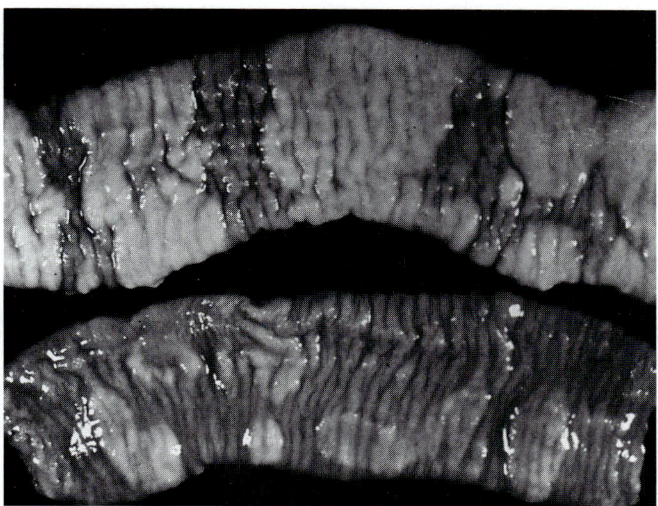

Fig. 1-59 Small intestine; dog. Intestinal lymphangiectasia. Raised white zones and plaques are produced by mucosal edema. *Courtesy Dr. D.J. Meuten.*

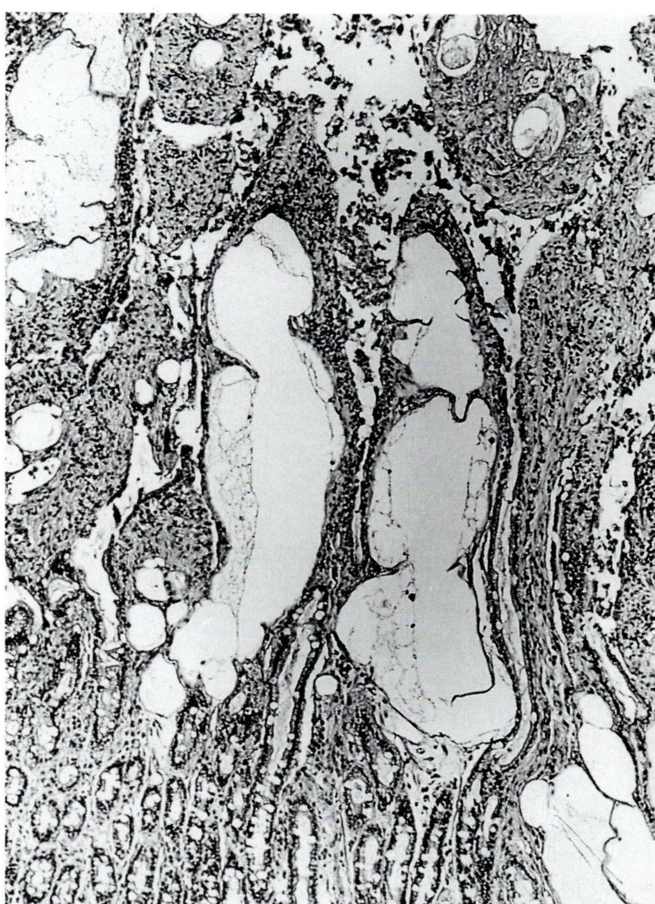

Fig. 1-60 Small intestine; dog. Intestinal lymphangiectasia. Lacteals are dilated and distorted as a consequence of lipogranulomatous lymphangitis. H & E stain.

variably thickened by edema, and patches of the mucosa appear lighter in color and raised above the more normal mucosa (Fig. 1-59). Villi grossly are yellow flecks on a red mucosal background, an effect created by the dilated lacteals. The mesentery to the affected segment has an opalescent appearance and, in chronic cases, may be thickened by fibrosis. Intralymphatic lipogranulomas are soap-white, smooth, oval granulomas, 1 to 5 mm in diameter, along the course of lymph vessels at the point of attachment of the mesentery to the intestine. The granulomas have been considered secondary to stagnated chyle, occurring in intestinal lymphangiectasia or so-called protein-losing enteropathy. However, lipogranulomas have never been reported in experimental intestinal lymph vessel obstruction in dogs, even when they were followed for 1 year.

Microscopically, intestinal lymph vessels and lacteals are markedly dilated (Fig. 1-60). There may or may not be an increase in the lymphocyte–plasma cell population of the mucosa. The lipogranulomas, when they occur, are located in submucosal, muscular, or subserosal lymph vessels, and are composed of a broad collar of lipophages surrounding centrally located amorphous lipid material (Fig. 1-61).

Regional enteritis

Canine regional enteritis closely resembles Crohn's disease in human beings. The lesions are segmental, often involving the distal ileum or a portion of the colon, and are transmural in their extent. A comparable disease of the pig is also called regional enteritis; this latter disease is caused by an intraepithelial *Campylobacter*-like organism. Clinically, animals have chronic diarrhea, weight loss,

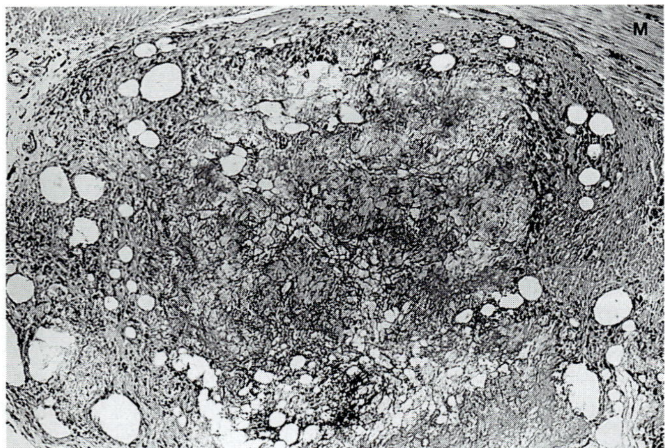

Fig. 1-61 Small intestine; dog. Lipogranulomatous lymphangitis. A subserosal lymph vessel is occluded by lipogranuloma. Amorphous lipid material at the center is surrounded by a collar of foamy macrophages (lipophages). *M*, tunica muscularis. *Van Kruiningen HJ, Lees GE, Hayden DW, Meuten DJ, Rogers WA. Vet Pathol 1984; 21:380.*

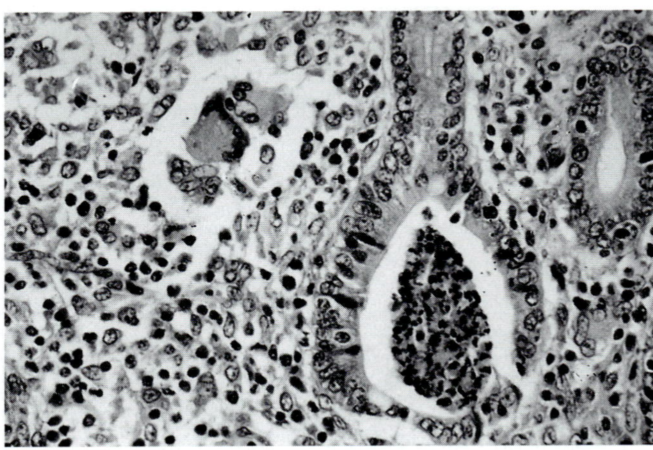

Fig. 1-62 Small intestine; pig. Regional enteritis. The lamina propria is infiltrated with mononuclear leukocytes, epithelioid cells, and giant cells. A crypt abscess is within the inflamed mucosa. *Rahko T, Saloniemi H. Nord Vet Med 1972; 24:132-138.*

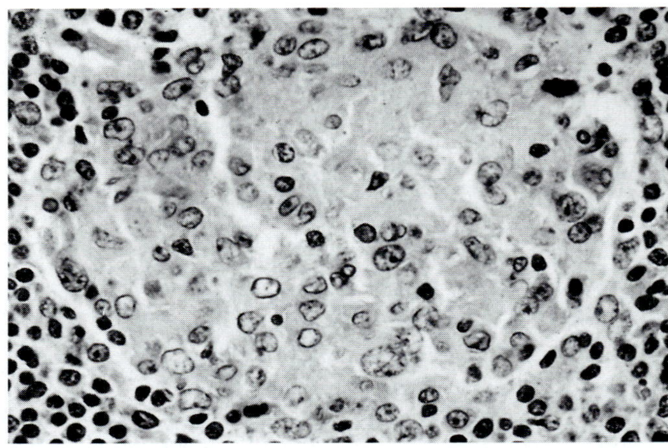

Fig. 1-63 Small intestine; pig. Regional enteritis. Epithelioid cell granuloma occurs within a lymphoid follicle of a Peyer's patch. *Rahko T, Saloniemi H. Nord Vet Med 1972; 24:132-138.*

variable eosinophilia, abdominal discomfort, palpable intestinal mass, and, sometimes, vomiting.

Affected intestines are firm, rigid, discolored dark red, thickened, and stenotic; the associated mesentery is thickened. Microscopically, the early lesions are characterized by infiltrates of eosinophils and other leukocytes, lymph stasis, and edema. Later, the lesions are characterized by lymphocytic infiltration, both follicular and scattered, plasmacytosis, inflammatory lymph vessel obstruction, and granulomas. The epithelium is usually focally ulcerated. Macrophage granulomas occur in the mucosa and submucosa and epithelioid cell granulomas with giant cells (sarcoid or tuberculoid) are seen in the deep submucosa, muscularis, and subserosa (Figs. 1-62 and 1-63). The disease process is transmural, as aggregates of lymphocytes, plasma cells, and granulomas extend through the tunica muscularis to the tunica serosa. Regional lymph nodes contain tuberculoid granulomas. In a small number of animals, focal lymphocytic aggregates or granulomas are present in the liver. Bacterial or mycotic organisms have not been found in these lesions except in the camphylobacteria-like organism (CLO)-induced disease of swine.

Equine granulomatous enteritis

This disease, characterized by chronic wasting, hypoalbuminemia, edema, and diarrhea, has been described in Standardbred and Thoroughbred horses in several different countries, most often in animals 1 to 5 years of age. Equine granulomatous enteritis should be considered when young horses have inexplicable weight loss, hypoalbuminemia, decreased activity, and poor hair coats. About half of affected horses have diarrhea, and some have repeated bouts of colic.

The gross lesions are characteristic and include diffuse or segmental granulomatous disease of the small intestine, particularly of the ileum and duodenum, with variable involvement of the large intestine. The lesions are raised, red, serosal nodules and plaques from 1 cm to several centimeters in diameter. In some horses, white fibrous plaques extend around the circumference of the small intestine; and, in other animals, raised, red, irregular plaques are confluent with one another, extending over several feet of the small intestine (Fig. 1-64). Adhesions of the omentum to the serosal lesions can be observed, and adjacent loops of

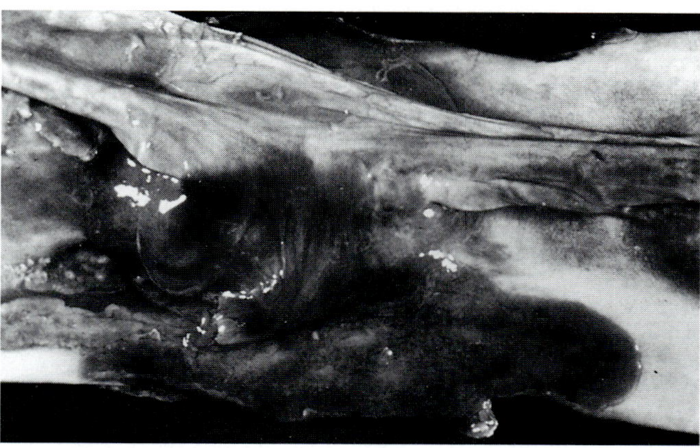

Fig. 1-64 Small intestine, serosal surface; horse. Equine granulomatous enteritis. The serosal surface has irregular, thickened, dark red plaques of inflammatory tissue. *Courtesy Dr. D.J. Meuten.*

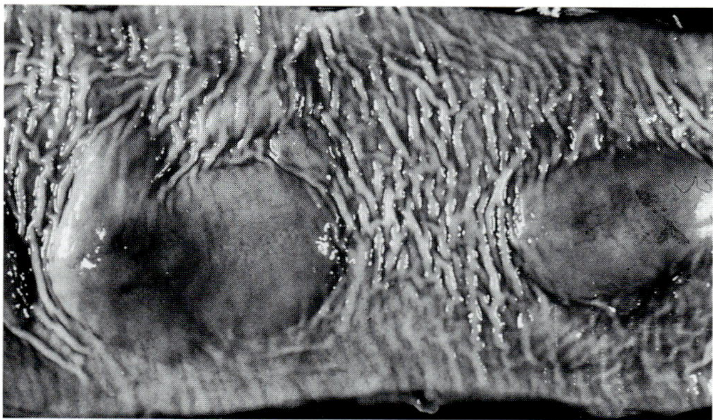

Fig. 1-65 Small intestine; horse. Equine granulomatous enteritis. The lesions are firm gray or white plaques that protrude above the surface of the mucosa. The plaque on the left has a central ulcer. *Courtesy Dr. D.J. Meuten.*

intestine may be adhered to one another. The wall of the large intestine is diffusely thickened and contains multiple, small granulomas. The mucosa is thickened, irregularly corrugated, and variably red, tan, or gray. A central ulceration occurs in some of the large, firm, fibrous plaques (Fig. 1-65). The mucosa of affected large intestine may contain protruding granulomas with white, tan, or brown cut surface. Ulcers appear as small craters at the centers of 5 to 8 mm diameter granulomas, or as variable-length, linear lesions of the mucosa. Regional lymph nodes are enlarged, swollen, wet on cut section, and variably reddened. Lymph nodes and the liver have grossly visible gray to tan nodules, some of which are gritty when cut.

Microscopically, granulomatous enteritis of the horse is characterized by a severe infiltration of lymphocytes, plasma cells, and histiocytes (Figs. 1-66 and 1-67), with giant cells in about half of the lesions. The inflammatory infiltrate is diffuse in the lamina propria, between intestinal crypts or in the cores of villi, and, thus, resembles a lymphosarcomatous infiltrate. The inflammatory process extends into the submucosa, transmurally in places, often with a perivascular arrangement. The liver in some horses has granulomatous inflammatory lesions, as do some of the regional lymph nodes. The macrophages, histiocytes, or giant cells in the granulomatous lesions do not contain stainable bacilli or acid-fast organisms.

The distribution and character of the lesions of equine granulomatous enteritis suggest that the lesions are caused by strongyle larvae. The fibrovascular serosal plaques resemble **hemomelasma ilei;** the raised mucosal nodules and central ulcers or cores of eosinophils suggest a parasitic etiology. Attempts to reproduce the disease have failed, and, although *Mycobacterium avium* has been isolated from a few cases, no etiologic agent has been identified.

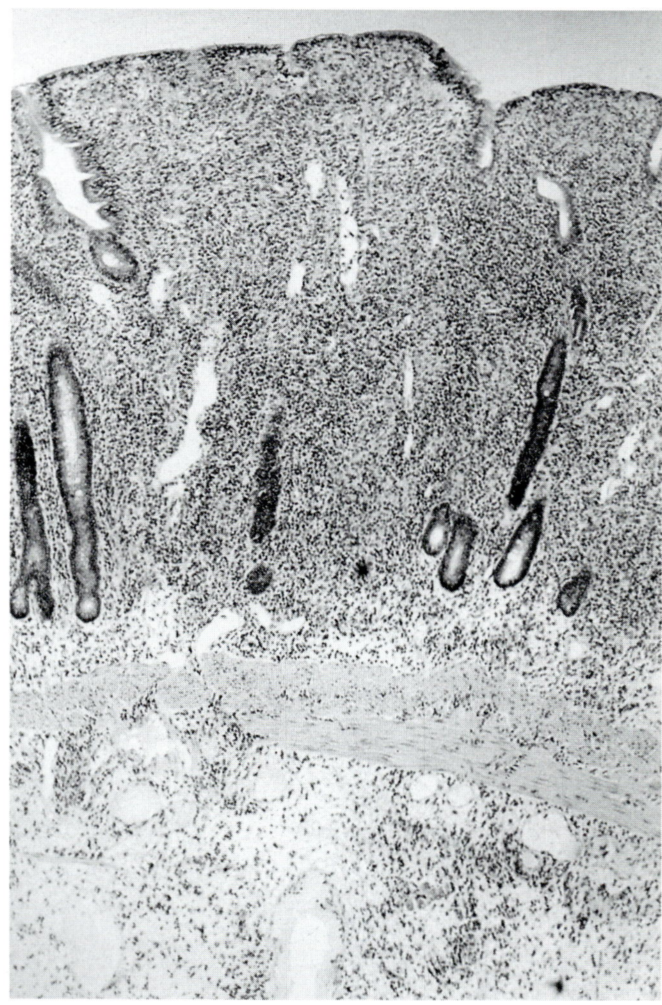

Fig. 1-66 Intestine; horse. Equine granulomatous enteritis. The mucosa and submucosa are diffusely infiltrated by a mixed population of inflammatory cells. *Meuten DJ, Butler DG, Thompson GW, Lumsden JH. J Am Vet Med Assoc. 1978; 172:330.*

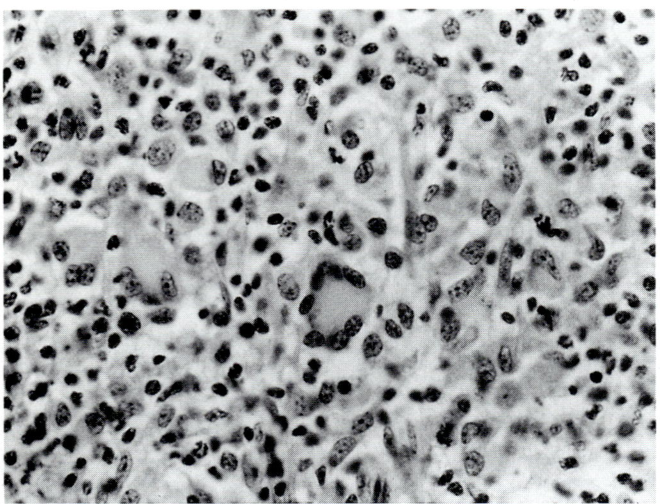

Fig. 1-67 Intestine; horse. Equine granulomatous enteritis. Mixed mucosal cellular infiltrate includes lymphocytes, plasma cells, macrophages, and giant cells. *Meuten DJ, Butler DG, Thompson GW, Lumsden JH. J Am Vet Med Assoc 1978; 172:330.*

Parasitic enteritis

Giardiasis occurs in many species, including human beings, dogs, cats, horses, cattle, rabbits, guinea pigs, hamsters, rats, mice, chinchillas, and parakeets. In clinical veterinary medicine, giardiasis is frequently recognized in puppies and kittens.

Giardiasis is caused by a unicellular flagellated protozoan. The pear-shaped organism has posterior flagella, a ventral sucker, and four nuclei, two of which resemble eyes (Fig. 1-68). *Giardia lamblia* inhabits the small intestine, particularly the duodenum, where the organisms attach to the microvillous border of epithelial cells producing craters in the surface.

When *Giardia* are present in small numbers, they produce no clinical illness. However, when in great numbers or in an immunologically deficient individual, diarrhea occurs. The parasites in large numbers inhibit the absorption of simple sugars and disaccharides, which are then fermented by bacterial flora, creating intestinal gas. The sugars also have an osmotic effect and draw water into the lumen. The result is distention of the small intestine with fluid and gas.

Clinically, animals with giardiasis have brown, fluid diarrhea, signs of abdominal discomfort without fever,

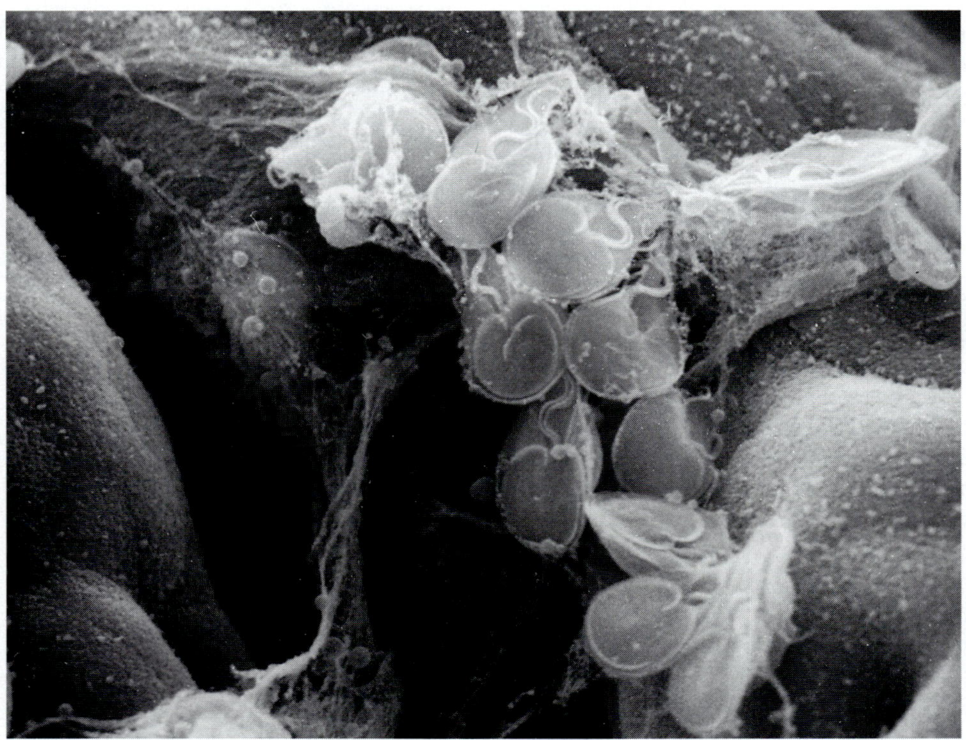

Fig. 1-68 Small intestine; man. Scanning electron micrograph. Giardiasis. *Giardia* trophozoites are attached to villous epithelium, their backs adherent to mucus. ×1800. *Poley JR, Rosenfield, S. J Pediatr Gastroenterol Nutr 1982; 1:63-80.*

weight loss, melena, or steatorrhea. The diagnosis is made by demonstrating *Giardia* in preparations of fresh feces.

The lesions of giardiasis are few. The diagnosis is made by searching the periphery of duodenal and jejunal villi, as the organisms are seen attached to villous epithelial cells or between villi. The parasites can be seen in H & E–stained sections, but are more readily identified in Giemsa-stained sections.

Cryptosporidiosis is being recognized with increasing frequency and has been reported in several animal species. It causes diarrhea and lesions in pigs, lambs, calves, foals, and human beings.

Cryptosporidia are very small coccidia that attach to surface epithelial cells of the stomach, small intestine, or colon (Fig. 1-69). The protozoa attach to the epithelial cells, displace the microvilli (Fig. 1-70), and are enclosed by surface cell membranes. Microgametes, macrogametes, schizonts, trophozoites, and oocytes can be demonstrated in the intestine adjacent to or attached to epithelial cells. Oocysts are 4 to 5 μm in diameter and are shed in the feces (Fig. 1-71). In fecal smears stained by the Giemsa method, the oocysts contain two to five dense red granules in a blue to blue-green cytoplasm. Oocysts can also be identified by a modified acid-fast stain and by immunofluorescence. The disease is transmitted by ingestion of oocysts and, experimentally, by the gavage administration of ileal scrapings or feces.

Clinically, cryptosporidiosis causes subacute or chronic watery diarrhea, sometimes tinged with blood, with an associated dehydration, loss of electrolytes, and, subsequently, weakness. Although the disease can be fatal, par-

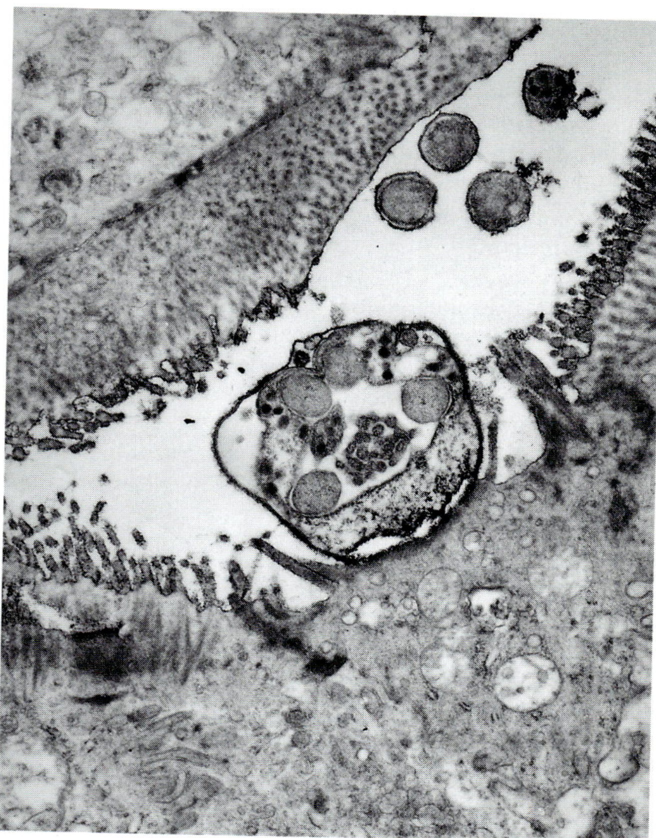

Fig. 1-70 Small intestine; calf. Cryptosporidiosis. Microvilli are displaced where *Cryptosporidium* is attached. *Courtesy Dr. D.J. Meuten.*

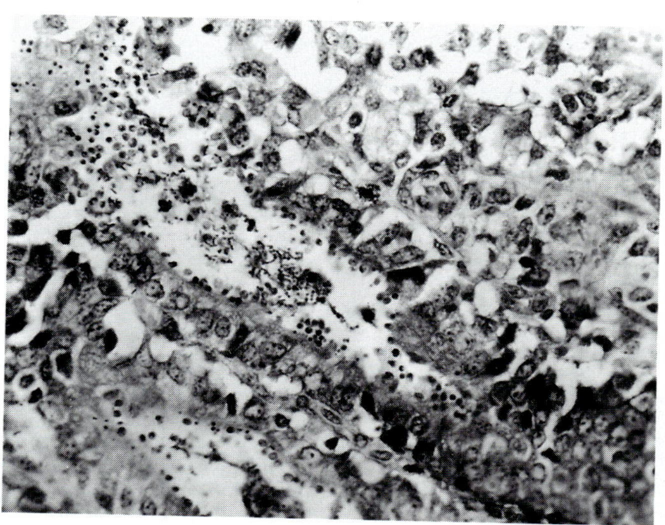

Fig. 1-69 Small intestine; calf. Cryptosporidiosis. Numerous dot and ring forms are attached to the villous surface epithelium. Wolbach-Giemsa stain. *Courtesy Dr. D.J. Meuten.*

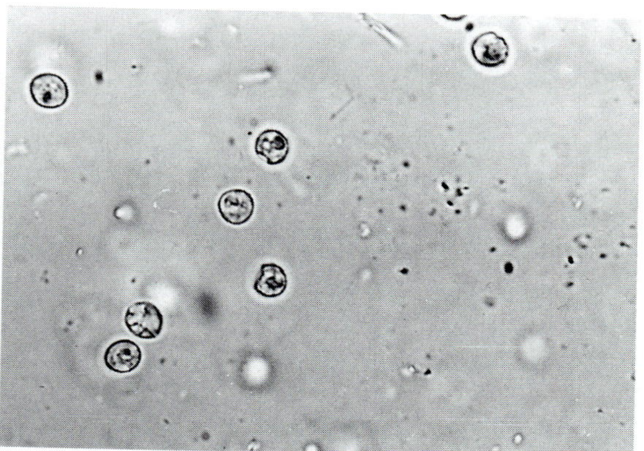

Fig. 1-71 Feces; human. Cryptosporidiosis. *Cryptosporidium parvum* oocytes, 4 to 5 μm in size, are demonstrated in a sugar flotation medium (sp. gr. 1.27). ×1280. *Anderson BC, Donndelinger T, Wilkins RM, Smith J. J Am Vet Med Assoc 1982; 180:408-409.*

ticularly in the presence of other pathogens, it is often self-limited in immunocompetent individuals, with the illness abating spontaneously in 6 to 8 days.

Grossly, affected portions of the GI tract are diffusely reddened and have fluid contents. Microscopically, in H & E–stained sections, the very small organisms appear as tiny blue dots attached to the epithelial cells of affected segments. In addition to the dot forms, ring- and banana-shaped organisms are readily seen in Giemsa-stained preparations. The lesions of the enteritis or colitis consist of decreased mucosal height, irregular mucosal thickness, cryptitis, hyperemia, and an increase in lymphocytes and plasma cells in the lamina propria (Fig. 1-72). Villi undergo atrophy and fusion.

Coccidiosis. Coccidia are protozoa that parasitize the intestinal mucosa of all animal species. Two genera of most concern are *Eimeria* and *Isospora.* Oocysts of the former genus develop at sporulation into four sporocysts, each with two sporozoites; whereas, those of the latter genus yield two sporocysts, each with four sporozoites. Oocysts are the product of the sexual cycle of these parasites; they are shed in the feces, are oval with refractile hyaline walls, and are tolerant of a wide range of environmental conditions. A new host acquires the infection by ingesting sporulated oocysts. Sporozoites liberated in the stomach penetrate intestinal epithelial cells to induce disease.

The various species of *Eimeria* and *Isopora* reside in very specific segments of intestine and are species-specific. Most infect villous or crypt epithelial cells; some species reside in the endothelium of lacteals; other species occur in the lamina propria; and, on occasion, some organisms reach the regional lymph nodes. The coccidia undergo one or more asexual reproductive cycles, with the resulting sporoziotes producing schizonts that contain from few to thousands of merozoites. The latter emerge and penetrate other cells. Within the sexual cycle, merozoites yield gamonts that differentiate into microgametes and macrogametes; the microgametes fertilize the macrogametes to yield zygotes, which develop into oocysts.

When a small number of coccidia parasitize the intestine of otherwise healthy young growing animals, little disease results. However, in animals under crowded conditions, when sanitation is not sound, fecal-oral transmission of large numbers of organisms may occur; particularly if accompanied by marginally deficient nutrition or concomitant parasitism, significant clinical disease can occur. With each cycle, sexual and asexual, epithelial cell lysis occurs; total damage is proportional to the environmentally acquired dose and the numbers generated endogenously. Young animals are most susceptible.

Clinically, coccidiosis is characterized by unthriftness and diarrhea. When the large intestine is diseased, streaks of red blood may color the feces and the animal may have tenesmus. Diagnosis is made by demonstrating oocysts in the feces; the size and internal features enable species identification (Fig. 1-73).

The gross lesions of coccidiosis are variable hyperemia and fluid distention of affected segments, often caudal small intestine and/or cecum and colon. If the infecting *Eimeria* generate large schizonts, 300 μm in size, pinpoint white foci are visible from both serosal and mucosal surfaces. The mucosa may appear normal, be raised in convoluted hyperplastic patches, or be variably eroded, with or without a fibrinonecrotic pseudomembrane. Erosion and fissuring of the mucosa of the large intestine may be accompanied by bleeding. The severity of the hyperemia, segmental demarcation, and surface bleeding vary considerably among coccidial species.

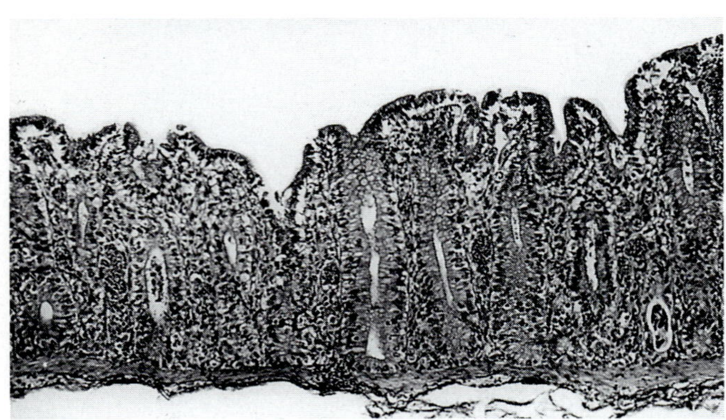

Fig. 1-72 Colon; calf. Cryptosporidiosis. Mucosal height is reduced, epithelium is tattered, there has been a loss of crypts, leukocytes of the lamina propria are increased, and there is scattered cryptitis. Wolbach-Giemsa stain. *Meuten DJ, Van Kruiningen HJ, Lein DH. J Am Vet Med Assoc 1974; 165:914-917.*

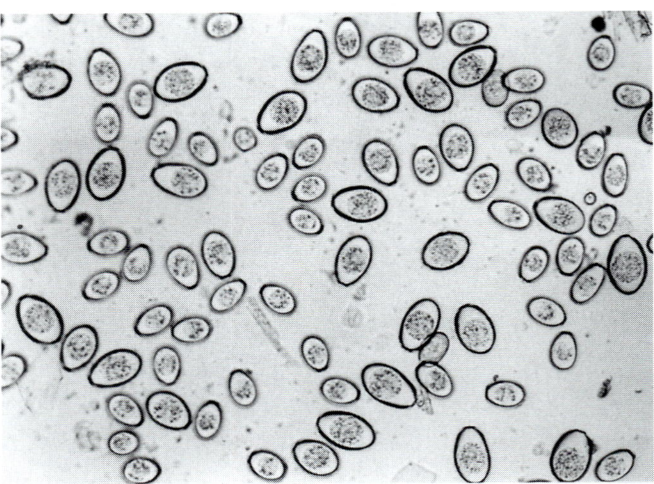

Fig. 1-73 Feces; goat. Coccidiosis. Oocysts of two species of *Eimeria* are abundant in this fecal preparation.

Microscopically, coccidiosis is characterized by necrosis of villous or crypt epithelium, hyperemia, and a moderate inflammatory response in the lamina propria. The infiltrate usually consists of lymphocytes and plasma cells, but, sometimes, eosinophils are numerous. Globule leukocytes increase in number. The loss of epithelial cells may result in villous atrophy, collapse of the glandular mucosa, or pseudomembrane formation. In some chronic infections, the epithelium is hyperplastic, and this proliferation produces an adenomatous mucosal surface. The coccidia are readily recognized (Fig 1-74). The schizonts are oval and filled with basophilic, banana-shaped merozoites; oocysts are oval and have refractile walls; macrogametes are large cells with refractile, eosinophilic, red ''plastic granules''; and gamonts are round to oval with uniformly eosinophilic staining and a dotlike nucleus.

Ascariasis. Ascarids are long, smooth, white roundworms that vary in size from 3 to 4 cm in small animals up to 40 to 50 cm in pigs and horses. They reside in the upper small intestine. Common species include *Ascaris suum* of pigs, *Parascaris equorum* of horses, *Toxocara canis* of dogs, *T. cati* of cats, and *T. lumbricoides* of human beings. Young animals acquire ascarids by one of several routes. Intrauterine transmission of larvae occurs during the last 7 to 10 days of gestation. Larvae may be transmitted via the milk of the dam, and, later in life, embryonated eggs are ingested as a consequence of fecal contamination of the mammary gland, through feed, or via coprophagy. Transmission can also occur via paretenic hosts. Infective larvae penetrate the intestine and migrate to the liver via the portal circulation. From the liver, the larvae travel via the vena cava to the lungs, where they break out of alveolar capillaries, undergo development, and migrate up the trachea or are coughed up. Larvae are swallowed and pass to the intestine for development to adults. Ova are passed with the feces. *Toxascaris leonina,* another ascarid of dogs, is transmitted via ingestion and through an intermediate host; hepatopulmonary migration does not occur. The larvae of ascarids produce eosinophilic gastroenteritis when trapped in the submucosa of the stomach or intestine; they are responsible for eosinophilic granulomas of mesenteric lymph nodes, kidneys, and, rarely, the retina or other tissues. Larvae produce eosinophilic tracts, granulomas, periportal infiltrates, and focal fibrosis in the liver; the larvae cause focal hemorrhages, eosinophilic infiltrates, and granulomas of the lungs. In aberrant hosts, the larvae appear to wander with less direction, often producing neurologic disease, ocular granulomas, visceral larva migrans, and acute interstitial pneumonia.

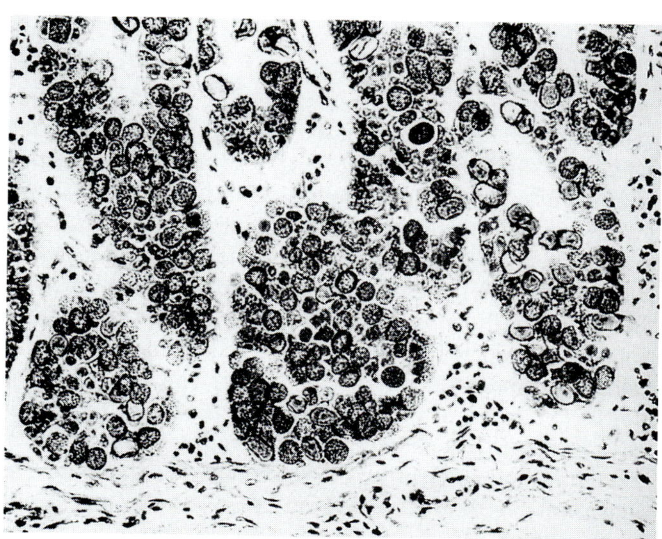

Fig. 1-74 Intestine; goat. Coccidiosis. Virtually every epithelial cell contains stages of the *Eimeria* life cycle. H & E stain.

Adult ascarids apparently produce clinical disease by their physical presence and by inducing moderate malabsorption. Affected animals have less-than-normal weight gains, lassitude, pendulous abdomen, partial anorexia, and intermittent vomiting or diarrhea. Coughing and labored respiration called ''thumping'' are signs of pulmonary larva migrans. Eosinophilia occurs during the larval migration.

Adult ascarids are readily observed in the upper small intestine at necropsy (Fig. 1-75). They produce no gross lesions other than an occasional perforation or intussusception, when large masses occlude the lumen. Sometimes, the ascarids find their way into the bile duct or pancreas, where they cause obstruction and inflammation. Microscopically, parasites in the lumen of the intestine may produce no lesions or increased mucosal eosinophils or globule leukocytes. Pigs develop hypertrophy of the intestinal tunica muscularis.

Hookworm disease. Hookworms are short, stocky worms, 1 to 1.5 cm long, that inhabit the proximal small intestine of a number of animal species. Some of the commonly occurring species include *Ancylostoma caninum* and *Uncinaria stenocephala* of dogs, *Bunostomum* species of ru-

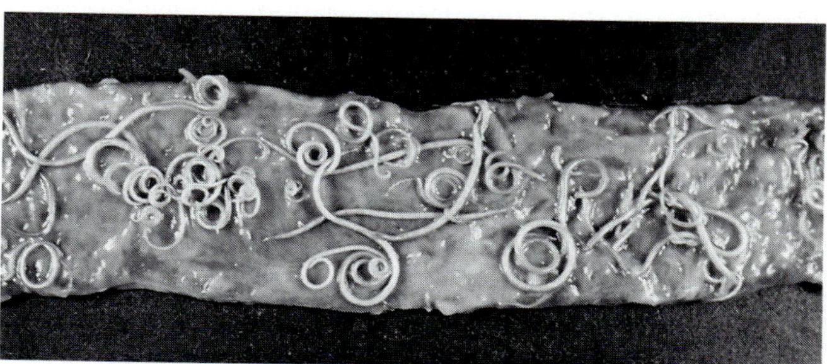

Fig. 1-75 Small intestine; dog. Ascariasis. Ascarids are abundant in the lumen of the proximal jejunum.

minants, and *Ancylostoma duonenale* and *Necator americanus* of human beings. The canine hookworm, *A. caninum,* is transmissible to human beings, causing eosinophilic enteritis and obscure abdominal pain. Hookworm eggs, discharged from females living in the small intestine, are passed in the feces. Under satisfactory environmental conditions, development outside the host progresses to third-stage infective larvae that enter the host by cutaneous penetration or by ingestion. Depending on species and portal of entry, the larvae may move directly to the small intestine, or they may follow a transpulmonary route. Development continues through fourth- and fifth-stage larvae to adults that attach to the intestinal mucosa. Larvae of the canine hookworm, *A. caninum,* are transmitted in utero and via mammary secretion. These routes of transmission are responsible for the unusual occurrence of hookworm larvae in premature or stillborn puppies and the presence of hookworm eggs in the feces of puppies.

Hookworms are prevalent in animals occupying a warm, wet climate, particularly climates that are above freezing for most of the year. Larval development is inhibited by temperatures below 10° C or above 40° C, by sunlight, by abrupt changes in temperature, and by dessication. Some species of hookworms have seasonal variation in egg output, an adaptation favoring survival.

Hookworm disease affects primarily the young of all host species. The young are also at risk from intrauterine or mammary transmission and are most likely to encounter oral or cutaneous contact with feces. Infections occur more commonly and are more severe under circumstances of poor sanitation, malnutrition, and multiple parasitisms. The canine hookworm, *A. caninum,* can be disseminated by the housefly, *Musca domestica.*

Once larval migration has been completed, adult hookworms reside in the small intestine, the organ generally considered the site of hookworm disease. However, in at least a few species, adults are found in the caudal intestine to the level of the colon and rectum and make their way cranially. Lacerations of 1 to 2 mm are found where the parasites have attached. In the colon, cecum, and rectum, lacerations with hemorrhages, usually 2 to 3 mm, occur focally or in rows on mucosal folds; the lacerations are frequently present in the mucosa around solitary lymphoid follicles and along the edge of the ileocolic valve. This latter lesion, an ileocolic valvulitis, has been observed in young dogs at necropsy, sometimes in several of a litter. The edge of the ileocolic valve contains several raised, glistening, black-red mucosal nodules, 2 to 4 mm in diameter; a hookworm is rarely found attached. Microscopically, the colonic mucosa lining the edge of the valve is moderately hyperplastic, and the lamina propria contains a few aggregates of lymphocytes and plasma cells, and sometimes a few eosinophils, a few siderocytes, and hemorrhage.

Hookworms coil in preparation for attachment and then thrust their heads into the villus. The worm penetrates the epithelium and sucks up a wedge-shaped portion of the villous core. Vessels of the lamina propria immediately engorge, and a red disc appears at the point of attachment. The worm makes vigorous sucking movements, ingesting tissue fluid, mucus, and boluses of mucosa, as well as blood. The wound left by the bite, after the worm shifts from one point of attachment to another, continues to ooze blood for as long as 30 minutes. The blood loss that occurs in hookworm disease is the result of blood ingestion by the parasites and multifocal intestinal laceration. The magnitude of the blood loss varies among species, from 0.07 ml per worm per day for *A. caninum* up to 0.2 ml per worm per day for *A. duodenale.* Boring, twisting movements help the worm to thrust its head deeper along the villous margin toward the intestinal crypts.

The hookworm usually produces damage over an area of two to three villi, but may injure many more. Grossly, the points of attachment may be seen as punctiform hemorrhages or ulcerations. Microscopically, mucosal lymphocytes appear increased in the vicinity of hookworms, and granulocytes occur at the sites of attachment. There is increased activity of intestinal mucous cells.

Clinically, canine hookworm disease is characterized by unthriftiness, lethargy, weight loss, poor hair coat, anemia, diarrhea, variable appetite, and dehydration. Death commonly follows heavy infections in puppies. The feces may be dark brown, olive-green, or black and variable in consistency. Infrequently, dogs with hookworms may pass red blood. Laboratory findings include hypochromic, microcytic anemia, eosinophilia, hypoalbuminemia, occult fecal blood, and characteristic ova. Rectal involvement may provoke rectal pruritis or tenesmus. Ileocolic valvulitis is manifested by streaks of red blood mixed with, or on the surface of, formed feces. Cats, cattle, sheep, and swine have lethargy, weight loss, poor hair coat, diarrhea, and weakness.

Stronglyoidosis. Stronglyoidosis is recognized infrequently. The enteritis induced can be severe; larvae or larvated eggs are recognized in the feces of infected animals. The canine and primate parasite, *Strongyloides stercoralis,* is transmissible to human beings. Other species of *Strongyloides* infect horses, pigs, and cats. Parasitism occurs in the upper small intestine, where parthenogenic females, 2 to 9 mm in length, reside in shallow epithelial tunnels at the base of villi. In the case of *S. stercoralis,* "autoinfection" is possible; i.e., eggs discharged from females develop into larvae without exiting the host and, in turn, reinfect the intestine of their host. Larvae (rhabditiform) that leave the host with the feces develop into free-living males and females, the offspring of which may become parasitic (filariform), or they may develop into infective (filariform) larvae directly. Infective larvae penetrate the skin or are ingested and penetrate the gastrointestinal mucosa. The larvae travel in the circulation to the lungs, enter the alveoli, are coughed up and then swallowed, and come to reside in the small intestine. Some species of *Strongyloides* are transmitted in utero and through mammary secretions. Clinically, affected animals have diarrhea, weight loss, dehydration, hypoproteinemia, eosinophilia, anorexia, and debility. Larvae or eggs are demonstrable in the feces.

Grossly, the affected intestine may be hyperemic and fluid-filled. Microscopically, the nematodes occur in the epithelium, which may be ulcerated or hyperplastic (Figs. 1-76 to 1-78). Villi are reduced, cells of the crypts are hyperactive, and the lamina propria has increased numbers of lymphocytes and plasma cells, as well as eosinophils. Serum components and granulocytes are lost into the lumen.

Trichostrongylosis. Trichostrongyles are small nematodes that parasitize the duodenum and jejunum of sheep, goats, cattle, and other ruminants. Three genera of the family *Trichostrongylidae* are significant: *Nematodirus,* which are 2 to 3 cm long; *Cooperia,* 1 cm long; and *Trichostrongylus,* 5 to 8 mm long. These parasites all have a direct life cycle; eggs are passed in the feces and larvae are acquired by ingestion. Prepatent periods are 3 to 4 weeks, 2 to 3 weeks, and 2 to 3 weeks, respectively. Young animals are most susceptible; crowding, poor sanitation, and inadequate nutrition increase susceptibility.

Clinically, trichostrongylosis is characterized by weight loss, diarrhea, poor hair coat, dehydration, sunken eyeballs, anorexia, anemia, intermandibular edema, and recum-

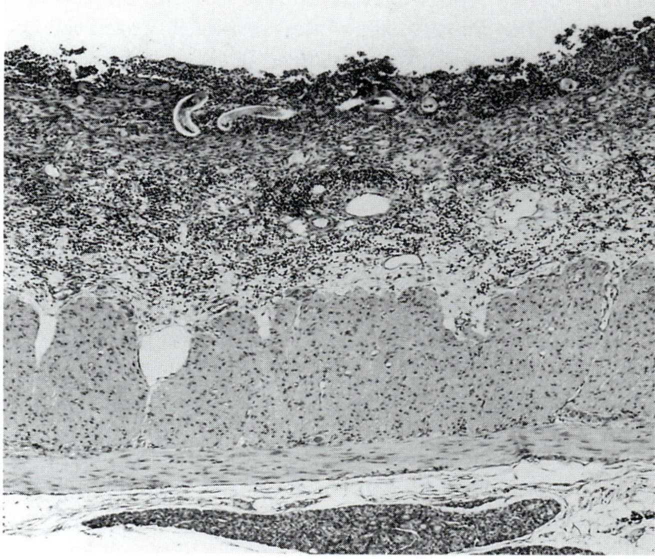

Fig. 1-77 Small intestine; patas monkey. Strongyloidosis. *Strongyloides* are present within the inflammatory response beneath a focus of ulceration. *Harper JS III, Genta RM, Gam A, London WT, Neva FA Am J Trop Med Hyg 1984; 33:431-443.*

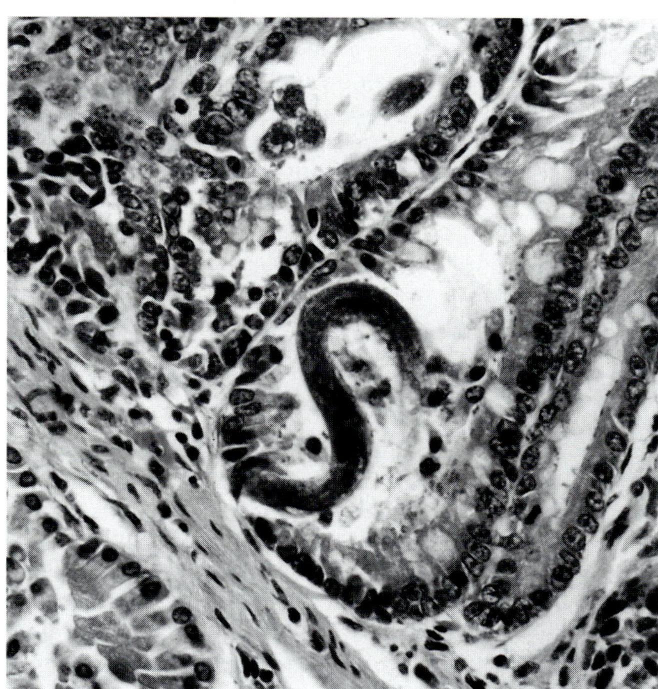

Fig. 1-76 Small intestine; patas monkey. Strongyoidosis. *Strongyloides stercoralis* resides within an intestinal crypt. *Courtesy Dr. J.S. Harper III.*

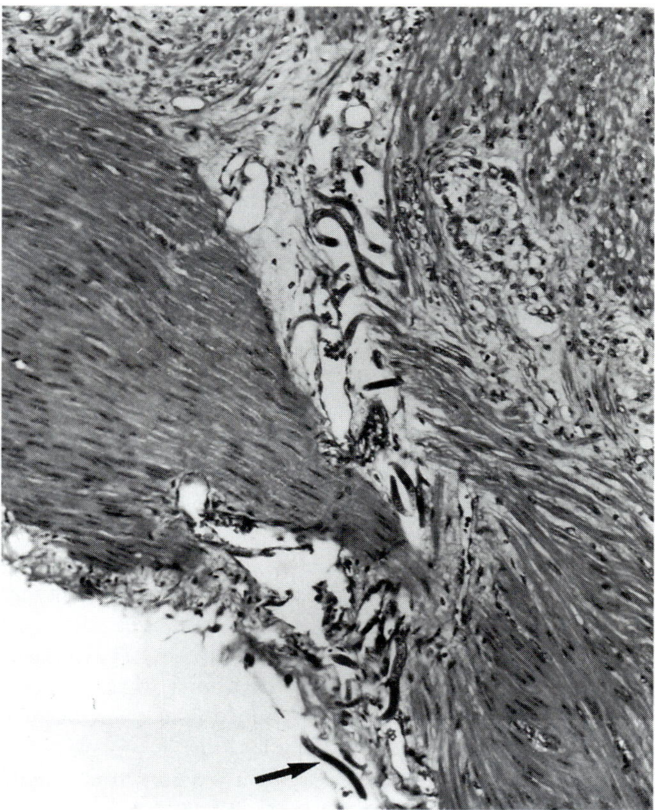

Fig. 1-78 Colon; patas monkey. Strongyloidosis. *Strongyloides* are within a lymphatic between inner and outer muscle coats, and in subserosa *(arrow). Courtesy Dr. J.S. Harper III.*

bency. Malabsorption and enteric protein loss are variable. The feces may be formed but more commonly are fluid and dark. Laboratory findings include decreased hemoglobin concentrations and hypoalbuminemia. Parasite eggs can be identified in the feces.

An animal that is heavily parasitized has stunted growth, pendulous abdomen, and fecal staining of the hair or wool of the perineum. Intermandibular edema, pale tissues, and serous atrophy of fat may be present at necropsy. The intestines have variable hyperemia, dark brown or green fluid contents, and a delicate, grayish-white film of exfoliated cells, albumin, and fibrin on the villous surface. The parasites can be recognized on the mucosal surface, but recognition is enhanced by screening of intestinal contents.

Microscopically, adults of the *Trichostrongylus* species are found in shallow epithelial tunnels, whereas the adults of *Nematodirus* and *Cooperia* are entwined among the villi. How the parasites induce damage is not totally clear. They cause tunnels and creases in the margins of villi; villous epithelium may have damaged microvilli and reduced activity of brush border enzymes. Crypt epithelium has increased numbers of globule leukocytes and mitotic figures, and the lumens are deeper than normal. The lamina propria is infiltrated by lymphocytes, plasma cells, and eosinophils. Villous atrophy varies in severity, and erosions may develop.

Viral enteritis

Transmissible gastroenteritis of pigs. Transmissible gastroenteritis of pigs is well recognized in swine-producing areas throughout the world, appears most frequently in midwinter to spring, and tends to have cyclic recurrences. Classically, transmissible gastroenteritis occurs in epizootics. Morbidity is high, and essentially all pigs under 10 to 14 days of age become affected. In herds that have not experienced this disease before, animals of other age groups, including sows, are affected. Mortality is high in 2 to 3 days and may reach almost 100% in young pigs. The outbreak ends in 3 to 5 weeks, and an immunity is produced that lasts for 3 to 6 years. The duration of this immunity explains the cyclic occurrence of the disease in a particular area.

Transmissible gastroenteritis is caused by an epitheliotropic coronavirus. The virus invades and destroys mature epithelial cells of the intestinal villi of the lower portion of duodenum, jejunum, and, sometimes, ileum. The virus is readily transmitted from animal to animal by aerosol and by feces. The disease is readily transported from farm to farm by carrier animals and vehicles.

Pigs infected at less than 2 weeks of age become ill and have diarrhea within 24 hours of exposure to the virus. Epithelial cells contain virus particles, and diseased pigs become shedders immediately, thus promoting transmission. The virus kills villous epithelial cells. Inclusion bodies do not occur. There is karyorrhexis, lysis, and sloughing of epithelial cells along the lateral borders and tips of villi. Crypt epithelial cells are spared and undergo hyperplasia to replace lost villous epithelial cells. The rapid destruction of large numbers of epithelial cells causes immediate osmotic diarrhea and malabsorption. Within a few days, the villi become atrophic. The pig suffers malabsorption of nutrients as well as fluid and electrolyte disturbances.

Clinically, transmissible gastroenteritis is characterized by a sudden onset of vomiting and diarrhea. The diarrhea is profuse, contains white, undigested milk, and has an offensive odor. Dehydration is pronounced. Young pigs may have only a transitory fever, whereas affected sows are febrile for several days. Weakness and emaciation are progressive to death from the second to the fifth day of illness. Pigs that survive grow poorly because of continued intestinal malabsorption and may never recover completely. In affected sows, the illness lasts up to 10 days with signs of inappetence and agalactia. In growing and fattening swine, transmissible gastroenteritis usually occurs as a transient, watery diarrhea, mild anorexia, some weight loss, and dehydration for 2 to 4 days. Laboratory findings include transient, mild leukopenia early in the disease and leukocytosis later.

At necropsy, young pigs that have died of transmissible gastroenteritis are dehydrated, and their caudal parts are stained with fluid feces. The small intestine is ballooned and is filled with a copious yellow fluid. The walls of the small intestine appear thin and translucent. Mesenteric blood vessels may appear congested, giving variable light redness to some portions of the intestine. Mesenteric lymph vessels are notably empty of chyle. The stomach may have patchy vascular engorgement. Microscopically, the diagnosis is based on the demonstration of villous atrophy (Fig. 1-79). The villous height: crypt depth ratio is reduced from 7:1 in normal pigs to 1:1 in infected animals (Figs. 1-80 and 1-81). The lesion is not accompanied by great infiltration of inflammatory cells; however, this aspect varies from one outbreak to the next and is influenced by secondary bacterial infections. Accumulations of neutrophils and lymphocytes occur where the mucosa is denuded. Epithelial cell necrosis and villous atrophy are the major lesions of transmissible gastroenteritis, but are not pathognomonic. Colibacillosis, coccidiosis, and certain other virus infections may also result in villous atrophy.

Feline panleukopenia. Feline panleukopenia occurs worldwide and is one of the most important causes of disease in cats. Feline panleukopenia is caused by a parvovirus that infects young animals, including young mink and raccoons. Kittens that reach 6 weeks of age are likely to have the disease unless vaccinated.

Clinically, the disease affects young cats most often, although unvaccinated animals of all ages are susceptible.

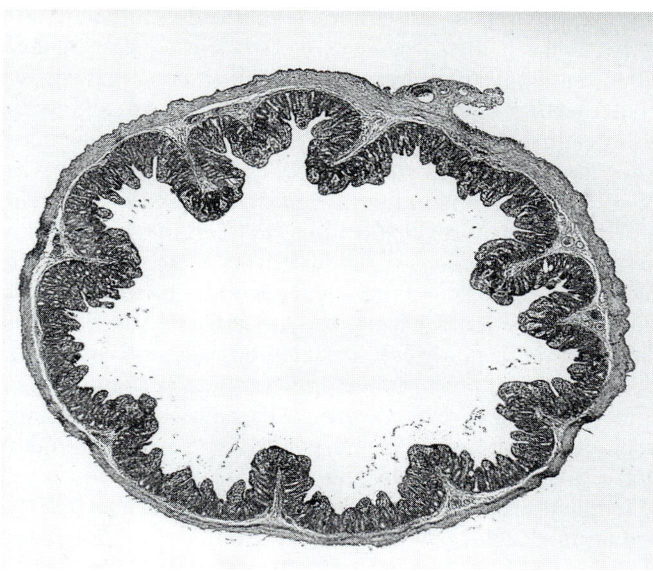

Fig. 1-79 Small intestine; newborn pig. Transmissible gastroenteritis. Extensive villous atrophy is present throughout the circumference of the mucosa in this transverse section of proxima jejunum. *Moon HW. J Am Vet Med Assoc 1969; 155:1853-1859.*

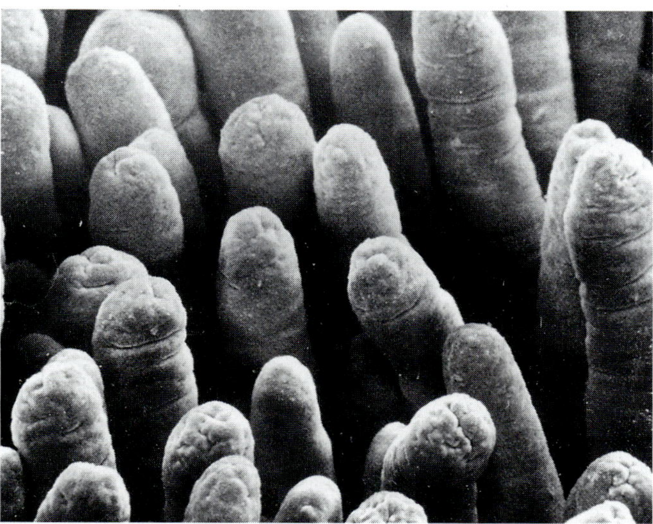

Fig. 1-80 Small intestine; pig. Normal villi. Scanning electron micrograph. Note the tall, lightly scalloped, fingerlike villi of the normal intestine. *Moon HW. Intestine. In: Cheville NF, ed. Cell Pathology. 2nd ed. Ames, IA: Iowa State University Press, 1983: 503.*

The signs include anorexia, vomiting, prostration, diarrhea, and dehydration. Affected cats often crouch over their food or water dish. Mortality varies from 65% to 90%. A profound leukopenia is usually present.

At necropsy, the dilated, fluid-filled, flaccid small intestine is quite characteristic. There is little hyperemia, however. The small intestine may contain brown to red-brown fluid, fibrinous exudate, and/or hemorrhage. Mesenteric lymph nodes may be enlarged and have a variegated, red discoloration. The bone marrow is semiliquid and yellow-gray.

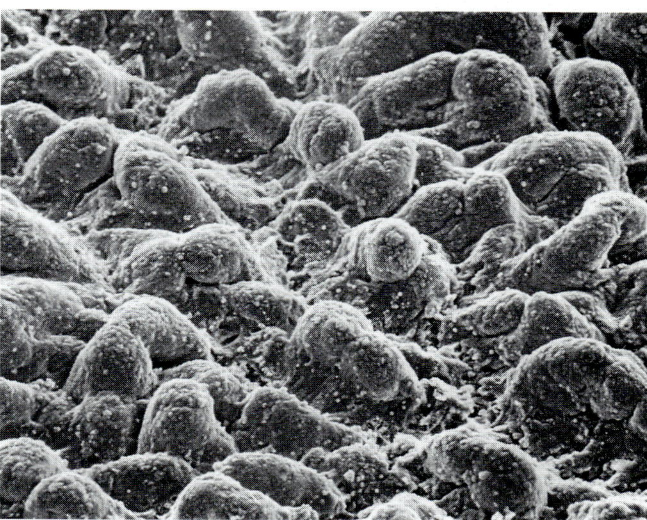

Fig. 1-81 Small intestine; pig. Transmissible gastroenteritis. Scanning electron micrograph. Villi are reduced to atrophic nubbins as a consequence of viral epithelial damage. *Moon HW. Intestine. In: Cheville NF, ed. Cell Pathology. 2nd ed. Ames, IA: Iowa State University Press, 1983:503.*

Microscopically, the intestinal lesion is characterized by necrosis of crypt epithelial cells. Necrotic cell fragments appear in the intestinal glands. Surviving epithelial cells become cuboidal or squamous and stretch over the surface of the crypt. After several days, loss of epithelium occurs along the margins of the villi as the crypts fail to supply cells. Severe lesions consist of partially denuded small villi over a series of damaged crypts, some of which lack epithelial cells completely. Other crypts are lined by squamous epithelial cells; some have a hyperplastic response (Fig. 1-82). The lamina propria is collapsed, and the denuded surface may be covered by a mat of bacteria or fungi (Fig. 1-83). Characteristic basophilic intranuclear inclusion bodies can be demonstrated in the crypt epithelial cells approximately 5 to 7 days after infection. These inclusion bodies are best demonstrated in tissues fixed in acidic fixatives, such as Bouin's or Zenker's. Loss of lymphocytes occurs in germinal centers of intestinal lymphoid follicles, resulting in the normally obscured reticular cells being prominent. Mesenteric lymph nodes may have hemorrhages, and macrophages filled with erythrocytes are common. Usually, inclusion bodies are not present in lymphoid tissues. Bone marrow smears or sections have normal erythropoiesis but an absence of granulopoiesis. The colon

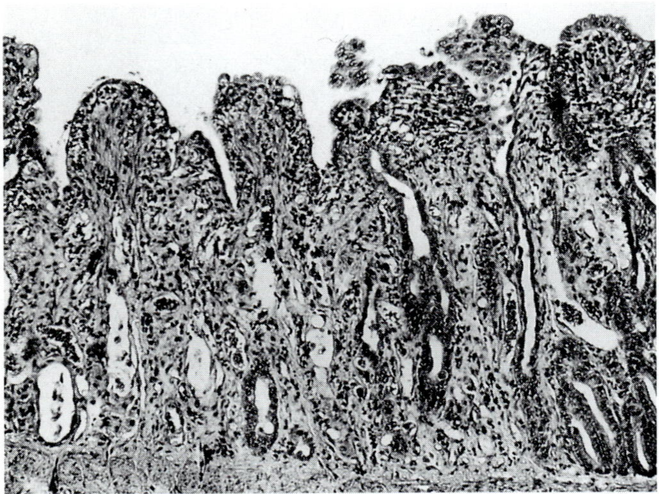

Fig. 1-82 Small intestine; cat. Feline panleukopenia. Villi are denuded of epithelium and reduced in size. Some crypts are absent, others dilated. Note the squamous epithelial cells in some crypts and hyperplasia in others. H & E stain.

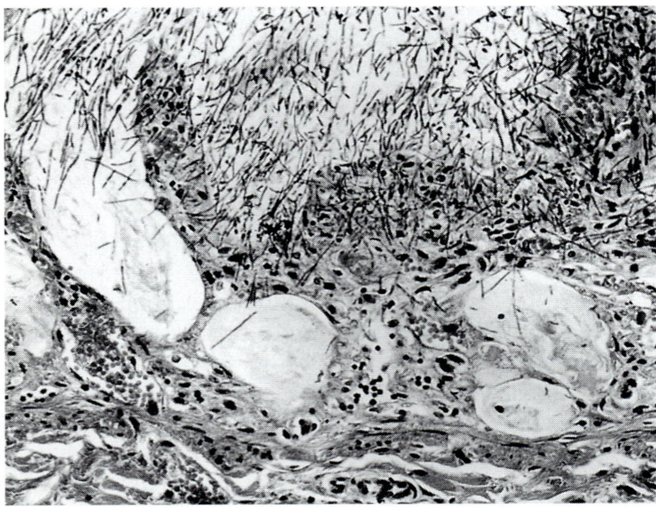

Fig. 1-83 Intestine; cat. Feline panleukopenia. Surface epithelium is lost and few remnants of intestinal crypts remain. *Candida albicans* coats the damaged surface. H & E stain.

has lesions as well, but these are usually focal and less severe, and seldom receive much attention because of the more severe damage of the small intestine.

Canine parvovirus enteritis. Canine parvovirus enteritis first appeared in North America in 1978 and spread through the canine population. It was characterized by acute bloody diarrhea, fever, dehydration, shock, and death. Shortly after its recognition, the similarity of the lesions of this new canine disease to those of feline panleukopenia was recognized, and a parvovirus was demonstrated by electron microscopy and tissue culture. The close antigenic similarity to the panleukopenia virus was subsequently quantified, antibody titers were recognized in dogs that recovered, electron microscopic recognition of the virus in feces or intestinal contents became routine, and feline panleukopenia vaccine was soon used to immunize dogs. It was then recognized that milder forms of the disease occurred, and that a parvovirus myocarditis occurred in puppies from kennels with the enteric disease. Within a few years, canine parvovirus disease was much reduced in incidence, partially the result of widespread natural exposure, which caused little or no disease in many dogs, and partially the consequence of prompt development and application of canine-strain parvovirus vaccines. The disease still occurs sporadically in unvaccinated populations; foxes, coyotes, and wolves are also susceptible.

Clinically, canine parvovirus enteritis is characterized by vomiting, diarrhea, anorexia, fever, panleukopenia, and dehydration. Those dogs with the hemorrhagic form of disease have bloody diarrhea and die a shocklike death in 24 hours. Puppies with viral myocarditis are severely ill, and most die.

Although canine parvovirus enteritis has many similarities to panleukopenia and the sequence of tissue events is virtually the same, there are some differences. The gross lesion in the canine disease is segmental or diffuse hemorrhagic enteritis. The affected segment is hyperemic, congested, and blood-filled (Fig. 1-84). It has not been possible to reproduce this form of the disease experimentally by giving canine parvovirus to young dogs. This suggests participation by another pathogen in those natural cases characterized by hemorrhagic diarrhea. The segmental vascular engorgement and mucosal hemorrhages are reminiscent of what occurs in *Clostridium perfringens* enterotoxemias.

Microscopically, the lesions that occur in the intestinal crypts are identical to those of feline panleukopenia, including the presence of viral inclusion bodies. In addition, coagulation necrosis involves the lymphoid tissue of Peyer's patches and regional lymph nodes, a lesion not seen in panleukopenia. This latter change can be diagnostic, even when the intestinal mucosa has been effaced by autolysis.

Calfhood rotavirus enteritis. Rotavirus enteritis of calves was first described in 1969. Using gnotobiotic calves inoculated with cell-free fecal filtrates, the lesions and clinical disease were defined. Subsequently, the virus was recovered and named neonatal calf diarrhea virus. The calf rotavirus is 65 to 75 nm in diameter and composed of double-stranded RNA with a hexagonal core and radiating capsomeres. Morphologically similar and antigenically related viruses cause diarrhea in human infants, suckling mice, foals, lambs, nonhuman primates, pigs, and rabbits. Calves up to 21 days of age are most susceptible. The severity of the infection is influenced by serotype of virus, prior in-

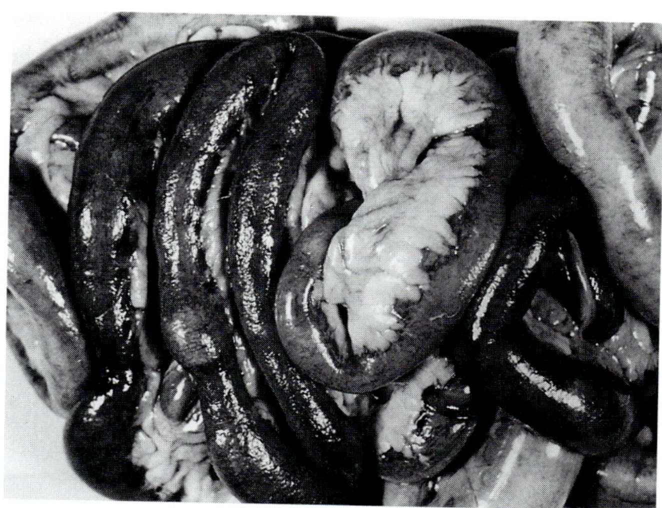

Fig. 1-84 Small intestine; dog. Parvovirus enteritis. Affected segments of small intestine are diffusely reddened, and the serosa is faintly granular.

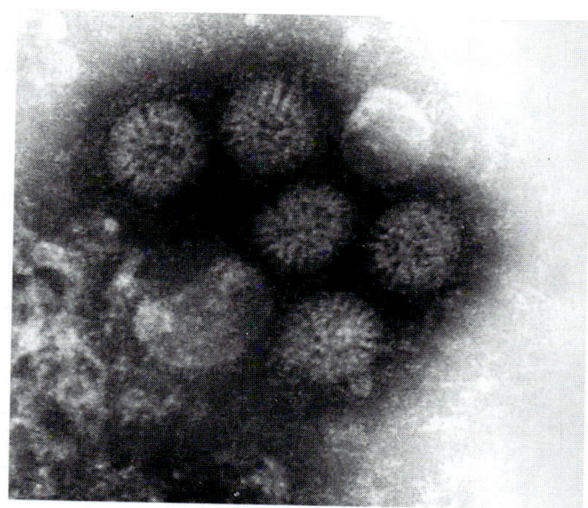

Fig. 1-85 Intestinal contents; calf. Rotavirus. Electron micrograph. Negatively stained rotavirus particles are 60 nm in diameter.

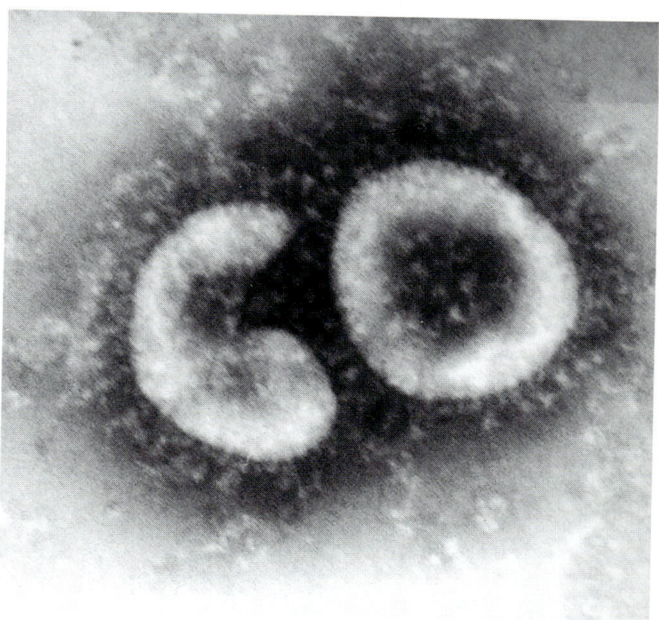

Fig. 1-86 Intestinal contents; calf. Coronavirus. Electron micrograph. Negatively stained coronavirus particles are 115 nm in diameter, with 35-nm peplomeres.

gestion of colostral antibody, and the presence of concomitant disease. Calves are often concomitantly infected with coronavirus, enterotoxigenic *E. coli,* or cryptosporidia.

Affected calves have a yellow, fluid diarrhea, are reluctant to stand and nurse, appear depressed, and, sometimes, have a few strings of thick saliva hanging from their lips. Calves that have died of rotavirus enteritis are often less than 72 hours old, are dehydrated, and have a "tucked-up" abdomen and sunken eyeballs. The intestines are moderately distended with yellow fluid, some loops appearing thin and transparent. Microscopically, the epithelial cells over the distal two thirds of the affected villi of the proximal small intestine are infected first; this event coincides with the onset of diarrhea. Within hours, desquamation of villous cells is followed by accelerated migration of remaining cells toward the villous tips. The infection progresses to the villous epithelial cells of the middle and distal small intestine. Within hours of the onset of diarrhea, all virus-containing cells (demonstrated by immunofluorescence) have been shed and replaced by cuboidal to squamous cells. The villi are shortened and have irregular surfaces. Rotavirus can be demonstrated in intestinal contents or feces for 5 or 6 days after the onset of illness (Fig. 1-85).

Calfhood coronavirus enteritis. In 1971, a coronavirus that also was responsible for calfhood enteritis was discovered. The virus was characterized, and, by using gnotobiotic calves, the pathogenesis of the disease was elucidated. The virus, 100 to 120 nm in diameter, is composed of single-strand RNA and has projecting peplomeres (Fig. 1-86). Calves up to 21 days of age (usually 4 to 6 days old) are susceptible. Severity of infection is influenced by serotype of the virus, ingestion of colostral antibody, and the presence of concomitant disease. The incubation period is 36 to 60 hours. Clinically, the disease is characterized by yellow, fluid, sometimes bloody, diarrhea, depression, reluctance to nurse, dehydration, and weakness.

The course of infection, clinical signs, and tissue damage are more prolonged in coronavirus enteritis than in rotavirus-induced disease, and death occurs after 2 to 4 days of diarrhea. The gross lesions are indistinguishable from those of rotavirus enteritis or enterotoxigenic colibacillosis. The small and large intestines are moderately distended with yellow fluid. Microscopically, the coronavirus infection is first apparent in villous epithelial cells of the proximal small intestine and, subsequently, in the caudal small intestine and colon. Immunofluorescence for viral antigen is present in all the cells lining the villi at the onset of diarrhea. In the colon, virus is present in surface cells and cells in the crypts. Antigen persists in crypt cells for 3 to 4 days after the onset of diarrhea. During the first 48 to 96 hours after the onset of the illness, epithelial cells are necrotic and are replaced by immature cuboidal or squamous cells, covering markedly shortened or fused villi. In the colon, surface cells are lost and replaced by less mature cells. Crypt lumina contain degenerate and necrotic cells. Focally, crypt epithelium is hyperplastic, and the lamina propria near the surface contains increased numbers of lymphocytes and plasma cells. Cells of the lamina propria, including fibroblasts, histiocytes, and endothelial cells, are infected; these undergo necrosis, producing a focal loss of cells. The paracortical sinuses of regional lymph nodes are filled with lymphocytes and plasma cells, as well as with macrophages that contain nuclear fragments. A hemorrhagic form of coronavirus enterocolitis is recognized in which virtually all colonic crypts are damaged throughout their length (Figs. 1-87 and 1-88). A bloody, fibrinonecrotic pseudomembrane covers the denuded colonic mucosa. It is not known if this form of the disease represents infection with a more virulent strain of virus or an interaction of the virus with other pathogens.

Bovine virus diarrhea. Bovine virus diarrhea is an acute infectious disease of cattle caused by a togavirus (Fig. 1-

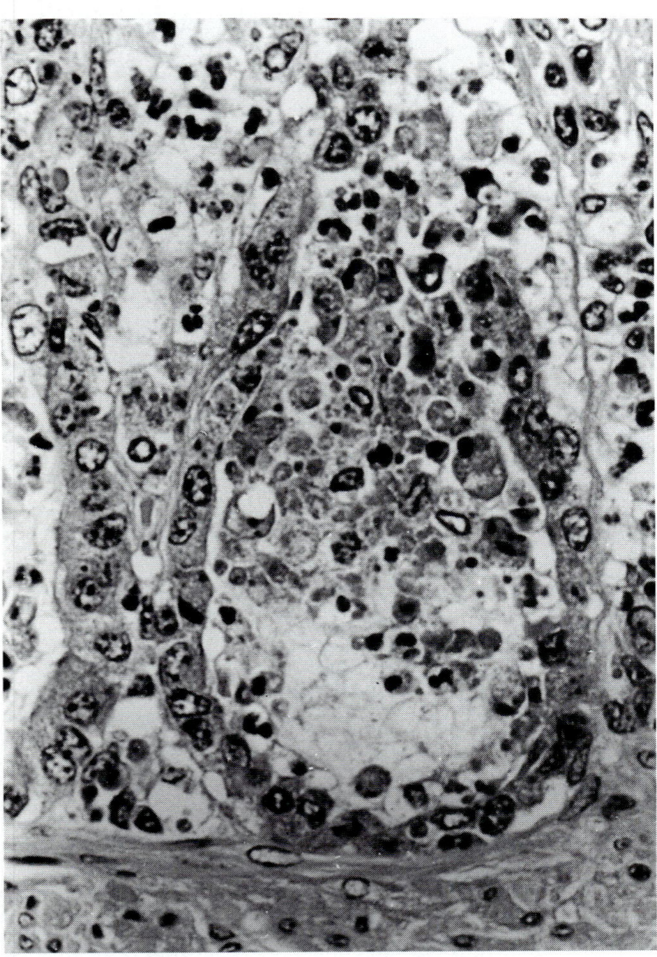

Fig. 1-87 Colon; calf. Coronavirus enterocolitis. Crypt epithelium has undergone extensive degeneration, pyknosis, and karyorrhexis. There is lysis of cells in the lamina propria as well. H & E stain.

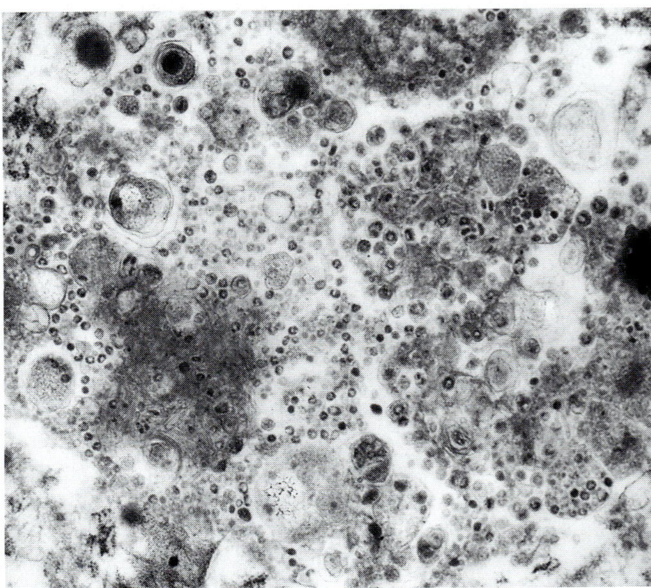

Fig. 1-88 Colon; calf. Coronavirus enterocolitis. Electron micrograph. The cytoplasm of damaged epithelial cells is filled with 80- to 120-nm, doughnut-shaped coronavirus particles.

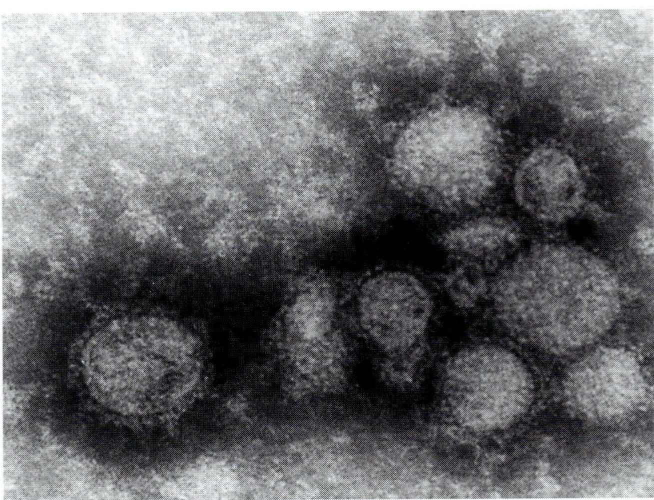

Fig. 1-89 Intestinal contents; calf. Bovine virus diarrhea virus. Electron micrograph. Negatively stained virus particles are roughly round in shape, vague in structure, and 45 to 90 nm in diameter.

89). The disease was first described in 1946 in New York State. Shortly thereafter, a similar disease recognized in the Midwest was designated mucosal disease. The mucosal disease variant of bovine virus diarrhea appears to be the product of simultaneous infection with two bovine virus diarrhea viruses, one cytopathic and the other noncytopathic, carried in a persistently infected animal. This dual infection causes greater severity of the ulcerative aspects of this disease, greater propensity for cutanous lesions and lameness, and greater potential for death or chronicity.

When first described in populations with few resistant animals, the disease occurred as epizootics with high morbidity (33% to 88%) and low mortality (4% to 8%). In recent years, because the virus(es) and the antibody to them are so widespread, cases are sporadic and mortality is greater. Outbreaks of disease have occurred following administration of modified live bovine virus diarrhea vaccines.

Young animals, less than 2 years of age, without maternal antibody are most susceptible to the disease. Transmission may occur through inhalation or ingestion of infected saliva, oculonasal discharge, urine, and feces. The incubation period is 7 to 9 days. The initial sign of high fever is accompanied by leukopenia (which actually precedes clinical signs by 3 or 4 days), lasts 3 to 6 days, and may be biphasic in some animals. The several disease syndromes encompassed by bovine virus diarrhea include (1) acute virus diarrhea in immunologically incompetent and persistently infected cattle, without and with interdigital and coronary band lesions, respectively; (2) chronic virus diarrhea, with more extensive cutaneous lesions, chronic ocular and nasal discharge, chronic rumen atony, diarrhea, and progressive emaciation; (3) reproductive failures, abortions, or teratogenic disease; (4) fatal enteritis in neonatal calves; and (5) viral pneumonia in calves and young stock.

Clinical signs of bovine virus diarrhea include anorexia, depression, profuse diarrhea, cessation of milk production, fever, rumen atony, salivation, lacrimation, mucopurulent nasal discharge, and erosions and ulcers of the muzzle and oral cavity. The feces are fetid and may contain mucus and variable quantities of blood. In some cases, animals are lame. Erosive cutaneous lesions involve the interdigital cleft and the coronary band. Pregnant cows may abort, sometimes as long as 3 months after apparent recovery. A profound leukopenia and dehydration are defined by laboratory tests.

The sum total of the very characteristic lesions in bovine virus diarrhea is clearly diagnostic. Squamous epithelium of the upper alimentary tract has sharply demarcated, pink ulcers. These round, oval, or irregular lesions occur on the dental pad, palate (Fig. 1-90), ventral and lateral surfaces of the tongue, the gums above the incisors, the buccal surface of the cheeks, the muzzle, and the rostral nares. Similar ulcers sometimes occur, though less frequently, in the pharynx. In the esophagus, small, irregular ulcers often coalesce in a linear fashion. Ulcers also occur on the pillars of the rumen and leaves of the omasum. The bases of ulcers that occur in the rumen and omasum are hyperemic and sometimes hemorrhagic. The mucosa of the abomasum is usually diffusely hyperemic, with many small petechiae and, often, small, round ulcers surrounded by pink rims of hyperemia (Fig. 1-91). The small intestine is hyperemic, is finely peppered with petechiae, and has fluid contents, often admixed with shreds of mucus and desquamated epithelial cells. Peyer's patches are sunken, bright red, and often covered by mucus or a fibrinonecrotic exudate. Typhlitis and colitis vary in severity but, in some animals, are hemorrhagic.

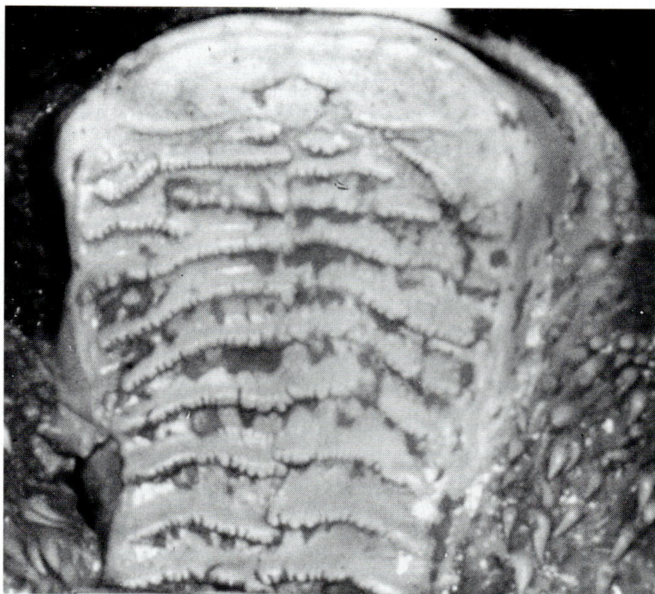

Fig. 1-90 Hard palate; cow. Bovine virus diarrhea. Multiple, shallow, pink erosions are present among the mucosal ridges of the palate.

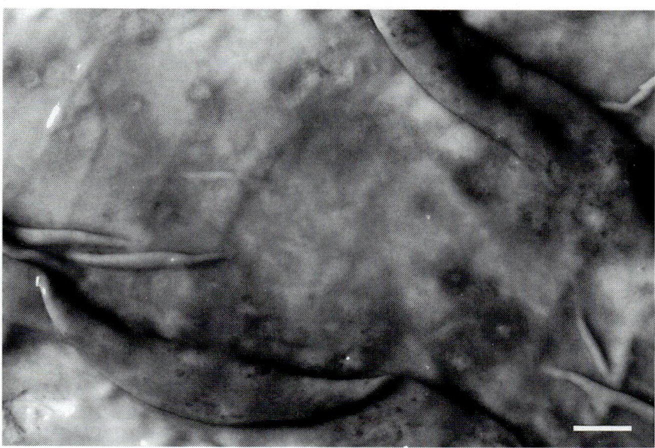

Fig. 1-91 Abomasum; cow. Bovine virus diarrhea. The mucosa contains multiple, 2 to 3 mm, shallow ulcers with hyperemic rims. Bar = 1 cm. *Courtesy Dr. M.D. McGavin.*

Microscopically, the lesions in the stratified squamous epithelia begin focally with hydropic degeneration and necrosis of the stratum spinosum. This is followed by erosion and ulceration, with hyperemia and influx of granulocytes at the margins and base of the lesions. In the abomasum, small intestine, cecum, and colon, the villous and crypt epithelium is necrotic. Loss of epithelium is extensive; cells that survive are spread thin, and there is dilatation of some intact crypts. The lamina propria is collapsed and infiltrated by a variety of acute and chronic inflammatory cells. Necrosis of lymphocytes is extensive within the germinal centers of Peyer's patches. These lymphoid follicles often have acellular centers that have cystic crypt epithelium or necrotic debris and mucus. A fibrinonecrotic or fibrinohemorrhagic pseudomembrane may cover Peyer's patches, the ileum, and large intestine.

Bacterial and mycotic enteritis

Colibacillosis. Colibacillosis is one of the most significant diseases in veterinary medicine. *E. coli* is the cause, and infant animals less than 3 weeks of age are the most susceptible. Although all species are affected, the greatest economic losses occur in calves and pigs. The bacterium is among the first of the intestinal flora acquired after birth and comprises a part of that flora in virtually all animals. Various serotypes induce disease by a variety of means, especially in the young of each species. The propensity for disease can be reduced by genetic resistance, maternal antibodies, a high plane of hygiene, and high-quality nutrition. In contrast, a heavily contaminated environment, failure to consume colostrum, formula feeding rather than maternal nursing, cold stress, and crowding increase the susceptibility of animals for colibacillosis. *E. coli* often occur in combined infections with rotavirus, coronavirus, or cryptosporidia. In farms and kennels, particular serotypes sometimes become endemic, seeming to increase in number or pathogenicity, so that virtually no new offspring escape the disease. Under such circumstances, morbidity and mortality can approximate 100%. Animals healthy through 3 weeks of age have, for the most part, survived the threat of colibacillosis.

Three mechanisms by which *E. coli* produce diarrhea have been defined:

1. Enterotoxigenic *E. coli* adhere to the surface of intestinal epithelial cells and produce heat-labile (LT) and heat-stable (ST) enterotoxins that cause a secretory diarrhea. These *E. coli* induce a biochemical lesion rather than a morphologic one. Villous atrophy occurs in ligated loops in response to heat-stable enterotoxin B.
2. Enteroinvasive *E. coli* invade, multiply in, and destroy epithelial cells, with partial loss of villous cells, exudation of serum, and villous atrophy. Enteroinvasive *E. coli* cause acute exudative enteritis, endotoxemia, and septicemia.
3. Attaching and effacing *E. coli* embed themselves into enterocyte cell membranes, efface microvilli, and produce a Shiga-like toxin (Vero toxin). The Shiga-like toxin is responsible for the rather severe enteritis or bloody colitis that occurs, which is characterized by epithelial cell necrosis, hemorrhage, exudation of granulocytes, and mucosal and submucosal edema.

Two other diseases are encompassed under the term colibacillosis. **Edema disease** of growing, weaned pigs is caused by a neurotoxin (similar to *Shigella* neurotoxin) that is elaborated by *E. coli,* adhered to and colonizing the small intestine. Edema disease, an enterotoxemia, affects pigs between 6 and 14 weeks of age, occurs in the largest, fastest-growing individuals, can affect few or many, and often follows an increase or change in feed. **Septicemic colibacillosis** results from systemic infection by particular serotypes of *E. coli.* Infection occurs as an extension of enteroinvasiveness and via the umbilicus, respiratory tract, and tonsils.

Clinically, enterotoxigenic colibacillosis is common in animals 2 days to 3 weeks of age. The feces are profuse, yellow to white, and watery to pasty. The temperature may be normal or elevated (depending on other factors). Anorexia may be partial or total. The animals are dehydrated, with abdomen "tucked up" and eyeballs sunken. Septicemic colibacillosis has similar signs; however, fever is always present, except just before death. The hocks or carpi are often swollen, and a fibrinopurulent exudate may be present in the anterior chamber of one or both eyes; meningitis may occur. Dysentery, a rare finding in neonatal animals, suggests the presence of Shiga-like, toxin-producing, adhering/effacing *E. coli.*

Animals that die of enterotoxigenic *E. coli* infection are severely dehydrated, often emaciated, have sunken eyeballs, and have diarrheic feces pasted about the rear parts. The small intestine is dilated, flaccid, and filled with translucent fluid. Enterotoxigenic strains from calves have the K-99 antigen, whereas many of the porcine strains have the K-88 antigen; these antigens are associated with the ability of the strains to adhere (pili). In a standard H & E–stained section, *E. coli* can be found attached to the intestinal villi. Immunofluorescent methods are available for identifying the K-99 or K-88 antigens.

In invasive colibacillosis that has terminated in septicemia, the lesions include mucosal hyperemia of the stomach and small intestine, dilatation and fluid accumulation in the small intestine, and variable petechial hemorrhages occurring subserosally over a number of organs. Fibrinous exudates may be demonstrated in the hock joints, in the anterior chamber of the eye, or in the meninges.

In some animals, there may be peritonitis. The *E. coli* in pure culture can be recovered from the spleen, heart blood, synovial fluid, or meninges. The *E. coli* can be demonstrated microscopically in foci of inflammation at these extraintestinal sites.

Edema disease is characterized by incoordination of the hind legs, sagging and swaying, difficulty in rising, irritation, muscle tremor, aimless wandering, and clonic convulsions. The lesions of edema disease include edema of the eyelids, the gastric wall, and the mesentery of the spiral colon (Fig. 1-92). Pleural, peritoneal, and pericardial fluid may be excessive. Skeletal muscles are pale. Microscopically, the lesions include mural edema (Fig. 1-93), hyaline degeneration, and fibrinoid necrosis of arteries and arterioles, which in the brain can result in focal infarcts.

Clostridial enterotoxemia. Clostridial enterotoxemia occurs worldwide and probably affects all species of warm-blooded animals. Various names—overeating disease of lambs; lamb dysentery; pulpy kidney disease; struck of sheep; neonatal hemorrhagic enterotoxemia of calves, foals, and lambs; necrotic enteritis of human beings and fowl—have been attached to some of the diseases produced by clostridial enterotoxins.

The disease is caused by *Clostridium perfringens,* a gram-positive, anaerobic rod that is a normal inhabitant of the GI tract. These bacilli are spore-formers under adverse circumstances and produce toxins in the presence of large quantities of nutrients that favor their proliferation. The *C. perfringens* species is a very heterogeneous group of organisms and has been divided into five types, from A to E, based on the production of one or more of the four major lethal toxins. *C. perfringens* type A produces the alpha toxin; type B produces alpha, beta, and epsilon toxins; type C produces alpha and beta toxins; type D produces epsilon toxin; and type E produces alpha and iota toxins. The identified toxins are protein exotoxins, some of which are proenzymes, and many have enzymatic activity. In addition, some strains of types A, C, and D produce an enterotoxin that is released upon lysis during sporulation.

Enterotoxigenic strains of *C. perfringens* are responsible for clostridial food poisoning in any species. Most cases of clostridial food poisoning occur because of the consumption of cold or warmed-up poultry or other meat cooked the previous day or even a few hours before consumption and allowed to cool slowly. Cooking kills the vegetative cells of *C. perfringens,* but activates surviving spores that can eventually germinate and multiply in the low redox environment of the cooked food. Enterotoxin produced by sporulating *C. perfringens* is responsible for the poisoning.

Enterotoxemia is produced by one of the five *C. perfringens* types elaborating the classic exotoxins. *C. perfringens* type D is often incriminated. Clostridial enterotoxemia most often affects young fat animals. Outbreaks often follow a change in feed or an increase in carbohydrate content, as when an animal is fed for sale or slaughter. In foals, it has been associated with increased feeding of readily available carbohydrates and soybeans found in high protein feeds for pet horses. A change in feed or overfeeding precipitates an alteration in the balance within the bacterial flora. The *C. perfringens* have an opportunity to overgrow, and toxin production is abundant.

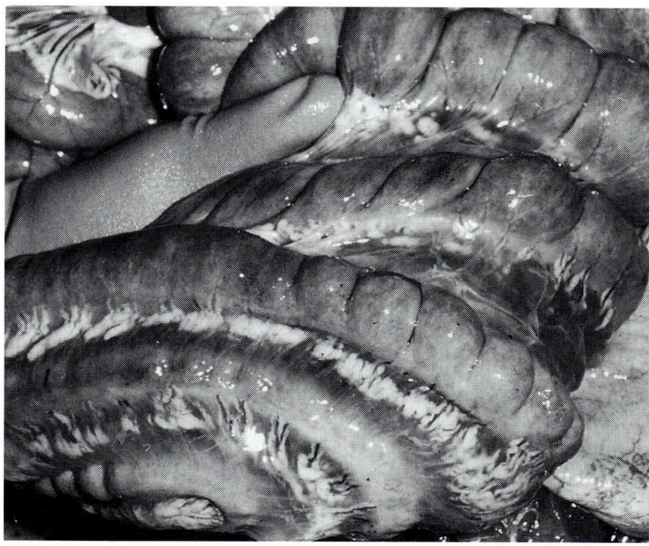

Fig. 1-92 Spiral colon; pig. Edema disease. Gelatinous edema occurs in the mesocolon between loops of colon. *Courtesy Dr. M.D. McGavin.*

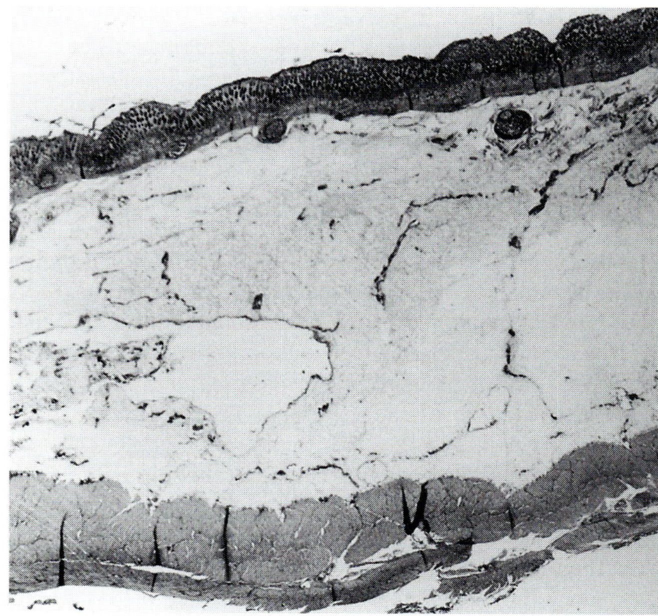

Fig. 1-93 Stomach; pig. Edema disease. Submucosa is distended with a thick layer of edema. H & E stain. *Courtesy Dr. R.G. Thomson.*

Clinical signs of enterotoxemia include diarrhea, which may be brown, black, or bloody fluid, anorexia, lethargy, increased heart rate, dilated atonic abdomen, dehydration, prostration, and death. Some animals die peracutely without diarrhea. Affected lambs have glucosuria, a feature not seen in other species.

Acute hemorrhagic gastroenteritis of dogs appears to be a clostridial enterotoxemia. *C. perfringens* has been recovered from some cases. However, canine hemorrhagic gastroenteritis may also be caused by Shiga-like toxin-producing *E. coli,* such as the S102-9 or 0157:H7. The disease, occurring in miniature Schnauzers, miniature and toy poodles, German shepherd dogs, and Great Danes, is characterized by vomiting and severe bloody diarrhea.

In clostridial enterotoxemia, the small intestine is the target organ, with lesions of patchy, focal, or diffuse reddening. Congestion and blood extravasation take the forms of petechiae, ecchymoses, paint-brushed hemorrhages, or diffuse hemorrhage that appears grossly similar to that of intestinal strangulation. The intestines are flaccid, thin-walled, dilated, and, often, gas-filled. Gas bubbles may occur in the wall of the affected intestine. Intestine may rupture as a result of the thinning of the wall and gas entrapment. The intestinal changes are often accompanied by hypermia of the stomach, excessive pericardial or abdominal fluid, and, sometimes, a cooked appearance of skeletal musculature. The spleen is enlarged and pulpy as a result of congestion. Lambs dying of clostridial enterotoxemia have pulpy kidneys, a softening and dark discoloration of the kidneys that is readily confused with postmortem autolysis.

Microscopically, the toxins produced by the *C. perfringens* damage intestinal villi in a fashion similar to an acid burn. Within a few minutes of exposure, epithelial cells at the tip of the villus undergo degeneration and separate from the basement membrane. These changes are followed shortly thereafter by extensive desquamation of cells. These lesions progressively extend down the villus, with successive degeneration and necrosis of epithelial cells. There is edema and transient leukocyte infiltration of the lamina propria, followed by necrosis. After 6 to 8 hours, one third or more of the villus has been damaged. This results in exudation of serum, inflammatory cells, and blood. Microscopically, villi that have been damaged by *C. perfringens* exotoxins are faded and acellular, with only shriveled cores apparent. This change resembles autolysis; therefore, knowledge of the postmortem interval is important. Coagulation necrosis may destroy half or more, and in many instances, the entire villous layer of the small bowel mucosa. The crypts usually remain intact, but may appear dilated. Intestinal submucosa may be edematous, hemorrhagic, or filled with an acute leukocyte response. Muscle layers are stretched thin and contain congested vessels. Death occurs 24 to 36 hours after the onset of clinical signs.

Tyzzer's disease. Tyzzer's disease was first described in 1917 as a cause of diarrhea and death of Japanese waltzing mice. Since that discovery, Tyzzer's disease has been described in a variety of animal species, including laboratory mice, rats, hamsters, guinea pigs, Mongolian gerbils, laboratory rabbits, cottontail rabbits, dogs, coyotes, cats, calves, horses, nonhuman primates, muskrats, and foxes.

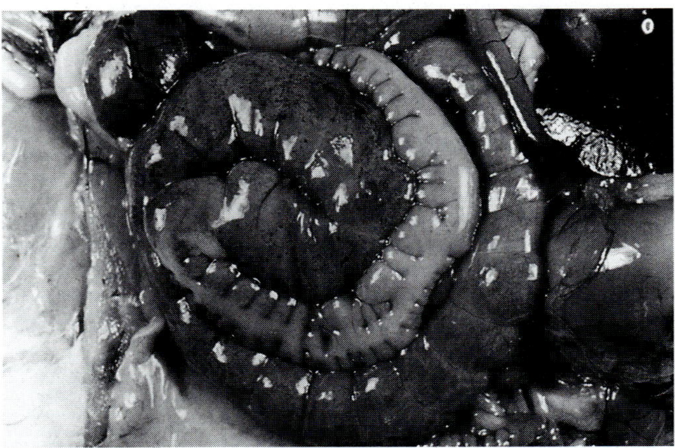

Fig. 1-94 Intestines; rabbit. Tyzzer's disease. The cecum is congested, edematous, and speckled with clusters and linear aggregates of petechiae. The proximal 2 cm of sacculated colon is reddened also, and there is abrupt transition to normal colon. *Van Kruiningen HJ, Blodgett SB. J Am Vet Med Assoc 1971; 158:1207.*

In animals held in colonies, epizootics have resulted in illness and death in 50% to 100%. The young of each species appear more susceptible than adults. Latent infection in newly purchased laboratory animals may become clinically manifest following the stress of shipping, housing in new quarters, change in feed, or the administration of corticosteroids.

The causative organism is *Bacillus piliformis,* a slender, gram-negative rod which may be up to 20 μm in length and 0.3 to 0.5 μm in diameter. The *B. piliformis* is a flagellated bacterium that is rather fastidious in its growth requirements. It has been recovered in chicken embryos and, in limited fashion, in tissue culture. Sporulation occurs within host cells, with the spores forming at the poles of the rods. The organism is transmitted by ingestion and gains access to the host via uptake or penetration of the ileum, cecum, or colon.

In all animal species, Tyzzer's disease is characterized by diarrhea, fever, wasting, prostration, and death within 24 to 36 hours.

The intestinal lesion of Tyzzer's disease is very characteristic. The affected segment, usually the distal ileum, cecum, and proximal colon, is intensely hyperemic and has multiple petechiae or paint-brushed hemorrhages (Fig. 1-94). The wall is thickened and the serosa opalescent because of edema. Microscopically, mucosal necrosis is accompanied by edema of the lamina propria, submucosa, and serosal mesenteric attachments and necrosis of smooth muscle cells of the muscularis mucosae (Fig. 1-95). The earliest mucosal lesion is a focal one, characterized by numerous damaged epithelial cells with karyorrhectic fragments (Fig. 1-96). Cells of the lamina propria have similar karyorrhexis. The causative bacilli are not found in necrotic cells, but are demonstrated by special silver stains

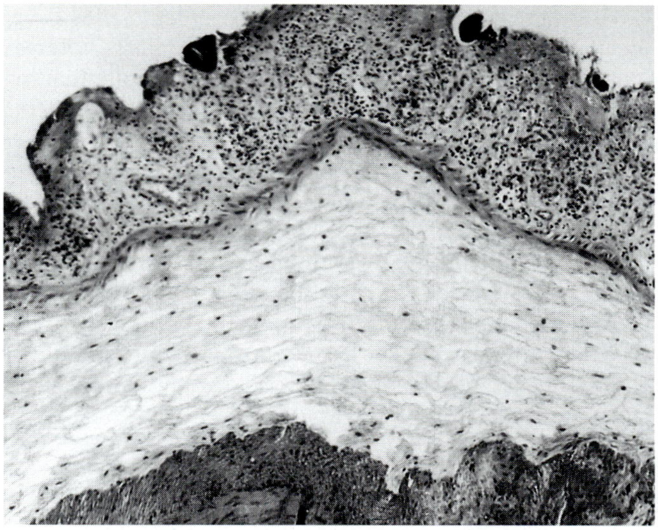

Fig. 1-95 Cecum; rabbit. Tyzzer's disease. This advanced lesion has extensive necrosis of mucosal epithelial cells, few remaining crypts, and submucosal edema. H & E stain.

in the adjacent viable epithelium. Focal necrosis of epithelium is followed by ulceration. Edema and cellular infiltration of the lamina propria are severe. Tyzzer's bacillus also may be demonstrated in myocytes of the muscularis mucosae in the areas of mucosal necrosis.

A common lesion in animals with Tyzzer's disease, and one reported in all affected species, is focal hepatic necrosis. The foci can be numerous and grossly obvious as opaque, gray, 1 to 2 mm spots. Microscopically, these foci are composed of necrotic hepatocytes. The Tyzzer's bacillus can be demonstrated in viable hepatocytes adjacent to the foci of necrosis (Fig. 1-97). In some species, focal myocardial necrosis also occurs. The myocardium is flecked or streaked with off-white foci. *B. piliformis* can be demonstrated in the viable myocytes surrounding necrotic foci. The Warthin-Starry silver stain or the Giemsa stain readily reveals the Tyzzer's bacilli in viable epithelial cells or myocytes. The long, thin bacilli lie in parallel arrays or like crisscrossed sticks in the cytoplasm of affected cells.

Although these are the characteristic lesions of Tyzzer's disease (i.e., segmental ileocolitis or ileotyphlitis and colitis, focal hepatic necrosis, and focal myocardial necrosis), not all affected animals have each of the lesions. The initial damage and entrance of the organism occur in the ileum, cecum, or colon; the liver is affected secondarily, with bacteria carried via the portal circulation. In some animals, the myocardial necrosis is an additional event associated with septicemia.

Campylobacter enteritis

Campylobacter jejuni. The campylobacters are gram-negative, curved or spiral rods that vary in length from 1.5 to 3.5 μm and in width from 0.2 to 0.4 μm. They move rapidly in liquid media by means of one or more flagella.

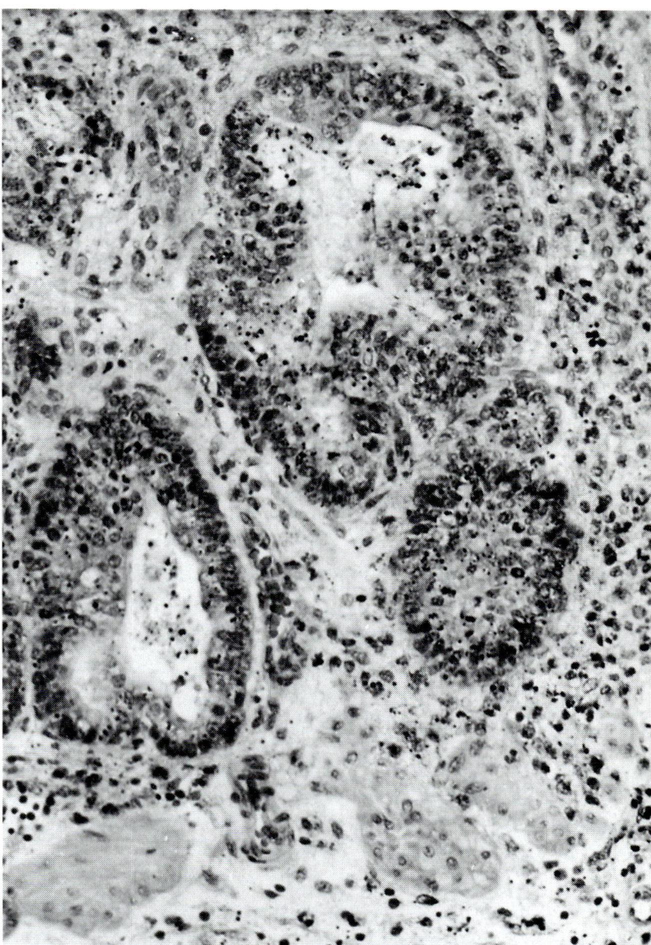

Fig. 1-96 Colon; rabbit. Tyzzer's disease. Karyorrhexis of epithelial cells and cells of the lamina propria is characteristic. H & E stain.

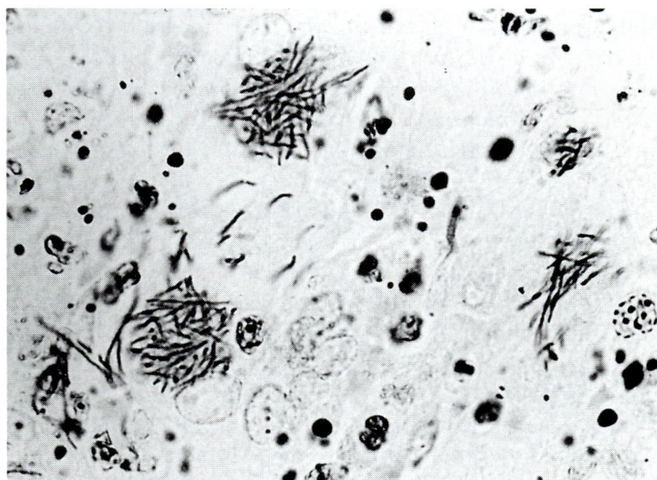

Fig. 1-97 Liver; rabbit. Tyzzer's disease. Hepatocytes adjacent to foci of necrosis contain crisscrossed *Bacillus piliformis.* Warthin-Starry stain.

Campylobacter grow best in microaerobic environments, i.e., 5% to 10% oxygen, 3% to 10% CO_2 and at 42° C. Infection with *Campylobacter* occurs by ingestion, most often of contaminated foods. Unpasteurized raw milk is a source of infection for human beings. *C. jejuni* is a common inhabitant of the GI tract of poultry, cattle, other farm animals, and, on occasion, dogs and cats. Zoonotic transmission from pets with diarrhea to human beings has been recognized. Once the organism has gained entrance to the intestine, disease may be produced by one of several mechanisms. The *Campylobacter* may colonize the intestine and elaborate a toxin that results in a secretory diarrhea similar to that of enterotoxogenic colibacillosis and cholera. Toxin production is the proposed mechanism in animals with acute, watery diarrhea. A second mechanism involves penetration and proliferation within the intestinal epithelium, particularly that of the ileum and colon, and the production of a cytotoxin; this results in bloody diarrhea. The third mechanism of disease has been called "translocation" and is similar to what occurs in *Salmonella* and *Yersinia* infections. The organisms penetrate the mucosa, proliferate in the lamina propria, and are transported by macrophages to the regional lymph nodes, where they produce mesenteric lymphadenitis.

C. jejuni has been associated with spontaneous disease in dogs, manifesting as diarrhea of 5 to 15 days' duration. The diarrhea is mucus-laden or watery, with or without blood, and accompanied by partial anorexia, vomiting, and slight fever. Although limited microscopic studies have been done in spontaneous cases, hyperplasia of the colonic mucosa has been documented. Lymphocytes of the lamina propria are increased. With Warthin-Starry staining, *Campylobacter* organisms are demonstrated attached to colonic epithelium, but not within epithelial cells. Lesions of the ileum consist of focally damaged crypts and blunt and irregular villi that are occasionally fused.

Clinically, *C. jejuni* enteritis is often characterized by self-limited, fluid diarrhea lasting 7 to 10 days. Excretion of the organisms persists from 2 weeks to 3 months. A dysentery-like syndrome mimicking mucosal colitis also occurs. The mesenteric lymphadenitis form of *C. jejuni* infection in human beings is sometimes mistaken for appendicitis.

The gross lesions in *C. jejuni* enteritis or enterocolitis vary with the mechanism of damage. When the effect is mediated by enterotoxin, the affected segments are dilated and fluid-filled. In those cases when cytotoxin production occurs, hyperemia is obvious, and the mucosal surface is friable and bloody. Microscopically, there is little or no damage when enterotoxin has produced a secretory diarrhea. However, when invasiveness and cytotoxicity have been expressed, the lesions are those of acute ileitis or colitis. The surface is irregular, and the epithelium is focally ulcerated. The lamina propria is edematous and has numerous congested blood vessels. Lymphocytes and plasma cells are greatly increased in number; granulocytes occur focally in the lamina propria and in the crypts. Affected mucosa has decreased goblet cells and focal epithelial hyperplasia. *C. jejuni* can be demonstrated between epithelial cells, but only rarely within them.

Campylobacter sputorum. For a number of years, *C. sputorum* subsp *mucosalis* was regarded as the causative agent of intestinal adenomatosis or proliferative ileitis of swine. The organism cultured from diseased intestines, is similar to the curved bacteria seen in the apical cytoplasm of villous epithelial cells in diseased segments of intestine (Fig. 1-98). Proliferative ileitis has been repeatedly reproduced with mucosal homogenates, even frozen homogenates; however, there are few reports, and these questionable, of pure cultures of *C. sputorum* reproducing the disease. Immunofluorescence microscopy has produced confusing results, in that both *C. sputorum* and *C. hyointestinalis* were demonstrated in proliferating epithelium. Now it appears, after DNA and immunologic studies, that the intracytoplasmic bacterium responsible for this disease belongs to a new taxon within the delta group of the proteobacteria. The name *Ileal symbiont intracellularis* has been proposed. This latter agent reliably reproduces proliferative ileitis in conventional swine, but not in gnotobiotic animals.

A variety of names have been given to the various dis-

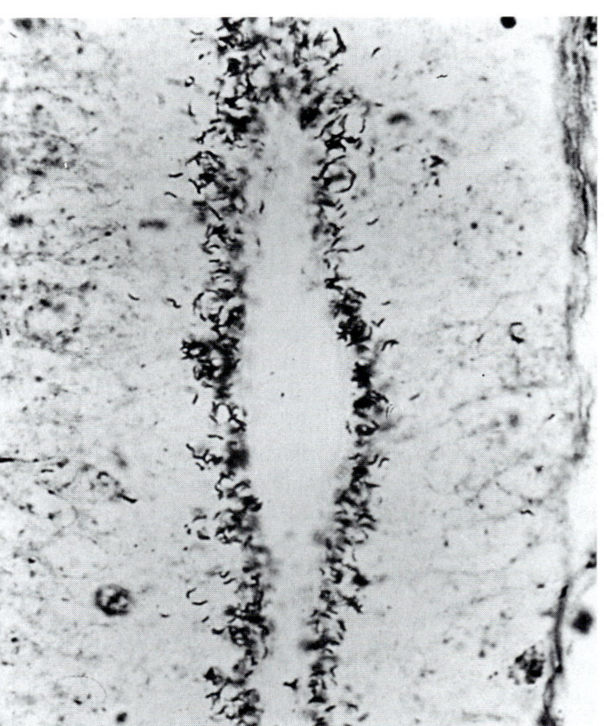

Fig. 1-98 Ileum; pig. Proliferative ileitis. Curved *Campylobacter*-like organisms, now called *Ileal symbiont intracellularis,* are present in the apical cryptoplasm of epithelial cells of two parallel villi. Warthin-Starry stain.

orders associated with the intracellular campylobacter-like organisms. These include intestinal adenomatosis, proliferative enteropathy, necrotic proliferative enteritis (Fig. 1-99), and regional ileitis or enteritis of swine. Clinically, there is reason to believe that a mild or acute diarrhea precedes the features associated with the proliferative lesion. In some instances, the disease occurs epizootically. Pigs with proliferative enteritis have diarrhea, intestinal obstruction, and anorexia. Pigs with hemorrhagic proliferative enteropathy bleed profusely or pass black, bloody material and may die of intestinal exsanguination. There is usually no fever associated with these disorders, unless secondary bacteria, such as the *Salmonella,* produce superficial necrosis. The necrotic components that sometimes complicate proliferative enteritis appear to result from secondary infections, particularly those due to *Salmonella choleraesuis* and *Fusobacterium necrophorum.* When pigs inadvertently received an inoculum that contained *S. choleraesuis,* fibrinonecrotic pseudomembranous casts and necrosis of the proliferative surface occurred in diseased segments of intestine.

Microscopically, this disease is characterized by hyperplasia of crypt epithelium, resulting in folded crypts and hyperplastic villous fronds as well as downgrowth of crypt epithelium. This downgrowth extends into lymphoid follicles of the submucosa, creating mucus-filled cysts (enteritis cystica profunda). Bacteria and intestinal contents are present within the cysts. Rupture of such cysts generates a pyogranulomatous response. The thickening of affected segments occurs as a result of proliferative hyperplasia of the epithelium, variable lymphocytic and plasmacytic inflammatory response in the lamina propria and submucosa, pyogranulomatous response adjacent to foci of cystic epithelial downgrowth, and muscular hyperplasia. Clusters of hyperplastic epithelium occur infrequently in regional lymph nodes.

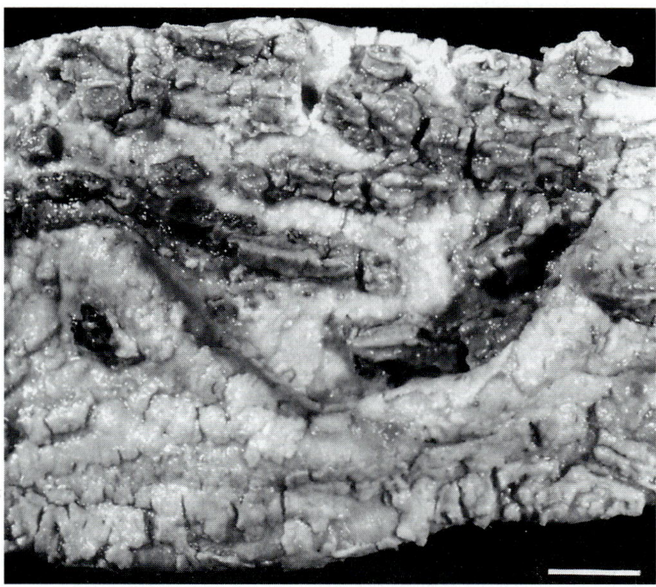

Fig. 1-99 Ileum; pig. Necrotic proliferative ileitis. The mucosa is raised and hyperplastic, and partially coated by aggregated necrotic epithelium. Bar = 1 cm. *Courtesy Dr. M.D. McGavin.*

Chlamydial enterocolitis. The *Chlamydia* are small, 300 to 800 nm, coccoid bacteria that are obligate intracellular parasites. Their cell envelopes resemble those of gram-negative bacteria. These bacteria include two species: *Chlamydia psittaci,* which occurs mostly in mammals and birds, and *Chlamydia trachomatis,* which affects human beings. The organisms are detectable by light microscopy in cells stained by the Giemsa method. In the case of *C. trachomatis,* the organisms are clumped in the form of a cytoplasmic inclusion body, which contains glycogen. *C. trachomatis* inclusions (organisms) stain with iodine, whereas *C. psittaci* inclusions do not.

Bovine chlamydias (strains of *C. psittaci*) have been recovered from a spontaneous enteritis of young calves. Clinically affected calves have diarrhea, fever, anorexia, and depression. Following experimental inoculation, newborn calves develop fever and diarrhea within 24 hours and become moribund within 4 to 5 days. Grossly, the ileum is most severely affected, but the jejunum and large intestine have lesions as well. Diseased segments have hyperemia, congestion, and petechiae. The wall and mesentery are edematous. The lumen contains watery, yellow fluid mixed with yellow, tenacious, fibrin-rich material attached to the surface. Colonic ridges are reddened by hyperemia and have small erosions. Bleeding from petechiae and ecchymoses of the colonic or rectal ridges occurs infrequently. Regional lymph nodes are enlarged.

Microscopically, villous epithelial cells, macrophages of the lamina propria, endothelial cells of lacteals, and enterochromaffin cells, goblet cells, and fibroblasts are parasitized by the *Chlamydia.* In the epithelial cells, the *Chlamydia* are located in the apical cytoplasm. The *Chlamydia* are adsorbed to the brush border, taken up by endocytosis, multiply in epithelial cell apices, and are subsequently liberated into the lamina propria and its cells. Villi are enlarged by dilated lacteals and infiltrates of mononuclear cells and neutrophils. Crypts of both small and large intestine are dilated and contain desquamated epithelial cells and inflammatory exudate **(colitis cystica superficialis).** The centers of lymphoid follicles of Peyer's patches are necrotic. The mucosa and submucosa are thickened by a diffuse granulomatous reaction. The abomasum also has lesions, and, in some calves, foci of inflammation extend transmurally, thereby initiating focal peritonitis.

Salmon poisoning. Salmon poisoning is an acute granulomatous enterocolitis of the dog and fox. Animals that eat salmon carrying the fluke *Nanophyetus salmincola* are affected. This small trematode is the bearer of *Neorickettsia* *helminthoeca,* a 0.3 μ, coccoid rickettsia. Six to 8 days after eating parasitized fish, dogs become acutely ill, febrile, and depressed. Affected animals have ocular and nasal discharge, severe diarrhea, vomiting, complete anorexia, and enlarged tonsils, spleen, and lymph nodes. Untreated animals die within 6 to 10 days of the onset of signs.

Hemorrhagic inflammation of the intestine that can extend from the pylorus to the anus is the most characteristic gross lesion of salmon poisoning. The primary lesions are in the lamina propria and submucosa of the intestine and consist of hemorrhage, necrosis, and infiltrates of lymphocytes, plasma cells, macrophages, and neutrophils. The macrophages contain large numbers of rickettsial elementary bodies demonstrated by the Giemsa stain. The Peyer's patches and solitary lymphoid follicles of the intestine are hyperplastic, as are the mesenteric, colic, portal, and iliac lymph nodes. Lymphoid hyperplasia causes enlarged cortical nodules, and sinuses contain neutrophils and macrophages. Peripheral lymph nodes are affected, but less severely than the regional nodes of the intestine. The characteristic macrophages containing Giemsa-stained elementary bodies occur in peripheral lymph nodes, spleen, liver, lungs, and blood, and in intracerebral lesions.

***Rhodococcus equi* enterocolitis of foals.** *Rhodococcus equi* is a large, gram-positive rod that occurs as a soil saprophyte. The organism survives in soil for up to 12 months. *Rhodococcus equi* has a predilection for the respiratory system. Most affected foals have pneumonia characterized by multiple, variably sized abscesses. Infection occurs by way of the respiratory system; however, the frequent concomitance of helminthiasis and *R. equi* infection suggest that migrating larvae may participate in distributing the bacterium through the body of the foal. Helminth control appears to bring about great reduction or elimination of *R. equi* infection.

On some farms, *R. equi* infection occurs sporadically; on others, infection is endemic. The disease occurs in foals less than 6 months of age and is characterized by nonresponsive diarrhea or respiratory signs, suppurative arthritis, or subcutaneous abscesses. The course of the disease is 30 to 40 days, with a 64% mortality. Foal losses on any given farm may total 10% to 15%. The classic manifestations of *R. equi* infection are abscesses in the lungs. Gray-white abscesses vary in diameter from less than 1 cm to several cm, and many or few are scattered through the lungs. Secondary involvement of regional lymph nodes is common. Some animals may have pleurisy, ulcerative lymphangitis, abscesses of the intestines or mesentery, suppurative arthritis, or subcutaneous abscesses.

Enteric lesions that sometimes occur in *R. equi* infections involve segments of the small intestine as well as the cecum and colon. These segments have greatly thickened, corrugated mucosa, 2 to 5 cm thick, which is mottled red, white, and tan. Multiple, irregularly shaped, soft, well-defined, necrotic foci, 1 to 3 cm in diameter, may occur in the mucosal surface of the colon along with multiple, small ulcers. Mesenteric, cecal, and colic lymph nodes are enlarged and firm. On incision, the lymph nodes contain masses of homogeneous gray tissue and abscesses.

Microscopically, the enterocolitis is characterized by a diffuse granulomatous inflammation. The mucosa of the small intestine, colon, and cecum is distended by large macrophages filled with gram-positive causative bacilli 1 to 2 μm in length and 0.25 μm in diameter. The accumulations of large, bacteria-filled macrophages and multinucleated giant cells involve the lamina propria, distort the shapes of villi, and displace intestinal glands or colonic and cecal crypts. Sharply demarcated foci of coagulation necrosis may occur, and the mucosal surface may be ulcerated. Affected lymph nodes have masses of the bacteria-filled, PAS-positive macrophages, as well as multinucleated giant cells. Portions of the cortex of lymph nodes have foci of coagulation necrosis as well.

Johne's disease. Johne and Frothingham, in Germany in 1895, described the presence of acid-fast organisms in tissues of cattle affected with a chronic disease that later became known as Johne's disease. The disease now occurs throughout the world. Besides cattle, Johne's disease has been described in sheep, goats, and a variety of wild and exotic ruminants. The causative bacterium, *Mycobacterium paratuberculosis,* can be isolated from feces of affected animals, from diseased intestine and lymph nodes, and, sometimes, from a variety of other tissues and fluids, including the liver, uterus, fetus, milk, urine, and semen.

Transmission is via the fecal-oral route. Most animals are infected before they are 6 months of age. The portals of entry are the tonsils and Peyer's patches. The disease may be clinically silent for 6 months to 3 years. During this time, the bacterium is, for the most part, contained intracellularly in macrophages of the GI tract and regional lymph nodes. A host-parasite balance is never quite achieved, as this insidious disease becomes progressively worse over a period of months.

Clinically, some cattle with Johne's disease appear ill, whereas others do not. Epidemiologically, cattle in an infected herd fall into four categories: those that are infected and have clinical signs, asymptomatic shedders, carriers (nonshedders) without clinical disease, and the noninfected. Immunologically, the latter have no response; some affected animals have detectable humoral immunity; some have cellular immunity; some have a lepromatous granulomatous disease indicative of the infection-tolerant state, whereas others have a tuberculoid response that suggests an infection-resistant state. There are also intermediate variants.

Clinically, Johne's disease presents as chronic diarrhea, weight loss, wasting, and decreased productivity, usually in one animal in a herd. Though only 1% to 2% of a herd appear ill, 4% to 100% may be infected. Bacteriologic isolation of the organism from feces is currently the most reliable diagnostic method; however, it has the disadvantage of taking 2 to 4 months from the time of sampling to the final result. Also, infected animals must be shedding at least 100 organisms per gram of feces before they can be detected by culture. An absorbed ELISA, i.e., an ELISA conducted on sera that have been preabsorbed to remove *M. phlei* cross-reactivity, is currently the most cost-effective serologic herd screening test, with a sensitivity of 45.5% ± 6.7% for preclinical cases and 99.7% ± 0.3% specificity. When combined with fecal culture, sensitivity for detection of preclinical cases reaches 69%.

The lesion in Johne's disease is a chronic, segmental thickening of the caudal small intestine, cecum, and proximal colon. Peyer's patches of the distal ileum are the primary sites of disease. Affected segments have a corrugated mucosa that is focally ulcerated. Mesenteric lymph nodes are greatly enlarged. Granulomas of the liver are rare. In animals with significant wasting, calcified plaques may occur in the aorta, vena cava, or endocardium. Microscopically, the lamina propria and submucosa of affected portions of the intestines are distended and distorted by a granulomatous infiltrate (Fig. 1-100). The cells that characterize the response vary with strain of organism, host, and duration of infection. Macrophage invasion occurs, most commonly constituting a lepromatous reaction. The macrophages are large and eosinophilic, have foamy cytoplasms, and contain large numbers of acid-fast organisms. In contrast, other animals have a tuberculoid response (sometimes with central necrosis). These lesions are composed of well-differentiated epithelioid cells in a whorled pattern and a variable number of Langhans'-type giant cells (Fig. 1-101). Organisms are few. Granulomas of either type occur in the regional lymph nodes (Figs. 1-102 and 1-103). The rectum is affected only in 25% of cases, a finding that implies that rectal biopsy may be a poor diagnostic procedure.

Intestinal tuberculosis and *Mycobacterium avium* infections. Intestinal tuberculosis of human beings is caused by *M. tuberculosis* or *M. bovis*. In animals, intestinal *M. avium* infections have in the past been called avian tuberculosis. There is a strong consensus presently, particularly in view of the increasing numbers of *M. avium* infections in human patients with acquired immune deficiency syndrome, to refer to the latter infections as *M. avium-intracellulare* infection (MAI). The *M. avium-intracellulare* bacteria are environmental microorganisms that are often pathogenic in fowl, pigs, and nonhuman primates, but rarely so in other species unless their immunity is compromised.

The *M. tuberculosis* and *M. bovis* are acquired by the respiratory or gastrointestinal route. Intestinal tuberculosis occurs rarely in cattle, nonhuman primates, and human beings. The portal of entry appears to be the lymphoid tissue of the intestinal tract, where the bacilli are phagocytosed by M cells of Peyer's patches. The most common site of

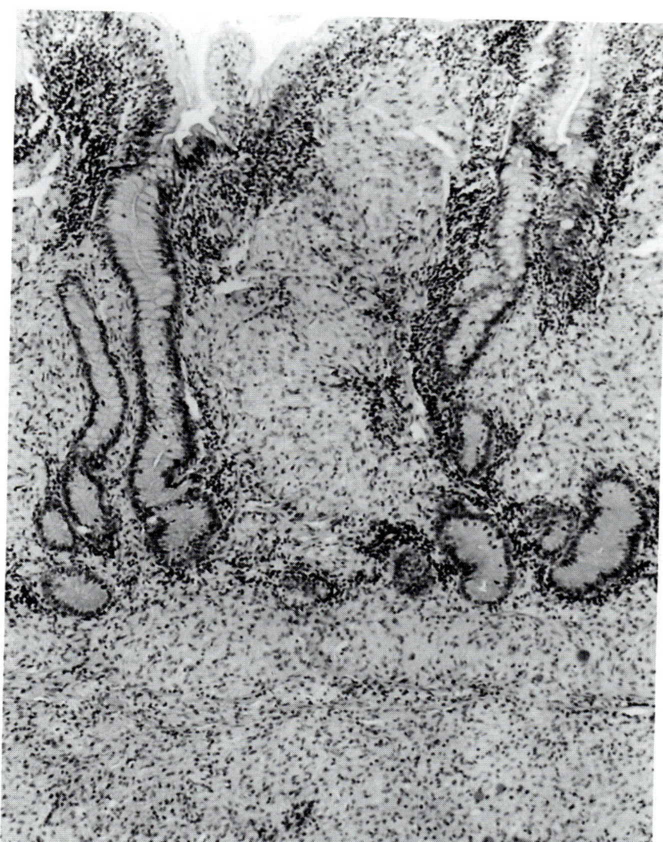

Fig. 1-100 Small intestine; cow. Johne's disease. Macrophages distend the lamina propria of the villi and submucosa, a lepromatous granulomatous response.

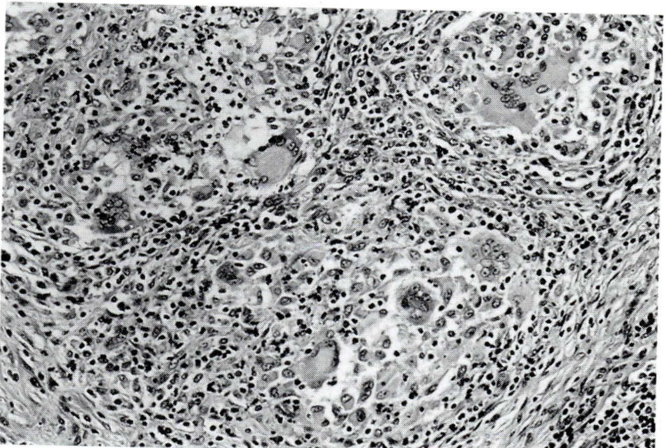

Fig. 1-101 Small intestine; goat. Johne's disease. Tuberculoid, epithelioid and giant cell granulomas, with collars of lymphocytes, in a Peyer's patch of a goat that had been inoculated with *Mycobacterium paratuberculosis* 5 months previously. These granulomas contained no acid-fast bacilli. H & E stain.

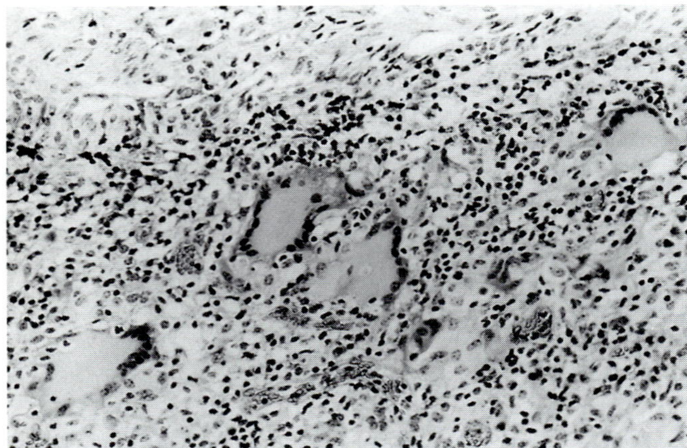

Fig. 1-102 Mesenteric lymph node; cow. Johne's disease. Giant cells are numerous in the cortex. H & E stain.

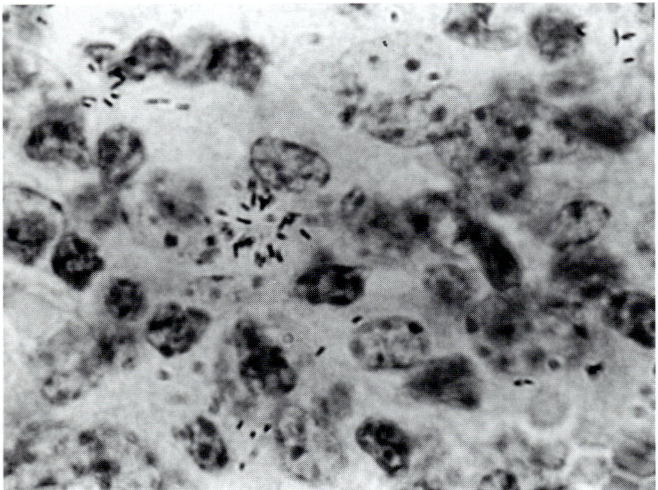

Fig. 1-103 Mesenteric lymph node; cow. Johne's disease. Note the acid-fast mycobacteria within macrophages. Ziehl-Neelsen stain.

disease is the distal ileum, and "skip" lesions occur, apparently corresponding to the location of patches.

Clinically, animals with intestinal tuberculosis suffer with chronic diarrhea, lower abdominal pain, and chronic weight loss. If a portion of the small intestine has become stenotic, vomiting may be a clinical sign. In some species, such as the dog, it may be possible to palpate a thickened, firm, hoselike segment of intestine through the abdominal wall. In large animals, thickened, firm loops of intestine may be recognized at rectal examination. Intradermal tuberculin tests are used to confirm a diagnosis.

The affected segment is thickened, and the mucosa is corrugated and may be ulcerated. Regional lymph nodes have granulomas and calcification. The tuberculous lesion consists of numerous epithelioid granulomas with necrotic centers. Swirled arrangements of epithelioid cells and giant cells infiltrate the lamina propria and the submucosa. The affected mucosa and submucosa are distended by the tuberculoid granulomatous lesion and have prominent infiltrates of lymphocytes and plasma cells as well.

In some animals, *Mycobacterium avium* infections result in lesions very similar to those of *M. tuberculosis,* complete with caseation necrosis, and calcification. However, in most spontaneous *M. avium*–induced disease, a lepromatous granulomatous inflammation occurs, similar to that of Johne's disease. Such lesions are described in dogs, pigs, horses, rhesus monkeys, AIDS patients, and exotic birds. The lesion consists of sheets of macrophages, 10 to 40 cells deep in the mucosa and up to 200 cells deep in the submucosa, and occurs over a large segment of the small intestine, colon, or both. Ziehl-Neelsen staining of these tissues demonstrates large numbers of intracellular acid-fast bacilli.

Intestinal histoplasmosis. Histoplasmosis occurs rarely as an intestinal infection in human beings and the dog, but has not often been documented in other species. The disease occurs worldwide and is prevalent in the north central United States.

The cause is *Histoplasma capsulatum,* a small, oval, intracellular fungus. The reservoir for this organism is bird droppings or soil. The disease is transmissible from animals to human beings. Histoplasmosis has been well studied in the dog, where the pulmonary form occurs more frequently than the intestinal form. The organisms may be acquired by inhalation or by ingestion. The yeast invades tissue, causes necrosis, and attracts macrophages, resulting in granulomatous lesions of the lungs, GI tract, lymph nodes, and liver. Clinically, dogs with intestinal histoplasmosis suffer with intractable chronic diarrhea, progressive weight loss, anorexia, lassitude, poor hair coat, and anemia. Respiratory signs and peripheral lymphadenitis are present in some dogs.

The small intestine has a corrugated mucosa and ulcers. Mesenteric lymph nodes are enlarged and firm. The liver is enlarged and mottled. The lungs have areas of gray or red consolidation. The colonic wall is thickened, and colonic mucosal folds are prominent. In the small intestine, macrophages engorged with *H. capsulatum* fill the lamina propria and submucosa. The macrophages are unable to digest the ingested fungi, and large numbers accumulate to cause corrugation of the mucosal surface. Extension of the inflammation may occur through the muscle layers and into lymph vessels and the subserosa. Regional lymph nodes have large masses of macrophages in the cortex and medullary sinuses. In the liver, numerous clusters of yeast-filled macrophages occur throughout.

Neoplasia

Intestinal lymphosarcoma

Primary intestinal lymphosarcoma occurs in dogs, cattle, cats, horses, poultry, and human beings. A C-type oncornavirus has been established as the cause in some animals.

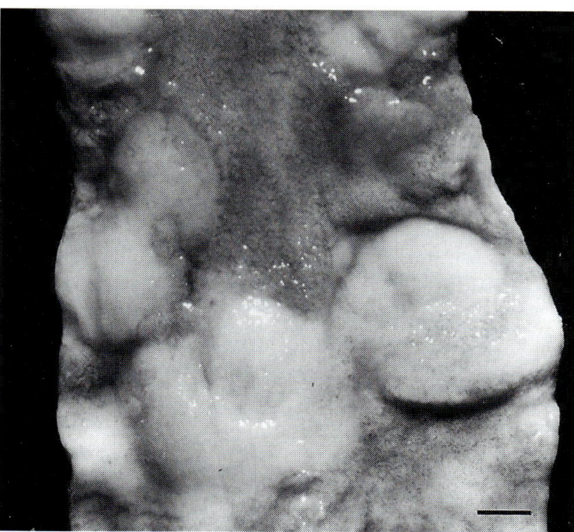

Fig. 1-104 Ileum; dog. Intestinal lymphosarcoma. Multiple white plaques of lymphosarcoma protrude from the mucosal surface. Bar = 5 mm. *Courtesy Dr. M.D. McGavin.*

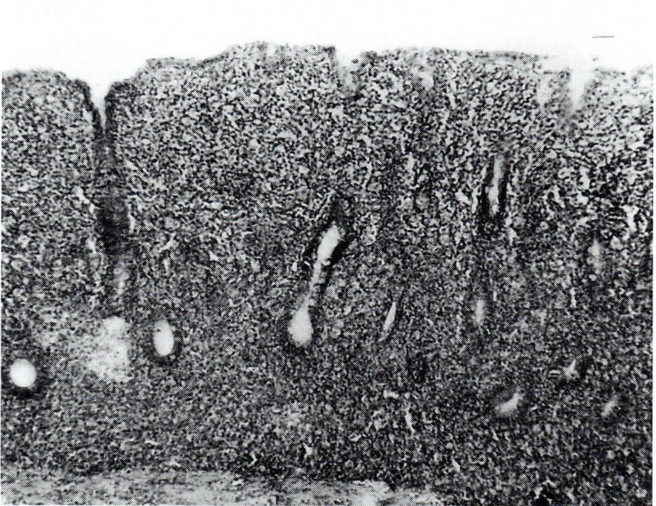

Fig. 1-105 Intestine; dog. Intestinal lymphosarcoma. A homogeneous population of malignant lymphocytes has obliterated the intestinal architecture. H & E stain.

Clinically, animals with the diffuse type of intestinal lymphosarcoma often present with chronic diarrhea, steatorrhea, malnourishment, and weight loss. When the disease is segmental, a thickened intestinal segment may be palpated. Some animals, such as dogs and cats, may vomit because of partial obstruction. Ventral edema occurs when there has been significant plasma protein leakage from the diseased intestine.

This neoplasm arises from the lymphocytes of the lamina propria or the lymph nodes of the intestinal tract. Intestinal lymphosarcoma may be segmental or diffuse (Fig. 1-104). This latter form occurs more commonly in the dog. Proliferation of lymphoblasts or lymphocytes occurs in such proportions that the normal architecture is obliterated (Fig. 1-105). The lamina propria and submucosa become distended with malignant lymphocytes. Lacteals and blood supply are crowded out, the villi are distended, and the animal has either segmental obstruction of the intestine or, with the diffuse type, malabsorption. Microscopically, the lymphocytes of lymphosarcoma are distinctly different from the usual population found in the villi or submucosa. They are less mature and larger, and have more active-appearing nuclei and nucleoli. Mitotic figures are common. A homogeneous population of such immature lymphocytes or lymphoblasts is diagnostic. Mucosa in diseased segments may become ulcerated because of secondary ischemia. Regional lymph nodes are often affected after the initial disease process in the small intestine.

LARGE INTESTINE

Obstructions and Functional Disorders

Enteroliths

Enteroliths are hard, round concretions that form in the large colon of the horse and sometimes in other species. Animals 6 to 14 years of age are affected, and a disproportionate number of cases have occurred in Arabian horses.

Enteroliths form around a nidus, usually an ingested particle or object. Items found at the core include nails, pins, needles, coins, pebbles, grit, metal fragments, horse hair, cloth, chert, and glazier's points. Ammoniomagnesium phosphate (struvite) is deposited around the nidus, thereby progressively enlarging the calculus. A mass, the size of a man's fist, may be generated in 1 year's time. Diets with high concentrations of magnesium and phosphorus enhance enterolith formation. In the past, miller's horses were frequently fed large amounts of bran and had an increased incidence of enteroliths. The frequency of enteroliths has been reduced by using magnets to remove metals from grain and by reducing the concentration of dietary bran fed. The feeding of alfalfa hay, which is high in protein, and the greater-than-average magnesium content of California hay may have contributed to the increased incidence of enteroliths in pleasure horses in that state.

Enteroliths may be solitary and round or multiple; in the latter case, they are often faceted. They generally weigh between 200 to 1500 g, but enteroliths weighing up to 12 kg have been recorded. Enteroliths produce recurrent colic by causing obstruction. The most common sites for lodgment in horses are the pelvic flexure and beginning of the small colon.

Congenital aganglionic megacolon

Congenital megacolon occurs in several species of animals and in human beings, in whom it is called Hirschsprung's disease. It is defined as the absence of intramuscular and submucosal ganglia from the rectum and a varying, but continuous, length of colon. The primary lesion occurs in the contracted segment; however, the disease has been named for the dilated proximal portion. Congenital megacolon occurs in white foals produced by breeding horses with the overo pattern of spotting. This is characterized by white patches on the ventral or lateral midsection that extend dorsally up to, but not including, the midline of the back. White also occurs on the lateral neck and flank. At least one, and usually all four legs are colored, i.e., not white. Affected foals appear normal at birth, but fail to pass meconium, develop colic, and die.

Hirschsprung's disease is the result of an interference with the migration of neuroblasts from the embryonic craniocervical neural crest to the myenteric plexus region of the colon and rectum. Neuroblasts destined to compose Auerbach's myenteric plexuses of the gut migrate between the sixth and twelfth weeks of human embryonic development. Migration of neuroblasts to the terminal colon takes considerably longer than migration to stomach and small intestine. Neuroblasts destined to form Meissner's plexuses migrate from the myenteric populations, through inner muscle layer to submucosa; completion of plexuses here lags by 1 week. Interruption of migration during the seventh week causes aganglionosis of the ileum and entire colon; during the eighth week, aganglionosis of colon; during the ninth, aganglionosis of descending colon and rectum; and during weeks 10 through 12, aganglionosis of the sigmoid colon or rectum.

The gross lesion in congenital aganglionic megacolon is a contracted, nonperistaltic segment of rectum or rectum and contiguous colon, the so-called contracted distal segment. In foals, the abnormality is confined to the rectum and small colon or rectum and the entire colon.

Microscopically, this disease is characterized by an absence or paucity of ganglion cells from the intermuscular and submucosal plexuses and by the presence of excessive, tortuous, large, nonmedulated nerve fibers in the intermyenteric zone. These nerves are known to be postganglionic parasympathetic and sympathetic fibers in disarray. Histochemically, acetylcholinesterase activity is greater than normal in these parasympathetic fibers.

Volvulus of the large intestine

Volvulus of the large intestine is recognized with some frequency in horses, cattle, and human beings. A volvulus is a twist of a segment of intestine on its mesenteric axis and results in occlusion of the blood supply. Torsion, on the other hand, is a twist of a part on its longitudinal axis. Bulky, high-residue diets and diets consisting largely of cereals and vegetables, often taken as a single large meal once daily, have been incriminated in volvulus of human beings. Long-term enlargement of the part, coupled with stretching of the mesentery and excessive mobility, appear contributory. Distention and exaggerated peristalsis, with or without a partial obstruction distal to the site, are probably necessary for the development of volvulus.

Cattle suffer with volvulus of the cecum, spiral colon, and terminal ileum. In this species, volvulus probably represents the most severe stage of what began as cecal dilatation and torsion. This latter disorder occurs in intensively reared dairy cattle that have been fed large amount of grain, and it is associated with ketosis. Such elements suggest a metabolic induction of cecal malfunction; one hypothesis suggests that the feeding of high concentrations of grain increases circulating volatile fatty acids, which inhibit cecal motility. Torsion obstructs the cecum, whereas additional twisting results in cecal-spiral colon volvulus and obstruction of the ileum and colon.

In cattle, cecal dilatation, torsion, or volvulus is characterized by anorexia, decreased milk production, right-sided tympany, malaise, congested membranes, "quiet" rumen, lack of feces, treading, restlessness, kicking at the abdomen, moaning, and tenesmus. Horses with volvulus of the left colon have colic, but it is often less intense than other forms, e.g., small bowel incarceration. Horses roll, paw at the ground, sweat, and appear restless. Abdominal distention may be obvious, and the horses often assume a stretched-out "sawhorse" stance and turn to look at their flanks.

The most common site of large bowel volvulus of the horse is the left colon. In this species, the colon extends from the cecum forward on the right, then across the ventral abdomen at the diaphragm to form the (sacculated) left ventral colon, then pelvic flexure, to form the left dorsal (nonsacculated) colon. This left side loop undergoes volvulus of 180 degrees or more. Although often referred to as torsion, the twist in this horizontally held reflection of the colon occurs around its mesenteric axis, quite analogous to volvulus that occurs in vertically suspended loops and with the same ischemic consequences. The twist is thought to be caused by overfilling, especially disproportionate filling, of the left dorsal colon with feces or sand. Most often in this disorder, the dorsal left colon is displaced medially, while the ventral left colon moves laterally. The reverse twist, counterclockwise, occurs less frequently. At necropsy, that portion of the colon beyond the twist is black and its wall blood-filled, the result of the occlusion of veins prior to the occlusion of arteries.

Injuries and Inflammation

Canine mucosal colitis

Canine mucosal colitis occurs infrequently. It is recognized sporadically in such breeds as the Belgian Tervuren, dachshund, German shepherd dog, Old English sheepdog, and collie. Adult dogs, 3 to 6 years of age, are affected, and males appear to be disproportionately affected. The cause of mucosal colitis is unknown. On evaluation of the lesions, it appears that an inciting agent damages colonic epithelium, and, subsequently, the lesion is perpetuated by continued presence of an antigen, the microbiologic flora, or immunologic events.

Dogs with mucosal colitis are usually afebrile, have chronic diarrhea, and pass fresh blood. There may not be weight loss. If the colitis is severe, however, secondary effects contribute to ill health and anorexia, and weight loss does occur. Tenesmus is a prominent clinical feature if the rectum is affected. Granulocytes can be demonstrated in the feces in some varieties of mucosal colitis.

The gross lesions of the colon include hyperemia, granularity, friability, and multifocal ulceration. Some forms of canine mucosal colitis have a diffuse distribution affecting the entire colon and rectum, whereas other forms are segmental. Microscopic lesions involve the colonic epithelial cells. They have degeneration and necrosis, granulocytes are attracted into the colonic crypts, and a variety of inflammatory cells infiltrate the lamina propria between the crypts. The epithelium often undergoes regenerative hyperplasia (Fig. 1-106). Crypt abscesses occur in one, several, or many colonic crypts (Fig. 1-107). Granulocytes are discharged onto the luminal surface. Other mucosal changes include congestion and hemorrhages in the lamina propria, increased numbers of lymphocytes and plasma cells in the lamina propria, and hyperplastic regenerative downgrowths of epithelium into the lymphoid follicles of the submucosa. Ulcers may occur and be round, stellate, or serpiginous and coated with fibrinopurulent tags. The ulcers may coalesce, crisscross one another, and isolate islands of healthy mucosa. Eosinophils often comprise a moderate part of the inflammatory cell infiltrate in canine mucosal colitis, and increased numbers of mast cells occur in these areas as well. These forms of colitis are limited to the mucosa and superficial portions of the submucosa.

Parasitic colitis

Amebiasis. Amebiasis is an acute or chronic disease caused by the single-cell protozoan *Entamoeba histolytica*. Dogs, nonhuman primates, and human beings have colitis and amebic abscesses.

E. histolytica is found in intestinal contents; the trophozoites are transparent; contain an eccentric nucleus and, sometimes, erythrocytes; are three to five times the diameter of erythrocytes; and are noted by ameboid movement. Trophozoa parasitize intestinal mucosa; under unfavorable

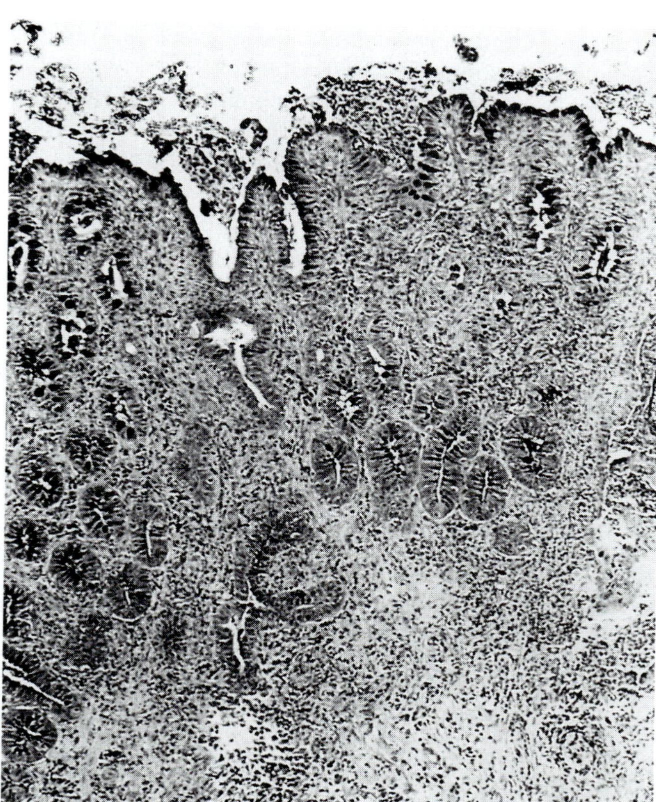

Fig. 1-106 Colon; dog. Mucosal colitis. The surface is irregular, with granulocytes exuding from crypts. PAS staining demonstrates reduced mucus in glands at the center, which are hyperplastic and surrounded by an acute inflammatory cell infiltrate. PAS stain.

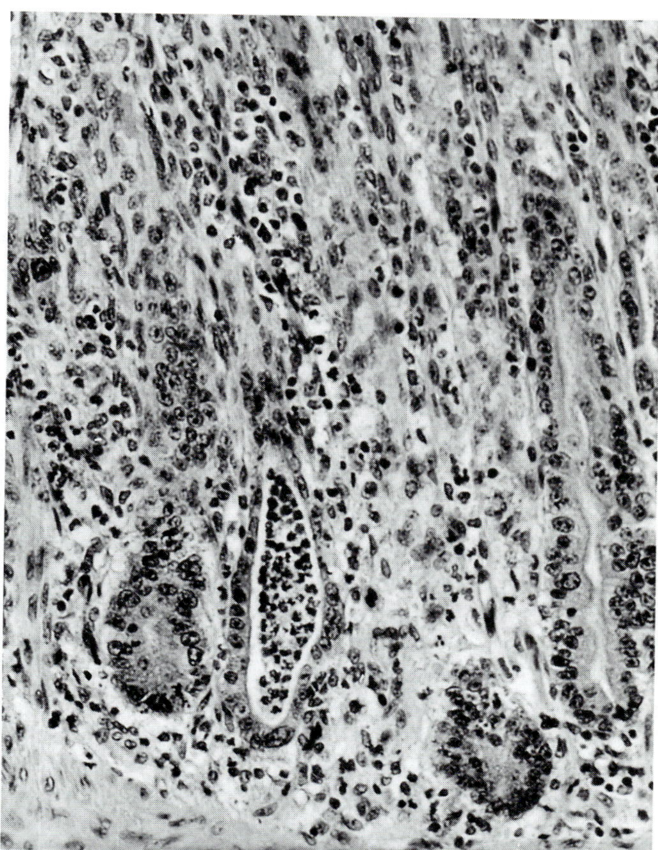

Fig. 1-107 Colon; marmoset. Colitis. Colon glands are separated by mononuclear leukocytes, and one crypt is abscessed. H & E stain.

circumstances, trophozoites encyst. The cysts, infectious forms of the agent, survive outside the body for as long as 10 days. A cyst ingested with feed or water undergoes cell division, which results in eight trophozoites that are liberated into the lumen of the intestine.

Amebae invade intact mucosa by means of lysozymes liberated at their surface. With continued cellular destruction, a punctiform ulcer with characteristic undermined edges is formed. Eventually, a flask-shaped ulcer extends into the submucosa and, sometimes, into the muscle layers. In the mucosa, the amebae create a colony, but do not stimulate an inflammatory response. Ulcers may be covered by a small amount of yellow, fibrinopurulent exudate or have an exposed and bleeding surface. Amebae that enter the portal circulation become disseminated systemically. The organ most often secondarily infected is the liver, and it has amebic abscesses or granulomas.

Clinically, amebiasis is characterized by abdominal pain, intermittent diarrhea, anorexia, and malaise. These signs may wax and wane for weeks or months. Diarrhea is the most common feature, and the feces often contain blood and mucus. If the parasites have extended into the rectum, tenesmus is observed.

Grossly, the affected colon contains numerous, randomly scattered punctiform ulcers, varying from pinhead to 2 cm in diameter. In severe cases, greater denudation of the surface and pseudomembrane formation occurs.

Microscopically, punctiform ulcers containing the unicellular protozoa are diagnostic. Amebae are numerous in these areas and are unaccompanied by necrosis, eosinophils, or granuloma formation. In some individuals, a mild lymphocyte–plasma cell infiltrate is present. The protozoa may be recognized in H & E–stained sections, but details are more readily discerned in Giemsa-stained sections.

Trichuriasis. Trichuriasis occurs worldwide among several animal species and in human beings. The parasites most commonly involved in disease are *Trichuris vulpis* of the dog, *T. suis* of the pig, and *T. trichiura* of human beings. The trichurids, 3 to 5 cm in length, are whip-shaped parasites, with a long and slender anterior two thirds, like the lash of a whip, joined to the stouter hind end, the whip handle. The life cycle is direct. Eggs, discharged in the feces of a parasitized host, embryonate in damp, shady environments, and infection is acquired by ingestion. In the digestive tract, larvae emerge from the eggs and penetrate the small intestinal mucosa, where they reside for a short time. They emerge, undergo several stages of development, and then attach to the mucosa of the cecum and colon. The prepatent period is 4 to 5 weeks.

The trichurids damage the mucosa of cecum, colon, and rectum by the tunneling produced as the parasites burrow into the superficial lamina propria. The tunnels are composed of greatly attenuated surface epithelial cells that form a thin covering. The tunnels have an undulating pattern consistent with the way the worm burrows through the surface mucosa. When few parasites are present, the animal experiences no clinical signs. When great numbers of parasites are present, diarrhea results.

Clinically, *Trichuris* infection in the dog causes chronic diarrhea, which most often is bloodless. Less frequently, the feces contain blood and mucus. Weight loss is minimal, but some dehydration occurs. Laboratory findings include hypoalbuminemia, hyperglobulinemia, anemia, and electrolyte disturbances. The eggs of *Trichuris* are characteristic: lemon-shaped with an operculum on both ends. Dogs with trichuriasis sometimes have clinical signs indicative of typhlitis. They suck their flank or turn in circles trying to gnaw at their flank. In the pig, trichuriasis is characterized by anorexia, diarrhea, mucus and blood in the feces, anemia, fever, labored respiration, incoordination, emaciation, retardation of growth, and death.

The entire surface of the cecum may be covered by these parasites; they may extend to cover the surface of the proximal colon; and in some species such as the dog, the parasites, when numerous, may extend to the rectum (Fig. 1-108). Microscopically, thin-walled tunnels encase the esophageal end of the trichurids, but little tissue damage is evident. The parasites induce little leukocytic infiltration and no necrosis. In heavy infections, a few parasites migrate into the deeper layers of the intestine and incite a granulomatous inflammation.

Oesophagostomiasis. Oesophagostomiasis occurs in sheep, cattle, and pigs. The most important species include *Oesophagostomum columbianum, O. radiatum,* and *O. dentatum.* Third-stage larvae are ingested, penetrate the mucosa of the distal small intestine or cecum and colon, reside there for a time, and then exit to develop into adults, 1 to 2 cm in length, that live on the mucosal surface of the cecum and colon. Here, they stimulate a response of eo-

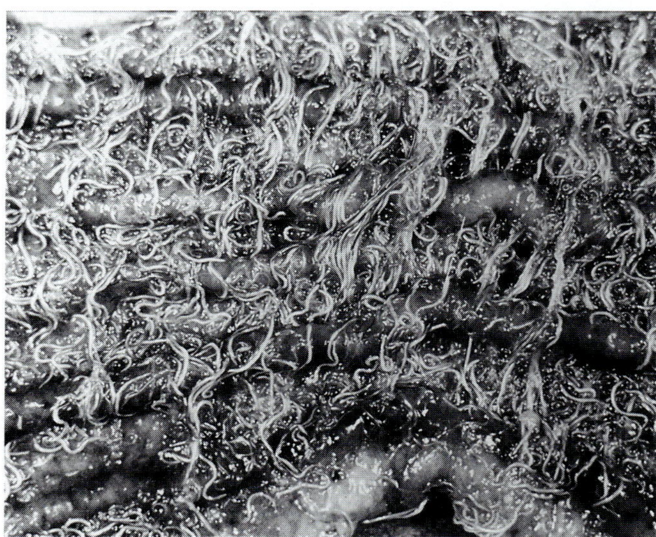

Fig. 1-108 Colon; dog. Trichuriasis. *Trichuria vulpis* coat the entire mucosal surface.

sinophils and globule leukocytes. Clinically, *Oesophagostomum* sp are responsible for moderate electrolyte and protein loss, diarrhea, anemia, and unthriftiness.

The lesion seen most frequently at necropsy is a granulomatous nodule, 0.5 to 1.5 cm in diameter, produced by penetration of the cecal and colonic wall by fourth-stage larvae. Very few sheep are free of these lesions, which protrude from the serosa of the intestines (Fig. 1-109) and which, on incision, contain a gritty, yellow to green, necrotic center. Nodules may number 50 to 100; some occur in the mesentery, mesenteric lymph nodes, liver, and lungs as well. Microscopically, the *Oesophagostomum* nodules contain parasite fragments and central, caseous, necrotic material; eosinophils; and a granulomatous encasement, complete with Langhans' giant cells.

Equine thromboembolic colic. One of the most significant parasites in veterinary medicine is *Strongylus vulgaris,* a stocky, dusky-red nematode of 2 to 3 cm length that resides in the large intestine of the horse. The adults produce little disease per se, but when combined with other *Strongylus* species and small strongyles, the parasite contributes to unthriftiness, weight loss, and anemia. Of greater concern is the damage induced by the larval stages of *S. vulgaris.*

Eggs produced by adults in the colon are discharged with the feces, embryonate on pasture, and, in less than 2 weeks, develop into third-stage infective larvae. These, ingested with forage, penetrate the intestinal mucosa to the submucosa, where they moult and gain access to submucosal arteries. In these arteries, they migrate along the endothelium to the cranial mesenteric artery. After a developmental period of 3 to 4 months, larvae exsheath and migrate as young adults down the lumen of arteries to the intestines. Subsequently, young adults are trapped in intramural nodules that ultimately rupture to the intestinal lumen. Larvae that journey beyond the cranial mesenteric artery take up residence in the aorta or major abdominal branches. The prepatent period is 6 months or longer.

Wherever the larvae reside, they produce verminous arteritis, thrombosis, arterial thickening, and aneurysms. The cranial mesenteric artery is enlarged, saccular, and thickened. Larvae, 1 cm in length, adhere to or penetrate the intima and may number a few to several hundred. The arterial surface is rough and covered by layered thrombi in which the parasites are partially embedded. Chronically affected sites have degeneration of elastic laminae and muscle fibers. Until recently, it was said that 95% of horses had *Strongyle*-induced vascular lesions and 90% to 95% had aneurysms. Earlier writers estimated that 80% of colics were caused by *Strongylus* larvae. Since the introduction and widespread use of ivermectin, an orally administered vermifuge with broad systemic larvacidal activity, this is no longer true.

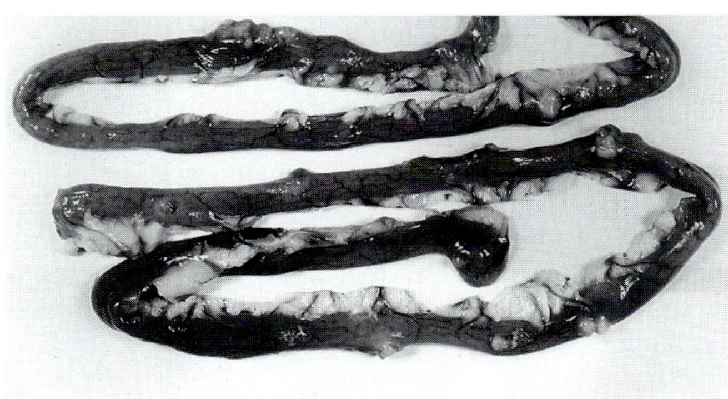

Fig. 1-109 Small intestine; sheep. Oesophagostomiasis. Multiple, firm nodules protrude from the serosal surface.

Clinical signs include recurrent bouts of colic, failure to thrive, weight loss, variable appetite, and poor hair coat. Attacks of colic may be severe, accompanied by fever, anorexia, dullness, sternal recumbency, looking at the flank, discomfort on lying down, kicking at the abdomen, sweating and rolling, increased intestinal sounds, and the passage of soft feces. The detection on rectal examination of a large (6-cm diameter or greater), firm, tortuous mass at the site of the cranial mesenteric artery may be taken as evidence of parasitic arteritis. Laboratory findings include leukocytosis, neutrophilia, eosinophilia, normocytic anemia, hypoalbuminemia, and elevated beta globulins. Death occurs when strongyle-induced thrombi or emboli occlude branches of major arteries to the cecum, colon, or, less frequently, the small bowel, with resultant infarction. At necropsy, the affected bowel is black, blood engorged, and friable. Often perforation has occurred and caused a terminal peritonitis.

Viral colitis

Winter dysentery. Winter dysentery is an acute gastrointestinal disorder of adult cattle, particularly dairy cattle, of the northern United States. A similar, if not identical, disease has been reported in Canada, England, Australia, New Zealand, France, Israel, and Sweden. The disease occurs in epidemic proportions from November to March and is highly contagious within a farm or community. The illness is characterized by acute onset of profuse diarrhea, severe decrease in milk production, variable depression and anorexia, and, sometimes, a mild cough. Fever, leukocytosis, and leukopenia are notably absent at the onset of diarrhea. The feces can be dark brown, dark green, or black (melena) and often are flecked or streaked with blood or mucus and have a characteristic fetid odor. At the onset of winter dysentery, 5% to 10% of a herd are ill. By the second day, 30% to 50% are affected; morbidity reaches 100% by the third day. The course of the illness is 1 to 4 days. Postparturient individuals are affected most severely, heifers experience mild disease, and calves less than 4 to 6 months old apparently are unaffected. Mortality is less than 1%, but milk production losses are severe. Cattle that have had the disease cannot be reinfected for several years.

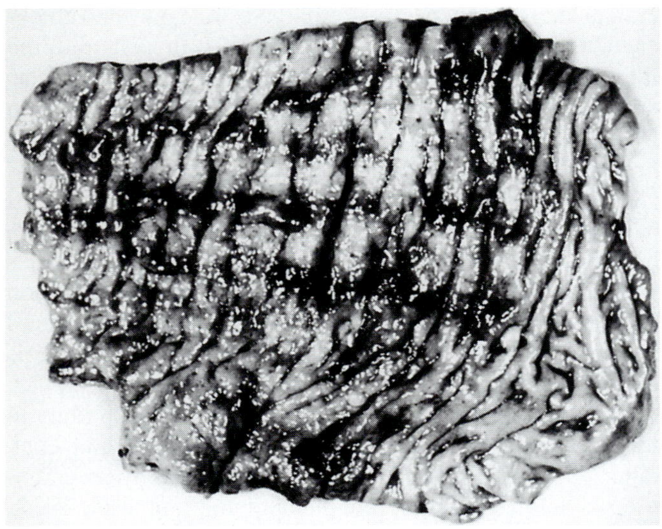

Fig. 1-110 Colon; cow. Winter dysentery. Linear mucosal hemorrhages occur in a lymphoid patch of the proximal colon. *Van Kruiningen HJ, Hiestand L, Hill DL, Tilton RC, Ryan RW. Compend Cont Educ Pract Vet 1985; 7:5591-5598.*

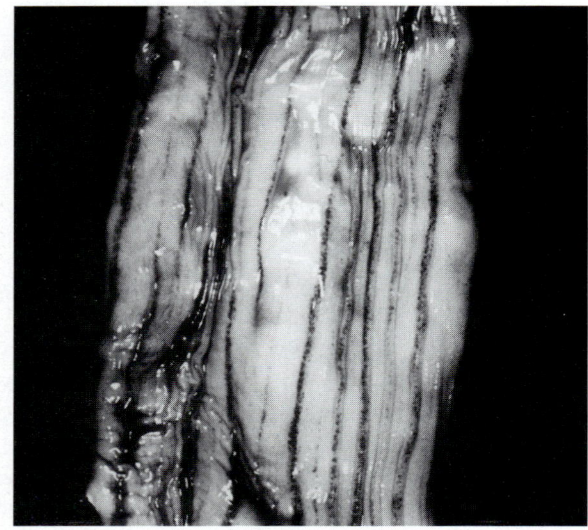

Fig. 1-111 Colon; cow. Winter dysentery. Petechiae occur in linear array in the crests of distal colonic mucosal folds. *Van Kruiningen HJ, Hiestand L, Hill DL, Tilton RC, Ryan RW. Compend Cont Educ Pract Vet 1985; 7:5591-5598.*

Following the initial definition of winter dysentery in 1931, *Vibrio jejuni* (later named *Campylobacter jejuni*) was considered the causative agent; however, this was refuted by subsequent studies. The disease was reproduced with cell-free filtrates as early as 1957, but attempts at virus isolations were only partially successful. Recently, coronavirus-like agents have been demonstrated in the feces of adult cattle with "epizootic diarrhea" in Japan and winter dysentery in France, as well as in feces from healthy adult dairy cows in the United States. The histologic features of winter dysentery were characterized for the first time in 1985. The spiral colon was defined as an important target organ, and, subsequently, coronavirus was demonstrated in the lesions.

At necropsy, the abomasal mucosa is reddened, and the small intestine is segmentally hyperemic and variably dilated and flaccid. The contents have the consistency of thin paint and are gray, tan, or olive green. Peyer's patches have a variegated appearance. The cecum is unaffected. The spiral and distal colon are empty or contain a thin fluid. The mucosal surface is moist and shiny, without necrosis or pseudomembranes, and streaked segmentally with linear aggregates of petechiae. The latter course irregularly over colonic lymphoid patches or in parallel rows along colonic ridges ("zebra striping") (Figs. 1-110 and 1-111).

Microscopically, the lesions of the colon consist of focal crypt epithelial damage and necrosis of cells of the lamina propria. Damaged crypts contain clusters of cells with pyknosis, karyorrhexis, and granular, hydropic and hyaline droplet degeneration (Fig. 1-112). Similar fragmented and pyknotic nuclei occur in the lamina propria, where the lysis of cells creates a "moth-eaten" appearance. Capillary beds near the surface of colonic ridges are the source of petechial hemorrhage and luminal bleeding. The coronavirus of winter dysentery can be demonstrated in damaged crypt epithelium by immunoperoxidase and electron microscopic methods (Figs. 1-113 and 1-114).

Colitis of feline infectious peritonitis. Feline infectious peritonitis (FIP) is a transmissible disease of young cats caused by a coronavirus, a pleomorphic RNA virus, 75 nm in diameter. The peritonitis is serofibrinous, accompanied by large volumes of transudate, and is characterized by military granulomas of the serosal surfaces of viscera, particularly the liver and intestines. Granulomatous lesions occur elsewhere, such as the lungs, central nervous system, eyeballs, kidneys, liver, or visceral lymph nodes. An immune component to FIP is suggested by the observations that the disease occurs more rapidly and more extensively in seropositive cats than in seronegative ones, lesions develop experimentally only after serum antibody is demonstrable, and virus antigen and IgG antibody occur in focal areas of necrosis. In the presence of a strong immune response, phlebitis, thrombophlebitis, and thrombosis occur in several organ systems, including the intestines.

The "wet form" of FIP is characterized by large volumes of yellow peritoneal transudate that contains flecks or strands of fibrin and by multiple granular, glistening granulomas along the serosa of abdominal viscera. The granulomas are translucent and less than 2 mm in diameter. The "dry form" of the disease, on the other hand, consists of localized, firm, gray to white masses. These sometimes occur as 1- to 2-cm nodules in the kidneys. The localized

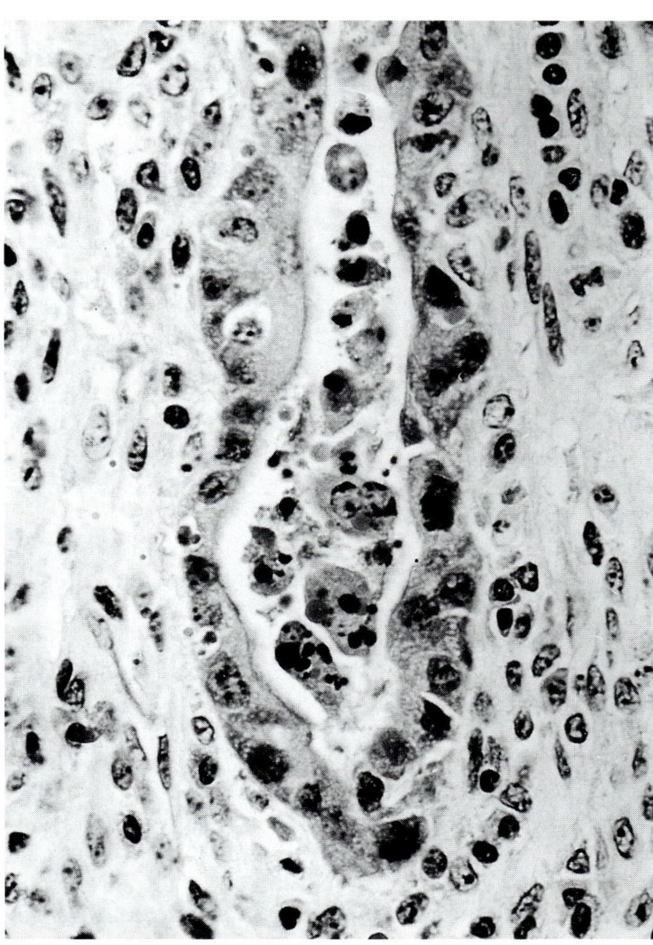

Fig. 1-112 Colon; cow. Winter dysentery. Virus-induced colonic crypt damage is extensive. Degenerate and necrotic cells in the lumen have hyaline droplet degeneration, pyknosis, and karyorrhexis. Those still attached have similar changes and are hyperplastic. H & E stain. *Van Kruiningen HJ, Hiestand L, Hill DL, Tilton RC, Ryan RW. Compend Cont Educ Pract Vet 1985; 7:5591-5598.*

''dry form'' of FIP causes segmental granulomatous disease of the ileum, cecum, or colon. The affected bowel wall is thickened, firm, and fibrotic, and the lumen is stenotic. The granulomatous ileal or colonic lesions have insidious and progressive clinical effects on the cat. Signs include unthriftiness, weight loss, constipation, obstipation, vomiting, and palpable abdominal mass.

The microscopic lesions of colonic granulomatous FIP occur segmentally, originate in the submucosa or subserosa, and extend transmurally to the mucosa or along vascular channels through the tunica muscularis. The deeper layers of the colon are thickened by multifocal granulomas, accompanied by an intense mononuclear infiltration. Connective tissue fibroplasia, lymphangiectasia, edema, and muscular hypertrophy contribute to the mural thickening. Neuronal plexuses are accentuated in the diseased sub-

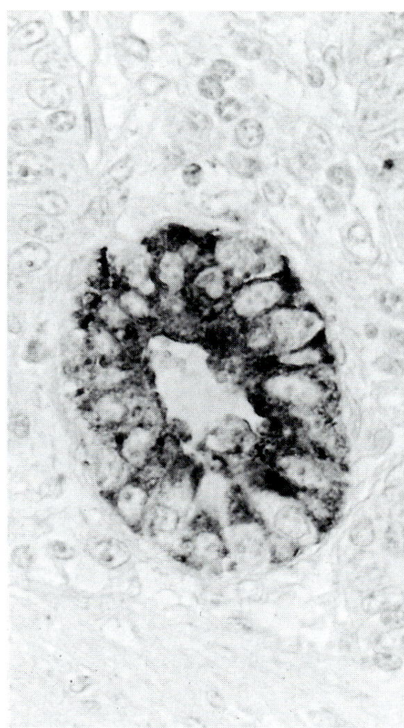

Fig. 1-113 Spiral colon; cow. Winter dysentery. Immunoperoxidase reactivity demonstrates coronavirus antigen in crypt epithelial cells.

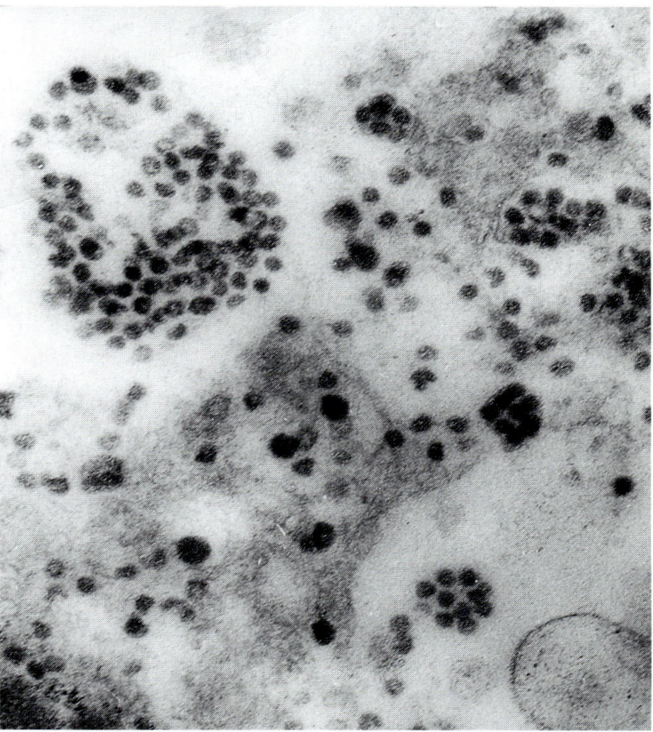

Fig. 1-114 Colon; cow. Winter dysentery. Electron micrograph. Coronavirus particles and ''virus factories'' are abundant within a degenerate epithelial cell from damaged colonic mucosa.

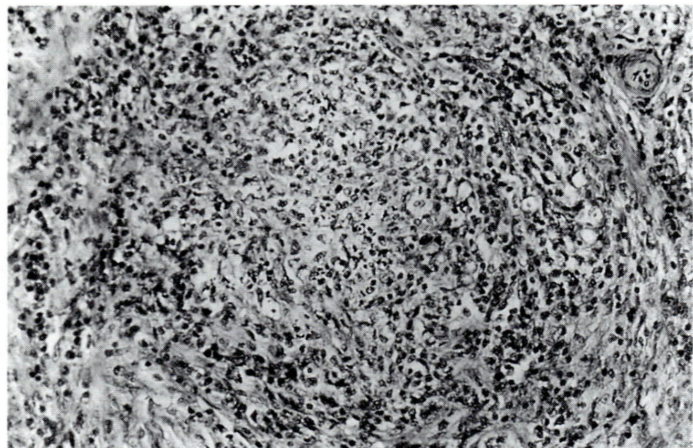

Fig. 1-115 Colon, subserosa; cat. Feline infectious peritonitis. The granuloma has a few granulocytes at the center which lie among and are surrounded by histiocytes. Outside of these is a collar of lymphocytes and plasma cells. H & E stain.

mucosa and muscularis. Mucosal glandular architecture is, for the most part, preserved, although focally or segmentally the lamina propria has excessive mononuclear cells. Focally, granulomatous nodules of the submucosa are confluent with areas of intense mononuclear reaction in the mucosa, with concomitant disruption of glandular architecture and occasional crypt abscesses.

The submucosal and subserosal granulomas are of three types. Some of the granulomas are composed of whorled, small, stellate or pleomorphic histiocytes with a few necrotic cell fragments at the center; others consist of whorled granuloma cells surrounding lymphoid aggregates; and a third type has whorled histiocytes around a central microabscess (Fig. 1-115). Characteristic FIP granulomas occur in other tissues as well, including lungs, liver, pancreas, kidneys, and mesentery. Regional lymph nodes have follicular hyperplasia, often with necrotic and purulent or hyalinized germinal centers.

Bacterial colitis

Salmonellosis. Salmonellosis is a significant cause of acute and chronic diarrhea and death in numerous animal species and in human beings. In veterinary medicine, salmonellosis can occur epizootically, enzootically, or sporadically. The species that are of major disease significance include *Salmonella typhimurium, S. enteritidis, S. dublin, S. cholerae-suis,* and *S. typhosa.* The *Salmonellae* are gram-negative, motile bacilli, 0.5 to 0.8 μ in diameter and 1 to 3.5 μ in length. The bacteria are aerobes or facultatively anaerobes. *Salmonella* reside in the gallbladder and intestinal tracts of carrier animals. Infection is produced by ingestion of fecally contaminated material. Contaminated feed and water are important sources of infection in all species. The disease may be transmitted by the fingers, flies, and fomites, and is transmissible between animals and human beings. Fatal salmonellosis of horses and cats has occurred in veterinary hospitals following the stress of surgery and antibiotic treatment.

Salmonella infections are acquired by ingestion. The tonsils and Peyer's patches are portals of entry for some species, whereas other species colonize the intestine, are invasive, and enter epithelial cells and, subsequently, macrophages of the mucosa. *Salmonella* produce disease via enterotoxins, cytotoxins (Vero toxins), and endotoxins. Once they are in contact with macrophages of the lamina propria or Peyer's patches, the organisms are phagocytosed and then transported to regional lymph nodes and, by way of the portal circulation, to the liver. The organisms colonize the small intestine, colon, lymph nodes, and the gallbladder. The latter location is the site from which organisms are shed during the asymptomatic carrier state. Salmonellosis affects the young more frequently and more severely than adults, and the young are more likely to succumb to septicemia.

Clinically, the signs of salmonellosis vary from species to species and with age. The horse suffers an acute fatal colitis. The cow has lingering febrile diarrhea with the passage of pseudomembranes, and calves have an acute diarrhea. Dogs have sudden bouts of acute, but not life-threatening, diarrhea. Cats succumb to febrile enterocolitis. Pigs die of septicemia or enterocolitis. A sequel to salmonellosis in the pig is the "anal stricture syndrome," a segmental scarring secondary to ulcerative proctitis and thrombosis of hemorrhoidal vessels. Such pigs are stunted and obstipated, and have a pendulous abdomen due to fecal retention.

Salmonellosis often produces an enterocolitis. Lesions occur in the villi of the small intestine, lymphoid tissues, and colonic mucosa. The invasive *Salmonella* have a cytotoxic effect on epithelial cells, cause their dissociation and desquamation, and induce a cellular response in the lamina propria. Initially, granulocytes occur as infiltrates in the lamina propria and as a focal cryptitis. Later, diphtheritic pseudomembranes form at the mucosal surface. Macrophages of the mucosa have the organisms in their cytoplasm and are accompanied by plasma cells and lymphocytes. In the basal mucosa and submucosa, additional lesions include vasculitis, perivasculitis, and thrombosis. The gross and microscopic hallmark of salmonellosis is the enlargement of Peyer's patches and the lymphoid follicles of the cecal and colon with necrosis of surface epithelium. In the ileum of the pig, the oval, elongated Peyer's patches are ulcerated and coated with necrotic pseudomembrane; in the colon, the solitary follicles are raised and ulcerated, creating so-called "button ulcers" (Figs. 1-116 and 1-117).

Mesenteric lymph nodes are enlarged, swollen, and edematous and may have foci of necrosis. The hepatic lesions are focal necrosis and/or microgranulomas; the latter are small clusters of macrophages (the "paratyphoid gran-

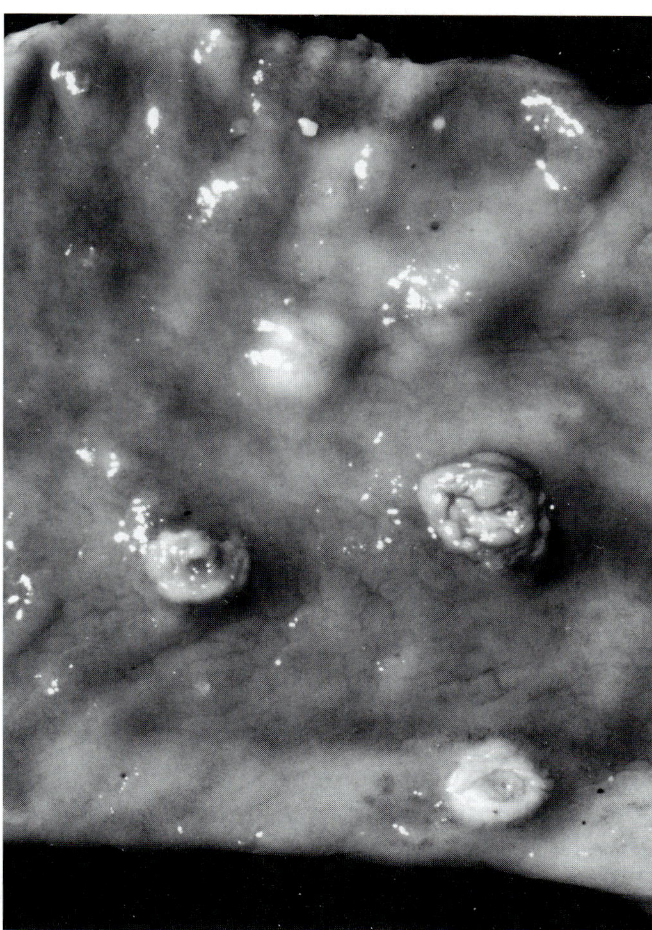

Fig. 1-116 Colon; pig. Salmonellosis. Necrotic "button ulcers" are raised above the mucosal surface. *Courtesy Dr. M.D. McGavin.*

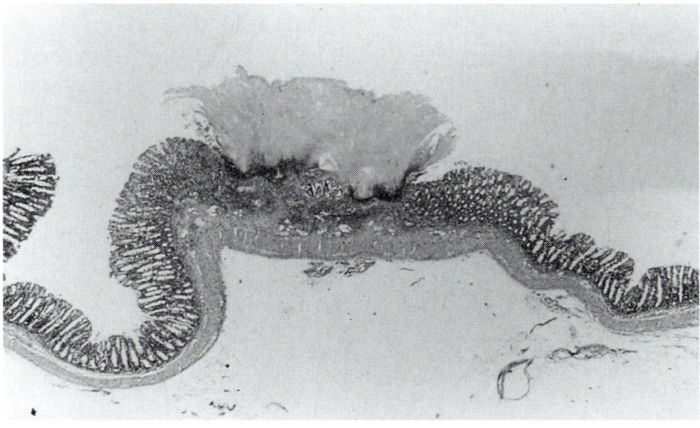

Fig. 1-117 Colon; pig. Salmonellosis. Necrotic material protrudes within the "button ulcer" originating in lymphoid tissue of the colon. H & E stain. *Courtesy Dr. M.D. McGavin.*

uloma") that are a response to the seeding of bacterial emboli. In the septicemic form, *Salmonella* disseminate to other tissues to produce, in some animals, focal meningoencephalitis, suppurative bacterial arthritis, or renal infarcts. In pigs, septicemic salmonellosis is often accompanied by violet discoloration of the skin and extensive petechiae of the kidneys ("turkey egg kidney").

Colitis X of horses. "Colitis X" is an acute, fulminating disease of young horses stressed physically or by an upper respiratory infection. The colitis is manifested clinically by severe, profuse, dark brown, fluid diarrhea; severe progressive dehydration; fever; leukopenia; discolored membranes; cyanosis; increased respiratory and cardiac rates; colic; prostration; and, finally, death. The course of the disease is usually less than 48 hours.

Colitis X is very similar in clinical appearance to acute salmonellosis. The diagnosis is made after salmonellosis has been eliminated from consideration by failure to recover the bacterium from diseased intestines. At the time colitis X was first recognized in horses (the 1960s), a life-threatening colitis occurred with alarming frequency in human beings. The latter was subsequently identified as an antibiotic-induced *Staphylococcus aureus* colitis. Human patients treated with antibiotics developed a life-threatening, pseudomembranous colitis from which pure cultures of an antibiotic-resistant staphylococcus were recovered. It is curious that endemic staphylococcal pseudomembranous colitis in human beings decreased in incidence at about the same time that the incidence of colitis X in horses declined.

In recent years, a new wave of antibiotic-induced colitis has been recognized in human beings. The lesion is a focal pseudomembranous colitis, and the causative agent has been identified as a toxigenic *Clostridium difficile.* The toxin produces mucosal necrosis and can be recovered from the colonic contents of patients with the disease. In both the human and equine diseases, no evidence is available to suggest that antibiotics are toxic to the colonic mucosa. Instead, the evidence indicates that antibiotics suppress competitive, normal flora and allow overgrowth of potential pathogens. Each case should be examined selectively for the presence of *S. aureus, C. difficile, C. perfringens, Salmonella* species, *Campylobacter* species, and *Yersinia* species.

From the various published descriptions of colitis X, it is not clear to what extent toxic megacolon or, alternatively, pseudomembranous colitis occurs. Because of the great size of the equine colon and cecum, inflammatory diseases of the mucosa rapidly reach devastating proportions. Whichever organisms appear responsible, toxic products produce diffuse mucosal necrosis, edema of the mucosa and submucosa, diapedesis, hemorrhage, venous engorgement, vascular collapse, ileus, and stagnation of intestinal contents. The result is toxic megacolon, with or without the development of pseudomembranes.

At necropsy, the large intestine is an enlarged, flaccid,

bluish, fluid-filled sac obviously thickened by edema. The mucosal surface is red-black; is irregularly lightly coated by thin, shaggy, necrotic, gray-to-black pseudomembranes; and has multiple small, round or stellate ulcers. Colic lymph nodes are enlarged, turgid, and hemorrhagic. In some cases, the adrenal cortices are red with hemorrhages, suggesting Waterhouse-Friderichsen syndrome. The mucous membranes of the conjunctiva and oral cavity are muddy red or bluish and dry. Ecchymoses and petechiae occur epicardially, in the parietal pleura, on the diaphragm, in the serosa of the small intestine, and in the spleen. Microscopically, the epithelium of the large intestine is often separated or disintegrated, sometimes with the formation of necrotic pseudomembranes. Mucosal venous dilatation and arterial constriction are widespread, accompanied by edema, hemorrhages, and degeneration or necrosis of lymphocytes in the submucosal lymphoid follicles (Fig. 1-118). These lesions occur on a background of the usual population of lymphocytes, plasma cells, and eosinophils found in the lamina propria and superficial submucosa of the equine colon.

Potomac horse fever. Potomac horse fever is a disease of the horse that is clinically and pathologically similar to salmonellosis and colitis X. First described from the Potomac River Valley in Maryland, the disease has since been recorded in 14 other states. It is characterized by fever, depression, diarrhea, anorexia, leukopenia, and 30% mortality. The disease's course is several days to weeks. Potomac horse fever has a seasonal incidence and occurs more commonly from June to September. The disease is more frequent in older horses and is seldom seen in foals and weanlings.

Shortly after the disease was recognized, it was transmitted by inoculating whole blood from an infected horse; antibodies to *Ehrlichia* sp were recognized, and, later, *Ehrlichia* organisms were cultured from experimentally infected horses. The same organism was used to reproduce the disease in susceptible ponies, with an incubation period of 9 to 14 days. The causative agent, a rickettsia, *Ehrlichia risticii,* is an obligate, intracellular, coccobacillary parasite. Two sizes of organisms have been identified ultrastructurally; the smaller is 0.2 to 0.4 μm in diameter and the larger, 0.6 to 1.5 μm. In the horse, blood monocytes, colonic epithelial cells, mucosal mast cells, and macrophages contain the *Ehrlichia* organisms.

The gross lesions of Potomac horse fever occur primarily in the cecum and colon; however, the small intestine may have lesions as well. Diseased segments are bright pink and have petechiae. Small segments (4 to 8 cm) of the small intestine and large patches of the cecum or colon (5 to 20 cm) have patchy mucosal hyperemia with petechiae; less frequently, ecchymoses; and scattered 1- to 2-mm ulcers (Fig. 1-119). Intestinal contents are fluid, pale brown, and fetid.

Microscopically, in the cecum and colon, the mucosa is reduced in thickness with loss of surface epithelium, a marked decrease in the number of intestinal crypts, and collapse of the lamina propria (Fig. 1-120). Capillaries and veins of mucosa are engorged with blood. The remaining intestinal crypts have intact epithelium, and a few have necrotic debris. Pseudomembranes are focal and consist of fibrin, necrotic cells, and bacteria. The lamina propria is hypercellular, most severely at the base of the intestinal crypts. Macrophages are prominent both in the lamina propria and in the edematous submucosa. The germinal centers of the lymphoid follicles of Peyer's patches are depleted of lymphocytes and contain karyorrhectic nuclei. Clusters of the *Ehrlichia* are readily demonstrated in macrophages of the basal lamina propria and submucosa (Fig. 1-121) in sections stained with a modified Steiner's or Dieterle's silver stain.

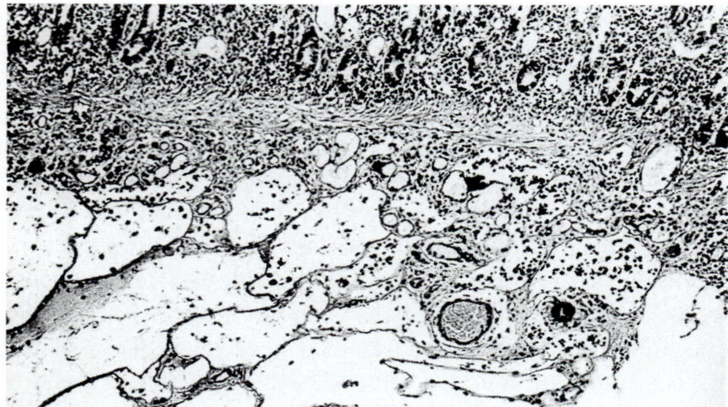

Fig. 1-118 Colon; horse. Colitis X. There has been a loss of mucosal glands and an influx of inflammatory cells in the lamina propria. The submucosa is edematous and has constricted arterioles and dilated venules. H & E stain.

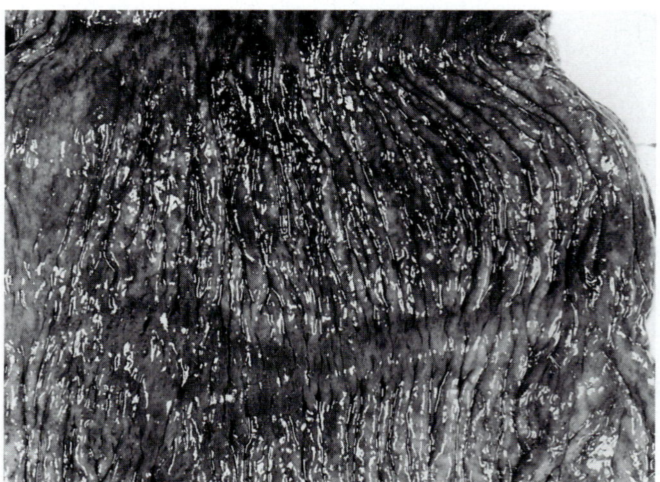

Fig. 1-119 Colon; horse. Potomac horse fever. The mucosa contains patchy areas of congestion and hyperemia. *John GA, Van Kruiningen HJ, Reim D, Wachtel AW. J Equine Vet Science 1989; 9:250-252.*

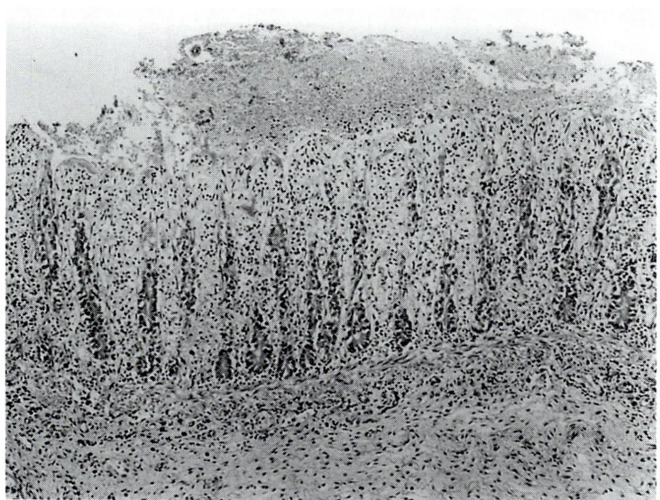

Fig. 1-120 Cecum; horse. Potomac horse fever. Necrosis of epithelium contributes to a surface pseudomembrane. Crypts are decreased in number. Mononuclear leukocytes, including macrophages, occur in submucosa just beneath muscularis mucosae. H & E stain. *John GA, Van Kruiningen HJ, Reim D, Wachtel AW. J Equine Vet Science 1989; 9:250-252.*

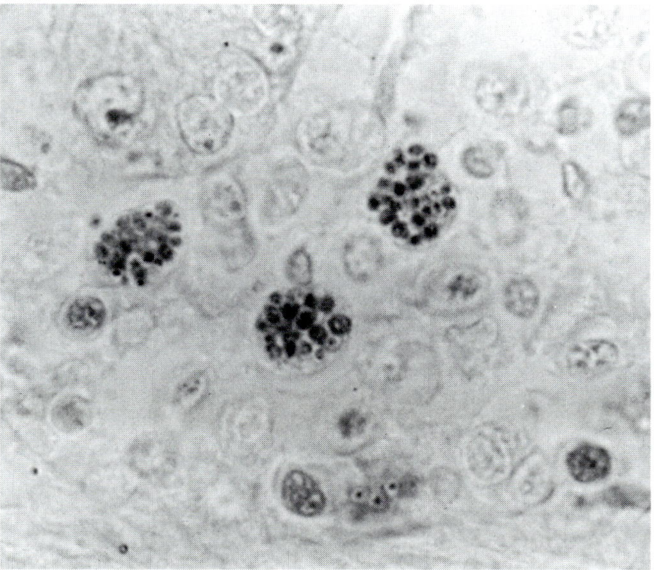

Fig. 1-121 Cecum; horse. Potomac horse fever. Clusters of *Ehrlichia* are present in macrophages of the basal lamina propria adjacent to intestinal crypts. Steiner's silver stain. *John GA, Van Kruiningen HJ, Reim D, Wachtel AW. J Equine Vet Science 1989; 9:250-252.*

Pseudomembranous colitis. Pseudomembranous colitis occurs in several species of animals and in human beings. The disease may take a diffuse form or be multifocal in nature. **Swine dysentery** is a pseudomembranous colitis of the diffuse type that occurs in feeder pigs 8 to 14 weeks of age. Synonyms include diphtheritic colitis and necrotic or necrotizing colitis.

Pseudomembranous colitis occurs in swine dysentery when a pathogen, *Serpulina hyodysenteriae,* acts in concert with several species of the endogenous gut flora to cause superficial damage to the colonic mucosa. The pathogens *S. hyodysenteriae, Salmonella,* and *Shigella* can induce pseudomembranous colitis without the need for alteration in the intestinal flora. However, antibiotics that suppress competitive flora or enhance synergistic pathogens, such as the *Bacteroides, fusobacteria,* and *clostridia,* contribute to the induction of more severe disease.

Swine dysentery may occur in epizootics or enzootics and is readily transmissible using feces or pure cultures. Blood and mucus are prominent in the feces, and the spirochetes can be demonstrated by darkfield or phase microscopy.

Grossly, diffuse pseudomembranous colitis is characterized by a tan, brown, or yellow, shaggy, fibrinonecrotic coating on the surface of a red, raw, damaged colonic mucosa (Figs. 1-122 and 1-123). Microscopically, the luminal third of the mucosa is necrotic, and covered by an attached pseudomembrane composed of fibrin, albumin, mucus, desquamated epithelial cells, necrotic cells, and granulocytes. The lamina propria beneath the damaged zone has a mixed inflammatory cell infiltrate. Crypts either appear relatively undamaged or are dilated and mucus-filled. In swine dysentery, the causative spirochetes, 6 to 8 μm long, can be demonstrated in sections stained by the Warthin-Starry silver stain.

Granulomatous colitis of boxer dogs. Granulomatous colitis of boxer dogs has been reported from several states in the United States and from Canada, England, Australia, and Holland. It is a disease of young dogs, from 2 months to 4 years of age, and occurs equally in males and females. The disease is endemic in some kennels.

Granulomatous colitis of boxer dogs is characterized by a granulomatous inflammation. The similarity of this disorder to Whipple's disease, Johne's disease, and intestinal malacoplakia and the response of less severe cases to long-

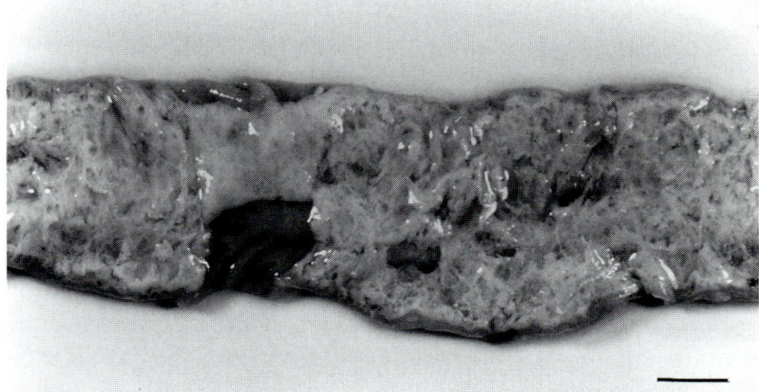

Fig. 1-122 Intestine; cow. Pseudomembranous enteritis. The diffuse pseudomembrane can be peeled from mucosa beneath. Bar = 1 cm. *Courtesy Dr. M.D. McGavin.*

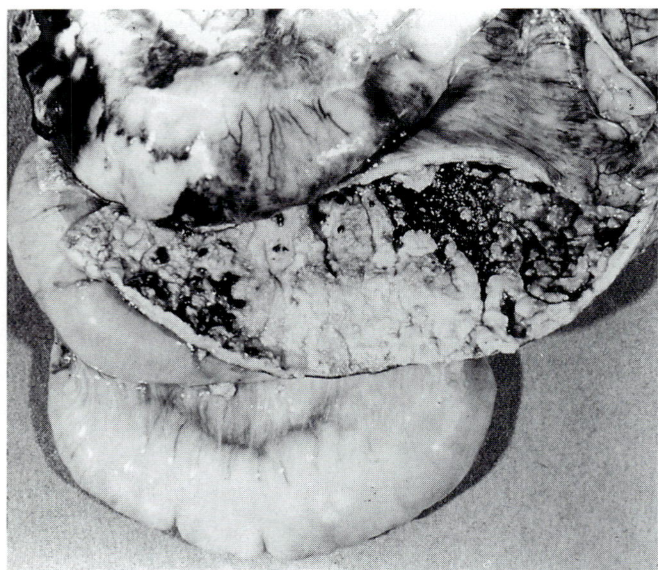

Fig. 1-123 Colon; pig. Pseudomembranous colitis. A diffuse pseudomembrane coats the necrotic hemorrhagic mucosa beneath. This animal had been inoculated with *Salmonella typhimurium* 6 days earlier. *Courtesy Dr. R.G. Thomson.*

term treatment with broad-spectrum antibiotics have long suggested that the disease is infectious.

Some of the macrophages in this disease contain bacteria of size and structure consistent with the coliforms (Figs. 1-124 and 1-125). Coliform bacilli have been demonstrated in malacoplakia, and electron microscopic and histochemical studies suggest that the macrophages in this disease are filled with glycolipid breakdown products of these bacteria. Malacoplakia has been experimentally induced by injecting endotoxin-antigen complex of *E. coli* 075 into the tissues of rats. Recently, immunocytochemistry has demonstrated that the macrophages in granulomatous colitis of boxer dogs are filled with *E. coli* antigen. When colic lymph nodes from affected dogs were taken aseptically, triturated, and cultured, *E. coli* were recovered in seven of eight cases examined.

Dogs with granulomatous colitis have intractable bloody diarrhea. Most show no weight loss; have healthy skin and hair coats; are afebrile, bright, and alert; and have a good appetite. More severely affected dogs are thin, or emaciated, have enlarged lymph nodes, may be anemic, and often have an unhealthy skin and hair coat. Defecation occurs 8 to 15 times daily and is often followed by tenesmus and the passage of blood. Stools are malodorous, tan to light brown, blood-streaked to bloody, and liquid. They often contain mucus. Coprophagia is common. In laboratory tests, serum albumin is reduced, and globins are elevated.

Grossly, the luminal surface of diseased segments is irregular, corrugated, and ulcerated (Fig. 1-126). Affected

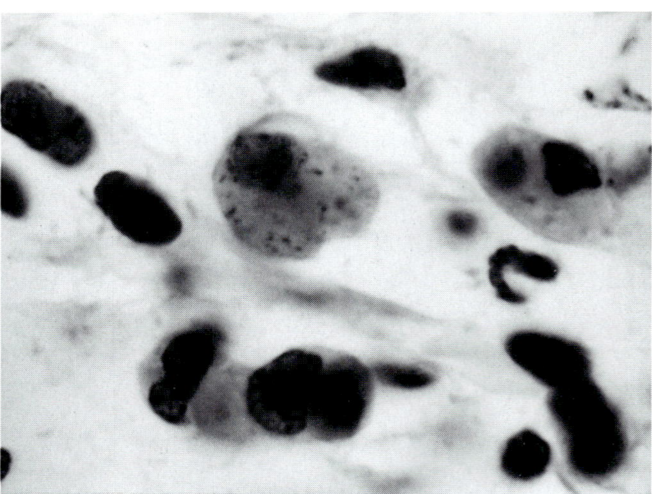

Fig. 1-124 Colon; dog. Granulomatous colitis of boxer dogs. Some of the macrophages of the lamina propria contain bacteria. Brown and Brenn (Gram) stain.

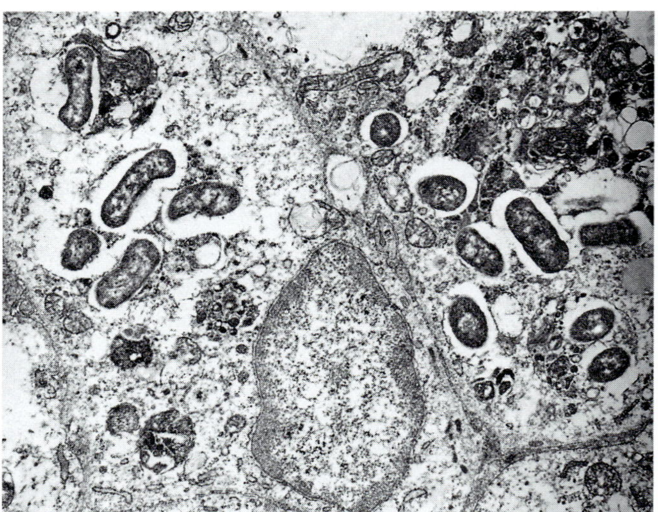

Fig. 1-125 Colon; dog. Granulomatous colitis of boxer dogs. Electron micrograph. The bacteria are bacilli 2.2 μm in length and 0.7 μm in diameter.

areas become eccentrically thickened, the luminal diameter is eccentrically reduced, elasticity and motility are lost, and the segment becomes shortened. In the most severe cases of granulomatous colitis, the colons are almost completely devoid of mucosa and only a few islands of intact mucosa remain (Fig. 1-127). The cecum undergoes changes that are similar, but the process usually is less severe. The rectum is diseased in approximately 50% of cases.

The earliest recognized lesion is the presence of large, foamy macrophages with abundant eosinophilic cytoplasm scattered in the basal lamina propria and superficial submucosa. In some dogs, lymphocytes and plasma cells of

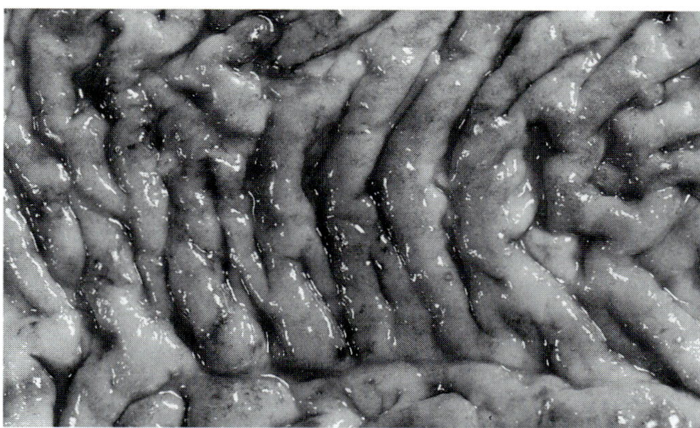

Fig. 1-126 Colon; dog. Granulomatous colitis of boxer dogs. Mucosa is thickened and corrugated and has several round to stellate ulcers. *Van Kruiningen HJ. Proc 16th Gaines Vet Symp 1966; 20.*

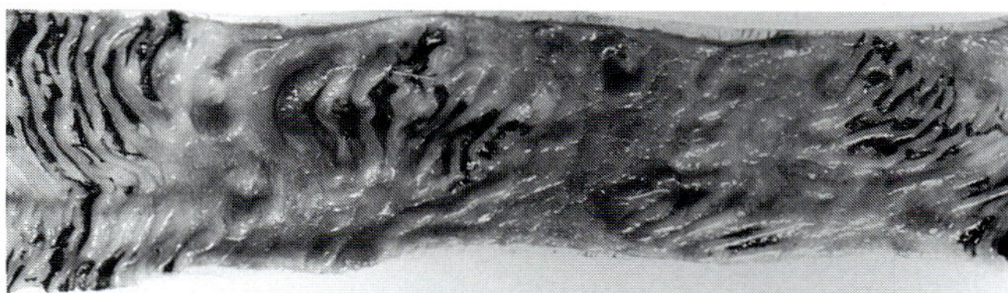

Fig. 1-127 Colon; dog. Granulomatous colitis of boxer dogs. Intact islands of mucosa with thickened folds are separated from one another by areas devoid of mucosa that have a beaded or granular, glistening surface. A few *Trichuris* are attached. *Van Kruiningen HJ. Proc 16th Gaines Vet Symp 1966; 19-26.*

the mucosa are increased, but, in most dogs, the infiltrate is composed exclusively of macrophages. These cells apparently phagocytose bacteria to capacity, and accumulate in numbers sufficient to distort the mucosa and submucosa. The colonic glands are obliterated by lateral compression or appear lifted from their basal attachments by a mantle of cells in the basal lamina propria (Fig. 1-128). In severe lesions, the macrophages are 10 to 12 cells deep in the mucosa and 50 to 200 cells deep in the submucosa. The macrophages are 11 to 17 μm in diameter, are round to oval, and have abundant eosinophilic cytoplasm and prominent eccentric nuclei (Fig. 1-129). The macrophage cytoplasm is strongly PAS-positive, and a few macrophages have cytoplasmic bacilli demonstrable with the Brown and Hopps modification of the Gram stain.

Lymph nodes that drain the colon, cecum, or rectum and those that receive afferent lymphatics from colic lymph nodes are enlarged and have lymphoid hyperplasia. Macrophages aggregate in the cortex or medullary cords. In severely affected dogs, lymphadenopathy is generalized, and macrophages are found in many peripheral lymph nodes.

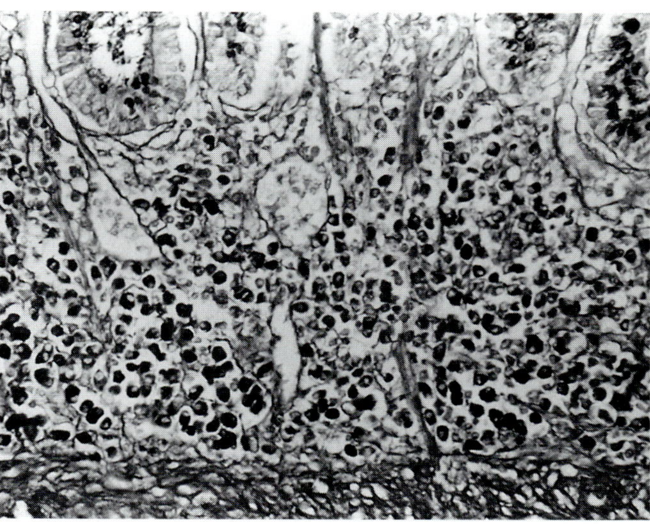

Fig. 1-128 Colon; dog. Granulomatous colitis of boxer dogs. A mantle of PAS-positive macrophages, 20 cells deep, displaces colonic glands (above) from muscularis mucosae (beneath). PAS stain. *Van Kruiningen HJ. Gastroenterology 1967; 53:114-122.*

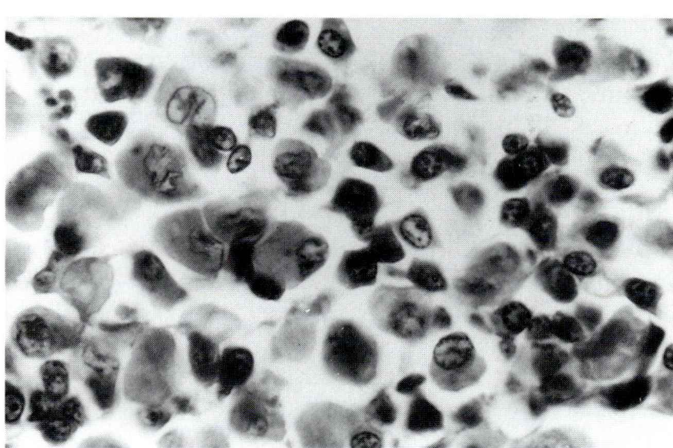

Fig. 1-129 Colon: dog. Granulomatous colitis of boxer dogs. Large, eosinophilic macrophages characterize the colitis of boxer dogs and are accompanied by scattered lymphocytes and plasma cells. H & E stain. *Van Kruiningen HJ, Montali RJ, Strandberg JD, Kirk RW. Pathol Vet 1965; 2:521-544.*

Neoplasia

Colorectal polyps and adenomas

Masses that protrude above the mucosa of the colon and rectum have traditionally been called **polyps.** Polyps may be either small or large and either pedunculated or sessile. They can also be categorized as either nonneoplastic or neoplastic. The distinction between nonneoplastic and neoplastic lesions is sometimes difficult. Colorectal adenomas have been recognized in the dog and, less frequently, in the cat. The clinical signs include dyschezia, periodic intermittent diarrhea, sometimes melena, and often rectal prolapse of the adenoma.

In veterinary medicine, the nonneoplastic types of polyps that occur in the colon or rectum include the inflammatory or regenerative polyp and the benign lymphoid polyp. The term **inflammatory** or **regenerative** polyp designates a protrusion produced by regenerative hyperplasia of the colonic epithelium, so that there is too much tissue focally. The cause for such a lesion is not known. The regenerative or inflammatory polyp is characterized by hyperplasia of the colonic epithelium, usually with normal differentiation into goblet cells, some infolding of the hyperplastic epithelium, often cystic dilatation of crypts, edema of the lamina propria, and infiltrates of inflammatory cells, particularly lymphocytes and plasma cells but sometimes including clusters of granulocytes.

The second type of nonneoplastic polyp is the **benign lymphoid polyp** that develops from reactive hyperplasia in one or more of the lymphoid follicles. With subsequent protrusion into the lumen, the polyp is drawn into the stream of contents, becomes enlarged, and undergoes secondary inflammation.

The neoplastic protrusions of colonic or rectal mucosa are adenomas or adenocarcinomas. Adenomas of the colon and rectum are categorized as tubular, villous, or tubulovillous. The **tubular adenoma** (adenomatous polyp) consists of dysplastic tubules of colonic or rectal epithelium with very little lamina propria, crowding of tubules, and lateral branching and extension of the tubules parallel to the muscularis mucosae. Tubular adenomas are usually small, spherical, and pedunculated and have a smooth surface. The **villous adenoma** consists of fingerlike processes made up of cores of lamina propria covered by dysplastic epithelium. The villouslike fronds extend perpendicular to the muscularis mucosae and give the surface a shaggy appearance. The villous adenoma is usually large and sessile. Neoplasms with both patterns of cellular growth are called tubulovillous adenomas.

Microscopically, the epithelial cells are hyperchromic and crowded. The nuclei have lost their polarity, and there is pseudostratification of nuclei. Mucus content of neoplastic cells is decreased. Mitotic figures are numerous. Severe dysplasia is synonymous with carcinoma-in-situ. The latter identifies carcinoma originating in a focus, which has not yet invaded beyond the limits of the muscularis mucosae. Frequently, entrapment of dysplastic epithelium may occur in the stalk of a pedunculated adenoma. Such a change is called pseudocarcinomatous invasion and should be differentiated from carcinoma.

In human medicine, it has been established that three factors are correlated with malignant potential: size of the adenoma, histologic growth pattern, and the degree of epithelial dysplasia. Most adenomas do not grow appreciably and may never reach sufficient size to become significantly at risk for malignant change. As adenomas grow, cancer risk rises. The villous pattern has a higher malignant potential than the tubular. Histologic pattern and size are intimately related. Even small villous tumors have a malignant potential 10 times greater than tubular adenomas of the same size. Lastly, malignant potential increases with increasing degrees of atypia. Separation of adenoma from adenocarcinoma of the colorectum is essentially made on the basis of invasion by carcinoma of tissue spaces and blood and lymph vessels of the stalk of the polypoid neoplasms (Fig. 1-130).

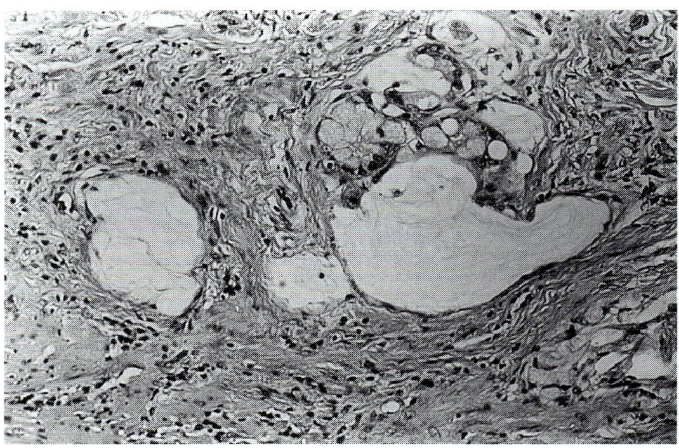

Fig. 1-130 Colon; dog. Colonic adenocarcinoma. Signet ring (tumor) cells and pools of mucus have infiltrated into the submucosa. H & E stain.

Acknowledgments

Grateful acknowledgment is expressed to Lynelle Hengen for manuscript preparation, to Dr. A. Brian West for review, and to my colleagues at other universities for contributing photographs.

Suggested Readings

Baker GJ. Oral anatomy of the horse. In: Harvey CE, ed. Veterinary Dentistry. Philadelphia: Saunders, 1985:203-216.

Barker IK, Van Dreumel AA. The alimentary system. In: Jubb KVF, Kennedy PC, Palmer N, eds. Pathology of Domestic Animals. 3rd ed. New York: Academic Press, 1985: 2:1.

Batt RM, McLean L, Carter MW. Sequential morphologic and biochemical studies of naturally occurring wheat-sensitive enteropathy in Irish Setter dogs. Dig Dis Sci 1987; 32:184-194.

Batte EG, McLamb RD, Muse KE, Tally SD, Vestal TJ. Pathophysiology of swine trichuriasis. Am J Vet Res 1977; 38:1075-1079.

Bentinck-Smith J. Feline panleukopenia (feline infectious enteritis): A review of 574 cases. North Am Vet 1949; 30:379-384.

Brown PJ, Clayton HM. Hepatic pathology of experimental *Parascaris equorum* infection in worm-free foals. J Comp Pathol 1979; 89:115-123.

Burrows CF. Canine hemorrhagic gastroenteritis. J Am Anim Hosp Assoc 1977; 13:451-458.

Carpenter JL, Roberts RM, Harpster NK, King NW. Intestinal and cardiopulmonary forms of parvovirus infection in a litter of pups. J Am Vet Med Assoc 1980; 176:1269-1273.

Cheville NF, Olson C. Cytology of the canine oral papilloma. Am J Pathol 1964; 45:849-872.

Chiodini RJ, Van Kruiningen HJ, Merkal RS. Ruminant paratuberculosis (Johne's disease): The current status and future prospects. Cornell Vet 1984; 74:218-262.

Cimprich RE. Equine granulomatous enteritis. Vet Pathol 1974; 11:535-547.

Cimprich RE, Rooney JR. *Corynebacterium equi* enteritis in foals. Vet Pathol 1977; 14:95-102.

Cordes DO, Perry BD, Rikihisa Y, Chickering WR. Enterocolitis caused by *Ehrilichia sp.* in the horse (Potomac horse fever). Vet Pathol 1986; 23:471-477.

Cordy DR, Gorham JR. The pathology and etiology of salmon disease in the dog and fox. Am J Pathol 1950; 26:617-637.

Croese J, Loukas A, Opdebeeck J, Prociv P. Occult enteric infection by *Ancylostoma caninum:* A previously unrecognized zoonosis. Gastroenterology 1994; 106:3-12.

Doughri AM, Young S, Storz J. Pathologic changes in intestinal chlamydial infection of newborn calves. Am J Vet Res 1974; 35:939-944.

Dubielzig RR, Adams WM, Brodey RS. Inductive fibroameloblastoma: An unusual dental tumor of young cats. J Am Vet Med Assoc 1979; 720-722.

Dubielzig RR, Goldschmidt MH, Brodey RS. The nomenclature of periodontal epulides in dogs. Vet Pathol 1979; 16:209-214.

Dubielzig RR, Higgins RJ, Krakowka S. Lesions of the enamel organ of developing dog teeth following experimental inoculation of gnotobiotic puppies with canine distemper virus. Vet Pathol 1981; 18:684-689.

Dubielzig RR, Thrall DE. Ameloblastoma and keratinizing ameloblastoma in dogs. Vet Pathol 1982; 19:596-607.

Dubielzig RR, Wilson JW, Beck KA, Robbins T. Dental dysplasis and epitheliogenesis imperfecta in a foal. Vet Pathol 1986; 23:325-327.

Eisner ER. Chronic subgingival tooth erosion in cats. Vet Med 1989; 84:378-387.

Fox JG, Krakowka S, Taylor NS. Acute-onset *Campylobacter*-associated gastroenteritis in adult Beagles. J Am Vet Med Assoc 1985; 187:1268-1270.

Gebhart CJ, Barns SM, McOrist S, Lin GF, Lawson GHK. Ileal symbiont intracellularis, an obligate intracellular bacterium of porcine intestines showing a relationship to *Desulfovibrio* species. Int J Syst Bacteriol 1993; 43:533-538.

Griesemer RA, Cole CR. Bovine papular stomatitis. II. The experimentally produced disease. Am J Vet Res 1961; 22:473-481.

Griesemer RA, Cole CR, Bovine papular stomatitis. III. Histopathology. Am J Vet Res 1961; 22:482-488.

Harris DL, Alexander TJL, Whipp SC, Robinson IM, Glock RD, Matthews PJ. Swine dysentery: Studies of gnotobiotic pigs inoculated with *Treponema hyodysenteriae, Bacteriodes vulgatus,* and *Fusobacterium necrophorum.* J Am Vet Med Assoc 1978; 172:468-471.

Harvey CE, Dubielzig RR. Anatomy of the oral cavity in the dog and cat. In: Harvey CE, ed. Veterinary Dentistry. Philadelphia: Saunders, 1985; 11-22.

Hayden DW, Fleischman RW. Schirrous eosinophilic gastritis in dogs with gastric arteritis. Vet Pathol 1977; 14:441-448.

Hayden DW, Van Kruiningen HJ. Eosinophilic gastroenteritis in German Shepherd dogs and its relationship to visceral larva migrans. J Am Vet Med Assoc 1973; 162:379-384.

Holland CJ, Ristic M, Cole AI, Johnson P, Baker G, Goetz T. Isolation, experimental transmission, and characterization of causative agent of Potomac horse fever. Science 1985; 227:522-524.

Hooper BE, Haelterman EO. Lesions of the gastrointestinal tract of pigs infected with transmissible gastroenteritis. Can J Comp Med 1969; 33:29-36.

Jonsson L, Martinsson K. Regional ileitis in pigs: Morphological and pathogenetical aspects. Acta Vet Scand 1976; 17:223-232.

Krook L, Maylin GA, Lillie JH, Wallace RS. Dental fluorosis in cattle. Cornell Vet 1983; 73:340-362.

Lindberg R. Pathology of equine granulomatous enteritis. J Comp Pathol 1984; 94:233-247.

Lloyd K, Hintz HF, Wheat JD, Schryver JF. Enteroliths in horses. Cornell Vet 1987; 77:172-186.

McOrist S, Jasni S, Mackie RA, MacIntyre N, Neef N, Lawson GHK. Reproduction of porcine proliferative enteropathy with pure cultures of *Ileal Symbiont intracellularis.* Infect Immun 1993; 61:4286-4292.

Mebus CA, Stair EL, Rhodes MB, Twiehaus MH. Pathology of neonatal calf diarrhea induced by a coronavirus-like agent. Vet Pathol 1973; 10:45-64.

Mebus CA, Stair EL, Underdahl NR, Twiehaus MJ. Pathology of neonatal calf diarrhea induced by a reo-like virus. Vet Pathol 1971; 8:490-505.

Meunier PC, Cooper BJ, Appel MJG, Lanieu ME, Slauson DO. Pathogenesis of canine parvovirus enteritis: Sequential virus distribution and passive immunization studies. Vet Pathol 1985; 22:617-624.

Montali RJ, Strandberg JD. Extraperitoneal lesions in feline infectious peritonitis. Vet Pathol 1972; 9:109-121.

Morin M, Morehouse LG, Solorzano RF, Olson LD. Transmissible gastroenteritis in feeder swine: Clinical, immunofluorescence, and histopathological observations. Can J Comp Med 1973; 37:239-248.

Murray M, Robinson PB, McKeating FJ, Baker GJ, Lauder IM. Peptic ulceration in the dog: A clinico-pathological study. Vet Rec 1972; 91:441-447.

Navin TR, Juranek DD. Cryptosporidiosis: Clinical, epidemiologic, and parasitologic review. Rev Infect Dis 1984; 6:313-327.

Patnaik AK, Hurvitz AI, Johnson GF. Canine gastric adenocarcinoma. Vet Pathol 1978; 15:600-607.

Pospischil A, Mainil JG, Baljer G, Moon HW. Attaching and effacing bacteria in the intestines of calves and cats with diarrhea. Vet Pathol 1987; 24:330-334.

Provenza DV. Fundamentals of Oral Histology and Embryology. Philadelphia: Lippincott, 1972.

Rikihisa Y, Perry BD, Cordes DO. Ultrastructural study of ehrilichial organisms in the large colons of ponies infected with Potomac horse fever. Infect Immun 1985; 49:505-512.

Robertson JM. Left displacement of the bovine abomasum: Epizootiologic factors. Am J Vet Res 1968; 29:421-434.

Sander CH, Langham RF. Canine histiocytic ulcerative colitis. Arch Pathol 1968; 85:94-100.

Seiler RJ. Colorectal polyps of the dog: A clinical pathologic study of 17 cases. J Am Vet Med Assoc 1979; 174:72-75.

Sheaser TR, Kostad DL, Suttie JW. Bovine dental fluorosis: Histologic and physical characteristics. Am J Vet Res 1978; 39:597-602.

Strand EA, Sommers SC, Petrak M. Regional enterocolitis in Cocker Spaniel dogs. Arch Pathol 1954; 57:357-362.

Torres-Medina A, Schlafer DH, Mebus CA. Rotaviral and coronaviral diarrhea. Vet Clin North Am Food Anim Pract 1985; 1:471-493.

Turk MAM, Gallina AM, Perryman LE. *Bacillus piliformis* infection (Tyzzer's disease) in foals in Northwestern United States: A retrospective study of 21 cases. J Am Vet Med Assoc 1981; 178:279-281.

Van Kruiningen HJ. Canine colitis comparable to regional enteritis and mucosal colitis in man. Gastroenterology 1972; 62:1128-1142.

Van Kruiningen HJ, Gregoire K, Meuten DJ. Acute gastric dilatation: A review of comparative aspects, by species, and a study in dogs and monkeys. J Am Anim Hosp Assoc 1974; 10:294-324.

Van Kruiningen HJ, Hiestand L, Hill DL, Tilton RC, Ryan RW. Winter dysentery in dairy cattle: Recent findings. Comp Cont Educ Pract Vet 1985; 7:S591-S598.

Van Kruiningen HJ, Lees GE, Hayden DW, Meuten DJ, Rogers WA. Lipogranulomatous lymphangitis in canine intestinal lymphangiectasia. Vet Pathol 1984; 21:377-383.

Van Kruiningen HJ, Montali RJ, Strandberg JD, Kirk RW. A granulomatous colitis of dogs with histologic resemblance to Whipple's disease. Path Vet 1965; 2:521-544.

Van Kruiningen HJ, Wojan LD, Stake PE, Lord PF. The influence of diet and feeding frequency on gastric function in the dog. J Am Anim Hosp Assoc 1987; 23:145-153.

Van Kruiningen HJ, Khairallah LH, Sasserville VG, Wyand MS, Post JE. Calfhood coronavirus enterocolitis: A clue to the etiology of winter dysentery. Vet Pathol 1987; 24:564-567.

Verstraete, FJM, Ligthelm AG, Weber A. The histological nature of epulides in dogs. J Comp Path 1992; 106:169-182.

Vonderfecht SL, Trommershausen Bowling A, Cohen M. Congenital intestinal aganglionosis in white foals. Vet Pathol 1983; 20:65-70.

Walker RI, Caldwell MB, Lee EC, Guerry P, Trust TJ, Ruiz-Palacios GM. Pathophysiology of *Campylobacter* enteritis. Microbiol Rev 1986; 50:81-94.

Wilcock BP, Olander HJ. The pathogenesis of porcine rectal stricture. I. The naturally occurring disease and its association with salmonellosis. Vet Pathol 1977; 14:36-42.

CHAPTER

2

Liver, Biliary System, and Exocrine Pancreas

N. JAMES MACLACHLAN
JOHN M. CULLEN

LIVER AND BILIARY SYSTEM

Structure and Function

The normal liver consists of friable red-brown tissue and has a smooth capsular surface. Its location within the cranial abdomen varies somewhat among the domestic species; in ruminants, the liver is displaced to the right side of the abdomen by the forestomachs. Also, gross subdivision of the liver into lobes differs among the domestic species.

The traditional functional subunit of the liver is the hepatic lobule, which is a hexagonal structure, 1 to 2 mm wide with a terminal hepatic venule (synonym: central vein), a tributary of the hepatic vein, at the center and portal tract at the angles of the hexagon (Fig. 2-1). Within the portal tracts are bile ducts, lymph vessels, and branches of the portal vein and the hepatic artery.

A more functionally precise anatomic subunit is the acinus, a diamond-shaped structure that centers on the terminal branches of the portal vein. Thus, branches of the portal vein and hepatic artery are at the center of the acinus, and the terminal hepatic venule (central vein) is located at the periphery. Each terminal hepatic venule receives blood from several acini. Also, the acinus more accurately reflects the nature of the liver as a gland. Its secretion, bile, flows from the hepatocytes through the bile canaliculi into the bile duct in the portal tract. The pathophysiologic features of toxic and ischemic injury to the liver are most readily explained on the basis of the acinus. Within the lobule (or acinus), hepatocytes are arranged into branching plates, which are separated by sinusoids that are arranged radially around the terminal hepatic venule. Blood flows from the branches of the hepatic artery and portal vein from the portal tracts through the sinusoids to the terminal hepatic venule. Sinusoids are lined by a highly fenestrated endothelium and numerous fixed macrophages (Kupffer cells). The hepatocytes and sinusoidal endothelial cells are separated by the space of Disse, in which specialized perisinusoidal lipocytes (lipid-containing cells also called stellate cells or Ito cells) are scattered. These specialized lipocytes are important for storage of vitamin A and for production of collagen, and, thus, have a central role in the development of hepatic fibrosis.

The biliary system commences as canaliculi within the centrolobular (periacinar) areas of the hepatic lobule. The wall of the canaliculus is formed entirely by the cell membranes of adjacent hepatocytes (Fig. 2-2). Bile flows within the lobule in the opposite direction to blood flow; that is, bile is secreted into the bile canaliculi and reaches the bile ducts within the portal tracts via the cholangioles (also known as the canals of Hering) present at the periphery of the lobule (periportal or centroacinar). The bile ducts converge into larger intrahepatic ducts, and the main hepatic ducts unite to form the common bile duct by which bile is carried to the intestine. The gallbladder is responsible for storage and concentration of bile.

The liver performs many critical functions, some of which include the following:

1. The smooth endoplasmic reticulum of the hepatocyte is responsible for synthesis of cholesterol and bile acids, degradation of glycogen, and the metabolism and conjugation of bile pigments, xenobiotics or ingested substances, and steroid hormones before their excretion in bile or urine.
2. The rough endoplasmic reticulum of the hepatocyte produces plasma proteins such as albumin and fibrinogen; clotting Factors V, VII, VIII, IX, and X; and a variety of alpha and beta globulins.
3. Hepatocytes are responsible for the production of bile, and specialized portions of their cell membranes form the walls of the canaliculi that carry bile from centrilobular areas to bile ducts within the portal areas. Bile consists of water, cholesterol, bile acids, bilirubin, and other constituents.

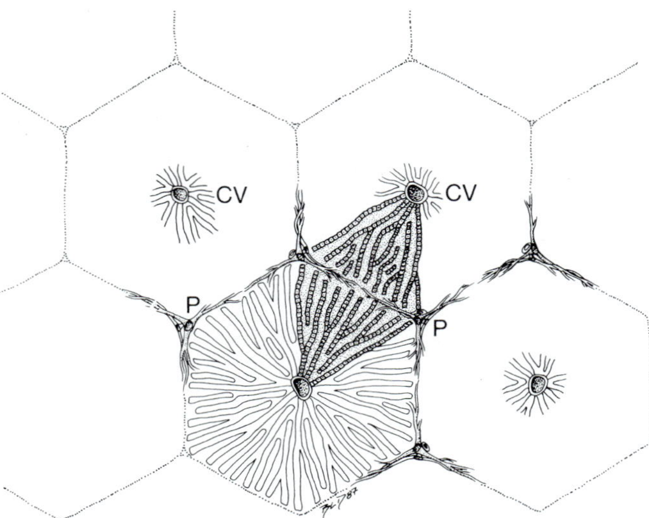

Fig. 2-1 Schematic diagram of liver lobules. Blood flows from branches of the portal vein and hepatic artery present within portal tracts (*P*), through the sinusoids to the terminal hepatic venule (central vein *CV*). Bile flows in the opposite direction to blood and commences in periacinar areas (adjacent to the terminal hepatic venule) and flows to the bile ducts within portal tracts.

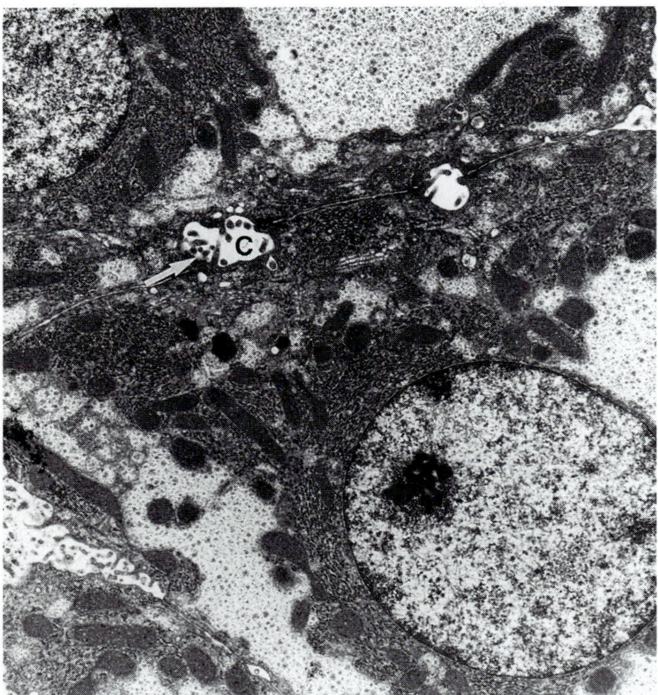

Fig. 2-2 Transmission electron micrograph. Liver; normal pig. A bile canaliculus (*C*) is between two adjacent hepatocytes, and microvilli (*arrow*) line the lumen of the canaliculus.

4. The liver provides a vast filter for blood entering the liver via the portal vein. Fixed macrophages (Kupffer cells) lining the sinusoids can phagocytose potentially injurious infectious agents before they can gain access to the systemic circulation. Kupffer cells serve as the major site of clearance of foreign material in the bloodstream of all domestic species except members of the family Artiodactyla (swine, goats, and cattle). Hepatocytes can metabolize and render inactive many toxins absorbed into the portal circulation.
5. Mitochondria within hepatocytes produce energy by oxidative phosphorylation and oxidation of fatty acids. Hepatocytes store glycogen as a readily available energy source.

Hepatic Dysfunction and Failure

The liver possesses considerable functional reserve and regenerative capacity. In healthy animals, more than two thirds of the hepatic parenchyma can be removed without significant impairment of hepatic function, and normal hepatic mass can be regenerated in a matter of days. In all species, hepatic derangements, regardless of cause, tend to produce similar signs, but these are manifest only when the liver's considerable reserve and regenerative capacity are overwhelmed or when biliary outflow is obstructed. Only lesions that affect the majority of the hepatic parenchyma are likely to produce the signs of hepatic failure because focal lesions rarely destroy sufficient parenchyma to overwhelm the liver's reserve. The term **hepatic failure** implies loss of normal hepatic function as a consequence of either acute or chronic hepatic damage; however, all hepatic functions are not usually lost at the same time. The potential consequences of hepatic dysfunction and failure include cholestasis and icterus, hepatic encephalopathy, a variety of metabolic perturbations, vascular and hemodynamic alterations, and photosensitization in herbivores.

Cholestasis and icterus

Bilirubin is produced from the metabolic degradation of hemoglobin and, to a lesser extent, other heme proteins, including myoglobin and the cytochromes. The majority of bilirubin is derived from normal extravascular breakdown of senescent erythrocytes. Erythrocytes normally are phagocytosed by macrophages of the spleen, bone marrow, and liver. Within the phagocyte, the heme portion of hemoglobin is first converted to biliverdin and subsequently to bilirubin, which is then released into the blood in its unconjugated form. Unconjugated bilirubin circulates in plasma, bound to albumin. Bilirubin is then taken up by hepatocytes, conjugated principally with glucuronic acid, and secreted in bile. Conjugated bilirubin is converted to urobilinogen within the gastrointestinal (GI) tract, and a portion of the urobilinogen is reabsorbed into the portal blood during the **enterohepatic circulation** of bile salts. The majority of urobilinogen absorbed from the GI tract is resecreted into bile. Urobilinogen has a small molecular weight and is freely filtered through the glomerulus; small amounts are normally found in the urine. Urobilinogen that is not absorbed from the intestine oxidizes to stercobilin, which colors the feces.

Increased concentrations of conjugated or unconjugated bilirubin in blood are called hyperbilirubinemia. High concentrations can produce icterus (jaundice), a yellow discoloration of tissues especially evident in those tissues rich in elastin, such as the aorta and sclera. The level of serum bilirubin that produces icterus varies between species such that it is possible for an animal to be hyperbilirubinemic before icterus is apparent.

The causes of hyperbilirubinemia include the following:

1. Overproduction of bilirubin as a consequence of hemolysis, particularly, severe intravascular hemolysis, which overwhelms the liver's capacity to remove bilirubin from the plasma and to secrete conjugated bilirubin into bile. Secretion of conjugated bilirubin into bile canaliculi is an energy-dependent process and is the rate-limiting step in bilirubin excretion in most species.
2. Decreased uptake, conjugation, or secretion of bilirubin by hepatocytes as a consequence of diffuse, severe hepatic disease, whether acute or chronic.
3. Reduced outflow of bile **(cholestasis).** Cholestasis refers to reduced canalicular flow of bile, which occurs as a consequence of either obstruction of the bile ducts (extrahepatic cholestasis) or impairment of bile flow within canaliculi (intrahepatic cholestasis). **Extrahepatic cholestasis** is a consequence of mechanical obstruction of bile flow, as can occur with choleliths or foreign body obstructions (such as a parasite within the bile duct), neoplasms that compress or constrict the duct, or inflammatory or reparative processes that result in fibrosis that subsequently constricts the lumen of the duct and reduces or prevents outflow of bile. Extrahepatic obstruction initially leads to distention of the bile ducts proximal to the obstruction, and eventually, to progressive retrograde distention of the intrahepatic ductal system. Within the lobule, changes are first obvious within the portal tracts and only later does plugging of canaliculi and stasis of bile occur within the cytoplasm of hepatocytes. Chronic extrahepatic cholestasis may result in extensive hepatic fibrosis (biliary fibrosis) that is centered on the portal tracts (Fig. 2-3). Distention of canaliculi may, on occasion, lead to rupture and extravasation of bile, thereby resulting in focal areas of hepatocellular necrosis. In contrast, **intrahepatic cholestasis** is commonly associated with a variety of disorders of hepatocytes, because these cells form the walls of the canaliculus. Intrahepatic cholestasis commences where bile flow originates, that is, in centrilobular areas; and as bile accumulates, the canaliculi become distended and bile pigments discolor the cytoplasm of adjacent hepatocytes (Fig. 2-4). In domestic animals, intrahepatic cholestasis usually results from hepatocyte dysfunction as a consequence of a wide variety of insults (toxic, infectious, metabolic, and ischemic), all of which can inhibit membrane-bound and cytoplasmic enzymes that facilitate metabolism of either bile acids or bilirubin and secretion of bile.

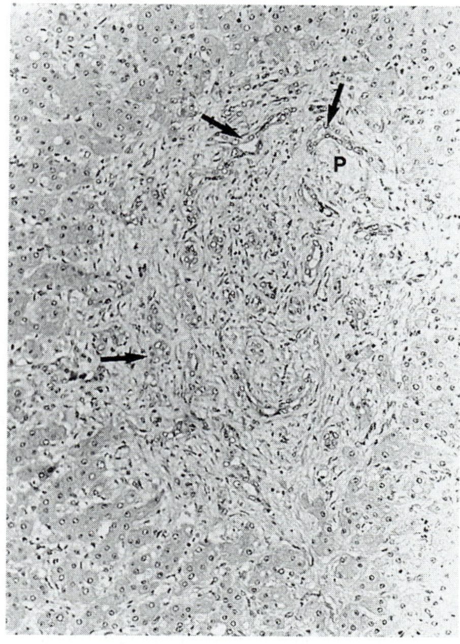

Fig. 2-3 Liver; horse. Chronic extrahepatic cholestasis caused by cholelithiasis. There is reduplication of bile ducts (*arrows*) and extensive fibrosis (biliary fibrosis) throughout the portal tract (*P*) as a consequence of prolonged stasis and subsequent leakage of bile. Hematoxylin-eosin (H & E) stain.

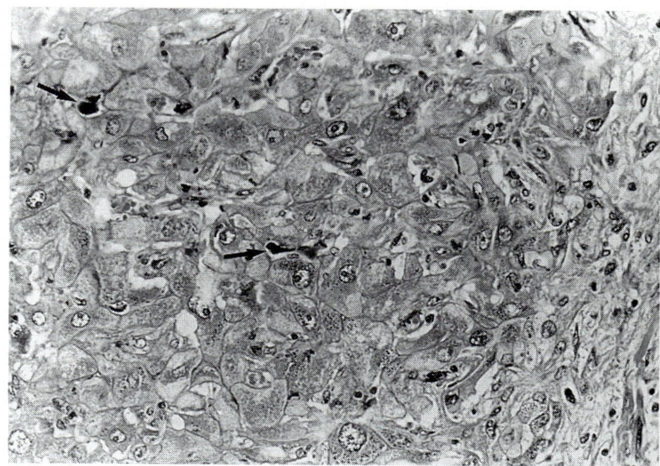

Fig. 2-4 Liver; horse. Intrahepatic cholestasis associated with pyrrolizidine alkaloid intoxication. Note that the canaliculi are grossly distended with bile (*arrows*). H & E stain.

Obviously, hepatic dysfunction is not the only cause of hyperbilirubinemia and icterus. In fact, icterus in ruminants is usually a consequence of severe intravascular hemolysis and, less often, a sequela to hepatic damage. Horses, however, often manifest icterus with acute hepatic dysfunction, but icterus may or may not occur in horses with chronic hepatic disease. Interestingly, "physiologic icterus" is also common in the horse, and deprivation of feed for relatively short intervals can produce icterus because of decreased uptake of bilirubin by hepatocytes. Icterus in carnivores occurs as a consequence of either hemolysis or hepatic dysfunction. Complete obstruction of bile outflow in any species can lead to extrahepatic cholestasis and icterus. However, in the dog, obstruction of the common duct does not always lead to icterus because of the supernumerary ducts.

Hepatic encephalopathy

Hepatic failure as a consequence of hepatic dysfunction can result in a metabolic disorder of the central nervous system that is termed hepatic encephalopathy (synonym: hepatic coma or **portosystemic encephalopathy**). Neurologic manifestations vary from depression and other behavioral changes to mania and convulsions. Undetermined as yet are the specific metabolites that cause the neurologic dysfunction, but amines absorbed from the GI tract are probably responsible. These products are absorbed from the intestines into the portal blood, but if they gain access to the systemic circulation, they can exert toxic effects on the brain. Failure of the liver to remove these toxic metabolites may result from either hepatic failure or shunting of portal blood directly into the systemic circulation without passage through the liver. Hepatic encephalopathy is common in ruminants and horses with hepatic failure and in dogs with congenital portosystemic shunts.

Metabolic disturbances of hepatic failure

Animals with hepatic failure can manifest a variety of metabolic disturbances. These may be influenced by the type and duration of the hepatic disorder.

Bleeding tendencies. Bleeding tendencies (hemorrhagic diathesis) sometimes accompany hepatic failure, as fibrinogen, prothrombin, and several other clotting factors are manufactured by the liver. The half-life of these factors is relatively short, so hemorrhage can occur as a consequence of acute hepatic failure. Acute hepatic failure may also precipitate disseminated intravascular coagulation that can itself cause hemorrhagic diathesis. Acute hepatic failure in the horse, and perhaps in other species, is sometimes accompanied by severe intravascular hemolysis, the cause of which is undetermined.

Hypoalbuminemia. Hypoalbuminemia can occur in association with severe, diffuse hepatic disease as a consequence of both decreased hepatic production of albumin and, because of portal hypertension, increased loss of albumin in ascitic fluid or into the intestinal tract. Hypoalbuminemia, as a consequence of hepatic dysfunction, usually reflects severe chronic liver disease, because of the relatively long half-life of plasma albumin (which ranges from 8 days in dogs to 21 days in cattle) and the time necessary for portal hypertension to develop.

Vascular and hemodynamic alterations of hepatic failure. Chronic hepatic injury typically is accompanied by extensive diffuse fibrosis of the liver, which increases resistance to blood flow through the liver. This, in turn, elevates pressure within the portal vein (portal hypertension). With time, collateral vascular channels open to allow blood in the portal vein to bypass the abnormal liver (acquired portosystemic vascular anastomoses that connect the portal vein and its tributaries to the systemic venous circulation). In addition, in some species, the increased pressure within the hepatic vasculature causes transudation of fluid (modified transudate) into the peritoneal cavity to produce ascites. Transudation of fluid into the peritoneal cavity is enhanced by the decreased colloid osmotic pressure of plasma that accompanies hypoalbuminemia as a consequence of accelerated loss and reduced hepatic synthesis of plasma proteins. Ascites associated with chronic liver disease (end-stage liver disease) occurs most commonly in dogs and cats, occasionally in sheep, and rarely in horses and cattle.

Photosensitization. Injury to the cutaneous tissues resulting from activation of photodynamic pigments by ultraviolet light present in the sun's rays is called photosensitization. Cutaneous lesions typically are limited to hairless skin, and to lightly or nonpigmented areas of skin in particular. Sources of photodynamic pigments that can induce photosensitization include those from plants and certain drugs, and only in hepatogenous (secondary) photosensitization is hepatic dysfunction responsible for photosensitization.

1. **Primary photosensitization** is the disease that occurs after some primary (preformed) photodynamic agent is deposited in tissues following its absorption into the blood after ingestion. Certain plants such as Saint-John's-wort (*Hypericum perforatum*) and pharmaceutic agents such as phenothiazine contain compounds that are photodynamic. Lesions are described in Chapter 11.
2. **Hepatogenous** or **secondary photosensitization** occurs in herbivores when hepatic dysfunction or biliary obstruction impairs normal excretion of phylloerythrin in bile. Phylloerythrin, a photodynamic agent, is produced from the chlorophyll contained in ingested plants by microflora of the GI tract of herbivores. Phylloerythrin is normally absorbed from the intestines and excreted in bile, using the same pathway as bilirubin; thus, hepatocellular dysfunction or biliary obstruction prevents normal excretion and allows high concentrations of phylloerythrin to accumulate in blood and cutaneous tissues. Hepatic pho-

tosensitivity is a consequence of the increased serum concentration of phylloerythrin, and this may occur in either acute or chronic hepatic disease.

3. **Congenital porphyria** is a metabolic disorder that occurs in several species, including cattle and cats, that results in accumulation of porphyrins, which are themselves photodynamic.

Developmental Anomalies and Incidental Findings

Developmental anomalies of the liver occur in domestic animals, although most are of little consequence.

Congenital cysts

These cysts can be found within the livers of all domestic species, and are usually an incidental finding. The potential origins of congenital cysts include the intrahepatic bile ducts and the hepatic capsule. Although these cysts are considered to be congenital anomalies, they can be found in animals of any age (Fig. 2-5). There is some uncertainty as to whether cysts that occur within the liver of adult cats, which typically are multiple and affect extensive areas of the liver, are developmental anomalies or benign cystic neoplasms (Figs. 2-5 and 2-6). Congenital polycystic liver disease, characterized by numerous epithelial-lined cysts in the liver and kidneys, occurs in the dog, and the Cairn terrier is predisposed. Congenital cysts must be distinguished from parasitic cysts, particularly cysticerci.

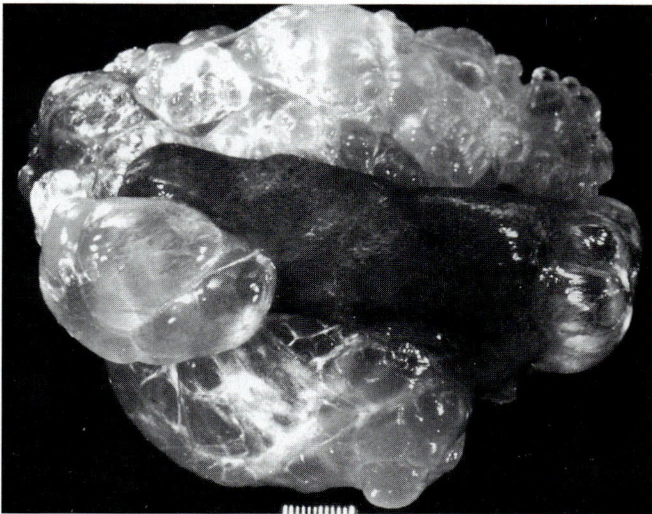

Fig. 2-5 Liver; cat. Multilobular biliary cysts have replaced much of the parenchyma in the affected portion of liver.

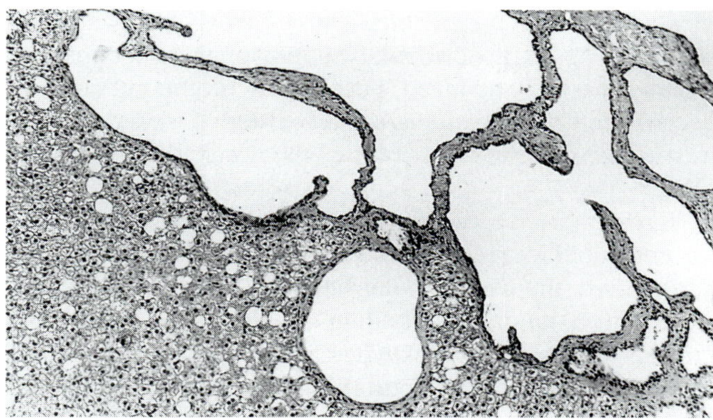

Fig. 2-6 Liver, biliary cysts; cat. Note that the biliary cysts are lined by a single layer of biliary epithelium. H & E stain.

Hepatic displacement

Displacement of the liver into the thoracic cavity is encountered in congenital diaphragmatic hernias but can be a sequela to trauma.

Tension lipidosis

Discrete, pale areas of parenchyma at the liver margins are common in cattle and horses (Figs. 2-7 and 2-8). These foci typically occur adjacent to the insertion of a ligament (serosal) attachment, and it is proposed that these attachments impede blood supply to the subjacent hepatic parenchyma by exerting tension on the capsule. Affected hepatocytes most probably accumulate fat within their cytoplasm (fatty degeneration) as a consequence of hypoxia.

Capsular fibrosis

Discrete fibrous tags or plaques are frequently present on the diaphragmatic surface of the liver and on the adjacent diaphragm of the horse (Fig. 2-9). Resolution of nonseptic peritonitis, rather than of parasitic nematode migration tracts, has been proposed as the cause of these regions of capsular fibrosis.

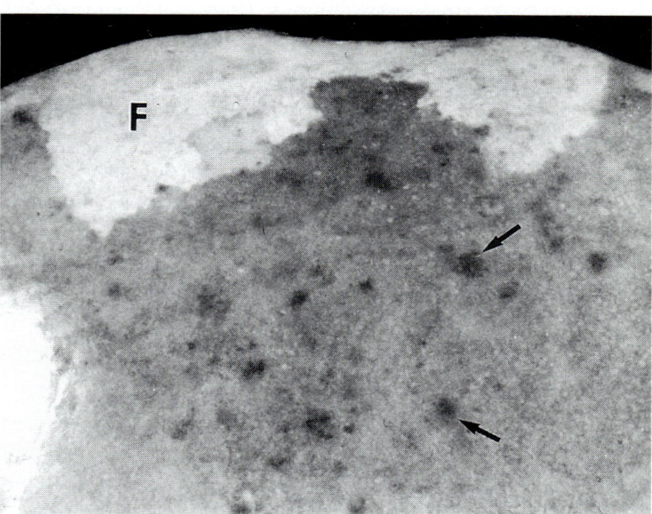

Fig. 2-7 Liver, capsular surface; cow. Tension lipidosis. Note the pale area of fatty infiltration (*F*) and scattered areas of telangiectasis (*arrows*).

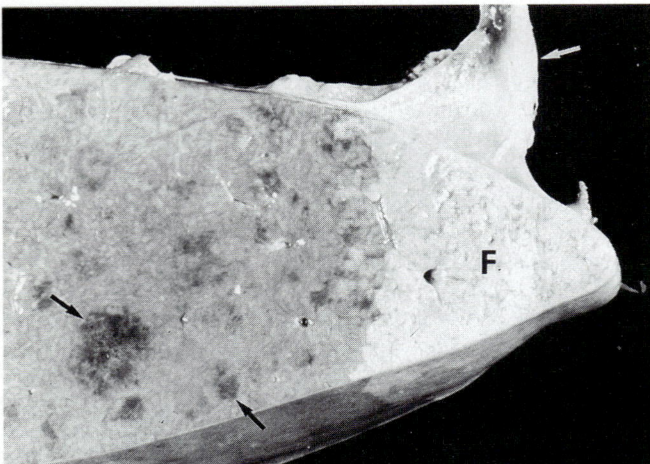

Fig. 2-8 Liver, cut surface; cow. Tension lipidosis. Area of fatty infiltration (*F*) adjacent to mesenteric attachment adjacent to the affected portion (*white arrow*). Areas of telangiectasis are indicated by the black arrows.

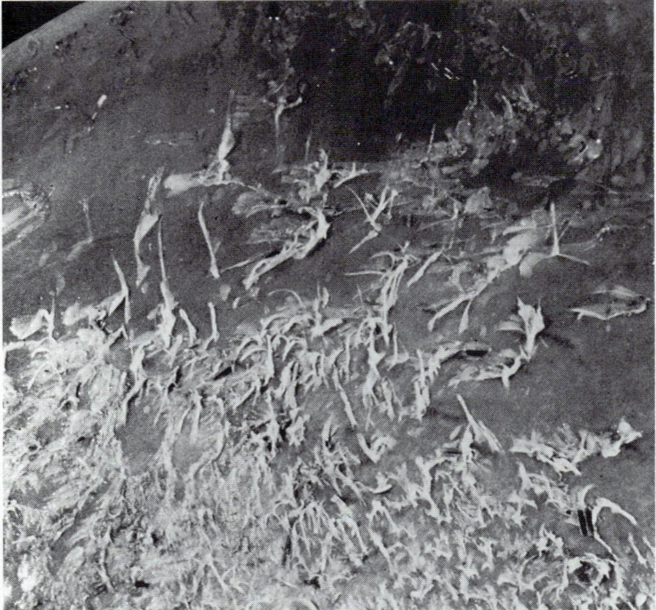

Fig. 2-9 Liver, diaphragmatic surface; horse. Capsular fibrosis. Note the fibrous tags scattered across the capsule.

Postmortem Change

Autolysis of the liver occurs rapidly and can be advanced before it is obvious in most other tissues. Bacteria released from the GI tract rapidly proliferate in the liver after death. This process is especially rapid in large animals, particularly cattle and pigs during hot weather. Pale areas appear on the capsular surface as bacterial degradation begins. In time, the organ becomes a green-blue as bacteria degrade blood pigments to hydrogen sulfide. The liver near the gallbladder is quickly discolored by bile pigment. The normal consistency of the organ is rapidly lost, and gas bubbles may form beneath the capsule and in the parenchyma from bacterial fermentation.

Hemodynamic and Vascular Disorders of the Liver

The liver has high metabolic activity, which renders it susceptible to anoxia. Oxygen is carried to the liver by both the portal vein and hepatic artery. Although approximately 80% of the hepatic blood supply derives from the portal vein and 20% via the hepatic artery, the oxygen supply is approximately equal from the two sources.

The liver and anemia

The centrilobular (periacinar) region receives blood last; thus, it is the least oxygenated, and the effects of hypoxia are usually manifested first in this area. Acute severe anemia, regardless of cause, can cause centrilobular degeneration and even necrosis of hepatocytes. This typically occurs in severe anemias of precipitous onset. Chronic anemia can result in atrophy of centrilobular hepatocytes with accompanying dilatation and congestion of sinusoids. Livers from animals with severe anemia, whether acute or chronic, typically have an enhanced lobular pattern (see Figs. 2-21 and 2-22) that is evident on both the capsular and cut surfaces of the organ (see description of enhanced lobular pattern in the next section).

Passive hepatic congestion

Right-sided heart failure produces elevated pressure within the caudal vena cava and, subsequently, the hepatic vein and its tributaries. Passive congestion may be either acute or chronic, and the appearance of the liver differs with the duration and severity of the congestion. Passive congestion initially causes distention of central veins and centrilobular sinusoids. Persistent centrilobular hypoxia leads to atrophy or loss of hepatocytes and, eventually, to fibrosis about central veins.

Acute congestion of the liver produces slight enlargement of the organ, and blood flows freely from any cut surface. The intrinsic lobular pattern of the liver may be slightly more pronounced, particularly on the cut surface, because centrilobular areas are congested (dark red) in contrast to the more normal color of the remainder of the lobule.

Chronic passive congestion leads to persistent hypoxia in centrilobular areas, and, because of oxygen and nutrient deprivation, the centrilobular hepatocytes atrophy, degenerate, or eventually may undergo necrosis. As a result, sinusoids in these areas are dilated and congested and grossly appear red, whereas periportal hepatocytes frequently undergo fatty degeneration because of hypoxia, thereby causing this area of the lobule to appear yellow. The result is accentuation of the lobular pattern of the liver, referred to

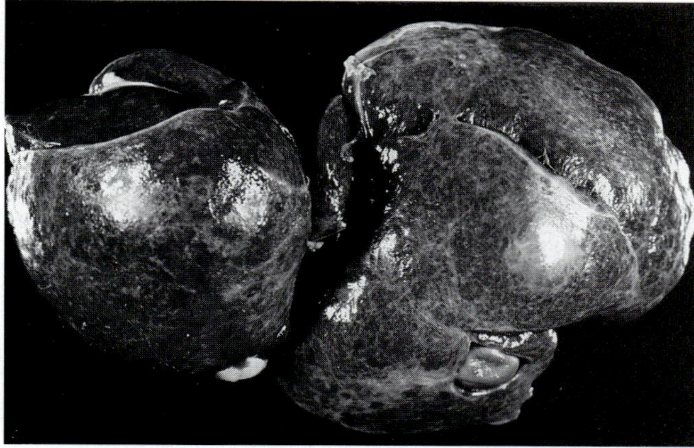

Fig. 2-10 Liver, diaphragmatic surfaces, dog. Chronic passive hepatic congestion. The liver is enlarged and has rounded margins. *Courtesy Dr. K. Sokoe*

as an enhanced lobular or reticular pattern. It is especially evident on the cut surface of the liver, and the enhanced lobular pattern that occurs with severe chronic passive congestion has been likened to the appearance of the cut surface of a nutmeg, and so is termed the **nutmeg liver.** This pattern is not unique to passive congestion, however, and is encountered with other processes, such as zonal hepatic necrosis. In addition to an enhanced lobular pattern, chronic passive congestion is characterized by rounding of the margins of the liver, focal fibrous thickening of the capsule, and, in severe cases, widespread hepatic fibrosis, particularly around central veins (Figs. 2-10 to 2-12).

Passive congestion of the liver can occur in any species and is almost always the consequence of cardiac dysfunction. Chronic passive congestion is particularly common in aged dogs and occurs in association with endocardiosis (mucoid degeneration) of the right atrioventricular valve. Acute passive congestion, on the other hand, can occur as a consequence of acute right heart failure, which has a wide variety of causes. Far less common is passive congestion of the liver occurring as a result of partial or complete occlusion of the hepatic veins (Budd-Chiari syndrome) or the adjacent caudal vena cava.

Portosystemic shunts

Portosystemic vascular anastomoses or "shunts" can be either congenital or acquired and intrahepatic or extrahepatic in location. Shunts are vascular channels that allow blood within the portal venous system to bypass the liver and to drain into the systemic circulation. Thus, blood within the portal vein drains, indirectly or directly, into either the caudal vena cava or the azygous vein. Acquired portosystemic shunts are a consequence of persistent portal hypertension, usually as a sequela to advanced hepatic disease or, less often, to portal vein obstruction. In severe cases, numerous distended, thin-walled veins may connect the mesenteric veins and the caudal vena cava (Fig. 2-13).

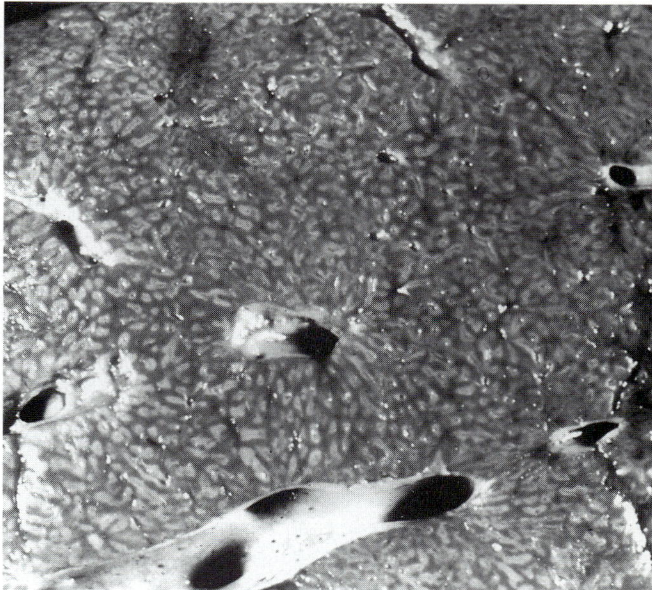

Fig. 2-11 Liver, cut surface; cow. Chronic passive hepatic congestion secondary to severe fibrinous pericarditis. Note enhanced lobular (nutmeg) pattern. The irregular light gray foci are portal tracts. The hepatic parenchyma between the portal tracts is congested. *Courtesy Dr. C. Miller*

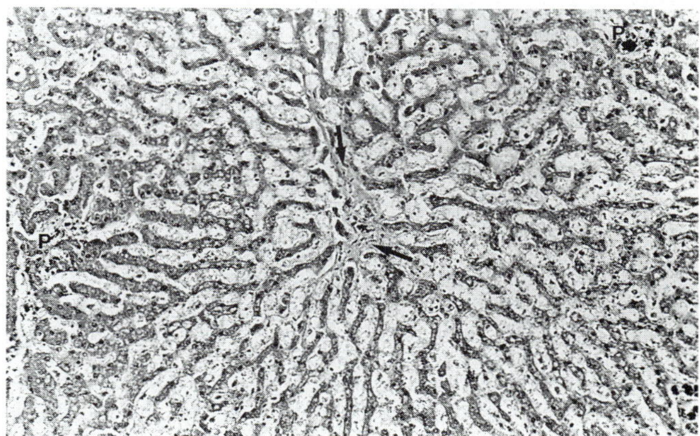

Fig. 2-12 Liver; dog. Chronic passive hepatic congestion. Hepatic fibrosis is most severe in centrilobular areas (*arrows*). The central vein is encircled with connective tissue. Adjacent hepatic plates are atrophic, and sinusoids are excessively dilated. Hepatic plates are of relatively normal thickness around the portal tracts (*P*). H & E stain.

Congenital portosystemic shunts have been described in several species, but occur most commonly in the dog and cat. A variety of different shunts have been described, including persistence of the fetal ductus venosus, portal vein to caudal vena cava anastomoses, and portal vein to azy-

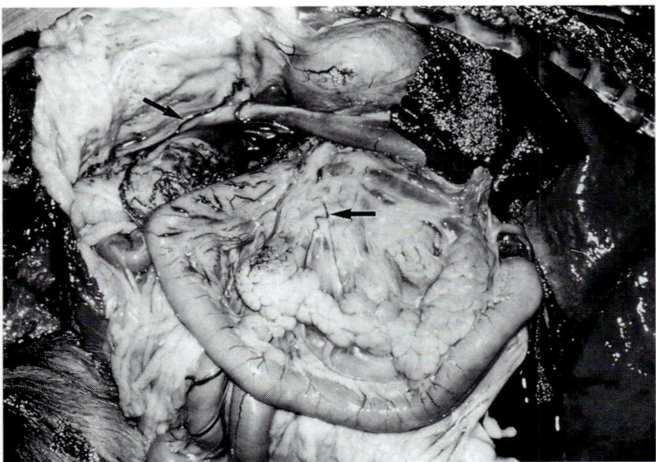

Fig. 2-13 Abdomen; dog. Acquired portosystemic anastomoses secondary to portal hypertension and subsequent to chronic passive congestion. Numerous prominent veins (*arrows*) within the mesentery allow blood in the portal venous system to bypass the liver and directly enter the systemic circulation. *Courtesy Dr. R. Fairley*

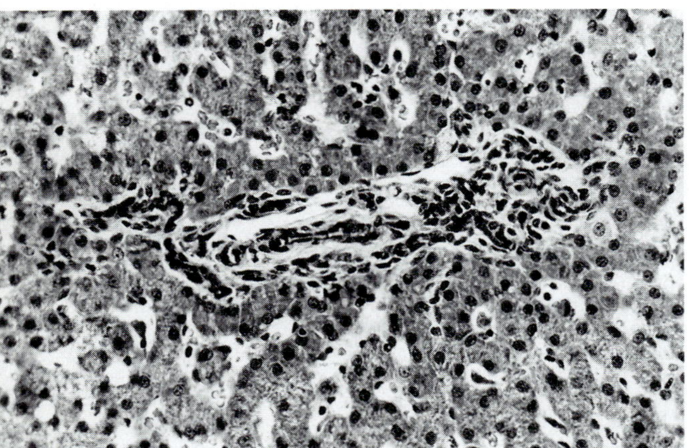

Fig. 2-14 Liver; dog. Congenital portosystemic vascular anastomosis. Numerous unperfused blood vessels are present within the portal tract. H & E stain.

gous vein anastomoses. Affected animals are typically stunted and frequently have signs of hepatic encephalopathy. The liver is small and may have a characteristic histologic appearance of lobular atrophy and reduplication of arterioles and small veins located within the portal triads (Fig. 2-14). The vascular anastomoses are often difficult to identify without benefit of antemortem radiographic studies.

Arterioportal shunts (anastomoses)

Arterioportal shunts, either acquired or congenital, occur in the dog and cat, are direct communications between the hepatic artery and branches of the portal vein, and may occur anywhere within the liver. Shunting of blood may lead to portal hypertension and subsequent development of acquired portocaval shunts and ascites; clinical signs are probably the result of the portosystemic shunting of blood.

Telangiectasis

Telangiectasis means the marked dilatation of sinusoids in areas where hepatocytes have been lost. These areas appear as variably sized dark blue foci within the liver (see Figs. 2-7 and 2-8). Telangiectasis is particularly common in cattle and, apparently, is of no clinical significance.

Infarction

Infarction of the liver occurs infrequently because of the organ's dual blood supply from the hepatic artery and portal vein. Infarcts are usually sharply delineated and may be either dark red or pale. They tend to occur at the margins of the liver. Torsion of individual lobes of the liver also occurs infrequently, and the resultant vascular occlusion produces infarction of the affected lobe.

Hepatic venoocclusive disease

The distinctive lesion of this syndrome is characterized by intimal thickening and occlusion of the central vein by fibrous connective tissue. The consequence is passive hepatic congestion and resultant hepatic injury, which may progress to hepatic failure and its associated constellation of signs. The lesion is not etiologically specific, but can follow pyrrolizidine alkaloid or aflatoxin-induced hepatic injury. An extremely high incidence is recognized in captive exotic cats such as cheetahs, possibly because of the ingestion of large amounts of vitamin A.

Metabolic Disturbances and Hepatic Accumulations

Hepatic lipidosis or fatty liver

Lipids are normally transported to the liver from adipose tissue and the GI tract in the form of either free fatty acids or chylomicrons, respectively. Within hepatocytes, free fatty acids are esterified to triglycerides that are complexed with apoproteins to form low-density lipoproteins, and these are released into the plasma as a readily available energy source for a variety of tissues. Some oxidation of fatty acids for energy production occurs within hepatocytes, and some fatty acids are converted to phospholipid and cholesterol esters. With the exception of that of ruminants, the liver also actively produces lipids from amino acids and glucose.

The presence of excessive lipid within the liver is termed hepatic lipidosis or fatty liver and occurs when the rate of triglyceride accumulation within hepatocytes exceeds either their rate of metabolic degradation or their release as lipoproteins. Fatty liver is obviously not a specific disease entity, but can occur as a sequela to a variety of perturbations of normal lipid metabolism. The potential mechanisms responsible for excessive accumulation of fat within the liver include the following:

1. Excessive entry of fatty acids into the liver, which occurs as a consequence of excessive dietary intake of fat or increased mobilization of triglycerides from adipose tissue due to increased demand (e.g., lactation, starvation, and endocrine abnormalities)
2. Abnormal hepatocyte function leading to accumulation of triglycerides within hepatocytes as a result of decreased oxidation of fatty acids within hepatocytes
3. Excessive dietary intake of carbohydrates resulting in the synthesis of increased amounts of fatty acids with formation of excessive triglycerides within hepatocytes
4. Increased esterification of fatty acids to triglycerides
5. Decreased apoprotein synthesis and subsequent decreased production and export of lipoprotein from hepatocytes
6. Impaired secretion of lipoprotein from the liver

It must be stressed that these are potential mechanisms (some being more significant than others) and that more than one defect might occur in any given hepatic disorder. Regardless of cause, the gross appearance of the fatty liver is highly characteristic. With progressive accumulation of lipid, the liver enlarges and becomes yellow (Fig. 2-15). In mild cases, lipids may accumulate only in specific portions of each lobule, such as centrilobular regions, thereby imparting an enhanced lobular pattern to the liver. In extreme cases, the entire liver is affected, and the organ may become considerably enlarged and have an extremely greasy texture. Lipid vacuoles are readily detected within the cytoplasm of hepatocytes (Fig. 2-16).

Specific causes and syndromes of fatty liver in domestic animals include the following:

1. Dietary causes of fatty liver include simple dietary excess in monogastric animals, such as a high-fat/high-cholesterol diet. Fatty liver is especially common in ruminants with high energy demands, such as those in peak lactation or late gestation, which reflects increased entry of lipids into the liver as a result of increased mobilization of lipids from adipose tissue. Obese animals are particularly predisposed to develop fatty livers as a consequence of dietary restriction. Deficiencies of cobalt and vitamin B_{12} have been implicated as causes of fatty liver in sheep and goats.
2. Toxic and anoxic causes of fatty liver are common. Sublethal (reversible) injury to hepatocytes frequently results in accumulation of lipid within the affected cell. Injury to hepatocytes can lead to accumulation of lipids because of decreased formation and/or export of lipoproteins by hepatocytes and decreased oxidation of fatty acids within hepatocytes.
3. Ketosis is a metabolic disease that results from impaired metabolism of carbohydrate and volatile fatty acids. Ketone bodies are derived from acetyl coenzyme A (acetyl-CoA), which is a normal intermediate in the oxidation of fatty acids. In pregnant and lactating animals, there is a continuous demand for glucose and amino acids, and ketosis results when fat metabolism, which occurs in response to the increased energy demands, becomes excessive. Ketosis is characterized by increased concentrations of ketone bodies in blood (hyperketonemia), hypoglycemia, and low concentrations of hepatic glycogen. Ketosis is common in ruminants and usually occurs during peak lactation whereas ketosis of sheep usually occurs in late gestation, particularly in ewes carrying twins; this latter disease is known as pregnancy toxemia.

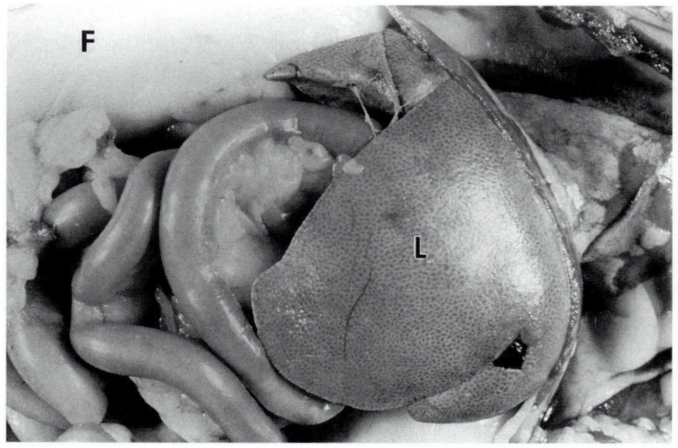

Fig. 2-15 Abdomen; cat. Idiopathic fatty liver syndrome. The liver (*L*) is swollen and yellow, and the animal has extensive fat deposits (*F*).

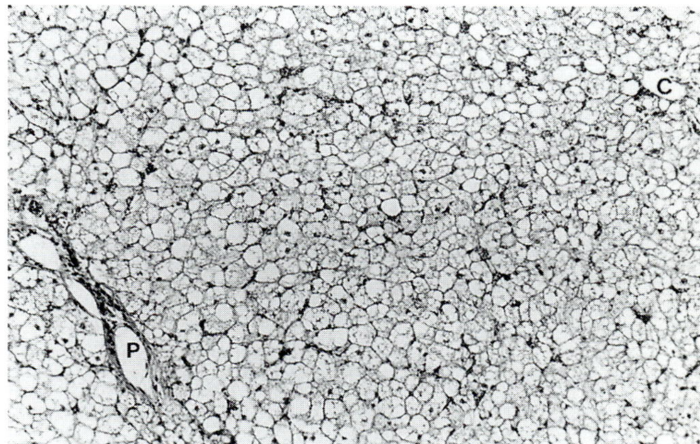

Fig. 2-16 Liver; cow. Ketosis. Diffuse cytoplasmic accumulation of lipid is evident within the hepatocytes throughout the liver. Terminal hepatic venule (*C*); portal tract (*P*). H & E stain.

4. Bovine fatty liver syndrome, also known as fatty liver disease, is mechanistically similar to ketosis. In dairy cattle, the disease is usually encountered in obese animals within a few days after parturition and is often precipitated by an event that causes anorexia such as retained placenta, metritis, mastitis, abomasal displacement, or parturient paresis. Typically, affected beef cattle are obese and the disease occurs within a few days before parturition. Accumulation of lipid within the liver is the result of both increased mobilization of lipids from adipose tissue, which results in increased influx of fatty acids to the liver, and decreased export of lipoprotein from the liver.
5. Feline fatty liver syndrome is a distinct syndrome of idiopathic hepatic lipidosis recognized in cats. Typically affected cats are obese and anorectic and have no other diseases that could cause hepatic lipidosis. Cats with this type of hepatic lipidosis (see Fig. 2-15) frequently develop hepatic failure, icterus, and subsequent hepatic encephalopathy.
6. Endocrine disorders, such as diabetes mellitus and hypothyroidism, can produce hepatic lipidosis in a variety of species. In these cases, hepatic lipidosis is obviously but one manifestation of abnormal metabolism. The accumulation of lipids in the liver in the diabetic animal is the result of increased fat mobilization and decreased utilization of lipids by injured hepatocytes.

Glycogen accumulation

Glucose is normally stored within hepatocytes as glycogen and is often present in large amounts after feeding. Excessive hepatic accumulation of glycogen occurs with the metabolic perturbations associated with diseases such as diabetes mellitus and the glycogen storage diseases, but, in these instances, hepatic involvement is just one manifestation of a systemic disease process.

Glucocorticoid-induced hepatocellular degeneration is a specific disorder characterized by excessive hepatic accumulation of glycogen. Excessive amounts of endogenous or exogenous glucocorticoids cause extensive swelling of hepatocytes owing to accumulation of glycogen. Glucocorticoids induce glycogen synthetase and so enhance hepatic storage of glycogen. Glycogen accumulation leads to pronounced swelling of hepatocytes (up to 10 times normal volume), particularly those in the midzonal areas (Fig. 2-17). In severe cases of glucocorticoid-induced hepatocellular degeneration (often referred to as steroid-induced hepatopathy), the liver is enlarged and pale, but otherwise unremarkable. The disorder occurs in dogs, and frequently is iatrogenic, but can also be a consequence of hyperadrenocorticism. The diagnosis can be confirmed on the basis of the characteristic microscopic appearance of the liver and identification of the source of the excess glucocorticoids.

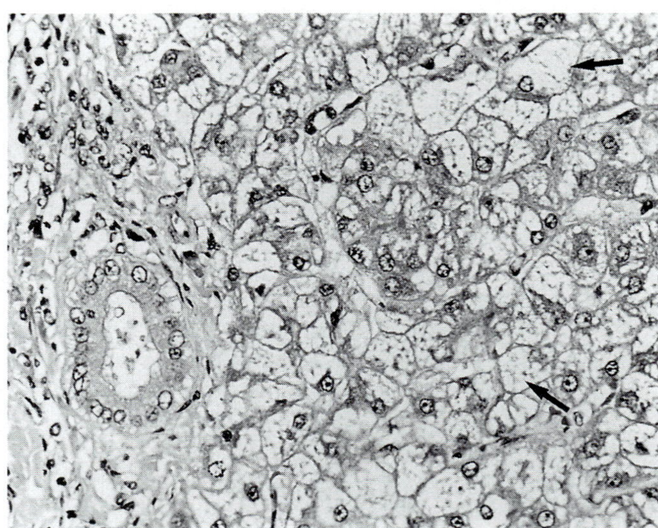

Fig. 2-17 Liver; dog. Glucocorticoid-induced hepatopathy. The swollen hepatocytes (*arrows*) have extensive cytoplasmic vacuoles. H & E stain.

Amyloidosis

Amyloid is a protein that consists of β-pleated sheets of nonbranching fibrils. Several distinct protein precursors of amyloid have been identified, but amyloid deposited in the liver is usually derived from either immunoglobulin light chains (amyloid AL) or a serum protein synthesized by the liver (amyloid AA). Hepatic amyloidosis probably occurs in most species of domestic animals. Hepatic amyloidosis usually occurs as a consequence of prolonged antigenic stimulation such as chronic infection or repeated inoculations of an antigen, and it usually accumulates in the space of Disse.

Amyloid deposits can produce varying degrees of hepatomegaly, and extensive accumulations cause the liver to appear pale. In severe cases, affected animals may have clinical signs of either hepatic dysfunction or failure. Frequently, amyloid is also deposited within the kidneys. Renal failure may occur before signs of hepatic dysfunction are manifested.

Copper accumulation

Copper poisoning is included as a metabolic disorder because hepatic injury in copper poisoning of domestic animals frequently is the result of progressive accumulation of copper within the liver. This occurs in domestic animals, especially sheep, in which storage of copper is poorly regulated. Also, hereditary disorders of copper metabolism have been described in dogs.

Copper is an essential trace element of all cells, but even a modest excess of copper can be life threatening because copper must be properly sequestered to avoid toxicosis. In domestic animals, copper toxicosis usually occurs as a consequence of one of the following:

1. Simple dietary excess in ruminants, occurring, for example, from excessive dietary supplementation as an overcorrection for copper deficiency or from contamination of pasture with copper from sprays or fertilizer.
2. Grazing animals on pastures with normal concentrations of copper, but with inadequate concentrations of molybdenum.
3. Pasturing herbivores on fields with plants that contain hepatotoxic phytotoxins, usually pyrrolizidine alkaloids. *Heliotropium* and *Senecio* species are common examples of such plants. Copper is excreted in the bile, and hepatic diseases that result in cholestasis are particularly likely to produce excessive accumulation of copper within the liver, even when dietary intake of copper is not excessive.
4. Hereditary disorders of copper metabolism, as occur in Bedlington and West Highland white terriers. Impaired excretion of copper leads to its progressive accumulation within the liver.

The consequences of excessive accumulation of copper within the liver of domestic animals are species-dependent. In ruminants, particularly sheep, copper accumulates within the liver over a period of time (for one of the first three reasons listed above), but some event triggers sudden release of copper, which is followed by acute, severe intravascular hemolysis and hepatocellular necrosis. Necrosis of the liver is extensive and affects centrilobular and midzonal regions most consistently, but massive necrosis can occur. Despite the acute and fulminant nature of the terminal event, this process is referred to as **chronic copper poisoning** to distinguish it from disease associated with simple copper intoxication, which causes gastroenteritis. In contrast, copper continues to accumulate in the liver of dogs with hereditary metabolic disorders of copper metabolism and leads to ongoing necrosis of hepatocytes, chronic inflammation, replacement fibrosis, and eventually to an end-stage liver and signs of hepatic failure (see Fig. 2-26). Excessive concentrations of hepatic copper may be present in other breeds of dog with increased incidence of chronic liver disease, including the Doberman pinscher, Skye terrier, cocker spaniel, and Labrador retriever, although the significance of copper in the hepatic disease of these breeds of dog is uncertain. These diseases are discussed in the section on canine chronic-active hepatitis.

Pigment accumulation

Pigments are colored substances, some of which are normal cellular constituents, while others accumulate only in abnormal circumstances.

1. **Bile pigments** may accumulate in excessive amounts as a consequence of either extrahepatic or intrahepatic cholestasis and typically produce icterus and green discoloration of the liver.
2. **Hemosiderin** is an iron-containing, golden-brown, granular pigment derived from ferritin, the primary iron storage protein. As iron accumulates within the cell, degraded aggregates of ferritin molecules form hemosiderin. Most hemosiderin in Kupffer cells and other macrophages located in tissues throughout the body is derived from breakdown of erythrocytes, whereas most hepatocellular hemosiderin is derived from iron present in transferrin and to a lesser extent hemoglobin. Hemosiderin forms in the liver when there is local or systemic excess of iron such as when erythrocytic breakdown is excessive (e.g., hemolytic anemia), and within areas of hepatic necrosis. In contrast, hemochromatosis is an abnormal increased storage of iron within the body associated with hepatic dysfunction. Marked accumulation of iron can produce a dark brown or even a black liver.
3. **Lipofuscin** is an insoluble pigment that is yellow-brown to dark brown and is derived from incomplete oxidation of lipids such as those in cell membranes. Lipofuscin is progressively oxidized with time; thus, it actually is a group of lipid pigments, all of which consist of polymers of lipid, phospholipid, and protein. **Ceroid** is the earliest form of lipofuscin, and the least oxidized. Amounts of lipofuscin present in the liver tend to increase with age.
4. **Melanin** is an endogenous pigment that is dark brown or black. Benign disorders of melanin pigmentation are usually designated as **melanosis.** Congenital melanosis of the liver occurs in swine and ruminants and produces variably sized areas of discoloration of the liver. Acquired ''melanosis'' of sheep has been described in Australia and is associated with the ingestion of certain plants.
5. **Liver flukes** specifically produce a very dark excreta that contains a mixture of iron and porphyrin. This excreta produces the characteristic discoloration of bile that occurs in fascioliasis *(Fasciola hepatica),* and is especially pronounced in the migratory tracts produced by *Fascioloides magna.*

Hepatic Injury and Inflammation

The high metabolic rate of hepatocytes renders them extremely susceptible to cellular degeneration and necrosis. This section will consider the patterns of hepatic degeneration, responses of the liver to injury, and inflammation of the liver and will conclude with descriptions of various infectious and toxic disorders of the liver in domestic animals.

Patterns of hepatocellular degeneration and necrosis

Although the liver is subjected to a wide variety of different insults, resultant cellular degeneration and/or necrosis invariably occurs in one of three morphologic patterns.

Random hepatocellular degeneration and/or necrosis. This pattern is characterized by the presence either of single cell necrosis throughout the liver or multifocal aggregates of necrotic hepatocytes. These areas are scattered randomly throughout the liver; there is no predictable location within lobules. This pattern is typical of many infectious agents, including the protozoan *Toxoplasma gondii,* and certain viruses and bacteria. Lesions may be obvious grossly as discrete pale or, less often, dark red foci that are sharply delineated from the adjacent parenchyma (Figs. 2-18 to 2-20). The size of such foci is variable, ranging from tiny (<1 mm) to several centimeters. Hepatocytes in affected areas are either degenerated or necrotic.

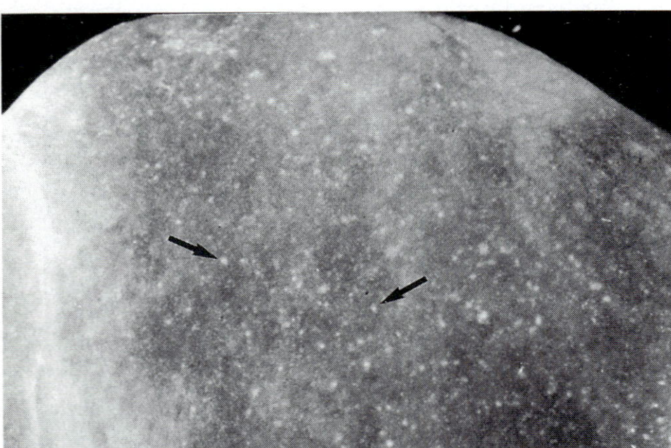

Fig. 2-18 Liver; foal. Random hepatic necrosis in a foal with septicemia caused by *E. coli.* Multiple pale foci of necrosis are evident on the capsular surface (*arrows*). *Courtesy Dr. K. Thompson.*

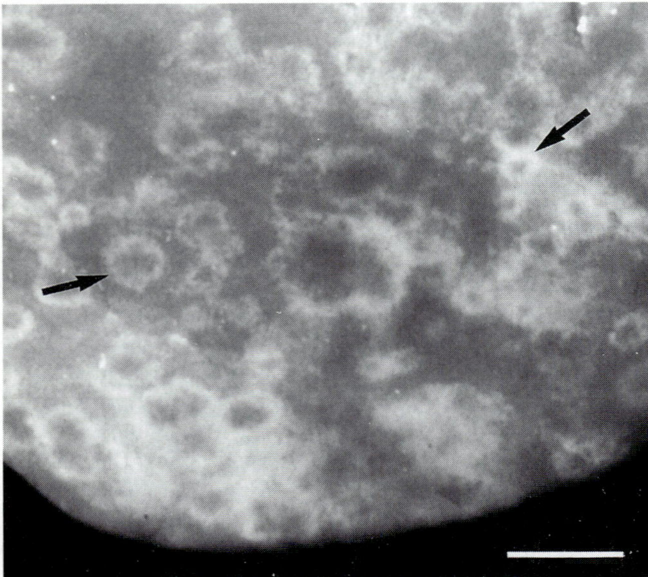

Fig. 2-19 Liver; lamb. Random hepatic necrosis in an aborted lamb caused by *Campylobacter fetus* infection. Arrows indicate areas of necrosis. Bar = 1 cm. *Courtesy Dr. B. Johnson.*

Zonal hepatocellular degeneration and/or necrosis. Zonal hepatocellular degeneration or, as it is more simply termed, zonal change, affects hepatocytes within defined areas of the hepatic lobule. The zones are centrilobular (periacinar), midzonal (between centrilobular and periportal areas), or periportal (centroacinar) areas. Extensive zonal change within the liver, regardless of location within the lobule, typically produces a liver that is pale and modestly enlarged with rounded margins, has increased friability, and characteristically, has an enhanced lobular pattern on the capsular and cut surface of the organ (Figs. 2-21 and 2-22). Degenerated hepatocytes swell, and, when the majority of hepatocytes in a zone are affected, that portion of the lobule appears pale. In contrast, necrosis of hepatocytes in a particular zone of the lobule results in dilatation and

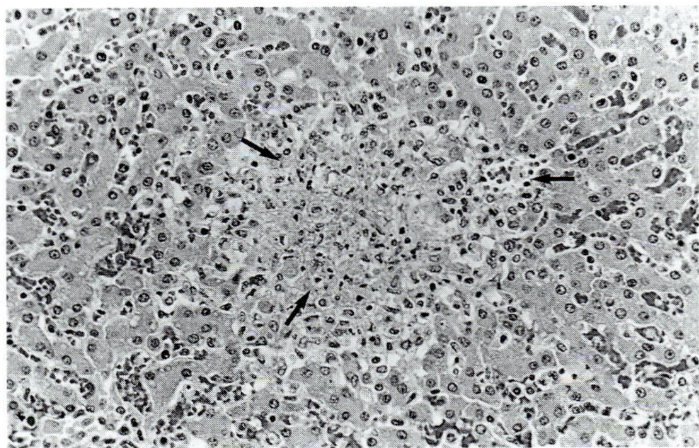

Fig. 2-20 Liver; horse. Random hepatic necrosis in an aborted fetus caused by equine herpesvirus. A focal area of necrosis is outlined by the arrows. H & E stain.

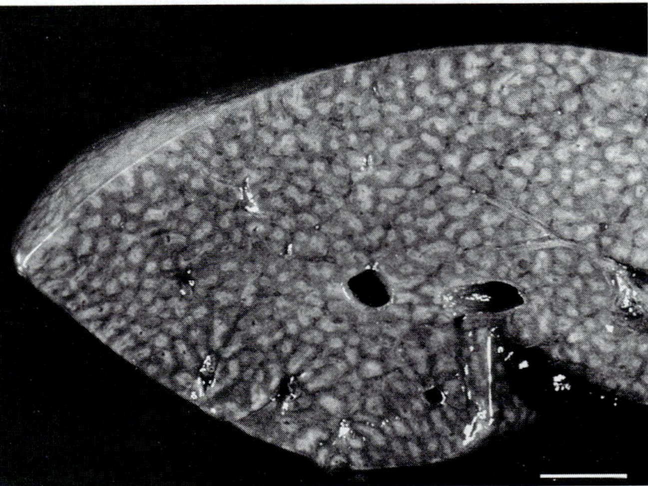

Fig. 2-21 Liver, cut surface; cat. Enhanced lobular pattern. Note accentuation of the normal lobular pattern. Bar = 5 mm. *Courtesy Dr. R. Fairley.*

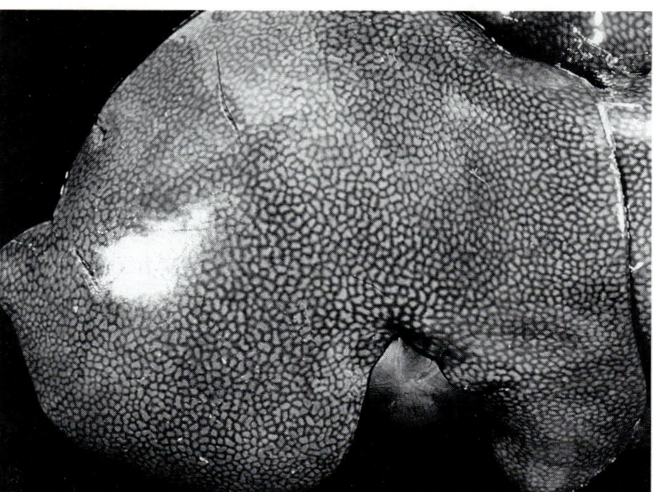

Fig. 2-22 Liver, diaphragmatic surface; cat. Enhanced lobular pattern. This is not a specific change, as it may be associated with zonal hepatocellular degeneration and/or necrosis (regardless of lobular location), passive congestion, and diffuse cellular infiltration within the liver (often reflecting disseminated cholangitis, diffuse portal hepatitis, or hepatic involvement with hematopoietic neoplasms, such as lymphosarcoma and myeloproliferative disorders).

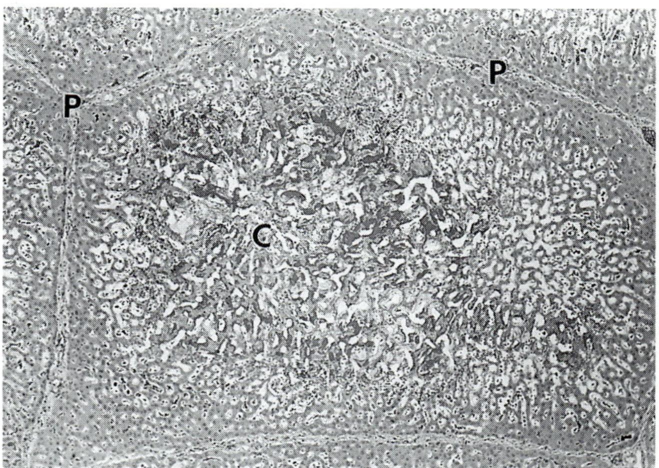

Fig. 2-23 Liver; pig. Centrilobular necrosis. Hepatocytes in centrilobular and midzonal areas have undergone coagulation necrosis (*C*), whereas those adjacent to portal tracts (*P*) appear normal. H & E stain.

congestion of sinusoids so that the affected zone appears red. Although zonal change typically produces an enhanced lobular pattern, microscopic examination is usually required to determine the type of zonal change. Specific forms of zonal change are described below.

1. **Centrilobular** degeneration and necrosis of hepatocytes are particularly common (Fig. 2-23), as this portion of the lobule receives the least oxygenated blood and is, therefore, susceptible to hypoxia, and it has the greatest enzymic activity (mono oxygenous) capable of activating compounds into toxic forms. Centrilobular necrosis can result from a precipitous severe anemia. Similarly, passive congestion of the liver produces stasis of blood and hypoxia of centrilobular areas.
2. Paracentral **(periacinar)** cellular degeneration is similar to centrilobular degeneration, but involves only a wedge around the central vein because only the periphery of one acinus is affected. As several acini border on a single central vein (terminal hepatic venule), changes induced by hypoxia may not be present equally in all acini, and, thus, hepatocytes at the periphery of one acinus can have more severe change than those in adjacent acini.
3. **Midzonal degeneration** and necrosis are unusual lesions in domestic animals but have been reported in pigs and horses with aflatoxicosis.
4. **Periportal degeneration** and necrosis are also uncommon, but may occur in certain toxic diseases such as phosphorus poisoning.

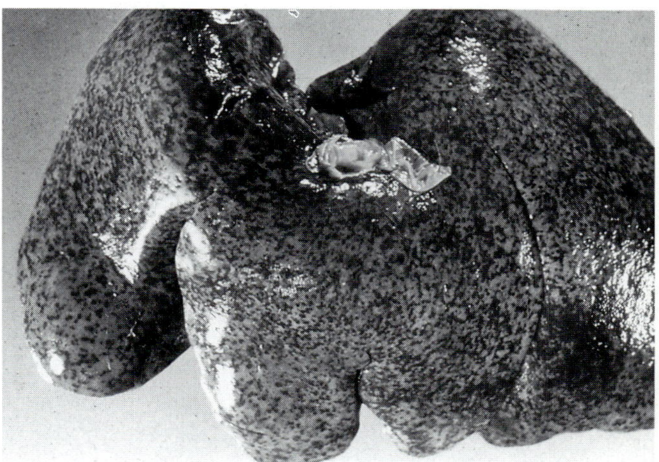

Fig. 2-24 Liver; pig. Hepatosis dietitica. Foci of massive necrosis appear as dark regions of different size that are scattered throughout the liver (*arrows*). *Courtesy Dr. R.L. Michel.*

5. **Bridging necrosis** is the result of confluence of areas of centrilobular necrosis (central bridging) or centrilobular areas to periportal areas.

Massive necrosis. This is not necessarily, as the name might be taken to imply, necrosis of the entire liver, but rather necrosis of an entire hepatic lobule or contiguous lobules. All hepatocytes are necrotic. The gross appearance of the liver varies. If the majority of the parenchyma is affected, the liver may be modestly increased in size with a smooth external surface and dark parenchyma because of extensive congestion. If the process is localized, the liver typically is small with a wrinkled capsule and depressed areas of parenchymal necrosis and vascular congestion scattered throughout the organ (Fig. 2-24). Microscopi-

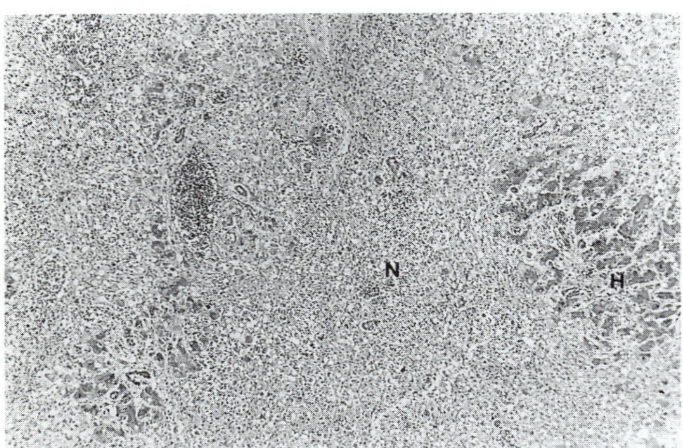

Fig. 2-25 Liver; dog. Massive hepatic necrosis in a dog with caval syndrome. Areas of complete hepatocellular necrosis (*N*) affecting entire lobules are adjacent to areas of viable hepatocytes (*H*). H & E stain.

cally, affected areas consist of blood-filled spaces within a connective tissue stroma devoid of hepatocytes (Fig. 2-25).

Response of the liver to injury

Following destruction of hepatic parenchyma, regeneration of parenchyma, replacement by fibrosis, and biliary hyperplasia may occur. The outcome of a given hepatic insult depends on the nature and duration of the insult, and if the host survives.

Regeneration. Regeneration is a common response because the liver has an enormous functional reserve and regenerative capacity. Experimentally, as much as two thirds of the liver can be excised from a healthy rat without signs of hepatic dysfunction and the liver is rapidly regenerated. Extensive hepatic necrosis is usually followed by parenchymal regeneration without scarring as long as the reticulin framework of the affected portion remains intact. However, in massive necrosis, the affected areas will collapse on removal of the dead hepatocytes, resulting in a scar (postnecrotic scarring). Even when necrosis of hepatocytes is continuous, the liver will attempt to regenerate its functional mass. However, prolonged regenerative effort often results in nodular proliferations of parenchyma that architecturally distort the liver.

Fibrosis. Fibrosis occurs in the liver as a response to necrosis and inflammation. Ongoing necrosis of hepatocytes that overwhelms the liver's regenerative capacity can be followed by replacement with fibrous tissue. Thus, fibrosis can be a sequela to chronic toxic injury, metabolic disorders of hepatocytes, or chronic inflammation. Chronic cholangitis and/or biliary obstruction can produce fibrosis that is most pronounced in portal tracts. Prolonged hypoxia, usually in centrilobular areas of the liver, as a consequence of chronic passive congestion can result in fibrosis. A single event of widespread hepatocellular necrosis is sometimes followed, not by the usual regenerative response, but by fibrosis and condensation of the preexisting connective tissue stroma, which results in formation of bands of dense connective tissue. This process is referred to as **postnecrotic scarring.**

Hepatic fibrosis may manifest in any one of several patterns, including diffuse hepatic fibrosis (affects all regions of the lobule and is present throughout the liver), biliary fibrosis (centered on bile ducts in the portal tracts), centrilobular (periacinar) fibrosis (centered on central veins), and focal or multifocal hepatic fibrosis (randomly scattered throughout the hepatic parenchyma). Different hepatic insults may produce different patterns of fibrosis, but when fibrosis is severe (end-stage liver disease), it frequently is impossible to determine either the cause or the initial pattern of fibrosis. **Bridging fibrosis,** which is analogous to bridging necrosis, implies fibrosis that extends from one portal tract to another or from portal tracts to central veins. Bridging fibrosis is more likely to be associated with impaired hepatic function than are other forms of hepatic fibrosis; however, all forms of hepatic fibrosis, if sufficiently severe, are associated with impaired hepatic function.

Biliary hyperplasia. Biliary hyperplasia, proliferation of new bile ducts within the portal tracts and periportal regions, results from a variety of insults to the liver (see Fig. 2-3). The mechanism responsible for this proliferation is unknown. Also, some hepatic disorders are characterized by the presence of tubular structures in periportal areas. The origin of cells that form these structures is uncertain, although bile duct epithelium, cholangioles, and hepatocytes have all been proposed.

End-stage liver or cirrhosis

The end-stage or cirrhotic liver is characterized by three of the features just described, specifically, nodular regen-

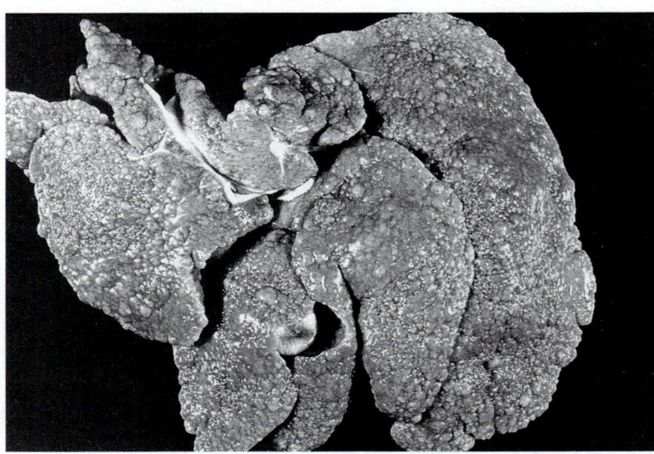

Fig. 2-26 Liver; dog, Doberman pinscher. End-stage liver with chronic-active hepatitis. The liver is small, firm, and irregular with nodules of regenerative parenchyma separated by tracts of connective tissue. *Courtesy Dr. S. Smith.*

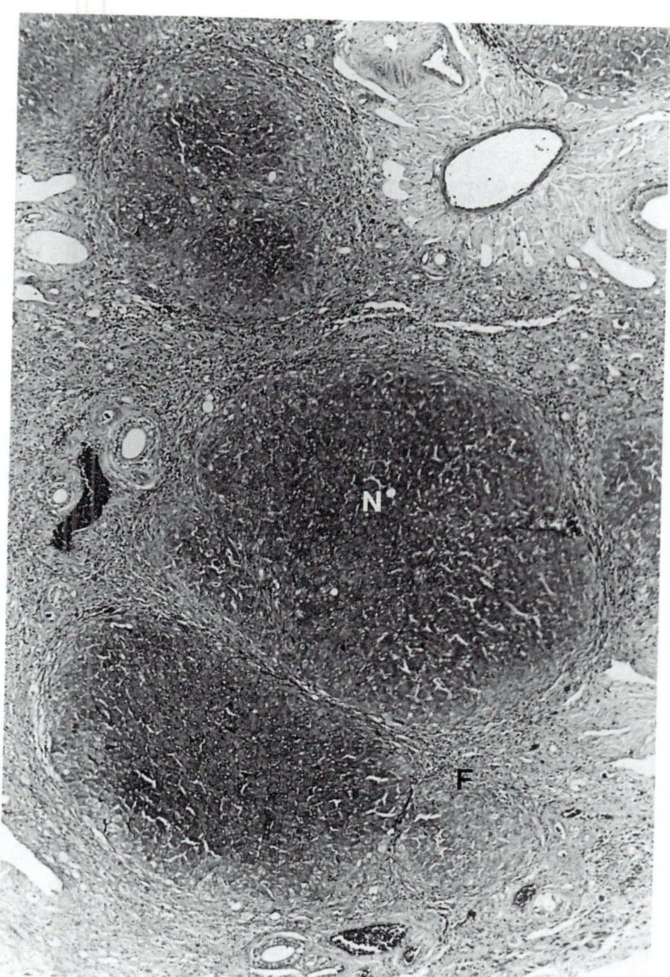

Fig. 2-27 Liver; dog. End-stage liver induced by chronic anticonvulsant therapy. Nodules of regenerative parenchyma (*N*) are separated by tracts of collapsed reticulin and fibrous connective tissue (*F*), which also contain numerous blood vessels and bile ducts. H & E stain.

eration of parenchyma, fibrosis, and, often, bile duct hyperplasia (Figs. 2-26 and 2-27). Abnormal arteriovenous anastomoses may form as a consequence of the increased portal pressure subsequent to parenchymal loss and hepatic fibrosis. As it is the final, irreversible result of any one of several different hepatic diseases, the term end-stage liver is appropriate, particularly since the term cirrhosis is neither descriptive nor precise in meaning and originally meant "tawny yellow." However, "cirrhosis" is still widely used, and one definition is that it is "a diffuse process characterized by fibrosis and conversion of normal liver architecture into structurally abnormal lobules." Another authority states that the hallmark is the total absence of any normal lobular architecture. The architecture of the liver is altered by loss of hepatic parenchyma, condensation of reticulin framework, and formation of tracts of fibrous connective tissue. Regeneration of hepatic tissue between fibrous bands leads to the formation of variably sized regenerative nodules. The entire liver is, thus, distorted and consists of nodules of regenerating parenchyma separated by fibrous bands that appear as depressions on the surface. The potential causes of an end-stage (cirrhotic) liver are numerous.

Chronic toxic insult results from the continued ingestion by herbivores of toxic plants such as those that contain pyrrolizidine alkaloids and the long-term administration of anticonvulsant drugs such as primidone to dogs. Chronic extrahepatic **biliary obstruction** and **cholestasis** lead to extensive fibrosis centering on the portal tracts, but the fibrosis can eventually extend into the adjacent hepatic parenchyma. Chronic inflammation of the liver (hepatitis) or biliary tract (cholangitis) may lead to an end-stage liver. Although infection of the liver typically is focal or multifocal, diffuse hepatitis and subsequent fibrosis occur in disease entities such as so-called canine **chronic-active hepatitis. Chronic passive hepatic congestion** eventually leads to fibrosis around central veins, which is sometimes termed **cardiac sclerosis.** The actual amount of fibrosis is usually small. Abnormal storage or metabolism of metals such as copper, as occurs in Bedlington and West Highland white terriers with hereditary copper accumulation, may produce an end-stage liver. A variety of more poorly defined disease entities can lead to progressive hepatocellular injury and hepatic fibrosis resulting in end-stage hepatic disease.

The end-stage liver obviously cannot perform its normal functions, so the clinical manifestations of hepatic failure invariably occur in affected animals. However, the cause of the hepatic damage that leads to the end-stage liver frequently cannot be determined at the time signs of hepatic failure are observed.

Inflammation of the liver (hepatitis)

Routes of infection into the liver are hematogenous, direct penetration, and ascending via the biliary system. The most common route is hematogenous because the liver receives both arterial blood via the hepatic artery and venous blood from the GI tract via the portal vein. Ascending biliary infections and direct penetration are less common. The nature and distribution of inflammatory lesions in the liver are usually dictated by the nature of the infectious agent, e.g., virus, bacterium, fungus, and any prediliction for a cell type in the liver.

Inflammation of the liver parenchyma is termed **hepatitis,** whereas inflammation of the biliary ducts (either intrahepatic or extrahepatic) is **cholangitis. Cholangiohepatitis** affects both the biliary ducts and the hepatic parenchyma. Other terms are occasionally used. **Pericholangitis** implies inflammation that surrounds, but does not encroach on, the biliary ducts; **portal hepatitis** refers to accumulation of inflammatory cells within the portal tract.

Acute hepatitis frequently accompanies hepatocellular necrosis. Inflammatory cells—initially neutrophils, and, subsequently, lymphocytes, plasma cells, and macrophages—surround and infiltrate areas of hepatocyte necrosis, particularly if an infectious agent is present. Inflammatory cells accumulate in response to the usual chemotactic stimuli. In time, if the animal survives, necrotic tissue is removed by phagocytes and replaced by regenerating parenchyma or fibrous tissue. If antigen persists, as occurs with some infectious agents (see below), an abscess or granuloma may form.

Grossly, acute inflammation is usually detected only if accompanied by hepatocellular necrosis. Characterization of the type of inflammation usually requires microscopic evaluation. A variety of patterns occur. Random foci of neutrophilic hepatitis as a consequence of embolic localization of bacteria are relatively common in all species. In neonates, especially calves, lambs, and foals, bacteria usually seed the liver via the umbilical vessels or the portal venous or hepatic arterial systems. Neutrophilic cholangitis and cholangiohepatitis typically result from ascending bacterial infection of the biliary system, often as a consequence of biliary obstruction by parasites or compression of the duct by either fibrous tissue or a neoplasm.

Chronic hepatitis results when there is continued inflammation due to persistence of an antigenic stimulus. In the absence of such a stimulus, inflammation rapidly resolves. Certain species of bacteria *(Mycobacterium)* and fungi *(Histoplasma capsulatum)* are particularly resistant to killing by phagocytic cells and induce chronic inflammation and granuloma formation. Other causes of chronic inflammation of the liver include chronic cholangiohepatitis from persistent infection of the biliary system, and so-called chronic-active hepatitis of the dog (see Canine Chronic-Active Hepatitis). Chronic inflammation is obvious grossly if it produces a discrete granuloma or abscess. Also, when chronic inflammation occurs throughout the liver, loss of hepatic parenchyma produces architectural distortion of the liver as a consequence of fibrosis and nodular parenchymal regeneration. Whereas acute hepatitis usually is characterized by accumulation of neutrophils, chronic hepatitis is characterized by fibrosis and accumulation of mononuclear inflammatory cells, including lymphocytes, macrophages, and plasma cells. Neutrophils often are present in chronic unresolved hepatic inflammation, such as that which characterizes canine chronic-active hepatitis. Focal lesions such as abscesses or granulomas often are sufficiently localized that they do not alter hepatic function. In contrast, diffuse and severe chronic hepatitis usually leads to end-stage hepatic disease with hepatic failure and its associated constellation of clinical signs.

Viral Diseases

Infectious canine hepatitis

This disease is caused by canine adenovirus 1 and now is uncommon in much of the world, probably because of widespread vaccination. The majority of infections are asymptomatic, and infections that result in disease may not be fatal. The virus has a predilection for vascular endothelium and hepatocytes; fulminant disease is characterized by hepatic necrosis and widespread hemorrhage, which can affect a variety of organs. Virus-induced endothelial damage may lead to disseminated intravascular coagulation and hemorrhagic diathesis.

Lesions of infectious canine hepatitis include widespread petechiae and ecchymoses, accumulation of clear fluid in the peritoneal and other serous cavities, the presence of fibrin strands on the surface of the liver, and enlargement and reddening of the tonsils and lymph nodes. The liver is moderately enlarged, friable, and may contain disseminated small foci of hepatocellular necrosis. An enhanced lobular pattern is sometimes evident, and reflects centrilobular hepatic necrosis. Characteristically, the wall of the gallbladder is thickened by edema.

The severity of microscopic lesions present in individual dogs may reflect the duration of the disease. Susceptible puppies rapidly succumb to infection and have only scattered foci of hepatocellular necrosis, whereas fulminant disease in older dogs often produces both randomly scattered foci of hepatocellular necrosis and widespread centrilobular necrosis. Large amphophilic intranuclear inclusions are found in vascular endothelium and hepatocytes. Zonal necrosis may reflect ischemic injury and not direct virus-mediated destruction of hepatocytes. Some dogs recovering from infectious canine hepatitis develop an immune complex uveitis (type III hypersensitivity), which produces degeneration of the corneal endothelium and corneal edema, clinically known as "blue eye."

Rift Valley fever

This is an acute, arthropod-transmitted zoonotic viral disease that principally affects ruminants, causing extensive mortality among calves and lambs and abortion of pregnant ewes and cows. The causative virus is a member of the Bunyaviridae, genus *Phlebovirus.* The disease occurs throughout much of Africa. Hepatic involvement is consistent in fulminant cases and is characterized by hepatic enlargement and orange-brown discoloration. Pale foci of hepatocellular necrosis that are randomly scattered throughout the parenchyma impart a mottled appearance and, sometimes, an enhanced lobular pattern because of the centrilobular hepatic necrosis. Diffuse petechiae and ecchymoses are also characteristic of the disease, as are edema and hemorrhages of the wall of the gallbladder. Disseminated intravascular coagulation probably contributes to the hemorrhagic diathesis and perhaps to the zonal hepatic necrosis.

Microscopic lesions are characterized by the presence of both randomly distributed foci of hepatocellular necrosis and more widespread zonal necrosis that ranges from centrilobular to massive. These lesions, particularly random hepatic necrosis, are more severe and widespread in young animals and aborted fetuses. Eosinophilic intranuclear inclusion bodies may be present in degenerate hepatocytes in areas of necrosis.

Wesselsbron disease

This disease, like Rift Valley fever, is a zoonotic arthropod-transmitted viral disease occurring in Africa; the virus occasionally causes disease in newborn lambs and abortion in ewes. The causative agent is a member of the Flaviviridae. Affected lambs have multifocal areas of hepatocellular necrosis, and icterus develops occasionally. Infected adult sheep usually survive infection, although they may develop focal areas of hepatocellular necrosis.

Herpesvirus infections

A variety of abortogenic herpesviruses are described, each animal species having a specific virus. The abortogenic herpesviruses characteristically induce multifocal, randomly distributed, small (<1 mm) areas of necrosis in several organs, including the liver (see Fig. 2-20). Similar lesions occasionally are present in neonates infected with abortogenic herpesviruses. Examples of these viruses include the abortogenic equine herpesvirus (equine herpesvirus 1), infectious bovine rhinotracheitis virus (bovine herpesvirus 1), caprine herpesvirus, feline viral rhinotracheitis virus, and pseudorabies virus. Canine herpesvirus can produce multifocal hepatic necrosis in neonatal pups, but foci of necrosis are more consistently present in the kidneys, lungs, and spleen.

Other viral infections

Certain viral diseases may involve the liver, but the hepatic involvement either does not occur invariably or is but one manifestation of a systemic process. Such diseases include feline infectious peritonitis, which is characterized by foci of pyogranulomatous inflammation or perivascular accumulations of lymphocytes and plasma cells within multiple organs, sometimes including the liver. Subacute and chronic forms of equine infectious anemia are characterized by cellular infiltration, particularly lymphocytes, in portal tracts of the liver. Systemic adenoviral infection of lambs, calves, and goat kids may produce multifocal areas of hepatocellular necrosis, cholangitis, and necrosis of biliary epithelium.

Bacterial Diseases

Liver abscess

Bacteria can reach the liver via a number of different routes and induce the formation of abscesses. These routes include the portal vein, the umbilical veins from umbilical infections in newborn animals, as part of a generalized bacteremia reaching the liver via the hepatic artery, as an ascending infection of the biliary system, by parasitic migration, and as a direct extension of an inflammatory process from tissues, such as the reticulum, immediately adjacent to the liver.

Bacterial infections of the liver and subsequent formation of hepatic abscesses are especially common in feedlot cattle. This usually occurs as a sequela to toxic rumenitis, because damage to the ruminal mucosa allows ruminal microflora, particularly *Fusobacterium necrophorum,* to enter the portal circulation. After initially localizing within the liver, bacteria proliferate and produce focal areas of hepatocellular necrosis and hepatitis that can, in time, develop into hepatic abscesses. Occasionally, fungi such as *Mucor* that proliferate in areas of ruminal ulceration invade the portal circulation and are carried to the liver and there cause extensive areas of necrosis.

Liver abscesses in cattle frequently are incidental lesions, but they can cause weight loss and decreased milk production. Less commonly, a hepatic abscess encroaches on the lumen of either a hepatic vein or the caudal vena cava. This can cause a phlebitis that results in mural thrombosis and, because of the obstruction of the outflow to the venous drainage of the liver, passive congestion of the liver and portal hypertension. Detachment of portions of these mural thrombi can produce septic thromboemboli that lodge in the lungs. Rupture of hepatic abscesses directly into the hepatic vein or into the caudal vena cava occurs sporadically in cattle and may result in death of the affected animal because of fatal septic embolization of the lungs. Sometimes, death can be sudden from the blockage of large areas of pulmonary capillaries by the exudate. Hepatic abscesses derived from bacteria in the portal vein may not be evenly distributed throughout the liver, possibly because of portal streaming.

Bacillary hemoglobinuria

This acute and highly fatal disease of cattle and sheep occurs in various areas of the world, typically in those regions in which liver fluke *(Fasciola hepatica)* infection also occurs. Spores of *Clostridium haemolyticum,* the causative agent of bacillary hemoglobinuria, are ingested and come to reside within Kupffer cells, but they proliferate only in areas of low oxygen tension. Migration of immature liver flukes or, less commonly, other parasites or an event, such as liver biopsy, produces a nidus of necrotic hepatic parenchyma in which bacterial spores can germinate. Bacteria proliferate and release toxins, the most important of which is phospholipase C, that induce the hepatocellular necrosis and intravascular hemolysis that characterize the disease. Affected animals have icterus, hemoglobinemia, and hemoglobinuria. The liver contains one or more discrete foci of hepatic necrosis in which causative organisms may be visible in histologic sections. Grossly, these foci are sharply delineated from the adjacent parenchyma, and usually are pale and surrounded by an intensely hyperemic zone. Migration tracts of the immature flukes that typically precipitate the disease may be present. Serous cavities (pleura, peritoneum, and pericardium) often contain excessive accumulation of red or straw-colored fluid that is sometimes flecked with fibrin.

Infectious necrotic hepatitis

Also known as black disease, infectious necrotic hepatitis is most common in sheep and cattle, but occurs in swine and horses. This disease is somewhat analogous to bacillary hemoglobinuria in that dormant spores of *C. novyi* (usually type B) germinate in areas of lowered oxygen tension and release toxins that produce discrete foci of coagulation necrosis within the liver and eventually death of the host. Germination of spores is usually initiated by hepatic necrosis caused by the migration of immature liver flukes; however, a variety of other initiating factors have been described. Affected animals typically have one or more areas of hepatocellular necrosis, which usually manifests as discrete, pale areas of variable size. A zone of intense hyperemia often surrounds these foci. Parasitic migration tracts are also usually present within the affected liver. Other lesions that may be present include diffuse venous congestion and accumulation of fluid within the pericardial sac and pleural and peritoneal cavities. The carcass of affected animals typically putrefies rapidly because of high fever prior to death.

Tyzzer's disease

This disease, caused by *Bacillus piliformis,* is well recognized in laboratory animals, but occurs only sporadically in domestic animals. It is most common in foals, but has been described in calves, cats, and dogs and many other species. Only very young or immunocompromised animals typically are affected. The disease is characterized by enlarged, edematous, and hemorrhagic abdominal lymph nodes, hepatic enlargement, and the presence of randomly distributed, pale foci of hepatocellular necrosis. Diagnosis requires the demonstration of the characteristic, elongated large bacilli within viable hepatocytes at the margins of necrotic foci.

Leptospirosis

The liver is often involved in acute, severe leptospirosis of all domestic species because of ischemic injury to centrilobular areas as a consequence of the intravascular hemolytic anemia that accompanies infection with some serovars. Furthermore, organisms are present in large numbers in the liver, although the direct effects of leptospira on hepatocytes are less well established. Infection of dogs with *Leptospira grippotyphosa* has been associated with chronic-active hepatitis, but it is not known whether leptospira are involved in the pathogenesis of the majority of spontaneous cases of chronic-active hepatitis.

Other bacterial infections

These include those that accompany bacteremia associated with systemic infection. A comprehensive list of systemic infections that may produce hepatocellular necrosis and hepatitis is beyond the scope of this chapter, but examples include *Yersinia tularensis (Francisella tularensis), Y. pseudotuberculosis, Haemophilus agni,* and *Pasteurella haemolytica* infection of sheep, *Salmonella* infection in many species (lesions present within the liver are discrete accumulations of mixed mononuclear inflammatory cells that often are referred to as "paratyphoid nodules"), *Actinomyces pyogenes (Corynebacterium pyogenes)* infection of the bovine fetus and neonate, *Actinobacillus equuli* infection of neonatal foals, and *Nocardia asteroides* infection of dogs. Bacterial infections such as these may produce lesions within the liver that range from small foci of hepatic necrosis to multiple, large abscesses (see Figs. 2-18 and 2-19; Figs. 2-28 and 2-29). Determination of the specific causative agent is often dependent upon bacterial isolation and characterization.

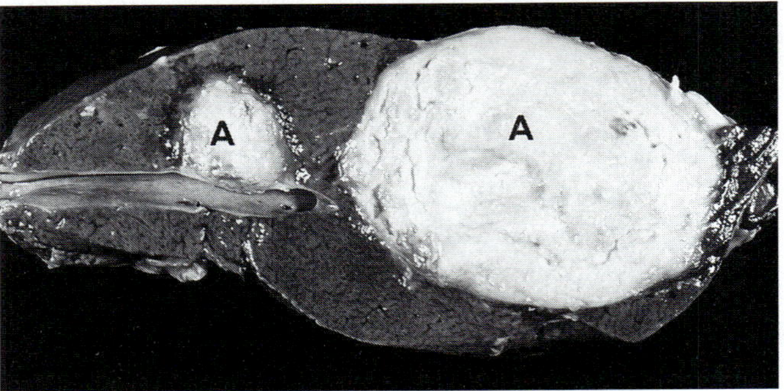

Fig. 2-28 Liver, cut surface; sheep. Two abscesses (*A*) caused by *Corynebacterium pseudotuberculosis. Courtesy of Dr. M. Leach.*

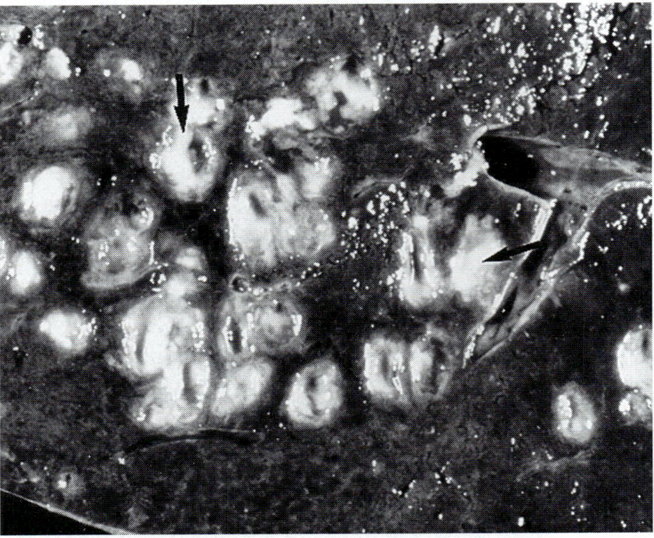

Fig. 2-29 Liver, cut surface; horse. Disseminated hepatic abscesses (*arrows*) caused by *Corynebacterium pseudotuberculosis. Courtesy of Dr. M. Leach.*

Parasitic Diseases

Nematodes

Migration of nematode larvae through the liver is a common occurrence in domestic animals. As larvae travel through the liver, they produce local tracks of hepatocel-

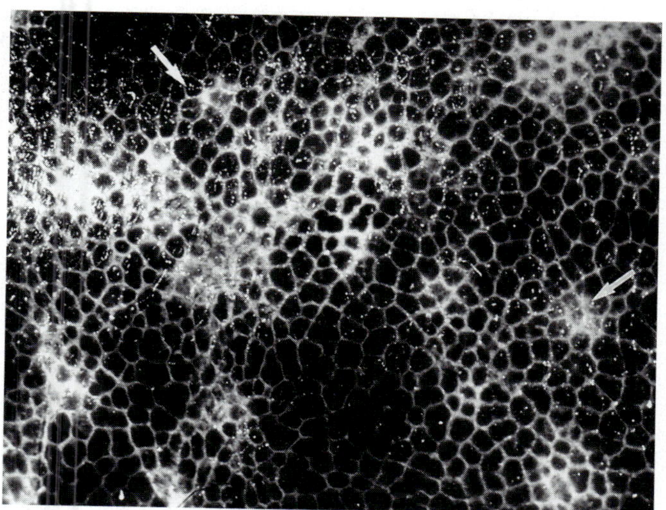

Fig. 2-30 Liver, diaphragmatic surface; pig. Capsular and portal fibrosis from parasitic migration (milk-spotted liver). Migration tracks and the fibrosis of adjacent portal areas are identified with arrows. *Courtesy Dr. M.D. McGavin.*

lular necrosis and accompanying inflammation. These tracks are eventually replaced with connective tissue to produce fibrous scars, which are especially prominent on the capsular surface (Fig. 2-30). These capsular scars appear as pale areas, and the term "milk spotted liver" has been used to describe livers in pigs scarred by migrating larvae of *Ascaris suum.* Larvae occasionally become entrapped within the liver or its capsule and are walled off within abscesses or granulomas. Examples of chronic hepatitis or hepatic scarring as a consequence of larval migration include that associated with migration of ascarids in several species of domestic animals, *Stephanurus dentatus* in swine, and *Strongylus* sp in the horse. Infestation of the liver with adult nematodes is considerably less common than larval migration. *Capillaria hepatica* occasionally may be found in the liver of dogs and cats.

Dogs with heartworm infection *(Dirofilaria immitis)* occasionally develop **vena caval syndrome,** also known as postcaval syndrome, which is characterized by disseminated intravascular coagulation, intravascular hemolysis, and acute hepatic failure. The syndrome typically occurs in dogs with large numbers of adult worms in the vena cava, as well as in the more usual location within the right heart and pulmonary artery. The liver is engorged with blood as a consequence of severe passive congestion from the partial blockage of the caudal vena cava. It is proposed that mechanical factors associated with the presence of large numbers of worms in the right atrium are the cause of the intravascular hemolysis that characterizes vena caval syndrome.

Cestodes

A number of cestodes occur within the hepatobiliary system of domestic animals. Those of greatest significance are the encysted forms of cestode parasites within the tissues of the intermediate hosts. The most important are larval cestodes of the genus *Taenia,* adults of which inhabit the GI tract of carnivores and which usually are innocuous to their definitive host. The ova ingested by an intermediate host develop into embryos, which penetrate the wall of the gut and, then, are distributed through the blood to virtually any site in the body. Parasitic cysts develop within the tissues of the intermediate host, and the life cycle of the parasite is completed when the cysts are ingested by the definitive host. Although the liver is but one organ in the intermediate host that may be affected, hepatic involvement is common since portal blood, in which embryos migrate, drains into the liver before flowing to the systemic circulation.

The cestode *Taenia hydatigena* occurs in dogs, whereas its intermediate stage, *Cysticercus tenuicollis,* occurs in the peritoneal cavity of a variety of species including horses, ruminants, and swine. Immature cysticerci migrate in the liver and can induce extensive damage if infection is heavy; lesions present are comparable with those induced by migration of immature *Fasciola hepatica.*

Hydatid liver disease is common in some countries. *Echinococcus granulosus* is a cestode that parasitizes canids, and hydatid cysts can develop in many different animal species, including human beings. The dog-sheep cycle is most important in many geographic areas. Pastured cattle are also commonly affected in some geographic locations. Embryos may develop into hydatid cysts in virtually any organ in the intermediate host, but the liver and lungs are commonly affected. These cysts are usually less than 10 cm in diameter, but can attain quite spectacular size, particularly in human beings. Hydatid cysts, even when present in large numbers, rarely cause overt clinical signs of disease in domestic animals.

Cestode worms that can occur within the hepatobiliary system include *Stilesia hepatica, S. globipunctata,* and *Thysanosoma actinoides,* all of which can inhabit the bile duct of ruminants. Infections with these parasites may result in chronic inflammation of the biliary tract, but they usually are not associated with clinical signs of hepatic dysfunction.

Trematodes

Liver fluke disease of sheep and cattle, and occasionally other species, most commonly is due to *Fasciola hepatica.* Hepatic fascioliasis occurs throughout the world in areas where climatic conditions (low swampy areas) are suitable for the aquatic snails that serve as intermediate hosts for the parasites. Adult *F. hepatica* are leaf-shaped parasites that inhabit the biliary system; their eggs pass via the bile to the intestinal tract and eventually are passed in the feces. Larvae then must develop in the snail intermediate host (genus *Lymnaea*). Cercariae that leave the snail encyst on herbage, where they develop into infectious metacercariae. Metacercariae are ingested by the ruminant host and penetrate the wall of the duodenum to enter the peritoneal cavity and, subsequently, enter the liver. They migrate within the liver before taking up residence within the bile ducts. Migration of immature flukes through the liver produces hemorrhagic tracks of necrotic liver parenchyma. These tracts are grossly visible and, in acute infestation, are dark red, but with time become paler than the surrounding parenchyma. Resolution is often by fibrosis. A variety of untoward sequelae can follow these migrations, including acute peritonitis; hepatic abscesses; the proliferation of spores of *Clostridium haemolyticum* or *C. novyi* in necrotic tissue and the subsequent development of bacillary hemoglobinuria or infectious necrotic hepatitis and death of the host as a consequence of acute, widespread hepatic necrosis associated with massive infiltration of immature flukes.

Mature flukes reside in the larger bile ducts and cause cholangitis or cholangiohepatitis. Chronic cholangitis and bile duct obstruction lead to ectasia and stenosis of the ducts, and periductular fibrosis that thickens the walls so the ducts become increasingly prominent. Bile within the distended ducts is brown. Obstruction of the ducts leads to extrahepatic cholestasis. Animals with chronic liver fluke disease are often in poor body condition.

Fasciola gigantica and *Fascioloides magna* are important causes of liver fluke disease of ruminants in some parts of the world. In contrast to both *Fasciola gigantica* and *F. hepatica,* the adults of which reside in the bile ducts, in aberrant hosts such as cattle and sheep, adult *Fascioloides magna* reside in the hepatic parenchyma. In cattle, the immature *F. magna* flukes cause extensive tissue damage as they migrate through the liver (Fig. 2-31), but the adults are enclosed by fibrous connective tissue in cysts containing a black fluid. In sheep, the flukes continuously migrate through the liver, causing extensive damage.

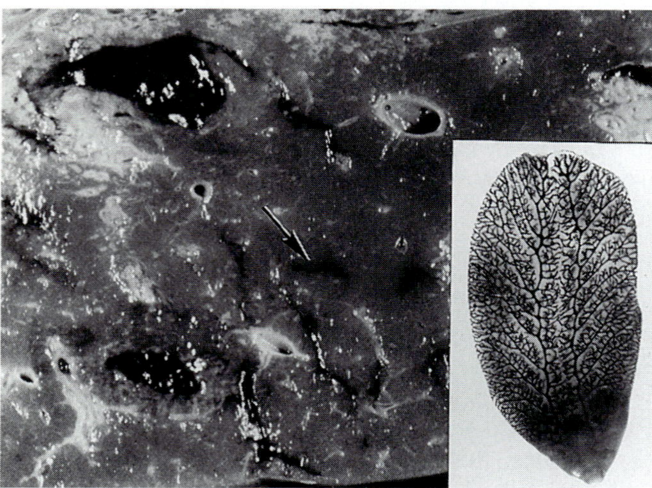

Fig. 2-31 Liver, cut surface; cow. Fascioliasis. Migration of *Fascioloides magna* through this bovine liver produced characteristic dark tracks (*arrow*) of hepatocellular necrosis. *Inset:* Adult *F. magna.* *Courtesy Dr. M. McEntee.*

Other trematodes that may inhabit the bile ducts include *Dicrocoelium dendriticum* in horses, ruminants, swine, dogs, and cats; *Eurytrema pancreaticum* and *E. coelomaticum* in ruminants; *Opisthorchis tenuicollis* in swine, dogs, and cats, and *O. viverrini* in dogs and cats; *Pseudamphistomum truncatum, Metorchis conjunctus, M. albidus, Parametorchis complexus, Concinnum procyonis,* and *Platynosum fastosum* in dogs and cats. All are capable of inducing changes similar to but usually considerably milder than those associated with *Fasciola hepatica.* In addition, they occasionally cause obstruction of the biliary ducts.

Nutritional Diseases

Hepatosis dietetica

Hepatosis dietetica (nutritional hepatic necrosis) is a syndrome of acute hepatic necrosis that occurs in young, rapidly growing swine. This is but one manifestation of a variety of disorders that are, at least in part, caused by deficiency of vitamin E and/or selenium. The pathogenesis of hepatosis dietetica is incompletely defined, although it is established that vitamin E and selenium-containing enzymes are antagonists of free radical formation and are, therefore, important for the maintenance of stability and integrity of cellular membranes.

Hepatosis dietetica is characterized by hemorrhagic centrilobular to massive hepatic necrosis (see Fig. 2-24). The appearance of the liver of individually affected swine reflects the extent of hepatic necrosis, the severity of the hemorrhages, and the duration of the deficiency. Regions of massive necrosis in the affected liver will initially be distended, deep red, and friable, and later collapse to form dense tracts of connective tissue (postnecrotic scarring) in some animals that survive the acute disease.

Toxic Liver Disease

The liver is the most common site of toxic injury for two reasons. First, the liver receives approximately 80% of its blood supply from the portal vein, which drains blood from the GI tract. Thus, ingested toxic substances, including plant, fungal, and bacterial products, as well as metals, minerals, and other chemicals that are absorbed into the portal blood, are transported to the liver. Second, the liver possesses the enzymes capable of biotransformation of a variety of endogenous and exogenous substances for elimination from the body; this process may also bioactivate some substances to a more toxic form, thereby causing hepatic injury.

Typically, during hepatic biotransformation, lipid-soluble compounds are made water soluble to facilitate their excretion into bile or urine. There are two stages or phases to this process. During phase 1 metabolism, polar groups are added to a compound or existing polar groups are exposed by oxidation, hydrolysis, or reduction. In phase 2, the product of phase 1 metabolism is conjugated to glucuronate, sulfate, or other groups, and this water-soluble form is then excreted in bile or urine. Phase 1 metabolism is usually performed by the mixed-function oxidase (MFO) system or, as it is also known, the cytochrome P-450 system. This is the major enzyme system of the liver involved with drug metabolism and is located in the smooth endoplasmic reticulum. Activity of this enzyme system is greatest in hepatocytes in centrilobular regions. The mixed-function oxidases are a collection of isoenzymes with different substrate specificities and can, therefore, oxidize a variety of chemicals. This enzyme system is inducible. Activities of these enzymes present within the liver increase in response to frequent exposure to substrates metabolized by this system, such as insecticides or phenobarbital. Amounts of smooth endoplasmic reticulum, and, thus, mixed-function oxidase activity, also vary between the sexes (males have more mixed-function oxidase activity than females) and with age (neonates have less activity than adults). Cytosolic enzymes also participate in biotransformation of some substances, particularly during phase 2 biotransformation.

Although hepatic biotransformation generally is a means of detoxifying and eliminating a variety of chemicals, biotransformation can also generate toxic metabolites. This process in which reactive metabolites are formed is termed bioactivation. These injurious metabolites are often free radicals. Free radicals can react with hepatocellular DNA, RNA, and proteins as well as produce oxidative stress within cells. Antioxidants, particularly reduced glutathione and vitamin E, afford some protection against oxidative injury to cell membranes or organelles. Animals deficient in antioxidants are especially predisposed to hepatocellular injury. Hepatocyte injury was once considered to result primarily from lipid peroxidation, but other factors such as oxidative stress, disruption of calcium homeostasis, and direct effects of certain chemicals on cellular and organelle membranes have come to be recognized as additional important pathways of cellular injury.

An individual compound may be simultaneously metabolized by several different pathways, and some of these pathways produce toxic intermediates, whereas others produce nontoxic compounds. The proportion of a compound metabolized by a particular pathway influences the degree of injury caused by the compound. For example, chemicals such as phenobarbital that induce formation of smooth endoplasmic reticulum and associated oxidases influence the toxicity of other compounds by altering the proportion of those compounds metabolized by mixed-function oxidases versus other metabolic pathways. A variety of factors influence the severity of injury induced by a toxin; these factors include age, sex, diet, endocrine function, genetic constitution, and diurnal factors. It is, therefore, not surprising that responses of individual animals exposed to the same toxin can vary considerably.

Toxic hepatic injury is best understood in terms of the acinus concept of hepatic microanatomy, although the site of injury is usually denoted based on the zones of the hepatic lobule. The site of toxic cellular injury within the hepatic acinus reflects the site of bioactivation of the chemical. For instance, carbon tetrachloride is metabolized by mixed-function oxidases to $CCl_3^{\cdot}$, a free radical. Lesions induced by carbon tetrachloride are most severe in the periacinar (centrilobular) areas, because this is the area where the smooth endoplasmic reticulum is most abundant and, therefore, where the active form of the chemical is present in greatest concentration. Conversely, allyl alcohol is activated by alcohol dehydrogenase, a cytosolic enzyme that is most abundant in centroacinar (periportal) areas; hepatocellular injury induced by allyl alcohol consequently is most severe periportally.

Toxic chemicals can be divided into two groups: those that cause predictable hepatic injury **(predictable hepatotoxins)** and those that do not, the latter being referred to as **idiosyncratic toxins.** Predictable hepatotoxins are those that, if given in a sufficient dose, produce hepatic injury in virtually all susceptible animals. The majority of recognized hepatotoxins in veterinary medicine fall into this category; carbon tetrachloride and pyrrolizidine alkaloids are examples of predictable hepatotoxins. Idiosyncratic toxins are those chemicals that cause hepatic injury in a minority of exposed individuals, usually only after prolonged or repeated exposure. The pathogenesis of idiosyncratic toxic injury to the liver is not well understood, and proof of the toxic effect of these chemicals is obviously more difficult to establish. An example of an idiosyncratic hepatotoxin is the inhalation anesthetic halothane.

The morphology of toxin-induced hepatic injury varies considerably with the type, dose, and duration of exposure to toxin, as well as with the other factors described above. Hepatocytic responses to acute toxic injury usually involve cellular swelling and accumulation of lipid (fatty degeneration or steatosis) with or without cholestasis. This may progress to necrosis if the toxicosis is sufficiently severe. Continuous or repetitive toxic injury to the liver is characterized by the three stereotypical responses of fibrosis, biliary hyperplasia, and parenchymal regeneration. Toxic hepatic injury can lead to an end-stage liver and, with toxins such as aflatoxins, to hepatic neoplasia. Both acute and chronic toxic injury to the liver can cause hepatic failure.

Toxic plants of great variety cause hepatic injury in domestic animals. A comprehensive discussion of each is beyond the scope of this chapter. The phytotoxins (Table 2-1) to be discussed represent three distinct types. The first of these are the preformed hepatic phytotoxins such as occur in blue-green algae. The second type, represented by pyrrolizidine alkaloids, must be metabolized to an active form in the liver. The third type are toxins that are deconjugated by bacteria within the digestive tract to release a factor that is subsequently bioactivated in the liver.

Table 2-1. Common hepatotoxic plants of veterinary importance

Plant family	Species affected	Toxic principle	Characteristic injury	Miscellaneous
Compositae *Xanthium* spp	Cattle, pigs	Carboxyatractyloside	Periacinar necrosis	Hypoglycemia and ascites in acute intoxication in pigs.
Myoporaceae *Myoporum* spp	Sheep, cattle, horses, pigs	Furanosesquiterperiod oils (ngaione)	Usually periacinar to variable zonal necrosis	Pulmonary injury also occurs in sheep.
Verbenaceae *Lantana camara* *Lippia* spp	Cattle, sheep, goats occasionally	Triterpens (lentadene A & B)	Megalocytosis, canalicular cholestasis, focal hepatocellular necrosis	Icterus and photosensitization common. Renal and myocardial injury also occur.
Compositae *Senecio* spp Leguminosae *Crotalaria* spp Boraginaceae *Heliotropium* spp *Echium* spp *Amsinki* spp	Pigs, horses, cattle, sheep, goats	Pyrrolizidine alkaloids	Megalocytosis, fibrosis, biliary hyperplasis	Pulmonary and renal injury also.
Leguminosae *Cassia* spp	Cattle	Unknown	Periacinar necrosis	Myocardial and skeletal muscle injury predominate in *C. occidentalis* intoxication.
Zygophyllaceae *Tribulus terrestris*	Sheep	Unknown	Crystalline material in bile ducts	Interaction with mycotoxin sporidesmin necessary to produce characteristic photosensitization (geeldikkop).
Ulmaceae *Trema aspera*	Cattle, sheep, goats	Trematoxin	Periacinar necrosis	Neuromuscular toxins also. Usually acute disease.
Solanaceae *Cestrum parqui*	Cattle, sheep	Unknown	Periacinar necrosis	Gallbladder edema and hemorrhage. Usually acute disease.
Asteroceae *Tetradymia glabrata*	Sheep	Tetradymol	Periacinar necrosis	Photosensitization is common.
Cyanophyceae (Blue-green algae) *Microcystis* *Aphanizomenon*	Cattle, sheep, horses, goats, dogs	Toxic polypeptide(s)	Periacinar to massive necrosis	Multiple toxins present. Can also cause death by neuromuscular injury.
Cycadales Zamiacea Cycadaceae Stangeriaceae	Cattle, sheep, goats	Methylazoxymethanol	Periacinar necrosis, megalocytosis, cholestasis	Toxin split from nontoxic glycoside. Neurotoxins also present. Chronic ingestation can cause paralysis in cattle.

Blue-green algae of several genera, including *Anabaena, Aphanizomenon,* and *Microcystis,* have been associated with lethal poisoning of livestock and, less commonly, small animals. Algal blooms usually occur in late summer or early fall, because of the warm temperatures, long hours of sunlight, and abundance of essential nutrients. Dead and dying algae that contain preformed toxins such as microcystin LR, a cyclic heptapeptide, accumulate on the surface of bodies of water and are ingested by livestock. Secondary bacterial growth in dying algae may contribute to toxin formation. Signs develop rapidly and include diarrhea, prostration, and death. Gross lesions include hemorrhagic gastroenteritis and zonal, or even massive, hepatic necrosis. Animals that survive the acute manifestations may develop signs of chronic liver disease. Other preformed toxins that affect different organ systems, including the nervous system, have also been identified in blue-green algae.

Pyrrolizidine alkaloids are found in many plant families, including Compositae, Leguminosae, and Boraginaceae, that occur throughout much of the world. The most important genera are *Senecio, Cynglossum, Amsinckia, Crotolaria, Echium, Trichodesma,* and *Heliotropium.* Approximately 100 different alkaloids are recognized; toxic effects depend upon which alkaloids are present within ingested plants. Ingested alkaloids are converted to pyrrolic esters by the hepatic mixed-function oxidase system. These esters are alkylating agents, which react with cytosolic and nuclear constituents. Swine are particularly susceptible to pyrrolizidine alkaloid intoxication, sheep considerably less

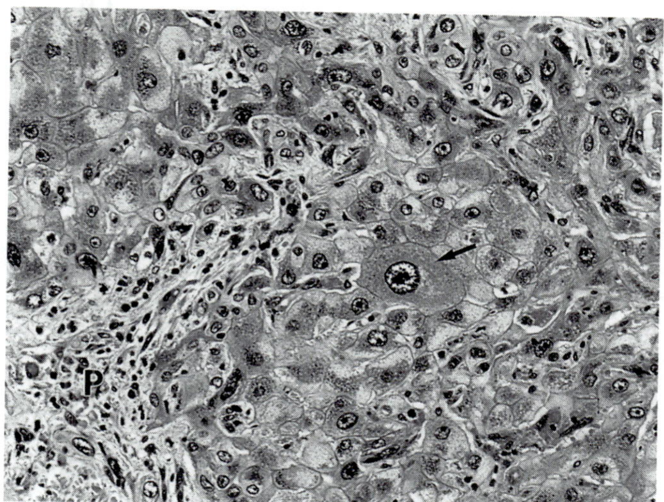

Fig. 2-32 Liver; horse. Pyrrolizidine alkaloid intoxication. Note the fibrosis and associated proliferation of bile ducts in portal tracts (*P*) and presence of a greatly enlarged hepatocyte (megalocyte) in the remaining lobular parenchyma (*arrow*). H & E stain.

so, and cattle and horses are intermediate in susceptibility. The characteristic lesion of pyrrolizidine alkaloid intoxication is the presence of megalocytes, which are hepatocytes with enlarged nuclei and increased cytoplasm. Megalocytes may be many times the size of normal hepatocytes (Fig. 2-32). Megalocytes result from the antimitotic effects of pyrrolizidine alkaloids, which prevent cell division but not DNA synthesis as the hepatocytes attempt to divide to replace those which have undergone necrosis. This change, although indicative of pyrrolizidine alkaloid intoxication, is not pathognomonic, since it occurs with other toxins such as aflatoxins and nitrosamines. Chronic intoxication is accompanied by the triad of hepatic fibrosis, biliary proliferation, and nodular regeneration of parenchyma. Chronic hepatic damage can lead to hepatic failure and its associated constellation of signs (described in detail earlier).

Cycads are primitive, palmlike plants that inhabit tropical and subtropical regions. They contain cycasin, a nontoxic glycoside that, following ingestion, is deconjugated by intestinal microflora to release a toxic metabolite, methylazoxymethanol. Hepatic metabolism of this compound produces alkylating agents leading to chronic hepatic lesions in cattle characterized by hepatocellular megalocytosis and nuclear hyperchromasia, and varying degrees of hepatic fibrosis. Acute intoxication is more common in sheep and produces acute GI dysfunction and periacinar hepatic necrosis. Chronic cycad poisoning in cattle causes a nervous disease with progressive proprioceptive deficits in the hind legs due to ''dying back'' of the spinocerebellar and corticospinal tracts. Table 2-1 summarizes some hepatotoxic plants of veterinary importance.

Mycotoxins are secondary metabolites of fungi; that is, their production is not necessary for the survival of the fungus. The amount of toxin synthesized by a given strain of fungus reflects the genetic constitution of the particular strain, presence of appropriate substrate, temperature, humidity, and available nutrients. Several hepatotoxic mycotoxins are of significance in veterinary medicine.

Aflatoxins are products of the fungi *Aspergillus flavus* and *A. parasiticus.* There are four major naturally occurring aflatoxins, B_1, B_2, G_1, and G_2. Aflatoxin B_1 is the most commonly occurring of the group and is also the most potent toxin and carcinogen. Aflatoxins are usually elaborated during storage of fungal-contaminated feed and may be present in many crops, including corn, peanuts, and cottonseed. Aflatoxins are converted to toxic intermediates by the smooth endoplasmic reticulum of hepatocytes. Carcinogenic, toxic, and teratogenic effects of aflatoxins reflect binding of the toxic intermediates to cellular DNA, RNA, or proteins. Pigs, dogs, horses, and cattle, especially younger animals, are sensitive to the toxic effects of aflatoxins, whereas sheep are more resistant. Acute intoxication is rare in domestic animals except dogs, because of the inordinately large amounts of contaminated feed that an animal would have to ingest at one time. Acute aflatoxicosis in dogs is characterized by hemorrhage and centrilobular to massive hepatocellular necrosis. Lipidosis and biliary proliferation also may occur. Chronic intoxication is more common and results in ill-thrift, increased susceptibility to infection, and, occasionally, signs of hepatic failure. Affected livers are firm and pale and, microscopically, are characterized by fatty degeneration and necrosis of hepatocytes, biliary hyperplasia, fibrosis, and cellular atypia of hepatocytes.

Facial eczema is caused by the mycotoxin sporidesmin, which is produced by *Pithomyces chartarum.* The fungus grows particularly well in dead rye grass (*Lolium perenne*), a common pasture plant in New Zealand and Australia. Ingestion of sufficient amounts of the toxin produces necrosis of the epithelium of the large intrahepatic and extrahepatic bile ducts and subsequent cholangiohepatitis. Cholestasis with failure to excrete phylloerythrin frequently leads to photosensitization with lesions of the head, thus the common name facial eczema. The disease is common in sheep and less so in cattle. Acute cases are characterized by a bile-stained liver with prominent bile ducts. In chronic cases of facial eczema, the bile ducts become thickened secondary to necrosis and subsequent inflammation (chronic cholangitis and cholangiohepatitis). Perhaps because of streaming of blood in the portal vein, the left lobe of the liver is usually most severely affected and, in severe cases, undergoes atrophy and fibrosis. A similar disease, **Geeldikkop,** which is characterized by hepatogenous photosensitization, occurs in sheep in South Africa. It is associated with ingestion of the plant *Tribulus terrestris,* and perhaps concurrent exposure to sporidesmin.

Phomopsins are products of the fungus *Phomopsis leptostromiformis,* which grows on lupins and produces hepatic injury in cattle, sheep, and, occasionally, horses that graze contaminated lupin stubble. Hepatic dysfunction is usually chronic and is characterized by hepatic atrophy and fibrosis. Signs of hepatic failure, including photosensitization, may occur in affected animals. Naturally occurring alkaloids in lupins are capable of inducing skeletal deformities but not obvious hepatic injury.

Other hepatotoxins

Primidone and phenobarbital toxicity has been described in dogs receiving these anticonvulsants for prolonged periods, either alone or in combination with phenytoin. The mechanism of hepatotoxicity is unknown. Only a small proportion of dogs receiving these drugs are affected, and these dogs frequently have signs of hepatic failure. The liver is small and has widespread hepatic fibrosis and nodular regeneration (end-stage liver).

Phosphorus occurs in two forms: red phosphorus and white phosphorus. Red phosphorus is unimportant as a toxin, but white phosphorus is occasionally used as a rodenticide. The mechanism of phosphorus toxicity is unclear, although it apparently is directly toxic. Poisoning is first indicated by signs of gastroenteritis and, subsequently, by microscopic lesions of fatty degeneration of hepatocytes and centroacinar (periportal) necrosis.

Metals also can cause toxic hepatic injury. Copper toxicity may present as an acute intravascular hemolytic anemia in ruminants or as chronic hepatic injury and end-stage hepatic disease in dogs. Two specific syndromes of iron poisoning are iron-dextran intoxication of piglets and ferrous fumarate intoxication of newborn foals. Severe cases of these two toxicities are characterized by massive hepatic necrosis. Ferrous fumarate intoxication in foals, which was associated with use of a specific dietary supplement, is also characterized by biliary hyperplasia, despite the short clinical course of the disease. Iron-dextran is frequently administered intramuscularly to suckling pigs to prevent anemia, but administration of iron-dextran has occasionally resulted in significant mortality and affected pigs die soon after injection. Inordinate iron supplementation of dogs and cats may result in excessive storage of iron and subsequently hepatic disease associated with iron overload, termed hemochromatosis.

Carbon tetrachloride is the classic example of a compound that must be bioactivated by the mixed-function oxidase system in order to become toxic. It is only occasionally used as an anthelmintic. Carbon tetrachloride produces centrilobular hepatic necrosis and fatty degeneration of surviving hepatocytes.

Cresols once were incorporated in clay pigeons and asphalt shingles. If these are ingested by swine, centrilobular to massive hepatic necrosis results.

Ingestion of the analgesic acetaminophen has been associated with hepatocellular necrosis in the cat. This is most likely because the cat's limited ability to conjugate and excrete toxic metabolites of acetaminophen leads to oxidative damage.

Diseases of Uncertain Etiology

Equine serum hepatitis

This disease was first described by Theiler in South Africa, but now is recognized in many countries. It frequently, but not invariably, occurs in horses that have received an injection of a biologic of equine serum origin; for instance, equine antisera such as tetanus antitoxin or pregnant mare serum gonadotropin. It appears that an infectious agent is responsible, although none has been identified. The incubation period is prolonged, but the clinical course of the disease is very rapid and is invariably fatal. Affected horses typically present with hepatic failure that manifests as hepatic encephalopathy and icterus. Intravascular hemolysis occurs in the terminal stages of the disease. The liver of affected animals is small and friable with an enhanced lobular pattern, because of diffuse centrilobular degeneration and necrosis of hepatocytes and subsequent congestion of these necrotic areas. Frequently, only a narrow rim of hepatocytes in portal areas survive, and these sometimes are accompanied by proliferating tubules or columns of cells that are speculated to have arisen from the cholangioles.

Canine chronic-active hepatitis

Chronic-active hepatitis is a chronic inflammatory and fibrosing hepatic disorder of human beings that may occur during chronic infection with the viruses of hepatitis B or hepatitis C. Hepatic disorders of the dog that have microscopic changes similar to those of the human disease have also been termed chronic-active hepatitis. The cause of most of the spontaneous cases of canine chronic-active hepatitis is undetermined, although some cases have been associated with leptospire infection and experimental infectious canine hepatitis virus infection. Chronic progressive hepatitis has been described in cases of hereditary copper toxicosis of Bedlington and West Highland white terriers and has been described above in the sections Metabolic Disturbances and Hepatic Accumulations. Familial chronic hepatitis, which often resembles chronic-active hepatitis, also is associated with excessive hepatic accumulation of copper in the Doberman pinscher (females are predisposed), Skye terrier, cocker spaniel, and Labrador retriever. Abnormal concentrations of hepatic copper in affected dogs of at least some of these breeds have been attributed to cholestasis and decreased hepatic excretion of copper. Many dogs with chronic-active hepatitis do not have elevated concentrations of hepatic copper, and a wide range of hepatic copper concentrations are present in clinically normal dogs. Thus, the precise role of copper in mediating chronic hepatic disease in breeds of dogs other than the Bedlington and West Highland white terrier remains

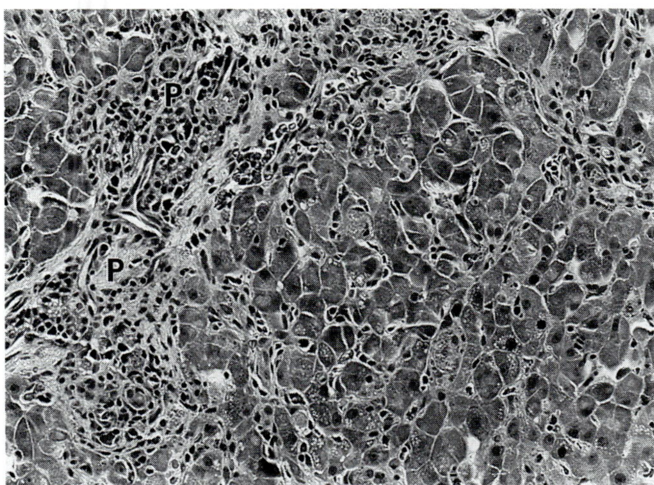

Fig. 2-33 Liver; dog, Doberman pinscher. Chronic active hepatitis. Note the fibrosis and accumulation of mononuclear and polymorphonuclear inflammatory cells within portal tracts (*P*). Inflammation and fibrosis also extend into the adjacent hepatic lobule. H & E stain.

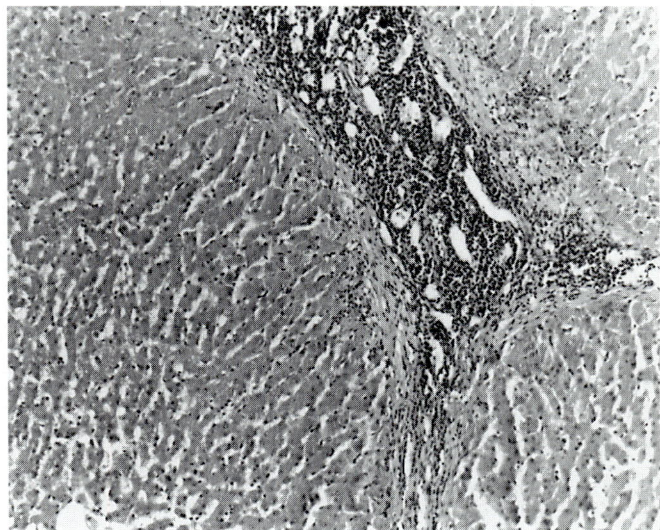

Fig. 2-34 Liver; cat. Feline lymphocytic cholangitis. Accumulation of large numbers of lymphocytes and plasma cells within the portal tracts. H & E stain.

uncertain. Given the uncertainties regarding etiology and the fact that many cases of chronic-active hepatitis in dogs and cats are diagnosed purely on microscopic criteria (i.e., they are proven to be neither chronic nor progressive), the use of the term may not be appropriate.

Chronic-active hepatitis is characterized by progressive destruction of individual hepatocytes, in association with infiltration of mononuclear inflammatory cells. For this reason, it is proposed that destruction of hepatocytes, which usually involves individual cells, is mediated by an immune mechanism. The liver in cases of chronic-active hepatitis is usually small, often with an accentuated lobular pattern; severely affected livers are characterized by architectural distortion that ranges from a coarsely nodular texture to an end-stage liver (see Fig. 2-26). The disorder is characterized microscopically by breaching of the limiting plate that delineates the periphery of the lobule from the portal tract by inflammatory cells, necrosis of individual hepatocytes (piecemeal necrosis), periportal fibrosis, accumulation of inflammatory cells, especially lymphocytes, in portal tracts and adjacent periportal areas of the lobule, and intrahepatic cholestasis (Fig. 2-33).

Chronic lymphocytic cholangitis of cats

Affected cats are usually older than 4 years of age and often present with icterus as a consequence of intrahepatic cholestasis. Extensive aggregations of inflammatory cells, typically lymphocytes and plasma cells, are present in portal tracts, particularly around bile ducts (Fig. 2-34). Inflammation usually is accompanied by biliary duct proliferation, hepatic or biliary fibrosis, and intrahepatic cholestasis. The cause or causes of this syndrome are unknown, but it should be distinguished from such known causes of cholangitis and cholangiohepatitis as ascending infection of the biliary system, cholelithiasis, pancreatitis, toxic injury, and parasitism or obstruction of the biliary system. The disease might have an immunologic basis and often is compared with primary biliary cirrhosis of human beings.

Hepatic injury as a consequence of systemic disease

A variety of extrahepatic disorders can result in hepatocellular injury and hepatic dysfunction. Acute hemorrhagic pancreatitis of dogs, for example, sometimes is accompanied by icterus and increased activities of hepatic enzymes in serum. The liver is showered by the release of various toxins and inflammatory mediators from the injured pancreas into the portal vein. Similarly, movement of potentially hepatotoxic substances into the portal vein can occur as a consequence of intestinal disease. Accumulation of inflammatory cells within the portal tracts may accompany blood-borne infection or abdominal sepsis.

The liver is particularly susceptible to the effects of hypoxia; thus, any disease that causes anemia can produce centrilobular degeneration and necrosis. Also, the liver, in cases of hemolytic anemias, must remove and conjugate the increased amounts of circulating bilirubin, and Kupffer cells remove either erythrocytes during extravascular hemolysis or erythrocytic fragments during intravascular hemolysis.

Hyperplasia and Neoplasia

Primary hyperplastic and neoplastic proliferations of the hepatobiliary system can arise from hepatocytes (hepatocellular), epithelium of the bile ducts (cholangiocellular) or gallbladder (adenoma and adenocarcinoma), and mesenchymal elements such as connective tissue and blood vessels. The liver is a common site of metastasis for many malignancies; in fact, the majority of neoplasms within the liver are metastases from other organs.

Hepatocellular nodular hyperplasia

Hepatic nodular hyperplasia is common only in the dog. Incidence increases with age, without predilection for either sex or breed. Nodular hyperplasia is not associated with significant hepatic dysfunction, but nodular hyperplasia must be distinguished from hepatic neoplasms, with which they are often confused, and regenerative nodules. Multiple nodules are frequently present. The nodules typically are raised and hemispherical, yellow to tan, 0.5 to 3.0 cm in diameter, and more friable than normal liver. On cut surface, the hyperplastic nodules are well demarcated from normal parenchyma and usually compress adjacent parenchyma (Figs. 2-35 and 2-36). Hyperplastic nodules contain all the elements of normal liver but with loss of normal architecture; thus, they consist of disorganized plates of hepatocytes and contain decreased numbers of portal tracts and central veins. Hepatocytes are variably sized and frequently contain cytoplasmic lipid vacuoles.

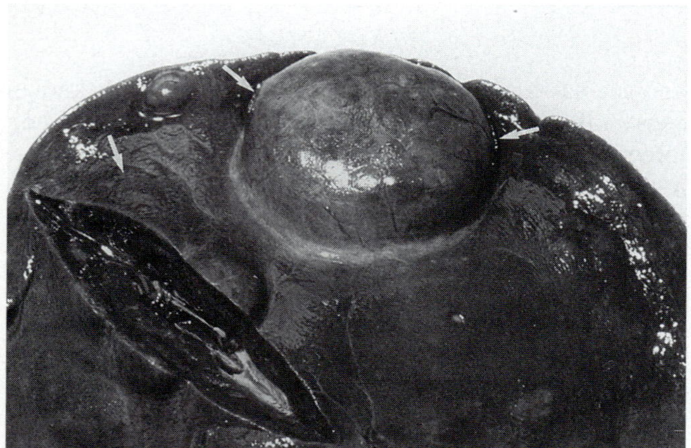

Fig. 2-35 Liver, visceral surface; dog. Nodular hyperplasia. Two nodules (*arrows*) protrude above the surface of the adjacent, normal parenchyma. *Courtesy Dr. M.D. McGavin.*

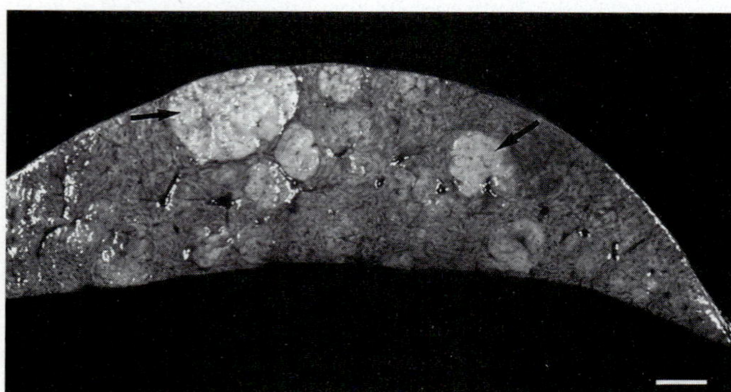

Fig. 2-36 Liver, cut surface; dog. Nodular hyperplasia. Several hyperplastic nodules are indicated by arrows. Bar = 5 mm. *Courtesy Dr. R. Fairley.*

Hepatocellular adenoma

Hepatocellular adenoma is a benign neoplasm of hepatocytes. The neoplasms usually are single, unencapsulated, variably sized masses of red or brown tissue and consist of well-differentiated hepatocytes. Portal tracts and central veins are scarce within the neoplasm. Hepatocellular adenoma has been most commonly described in young ruminants. It may be difficult in some cases to distinguish adenomas from well-differentiated hepatocellular carcinomas.

Hepatocellular carcinoma

Hepatocellular carcinoma is a malignant neoplasm of hepatocytes. It is uncommon in all domestic species, but may occur more frequently in ruminants, particularly sheep. Neoplasms are usually solitary, often involving an entire lobe, and are well demarcated. They typically consist of friable, gray-white or yellow-brown tissue that is subdivided into lobules by multiple fibrous bands (Fig. 2-37). Malignant hepatocytes characteristically form irregular trabeculae two or more cells thick, and vascular spaces are present between the trabeculae (Fig. 2-38). Crude acini or aggregates of neoplastic cells are sometimes present. Cells present in the neoplasm range from well-differentiated hepatocytes to atypical or bizarre forms. In the absence of metastasis, which is obviously indicative of malignancy, distinction of well-differentiated carcinoma and adenoma is difficult. Metastasis to a variety of tissues may occur,

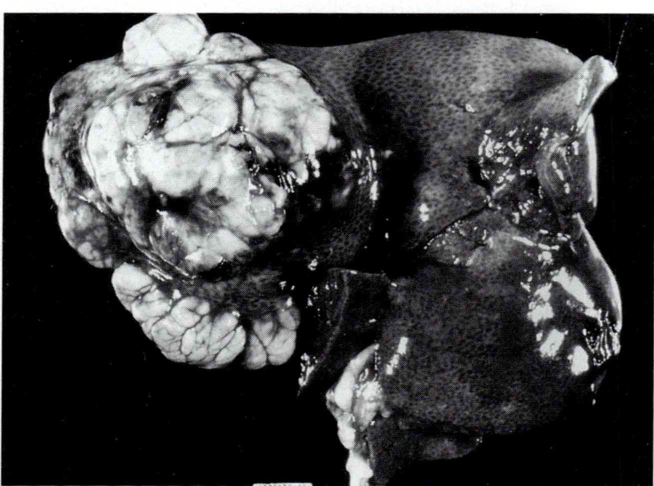

Fig. 2-37 Liver; cat. Hepatocellular carcinoma. Multilobular mass that has replaced much of the normal liver.

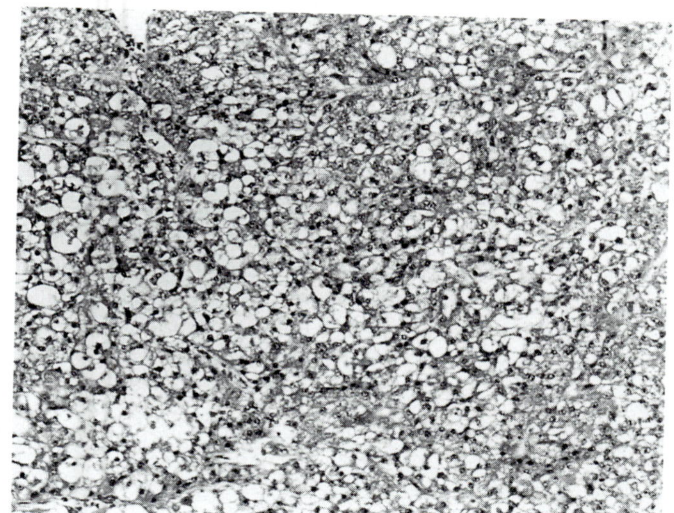

Fig. 2-38 Liver; dog. Hepatocellular carcinoma. Note the irregular lobules of hepatocytes that lack the normal microanatomic appearance of liver tissue. H & E stain.

particularly to lymph nodes within the cranial abdomen and lungs, and seeding into the tissues in the peritoneal cavity. Some hepatocellular carcinomas extensively spread within the liver (intrahepatic metastasis).

Cholangiocellular (bile duct) hyperplasia

Hyperplasia of bile ductules commonly occurs as a nonspecific response to a variety of hepatic injuries and has been described in the section Response of the Liver to Injury. Reactive proliferation of the ductular elements of the liver must be distinguished from neoplastic proliferations.

Cholangiocellular (bile duct) adenoma

Adenomas of the bile ducts are uncommon. They are usually discrete, firm, gray or white masses comprised of well-differentiated biliary epithelium. In cats, large cystic cavities that are lined by flattened biliary epithelium are regarded as adenomas by some investigators, whereas others consider them to be congenital malformations (see Figs. 2-5 and 2-6). Some of these lesions are multiloculated and can involve extensive areas of the liver. A similar, but clearly congenital, polycystic hepatic disease also occurs in dogs. It is likely that the proliferative ductular elements in affected dogs and cats represent abnormal cellular proliferations, rather than simple congenital anomalies of the ductular system.

Cholangiocellular (bile duct) carcinoma

Cholangiocellular carcinomas are malignant neoplasms of biliary epithelium that usually arise from the intrahepatic ducts. These neoplasms occur in all species. A large single mass or multiple nodules may be present within the liver; these typically are firm, raised, often with a central depression (umbilicated), pale gray to tan, and unencapsulated (Fig. 2-39). Neoplasms consist of ductules or crude acini of biliary epithelium (Fig. 2-40), which are separated by a fibrous stroma that is responsible for the characteristic firm texture of the neoplasm. Metastasis to extrahepatic sites is common, particularly to the adjacent lymph nodes of the craniad abdomen, lungs, or by seeding into the abdominal cavity. Metastasis into the peritoneal cavity can produce variably sized nodules within the mesentery and on the serosal surface of the abdominal viscera.

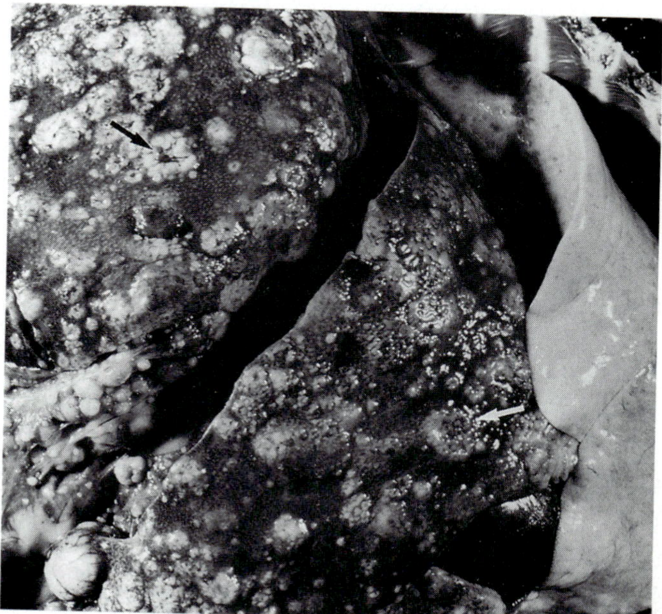

Fig. 2-39 Liver; dog. Cholangiocellular carcinoma. Multiple nodules of tumor, some of which have an umbilicated appearance (*arrows*). H & E stain. *Courtesy Dr. M.D. McGavin.*

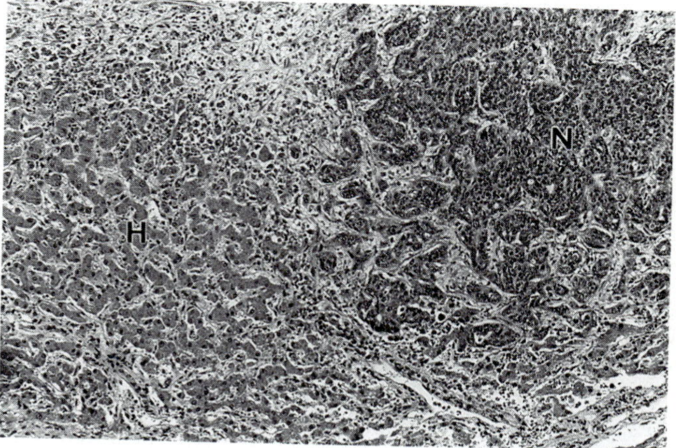

Fig. 2-40 Liver; cat. Cholangiocellular carcinoma. Cords and acini of neoplastic cells (*N*) are adjacent to persisting hepatic parenchyma (*H*). H & E stain.

Miscellaneous primary neoplasms of the liver

Primary neoplasms can arise from any of the cellular constituents of the liver, including mesenchymal neoplasms derived from the liver's connective tissue (fibrosarcoma, leiomyosarcoma, osteosarcoma) and endothelium (hemangioma and hemangiosarcoma), and carcinoids, which are neoplasms of neuroendocrine cells. Hemangiosarcoma primary to the liver is well recognized in dogs, although it is a relatively uncommon site of origin for this neoplasm as compared with the subcutis, heart and spleen. Primary mesenchymal neoplasms of the liver must be distinguished from those that are metastatic; the presence of disseminated masses throughout the liver is more typical of metastatic sarcoma than of primary hepatic sarcomas.

Metastatic neoplasms

Metastasis of neoplasms to the liver is common, and metastatic neoplasms must be distinguished from primary hyperplasia or neoplasia of the hepatobiliary tissues. It is important, therefore, when examining a neoplasm within the liver to determine if a neoplasm present at some extrahepatic site might be the primary neoplasm.

Some metastatic neoplasms have a typical appearance within the liver; for example, melanomas frequently are black because of the presence of melanin, and hematopoietic neoplasms such as lymphosarcoma and the myeloproliferative disorders can diffusely infiltrate the liver, thereby producing hepatomegaly and an enhanced lobular pattern on the cut surface (attributable to centrilobular hepatocellular degeneration because of anemia and sometimes because of zonal accumulation of neoplastic cells). The umbilicated appearance that is typical of cholangiocellular carcinoma may also occur with some metastatic carcinomas, but rarely is it a feature of sarcomas.

GALLBLADDER

Structure and Function

The gallbladder stores and concentrates bile. Considerable concentration (20- to 30-fold) of bile can occur within the gallbladder of the dog and cat, whereas little concentration occurs in swine and ruminants. The horse lacks a gallbladder and continuously releases bile into the duodenum.

The structure of the gallbladder and major ducts of the biliary system is similar in all species, consisting of a muscular wall (tunica muscularis) and a mucosa lined by simple columnar epithelium. The epithelium and muscularis are separated only by the lamina propria as the gallbladder lacks a muscularis mucosae. Hepatic bile ducts carry bile from different lobes of the liver; these ducts and the cystic duct from the gallbladder unite to form the common bile duct.* Location of the opening of the common bile duct into the intestine differs somewhat among the domestic species; it is as little as 2 cm from the pylorus in the pig to as much as 70 cm from the pylorus in the cow.

Bile consists of water, cholesterol, bile acids, bilirubin, inorganic ions, and a variety of other constituents. Secretion of bile provides (1) bile acids that are necessary for digestion of dietary fats, (2) an excretory route for various metabolites and drugs, and (3) buffers to neutralize the acid pH of the ingesta.

Bile acids are critical for normal digestion and absorption of fats and fat-soluble vitamins; however, the quantities of bile acids required far exceeds the liver's capacity to produce them. For this reason, bile acids are reabsorbed from the intestine and resecreted into bile. This is referred to as the **enterohepatic circulation** of bile acids; interruption of this process results in fat malabsorption and deficiency of fat-soluble vitamins.

Biliary Obstruction, Cholelithiasis, and Inflammatory Disorders

Biliary obstruction

Obstruction of the bile ducts occurs in domestic animals in association with cholelithiasis, foreign bodies such as parasites within the bile ducts, and stenosis of the ducts as a consequence of external compression by a neoplasm or periductular fibrosis associated with inflammation, as may follow pancreatic inflammation. Complete obstruction of major ducts may lead to extrahepatic cholestasis and jaundice. Prolonged extrahepatic cholestasis causes hepatocellular injury. The leakage of bile into portal areas causes inflammation and fibrosis that can progress to extensive scarring of the liver (biliary fibrosis) (see Fig. 2-3).

Cholelithiasis

Gallstones, as choleliths are commonly called, are concretions of normally soluble components of bile. They occur, apparently uncommonly, in all the domestic species, and are especially well described in ruminants. Stones form when these components become supersaturated and precipitate. Gallstones usually do not become clinically significant until they obstruct the biliary system.

Cholecystitis

Cholecystitis is inflammation of the gallbladder and can be acute or chronic. The gallbladder may be affected by viral infections such as infectious canine hepatitis (edema and hemorrhages) and Rift Valley fever. Fibrinous cholecystitis may occur in calves with acute salmonellosis, particularly that caused by *Salmonella enteritidis,* serotype *dublin.* Chronic cholecystitis typically accompanies prolonged bacterial infection of the biliary tree or ongoing irritation from choleliths or parasites of the gallbladder.

Hyperplastic and Neoplastic Lesions of the Gallbladder

Hyperplasia

Diffuse thickening of the gallbladder mucosa with sessile or polypoid masses occasionally is found, particularly

*The N.A.V. term is *ductus choledochus.* As this would be translated *bile duct* and would be ambiguous we have retained the older term of *common bile duct.*

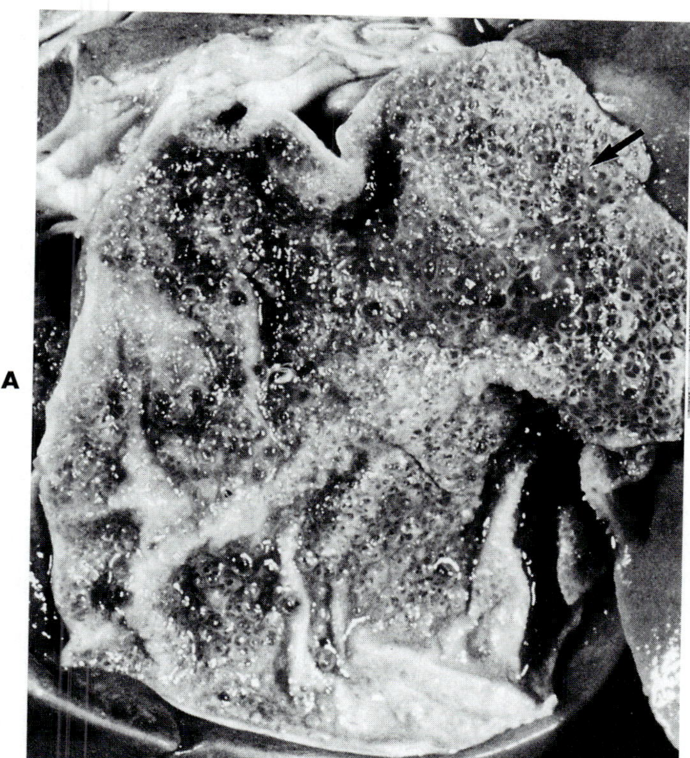

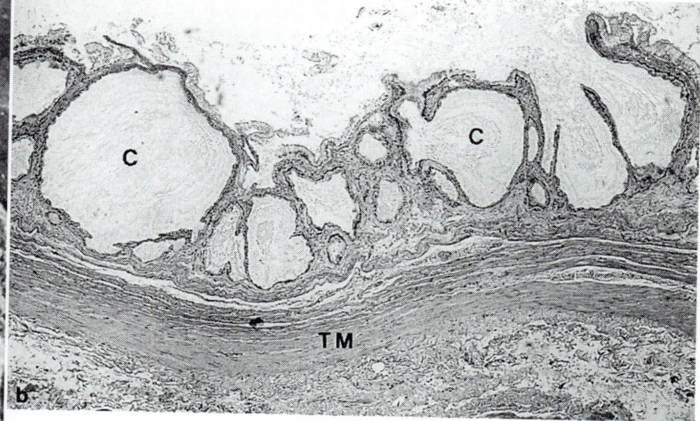

Fig. 2-41 Gallbladder; dog. Cystic mucosal hyperplasia of the gallbladder, **A**. The mucosa of the gallbladder contains numerous fluid-filled cysts that impart a bubbly appearance, **B**. The mucosa contains cysts (*C*) that are distended with mucus. Tunica muscularis (*TM*). H & E Stein. *Courtesy Dr. R. Fairley.*

in old dogs, and is referred to as cystic mucosal hyperplasia. The entire mucosa may be affected (Fig. 2-41). The mucosal masses consist of well-differentiated biliary epithelium and mucous glands. Multiple mucin-filled cysts may form within the wall of these masses. These lesions are usually of no significance to the host.

Adenoma

Adenomas of the gallbladder are rare neoplasms, but are most common in young cattle and have also been described in dogs and sheep. They are multinodular or papillary masses that protrude from the mucosal surface and consist of a loose connective tissue stalk that is lined by well-differentiated biliary epithelium.

Carcinoma

Malignant neoplasms of the gallbladder epithelium are rare in domestic animals, but have been described in dogs and cattle. They typically are composed of mucin-secreting epithelial cells and often have a papillary arrangement. Carcinoma of the gallbladder may invade the liver by direct extension and may metastasize to the hepatic lymph nodes and to more distant sites.

EXOCRINE PANCREAS

Structure and Function

The pancreas is a lobulated, pink to gray, tubuloalveolar gland, a large portion of which is located immediately adjacent to the duodenum. The blood vessels, nerves, and lymph vessels that serve the pancreas are located within the delicate connective tissue septa that separate the lobules of pancreatic tissue. The pancreas contains both endocrine and exocrine elements, the endocrine portion being the islets of Langerhans. The exocrine portion constitutes the majority of the pancreas and consists of acini composed of secretory cells. The ductal system, in which secretions of the exocrine pancreas are conveyed to the intestinal tract, commences as fine radicals within acini and progresses to intralobular and interlobular ducts. These small ducts eventually drain into the main pancreatic duct or ducts. The arrangement of the major pancreatic duct system varies considerably among the domestic species, and is particularly variable in the dog, in which at least five different anatomic arrangements are recognized.

The exocrine pancreas produces secretions that contribute to digestion in that they contain a variety of enzymes that break down dietary lipids (lipase and phospholipase), proteins (trypsin and chymotrypsin), and carbohydrates (amylase). The secretions also contain electrolytes that maintain the pH of the intestinal contents within a range that is optimal for enzymatic activity. Pancreatic enzymes act on the products of gastric digestion after they enter the duodenum. These enzymes often are released into secretions as inactive precursors (proenzymes), which help prevent degradation of the pancreas by its own digestive enzymes. These are activated within the intestine. In addition, inhibitors of pancreatic enzymes are present in the pancreatic tissue. Secretion is controlled by both neural and humoral factors.

Consequences of Dysfunction of the Exocrine Pancreas

The exocrine pancreas has considerable functional reserve; thus, only disorders that affect significant portions of this organ can cause the maldigestion that characterizes failure of exocrine pancreatic function. Maldigestion as a consequence of exocrine pancreatic insufficiency is most common in the dog, in which it usually is associated with either pancreatic atrophy or chronic pancreatitis. However, the disorder does occur sporadically in other species, including cattle, specifically in calves with pancreatic hypoplasia, and cats. Exocrine pancreatic insufficiency in small animals and calves is characterized by steatorrhea, diarrhea, and weight loss despite polyphagia. In contrast, horses with very little functional pancreatic tissue may develop hypoinsulism, but rarely develop the clinical signs that characterize exocrine pancreatic insufficiency in other species.

Developmental Anomalies

Pancreatic hypoplasia

Hypoplasia of the exocrine pancreas occurs sporadically in calves and is characterized by signs of exocrine pancreatic insufficiency. Pancreatic hypoplasia has also been described in the dog, but this disease entity is usually considered as pancreatic atrophy rather than true hypoplasia (described under Juvenile Pancreatic Atrophy). In cases of pancreatic hypoplasia, pancreatic tissue is difficult to identify; the amount is small and the persisting parenchyma is neither discrete nor lobulated like the normal gland.

Anomalies of the duct system

The arrangement of the major pancreatic duct or ducts varies between and within species, so a variety of normal arrangements occur. Sheep, for instance, have only one pancreatic duct draining into the common bile duct, whereas cattle and horses typically have two ducts, and several distinct arrangements of the pancreatic ducts have been described in dogs. Specific anomalies include congenital stenosis of the pancreatic ducts and cystic dilatation of the ducts. Congenital cysts within the pancreas occasionally occur in lambs.

Incidental Findings

Ectopic pancreatic tissue

Nodules of ectopic pancreatic tissue sometimes are present in the duodenum, stomach, spleen, gallbladder, and mesentery of the dog and cat.

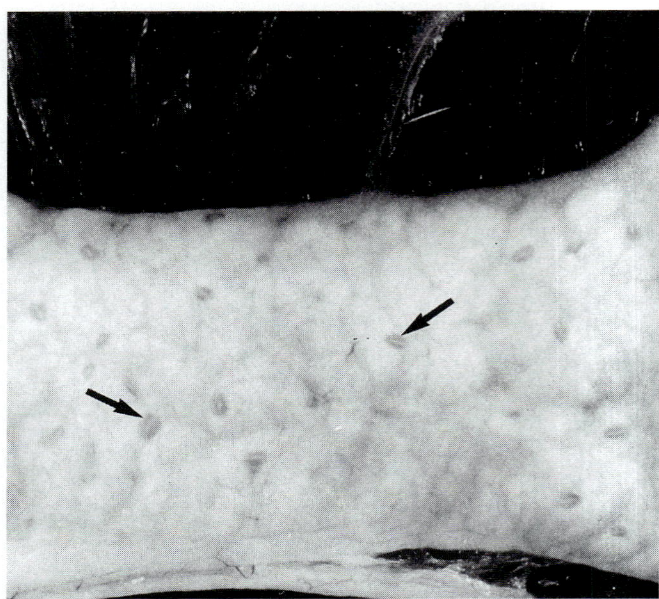

Fig. 2-42 Pancreas; cat. Pacinian corpuscles (*arrows*). The feline pancreas contains numerous pacinian corpuscles, which may be visible grossly.

Pacinian corpuscles

Pacinian corpuscles are normally present within the interlobular connective tissue of the pancreas of the cat and appear as discrete 1 to 3 mm nodules (Fig. 2-42). The corpuscles should not be mistaken for abnormal structures.

Autolysis

Autolysis of the pancreas is very rapid after death, particularly if the pancreas is traumatized. Thus, autolysis may be advanced in the pancreas before it is evident in other organs. As autolysis progresses, the color of the gland may change from its normal pink to dark red or green.

Pancreatic calculi

The formation of concretions or ''stones'' within the pancreatic duct system is termed **pancreolithiasis,** and occurs uncommonly in cattle. It is usually an incidental finding at slaughter, and apparently is slightly more common in cattle greater than 4 years of age.

Stromal fat cell infiltration

Fat cell infiltration of the interstitial connective tissue of the pancreas occurs occasionally, especially in obese cats. The pancreas itself is usually unaffected, so exocrine pancreatic function is normal, but the dispersion of the parenchyma creates the impression that the pancreas has been replaced by adipose tissue.

Pancreatic Degeneration, Necrosis, Inflammation, and Response to Injury

Pancreatic degeneration

Degeneration of the acinar cells of the exocrine pancreas is a nonspecific process that can occur as a consequence of a variety of local and systemic diseases. For instance, starvation results in loss of zymogen granules within the cytoplasm of acinar cells of the exocrine pancreas. Obstruction of the pancreatic ducts, whatever the cause, can also cause degeneration and atrophy of the exocrine pancreas. Obstruction of the pancreatic duct(s) can be caused by neoplasms or chronic inflammation and associated fibrosis that compress the duct, or by foreign bodies such as parasites or pancreoliths that occlude the ductal lumen. Pancreatic atrophy also may occur as a consequence of widespread interstitial fibrosis of the pancreas, as occurs, for example, in dogs with chronic pancreatitis.

Juvenile pancreatic atrophy

A distinct syndrome characterized by atrophy of the exocrine pancreas has been recognized in several breeds of dog. It is particularly common in the German shepherd dog, in which it appears to be inherited as an autosomal recessive trait. Young animals are affected, usually between 6 to 12 months of age. This lesion may be one of hypoplasia or atrophy. Affected dogs have signs typical of maldigestion secondary to exocrine pancreatic insufficiency and rapidly lose weight despite a voracious appetite. The pancreas in affected dogs is small (Fig. 2-43), but islands of normal exocrine pancreatic tissue are usually present.

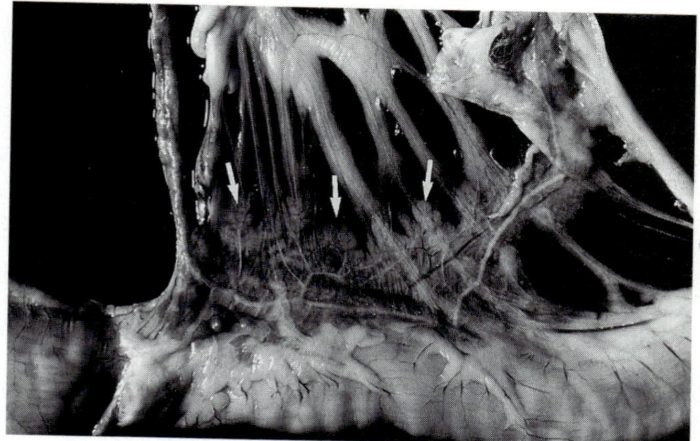

Fig. 2-43 Pancreas; dog. Pancreatic atrophy/hypoplasia. Virtually no pancreatic tissue is present in this case. Pancreatic remnant is identified with arrows. *Courtesy Dr. M.D. McGavin.*

Pancreatic necrosis, pancreatitis, and response to injury

Pancreatic necrosis and pancreatitis have been described in a variety of species, although the cause usually is different in each species. Causes of necrosis of acinar cells of the exocrine pancreas include *Cassia occidentalis* intoxication and T-2 toxin (a trichothecene mycotoxin) toxicosis of swine, as well as zinc toxicosis of veal calves and sheep. Undoubtedly, however, spontaneous necrosis and inflammation of the pancreas are most common in the dog. Pancreatic necrosis and pancreatitis may occur as either an acute or chronic disease process, and, although the pathogenesis is similar, the clinical signs and lesions of acute and chronic pancreatitis are distinct.

Acute pancreatitis, as either spontaneous or idiopathic pancreatitis, is particularly common in the dog, and obese, sedentary bitches are especially predisposed. Pancreatitis in dogs occurs as a consequence of release of activated pancreatic enzymes into the pancreatic parenchyma and adjacent tissues. These activated enzymes, particularly phospholipase A and elastase, digest pancreatic tissue, which in turn results in release of inflammatory mediators that further amplify the process and attract inflammatory cells. The mechanism responsible for the release of the potent pancreatic enzymes into these tissues is incompletely characterized and may involve more than one initiating event. Acute pancreatitis commonly occurs after dogs have consumed a meal high in fat.

Signs of acute pancreatitis include anorexia, vomiting, and abdominal pain. The lesions of acute pancreatitis are referable to proteolytic degradation of pancreatic parenchyma, vascular damage and hemorrhage, and necrosis of peripancreatic fat by lipolytic enzymes. Inflammation, characterized by the accumulation of leukocytes around the affected tissue, is rapidly superimposed upon the initial tissue necrosis. Mild cases of pancreatitis are characterized by edema of the interstitial tissue of the pancreas. Acute hemorrhagic pancreatitis is more severe and is characterized by a pancreas that is edematous and contains areas that are gray-white, reflecting coagulation necrosis, and other areas that are dark red or blue-black as a consequence of hemorrhage (Fig. 2-44). Areas of fat necrosis are manifested as chalky-white foci, due to saponification of necrotic adipose tissue in the mesentery adjacent to the pancreas. Portions of normal pancreatic parenchyma may be interspersed between affected portions. The peritoneal cavity frequently contains blood-stained fluid, which may contain droplets of fat. Peritonitis is manifested by fibrinous adhesions between the affected portions of the pancreas and adjacent tissues.

The microscopic appearance of acute hemorrhagic pancreatitis reflects the gross lesions just described. Characteristic lesions include focally extensive areas of coagulation necrosis of pancreatic parenchyma, accumulation of fibrinous exudate in the interlobular septa, hemorrhage, influx of leukocytes, and necrosis and inflammation of fat in

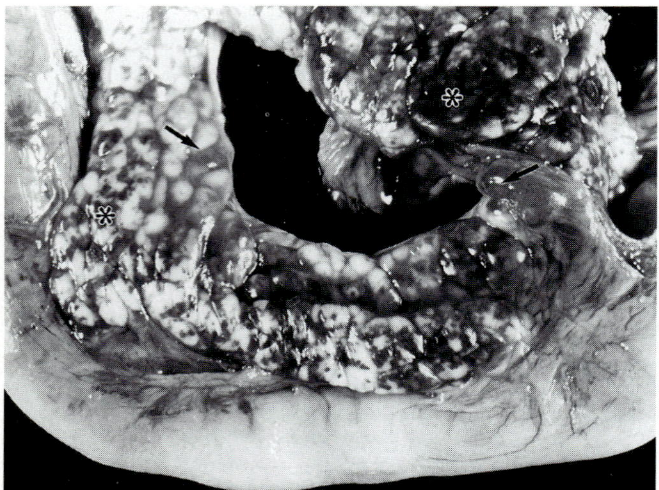

Fig. 2-44 Pancreas; dog. Acute hemorrhagic pancreatitis. Note areas of hemorrhage (*asterisks*) and edema (*arrows*) present throughout the pancreas. *Courtesy Dr. R. Fairley.*

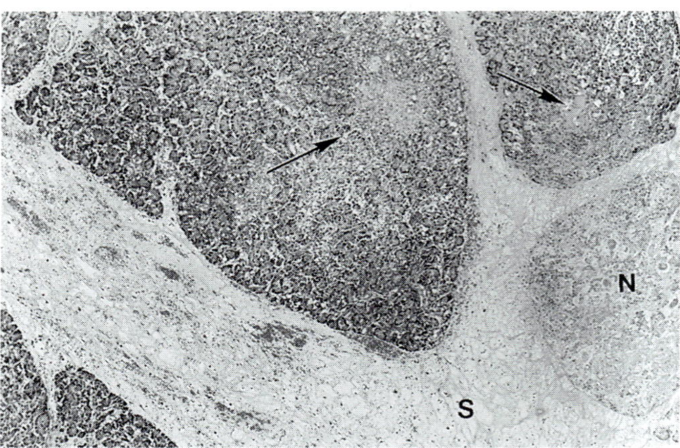

Fig. 2-45 Pancreas; dog. Acute hemorrhagic pancreatitis (histologic appearance of the pancreas depicted in Fig. 2-44). Note the accumulation of fibrinous exudate within the interlobular septa (*S*) and coagulation necrosis of one lobule (*N*) and portions of others (*arrows*). H & E stain.

the mesentery adjacent to the affected portions of pancreas (Figs. 2-45 and 2-46).

Acute, severe pancreatitis produces systemic effects in affected dogs. The release of inflammatory mediators and activated enzymes from the damaged pancreas may produce widespread vascular injury and subsequent widespread hemorrhage, shock, and disseminated intravascular coagulation. The liver also is affected in many cases of pancreatitis, as indicated by elevation in the activities of serum hepatic enzymes (such as alanine aminotransferase), and even focal hepatic necrosis.

Pancreatitis is occasionally initiated by trauma, usually in small animals as a consequence of some crushing or impact injury to the abdomen. Leakage of enzymes from the pancreas, as a result of trauma, initiates necrosis and inflammation of the pancreas and adjacent tissues in the same manner as previously described for pancreatitis in the dog.

Acute pancreatitis that is sufficient to cause clinical disease apparently is considerably less common in species other than the dog. Acute pancreatic necrosis occurs sporadically in cats. Acute pancreatic necrosis and pancreatitis also have been described in the horse; the pathogenesis of pancreatitis in this species differs from that in the dog and cat, because necrosis and inflammation are likely initiated by migration of strongyle larvae through the pancreas. Subsequent release of pancreatic enzymes results in enzymatic digestion of the pancreas and surrounding tissues.

Chronic pancreatitis is typically accompanied by fibrosis and parenchymal atrophy. Chronic inflammation of the pancreas is most common and important in the dog. Chronic pancreatitis does occur in other species, including cats, horses, and cattle, but rarely is of clinical significance in these species. In the dog, pancreatic fibrosis and chronic

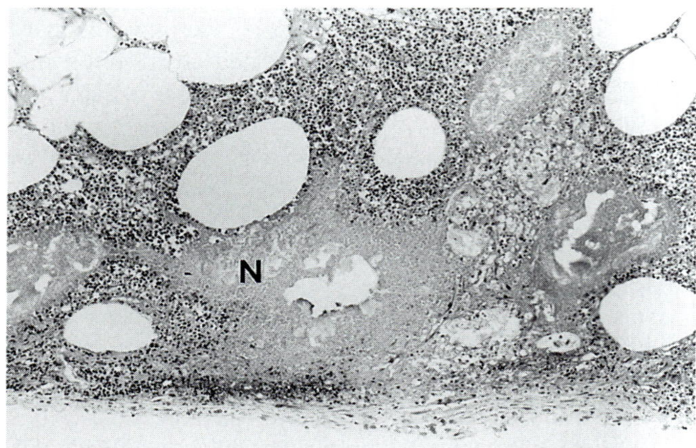

Fig. 2-46 Pancreas; dog. Acute hemorrhagic pancreatitis. Necrotic fat (*N*) in the mesentery adjacent to the pancreas is surrounded by degenerated neutrophils. H & E stain.

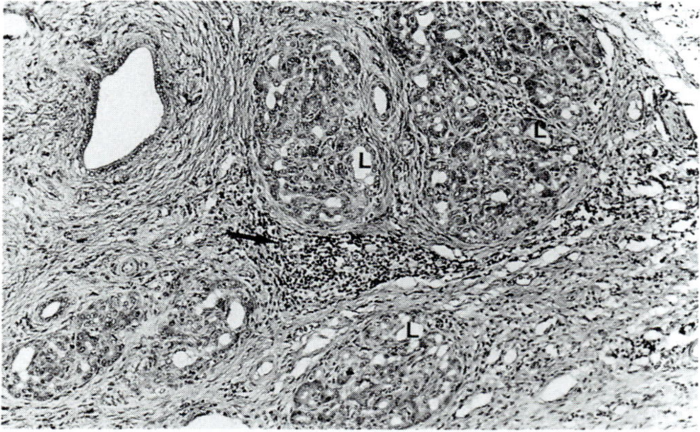

Fig. 2-47 Pancreas; cat. Chronic pancreatitis. Note the atrophic lobules (*L*) separated by fibrous connective tissue that contains lymphocytes (*arrow*). H & E stain.

pancreatitis are consequences of progressive destruction of the pancreas by repeated mild episodes of acute pancreatic necrosis and pancreatitis. The pancreas apparently has poor regenerative capacity and responds to injury with replacement fibrosis and atrophy of persisting parenchyma. Thus, ongoing destruction of pancreatic tissue will cause progressive loss of glandular tissue without replacement (Fig. 2-47). If a significant portion of the pancreas is affected, dogs may develop signs of exocrine pancreatic insufficiency, with or without signs of endocrine pancreatic insufficiency (diabetes mellitus). The pancreas in affected animals is severely distorted and becomes a shrunken and nodular mass; fibrous adhesions of the pancreas to adjacent tissues are often present. Destruction of pancreatic tissue frequently is not of sufficient magnitude to cause exocrine pancreatic insufficiency, because areas of pancreatic fibrosis are sometimes found as incidental lesions at necropsy of dogs with apparently normal digestive function. Pancreatic fibrosis also occurs in dogs and in sheep with zinc toxicosis.

Chronic pancreatitis and replacement fibrosis also occur in the horse, usually as a consequence of either parasitic migration or from ascending bacterial infection of the pancreatic ductal system. In addition, pancreatitis may occur in horses with chronic eosinophilic gastroenteritis. However, chronic pancreatitis usually is not clinically apparent in the horse, as signs of exocrine pancreatic insufficiency rarely, if ever, occur in this species.

Parasitic Infections

A variety of parasites may inhabit the pancreatic ducts of domestic animals. Parasitic infections of the pancreatic ducts are important if they occlude the ducts, either by direct physical obstruction or by inducing inflammation within and around ducts. Examples include flukes of the families Opisthorchidae *(Opisthorchis tenuicollis, O. viverrini, Clonorchis sinensis, Metorchis albidus, M. conjunctus)* and Dicrocoelidae *(Eurytrema pancreaticum, Concinnum procyonis, Dicrocoelium dendriticum)* that may inhabit the pancreatic ducts of a variety of animal species. Nematodes, particularly ascarids, and cestodes are common gastrointestinal parasites of the domestic species; occasionally, they may lodge within the pancreatic ducts.

Hyperplasia and Neoplasia

Pancreatic nodular hyperplasia

Nodular hyperplasia of the exocrine pancreas occurs in dogs, cats, and cattle. It is especially common in older dogs and cats. The lesion is of no clinical significance, but it must be distinguished from neoplasms of the endocrine and exocrine pancreas.

Hyperplastic nodules typically are multiple, raised, smooth, and a uniform gray or white on cut surface (Fig. 2-48). The nodules may be firmer than adjacent normal pancreas. Microscopically, these nodules consist of unencapsulated aggregates of acinar cells. The distinction between hyperplasia and adenoma of the exocrine pancreas is poorly defined in domestic animals.

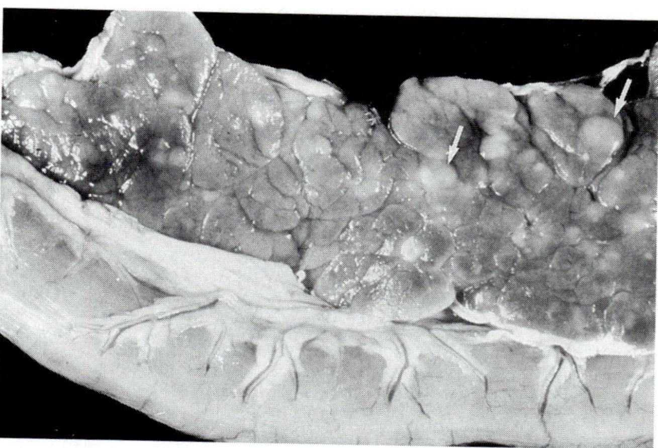

Fig. 2-48 Pancreas; dog. Nodular hyperplasia of exocrine pancreas. Hyperplastic nodules (*arrows*) are pale and project above the surface.

Pancreatic adenoma

Adenomas of the exocrine pancreas are extremely rare, but have been described in the cat (Fig. 2-49). Those of acinar cell origin share all the features of hyperplastic nodules, but are single and larger than normal pancreatic lobules, whereas hyperplastic nodules are not larger than normal lobules; this distinction clearly is somewhat arbitrary.

Pancreatic carcinoma

Carcinoma of the ductular epithelium or acinar cells of the exocrine pancreas is uncommon in all species. It is most often reported in the dog and cat. The neoplasms may consist of single or multiple nodules of variable size within the pancreas, each of which consists of gray or yellow tissue. Areas of hemorrhage or necrosis may be present within the neoplasm. The neoplasm is usually firmer than the adjacent pancreas because of proliferation of fibrous connective tissue. Adhesion of the affected pancreas to adjacent tissues may occur. This neoplasm often invades adjacent tissues and the peritoneal cavity. Peritoneal implants form nodules over the mesentery, omentum, and serosa of the abdominal viscera (Fig. 2-50). Metastasis to the abdominal lymph nodes adjacent to the pancreas is also common, and some carcinomas metastasize widely.

Microscopic features of carcinomas of the exocrine pancreas range from well-differentiated adenocarcinomas with tubular patterns to undifferentiated carcinomas with solid patterns. The amount of fibrous stroma varies considerably and, usually, is greatest in poorly differentiated neoplasms. Zymogen granules similar to those present in normal acinar cells of the pancreas are often absent within the cytoplasm of the neoplastic cells.

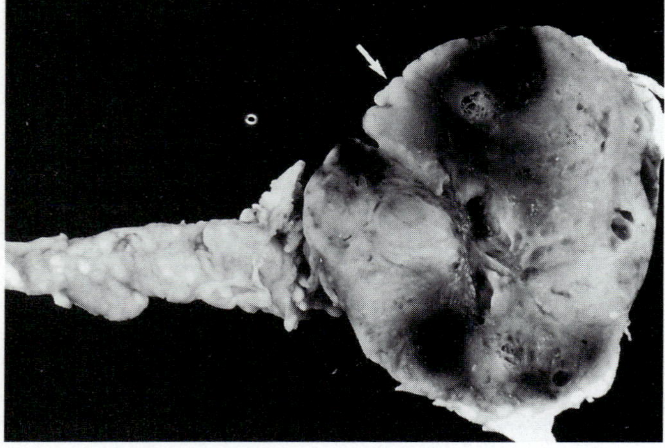

Fig. 2-49 Pancreas; cat. Pancreatic adenoma. This is a single large mass within the pancreas (*arrow*).

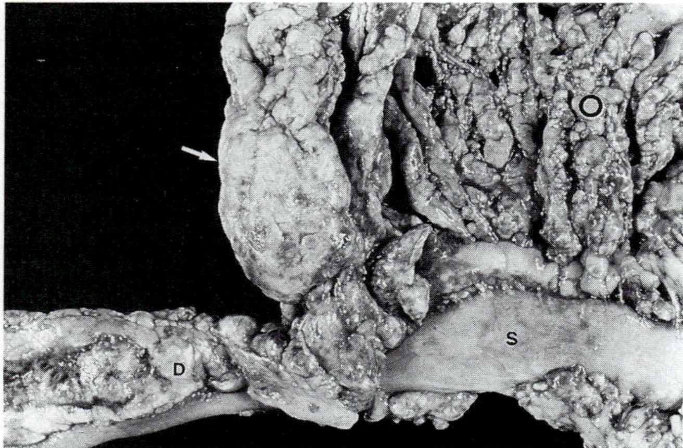

Fig. 2-50 Pancreas; dog. Pancreatic carcinoma with metastasis into the peritoneal cavity. The primary tumor is present in the pancreas (*arrow*), and tumor implants are present on the serosal surface of the stomach (*S*), duodenum (*D*), and omentum (*O*).

Acknowledgments
The authors gratefully acknowledge the following individuals who have generously contributed photographs or material used in the figures contained in this text: Drs. R. Fairley, B. Johnson, J. King, M. Leach, M. McEntee, R.L. Michel, S. Smith, and K. Sokol.

GLOSSARY

Acinus structure that depicts hepatic glandular microanatomy. The acinus is a diamond-shaped structure that centers on the portal tract so that the terminal branches of the portal vein and hepatic artery are at the center of the acinus and terminal hepatic venules are at the periphery.

Bioactivation process by which hepatic biotransformation of chemicals produces reactive metabolites that mediate hepatic injury.

Biotransformation process by which endogenous and exogenous substances are metabolized by the liver for excretion.

Bridging hepatic necrosis or fibrosis necrosis or fibrosis that connects terminal hepatic venule to terminal hepatic venules or other portal tracts.

Centroacinar that portion of the acinus that centers on the portal triad.

Centrilobular that portion of the hepatic lobule that is adjacent to the terminal hepatic venule.

Cholangiohepatitis inflammation that often centers on the biliary system but extends into the hepatic parenchyma.

Cholecystitis inflammation of the gallbladder.

Cholelithiasis the presence of ''stones'' within the biliary tree.

Cholestasis reduced canalicular flow of bile.

Cirrhosis synonymous with end-stage liver; a liver characterized by diffuse fibrosis and nodular parenchymal regeneration leading to severe architectural distortion of the liver.

Enterohepatic circulation reabsorption of materials, particularly bile acids, from the intestine for resecretion into the intestine via the hepatobiliary system.

Hemochromatosis iron overload disorder; a condition characterized by abnormal accumulation of iron in hepatocytes, associated with liver dysfunction.

Hemosiderosis condition characterized by excess hemosiderin in the liver.

Hepatic encephalopathy metabolic disorder of the central nervous system which occurs as a consequence of liver failure.

Hepatic lipidosis excessive accumulation of lipid within hepatocytes.

Hepatitis inflammation of the liver.

Icterus (synonym: jaundice) yellow discoloration of tissues, especially those rich in elastin, as a consequence of hyperbilirubinemia.

Idiosyncratic toxic hepatic injury that does not occur in the majority of animals exposed to a particular agent and is therefore not predictable.

Massive necrosis hepatic necrosis that affects entire lobules.

Midzonal necrosis that affects only the portion of the lobule between the periportal and centrilobular regions.

Mixed-function oxidases (MFOs) hepatic enzymes responsible for much of the biotransformation of chemicals which occurs in the liver.

Mycotoxin toxin produced by a fungus.

Pancreatitis inflammation of the pancreas; often used interchangeably with acute hemorrhagic necrosis of the canine pancreas.

Paracentrovenular synonymous with periacinar.

Passive hepatic congestion hepatic congestion secondary to increased pressure within the hepatic vein.

Periportal area of the hepatic lobule adjacent to the portal tract.

Periacinar area of the acinus adjacent to the central vein.

Photosensitization cutaneous injury resulting from the action of ultraviolet light on accumulated photodynamic pigments.

Phytotoxin plant toxin.

Reticular pattern enhancement of the liver's normal lobular pattern reflecting any one of a variety of different possible causes (ischemia, toxic injury, lipid accumulation, etc.); also known as enhanced lobular pattern and "nutmeg liver" if associated with passive hepatic congestion.

Tension lipidosis focal accumulation of fat at the margins of the liver, typically at the sites of mesenteric attachments; the condition likely is due to impaired blood flow to the affected portion of the liver.

Zonal change degeneration or necrosis affecting one or more zones of the hepatic lobule or acinus throughout the liver.

Suggested Readings

Acland HM, Mann PC, Robertson JL, Divers TJ, Lichensteiger CA, Whitlock RH. Toxic hepatopathy in neonatal foals. Vet Pathol 1984; 21:3-9.

Anthony PP, Ishak KG, Nayak NC, Poulsen HE, Scheuer PJ, Sobin LH. The morphology of cirrhosis: definition, nomenclature, and classification. Bull WHO 1977; 55:521-540.

Bergman JR. Nodular hyperplasia in the liver of the dog: An association with changes in the Ito cell population. Vet Pathol 1985; 22:427-438.

Bunch SE, Castleman WL, Hornbuckle WE, Tennant BC. Hepatic cirrhosis associated with long-term anticonvulsant therapy in dogs. J Am Vet Med Assoc 1982; 181:357-362.

Buoro IBJ, Atwell RB. Development of a model of caval syndrome in dogs infected with *Dirofilaria immitis*. Aust Vet J 1984; 61:267-268.

Center SA. Feline liver disorders and their management. Comp Cont Educ Pract 1986; 8:889-901.

Cornwell HJC, Wright NG. The pathology of experimental infectious canine hepatitis in neonatal puppies. Res Vet Sci 1969; 10:156-160.

Cullison RF. Acetaminophen toxicosis in small animals: Clinical signs, mode of action and treatment. Comp Cont Educ Pract 1984; 6:315-321.

Dillon R. The liver in systemic disease. Vet Clin North Am 1985; 15:97-117.

Ewing GO, Suter PF, Bailey CS. Hepatic insufficiency associated with congenital anomalies of the portal vein in dogs. J Am Anim Hosp Assoc 1974; 10:463-476.

Fittschen C, Bellamy JEC. Prednisone-induced morphologic and chemical changes in the liver of dogs. Vet Pathol 1984; 21:399-406.

Haywood S, Rutgers HC, Christian MK. Hepatitis and copper accumulation in Skye terriers. Vet Pathol 1988; 25:408-414.

Higgins R. A minireview of the pathogenesis of acute leptospirosis. Can Vet J 1981; 22:277-278.

Hill RC, Van Winkle TJ. Acute necrotizing pancreatitis and acute suppurative pancreatitis in the cat: A retrospective study of 40 cases (1976-1989). J Vet Int Med 7:25-33, 1993.

Kelly WR. The liver and biliary system. In: Jubb KVF, Kennedy PC, Palmer N, eds. Pathology of Domestic Animals. 4th ed. New York: Academic Press, 1985:239.

Kingsbury JM. Poisonous Plants of the United States and Canada. Englewood Cliffs, NJ: Prentice-Hall, 1964.

Kircher CH, Nielsen SW. Tumors of the pancreas. Bull WHO 1976; 53:195-202.

Moore PF, Whiting PG. Hepatic lesions associated with intrahepatic arterioportal fistulae in dogs. Vet Pathol 1986; 23:57-62.

Moore RP. Pathophysiology of canine exocrine pancreatic insufficiency. Comp Cont Educ Pract 1980; 2:657-660.

Newberne PM, Butler WH. Acute and chronic effects of aflatoxin on the liver of domestic and laboratory animals: A review. Cancer Res 1969; 29:236-250.

Ponomarkov V, Mackey LJ. Tumors of the liver and biliary system. Bull WHO 1975; 53:187-194.

Popp JA. Tumors of the liver, gall bladder, and pancreas. In: Moulton JE, ed. Tumors in Domestic Animals. 3rd ed. Berkeley: University of California Press, 1990.

Prentice DE, James RW, Wadsworth PF. Pancreatic atrophy in young beagle dogs. Vet Pathol 1980; 17:575-580.

Rowe LD, Corrier DE, Reagor JC, Jones LP. Experimentally induced *Cassia roemeriana* poisoning in cattle and goats. Am J Vet Res 1986; 48:992-997.

Scarratt WK, Saunders GK. Cholelithiasis and biliary obstruction in a horse. Comp Cont Educ Pract 1985; 7:S428-S431.68.

Schiff L, Schiff ER. Diseases of the Liver. 6th ed. Philadelphia: Lippincott, 1987.

Seawright AA. Animal Health in Australia. Vol. 2. Chemical and plant poisons. Canberra: Australian Government Printing Service, 1982.

Seawright AA, Allen JE. Pathology of the liver and kidney in Lantana poisoning of cattle. Aust Vet J 1972; 48:323-331.

Sherding RG. Acute hepatic failure. Vet Clin North Am 1985; 15:119-133.

Sipes IG, Gandolfi AJ. Biotransformation of toxicants. In: Klassen CD, Amdur MO, Doull J, eds. Casarett and Doull's Toxicology. 3rd ed. New York: Macmillan, 1986:64.

Stogdale L, Booth AJ. Bacillary hemoglobinuria in cattle. Comp Cont Educ Pract 1974; 6:S284-S290.

Tennant B, Evans CD, Schwartz LW, Gribble DH, Kanecko JJ. Equine hepatic insufficiency. Vet Clin North Am 1973; 3:279-289.

Thompson KG, Lake DE, Cordes DO. Hepatic encephalopathy associated with chronic facial eczema. N Z Vet J 1979; 27:221-223.

Thomson GW, Wilson RW, Hall EA, Physick-Sheard P. Tyzzer's disease in the foal: Case reports and review. Can Vet J 1977; 18:41-43.

Thornburg LP, Shaw D, Dolan M, Raisbeck M, Crawford S, Dennis GL, Olwin DB. Hereditary copper toxicosis in West Highland white terriers. Vet Pathol 1986; 23:148-154.

Trigo FJ, Thompson H, Breeze RG, Nash AS. The pathology of liver tumors in the dog. J Comp Pathol 1982; 92:21-39.

Twedt DC, Sternlieb I, Gilbertson SR. Clinical, morphologic and chemical studies on copper toxicosis of Bedlington terriers. J Am Vet Med Assoc 1979; 175:269-275.

Wigton DH, Kociba GJ, Hoover EA. Infectious canine hepatitis: Animal model for viral-induced disseminated intravascular coagulation. Blood 1976; 47:287-296.

CHAPTER

3

Respiratory System

ALFONSO LÓPEZ

Diseases of the respiratory system are some of the leading causes of morbidity and mortality in large domestic animals and a major source of economic loss to farmers. Thus, veterinarians are routinely called to diagnose and treat and to implement health management practices aimed at reducing the impact of these diseases in food animals. In companion animals, diseases of the respiratory tract are also very common, perhaps with little economic significance but with enormous importance to clinicians.

STRUCTURE AND FUNCTION

To facilitate the understanding of structure and function, it is convenient to arbitrarily divide the respiratory system into conductive, transitional, and gas exchange systems. The **conductive system** includes the nasal cavity, pharynx, larynx, trachea, and bronchi, all of which are largely lined by pseudostratified, ciliated, columnar cells plus a variable proportion of secretory goblet (mucous) and serous cells (Figs. 3-1 and 3-2). The **transitional system** of the respiratory tract is composed of bronchioles, which serve as a transition zone between the conductive system (ciliated) and the exchange (alveolar) system. The disappearance of cilia in the transitional system is not abrupt; the ciliated cells in the proximal bronchiolar region become scarce and progressively attenuated until the point where distal bronchioles no longer contain ciliated cells. Bronchioles also lack goblet cells, but instead contain other types of secretory cells, notably the Clara cell. These cells are highly metabolic and play an important role in detoxification of

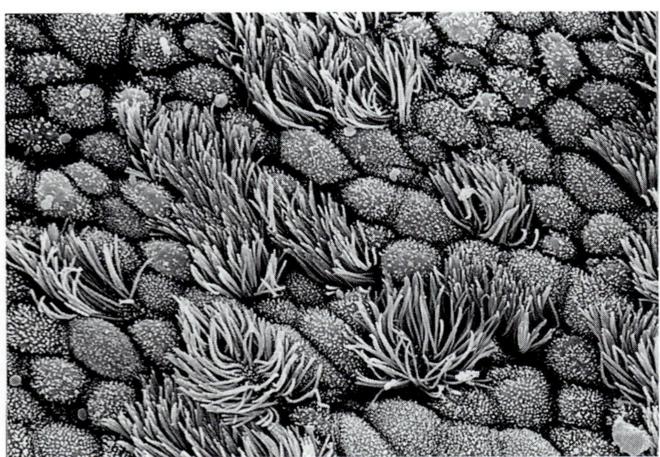

Fig. 3-1 Scanning electron micrograph. Bronchus; rat. Normal bronchial mucosa. Mucous layer was removed before fixation to expose the external surface of the epithelium. Mucosa is composed of ciliated and nonciliated secretory cells. Ciliated cells have numerous slender cilia. Nonciliated secretory cells have a dome-shaped surface with abundant microvilli. The proportion of ciliated to nonciliated cells varies depending on the level of airways. Ciliated cells are more abundant in proximal airways, whereas secretory cells are more numerous in distal portions of the conductive and transitional systems.

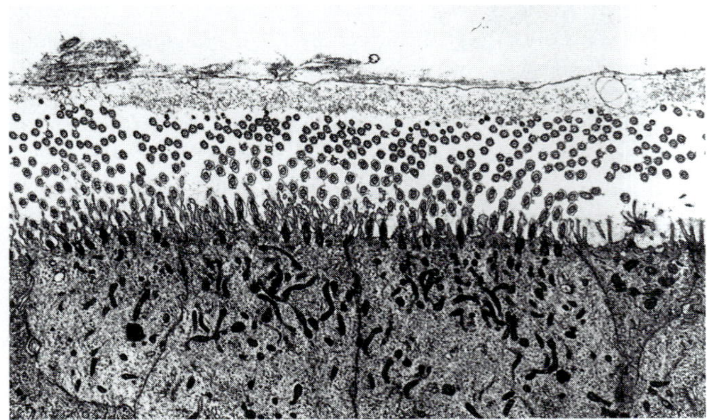

Fig. 3-2 Transmission electron micrograph. Trachea; cow. Cross-sectional view of cilia. Normal ciliated epithelium. This trachea was specially fixed in order to preserve the mucous lining. The mucous layer is composed of an internal, clear, hypophase-fluid layer (not visible) surrounding microvilli and kinocilia and an external mucous epiphase at the level of the tips of the kinocilia (X 5000). *Sims et al. Biotechnol Histochem 1991; 66:173-180.*

Table 3-1. Common pathogens, allergens, and toxic substances present in air

Microbes	Viruses, bacteria, fungi, protozoa
Plant dust	Grain, flour, cotton, wood
Animal products	Dander, feathers, mites, insect chitin
Toxic gases	Ammonia (NH_3), hydrogen sulfide (H_2S), nitrogen dioxide (NO_2), sulfur dioxide (SO_2), chlorine
Chemicals	Organic and inorganic solvents, herbicides, asbestos, nickel, lead

xenobiotics (foreign substances), similar to the role hepatocytes play in the liver. In carnivores and monkeys, and to a much lesser extent in horses and human beings, the most distal portion of the bronchiolar lining is repeatedly interrupted by alveolar structures giving origin to the respiratory bronchioles. The **gas exchange system** of the respiratory tract in all mammals is formed by millions of alveoli, which are superficially lined by two distinct types of epithelial cells known as pneumonocytes type I (membranous) and pneumonocytes type II (granular).

All three—the conductive, transitional, and exchange systems of the respiratory system—are vulnerable to injury due to constant exposure to air containing a myriad of microbes, particles, fibers, toxic gases, and vapors. Vulnerability of the respiratory system to aerogenous (airborne) injury is primarily due to (1) the extensive interface between the respiratory system and inspired air, (2) the large volume of air passing continuously into the lungs, and (3) the high concentration of noxious elements that can be present in the air (Table 3-1). For human beings, it has been estimated that the surface of the respiratory tract is approximately 200 square meters (m^2), roughly the area of a tennis court. It has also been estimated that the volume of air reaching the human lungs every day is around 10,000 L (liter), roughly the volume of a medium-sized swimming pool. In the horse, the surface of the lungs is estimated to be around 2000 m^2.

Lungs are also susceptible to hematogenously borne microbes, toxins, and emboli. This is not surprising since the pulmonary capillary bed is the largest in the body, with a surface area of 70 m^2 in the adult human being; this translates to 2400 km (kilometer) of capillaries, with 1 ml of blood occupying up to 16 km of capillary bed.

NORMAL FLORA OF THE RESPIRATORY SYSTEM

The respiratory system has its own normal bacterial flora as does any other body system in contact with the external environment. If a swab is passed deep into the nasal cavity of any healthy animal and is sent for microbiologic culture, various species of bacteria will be identified. This population of organisms constitutes the normal flora of the respiratory tract, which is restricted only to the most proximal region of the conductive system (nasal cavity, pharynx, larynx). The thoracic portions of the trachea, bronchi, and lungs are considered to be sterile. The types of bacteria present in the nasal flora vary considerably among animal species. Some bacteria present in the nasal flora are pathogens associated with important respiratory infections. For instance, *Pasteurella haemolytica* is part of the bovine nasal flora, yet this bacterium causes a devastating disease in cattle, pneumonic pasteurellosis (shipping fever pneumonia). Experimental studies have established that microorganisms from the nasal flora are continuously carried into the lungs via tracheal air. In spite of this constant bacterial bombardment from the nasal flora and from contaminated air, normal lungs remain sterile due to their remarkably effective defense mechanisms.

DEFENSE MECHANISMS OF THE RESPIRATORY SYSTEM

It is axiomatic that a particle, microbe, or toxic gas must first gain entry to a vulnerable region of the respiratory system before it can have a pathologic effect. The characteristics of size, shape, and distribution of particles present in inspired air are studied in **aerobiology.** It is important to recognize the difference between deposition and retention of inhaled particles. **Deposition** is the process by which particles of various sizes and shapes are trapped within specific regions of the respiratory tract. **Clearance** is the process by which deposited particles are destroyed, neutralized, and removed from the mucosal surfaces. The main mechanisms involved in clearance are sneezing, coughing, absorption, mucociliary transport, and phagocytosis. The difference between what is deposited and what is cleared from the respiratory tract is referred to as **retention.** Abnormal retention of particles resulting from increased deposition, decreased clearance, or a combination of both is the underlying pathogenetic mechanism involved in many pulmonary diseases.

The anatomic configuration of the conductive system (nasal cavity and bronchi) plays a unique role in preventing or reducing the penetration of noxious material into the lungs, especially into the alveolar region, which is the most vulnerable portion of the respiratory system. The coiled arrangement of the nasal conchae creates enormous turbulences of airflow and, as a result, centrifugal forces are created that forcefully impact particles larger than 10 μm (micrometer) onto the surface of the nasal mucosa. Although particles smaller than 10 μm could escape trapping in the nasal cavity, these medium-sized particles meet a second barrier at the bifurcation of the trachea and bronchi. Here, abrupt changes in the direction of air (inertia), occurring at the bifurcation of major airways, cause particles, the size of 2 to 10 μm, to impact onto the surface of the bronchial mucosa (Fig. 3-3). Since the velocity of inspired

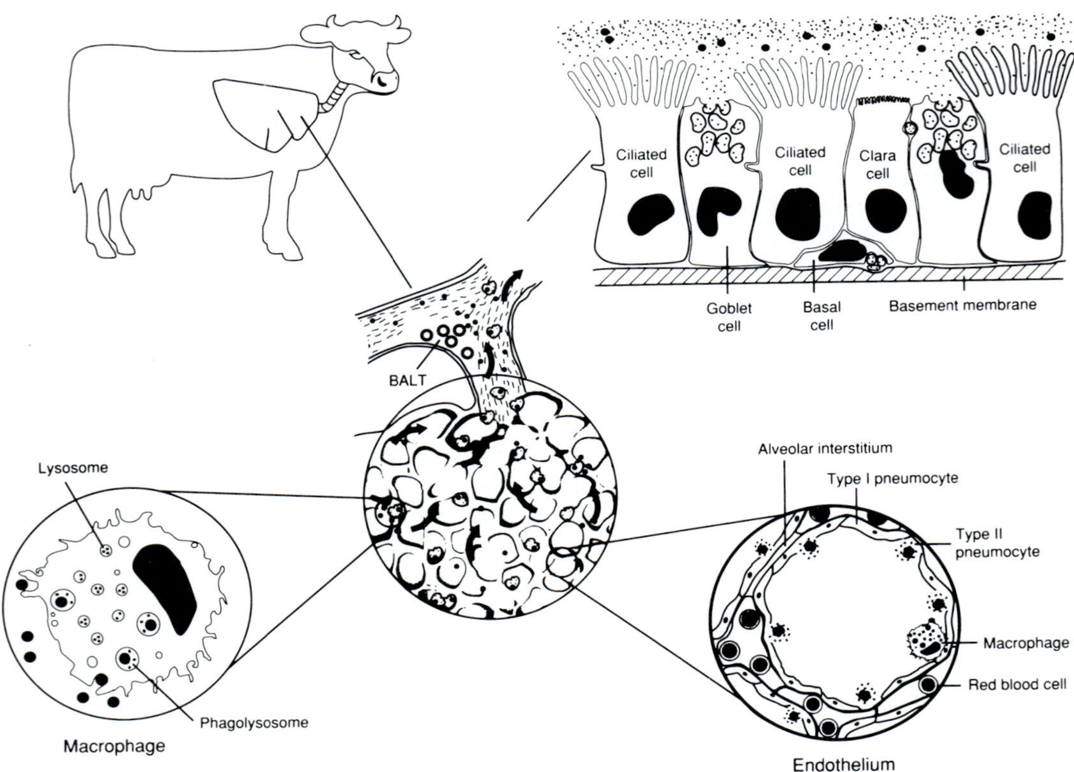

Fig. 3-3 Respiratory tract, schematic representation. The conductive system extending from nasal cavity to bronchi is lined by the mucociliary escalator, which is comprised of ciliated and nonciliated secretory cells and mucus. The large dots represent particles trapped by mucus. Bronchial associated lymphoid tissue (BALT) is strategically located at the bifurcation of airways. Particles reaching the transitional and exchange systems (bronchioles and alveoli) are ingested by the pulmonary alveolar macrophages, which exit the lung via the mucociliary escalator. The alveolar wall is comprised of capillaries, interstitium, and alveolar lining (type I and II pneumonocytes).

air at the level of small bronchi and bronchioles becomes rather slow, inertial and centrifugal forces no longer play a significant role in impacting inhaled particles onto the mucosal surface. Here, at the transitional (bronchiolar) and exchange (alveolar) regions, particles, 2 μm or smaller, may come into contact with respiratory mucosa by means of sedimentation due to gravitational force or by diffusion due to brownian movement. Infective aerosols containing bacteria and viruses are within the size range to gain access to the bronchiolar-alveolar region.

In addition to size, other factors such as shape, length, electrical charge, and humidity play an important role in deposition, retention, and pathogenicity of inhaled particles. For instance, particles longer than 200 μm may also reach the lower respiratory tract, provided the mean aerodynamic diameter of the airway is less than 1 μm. Asbestos is a good example of a large but slender fiber that can bypass the filtrating mechanisms by traveling parallel to the airstream. Once in the lungs, asbestos fibers cause asbestosis, a serious pulmonary disease in human beings. In summary, the anatomic features of the nasal cavity and airways provide an effective barrier, preventing the penetration of most large particles into the lungs.

Once larger particles are trapped in the mucosa of conductive airways and small particles are deposited on the surface of the bronchioalveolar mucosa, it is crucial that this exogenous material be removed to prevent or minimize injury to the respiratory system. For these purposes, the respiratory system is equipped with an array of defense mechanisms, all of which are provided by specialized cells operating in a remarkably well-coordinated manner.

Mucociliary Defense Mechanisms (Conductive System)

Mucociliary clearance is the physical removal of deposited particles or dissolved gases from the respiratory tract. The mucociliary clearance is provided by the **mucociliary blanket (mucociliary escalator)** and is the main defense mechanism of the conductive system (nasal cavity, trachea, and bronchi) (see Fig. 3-2). The mucus is a complex mixture of water, glycoproteins, immunoglobulins, lipids, and salts produced by goblet (mucous) cells, serous cells, submucosal glands, and fluid from transepithelial ion and water transport. Once serous fluid and mucus are secreted onto the surface of the respiratory mucosa, a thin, double-layer film of mucus is formed on top of the cells. The outer layer of this film is in a viscous, gel phase, while the inner layer, which is in a fluid or sol phase, is directly in contact with the cilia. Mucus is then propelled by the movement of cilia (see Fig. 3-3). Each ciliated cell in the conductive system has around 250 cilia (6 μm in length) beating spontaneously at approximately 1000 strokes per minute and producing an estimated longitudinal movement of up to 20 mm per minute. Rapid and powerful movement of cilia creates a series of waves that, in a continuous and harmonious manner, propel mucus and trapped particles out of the respiratory tract. If mucus flow were to move at the same rate in all levels of the conductive system, a ''bottleneck'' effect would be created in major airways to which the minor but more numerous airways converge. For this reason, the mucociliary movement in proximal airways is physiologically faster than that of the distal ones. The mucociliary blanket of the nasal cavity, trachea, and bronchi also plays an important role in preventing injury from and removing toxic gases. If a soluble gas enters into contact with the mucociliary blanket, it mixes with the mucus, thus reducing the concentration of gas reaching deep into the alveolar region. In other words, mucus acts as a ''scavenger system'' where gases are solubilized and subsequently cleared from the respiratory tract via the mucociliary blanket.

In addition to the physical transport provided by the mucociliary escalator, other cells closely associated with ciliated epithelium contribute to the defense mechanism of the conductive system. Among the most notable ones are those present in the lymphoepithelium and underlying **bronchial associated lymphoid tissue (BALT).** These two specialized structures are strategically located at the corner of the dichotomic branching of bronchi and bronchioles, where inhaled particles often impact due to inertial forces (see Fig. 3-3). From here, inhaled particles and soluble antigens are phagocytosed and transported by macrophages and specialized dendritic cells into the BALT, thus providing a unique opportunity for lymphocytes to enter into close contact with potentially pathogenic substances. Chronic airway diseases, especially those of infectious etiology, are often accompanied by severe hyperplasia of the BALT. Lymphocytes of the BALT contribute to both cellular (cytotoxic, helper, suppressor T cells) and humoral immune responses; IgA and, to a lesser extent, IgG and IgM play significant roles in the local immunity of the conducting system, especially with regard to preventing attachment of pathogens to the mucociliary blanket.

The mucociliary clearance terminates at the pharynx, where mucus, propelled caudally from the nasal cavity and cranially from the tracheobronchial tree, is eventually swallowed and thus eliminated from the conductive system of the respiratory tract.

Phagocytic Defense Mechanisms (Exchange System)

Alveoli lack ciliated and mucus-producing cells; thus the defense mechanism against inhaled particles in the alveolar region cannot be provided by mucociliary clearance. Instead, the main defense mechanism of alveoli (exchange system) is phagocytosis furnished by the **pulmonary alveolar macrophages.**

These highly phagocytic cells are derived largely from blood monocytes and, to a much lesser extent, from a slowly dividing population of interstitial macrophages. After a temporary adaptive stage within pulmonary interstitium, blood monocytes modify their cellular and biochemical mechanisms to function in an aerobic rather than in an anaerobic environment. Pulmonary alveolar macrophages readily attach to and ingest bacteria and other particles reaching the alveolar region (see Fig. 3-3). The number of macrophages in the alveolar space is closely related to the number of particles reaching the lungs. This ability to increase the number of available phagocytic cells within hours is vital in protecting the distal lungs against foreign material, particularly when the latter is excessive. Unlike that of tissue macrophages, the life span of alveolar macrophages in the alveoli is short, only a few days. Alveolar phagocytosis plays a particular role in the defense mechanism against inhaled bacteria. Bacteria reaching the alveoli are rapidly ingested, and bactericidal enzymes present in lysosomes are discharged into the phagosome containing the bacteria (see Fig. 3-3). Except for some facultative organisms that are resistant to intracellular killing (e.g., *Mycobacterium tuberculosis, Listeria monocytogenes*), most bacteria are rapidly destroyed by alveolar macrophages. Similarly, inhaled particles such as dust, pollen, spores, carbon, or erythrocytes from intraalveolar hemorrhage are all phagocytosed and eventually removed from alveoli by pulmonary alveolar macrophages.

Generally, most alveolar macrophages leave the alveoli by moving toward the bronchiolar (transitional) region until the mucociliary blanket is reached. Once there, pulmonary macrophages are dealt with in the same way as any other particle, that is, moved along the mucociliary flow to the pharynx and finally swallowed.

Pulmonary clearance by alveolar macrophages operates in a well-orchestrated manner with other cells and secretions of the distal lungs. These cell-to-cell interactions are complex and involve many cells, including pulmonary alveolar macrophages, lymphocytes, dendritic cells, and type II pneumonocytes. For instance, lymphokines produced by T-lymphocytes increase the phagocytic activity of pulmonary alveolar macrophages against some types of microorganisms. In addition, cytokines, such as interleukin-1 released by activated macrophages, promote the recruitment of lymphocytes and act as a maturation signal to prepare T cells to respond to antigenic stimulation. Humoral immune response also plays an important role in protecting the lungs against inhaled pathogens. Although IgA is the most common antibody in nasal and tracheal secretions, IgG is the most abundant antibody in the alveolar milieu and acts as an opsonizing antibody to promote uptake and destruction of inhaled pathogens. Other secretory products present in the alveolar lining material also provide protection against various types of infectious and chemical insults to the lungs (Table 3-2).

To facilitate phagocytosis and discriminate between "self" and "foreign" antigens, pulmonary alveolar macrophages are furnished with a wide variety of specific receptors on their cell surface. Among the most important ones are IgG and complement (C3b, C3a, C5a) receptors, which facilitate the phagocytosis of opsonized particles. "Scavenger receptors," which prompt recognition and uptake of foreign particulates such as dust and fibers, are also present on pulmonary alveolar macrophages.

Lungs are also susceptible to hematogenously borne microbes, toxins, or emboli. In dogs, laboratory rodents, and human beings, hepatic (Kupffer cells) and splenic macrophages are the primary cells responsible for removing circulating bacteria and other particulates from the blood. In contrast, removal of circulating pathogens and particles from the blood of ruminants, cats, and pigs is mainly dependent on **pulmonary intravascular macrophages,** a distinct population of phagocytes normally residing within the pulmonary capillaries and which in some species could be as numerous as Kupffer cells. In ruminants, intravenously injected tracer particles or bacteria are rapidly phagocytosed by these intravascular macrophages.

Existing in an oxygen-rich environment and being the site of numerous metabolic reactions, the lungs also require an efficient defense mechanism against oxidant-induced cellular damage. This form of damage can be caused by inhalation of oxidant gases (e.g., nitrogen dioxide, ozone, sulfur dioxide), by xenobiotic toxic metabolites produced locally or reaching the lungs via the bloodstream (e.g., 3-methylindole, paraquat), or by free radicals released by phagocytic cells during inflammation. Oxygen and free-radical scavengers such as catalase, superoxide dismutase, and vitamin E are largely responsible for protecting pulmonary cells against peroxidation.

In summary, the defense mechanisms are so effective in trapping, destroying, and removing bacteria that, under normal conditions, animals can be exposed to aerosols containing massive numbers of bacteria without any ill effects. If defense mechanisms are impaired, inhaled bacteria colonize, multiply, and produce infection, which, in some instances, results in fatal pneumonia. Similarly, when toxic gases, vapors, particles, or free radicals overwhelm the protective defense mechanisms, cells of the respiratory system can be injured, often causing serious respiratory disease.

Impairment of Defense Mechanisms in the Respiratory System

For many years, factors such as stress, viral infections, and pulmonary edema have been implicated in predisposing human beings and animals to secondary bacterial pneumonia. There are many pathways by which the defense mechanisms can be impaired, and only those relevant to veterinary species will be discussed here.

Viral infections

These are notorious for predisposing human beings and animals to secondary bacterial pneumonias by what is

Table 3-2. Defense mechanisms provided by some cells and secretory products present in the respiratory system

Cell/secretory product	Action
Alveolar macrophage	Phagocytosis, main line of defense against inhaled particles and microbial pathogens
Intravascular macrophage	Phagocytosis, removal of circulating particles, endotoxin, and microbial pathogens
Ciliated cells	Expell mucus, inhaled particles, and microbial pathogens by ciliary action
Clara cells	Detoxifies xenobiotics (mixed-function oxidases)
Mucus	Traps inhaled particles, microbial pathogens, and soluble gases
Surfactant	Protects alveolar walls and presumably enhances phagocytosis
Lysozyme	Antimicrobial enzyme
α_1-antitrypsin	Protects against the noxious effects of proteolytic enzymes release by phagocytic cells; also inhibits inflammation
Interferon	Antiviral and immune modulator
Complement	Chemotaxis and enhances phagocytosis
Antioxidants*	Prevent injury caused by superoxide anion, hydrogen peroxide, and free radicals generated during phagocytosis, during inflammation, or by inhalation of oxidant gases (ozone, NO_2, SO_2)

*Superoxide dismutase, catalase, glutathion peroxoidase, oxidant free-radical scavengers (tocopherol, ascorbic acid)

known as viral-bacterial synergism. A good example of this synergistic effect of combined viral-bacterial infections is documented from epidemics of human beings with influenza virus in which the mortality rate significantly increased due to secondary bacterial pneumonia. The most common viruses incriminated in predisposing animals to secondary bacterial pneumonia include influenza virus in pigs; *bovine herpesvirus* 1 (BHV-1), *parainfluenza*-3 *(PI-3), bovine respiratory syncytial virus* (BRSV) in cattle; and *canine distemper virus* in dogs. The mechanism of the synergistic effect of viral-bacterial infections was considered to be the destruction of mucociliary blanket and concurrent reduction of mucociliary clearance. However, in experimental studies, viral infections do not significantly reduce the physical removal of particles or bacteria from the lungs. Instead, it is now known that 5 to 7 days after a viral infection, the phagocytic function of pulmonary alveolar macrophages is notably impaired. Immunization against viral infections in many cases prevents or reduces the synergistic effect of combined viral-bacterial pneumonia. The mechanisms by which viruses impair defense mechanisms are multiple and remain not well understood (Table 3-3).

Toxic gases

Certain gases also impair respiratory defense mechanisms, rendering animals more susceptible to secondary bacterial infections. For instance, hydrogen sulfide and ammonia, frequently encountered in the farming environment, especially in areas with poor ventilation, can impair pulmonary bacterial clearance. The effects of environmental pollutants on the defense mechanisms of animals living in crowded and polluted cities remain to be determined.

Table 3-3. Postulated mechanisms by which viruses may impair the defense mechanisms of the respiratory tract

Changes in mucociliary clearance
Injured epithelium enhances attachment of bacteria
Enhanced bacterial attachment predisposes to colonization
Decreased mucociliary clearance prolongs resident time of bacteria, favoring colonization
Injured epithelium prevents mucociliary clearance and physical removal of bacteria
Lack of secretory products facilitates further cell injury
Dysfunction of pulmonary alveolar macrophages
Consolidation of lung causes hypoxia, resulting in decreased phagocytosis
Infected macrophages fail to release chemotactic factors for other cells
Infected macrophages fail to attach and ingest bacteria
Lysosomes become disoriented and fail to fuse with phagosome-containing bacteria
Intracellular killing/degradation is decreased due to biochemical dysfunction
Macrophages expressing viral antigen on their surfaces are destroyed by the immune system

Uremia, endotoxemia, dehydration, starvation, hypoxia, acidosis, pulmonary edema, anesthesia, and stress

These are only some of the many other factors that have been implicated in impairing the respiratory defense mechanism and concurrently predisposing animals to secondary bacterial pneumonia. The mechanisms by which each of these factors suppresses pulmonary defenses are varied and sometimes not well understood. For instance, hypoxia and pulmonary edema decrease phagocytic function of pulmonary alveolar macrophages and alter the production of surfactant by type II pneumonocytes; dehydration is thought to increase the viscosity of mucus, which reduces or stops mucociliary action; anesthesia induces ciliostasis with concurrent loss of mucociliary function; starvation, hypothermia, and stress can reduce humoral and cellular immune response.

Immunodeficiency

This disorder, whether acquired or congenital, is often associated with increased susceptibility to viral, bacterial, and protozoal pneumonias. For instance, human beings with acquired immunodeficiency syndrome (AIDS) are markedly susceptible to the development of pneumonia caused by proliferation of *Pneumocystis carinii.* This ubiquitous organism, which under normal circumstances is not considered pathogenic, is also found in the pneumonic lungs of immunosuppressed pigs, foals, dogs, and rodents. Arabian foals born with combined immunodeficiency disease easily succumb to infectious diseases, particularly adenoviral pneumonia.

PATTERN OF INJURY AND HOST RESPONSE IN THE CONDUCTIVE SYSTEM

The conductive portion of the respiratory system (nasal cavity, larynx, trachea, and bronchi) is lined by ciliated epithelium and, to a much lesser extent, by olfactory and squamous epithelium. The pattern of injury, inflammation, and host response is characteristic for each of these three types of epithelium, independent of its anatomic location.

Pseudostratified ciliated epithelium, which lines most of the nasal cavity and nasopharynx, part of the larynx, and all the trachea and bronchi, is exquisitely sensitive to injury. When cell injury becomes biochemically irreversible, whether caused by a viral infection, trauma, or inhalation of toxic gases, ciliated cells swell and typically lose their attachment to the underlying basement membrane (Fig. 3-4). This loss of cellular attachment results in rapid exfoliation of cells and ulceration of the mucosa, followed by a

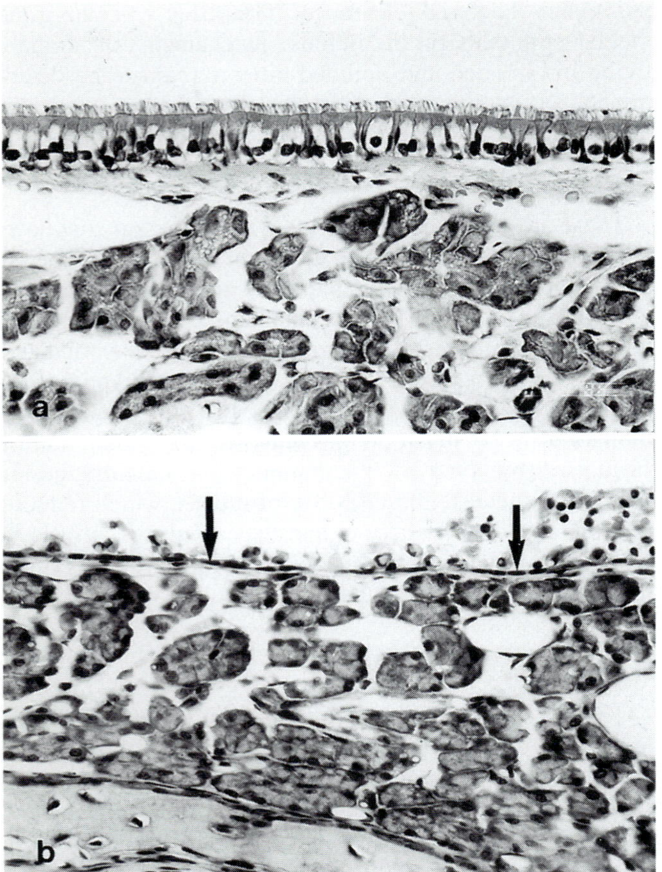

Fig. 3-4 Nasal conchae, histologic sections; rats. **A**, Ciliated epithelium, nasal mucosa; rat. The normal mucosal lining is predominantly comprised of tall columnar cells with numerous cilia projecting into the lumen. **B**, Histologic section of nasal mucosa; rat. Rat was exposed to an atmosphere containing an irritant gas (hydrogen sulfide) and euthanatized 2 hours after exposure. Note how extensive detachment and exfoliation of ciliated cells have left a denuded basement membrane *(arrows)*. This same type of lesion is seen in viral or mechanical injury to the mucosa of the conductive system. *López et al. Am J Vet Res 1988; 49:1107-1111.*

transient and mild exudation of plasma proteins and neutrophils. In the absence of complications or secondary bacterial infections, secretory cells present at the borders of the ulcers undergo mitosis and new cells attracted by chemotactic factors, such as fibronectins, move to cover the denuded basement membrane. The capacity of pseudostratified, ciliated epithelium to repair itself is remarkably effective. For instance, repair of an uncomplicated ulceration of the tracheal mucosa may be completed in only 7 days. This sequence of events with cell degeneration, exfoliation, ulceration, mitosis, and repair is typically found in many viral infections in which viruses replicate in nasal, tracheal, and bronchial epithelium. Examples of this type of transient infection include human colds (rhinoviruses), infectious bovine rhinotracheitis (*bovine herpesvirus* 1), feline rhinotracheitis (*feline herpesvirus* 1), canine infectious tracheobronchitis (*canine adenovirus* 2 and *canine parainfluenza*-2).

If damage to the mucociliary blanket becomes chronic, goblet cell hyperplasia results in concurrent excessive mucus production. In the most severe cases, prolonged injury causes squamous metaplasia of the underlying epithelium. Hyperplastic and metaplastic changes from persistent mucosal injury are considered a prelude to neoplasia in laboratory rodents.

The second type of epithelium lining the conductive system is the sensory **olfactory epithelium,** present in some parts of the nasal mucosa, particularly around the ethmoidal conchae. The patterns of degeneration, exfoliation, and inflammation in the olfactory epithelium are similar to those of the ciliated epithelium, except that olfactory epithelium has only limited capacity for regeneration. When olfactory epithelium has been irreversibly injured, olfactory cells swell, separate from adjacent sustentacular cells, and finally exfoliate into the nasal cavity. Once the underlying basement membrane of the olfactory epithelium is exposed, chemotactic factors are generated, and inflammatory cells move into the affected area. When damage is extensive, ulcerated areas of olfactory mucosa are replaced by ciliated and goblet cells or squamous epithelium, or by fibrous tissue, all of which eventually cause loss of olfactory function (anosmia).

Squamous epithelium is the third type of epithelium present in the conductive system, and compared with ciliated and olfactory epithelium, it is quite resistant to all forms of injury.

POSTMORTEM EXAMINATION OF THE RESPIRATORY TRACT

The respiratory tract should always be examined in a systematic fashion. To check whether negative pressure is present in the thoracic cavity, the diaphragm is punctured through the abdominal cavity before the thorax has been opened. In an animal that has not been dead for more than a few hours, the act of puncturing it results in loss of negative pressure which causes the dome of the diaphragm to drop back toward the abdominal cavity and at the same time to make an audible noise due to the inrush of air. Lack of movement may be an indication of advanced pneumothorax, pleural effusion, or presence of noncollapsible lungs due to pulmonary edema, pneumonia, or emphysema.

The rib cage must be removed in such a way that pleural adhesions and abnormal thoracic contents can be observed and grossly quantified (e.g., 200 ml of clear, yellow fluid, etc.). The tongue, pharynx, larynx, trachea, and thoracic viscera (lungs, heart, and thymus) should be removed as a unit and placed on the postmortem table.

The pharynx and esophagus are each opened by a single cut with scissors along the dorsal midline and inspected for ulceration, foreign bodies, and neoplasms. The larynx and trachea must be examined by opening both along the dorsal midline from cranial to caudal ends and then extending the incision into the large bronchi in the caudal lung lobes. Normal tracheobronchial mucosa has a smooth and glistening surface of pearl color, and lumina of airways should be empty. Presence of foamy fluid in airways indicates pulmonary edema. Feed particles may suggest bronchoaspiration; however, careful examination of the mucosa is required since passage of feed from stomach or rumen into the lungs commonly takes place at death.

Before incision to observe the parenchyma, the lungs should be carefully observed for external changes and presence of rib imprints on the pleural surface. In addition, the lungs should be inspected for changes in color, texture, and distribution of lesions. **Color** changes can be various shades of red, indicating congestion, hyperemia (acute pneumonia), and hemorrhage; dark collapsed lobules are indicative of atelectasis; pale pink to white lungs indicate fibrosis or emphysema. Lungs from exsanguinated and anemic animals are generally paler than normal due to reduced blood in the pulmonary tissue. A covering of yellowish material on the pleural surface indicates accumulation of fibrin. Since it is impossible to describe the texture of normal lungs, repeated palpation is required to understand the actual feeling of a normal lung. **Texture** is determined by gently palpating the surface and parenchyma of the lungs. Abnormal textures of the lungs include firm, hard, rubbery (elastic), or crepitant. Palpation of the lungs also permits detection of nonvisible nodules or abscesses in the parenchyma. Knowing the **distribution** of a lesion in the lungs also facilitates diagnosis since specific distributions are often associated with particular etiologic agents. Distribution of lesions is generally described as focal, multifocal, locally extensive, or diffuse. According to their topography, pulmonary lesions can also be classified as being cranioventral, dorsocaudal, and so on.

Postmortem reports must also contain an estimate of the extent of the pulmonary lesions, preferably expressed as a percentage (%) of the lungs affected. For instance, a report may read "cranioventral consolidation involving 40% of the lungs." If the lungs have focal lesions, a rough estimate of the number should also be included in the report. For instance, "numerous (approximately 25), small (1 to 2 cm in diameter), hard nodules were randomly distributed in all pulmonary lobes."

Two methods are used to examine the nasal structures. The first is by making a midsagittal cut through the head and removing the nasal septum; the second is by making several transverse sections of the nose. This latter method is preferred when examining pigs suspected of having atrophic rhinitis or in animals with suspected nasal neoplasms.

NASAL CAVITY AND SINUSES

Anomalies

Localized congenital anomalies of the nasal cavity are rare in domestic animals and are often merely part of a more extensive craniofacial deformity (e.g., cyclops) or a component of generalized malformation (e.g., chondrodysplasia). Congenital anomalies involving the nasal cavity and sinuses such as choanal atresia, some types of chondrodysplasia, and osteopetrosis are incompatible with life. Examples of nonfatal congenital anomalies include cystic nasal conchae, maxillary cysts, deviation of nasal septum, cleft upper lip (harelip, cheiloschisis), hypoplastic turbinates, and cleft palate (palatoschisis). Bronchoaspiration and pneumonia are common sequelae to cleft palate. As in other organs or systems, it is extremely difficult to determine the actual cause (genetic versus congenital) of anomalies based on pathologic examination.

Metabolic Disturbances of the Nasal Cavity

Metabolic disturbances in the nasal cavity and sinuses are also rare in domestic animals. **Amyloidosis,** the deposition of amyloid protein (fibrils with a β-pleated configuration) in various tissues, has been sporadically reported in the nasal cavity of horses. Affected horses have difficulty in breathing and show reduced athletic performance; on clinical examination, large nodules can be observed in the alar folds, rostral nasal septum, and floor of the nasal cavity. Microscopic lesions are similar to those seen in other organs and consist of a deposition of palely eosinophilic, amorphous material (Congo red-positive) in nasal mucosa. Unlike other cases of amyloidosis in domestic animals where amyloid is generally of the reactive type (amyloid AA), equine nasal amyloidosis appears to be of the immunocytic type (amyloid AL).

Circulatory Disturbances

Congestion and hyperemia

The nasal mucosa is extremely well vascularized and is capable of rather dramatic variation in blood flow, whether passively due to interference with venous return (congestion) or actively due to vasodilation (hyperemia). Congestion of the mucosal vessels is a nonspecific lesion commonly found at postmortem and presumably associated with circulatory failure preceding death (e.g., heart failure, bloat in ruminants). Hyperemia of the nasal mucosa is also associated with early stages of inflammation, whether caused by irritants (e.g., ammonia, feed regurgitation), viral infections, secondary bacterial infections, allergy, or trauma.

Hemorrhage. Epistaxis is the clinical term used to denote presence of blood flow from the nose (nosebleed) regardless of whether blood originates from the nasal cavity or from deep in the lungs. Unlike blood in the digestive tract, where the approximate anatomic location of the bleeding can be estimated by the color the blood imparts to fecal material, blood in the respiratory tract always is red. This is due to the rapid transport of blood out of the respiratory tract by the mucociliary blanket. Hemorrhages into the nasal cavity can originate from local trauma, erosions of submucosal vessels by inflammation, or neoplasms.

Inflammation

Rhinitis and sinusitis

Inflammation of the nasal mucosa is called **rhinitis** and that of the sinuses, **sinusitis.** These usually occur together, although mild sinusitis goes undetected.

The occurrence of infectious rhinitis presupposes an upset in the balance of the normal microbial flora of the nasal cavity. Innocuous bacteria are present normally, protecting the host through a process called **competitive exclusion,** whereby the numbers of potential pathogens are kept at harmless numbers. Disruption of this protective mechanism can be caused by respiratory viruses, pathogenic bacteria, irritant gases, environmental changes, immunosuppression, local trauma, stress, or prolonged antibacterial therapy.

Based on the nature of exudate, rhinitis can be classified into **serous, catarrhal, purulent, fibrinous,** or **granulomatous.** Other changes such as **hemorrhage, ulcers,** and **mucosal hyperplasia** can also be found in inflamed nasal mucosa. Rhinitis can also be classified according to the age of the lesions as acute, subacute, or chronic; to the severity of the insult as mild, moderate, or severe; and to the etiologic agent as viral, allergic, bacterial, mycotic, or toxic.

Serous rhinitis

This is the mildest form of inflammation and is characterized by hyperemia and increased production of a clear fluid locally manufactured by serous glands present in the submucosa. Serous rhinitis is of clinical interest only. It is caused by mild irritants or cold air, and it occurs during the early stages of viral infections, such as the common cold in human beings and upper respiratory infections in animals, or in mild allergic reactions.

Catarrhal rhinitis

This slightly more severe process has, in addition to serous secretions, a substantial increase in mucus production by increased activity of goblet cells and mucous glands. A mucus exudate is a thick, translucent or slightly turbid viscous fluid, sometimes containing a few leukocytes and cellular debris. In chronic cases, catarrhal rhinitis is characterized, microscopically, by marked hyperplasia of goblet cells.

Purulent (suppurative) rhinitis

This inflammation, characterized by a neutrophilic exudate, occurs when the nasal mucosa suffers a more severe injury and generally is accompanied by mucosal necrosis and secondary bacterial infection. Cytokines, leukotrienes, complement activation, and bacterial products cause exudation of leukocytes, especially neutrophils, which mix with nasal secretions including mucus. Grossly, the exudate in suppurative rhinitis is thick and opaque, but can vary from white to green to brown, depending on the types of bacteria and cells present in the exudate. In severe cases, the nasal passages are completely blocked by the exudate. Microscopically, neutrophils can be seen in the submucosa and mucosa and form plaques of exudate on the mucosal surface. Neutrophils are found between epithelial cells in their migration to the surface of the mucosa.

Fibrinous rhinitis

This reaction occurs when nasal injury causes notable alterations in vascular permeability, resulting in abundant exudation of plasma fibrinogen, which coagulates into fibrin. Fibrin accumulates on the surface and forms a distinct film of exudate (pseudomembrane) (Fig. 3-5). If this exudate can be removed, leaving an intact underlying mucosa, it is a **croupous** or **pseudodiphtheritic rhinitis.** Conversely, if removal of this membrane of exudate leaves an ulcerated mucosa, it is referred to as **diphtheritic** or **fibrinonecrotic rhinitis.** The term diphtheritic was derived from human diphtheria, which causes a severe and destructive inflammatory process of the respiratory mucosa. Microscopically, the lesions include a perivascular edema with fibrin, a few neutrophils infiltrating the mucosa, and plaques of exudate consisting of fibrin strands mixed with leukocytes and cellular debris on the affected epithelium.

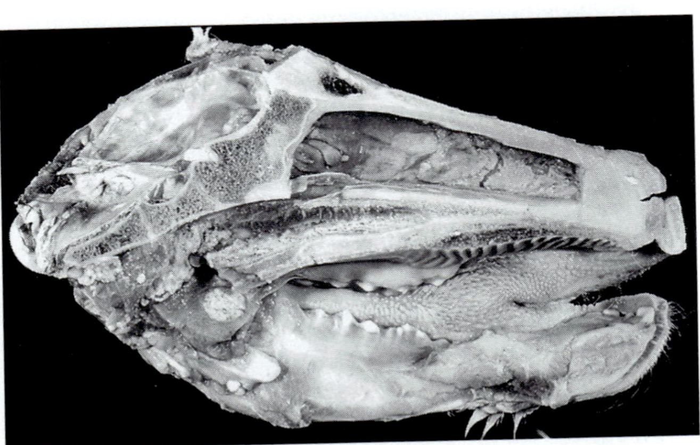

Fig. 3-5 Midsagittal section of head; neonatal calf. Infectious bovine rhinotracheitis (bovine herpesvirus 1). The nasal septum was removed to expose nasal conchae. The nasal mucosa is covered by diphtheritic membranes (fibrinonecrotic exudate). There is a large, round ulcer in the nasopharynx. *Courtesy of Western College of Veterinary Medicine.*

Granulomatous rhinitis

This reaction is characterized by infiltration of macrophages, lymphocytes, and plasma cells in the mucosa and submucosa. In some cases, inflammation leads to the formation of polypoid nodules that, in severe cases, are large enough to cause obstruction of the nasal passages. Granulomatous rhinitis is generally associated with specific organisms such as those of systemic mycoses (see Lungs), or tuberculosis, and with foreign bodies. In some cases, the etiology of granulomatous rhinitis cannot be determined.

Except for granulomatous rhinitis, inflammatory processes in the nasal cavity usually resolve completely. However, some potentially adverse sequelae include bronchoaspiration of exudate leading to bronchopneumonia and pulmonary abscesses. Also, there can be local extension into adjacent sinuses (sinusitis), into bone (facial osteomyelitis), or through the cribriform plate (meningitis).

Sinusitis occurs sporadically in domestic animals and is frequently combined with rhinitis or occurs as a sequela to septic wounds, improper dehorning in cattle (frontal sinus), or tooth infection in horses and dogs (maxillary sinus). Paranasal sinuses have poor drainage; therefore, exudate tends to accumulate, causing **mucocele** (accumulation of mucus) or **empyema** (accumulation of pus). Chronic sinusitis with extension may also be accompanied by osteomyelitis or meningitis.

SPECIFIC DISEASES OF THE NASAL CAVITY AND SINUSES

Bovine Diseases

Infectious bovine rhinotracheitis (IBR or "rednose")

This disease is of great importance in the cattle industry because of the synergism of the IBR virus with *Pasteurella haemolytica* in producing pneumonia, and its association with bovine abortion, systemic infections of calves, and infectious pustular vulvovaginitis (IPV). The causative agent, *BHV-1,* has probably existed as a mild venereal disease of cattle in Europe since at least the mid-1800s, but the respiratory form was not reported until intensive management feedlot systems were first introduced in North America around the 1950s. Typically, the disease is manifested as a transient, acute, febrile illness that only in very severe cases results in inspiratory dyspnea due to obstruction of airflow by exudate. Other forms of BHV-1 infection include nonsuppurative encephalitis, enteritis in calves, infertility, and, in experimental infections, mastitis, mammillitis, and necrosis of the ovaries. Except for the encephalitic form, the type of disease caused by BHV-1 relates more to the site of entry than to the viral strain. Like other herpesviruses, BHV-1 can also remain latent in nerve ganglia, with recrudescence following stress or immunosuppression.

The respiratory form of IBR is characterized by severe hyperemia and focal necrosis of nasal, pharyngeal, laryngeal, tracheal (Figs. 3-5 and 3-6), and, sometimes, bronchial mucosa. As in other respiratory viral infections, IBR lesions generally consist of necrosis and exfoliation of ciliated cells followed by repair. In some cattle, secondary bacterial infections in areas of necrosis result in the formation of a thick layer of fibrinonecrotic material on the airway mucosa. Fibrinonecrotic rhinotracheitis caused by a combined viral-bacterial infection is often seen at necropsy during outbreaks of IBR. Intranuclear inclusion bodies, commonly seen in herpesvirus infections, are rarely seen in field cases since they only occur during the early stages of the disease.

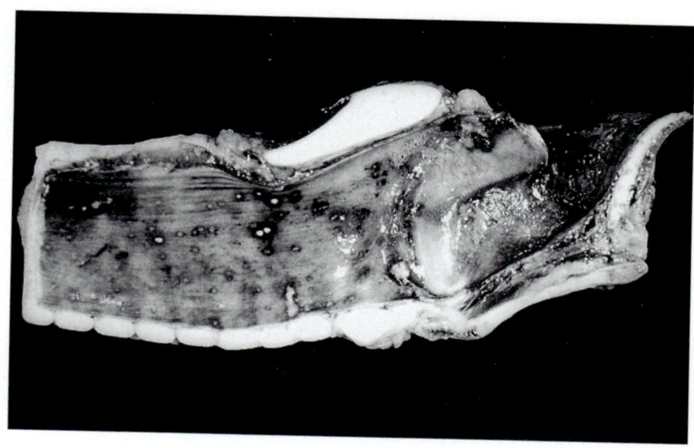

Fig. 3-6 Larynx and proximal trachea, mucosal surface; cow. Infectious bovine rhinotracheitis (IBR), multifocal necrotizing laryngitis, and tracheitis. Ten days before, this calf was exposed experimentally to an aerosol of bovine herpesvirus 1. *Courtesy Dr. G.A. Gifford.*

The most important sequela to IBR is pneumonia, which is caused either by direct aspiration of exudate from airways or as a result of an impairment in pulmonary defense mechanisms, thus predisposing the animal to secondary bacterial infection, most frequently *P. haemolytica.*

Porcine Diseases

Inclusion body rhinitis

This disease of young pigs, with high morbidity and low mortality, is caused by a porcine cytomegalovirus (herpesvirus) and is characterized by a mild rhinitis. This virus commonly infects the nasal epithelium of piglets less than 10 weeks of age and produces a mild and transient rhinitis, causing sneezing, nasal discharge, and excessive lacrimation. Since this disease is seldom fatal, lesions are seen only incidentally or in euthanatized animals. In uncomplicated cases, the gross lesion is hyperemia of the nasal mucosa, but, with secondary bacterial infections, mucopurulent exudate can be abundant. Microscopic lesions are typical and consist of a necrotizing, nonsuppurative rhinitis with giant, basophilic, intranuclear inclusion bodies in the epithelial cells of the mucosa and glands (Fig. 3-7). Pneumonia can

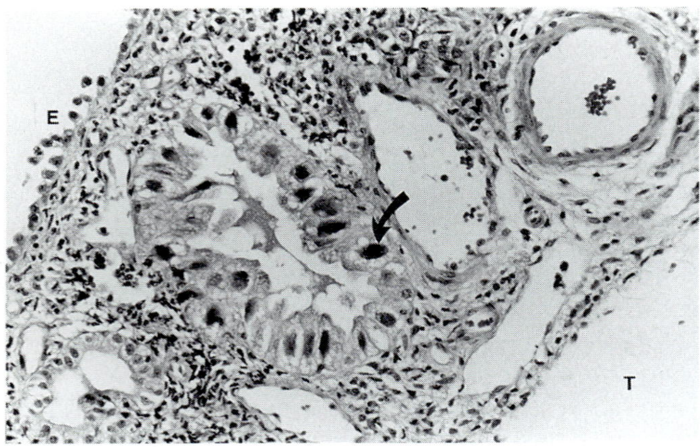

Fig. 3-7 Nasal conchae, histologic section; 4-week-old pig. Inclusion body rhinitis. Note the large intranuclear inclusion bodies *(arrow)* caused by cytomegalovirus infection in epithelial cells. The inclusions are in a submucosal gland between the epithelial surface (*E*) and the turbinate (*T*), which was removed during tissue processing. Hematoxylin-eosin (H & E) stain. *Courtesy of Western College of Veterinary Medicine.*

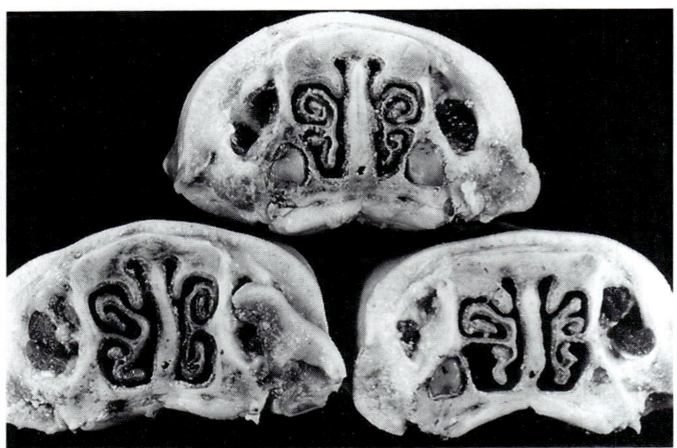

Fig. 3-8 Cross-section of nasal passages and sinuses at the level of the first and second premolar teeth; pigs. Atrophic rhinitis. Normal pig *(top)* and two pigs with atrophic rhinitis *(bottom).* The lower left shows deviation of the nasal septum, and the lower right shows septal deviation plus atrophy of a ventral concha (turbinate). *Courtesy of Western College of Veterinary Medicine.*

also be a complication of inclusion body rhinitis. Immunosuppressed piglets can develop a systemic cytomegalovirus infection characterized by necrosis of the liver, lungs, adrenal glands, and brain.

Atrophic rhinitis

A common worldwide disease of pigs, atrophic rhinitis is clinically characterized by sneezing, coughing, and nasal discharge as a result of inflammation and atrophy of nasal conchae (turbinates). In severe cases, atrophy of the conchae may cause a striking facial deformity due to deviation of the nasal bones. The etiopathogenesis of atrophic rhinitis is complex and has been a matter of controversy for many years. Pathogens historically associated with atrophic rhinitis include *Bordetella bronchiseptica, Pasteurella multocida, Haemophilus parasuis,* and viral infections such as porcine cytomegalovirus (inclusion body rhinitis). In addition, predisposing factors have included genetic makeup, environment, and nutritional deficiencies. Currently, the etiology of atrophic rhinitis is believed to be a combined infection of specific strains of *B. bronchiseptica* and some toxigenic strains of *P. multocida* (types D and A). Infection with *B. bronchiseptica* alone causes only mild to moderate and transient atrophy, but actively promotes the colonization of the nasal cavity by *P. multocida.* The toxigenic strains of *P. multocida* produce potent cytotoxins that inhibit osteoblastic activity in nasal bones, particularly in the ventral nasal conchae, where abnormal bone remodeling results in hypoplasia and atrophy of conchae.

The degree of conchal atrophy in pigs with atrophic rhinitis varies considerably, and, in most pigs, the severity of the lesions does not correspond to the severity of the clinical signs. The best diagnostic method of evaluating this disease is to make a transversal cross section of the snout between the first and second premolar teeth. In normal pigs, conchae are symmetrical and fill most of the cavity, leaving only narrow air spaces (meatuses) between coiled conchae. The normal nasal septum is straight and divides the cavity into two mirror-imaged cavities. In contrast, the septum in pigs with atrophic rhinitis is generally deviated, and the conchae appear smaller and asymmetrical (Fig. 3-8). Conchal atrophy causes meatuses to appear rather enlarged, and, in the most advanced cases, the entire nasal conchae may be missing, leaving a large, empty space. It may seem logical to assume that, after loss of conchae in an obligate nasal breather like the pig, the filtration defense mechanism of the nasal cavity would be impaired. However, the relationship between atrophic rhinitis, pneumonia, and growth rates in pigs is still controversial.

Obstruction of the nasolacrimal duct is common in pigs with atrophic rhinitis and results in accumulation of dust and dried lacrimal secretions on the skin below the medial canthus of the eye. Hypoplasia of cancellous bone is the key microscopic lesion in atrophic rhinitis. Depending on the stage of the disease, mucopurulent exudate may be found on the surface of the conchae, hyperplastic or metaplastic changes can occur in the nasal epithelium and glands, and infiltrates of lymphoplasmacytic cells can be present in the lamina propria. In summary, atrophic rhinitis is an important disease of swine worldwide; morphologic diagnosis is simple, but additional understanding in the pathogenesis will be necessary before effective preventive measures can be established.

Equine Diseases

Such viruses as *equine viral rhinopneumonitis virus, influenza virus, adenovirus,* and *rhinovirus* cause mild and generally transient respiratory infections in horses. All these infections are indistinguishable clinically and signs consist mainly of malaise, fever, coughing, and a nasal discharge varying from serous to purulent. Viral respiratory infections are common medical problems in adult horses.

Equine viral rhinopneumonitis (EVR)

This disease, caused by equine herpesvirus (EVH) may be manifested as a mild respiratory disease in weanling foals and racehorses (EHV-4) or as abortion in mares (EHV-1). The respiratory form of EVR is generally transient; thus, the primary viral-induced lesions in the nasal mucosa and lungs are rarely seen at necropsy unless complicated by secondary bacterial rhinitis, pharyngitis, or bronchopneumonia.

Equine influenza

This is a common upper respiratory infection of horses and occurs mainly in 2- to 3-year-old horses at the racetrack. It etiologically is associated with type A (A/equi-1 and -2) and possibly type B strains of influenza virus. As with human influenza, influenza in horses is usually a mild, self-limiting disease, but, occasionally, it can cause severe bronchointerstitial pneumonia with pulmonary edema. In other horses, viral infection is complicated by a secondary bacterial bronchopneumonia caused by opportunistic organisms found in the normal flora of the upper respiratory tract. Other viruses such as equine rhinovirus, adenovirus, and parainfluenza virus are also presumed to produce mild and transient upper respiratory infections in horses, unless complicated by secondary pathogens. Fatal adenoviral infections with severe pneumonia or enteritis occur commonly in immunocompromised horses, particularly in Arabian foals with inherited combined immunodeficiency disease.

Strangles *(Streptococcus equi),* glanders *(Pseudomonas mallei [Malleomyces mallei]),* and melioidosis *(Pseudomonas pseudomallei [Malleomyces pseudomallei])* of horses are all systemic bacterial diseases that cause purulent rhinitis and suppuration in various organs. These diseases are grouped as upper respiratory diseases because nasal discharge is often the most notable clinical sign.

Strangles

This infectious disease of equidae is caused by *S. equi* subsp *equi (S. equi).* It is characterized by suppurative rhinitis and lymphadenitis (mandibular and retropharyngeal) with occasional embolic dissemination to internal organs. Unlike *S. equi* subsp *zooepidemicus (S. zooepidemicus)* and *S. equisimilis, S. equi* is not part of the normal nasal flora; and infection occurs when susceptible horses come into contact with feed, exudate, or air-droplets containing the organism. After penetrating through the nasopharyngeal mucosa, *S. equi* disseminates to mandibular and retropharyngeal lymph nodes via lymph vessels. Clinically, the disease is characterized by nasal discharge, conjunctivitis, and marked swelling of lymph nodes.

The gross lesions correlate with clinical findings and consist of copious amounts of mucopurulent exudate in the nasal passages and marked hyperemia of nasal mucosa. Affected lymph nodes are enlarged and contain thick purulent exudate (purulent lymphadenitis). The term ''bastard strangles'' is used in cases where embolic dissemination of *S. equi* results in metastatic abscesses in such organs as the lungs, liver, spleen, kidneys, or brain or in the joints.

Common sequelae to strangles include bronchopneumonia due to aspiration of exudate; laryngeal hemiplegia (''roaring''), resulting from compression of the recurrent laryngeal nerves by enlarged retropharyngeal lymph nodes; facial paralysis and Horner's syndrome due to compression of cranial nerves; and purpura hemorrhagica as a result of vasculitis presumably caused by vascular deposition of *S. equi* antigen-antibody complexes. In severe cases, nasal infection extends directly into the paranasal sinuses or to the guttural pouches via the Eustachian tubes causing inflammation and accumulation of pus (empyema). Rupture of abscesses in the mandibular and retropharyngeal lymph nodes leads to suppurative inflammation of adjacent subcutaneous tissue (cellulitis).

Glanders

This infectious disease of equidae is caused by *P. mallei (M. mallei)* and can be transmitted to carnivores by consumption of infected horse meat. Human beings are also susceptible, and the infection is often fatal. In the past, it was found throughout the world, but today glanders has been eradicated from most countries, except for some areas in North Africa, Asia, and Eastern Europe. The pathogenesis of glanders is not fully understood. Results from experimental infections suggest that infection with *P. mallei* occurs via the ingestion of contaminated feed and water and, very rarely, via inhalation of infectious droplets. At the portal of entry, presumably the oropharynx or intestine, bacteria penetrate the mucosa and spread via lymph vessels to lymph nodes, and the bloodstream to the internal organs, particularly the lungs. Lesions in the nasal cavity start as pyogranulomatous nodules in the submucosa, and these subsequently ulcerate, releasing copious amounts of *P. mallei*–containing exudate into the nasal cavity. Finally, ulcerative lesions in conchal mucosa are replaced by typical stellate (star-shaped), fibrous scars. In some cases, the lungs also contain numerous gray, hard, small (2 to 10 mm), miliary nodules randomly distributed in one or more pulmonary lobes. Microscopically, these nodules are typical granulomas composed of a necrotic center, with or without calcification, surrounded by a thick band of connective tissue infiltrated with numerous macrophages, some giant cells, lymphocytes, and plasma cells. Cutaneous lesions, often referred to as *equine farcy,* are characterized by nodular thickening of extended segments of lymph vessels in the subcutaneous tissue of the legs and ventral abdomen. This thickening of lymph vessels results from severe suppurative lymphangitis, eventually leading to cutaneous fistulas that release large amounts of purulent exudate.

Melioidosis (pseudoglanders)

This is an important disease of horses, cattle, sheep, goats, pigs, dogs, cats, rodents, and human beings caused by *P. pseudomallei (M. pseudomallei).* This disease in horses is clinically and pathologically similar to glanders, hence the name pseudoglanders. In human beings, this infection can be fatal. Melioidosis is currently present in Southeast Asia and, to a much lesser extent, in some European countries and Australia, where the causative organism is frequently found in rodents, feces, soil, and water. Although the mode by which transmission occurs is not clear, ingestion of contaminated feed and water appears to be the main route of infection; direct transmission between infected animals and insect bites has also been postulated as a possible mechanism of infection. After gaining entrance to the animal, *P. pseudomallei* is disseminated by the bloodstream and causes suppuration and abscesses in most internal organs, the nasal mucosa, joints, brain and spinal cord, liver, spleen, and lymph nodes. The exudate is creamy or caseous and yellow to green. The pulmonary lesions in melioidosis are those of an embolic bacterial pneumonia with formation of pulmonary abscesses. Focal adhesive pleuritis develops where abscesses rupture through the pleura and heal.

Canine Diseases

Dogs have no specific infectious diseases affecting exclusively the nasal cavity or sinuses. Acute rhinitis occurs as part of general respiratory diseases caused by several distinct viruses such as *canine distemper virus, canine adenovirus 1 and 2, canine parainfluenza virus, reovirus,* and *canine herpesvirus.* The viral lesions in the respiratory tract are generally transient, but the effect of the virus on other tissues can be fatal, as in distemper encephalitis in dogs. As in other species, secondary bacterial rhinitis and sinusitis are possible sequelae of respiratory viral infections; *B. bronchiseptica, E. coli,* and *P. multocida* are the most common isolates in dogs with bacterial rhinitis.

Feline Diseases

Feline viral rhinotracheitis (FVR)

This common and important respiratory disease of cats is caused by a feline herpesvirus (FHV-1) and is characterized by oculonasal discharges, severe rhinitis, and conjunctivitis. The disease causes an impairment of pulmonary defense mechanisms, predisposing cats to secondary bacterial pneumonia. The virus also can remain latent in ganglia. The vast majority of cats that recover from FVR become carriers and shed FHV-1, either spontaneously or following stress. Susceptible animals, particularly kittens with low maternal immunity, become infected following exposure to a diseased or a carrier cat. Replication of FHV-1 in the nasal, conjunctival, pharyngeal, and, to a lesser extent, tracheal epithelium causes degeneration and exfoliation of cells. Lesions caused by FHV-1 are fully reversible, but secondary infections with bacteria such as *P. multocida, B. bronchiseptica, Streptococcus* sp. and *Mycoplasma felis* can cause a chronic, severe suppurative rhinitis and conjunctivitis. Intranuclear inclusion bodies are rarely seen in cats with FVR, because inclusions are only present during the early stages of infection and have disappeared by the time the cat is presented for diagnosis.

Respiratory sequelae to FVR can include chronic bacterial rhinitis and sinusitis with persistent purulent discharges, lytic changes of bone with loss of conchae, permanent damage to the olfactory apparatus, and secondary pneumonia. In addition to respiratory lesions, FVR also causes ulcerative keratitis, hepatic necrosis, emaciation, abortion, and stillbirths.

Feline calicivirus (FCV)

This disease is caused by different strains of feline calicivirus. It is an important infection of the respiratory tract of cats, and, depending on the virulence of the strain, lesions vary from a mild oculonasal discharge to severe rhinitis, conjunctivitis, and ulcerative stomatitis. Clinical and pathologic features of FCV disease are strikingly similar but not identical to those of FVR; these two viral infections account for 80% of all cases of feline respiratory disease. The lesions, in addition to rhinitis and conjunctivitis, include interstitial pneumonia, prominent ulcers of the tongue and hard palate, and acute arthritis. Primary viral lesions are generally transient, but secondary bacterial infections are a common complication. Carrier state and virus shedding are natural sequelae following recovery from the acute phase of the disease.

Feline chlamydiosis

This is a persistent respiratory infection of cats caused by *Chlamydia psittaci (felis).* Infection results in a mild conjunctivitis (similar to that of human trachoma) and rhinitis, but, in severe cases, it can also produce a mild, transient bronchointerstitial pneumonia (previously referred to as ''feline pneumonitis'').

Feline reovirus and *Mycoplasma* species can also cause a mild upper respiratory infection, with clinical signs and lesions overlapping those of feline viral rhinotracheitis, feline calicivirus infection, and chlamydiosis. Most respiratory tract infections in cats may be associated with the immunosuppressive effects of feline leukemia virus (FeLV).

Other Specific Types of Rhinitis and Sinusitis

Mycotic rhinitis

Cases of fungal-induced rhinitis occur in all species and are characterized by the formation of granulomatous nodules in the nasal mucosa. The most common mycotic infections in the nasal cavity are caused by *Aspergillus* sp. and *Penicillium* sp. in dogs, *Cryptococcus neoformans* in cats, and *Rhinosporidium seeberi* in horses, cattle, dogs, and cats. Gross lesions vary from barely visible granulomas to large polypoid nodules.

Parasitic rhinitis

Parasitism of the nasal passages and sinuses is seldom more than an incidental finding at necropsy.

***Oestrus ovis* (nasal bot).** This brownish fly, about the size of a honeybee, deposits first-stage larvae in the nostrils of sheep raised in most parts of the world. Microscopic larvae mature into large bots that spend most of their larval stages in nasal passages and sinuses, causing irritation, inflammation, and obstruction of airways. Matured larvae drop to the ground and pupate into flies. This type of parasitism in which living tissues are invaded by larvae of flies is known as myiasis. Although *O. ovis* is primarily a myiasis of sheep, it may sporadically affect goats and, sometimes, human beings. The presence of the larvae in nasal passages causes chronic irritation and erosive mucopurulent rhinitis; bots of *O. ovis* can be found easily if the head is cut to expose the nasal passages. Rarely, larvae of *O. ovis* penetrate the cranial vault through the ethmoidal plate, causing direct or secondary bacterial meningitis. The Russian gadfly, *Rhinoestrus purpureus,* is a related parasite afflicting horses.

Linguatula serrata. This highly specialized arthropod (pentastomid) parasite occurs primarily in carnivores, although herbivores and human beings may become aberrant hosts. The adult parasite is found throughout the nasal passages and, sometimes, can reach the sinuses and middle ear by moving through the eustachian tubes. In common with other nasal parasites, *L. serrata* acts as an irritant, causing catarrhal inflammation.

Capillaria aerophila. This nematode parasite of the nasal passages, sinuses, trachea, and bronchi of carnivores produces mild clinical signs and lesions. These are generally related to the local irritation, causing catarrhal to mucopurulent inflammation of airway mucosae.

Other parasites. The nasal cavity and sinuses can be infested with other parasites, including mites, occasionally seen in dogs *(Pneumonyssus caninum);* flukes *(Schistosoma nasalis),* which cause chronic rhinitis in ruminants and horses in Asia; and leeches, found in the upper respiratory tract of animals and human beings in North Africa.

Allergic rhinitis

Allergic rhinitis in domestic animals is rare and poorly documented. ''*Hay fever*'' (nasolacrimal urticaria), which is so common in human beings sensitized to pollens or allergens, has been reported only sporadically in dogs and cats. ''Hay fever'' in human beings and animals is a type I hypersensitivity reaction in which degranulation of mast cells results in an acute rhinitis and conjunctivitis clinically characterized by profuse serous nasal discharge and lacrimation. Microscopically, the nasal mucosa is edematous and infiltrated with numerous eosinophils, neutrophils, and some macrophages.

Another form of allergic rhinitis in animals is known as **''nasal granuloma,''** which occurs presumably as a result of repeated exposure to as-yet unidentified inhaled antigen. Nasal granulomas are reported mainly in cattle in Australia, where affected cattle develop multiple, small, polypoid nodules, starting in the nasal vestibule and, in time, extending into the caudal aspect of the nasal septum. These nodules are composed of granulation tissue covered by hyperplastic epithelium with abundant mast cells and eosinophils in the lamina propria. The microscopic features suggest that hypersensitivity type I, type III (immune complex), and type IV (delayed) may be involved in nasal granulomas of cattle. Bovine (idiopathic) nasal granuloma must be differentiated from nasal mycetomas, nasal rhinosporidiosis, and nasal schistosomiasis, which also cause the formation of nodules in the nasal mucosa of cattle.

Neoplasia of the Nasal Cavity and Sinuses

Neoplasms of the nasal cavity and sinuses may arise from any of the tissues forming these structures, including bone (osteoma or osteosarcoma), cartilage (chondroma or chondrosarcoma), connective tissue (fibroma or fibrosarcoma, myxoma or myxosarcoma), blood vessels (hemangioma or hemangiosarcoma), and from all the different types of cells of glands and lining epithelium (adenoma or carcinoma). In general, nasal neoplasms are rare, except for endemic ethmoidal neoplasms of sheep and cattle that can occur in several animals of a flock or herd.

In domestic animals, nasal neoplasms are seen most commonly in dogs, particularly in breeds such as the collie and German shepherd. The cat and the horse are significantly affected. The most common sites are the nasal passages for dogs, the nasal vestibule for cats, and the maxillary sinus for horses.

Nasal neoplasms become secondarily infected by bacteria, and clinical signs often overlap those of infectious rhinitis, including catarrhal or mucopurulent nasal discharge, periodic hemorrhage, increased lacrimation due to obstruction of nasolacrimal ducts, and sneezing. In some instances, it is not possible to clinically or grossly differentiate neoplasms from hyperplastic nodules or granulomatous rhinitis. Some neoplasms may infiltrate adjacent structures and produce notable facial deformities, loss of teeth, exophthalmus, and nervous signs. Large neoplasms also interfere with airflow, causing stertorous breathing (Fig. 3-9).

The majority of neoplasms in the nasal cavity are malignant. Benign nasal neoplasms (papilloma and adenoma) are rare and generally are either solitary or multiple, well-delineated nodules. In contrast, **nasal carcinomas** and **nasal sarcomas** are generally of larger but variable size, often pale and multilobulated masses composed of fleshy to friable tissue. Malignant neoplasms are locally invasive and tend to infiltrate sinuses, brain, nerves, and vessels, resulting in hemorrhage. Carcinomas vary from anaplastic (poorly differentiated) to more differentiated, in which cell and tissue morphology retains some glandular (adenocarcinoma) or squamous cell pattern.

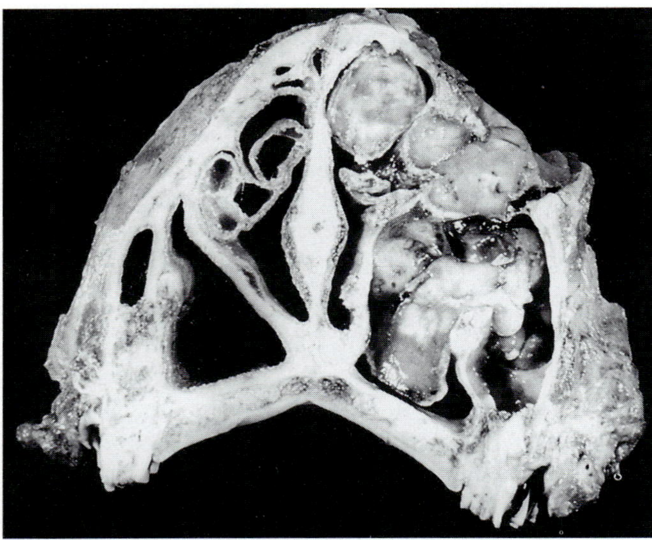

Fig. 3-9 Cross-section of nasal passages and sinuses; cow. Nasal neurofibroma. A swelling on the lateral aspect of the head was visible before slaughter. The tumor has destroyed bone dorsolaterally and has not yet invaded beyond the cartilaginous nasal septum. *Courtesy of Western College of Veterinary Medicine.*

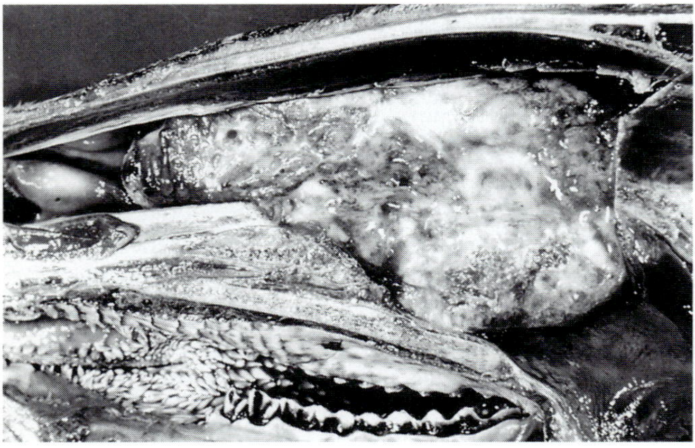

Fig. 3-10 Midsagittal section of the head; 2-year-old ewe. Nasal adenocarcinoma. The tumor has occluded the right nasal passage and posterior nares. The location and type of tumor are typical of a retrovirus-induced "enzootic nasal carcinoma." *Courtesy of Western College of Veterinary Medicine.*

Endemic ethmoidal neoplasms

A unique group of nasal carcinomas of sheep, goats, and cattle arise from the ethmoidal conchae (Fig. 3-10). These neoplasms tend to occur commonly in sheep in particular farming areas of Spain, France, Germany, Canada, and the United States. Ethmoidal neoplasms have been reported in goat herds in France, India, Spain, and Britain. These neoplasms are suspected of being of infectious origin, presumably caused by the retrovirus responsible for visna and maedi. Endemic carcinomas and sarcomas have also been reported sporadically in horses; attempts at transmission of this neoplasm to horses have not been successful. Endemic ethmoidal tumors are typically invasive, but do not metastasize.

Nasal polyps

Nonneoplastic masses that resemble neoplasms are common sequelae to chronic rhinitis in horses, cats, and, to a lesser extent, other species. In horses, polyps tend to form in the ethmoid region, whereas in cats, polyps are most frequently found in the nasopharynx and Eustachian tubes. Grossly, polyps appear as firm, pedunculated nodules of various sizes protruding from the nasal mucosa into the air passages; the surface may be smooth, ulcerated, secondarily infected, and hemorrhagic. Microscopically, polyps are characterized by a core of well-vascularized stromal tissue that contains inflammatory cells and is covered by pseudostratified or squamous epithelium.

PHARYNX, LARYNX, AND TRACHEA

Anomalies

Congenital anomalies of this region are rare in all species. Depending on their location and severity, they may be inconsistent with postnatal life, pose little or no problem, or manifest themselves in later life. If clinical signs of respiratory distress do occur, they are usually exacerbated by excitement, heat, stress, or exercise.

Brachycephalic airway syndrome

This clinical term refers to respiratory impairment caused by stenotic external nostrils and an excessive length of the soft palate. These abnormalities are present in brachycephalic canine breeds such as bulldogs, boxers, Boston terriers, pugs, Pekingese, and others. The defects are due to a mismatch of the ratio of soft tissue to cranial bone and the obstruction of airflow by excessive soft tissue. Secondary changes, such as nasal and laryngeal edema caused by forceful inspiration, eventually lead to severe upper airway obstruction and respiratory distress.

Hypoplastic epiglottis

This anomaly of horses leads to respiratory noise associated with dorsal displacement of the soft palate. An undersized epiglottis is prone to become trapped below the arytenoepiglottic fold, causing obstruction of the airways, exercise intolerance, respiratory noise, and cough. Epiglottic entrapment can also occur in horses with lateral deviation and deformity of the epiglottis, epiglottic cysts, or necrosis of the tip of the epiglottis. Hypoplastic epiglottis also occurs in pigs.

Subepiglottic and pharyngeal cysts

These types of anomalous lesions are occasionally seen in horses. These cysts occur most commonly in the subepiglottic area and to a lesser extent in the upper pharynx, larynx, and soft palate. Cysts are lined by squamous or pseudostratified epithelium and contain thick mucus.

Tracheal agenesis and tracheal hypoplasia

Tracheal hypoplasia occurs most often in English bulldogs, and the tracheal lumen is decreased throughout its length.

Tracheal collapse

This lesion occurs in toy and miniature breeds of dogs, in which it is also called **tracheobronchial collapse** or **central airway collapse.** The defect also occurs in horses, cattle, and goats. Grossly, there is dorsoventral flattening of the trachea with concomitant widening of the dorsal tracheal membrane, which may then prolapse ventrally into the lumen. Most commonly, the defect involves the entire trachea and only rarely affects the cervical portion alone. Areas with a compromised lumen may have froth and even a diphtheritic membrane. Tracheal collapse is presumed to be associated with a qualitative or quantitative defect in the tracheal cartilages. Tracheal collapse is usually diagnosed in mature, obese dogs that may have a superimposed, infectious respiratory disease.

Other tracheal anomalies include **scabbard trachea** in horses, in which there is lateral flattening, and **tracheoesophageal fistula** in dogs and cattle.

Degenerative Diseases

Equine laryngeal hemiplegia (paralysis)

This disease, sometimes called *roaring,* is a common, but obscure, disease of horses characterized by atrophy of the dorsal and lateral cricoarytenoid muscles (abductor/adductor of the arytenoid cartilage), particularly on the left side. Atrophy is due to denervation as a result of either a primary axonal disease (idiopathic) or secondary nerve damage caused by compression or inflammation of the left recurrent laryngeal nerve. The laryngeal nerve and retropharyngeal lymph nodes are located immediately beneath the floor of the guttural pouches. As a result of this close anatomic relationship, swelling or inflammation of the guttural pouches and retropharyngeal lymph nodes often results in secondary damage to the laryngeal nerve. Common causes of secondary nerve damage include guttural pouch mycosis, retropharyngeal abscesses, inflammation due to iatrogenic injection in perivascular tissues, neck injury, and neoplasms. The abnormal sounds (roaring) noted during exercise in horses with laryngeal hemiplegia are due to paralysis of the left dorsal and lateral cricoarytenoid muscles, which causes incomplete dilatation of the larynx, obstruction of airflow, and vibration of loose vocal cords. Grossly, affected laryngeal muscle is pale and smaller than normal. Microscopically, muscle fibers have lesions of denervation atrophy (see Muscular System).

Circulatory Disturbances

Laryngeal and tracheal hemorrhages

Hemorrhages in these sites usually occur as mucosal petechiae in septicemias such as hog cholera and porcine salmonellosis. Similarly, hemorrhages can be seen at slaughter as incidental findings relating to that process in cattle and pigs. Severe dyspnea prior to death can cause congestion and hemorrhages of the tracheal mucosa; this must be differentiated from postmortem imbibition of hemoglobin in autolysed carcasses.

Laryngeal edema

This lesion is a common feature of acute inflammation, but it is of particular importance because of the potential for obstruction of the laryngeal orifice and resultant asphyxiation. Laryngeal edema occurs in pigs with edema disease of swine, in horses with purpura hemorrhagica, in cattle with acute interstitial pneumonia, and in all species as a result of trauma, inhalation of irritant gases (e.g., smoke inhalation), local inflammation, allergy, or systemic anaphylaxis. Grossly, the walls of the larynx are swollen, and a thickened, edematous mucosa often protrudes onto the epiglottis.

Tracheal edema

Also known as the "honker" syndrome of feedlot cattle, this is a poorly documented, acute disease of unknown etiology, most often seen in heavy cattle during the summer months. Clinical signs include inspiratory dyspnea that can progress to oral breathing, recumbency, and death by asphyxiation. Severe edema and a few hemorrhages involve the mucosa and submucosa of the dorsal trachea extending caudally from the midcervical area to as far as the tracheal bifurcation.

Inflammation

Pharyngitis, laryngitis, and tracheitis

Inflammations of the pharynx, larynx, and trachea are important because of their potential to obstruct airflow and to lead to aspiration pneumonia. The pharynx is vulnerable to the maladies of both the upper respiratory and upper digestive tracts, and the trachea can be involved by extension from both the lungs and upper respiratory regions.

A number of nonspecific insults can cause lesions and clinical signs. Trauma may take the form of penetrating wounds in any species, perforation of the posterodorsal wall of the pharynx owing to the improper use of drenching or balling guns in sheep or cattle, choking injury due to use of collars in dogs and cats, and the shearing forces of bite wounds. The results of the trauma may be as minimal as local edema and inflammation or as serious as fatal cellulitis. Foreign bodies may occur anywhere in the region; the location and size determine the occurrence of dysphagia, regurgitation, dyspnea, or asphyxiation. Pigs have a unique structure known as the pharyngeal diverticulum (4 cm long in adult pigs), which is located in the pharyngeal wall rostral and dorsal to the esophageal entrance. It is important because barley awns may lodge in the diverticulum, causing an inflammatory swelling that affects swallowing. The diverticular wall may be perforated by awns or drenching syringes, which results in a cellulitis that can extend down the tissue planes of the neck. The pharynx of the dog may also be damaged by trauma from chicken bones, sticks, and needles resulting in the formation of a pharyngeal abscess.

More common than these intraluminal foreign bodies are those masses in surrounding tissues that obstruct the upper airway. Examples include neoplasms of the thyroid gland, thymus, and parathyroid glands, tonsils, lymph nodes, and esophagus; other esophageal lesions include those caused by *Spirocerca lupi,* lymph nodes swollen by hyperplasia or lymphadenitis, cysts, polyps, and abscesses. **Chronic polypoid tracheitis** occurs in dogs and cats, probably secondary to chronic infection. Laryngeal abscesses occur as a herd or flock problem in calves and sheep, presumably caused by a secondary infection by *Actinomyces pyogenes.*

Equine pharyngeal lymphoid hyperplasia

This very common and clinically significant disorder, particularly in 2- and 3-year-old racehorses, is the most common cause of partial upper airway obstruction in these animals. The etiology is undetermined, but chronic bacterial infection combined with environmental factors may cause the excessive lymphoid hyperplasia with clinical signs of stertorous inspiration and/or expiration. The gross lesions, viewed endoscopically, consist of variably sized white foci located on the dorsolateral pharynx and extending into the openings of the guttural pouches and onto the soft palate. Microscopically, the lesion is hyperplasia of lymphoid nodules.

Inflammation of guttural pouches

The guttural pouches of horses are large diverticula (300 to 500 ml) of the ventral eustachian tubes. They are, therefore, exposed to the same pathogens as is the pharynx and have drainage problems similar to those of sinuses. Although it is probable that various pathogens, including viruses, infect them, the lesions that are most often diagnosed are guttural pouch mycosis and guttural pouch empyema. Because of the close anatomic proximity of guttural pouches to the internal carotid arteries, cranial nerves (VI, IX, X, XI, and XII), atlantooccipital joint, and middle ears, disease of these diverticula may involve these structures and cause a variety of clinical signs in horses.

Guttural pouch mycosis occurs primarily in stabled horses and is caused by *Aspergillus fumigatus* and other *Aspergillus* species. Infection is usually unilateral, and presumably starts with the inhalation of spores from moldy hay. Grossly, the dorsal and lateral aspects of the guttural pouch are covered by a diphtheritic, fibrinonecrotic exudate. Microscopically, the lesions are severe necrotic inflammation of the mucosa and submucosa and widespread vasculitis with intralesional fungal hyphae. The necrotizing characteristics of this mycotic infection and the location of the internal carotid artery immediately adjacent to the roof of the guttural pouches explain why this disease is clinically characterized by epistaxis. Erosion of the internal carotid artery can lead to fatal bleeding into the guttural pouches or, in some other cases, to the release of mycotic thromboemboli into the carotid circulation, which generally results in multiple brain infarcts. Dysphagia, another clinical sign seen in guttural pouch mycosis, is associated with damage to the pharyngeal branches of the vagus and glossopharyngeal nerves, which lie on the ventral aspect of the pouches. Horner's syndrome results from damage to the cranial cervical ganglion and sympathetic fibers located in the caudodorsal aspect of the pouches. Finally, equine laryngeal paralysis can result from involvement of the laryngeal nerves (previously described under Laryngeal Hemiplegia).

Empyema of the guttural pouches occurs as a sequela to suppurative inflammation of the nasal cavity, most commonly to *Streptococcus equi* infection (strangles). It is clinically characterized by nasal discharge, enlarged retropharyngeal lymph nodes, parotitis, dysphagia, and respiratory distress. In severe cases, the entire guttural pouch can be filled with purulent exudate. With the exception of erosion of the internal carotid artery, empyema of guttural pouches causes clinical effects similiar to those of guttural pouch mycosis.

Necrotic laryngitis (calf diphtheria)

This is a common disease of feedlot cattle and cattle with intercurrent disease, with nutritional deficiency, or housed under unsanitary conditions. It also occurs in sheep. Necrotic laryngitis, caused by *Fusobacterium necrophorum,* is part of orolaryngeal necrobacillosis, which can include lesions of the tongue, gingivae, cheeks, palate, and pharynx. The bacterium produces several exotoxins and endotoxins after gaining entry either through lesions of viral

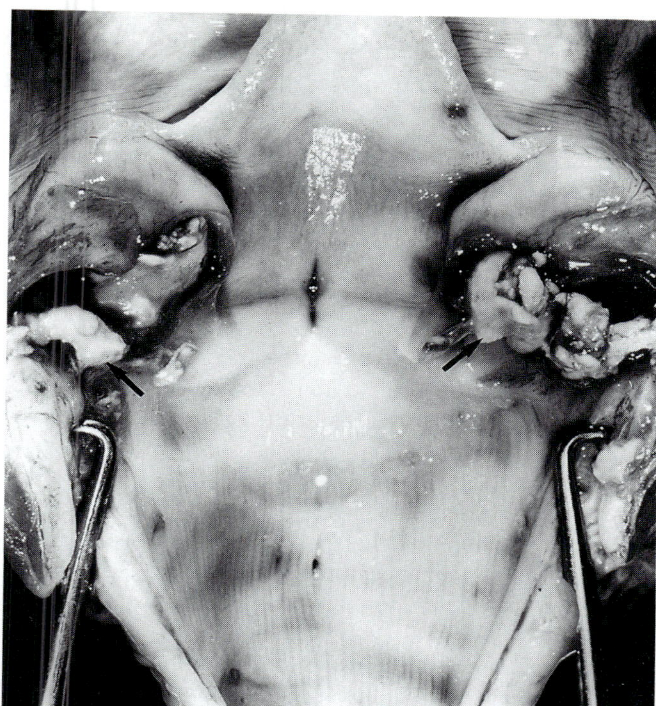

Fig. 3-11 Larynx and trachea; calf. Necrotic laryngitis, calf diphtheria *(Fusobacterium necrophorum)*. Plaques of fibrinonecrotic exudate *(arrows)* are present on the mucosal surface of the arytenoid cartilages. *Courtesy Dr. M.D. McGavin.*

infections such as IBR and papular stomatitis in cattle and contagious ecthyma in sheep or after traumatic injury produced by feed and careless use of specula or balling guns.

The clinical signs of necrotic laryngitis are fever; anorexia; depression; halitosis; moist, painful cough; dysphagia; and inspiratory dyspnea.

The gross lesions, regardless of location in the mouth or larynx, consist of well-demarcated, dry, yellow-gray, necrotic areas (Fig. 3-11) that, in the early stages, are bounded by a zone of hyperemia. Deep ulceration develops, and, if the lesion is not fatal, healing is by granulation tissue. Microscopically, large necrotic foci initially have hyperemic borders. Later, these are replaced by a band of leukocytes and, still later, by granulation tissue and fibrosis. The lesions can extend deep into the submucosal tissues, with bacteria evident at the advancing edge.

There are numerous important sequelae to calf diphtheria, the most serious being death due to toxemia or fusobacteremia. The exudate may be copious enough to cause asphyxiation or be aspirated to cause bronchopneumonia.

Laryngeal contact ulcers

These lesions found in feedlot cattle, grossly, are unilateral or bilateral circular ulcers (up to 1 cm in diameter) deep enough to expose the underlying arytenoid cartilages. The cause has not been established, and viral, bacterial, and traumatic etiologies have been proposed. These ulcers may be caused by increased frequency and rate of closure of the larynx (excessive swallowing and vocalization) when cattle are exposed to market and feedlot stresses, such as dust, pathogens, and interruption of feeding. Contact ulcers predispose calves to diphtheria and laryngeal papillomas. Ulceration of the mucosa and necrosis of the laryngeal cartilages have also been described in calves, sheep, and horses under the term **laryngeal chondritis.**

Canine infectious tracheobronchitis (kennel cough)

This highly contagious infection is clinically characterized by an acute onset of coughing notably exacerbated by exercise. The term is nonspecific, much like "common cold" in human beings or "shipping fever" in cattle. The infection occurs commonly as a result of mixing dogs from different origins, such as occurs at commercial kennels, animal shelters, and veterinary clinics.

The etiology of canine infectious tracheobronchitis is complex, and many pathogens and environmental factors have been incriminated. *Bordetella bronchiseptica, canine adenovirus 2* (CAV-2), and *canine parainfluenza virus* (CPV) are the most commonly reported. The severity of the disease is increased when more than one agent is involved or extreme environmental conditions add additional stresses. For example, dogs asymptomatically infected with *B. bronchiseptica* are more severely affected by superinfection with CAV-2 than those not carrying the bacterium. Other agents, sometimes isolated but of lesser significance, include CAV-1 (infectious canine hepatitis virus), reovirus type 1, canine herpesvirus, and *Mycoplasma* species.

Between bouts of coughing, most animals appear normal, although some may have rhinitis, pharyngitis, tonsillitis, or conjunctivitis; and some with secondary pneumonia become quite ill.

Depending on the agents involved, gross and microscopic lesions may be completely absent, or they may vary from catarrhal to mucopurulent tracheobronchitis with enlargement of the tonsils and regional lymph nodes. In dogs with *B. bronchiseptica* infection, the lesions are exudative suppurative rhinitis, tracheobronchitis, and bronchiolitis. In contrast, when lesions are purely viral, microscopic changes are focal necrosis of the tracheobronchial epithelium. Sequelae can include spread either proximally or distally into the respiratory tract, the latter possibly inducing chronic bronchitis and bronchopneumonia.

Parasitic Diseases

Parasitic infections of the pharynx, larynx, and trachea can have dramatic obstructive consequences, but burdens sufficient to cause such effects are not commonly seen.

Besnoitia bennetti

This coccidian, whose life cycle is still unknown, can cause papilloma-like lesions in the larynx of horses and has been reported from Africa, Central and South America, and Britain. Grossly, nodules up to 2 cm in diameter occur on most surfaces of the larynx; and these nodules, microscopically, consist of thick-walled parasitic cysts overlain by fingerlike projections that have acanthotic and, sometimes, ulcerated epithelium.

Syngamus laryngeus

This nematode is found in the larynx of cattle in tropical Asia and South America.

Filaroides osleri (oslerus osleri)

This parasite of dogs and other canidae forms characteristic protruding nodules at the tracheal bifurcation. In severe cases, these nodules can extend 5 cm above or below this site and even into primary and secondary bronchi. The disease occurs worldwide, and *F. osleri* is considered the most common respiratory nematode of dogs. Clinically, it can be asymptomatic, although it most often causes a chronic cough that can be exacerbated by exercise or excitement. Severe infestations can result in dyspnea, exercise intolerance, cyanosis, emaciation, and even death in young dogs.

The gross lesions are variably sized, up to 1 cm, submucosal nodules that extend up to 1 cm into the tracheal lumen (Fig. 3-12). Microscopically, the parasites are prominent in sections. A mild mononuclear cell reaction is present when parasites are alive, but with the death of the parasite, an intense foreign body reaction develops with neutrophils and giant cells.

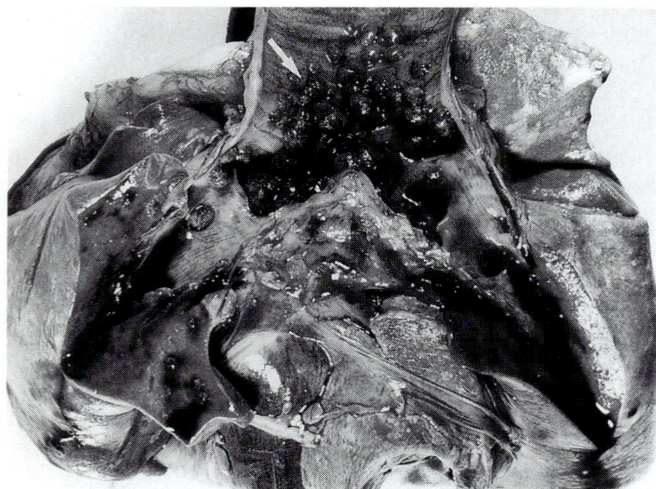

Fig. 3-12 Trachea, bronchi, and lungs; dog. Parasitic tracheobronchitis *(Filaroides osleri).* Note the numerous dark parasitic nodules *(arrow)* on the mucosal surface of distal trachea and bronchi. *Courtesy Dr. M.D. McGavin.*

Neoplasms of Guttural Pouches, Larynx, and Trachea

Neoplasms of the guttural pouches

These occur rarely in horses and are usually squamous cell carcinomas.

Neoplasms of the larynx and trachea

Laryngeal neoplasms are rare in dogs and extremely so in other species, although they have been reported in cats and horses.

When large enough to be obstructive, neoplasms may cause a change or loss of voice, cough, or respiratory distress with cyanosis, collapse, and syncope. Other signs include dysphagia, anorexia, and exercise intolerance. The neoplasm may be visible from the oral cavity and cause swelling of the neck. The prognosis is poor, as most lesions recur after excision.

The most common laryngeal neoplasm in dogs is **squamous cell carcinoma.** Others include **rhabdomyoma, rhabdomyosarcoma, mastocytoma, melanoma, leiomyoma, adenoma, adenocarcinoma, osteosarcoma,** and **chondrosarcoma.**

Tracheal neoplasms are even more uncommon than those of the larynx, but are similarly significant in clinical terms when they do arise. Giant cell tumor has been reported in the horse and adenocarcinoma in the dog. Tracheal cartilages can be the site of chondromas. **Lymphosarcomas** in cats can extend from the mediastinum to involve the trachea.

LUNGS

Species Differences

Each lung is subdivided into various numbers of **pulmonary lobes.** In the past, these were defined by anatomic fissures. However, in current anatomy, lobes are defined by the ramification of the bronchial tree. Following this criterion, the left lung of all species is composed of cranial and caudal lobes, while the right lung, depending on species, is composed of cranial, middle (absent in horse), caudal, and accessory lobes. Each pulmonary lobe is further subdivided by connective tissue into **pulmonary lobules,** which in some species are rather prominent and in others are much less conspicuous. From a practical point of view, identification of lungs among different species could be achieved by carefully observing the degree of lobation (external fissures) and the degree of lobulation (connective tissue between lobules). Cattle and pigs have well-lobated and very well lobulated lungs; sheep and goats have well-lobated but poorly lobulated lungs; horses have both poorly lobated and poorly lobulated lungs that resemble human lungs; finally, dogs and cats have very well lobated but not well-lobulated lungs. The degree of lobulation determines the degree of air movement between the lobules. This interlobular movement of air, together with the communications between alveoli (pores of Kohn) and the communication between bronchioles and alveoli, constitutes what is referred to as collateral ventilation. It is poor in cattle and pigs and good in dogs. The functional implications of collateral ventilation will be discussed in the section on Pulmonary Emphysema.

Congenital Anomalies

Congenital anomalies of the lungs are rare in all species but are most commonly reported in cattle. Compatibility with life largely depends on the type of structures involved and the proportion of functional tissue present at birth. **Accessory lungs** are one of the most common anomalies and consist of distinctively lobulated masses of incompletely differentiated pulmonary tissue present in the thorax, abdominal cavity, or subcutaneous tissue virtually anywhere in the trunk. Large accessory lungs can cause dystocia. **Ciliary dyskinesia (immotile cilia syndrome)** has been reported in dogs with chronic recurrent pneumonia and infertility, often associated with *situs inversus.* It is characterized by deficient ciliary movement due to a defect in the microtubules of all ciliated cells and, most important, in the ciliated respiratory epithelium and in spermatozoa. Ciliary dyskinesia reduces mucociliary clearance, leading to chronic rhinitis, sinusitis, bronchitis, bronchiectasis, and pneumonia. **Pulmonary agenesia, pulmonary hypoplasia, abnormal lobulation, congenital emphysema,** and **congenital bronchiectasis** are occasionally seen in domestic animals. **Congenital melanosis** is a common incidental finding in pigs and ruminants and is usually seen at slaughter. It is characterized by dark spots, often a few centimeters in diameter, in various organs, mainly the lungs, meninges, and aorta. Melanosis has no clinical significance, and the texture of pigmented lungs remains unchanged.

Metabolic Disturbances

Pulmonary calcification (''calcinosis'')

Calcification of the lungs occurs in some hypercalcemic states, generally associated with hypervitaminosis D or from ingestion of toxic plants such as *Solanum malacoxylon* (Manchester wasting disease) that contain vitamin D analogs. It is also a common sequela to pulmonary necrosis (dystrophic calcification) in most species and to uremia in dogs. Calcified lungs may fail to collapse when the thoracic cavity is opened and have a characteristic ''gritty'' texture. Microscopic lesions vary from mild calcification of the basement membranes to heterotopic ossification of the lungs. In most cases, pulmonary calcification in itself has little clinical significance, although its cause (e.g., uremia) may be very important.

Abnormalities of Inflation

To achieve gaseous exchange, balanced ratio of air to capillary blood must be present in the lungs (ventilation/perfusion ratio), and the two must be in close proximity across the alveolar membrane. This fails to occur if pulmonary tissue is either collapsed (atelectasis) or overinflated (emphysema).

Atelectasis

The term atelectasis means incomplete distention of alveoli and is used to describe lungs that have failed to expand with air at the time of birth (congenital atelectasis) or lungs that have collapsed after inflation has taken place (acquired atelectasis). During fetal life, lungs are not fully distended, contain no air, and are partially filled with a locally produced fluid known as **fetal lung fluid.** Not surprisingly, lungs of aborted and stillborn fetuses sink when placed in water, while those from animals that have breathed float. At the time of birth, fetal lung fluid is rapidly reabsorbed and replaced by inspired air, leading to the normal distention of alveoli. **Congenital atelectasis** occurs in newborns that fail to inflate their lungs after taking their first few breaths of air; it is caused by obstruction of airways, often as a result of aspiration of amniotic fluid (meconium aspiration syndrome) (Fig. 3-13). Congenital atelectasis also develops when alveoli cannot remain distended following initial aeration because of a defect in the pulmonary surfactant produced by type II pneumonocytes. This form of congenital atelectasis is referred to in human neonatology as **''acute respiratory distress syndrome''** or as **''hyaline membrane disease''** due to the clinical and microscopic features of the disease. It commonly occurs in babies that are premature or born to diabetic or alcoholic mothers and is occasionally found in animals,

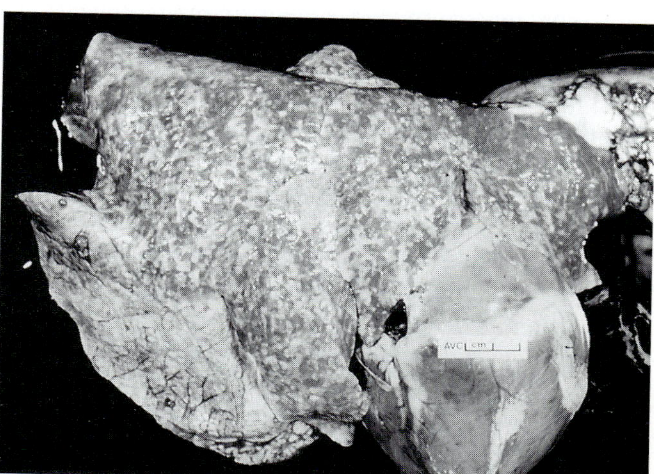

Fig. 3-13 Lung; 1-day-old calf. Multifocal neonatal atelectasis. Prominent mosaic pattern of normally inflated *(light)* and atelectatic, uninflated *(dark)* lobules. Atelectasis was due to aspiration of amniotic fluid, meconium, and squamous epithelial cells. All pulmonary lobes were involved. *López et al. Vet Pathol 1992; 29:104-111.*

particularly in foals and piglets. The pathetic, gasping attempts to breathe have prompted the use of the name "barkers" for affected foals and pigs; foals that survive may have brain damage and are referred to as "wanderers," owing to their aimless behavior and lack of a normal sense of fear.

Acquired atelectasis occurs in several ways. The simple physical presence of fluids, masses, or transferred pressures can cause **compressive atelectasis.** Examples include pneumothorax, hydrothorax, hemothorax, chylothorax, empyema, neoplasms, and bloat. **Obstructive atelectasis** occurs when an airway is blocked by exudates, aspirated foreign material, parasites, or neoplasms. Unlike the compression type, obstructive atelectasis often has a lobular pattern and is more common in species with poor collateral ventilation, such as cattle and sheep. **Hypostatic atelectasis** occurs when large animals are kept recumbent for prolonged periods, such as during surgery. The factors are a combination of blood-air imbalance, shallow breathing, failure of drainage, and inadequate surfactant production. **Massive atelectasis (lung collapse)** is usually the result of a pneumothorax. However, it can also be a sequela to the prolonged use of respirators in intensive care. In all types of atelectasis, the collapsed lung is prone to secondary infections.

In general, lungs with atelectasis of any type appear dark and collapsed and may be flabby or firm; they are firm if there is concurrent edema or other processes such as can occur in "shock" lungs. Distribution and extent vary with the process, being patchy (multifocal) in congenital atelectasis, lobular in the obstructive type, and of various degrees in between in the compressive type. Microscopically, the alveoli are collapsed or slitlike, giving prominence to the interstitial tissue even without any superimposed inflammation.

Pulmonary emphysema

Pulmonary emphysema, simply referred to as emphysema, is an extremely important primary disease in human beings, whereas in animals it is always a secondary lesion resulting from other types of pulmonary lesions. In human medicine, emphysema is strictly defined as an abnormal permanent enlargement of airspaces distal to the terminal bronchiole, accompanied by destruction of alveolar walls (alveolar emphysema). This definition separates it from simple airspace enlargement, in which there is no destruction and which can occur congenitally (Down's syndrome) or be acquired with age (aging lung, sometimes misnamed "senile emphysema"). The pathogenesis of emphysema in human beings is still controversial, but current thinking overwhelmingly suggests that destruction of alveolar walls is largely the result of an imbalance between proteases released by phagocytes and antiproteases produced in the lungs as a defense mechanism (the protease-antiprotease theory). The destructive process is markedly accelerated by any factor such as cigarette smoking, pollution, or defects in the synthesis of antiproteases in human beings that increases the recruitment of macrophages and leukocytes in the lungs. This theory originated when it was found that human beings with homozygous α_1-antitrypsin deficiency were remarkably susceptible to emphysema and that proteases (elastase) inoculated intratracheally into the lungs of laboratory animals produced lesions similar to those found in the disease. Over 90% of the problem relates to cigarette smoking. Airway obstruction is no longer considered to play a major role in the pathogenesis of emphysema in human beings.

Primary emphysema does not occur in animals, and, thus, no animal disease should be called simply emphysema. In animals, this lesion is always secondary to obstruction of outflow of air or agonal at slaughter. Depending on the area of the lung affected, emphysema can be classified into alveolar or interstitial. **Alveolar emphysema** occurs in all species, and it is characterized by distention and rupture of the alveolar walls forming variably sized air bubbles in pulmonary parenchyma (Fig. 3-14). **Interstitial emphysema** occurs mainly in cattle, presumably because lack of collateral ventilation in these species does not permit air to move freely into adjacent structures. As a result, accumulated air disrupts and forces its way into connective tissue, causing notable distention of the interlobular septa. Sometimes these air bubbles become confluent, forming large, several centimeters in diameter, pockets of air that are referred to as **bullae** (singular: bulla); the lesion is

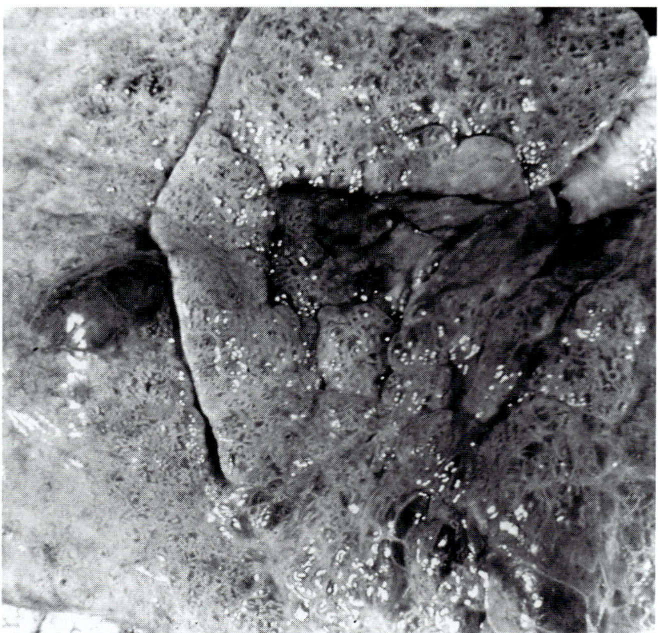

Fig. 3-14 Lung; cow. Bovine pulmonary edema and emphysema (fog fever). Emphysema, edema, and interstitial pneumonia involving all pulmonary lobes. Note variably sized air bubbles in pulmonary parenchyma and interlobular septa.

called **bullous emphysema.** This is not a specific type of emphysema and does not indicate a different disease process, but rather a larger accumulation of air at one focus. It should be noted that mild alveolar emphysema is difficult to judge at postmortem and by light microscopy unless special techniques are used. These include plugging of the trachea before opening the thorax to prevent collapse of the lungs when the thorax is opened.

Important diseases that cause secondary pulmonary emphysema in animals include **small airway obstruction** (such as **heaves**) in horses and **pulmonary edema and emphysema (fog fever)** in cattle.

Circulatory Disturbances of the Lungs

Lungs are extremely well vascularized organs with a dual circulation provided by pulmonary and bronchial arteries. Disturbances in pulmonary circulation have a notable effect on gaseous exchange, which may result in life-threatening hypoxemia and acidosis. In addition, circulatory disturbances in the lungs can impact on numerous organs due to passive congestion and generalized edema.

Hyperemia and congestion

Hyperemia is an active process that is part of acute inflammation, whereas congestion is the passive process resulting from decreased outflow of venous blood, as occurs in congestive heart failure. In the acute stages of pneumonia, the lungs appear notably red, and, microscopically, blood vessels and capillaries are engorged with blood from hyperemia. Pulmonary congestion is most frequently caused by heart failure, which results in stagnation of blood in the pulmonary vessels, leading to edema and egression of erythrocytes into the alveolar spaces. As with any other foreign particle, erythrocytes in the alveolar spaces are rapidly phagocytosed (erythrophagocytosis) by pulmonary alveolar macrophages. When extravasation of erythrocytes is severe, large numbers of macrophages with brown cytoplasm may accumulate in the bronchoalveolar spaces. The brown cytoplasm is the result of accumulation of considerable amounts of hemosiderin, and these macrophages are generally referred to as *"heart failure cells."* The lungs of animals with chronic heart failure usually have a patchy red appearance with foci of brown discoloration due to accumulated hemosiderin.

Pulmonary hemorrhage

Pulmonary hemorrhages can occur as a result of trauma, coagulopathies, pulmonary thromboembolism due to jugular thrombosis or hepatic abscess that has ruptured into the vena cava (cattle), disseminated intravascular coagulation, or septicemia. A finding that resembles pulmonary hemorrhage is the aspiration of blood after the carotid arteries and trachea have been cut at the time of slaughter. The lungs have a mosaic pattern of red discoloration.

Rupture of a major pulmonary vessel with resulting massive hemorrhage occurs occasionally in cattle when a growing abscess in a lung may invade and disrupt the wall of the vessel. In most cases, animals die rapidly, often with a spectacular hemoptysis. Massive amounts of blood are lost through the mouth and nostrils.

"Exercise-induced pulmonary hemorrhage" (EIPH) is a specific form of pulmonary hemorrhage in racehorses following exercise and clinically is characterized by epistaxis. Since only a small percentage of horses with bronchoscopic evidence of hemorrhage have clinical epistaxis, it is likely that EIPH goes undetected in many cases. The pathogenesis is still controversial, but current literature suggests asphyxia, bronchiolitis, laryngeal paralysis, and preexisting pulmonary injury as possible causes. EIPH is seldom fatal; postmortem lesions in affected horses are large areas of dark-brown discoloration, largely in the caudal lung lobes. Microscopically, lesions are alveolar hemorrhage, abundant macrophages containing hemosiderin (siderophages), and mild interstitial fibrosis.

Pulmonary edema

In normal lungs, fluid from the vascular space slowly but continuously passes into the interstitial tissues where it is rapidly drained by the lymph vessels. Edema develops when the rate of fluid transudation exceeds that of lymph removal. **Pulmonary edema** can be classified into hemodynamic or permeability types.

Hemodynamic pulmonary edema develops when there is an elevated rate of fluid transudation due to increased hydrostatic pressure in the vascular compartment or decreased osmotic pressure in the blood. Once lymph drainage has been overwhelmed, fluid accumulates in the perivascular spaces, causing distention of the interstitial tissue and eventually leaking into the alveolar spaces. Causes of hemodynamic pulmonary edema include congestive heart failure (increased hydrostatic pressure), disorders in which blood osmotic pressure is reduced such as in the hypoalbuminemia seen in some hepatic diseases, nephrotic syndrome, and protein-losing enteropathy. Hemodynamic pulmonary edema also occurs when lymph drainage is impaired and is generally associated with neoplastic invasion of lymph vessels.

Permeability edema occurs when there is excessive opening of endothelial gaps or damage to the air-blood barrier (type I pneumonocytes or to endothelial cells). This type of edema is an integral part of the inflammatory response, primarily due to the local release of inflammatory mediators such as leukotrienes, prostaglandins, platelet activator factor, cytokines, and vasoactive amines. In other cases, permeability edema results from direct damage to the endothelium and pneumonocytes. Since type I pneumonocytes are highly vulnerable to some pneumotropic viruses (influenza, BRSV), toxicants (NO_2, SO_2, H_2S, 3-methylindole), and especially to free radicals, it is not surprising that alveolar edema commonly accompanies many viral and toxic pulmonary diseases. Exposure to bacterial toxins (endotoxemia, septic shock, disseminated intravascular coagulation), anaphylactic shock, milk allergy, and adverse drug reactions are also important causes of permeability edema.

The concentration of protein in edematous fluid is greater in permeability edema (exudate) than in hemodynamic edema (transudate); this divergence has been used clinically in human medicine to differentiate one type of pulmonary edema from another. Microscopically, edematous fluid tends to stain more intensely eosinophilic in lungs with inflammation or damage to the air-blood barrier than that present with hemodynamic edema.

In the last few years, great attention has been given to a disease in human beings known as **adult respiratory distress syndrome (ARDS),** which is characterized by intravascular aggregation of neutrophils in the lungs, diffuse alveolar damage, permeability edema, and formation of hyaline membranes. This clinical syndrome is associated with a wide variety of insults such as septicemia, toxemia, burns, trauma, and pancreatitis. Although the pathogenesis of ARDS remains obscure, current literature indicates that diffuse alveolar damage is presumably caused by proinflammatory mediators and free radicals released by neutrophils and platelets in pulmonary capillaries. It is possible that a disease similar to ARDS occurs in domestic animals; this could help to explain why pulmonary edema is so common in animals dying of septicemia, toxemia, or other causes.

Grossly, edematous lungs are wet and heavy; the color varies depending on the degree of congestion or hemorrhage; and fluid may be present in the thoracic cavity. If edema is severe, bronchi and trachea contain considerable amounts of foamy fluid, which originates from the mixing of edema fluid and air (Fig. 3-15). In cattle and pigs, the lobular pattern becomes rather accentuated due to edematous distentions of interlobular septa (Fig. 3-16). Severe pulmonary edema may be impossible to differentiate from peracute pneumonia; this is not surprising since pulmonary edema is the very first stage of inflammation. Careful observation of lungs at the time of necropsy is critical, since diagnosis of pulmonary edema cannot be reliably performed microscopically. This is due in part to the loss of the edema fluid from the lungs during fixation with 10% neutral, buffered formalin and in part to the fact that the fluid itself stains very poorly because of its low protein content (hemodynamic edema). A protein-rich (permeability) edema is easier to visualize microscopically because it is deeply eosinophilic, particularly if a fixative such as Zenker's solution is used (Fig. 3-17).

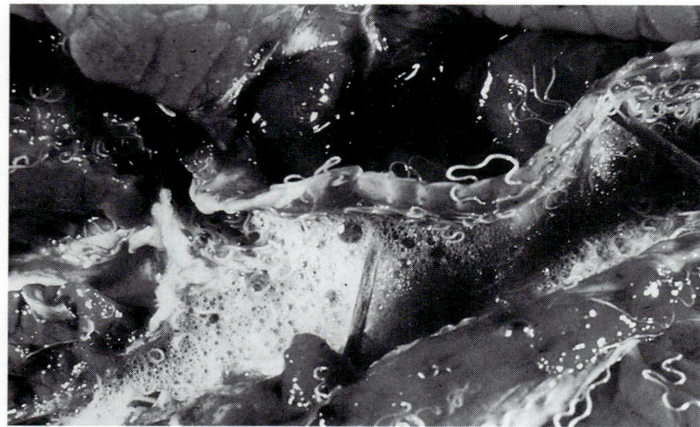

Fig. 3-15 Bronchus; calf. Verminous pneumonia *(Dictyocaulus viviparus)*. The bronchus contains large amounts of foamy edematous fluid and numerous slender lungworms.

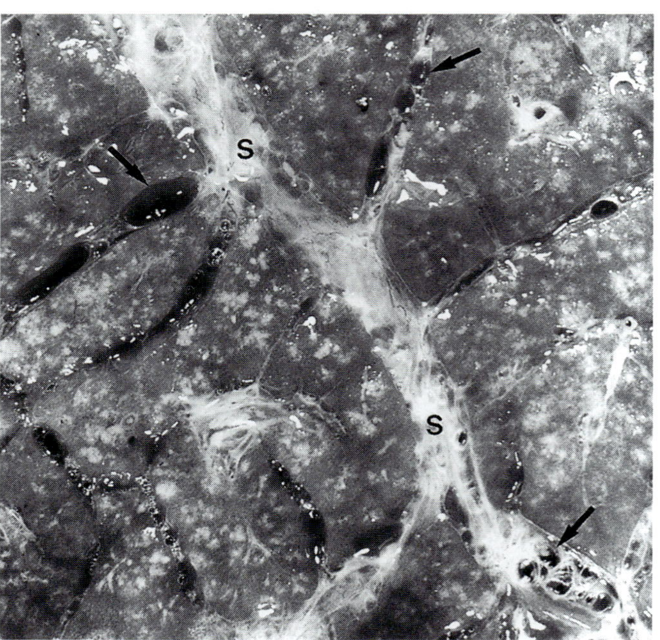

Fig. 3-16 Lung, cut surface; calf. Pulmonary edema. The lungs have a "wet appearance," because of the white froth exuding from the bronchioles, and the interlobular septa (*S*) are distended by accumulation of edematous fluid and emphysema *(arrows)*. *Courtesy Dr. M.D. McGavin.*

Embolism

With its vast capillary bed and position in the circulation, the lung acts as a safety net to catch emboli before they reach the brain and other tissues. However, this is often to its own detriment. The most common emboli found in domestic animals include thromboemboli, septic emboli, fat emboli, and tumor cell emboli.

Pulmonary **thromboembolism** generally originates from a thrombus present elsewhere in the venous circulation. Fragments released inevitably become trapped in pulmonary vasculature. Sterile thromboemboli are generally of little clinical or pathologic significance since they can be

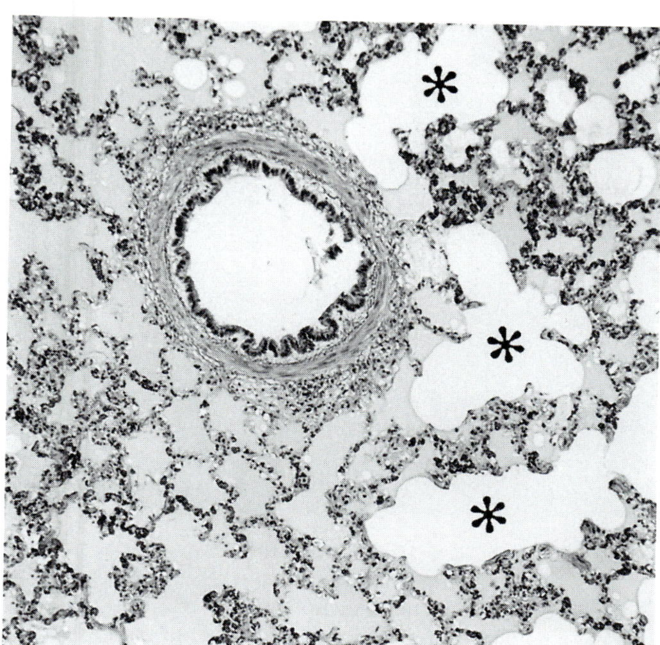

Fig. 3-17 Lung; horse. Pulmonary edema in the lungs of a healthy horse euthanatized with intravenous barbiturate. Note darker appearance of alveoli containing edematous fluid as compared with that of the alveoli filled with air *(asterisks)*. H & E stain.

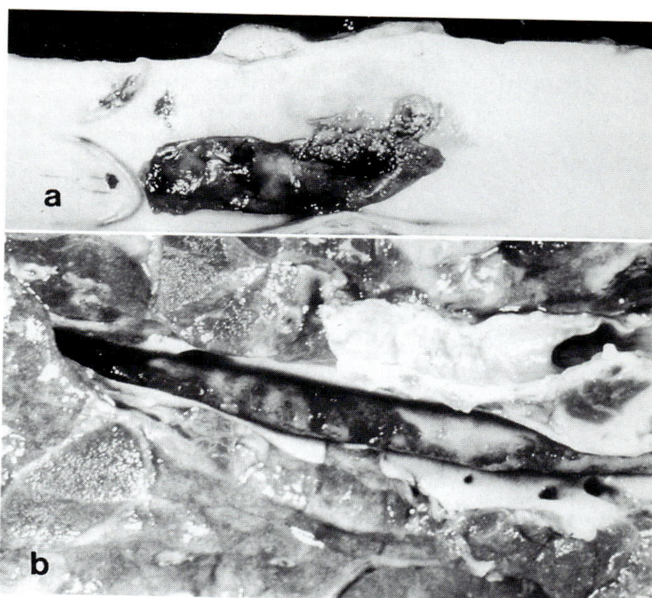

Fig. 3-18 Jugular vein and lung, cut surface; cow. Jugular thrombophlebitis and pulmonary thromboembolism. The jugular vein shows a large thrombus attached to the wall *(top)*. The pulmonary artery contains a large, well-organized thrombus *(bottom)*. These lesions were the consequence of prolonged catheterization of the jugular vein.

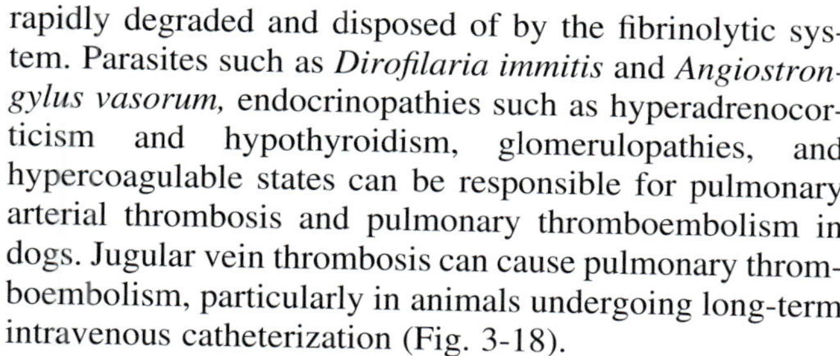

rapidly degraded and disposed of by the fibrinolytic system. Parasites such as *Dirofilaria immitis* and *Angiostrongylus vasorum,* endocrinopathies such as hyperadrenocorticism and hypothyroidism, glomerulopathies, and hypercoagulable states can be responsible for pulmonary arterial thrombosis and pulmonary thromboembolism in dogs. Jugular vein thrombosis can cause pulmonary thromboembolism, particularly in animals undergoing long-term intravenous catheterization (Fig. 3-18).

Septic emboli, pieces of thrombi contaminated with bacteria and broken free from infected mural thrombi, often eventually become entrapped in the pulmonary circulation. These emboli originate most commonly from bacterial endocarditis (right side) in all species, hepatic abscesses that have eroded into vena cava in cattle, and septic arthritis and omphalitis in farm animals. When present in large numbers, septic emboli may cause sudden death due to massive pulmonary edema; survivors generally develop arteritis, thrombosis, embolic (suppurative) pneumonia, and pulmonary abscesses.

Fat emboli can occur after bone fractures but are not as significant a problem in domestic animals as they are in human beings. At necropsy, **tumor emboli** (e.g., osteosarcoma in dogs, uterine carcinoma in cattle) can be numerous and striking and the ultimate cause of death in malignant neoplasia. In experimental studies, pulmonary inflammation generated chemotactic activity for tumor cells and promoted pulmonary metastasis.

Because of the dual arterial supply to the lung, **pulmonary infarction** is rare and generally asymptomatic. However, pulmonary infarcts can be readily caused when pulmonary thrombosis and embolism are superimposed on an already compromised pulmonary circulation, such as occurs in congestive heart failure. The gross features of infarcts vary considerably depending on the stage, and they can be red to black, swollen, firm, and cone- or wedge-shaped. In the acute stage, microscopic lesions are severely hemorrhagic with necrosis. In 1 to 2 days, a border of inflammatory cells develops. If sterile, they heal as fibrotic scars; if septic, an abscess may form.

Patterns of Injury and Host Response in the Lungs

Bronchi

The patterns of necrosis, inflammation, and repair in intrapulmonary bronchi are similar to those previously described for the nasal and tracheal epithelium. In brief, injury to ciliated bronchial epithelium may result in degeneration, detachment, and exfoliation of these cells. Under normal circumstances, this loss is promptly followed by exudative inflammation and repair. Depending on the type of exudate, **bronchitis** can be **fibrinous, catarrhal, purulent, fibrinonecrotic** (diphtheritic), and,

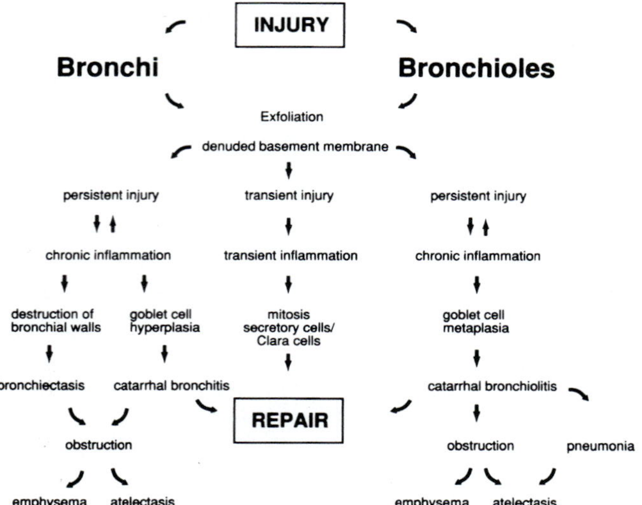

Fig. 3-19 Patterns of host response and possible sequelae to bronchial and bronchiolar injury.

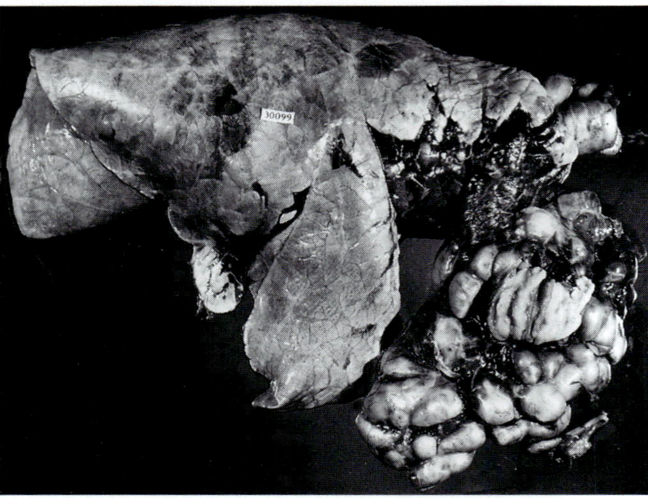

Fig. 3-20 Right lung; calf. Chronic suppurative bronchopneumonia with severe bronchiectasis. Note markedly distended (bosselated) cranioventral bronchi. The cut surfaces of affected bronchi are filled with purulent exudate. The surrounding parenchyma is partially atelectatic.

sometimes, **granulomatous.** When epithelial injury becomes chronic, production of mucus is increased via **goblet cell hyperplasia** (chronic catarrhal inflammation). This form of chronic bronchitis is well illustrated by habitual smokers who continuously need to cough out excessive mucous secretions (sputum). Unfortunately, in some cases excessive mucus cannot be effectively cleared from airways, and this leads to **chronic obstructive bronchitis** (Fig. 3-19). Chronic bronchial irritation can also cause **squamous metaplasia,** in which highly functional but vulnerable ciliated epithelium is replaced by a poorly functional, but more resistant, squamous epithelium. Squamous metaplasia has a calamitous effect on mucociliary clearance.

Bronchiectasis is one of the most devastating sequela that follows chronic bronchitis. It consists of a pathologic and permanent dilatation of a bronchus as a result of the accumulation of exudate in the lumen and partial rupture of bronchial walls. Destruction of walls occurs, in part, when proteolytic enzymes released from phagocytic cells during chronic inflammation degrade and weaken the smooth muscle and cartilage that help to maintain normal bronchial diameter. Bronchiectasis may be **saccular** when destruction affects only a small localized portion of the bronchial wall or **cylindrical** when destruction involves a large segment of a bronchus. Grossly, bronchiectasis is manifested by prominent lumps in the lungs resulting from dilatation of bronchi and concurrent (obstructive) atelectasis of surrounding parenchyma. The cut surfaces of dilated bronchi are filled with purulent exudate; for this reason, bronchiectasis is often mistaken for pulmonary abscesses (Fig. 3-20). Careful inspection, usually requiring microscopic examination, will confirm that bronchiectatic exudate is contained and surrounded by remnants of a bronchial wall. The exudate in a pulmonary abscess is confined by a true pyogenic membrane (connective tissue).

Bronchioles

The epithelial lining of the bronchiolar region (transitional zone) is exquisitely susceptible to injury, particularly to that caused by some respiratory viruses (PI-3, adenovirus, BRSV) (Fig. 3-21), oxidant gases (NO_2, SO_2, O_3), and toxic substances (3-methylindole). The precise explanation as to why bronchiolar epithelium is so prone to injury is still not clear, but it is presumably due in part to (1) its high vulnerability to oxidants and free radicals; (2) the presence of Clara cells rich in mixed-function oxidases, which locally generate toxic metabolites; and (3) the tendency for pulmonary alveolar macrophages and leukocytes to accumulate in this region of the lungs.

Once injury becomes irreversible, bronchiolar ciliated cells degenerate and exfoliate into the bronchiolar lumen, leaving a denuded basement membrane. Repair in the bronchiolar region is similar to but less effective than that in the tracheal or nasal mucosae. Under normal circumstances, recruited phagocytic cells remove exudate and cells debris from the lumina of affected bronchioles, thus preparing the basement membrane to be repopulated with new, undifferentiated cells originating from a rapidly dividing pool of Clara cells. After several days, these proliferating cells fully differentiate into normal bronchiolar ciliated cells.

In severe injury, exudate cannot be removed from the basement membrane of bronchioles. The exudate becomes

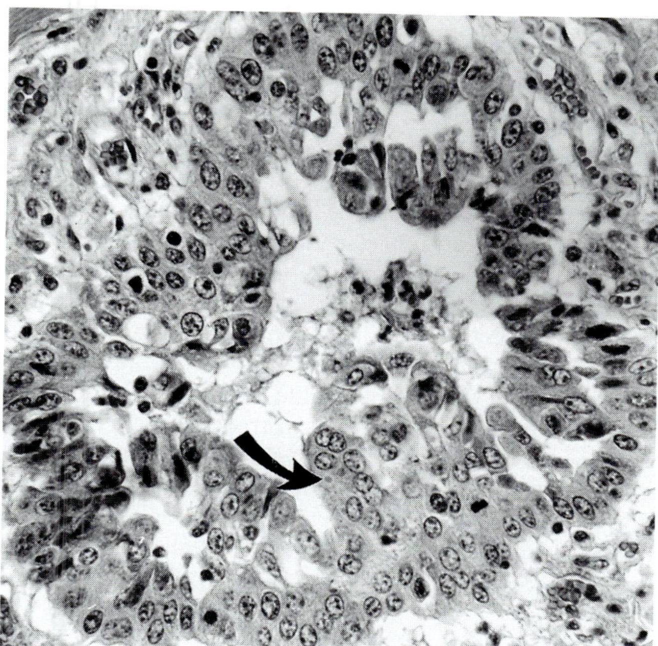

Fig. 3-21 Lung; 5-week-old calf. Acute necrotizing bronchiolitis. Bovine respiratory syncytial virus (BRSV). Bronchiolar cells are swollen and sloughed into the lumen. Inclusion bodies surrounded by a clear halo are present in the cytoplasm of bronchiolar epithelial cells *(arrow)*. H & E stain.

infiltrated by fibroblasts, which form small masses of fibrovascular tissue and develop into well-organized, microscopic polyps inside the bronchiolar lumen. Their external surface eventually becomes covered by ciliated cells. This lesion is commonly referred to as **bronchiolitis obliterans.**

On the other hand, if bronchiolar injury is mild but persistent, goblet cells normally absent from bronchioles proliferate, resulting in **goblet cell metaplasia** (Fig. 3-19) and alteration in the physicochemical properties of bronchiolar secretions. This is normally a serous type of fluid, produced by Clara cells, but becomes a tenacious material when mucus produced by goblet cells is added. As a result of increased viscoelasticity of the mucus, bronchiolar secretions cannot be removed effectively by ciliary action, leading to plugging and obstruction of distal airways. Under such conditions, often grouped together as **chronic obstructive pulmonary disease,** cough is required to clear mucus from obstructed bronchioles. Further sequelae to bronchiolar obstruction include pulmonary emphysema and atelectasis, and those are characteristically present in chronic obstructive pulmonary disease, such as "heaves" in horses.

Chronic obstructive pulmonary disease (COPD) of horses (chronic bronchiolitis-emphysema complex, heaves, chronic small airway disease, alveolar emphysema, "broken wind") is a common asthmalike syndrome of horses and ponies, clinically characterized by recurrent respiratory distress, chronic cough, and poor performance. The pathogenesis is still obscure, but genetic predisposition and airways exceptionally sensitive to environmental allergens (hyperreactive airways disease) have been postulated as the basic underlying mechanisms. What makes small airways hyperreactive to allergens is still a matter of controversy. Epidemiologic and experimental studies suggest that it could be the result of preceding bronchiolar damage caused by viral infections, ingestion of pneumotoxicants (3-methylindole), or prolonged exposure to environmental allergens (molds). Grossly, lungs are unremarkable, except for extreme cases in which alveolar emphysema may be present. Microscopically, the lesions include goblet cell metaplasia, plugging of airways with mucus mixed with a few eosinophils (Fig. 3-22), and hypertrophy of smooth muscle about airways. In severe cases, accumulation of mucus leads to the obstruction of small airways and concurrent alveolar emphysema.

"Airway hyperresponsiveness" is another sequela to bronchiolar injury. It develops in human beings and animals (experimentally) following a transient and often innocuous viral infection of the lower respiratory tract. Airway hyperresponsiveness is characterized by an exaggerated bronchoconstriction following exposure to mild stimuli such as cold air or after a challenge with aerosols of histamine or methacholine. Hyperreactive animals typically have an increased number of mast cells in the airway mucosa. Whether airway hyperreactivity is specifically associated with postviral bronchiolitis or is a nonspecific sequela to some types of bronchiolar injury remains to be elucidated.

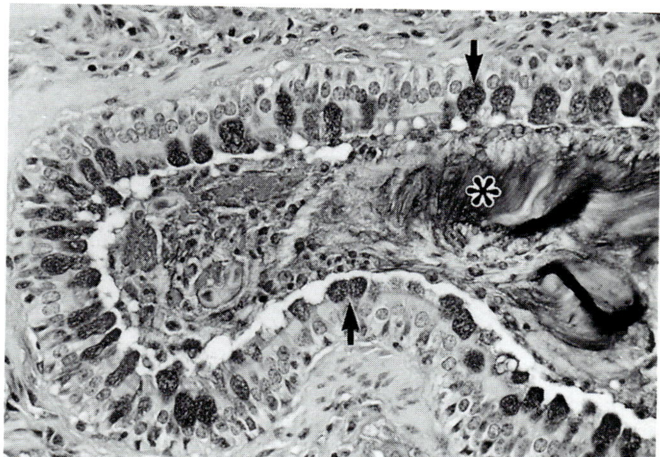

Fig. 3-22 Lung, histologic section; horse. Animal with a 3-year history of recurrent dyspnea and terminal pulmonary emphysema. Chronic obstructive pulmonary disease (COPD; heaves). Numerous goblet cells *(arrows)* in the bronchiolar epithelium (goblet cell metaplasia) are discharging mucus *(asterisk)* into the lumen, causing complete obstruction of the bronchiole. PAS-Alcian blue stain.

Alveoli

Due to their extremely delicate structure, alveoli are extremely vulnerable to injury once defense mechanisms have been overwhelmed. The alveolus has a thin, three-layered wall composed of **vascular endothelium, alveolar interstitium,** and **alveolar epithelium.** These three layers of cells constitute what is customarily referred to as the **air-blood barrier.** The epithelial side of the alveolus is primarily lined by rather thin **type I pneumonocytes,** which are arranged as a very delicate continuous membrane extending along the alveolar surface (see Fig. 3-3). Type I pneumonocytes are particularly susceptible to noxious agents that reach the alveolar region. Injury to type I pneumonocytes causes swelling and vacuolation of these cells. When cellular damage has become irreversible, type I cells detach, resulting in denudation of the basement membrane. Alveolar repair is possible as long as the basement membrane remains intact and lesions are not complicated by further injury or infection. Within 3 days, cuboidal **type II (granular) pneumonocytes,** which are more resistant to injury, undergo mitosis and provide a large pool of cells that replace necrotic **type I cells** and repave the denuded basement membrane. When alveolar injury is diffuse, proliferation of type II pneumonocytes becomes so spectacular that the microscopic appearance of the alveolus resembles that of a gland or a fetal lung, and the lesion has been termed **epithelialization** or **fetalization.** In uncomplicated cases, type II pneumonocytes eventually differentiate into type I pneumonocytes, thus completing the last stage of alveolar repair.

Injury to type I pneumonocytes is generally accompanied by alterations in the air-blood barrier, resulting in transient leakage of plasma fluid, proteins, and fibrin into the alveolar lumen. Under normal circumstances, these fluids and cell debris are rapidly cleared by pulmonary alveolar macrophages and leukocytes recruited to the area by cytokines and other inflammatory mediators. The regulation of leukocyte influx into the airspaces in pulmonary injury is a complex phenomenon. It is in part modulated by proinflammatory factors such as leukotrienes, interleukin-1, and tumor necrosis factor as well as by antiinflammatory factors such as cytokines, interleukin-6, and growth factor β.

In some cases, plasma proteins leaked into the alveoli mix with pulmonary surfactant, forming microscopic eosinophilic bands known as **"hyaline membranes."** These pseudomembranes are found in specific types of pulmonary inflammation, particularly in cattle with acute interstitial pneumonias such as **bovine pulmonary edema and emphysema** or **extrinsic allergic alveolitis.**

As long as alveolar injury is transient and there is no interference with the normal host response, the entire process of injury, degeneration, necrosis, inflammation, and repair can occur in less than 1 week. On the other hand, when alveolar injury becomes persistent or when the capacity of the host for repair is impaired, lesions can progress to an irreversible stage where restoration of pulmonary structure is no longer possible. In diseases such as allergic alveolitis, the constant release of proteolytic enzymes and free radicals by phagocytic cells during the inflammatory process tends to perpetuate alveolar damage. In other cases, such as in paraquat toxicity, the magnitude of alveolar injury can be so severe that type II pneumonocytes, basement membranes, and alveolar interstitium are so disrupted that the capacity for lung repair is lost. Chemical mediators such as fibronectins released from macrophages and other mononuclear cells at the site of chronic inflammation result in the recruitment, attachment, and proliferation of fibroblasts. In turn, these cells synthesize and release considerable amounts of extracellular matrix (collagen, elastic fibers, proteoglycans), eventually leading to fibrosis and total obliteration of normal alveolar architecture. In summary, in diseases in which there is chronic and irreversible alveolar damage, lesions invariably progress to a stage of terminal alveolar fibrosis.

Classification of Pneumonias

Few subjects in veterinary pathology have caused so much debate as the classification of pneumonias. Historically, pneumonias in animals have been classified or named based on (1) **presumed etiology,** with names such as viral pneumonia, pasteurella pneumonia, distemper pneumonia, verminous pneumonia, chemical pneumonia, hypersensitivity pneumonitis; (2) **type of exudation,** with names such as suppurative pneumonia, fibrinous pneumonia, pyogranulomatous pneumonia; (3) **morphologic features,** with names such as gangrenous pneumonia, proliferative pneumonia, embolic pneumonia; (4) **distribution of lesions,** with names such as focal pneumonia, cranioventral pneumonia, diffuse pneumonia, lobar pneumonia; (5) **epidemiologic attributes,** with names such as enzootic pneumonia, contagious bovine pleuropneumonia, shipping fever pneumonia; (6) **geographic regions,** with names such as Montana progressive pneumonia; and finally, (7) **miscellaneous attributes,** with names such as atypical pneumonia, cuffing pneumonia, progressive pneumonia, aspiration pneumonia, pneumonitis, farmer's lung, extrinsic allergic alveolitis. Until a universal and systematic nomenclature for animal pneumonias is established, veterinarians should be acquainted with this heterogenous list of names and should be well aware that one disease may be known by different names. In pigs, for instance, enzootic pneumonia, virus pneumonia, and mycoplasma pneumonia all refer to the same disease caused by *Mycoplasma hyopneumoniae.*

The word pneumonitis has been used by some as a synonym for pneumonia; however, others have restricted this term to chronic proliferative inflammation generally involving the alveolar interstitium and with little or no evidence of exudate. In this chapter, the word pneumonia will be used for any inflammatory lesion in the lungs, regardless of whether it is exudative or proliferative, alveolar or interstitial.

Pneumonias in domestic animals can be classified into four morphologically distinct types, namely, **bronchopneumonia, interstitial pneumonia, embolic pneumonia,** and **granulomatous pneumonia.** By using this classification, it is possible to predict with some degree of certainty the likely etiology (virus, bacteria, fungi, parasites), route of entry (aerogenous versus hematogenous), and possible sequelae to which each of these types of pneumonia may progress if the animal were to survive. However, overlapping of these four types of pneumonias is possible, and, sometimes, two morphologic types may be present in the same lung.

The criteria used to classify pneumonias into bronchopneumonia, interstitial pneumonia, embolic pneumonia, and granulomatous pneumonia are based on morphologic changes, including distribution, texture, color, and appearance of the affected lungs (Table 3-4). According to **distribution** of the inflammatory lesions in the lungs, pneumonias can be **cranioventral,** as in most bronchopneumonias; **focal,** as in embolic pneumonias; **diffuse,** as in interstitial pneumonias; or **locally extensive,** as in granulomatous pneumonias. **Texture** of pneumonic lungs can be **firmer** or **harder** (bronchopneumonias), more **elastic** (rubbery) than normal lungs (interstitial pneumonias), or have a nodular touch (granulomatous pneumonias).

Changes in the **appearance** of pneumonic lungs include abnormal color, presence of nodules or exudate, fibrous adhesions, and presence of costal imprints on serosal surface. On cut surface, pneumonic lungs may have exudate, necrosis, abscesses, bronchiectasis, granulomas, or pyogranulomas.

Bronchopneumonia

Bronchopneumonia is undoubtedly the most common type of pneumonia seen in domestic animals and is, with few exceptions, characterized by cranioventral consolidation of the lungs. The reason why bronchopneumonias in animals are almost always restricted to the cranioventral portions of the lungs is not well understood. Possible factors contributing to this topographic selectivity within the lungs include (1) shortness and abrupt branching of airways; (2) greater deposition of infectious organisms; (3) inadequate defense mechanisms; (4) reduced vascular perfusion; (5) gravitational sedimentation of exudate; and (6) regional differences in ventilation.

Bronchopneumonias are generally caused by bacteria and mycoplasmas or by bronchoaspiration of feed or gastric contents. As a rule, the bacterial pathogens causing bronchopneumonias arrive in the lungs via inspired air (aerogenous), either from infected aerosols or from the nasal flora. Before establishing infection, pathogens must overwhelm or evade the pulmonary defense mechanism. The initial injury in bronchopneumonias is centered on the bronchiolar-alveolar junction, and from there the inflammatory process can spread downward to distal portions of

Table 3-4. Different types of pneumonias in domestic animals

Type of pneumonia	Port of entry (e.g., pathogens)	Distribution of lesions	Texture of lung	Grossly visible exudate	Disease example	Common pulmonary sequelae
Bronchopneumonia						
Suppurative (lobular)	Aerogenous (bacteria and mycoplasmas)	Cranioventral consolidation	Firm	Yes, purulent exudate in bronchi	Enzootic pneumonia	Cranioventral abscesses, bronchiectasis, BALT hyperplasia
Fibrinous (lobar)	Aerogenous (bacteria and mycoplasmas)	Cranioventral consolidation*	Hard	Yes, fibrin in lung and pleura	Pneumonic pasteurellosis	"Sequestra," pleural adhesions, abscesses
Interstitial pneumonia	Aerogenous or hematogenous (viral, toxins, septicemias, allergens)	Diffuse	Elastic	Not visible, trapped in alveolar septa	Extrinsic allergic alveolitis Influenza	Edema, emphysema, type II alveolar hyperplasia, alveolar fibrosis
Granulomatous pneumonia	Aerogenous or hematogenous (*Mycobacteria,* systemic mycoses)	Focal	Nodular	(Pyo-)granulomas, caseous necrosis, or calcification	Tuberculosis Blastomycosis	Dissemination of infection to other organs
Embolic pneumonia	Hematogenous (septic emboli)	Focal	Nodular	Purulent foci surrounded by hyperemia	Vegetative endocarditis Ruptured liver abscess	Abscesses in all pulmonary lobes

*Porcine pleuropneumonia is an exception because it often involves the caudal lobes.

the alveoli and upward to the bronchi. Through the pores of Kohn, the infection can extend centripetally to adjacent alveoli until part or all of the alveoli in an individual lobule are involved. If the inflammatory process cannot control the inciting cause of injury, the lesions can spread rapidly from lobule to lobule until an entire lobe or large portion of a lung is involved.

At the early stages of bronchopneumonia, the pulmonary vessels are engorged with blood (hyperemia) and the bronchoalveolar space may contain some fluid (edema). In cases where pulmonary injury is mild to moderate, proinflammatory mediators cause leukotaxis with rapid recruitment of neutrophils and alveolar macrophages into bronchoalveolar spaces. When pulmonary injury is much more severe, proinflammatory mediators induce more pronounced vascular changes by further opening endothelial gaps and, thus, increasing vascular permeability. Alterations in permeability can be further exacerbated by structural damage to pulmonary capillaries and vessels directly caused by the infecting pathogens. The final result of these functional and structural changes is that blood vessels become markedly permeable and allow substantial leakage of plasma fluid and proteins (fibrinogen) into the alveoli. Filling of alveoli, bronchioles, and small bronchi with inflammatory exudate progressively obliterates airspaces, and as a consequence of this, portions of severely affected (consolidated) lungs sink to the bottom of the container when placed in fixative. The replacement of air by exudate also changes the texture of the lung and, depending on the severity of bronchopneumonia, the texture varies from firmer to harder than normal.

The term ''consolidation'' is used when the texture of pneumonic lungs becomes firmer or harder than normal as a result of loss of airspaces due to exudation and atelectasis. Inflammatory consolidation of lungs has been referred to in the past as ''hepatization,'' because the affected lungs have the texture of liver. The process was referred to as ''red hepatization'' in acute cases in which there was marked hyperemia and exudation of neutrophils; conversely, the process was referred to as ''gray hepatization'' in those chronic cases in which the hyperemia was no longer present and neutrophils were replaced by macrophages. This terminology, although used and applicable to human pneumonias, is rarely used in veterinary medicine primarily because the evolution of pneumonic processes in animals does not necessarily follow the red-to-gray hepatization pattern.

Bronchopneumonias can be arbitrarily subdivided into **suppurative bronchopneumonia** if the exudate is predominantly composed of neutrophils and **fibrinous bronchopneumonia** if fibrin is the predominant component of the exudate (see Table 3-4). It is important to note that some pathologists use the term ''fibrinous pneumonia'' or ''lobar pneumonia'' as a synonym for fibrinous bronchopneumonia, and ''bronchopneumonia'' or ''lobular pneumonia'' as a synonym for suppurative bronchopneumonia. Currently, the term ''bronchopneumonia'' is widely used for both suppurative and fibrinous consolidation of lungs, since both forms of inflammation have essentially the same pathogenesis. It must be emphasized that it is the severity and not the type of pulmonary injury that largely determines whether a bronchopneumonia becomes suppurative or fibrinous. In some instances, however, it is difficult to discriminate between suppurative and fibrinous bronchopneumonia since both types can coexist and one type can progress to the other.

Suppurative bronchopneumonia is characterized by cranioventral consolidation of lungs (Fig. 3-23), with typical presence of purulent or mucopurulent exudate in the airways. This can be best demonstrated by expressing intrapulmonary bronchi, thus forcing exudate out of the bronchi (Fig. 3-24). The inflammatory process in suppurative

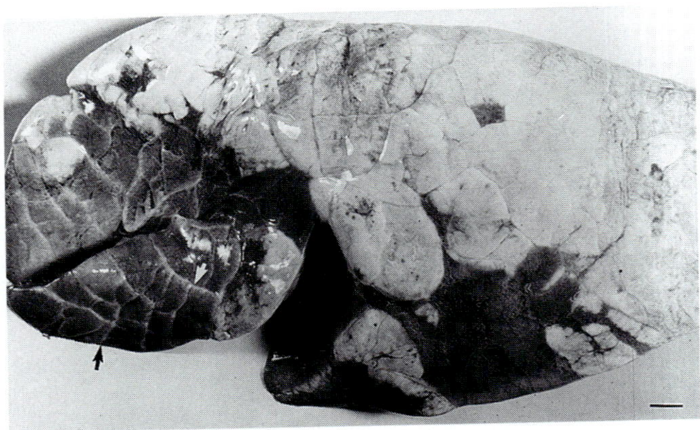

Fig. 3-23 Left lung; pig. Suppurative bronchopneumonia. Porcine enzootic pneumonia. Cranioventral consolidation of the lung involved approximately 40% of pulmonary parenchyma. The lobular pattern is accentuated due to widening of the interlobular septa *(arrows)*. Bar = 1 cm. *Courtesy Dr. M.D. McGavin.*

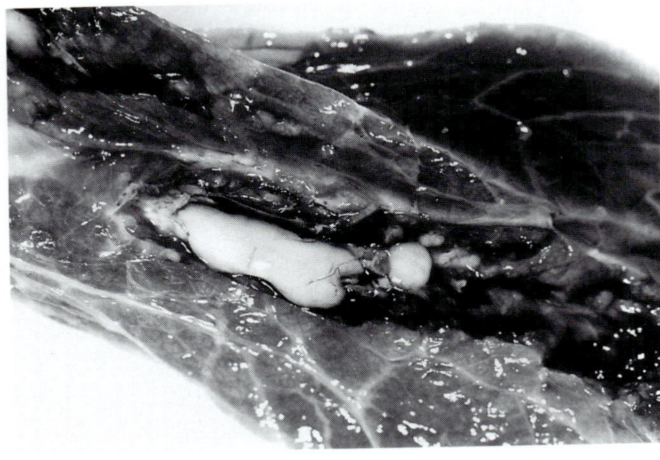

Fig. 3-24 Intrapulmonary bronchus; calf. Suppurative bronchopneumonia. Abundant purulent exudate appears in the bronchus when the lung is compressed.

bronchopneumonia is generally confined to individual lobules, and, as a result of this, the lobular pattern of the lung becomes markedly emphasized. This is particularly obvious in cattle and pigs, since these species have prominent lobulation of the lungs. The gross appearance often resembles an irregular checkerboard due to an admixture of normal and abnormal lobules (Fig. 3-23). Because of this typical lobular distribution, suppurative bronchopneumonias are also referred to as lobular pneumonias.

The color of consolidated lungs in suppurative bronchopneumonia varies considerably depending on the chronicity of the lesion. In acute cases, pneumonic lungs are red due to the hyperemic response that occurs during the early stages of inflammation. In subacute cases, the purulent exudate and the collapsed alveoli cause the lungs to be gray-pink. Finally, in the most chronic cases, the lungs take on a rather pale gray appearance similar to that of fish flesh. ''Enzootic pneumonias'' of ruminants and pigs are typical examples of chronic suppurative bronchopneumonias.

Microscopically, suppurative bronchopneumonias are characterized by abundant neutrophils, macrophages, and cellular debris within the lumen of bronchi, bronchioles, and alveoli (Fig. 3-25). Recruitment of leukocytes is promoted by cytokines, complement, and other chemotactic factors that are released in response to alveolar injury or by the chemotactic effect of bacterial toxins, particularly endotoxin. In most severe cases, purulent or mucopurulent exudate completely obliterates the entire lumen of bronchi, bronchioles, and alveoli.

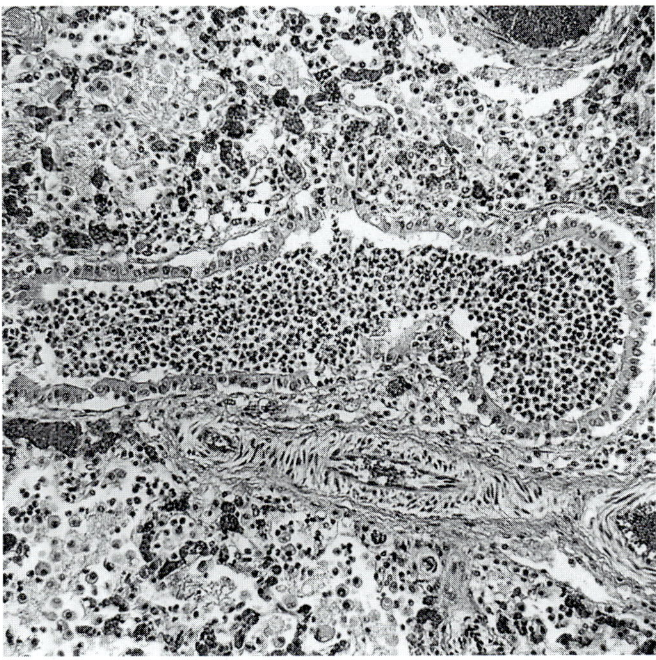

Fig. 3-25 Lung; calf. Suppurative bronchopneumonia. Note the extensive loss of airspaces due to infiltration of neutrophils and macrophages into the bronchoalveolar spaces. H & E stain.

If suppurative bronchopneumonia is merely the response to a transient pulmonary injury or a mild infection, lesions may resolve uneventfully. Within 7 to 10 days, cellular exudate can be removed from the lungs via the mucociliary escalator, and complete resolution may take place within 4 weeks. In other cases, if injury or infection is persistent, suppurative bronchopneumonia can become chronic, with goblet cell hyperplasia an important component of the inflammatory process. Depending on the proportion of pus and mucus, the exudate in chronic suppurative bronchopneumonia varies from mucopurulent to mucoid. Mucoid exudate is found in the more chronic stages when consolidated lung has the fish flesh appearance.

Hyperplasia of BALT is another change commonly seen in chronic suppurative bronchopneumonias; it appears grossly as conspicuous white nodules (cuffs) around bronchial walls (cuffing pneumonia). Further sequelae to chronic suppurative bronchopneumonia include bronchiectasis (Fig. 3-20), pulmonary abscesses, and pleural adhesions, as well as atelectasis and emphysema.

Clinically, suppurative bronchopneumonias can be acute and fulminating but are often chronic, depending on the etiologic agent, stressors affecting the host, and immune status. The most common pathogens causing suppurative bronchopneumonia in domestic animals include *Pasteurella multocida, Bordetella bronchiseptica, Actinomyces pyogenes, Streptococcus* spp., *E. coli,* and several species of mycoplasmas. Most of these organisms are secondary pathogens requiring a preceding impairment of the pulmonary defense mechanisms in order to colonize the lungs and establish an infection. Suppurative bronchopneumonia can also result from the aspiration of bland material.

Fibrinous bronchopneumonia is similar to suppurative bronchopneumonia except that the predominant exudate is fibrinous rather than neutrophilic. With only a few exceptions, fibrinous bronchopneumonias also have a cranioventral distribution (Fig. 3-26). However, exudation is not restricted to the boundaries of individual pulmonary lobules, as is the case in suppurative bronchopneumonias. Instead, the inflammatory process in fibrinous pneumonias involves numerous contiguous lobules and moves quickly through the pulmonary tissue until entire pulmonary lobes are affected. Because of the involvement of entire lobes, fibrinous bronchopneumonias are also referred to as lobar pneumonias. In general terms, fibrinous bronchopneumonias are the result of a more severe pulmonary injury and, thus, are more life threatening than suppurative bronchopneumonias. Even in cases where fibrinous bronchopneumonia involves 30% or less of total area, clinical signs and death can occur as a result of severe toxemia.

Grossly, acute fibrinous bronchopneumonias are characterized by severe congestion, hemorrhage, and massive exudation of fibrin, giving the affected lungs a characteristically intense red discoloration. Fibrin accumulates on the pleural surface, eventually forming thick yellow plaques. Because of this tendency of fibrin to deposit on

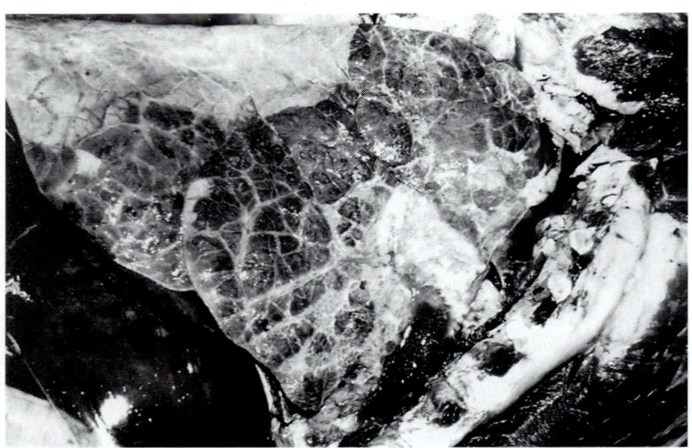

Fig. 3-26 Right lung; steer. Fibrinous bronchopneumonia (pleuropneumonia). Pneumonic pasteurellosis *(P. haemolytica).* Note the cranioventral distribution that affects approximately 80% of lung parenchyma. The lung is firm, swollen, and covered with fibrin, and interlobular septa are distended by edema and exudate. *Courtesy of Western College of Veterinary Medicine.*

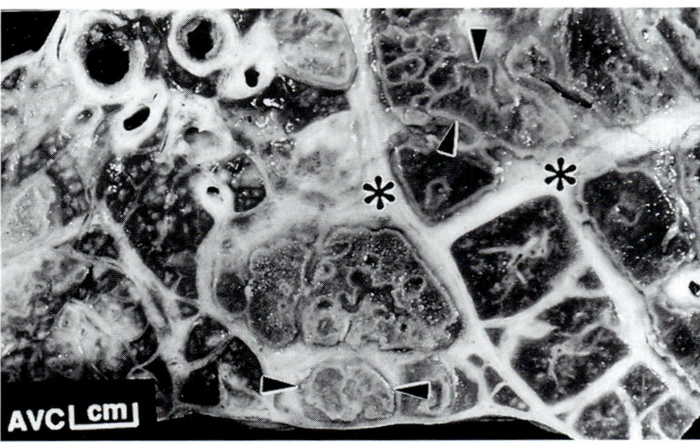

Fig. 3-27 Lung, cut surface; steer. Pneumonic pasteurellosis *(P. haemolytica).* Interlobular septa (*) are distended by edema and fibrin. Lung parenchyma has irregular areas of coagulative necrosis *(arrowheads)* surrounded by a rim of inflammatory cells.

the pleural surface, some pathologists use the term pleuropneumonia as a synonym for fibrinous bronchopneumonia. Fibrinous bronchopneumonias are generally accompanied by marked dilatation and thrombosis of lymph vessels, edema of interlobular septa, and accumulation of variable amounts of yellow fluid in the thoracic cavity. On cut surface, these changes in the interlobular septa give affected lungs a typical marbled appearance. Distinct focal areas of coagulative necrosis are also common in lungs with fibrinous bronchopneumonia (Fig. 3-27). In animals that survive the acute stage of fibrinous pneumonia, pulmonary necrosis often develops into pulmonary ''sequestra,'' which are pieces of necrotic lung encapsulated by connective tissue.

Microscopically, acute fibrinous bronchopneumonia is characterized by massive exudation of plasma proteins into the bronchioles and alveoli, and, as a result of this, most of the airspaces become obliterated by fluid exudate. Movement of plasma proteins into the alveolar lumen is primarily due to extensive disruption of the integrity of the blood-air barrier. Since fibrin is chemotactic for neutrophils, these types of leukocytes are always present in areas undergoing fibrinous inflammation. As inflammation progresses, fluid exudate is gradually replaced by a fibrinocellular exudate composed of fibrin, neutrophils, macrophages, and necrotic debris (Fig. 3-28). In chronic cases, fibroblasts can also infiltrate affected areas of the lungs and pleura, forming plaques of fibrovascular tissue.

In contrast to suppurative bronchopneumonia, fibrinous bronchopneumonia rarely resolves without leaving noticeable residual scars. The most common sequelae found in animals surviving an acute episode of fibrinous bronchopneumonia include bronchiolitis obliterans, gangrene, pulmonary fibrosis, pulmonary sequestra, abscesses, and chronic pleuritis. In some cases, pleuritis can be so extensive that fibrous adhesions extend onto the pericardial sac. Pathogens causing fibrinous bronchopneumonias in domestic animals include *Pasteurella haemolytica* (pneumonic pasteurellosis), *Actinobacillus pleuropneumoniae* (porcine pleuropneumonia), and *Mycoplasma mycoides* subsp *mycoides* small colony (contagious bovine pleuropneumonia). Fibrinous bronchopneumonia can also be the result of bronchoaspiration of irritant materials, such as gastric contents.

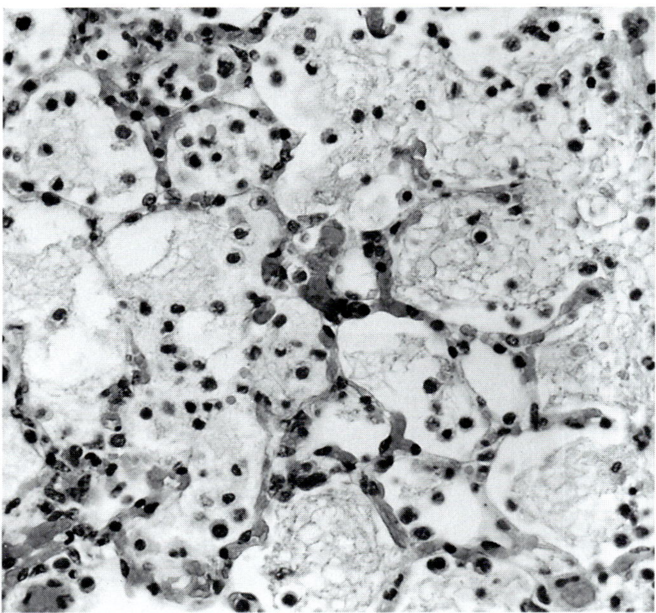

Fig. 3-28 Lung; calf. Pneumonic pasteurellosis *(P. haemolytica).* Alveoli contain abundant fibrin mixed with neutrophils and macrophages. H & E stain.

Interstitial pneumonia

Interstitial pneumonia refers to a particular type of pneumonia in which the inflammatory process takes place primarily in the alveolar walls and alveolar interstitium. This type of pneumonia is perhaps the most difficult one to diagnose at necropsy and generally requires microscopic confirmation. The pathogenesis of interstitial pneumonia is complex and can result from aerogenous injury to the alveolar epithelium (pneumonocytes I and II) or from hematogenous injury to the alveolar capillaries. Inhalation of toxic gases, toxic fumes, local generation of toxic metabolites by Clara cells, release of free radicals, and infection with pneumotropic viruses are just a few of the different agents that can damage alveolar epithelium. Injury to the vascular endothelium occurs in septicemias, in disseminated intravascular coagulation, from microembolisms, from circulating larval migrans, from toxins absorbed in the alimentary tract or toxic metabolites locally generated in the lungs, and from infections with endotheliotropic viruses. Damage to the alveolar wall can also occur when inhaled antigens such as fungal spores combine with circulating antibodies and form antigen-antibody complexes in the alveoli, which initiate a cascade of inflammatory responses and injury (allergic alveolitis). As are interstitial pneumonias in human beings, those of domestic animals are also subdivided, based on some morphologic features, into acute and chronic. It should be kept in mind, however, that not all acute interstitial pneumonias are fatal nor do they necessarily progress into the chronic form.

Acute interstitial pneumonias begin with injury to either type I pneumonocytes or alveolar endothelium, which provokes a disruption of the air-blood barrier and a subsequent exudation of plasma proteins into the alveolar space. This spillage of proteinaceous fluid into the alveolar lumen constitutes the **exudative phase** of acute interstitial pneumonias. In some cases, exuded plasma proteins mix with lipids and other components of pulmonary surfactant and form some elongated membranes that become partially attached to the alveolar and bronchiolar walls. These membranes are referred to as **hyaline membranes.** In addition to intraalveolar exudation of fluid, inflammatory edema and neutrophils accumulate in the alveolar interstitium and cause thickening of the alveolar walls. This acute exudative phase is generally followed a few days later by the **proliferative phase** of acute interstitial pneumonias characterized by hyperplasia of type II pneumonocytes. Hyperplastic type II pneumonocytes are, in fact, progenitor cells that differentiate and replace lost type I pneumonocytes (see Patterns of Alveolar Injury and Host Response). As a consequence, the alveolar walls become increasingly thickened. This is, in part, the reason why lungs become rubbery on palpation, what prevents their normal collapse after the thorax is opened, and why the cut surface of the lungs has a ''meaty appearance.''

Acute interstitial pneumonias are often mild and transient, especially those caused by some respiratory viruses. These mild forms of pneumonia are rarely seen in the postmortem room since they are not fatal and do not leave significant sequelae (see Alveolar Patterns of Injury and Host Response). In severe cases of acute interstitial pneumonias, animals may die of respiratory failure, usually as a result of a profuse exudative phase (leakage of proteinaceous fluid) leading to fatal pulmonary edema. Examples of this type of fatal acute interstitial pneumonia are bovine pulmonary edema and emphysema in cattle, ARDS in all species, and massive pulmonary migration of ascaris larvae in pigs.

When the source of alveolar injury persists, the proliferative and infiltrative lesions of acute interstitial pneumonia can progress into a different morphologic stage referred to as **chronic interstitial pneumonia.** The hallmark of chronic interstitial pneumonias is alveolar fibrosis and, in some cases, accumulation of inflammatory mononuclear cells in the interstitium and persistence of hyperplastic type II pneumonocytes. It should be emphasized again here that, although the lesions in interstitial pneumonia are centered in the alveolar walls and interstitium, a mixture of desquamated epithelial cells, macrophages, and mononuclear cells are usually present in the lumen of bronchioles and alveoli. Other concurrent changes that can accompany some forms of chronic interstitial pneumonia are formation of microscopic granulomas and hyperplasia of smooth muscle in airways or pulmonary vasculature. Ovine progressive pneumonia, hypersensitivity pneumonitis in cattle and dogs, and silicosis in horses are good veterinary examples of chronic interstitial pneumonia. Pneumoconioses (silicosis, asbestosis), paraquat toxicity, pneumotoxic antineoplastic drugs (bleomycin), and extrinsic allergic alveolitis (farmer's lung) are renowned examples of diseases that lead to chronic interstitial pneumonias in human beings.

In contrast to bronchopneumonias, where distribution of lesions is generally cranioventral, in acute or chronic interstitial pneumonias, lesions are more diffusely distributed and generally involve all pulmonary lobes, or, in some cases, they appear to be more pronounced in the dorsocaudal aspects of the lungs. Three important gross features of interstitial pneumonia are the failure of lungs to collapse when the thoracic cavity is opened, the occasional presence of costal impressions on the lung's pleural surface, and the lack of visible exudate unless complicated with secondary bacterial pneumonia. The color of the lungs varies from diffusely red to diffusely pale gray to a mottled appearance. The texture of lungs with uncomplicated interstitial pneumonia is typically elastic or rubbery, but definitive diagnosis based on texture alone is difficult due to the intrinsic subjectivity of palpation. The cut surface of the lungs may appear more ''meaty'' and have no evidence of exudates. It should be remembered, however, that acute interstitial pneumonias, particularly in cattle, are frequently accompanied by pulmonary edema (exudative phase) and inter-

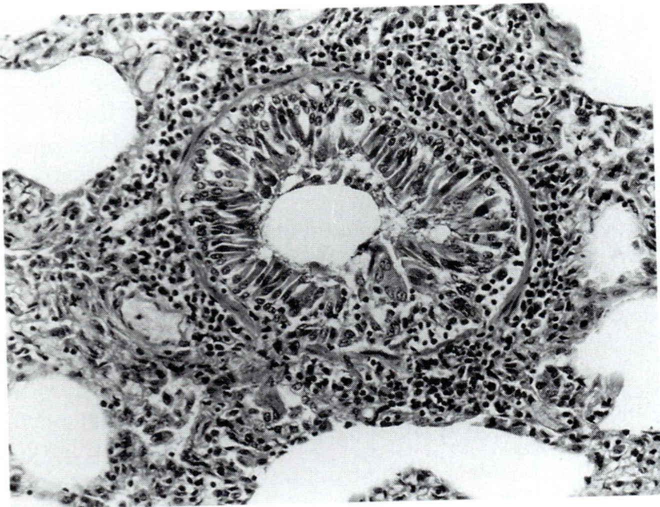

Fig. 3-29 Lung; horse. Bronchointerstitial pneumonia (unknown etiology). The bronchiolar epithelium is intact, but inflammatory cell infiltrate in the mucosa has extended peribronchially into alveolar interstitium. H & E stain. *Courtesy of Western College of Veterinary Medicine.*

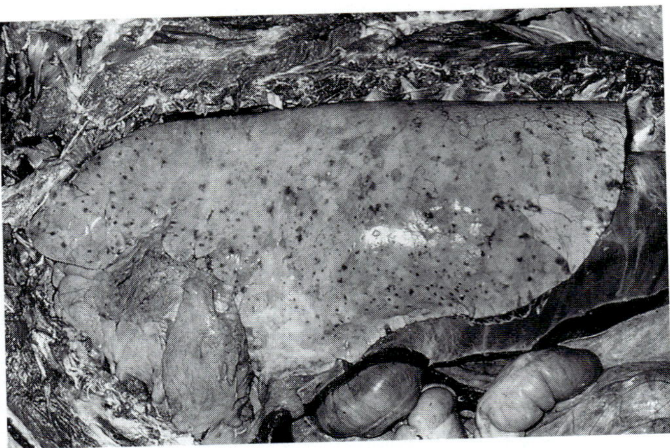

Fig. 3-30 Lung: foal. Acute embolic pneumonia. Note numerous small, dark foci of hemorrhage and inflammatory exudate randomly distributed in the pulmonary parenchyma.

stitial emphysema. Since edema tends to gravitate into the cranioventral portions of the lungs and emphysema is often more obvious in the dorsocaudal aspects, it is not rare that acute interstitial pneumonias in cattle have a gross cranioventral-like pattern that may resemble that of bronchopneumonia generally. The lungs are pale gray due to severe obliteration of alveolar capillaries (reduced blood/tissue ratio), especially when there is fibrosis. Lungs are notably heavy due to infiltrative and proliferative changes.

In the last few years, the term **"bronchointerstitial pneumonia"** has been introduced into veterinary pathology to describe cases in which pulmonary lesions share some histologic features of both bronchopneumonia and interstitial pneumonia. This combined type pneumonia is, in fact, frequently seen in many viral infections in which viruses replicate and cause injury in bronchial, bronchiolar, and alveolar cells. Damage to the bronchial and bronchiolar epithelium causes influx of neutrophils similar to what occurs in bronchopneumonias, and damage to alveolar walls causes proliferation of type II pneumonocytes, similar to what takes place in the proliferative phase of acute interstitial pneumonias. Examples of bronchointerstitial pneumonia include uncomplicated cases of respiratory syncytial virus infections in cattle and lambs, canine distemper, and porcine influenza (Fig. 3-29).

Embolic pneumonia

Embolic pneumonia is characterized by multifocal lesions randomly distributed in all pulmonary lobes, caused by entrapment of septic emboli. Lungs act as a biologic filter for circulating particulate matter. Sterile thrombi, unless extremely large, are rapidly dissolved and removed from the pulmonary vasculature by fibrinolysis, causing little if any ill effects. However, the results of experimental studies have confirmed that most types of bacteria injected intravenously (bacteremia) generally bypass the lungs and are finally trapped in the liver, spleen, joints, or other organs. To cause pulmonary infection, circulating bacteria must first attach to the pulmonary endothelium and then evade phagocytosis by intravascular macrophages or leukocytes. Infected thrombi promote entrapment of bacteria in the pulmonary vessels and provide a favorable environment to escape phagocytosis. Once trapped in the pulmonary vasculature, offending bacteria spread from the vessels to the interstitium and then to the surrounding lung, forming finally a nidus of infection. Early lesions in embolic pneumonia are grossly characterized by the presence of very small (1 mm), white foci in the lungs surrounded by a discrete, red, hemorrhagic halo (Fig. 3-30). Unless emboli arrive in massive numbers, causing fatal pulmonary edema, embolic pneumonia is seldom fatal; therefore, these acute lesions are rarely seen at postmortem examination. In most instances, acute lesions rapidly progress into the formation of pulmonary abscesses (Fig. 3-31) that are randomly distributed in all pulmonary lobes and are not restricted to the cranioventral aspects of the lungs, as is the case of abscesses developing from suppurative bronchopneumonia. The early inflammatory lesions in embolic pneumonias are always focal; thus, they differ from those of endotoxemia or septicemia, in which endothelial damage and interstitial reactions (interstitial pneumonia) are diffusely distributed in the lungs.

When embolic pneumonia or its sequelae (abscesses) are encountered, careful postmortem examination is required to locate the source of septic emboli. Most common causes include ruptured hepatic abscesses in cattle, omphalophlebitis in farm animals, and infected jugular catheter in all

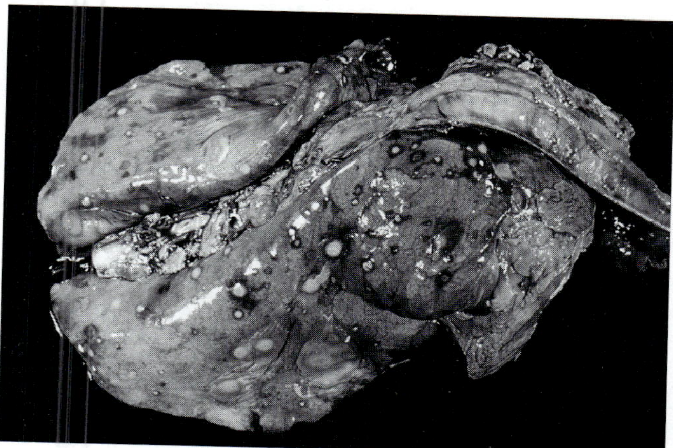

Fig. 3-31 Lungs; 3-week-old lamb. Embolic pneumonia *(Staphylococcus aureus)*. The lesions are spherical abscesses surrounded by a hyperemic border caused by septic emboli (pyemia). Heart, kidney, meninges, and joints were similarly affected. *Courtesy of Western College of Veterinary Medicine.*

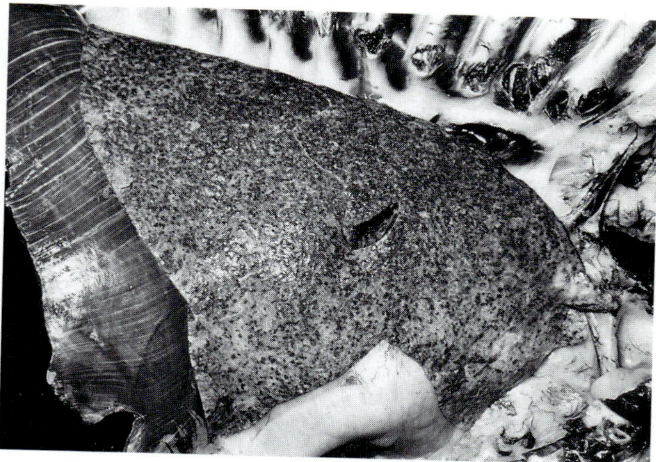

Fig. 3-32 Thoracic cavity, right lung; dog. Granulomatous pneumonia. Blastomycosis *(Blastomyces dermatitidis)*. The lungs contain large numbers of small granulomas distributed throughout all pulmonary lobes.

species. Valvular or mural endocarditis in the right side of the heart is also a usual source of septic emboli and embolic pneumonia in all species. Most frequent bacterial isolates from septic pulmonary emboli in domestic animals are *Actinomyces pyogenes, Fusobacterium necrophorum, Erysipelothrix rhusiopathiae, Staphylococcus aureus,* and *Streptococcus equi.*

Granulomatous pneumonia

Granulomatous pneumonia is characterized by the presence of variable numbers of caseous or noncaseous granulomas in the lungs (Figs. 3-32 and 3-33). On palpation, lungs have a typical nodular character given by well-circumscribed, variably sized nodules that, generally, have a firm texture, especially if calcification has occurred. During postmortem examination, granulomas in the lungs can be occasionally mistaken for neoplasms.

The pathogenesis of granulomatous pneumonia shares some similarities with those of interstitial and embolic pneumonias. Not surprisingly, some pathologists group granulomatous pneumonias within one of these types of pneumonias (e.g., granulomatous interstitial pneumonia). What makes granulomatous pneumonia a distinctive type is not so much the portal of entry or site of initial injury in the lungs, but the unique type of inflammatory response (granulomas), which can be easily recognized on gross and microscopic examination. The portal of agent entry into lungs can be aerogenous or hematogenous. As a rule, agents causing granulomatous pneumonia are resistant to phagocytosis and to the acute inflammatory response and persist in affected tissues for a long time.

The most common causes of granulomatous pneumonia in animals include systemic fungal diseases such as blastomycosis *(Blastomyces dermatitidis)*, cryptococcosis *(Cryptococcus neoformans)*, coccidioidomycosis *(Coccidioides immitis)*, histoplasmosis *(Histoplasma capsulatum)*, and bacterial diseases such as tuberculosis *(Mycobacterium bovis)*. Since most of these agents are usually part of a systemic infection, granulomatous lesions should also be expected in other organs, particularly the lymph nodes, liver, and spleen. Sporadically, aberrant parasites such as *Fasciola hepatica* in cattle and aspiration of foreign bodies can also cause granulomatous pneumonia. Feline infectious peritonitis is one of a few viral infections of domestic animals that may result in a granulomatous pneumonia. Lesions are caused by the deposition of antigen-antibody complexes in the vasculature of many organs, including the lungs.

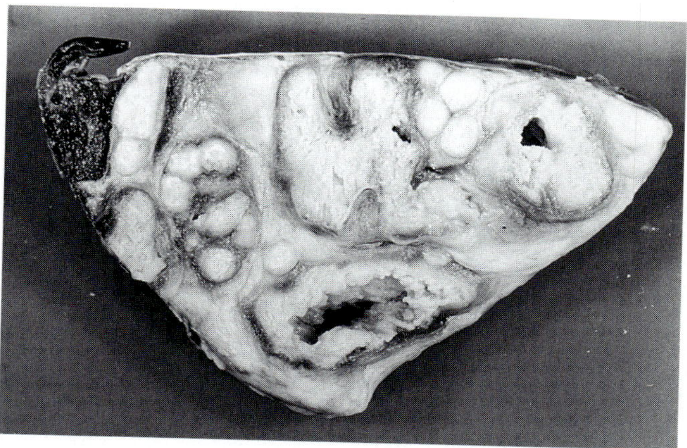

Fig. 3-33 Lung, cut surface; bison. Granulomatous pneumonia. Tuberculosis *(Mycobacterium bovis)*. Note discrete granulomas (tubercles) and larger confluent areas of caseous necrosis separated by fibrous connective tissue. *Courtesy Dr. S.V. Tessaro.*

Microscopically, pulmonary granulomas are composed of a center of necrotic tissue, surrounded by a rim of macrophages (epithelioid cells) and giant cells and an outer delineated layer of connective tissue commonly infiltrated by lymphocytes and plasma cells. Unlike other types of pneumonias, the causative agent in granulomatous pneumonia can, in many cases, be identified microscopically in sections stained by PAS or silver stains for fungal organisms or the acid-fast stain for mycobacteria.

Pneumonias of Cattle

Bovine respiratory disease (BRD)

This general term is often used by clinicians to describe acute and severe bovine respiratory illness of clinically undetermined etiology. This BRD complex includes enzootic pneumonia of calves (multifactorial etiology), bovine pneumonic pasteurellosis *(Pasteurella haemolytica),* respiratory hemophilosis *(Haemophilus somnus),* respiratory viral infections such as infectious bovine rhinotracheitis (IBR/BHV-1), parainfluenza-3 (PI-3) virus, bovine respiratory syncytial virus (BRSV), and noninfectious interstitial pneumonias such as bovine pulmonary edema and emphysema, reinfection syndrome, and many others.

Enzootic pneumonia, sometimes simply referred to as "calf pneumonia," is a disease caused by a variety of etiologic agents and with a variety of lesions in young, intensively housed calves. Morbidity is often great, but fatalities are uncommon unless management is poor or unless new, virulent pathogens are introduced by additions to the herd. Clinically, enzootic pneumonia is usually a mild respiratory disease.

Enzootic pneumonia is also called **viral pneumonia** because it often begins with an acute respiratory infection with PI-3 virus, BRSV, or possibly one or more of several others (adenoviruses, BHV-1, reoviruses, rhinoviruses). Mycoplasmas, notably *M. dispar, M. bovis,* and *Ureaplasma,* and possibly *Chlamydia,* may also be primary agents. Following infection with any of these agents, opportunistic bacteria such as *Pasteurella multocida, Actinomyces pyogenes, H. somnus,* and *E. coli* cause a secondary suppurative bronchopneumonia, the most serious stage of enzootic pneumonia. The pathogenesis of the primary invasion and how it predisposes the host to invasion by the opportunists are poorly understood, but it is likely that there is impairment of pulmonary defense mechanisms. Environmental factors, including poor ventilation, relative humidity, and animal crowding have been incriminated. The immune status of the calf also plays an important role in the development and severity of the disease.

Lesions are variable and depend largely on the agents involved as well as on the chronicity of the inflammatory process. In the acute phases, lesions caused by viruses are those of a bronchointerstitial pneumonia, which are generally mild and transient and, therefore, seen only sporadically at necropsy. Microscopically, the lesions are necrotizing bronchiolitis, necrosis of type I pneumonocytes with hyperplasia of type II pneumonocytes, and mild interstitial and alveolar edema. In the case of PI-3 and BRSV infection, intracytoplasmic inclusion bodies and formation of large multinucleated syncytia resulting from the fusion of infected epithelial cells can also be observed in the lungs. The mycoplasmas, too, can cause bronchiolitis, necrosis, and an interstitial reaction, but, in contrast to viral-induced pneumonias, mycoplasmal lesions tend to progress to a chronic stage characterized by striking peribronchiolar lymphoid hyperplasia (cuffing pneumonia). When complicated by secondary bacterial infections, viral or mycoplasmal lesions change from a pure bronchointerstitial to a suppurative bronchopneumonia (see Fig. 3-24). In late stages of bronchopneumonia, lungs contain creamy-mucoid exudate in airways and, often, have pulmonary abscesses or bronchiectasis. Airway hyperreactivity has been recently described in neonatal calves following BRSV infection; however, the significance of this syndrome in relation to enzootic pneumonia of calves is still under investigation.

It should be noted that the same viruses and mycoplasmas involved with the enzootic pneumonia complex can also predispose cattle to other diseases such as pneumonic pasteurellosis (shipping fever).

"Shipping fever" (transit fever) is a vague clinical term used in the past to denote acute respiratory diseases that occurred in cattle several days after shipment. The disease is characterized by a severe fibrinous bronchopneumonia. Because *P. haemolytica* and *P. multocida* are generally isolated from affected lungs, the name **pneumonic pasteurellosis** has been used synonymously. Currently, it is known that shipping fever can occur in animals that have not been shipped, and that organisms other than *Pasteurellae* can cause similar lesions. Therefore, the term "shipping fever" should be relinquished in favor of more specific names such as pneumonic pasteurellosis, respiratory hemophilosis, and others.

Pneumonic pasteurellosis (shipping fever) is the most important respiratory disease of cattle, particularly in feedlot animals that have been through the stressful marketing and assembly processes in North America. It is clinically characterized by acute fibrinous bronchopneumonia with toxemia.

P. haemolytica biotype A, serotype 1 is the etiologic agent responsible for the severe pulmonary inflammatory lesions. A few investigators still consider that *P. multocida* and other serotypes of *P. haemolytica* are also causes of this disease.

Even after many years of intense investigation, the pathogenesis of pneumonic pasteurellosis still remains incompletely understood. Experiments have established that *P. haemolytica A1* alone is usually incapable of causing disease, since it is rapidly cleared by pulmonary defense mechanisms. This may explain why *P. haemolytica A1,* in spite of being present in the nasal cavity of some healthy animals, only sporadically causes disease. For *P. haemolytica* to be established as a pulmonary infection, it is first required that stressors impair the defense mechanisms. These stressors include weaning, transport, fatigue, crowding, mixing of cattle from various sources, inclement weather, temporary starvation, and viral infections. Viruses that most commonly predispose cattle to pneumonic pasteurellosis include BHV-1, PI-3, BRSV, and several others. Once established in the lungs, *P. haemolytica* causes lesions by a combination of mechanisms that include endotoxin release, but the most important is probably the production of an exotoxin (leukotoxin) that kills bovine macrophages and neutrophils. The fact that this toxin exclusively affects ruminant leukocytes probably explains why *P. haemolytica* is a respiratory pathogen in cattle and sheep but not in other species.

Clinically, pneumonic pasteurellosis is characterized by a severe toxemia that can kill animals even when considerable parts of the lungs remain functional and structurally normal. Cattle usually become depressed, febrile, and anorexic and may have a productive cough, encrusted nose, mucopurulent nasal exudate, shallow respiration, or an expiratory grunt.

The gross lesions of pneumonic pasteurellosis are the prototype of fibrinous (lobar) bronchopneumonia with prominent fibrinous pleuritis (see Fig. 3-26) and pleural effusion. Lesions are always cranioventral and usually below a horizontal line through the tracheal bifurcation. The interlobular septa are distended by yellow, gelatinous edema and fibrin. The ''marbling'' of lobules is the result of areas of coagulation necrosis, interstitial edema, and congestion (see Fig. 3-27). The necrotic areas are typically bordered by a rim of elongated cells often referred to as ''swirling macrophages'' or ''oat-shaped cells,'' now known to be degenerated neutrophils mixed with a few alveolar macrophages. Edema and fibrin are the major components of the exudate in alveoli and interlobular septa. The extensive deposition of fibrin is the result of increased procoagulant activity and diminished profibrinolytic activity in the lungs. The conducting airways may also contain considerable amounts of exudates from deep within the lungs, but their walls are not particularly involved. Because of the necrotizing process, sequelae to pneumonic pasteurellosis can be serious and can include abscesses, sequestra, chronic pleuritis, fibrous pleural adhesions, and bronchiectasis.

Pneumonic pasteurellosis should not be confused with other forms of bovine pasteurellosis, such as **hemorrhagic septicemia** of ruminants caused by serotypes B and E of *P. multocida.* This disease does not occur in North America and currently is reported only from some countries in Asia and Africa. In contrast to pneumonic pasteurellosis, in which lesions are always confined to the lower respiratory tract, the bacteria in hemorrhagic septicemia always disseminate hematogenously to many organs. The disease is clinically characterized by a severe, acute septicemia, high fever, and rapid death. At necropsy, typically, numerous petechiae are present on serosal surfaces, in lungs, and in skeletal muscles. Lymph nodes are swollen and hemorrhagic. Variable lesions include fibrinohemorrhagic interstitial pneumonia, hemorrhagic enteritis, blood-tinged fluid in the thorax and abdomen, and subcutaneous edema.

Respiratory hemophilosis is part of the ''***Haemophilus somnus*** **disease complex**'' caused by *H. somnus,* which has different clinicopathologic forms, each one involving different organs. This complex includes septicemia, encephalitis known as infectious thromboembolic meningoencephalitis (ITEME), pneumonia (respiratory hemophilosis), pleuritis, myocarditis, arthritis, ophthalmitis, conjunctivitis, otitis, and abortion.

The respiratory form of bovine hemophilosis is the result of the bacterium's capacity to produce both suppurative and fibrinous bronchopneumonia. The latter is, in some cases, indistinguishable from that of pneumonic pasteurellosis. The pathogenesis of respiratory hemophilosis is still poorly understood, and the disease cannot be reproduced consistently by administration of *H. somnus* alone. Like *P. haemolytica,* it requires predisposing factors such as stress or a preceding viral infection. Mixed infections of *H. somnus,* pasteurellae, and mycoplasmas are fairly common.

Contagious bovine pleuropneumonia is of historical interest in veterinary medicine, as the object of an early control program for infectious disease. It was eradicated from North America in 1892 and from Australia in the 1970s, but it is still enzootic in large areas of Africa, Asia, Eastern Europe, and the Iberian Peninsula. The etiologic agent, *Mycoplasma mycoides* subsp. *mycoides* small colony, was the first mycoplasma isolated and is the most pathogenic of any that infect domestic animals. Pathogenetic mechanisms are still inadequately understood but are suspected to involve toxin production, effects on ciliary function, immunosuppression, and immune-mediated vasculitis. Vasculitis and thrombosis lead to parenchymal infarction.

The name of the disease is a good indication of the gross lesions. It is a severe, fibrinous bronchopneumonia (pleuropneumonia) similar to that of pneumonic pasteurellosis but having a more pronounced ''marbling'' of the lobules (different stages of inflammation), 60% to 79% of lesions in the caudal lobes (not cranioventrally), and more frequent and larger pulmonary sequestra (necrotic lung encapsulated by connective tissue). Microscopically, the appearance again is like that of pneumonic pasteurellosis, except that vasculitis and thrombosis of major pulmonary vessels and capillaries are much more obvious and are clearly the major cause of the infarction. *M. mycoides* remains viable in the sequestra for many years, and the organism may be expelled through respiratory secretions and become a source of infection for other animals.

Tuberculosis is an ancient, communicable, worldwide, chronic disease of human beings and domestic animals. It continues to be a major problem in human beings in underdeveloped countries, and it is on the rise in some industrialized nations, largely due to the immunosuppressive effects of AIDS. *Mycobacterium tuberculosis* is transmitted between human beings, but, where unpasteurized cow's milk is consumed, *M. bovis* from the milk of cattle with mammary tuberculosis is also important. Cattle can be infected with *M. bovis, M. tuberculosis,* and *M. avium-intracellulare* by several routes, but infection of the lungs by inhalation of *M. bovis* is the most common and significant. Infection usually starts when inhaled bacilli reach the alveoli and are phagocytosed by pulmonary alveolar macrophages. If these are successful in destroying the bacteria, infection is averted. However, *M. bovis* may multiply intracellularly, kill the macrophage, and start infection. From this first nidus of infection, bacilli spread via airways within the lungs and eventually to tracheobronchial and mediastinal lymph nodes via lymph vessels. The initial focus of infection at the portal of entry (lungs) plus the involvement of a regional lymph node is termed the *primary complex* of tuberculosis. If the infection is not contained within this primary complex, bacilli may disseminate again via lymph vessels to distant organs and other lymph nodes. Hematogenous dissemination occurs sporadically when the inflammatory process containing the organisms erodes the walls of blood vessels. If bacterial dissemination is sudden and massive, numerous small foci of infection develop in many tissues and organs and are referred to as **miliary tuberculosis.** The host becomes hypersensitive to the mycobacterium, which enhances the cell-mediated immune defenses in early or mild infections, but can result in host-tissue destruction in the form of caseous necrosis.

Clinically, the signs may relate to the dysfunction of a particular organ system or to a general debilitation and emaciation. In the pulmonary form, which is over 90% of bovine cases, there is a chronic, moist cough that can progress to dyspnea. Enlarged tracheobronchial lymph nodes can contribute to the dyspnea by impinging on airways, and the enlargement of caudal mediastinal nodes can compress the caudal thoracic esophagus and cause bloat.

Tuberculosis, the prototype for granulomatous pneumonia, is characterized by the presence of few to many caseated granulomas. The early gross changes are small foci *(tubercles)* most frequently seen in the dorsocaudal, subpleural areas. With progression, the lesions enlarge and become confluent with the formation of large areas of caseous necrosis (see Fig. 3-33). Single nodules or clusters may occur on the pleura and peritoneum, and this presentation has been termed *pearl disease.* Microscopically, the tubercle is composed of mononuclear cells of various types. In young tubercles, which are noncaseous, epithelioid and Langhans giant cells are at the center, surrounded by lymphocytes, plasma cells, and macrophages. Later, caseous necrosis is at the center, secondary to the effects of cell-mediated hypersensitivity, enclosed by the other cell types and with fibrosis at the periphery. Acid-fast organisms may be numerous but, more often, are difficult to find in histologic sections or smears.

Atypical interstitial pneumonia (AIP) is a vague clinical term well entrenched in veterinary literature, but one that has led to enormous confusion among veterinarians. It was first used to describe acute or chronic forms of bovine pneumonia that did not fit in any of the "classical" forms because of the lack of exudate. Microscopically, the criteria for diagnosis of AIP in cattle were based on the absence of obvious exudate and the presence of edema, interstitial emphysema, hyaline membranes, hyperplasia of type II pneumonocytes, and fibrosis of cellular infiltrates in the interstitium. At that time, any pulmonary disease or pulmonary syndrome that had a few of the above lesions was traditionally diagnosed as AIP, and grouping all these different syndromes together was inconsequential since their etiopathogeneses were then unknown.

Field and laboratory investigations have established that most of the syndromes previously grouped under AIP have rather different etiologies and pathogeneses. Further, what was "atypical" in the past has become so routine that it is fairly common nowadays to find "typical cases" of AIP. For all these reasons, investigators, largely from Britain, proposed that all these syndromes previously clustered into AIP should be named according to specific etiologies or pathogenesis. The most common bovine syndromes characterized by edema, emphysema, hyaline membranes, and hyperplasia of type II pneumonocytes include **bovine pulmonary edema and emphysema ("fog fever"), "extrinsic allergic alveolitis" (hypersensitivity pneumonitis), "reinfection syndrome" (hypersensitivity to** *Dictyocaulus* sp.), **milk allergy,** and others.

Acute bovine pulmonary edema and emphysema (ABPE), known in Britain as "fog fever" (no association with atmospheric conditions), occurs in cattle usually grazing "fog" pastures (that is, aftermath or foggage, regrowth after hay or silage has been cut). Epidemiologically, ABPE usually occurs in adult beef cattle in the fall when there is a change in pasture, from a short, dry grass to a lush, green grass. The probable, though unproven, pathogenesis is that L-tryptophan present in the pasture is metabolized in the rumen to 3-methylindole, which in turn is absorbed into the bloodstream and carried to the lungs. Mixed-function oxidases present in the nonciliated bronchiolar epithelial (Clara) cells metabolize 3-methylindole into a highly pneumotoxic compound that causes extensive necrosis of bronchiolar cells and type I pneumonocytes (Fig. 3-34). Clinically, severe respiratory distress develops within 2 weeks of the pasture change, and cattle develop expiratory

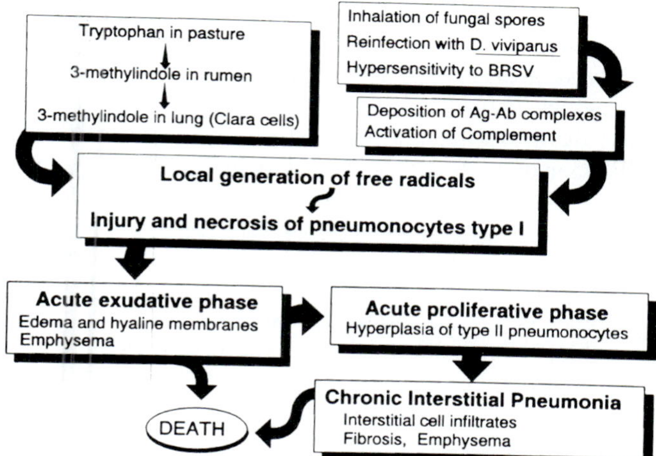

Fig. 3-34 Pathogenesis of toxic and allergic pneumonias (''atypical interstitial pneumonia'') in cattle.

dyspnea, oral breathing, and evidence of emphysema within the lungs and even subcutaneously along the back. The gross lesions are those of a diffuse interstitial pneumonia with severe alveolar and interstitial edema and interlobular emphysema (Fig. 3-35). The lungs are enlarged, pale, and rubbery in texture, and the lesions are most notable in the caudal lobes. Microscopically, the lesions are alveolar and interstitial edema and emphysema, formation of hyaline membranes within alveoli, and, in those animals that survive for several days, hyperplasia of type II alveolar epithelial cells.

A number of other agents cause virtually the same clinical and pathologic syndrome as is seen in ABPE. The pathogenesis is assumed to be similar, although presumably other toxic factors will be established specific for each syndrome. One of these pneumotoxic factors is 4-ipomeanol, which is found in moldy sweet potatoes contaminated with the fungus *Fusarium solani.* Mixed-function oxidases in the lungs activate 4-ipomeanol into a potent pneumotoxicant capable of producing irreversible injury to type I pneumonocytes and bronchiolar epithelial cells. Similarly, purple mint *(Perilla frutescens),* stinkwood *(Zieria arborescens),* and rapeseed and kale (*Brassica* species) also cause pulmonary edema, emphysema, and interstitial pneumonia.

Extrinsic allergic alveolitis (hypersensitivity pneumonitis) is a disease seen mainly in housed, adult dairy cows in winter. This condition shares many similarities with its human counterpart known as **farmer's lung,** which results primarily from a type III (Arthus) hypersensitivity reaction to inhaled fungal spores, mainly of the thermophilic actinomycete, *Micropolyspora faeni,* commonly found in moldy hay. Inhalation of these spores also causes extrinsic allergic alveolitis in cattle (bovine farmer's lung). Clinically, it can be acute or chronic; the latter has a cyclical

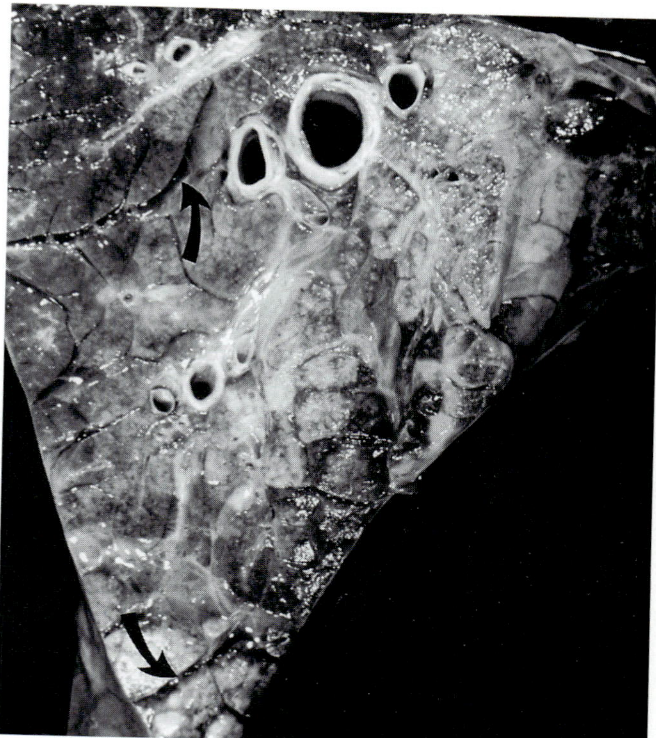

Fig. 3-35 Lung, cut surface; yearling calf. Interstitial pneumonia (unknown etiology). The lung was heavy, rubbery in texture, dark red-blue cranioventrally, and pale caudally. Interstitial emphysema and edema, both lesions characteristic of those of bovine pulmonary edema and emphysema, are evident in the interlobular septa *(arrows)* of the caudal lobes. *Courtesy of Western College of Veterinary Medicine.*

pattern of exacerbation during winter months. Weight loss, coughing, and poor exercise tolerance are clinical features. Grossly, the postmortem lesions vary from subtle, gray, subpleural foci (granulomatous inflammation) to severe, in which the lungs are firm and heavy and have a ''meaty appearance'' due to alveolar epithelial hyperplasia and fibrosis (see Fig. 3-34). Characteristically, discrete noncaseous granulomas are scattered throughout the lungs. Chronic cases of extrinsic allergic alveolitis can eventually progress into diffuse fibrosing alveolitis. Whether full recovery can occur in less severe cases is not known.

Other allergic syndromes manifested in the lungs include hypersensitivity to reinfection with larvae of *Dictyocaulus viviparus,* which causes signs and lesions indistinguishable from those of ABPE, with the exception of a component of eosinophils and possibly larvae seen microscopically in the exudate. Recently, it has been suggested that emphysema with proliferative alveolitis and formation of hyaline membranes can also occur in the late stages of BRSV infection in cattle. Presumably, this disease shares many similarities with severe infections occasionally seen in children with RSV (human strain), in which an immune-mediated mechanism has been implicated as the primary cause of the disease.

A type of systemic anaphylaxis (type I hypersensitivity) known as milk allergy can cause acute pulmonary congestion, edema, and even hemorrhage and emphysema in cows sensitized to their own milk casein and lactalbumin.

Inhalation of manure (''pit'') gases, such as hydrogen sulfide (H_2S) and ammonia (NH_3), and nitrogen dioxide (NO_2) from silos, can be a serious hazard to animals and human beings. At toxic concentrations, these gases cause necrosis of bronchiolar cells and type I pneumonocytes, fulminating pulmonary edema, asphyxiation, and rapid death. In addition, NO_2, like other oxidant gases, also causes bronchiolitis, edema, and interstitial pneumonia with fibrosis (''silo filler's disease'') in survivors.

Parasitic pneumonias of cattle

Pulmonary lesions in parasitic pneumonias (the word is used here in its restricted sense to mean helminth infestations of the lungs) vary from interstitial in larvae migration to chronic bronchitis caused by some intrabronchial adult parasites to granulomatous pneumonia caused by dead larvae, aberrant parasites, or eggs of parasites. In many cases, an ''eosinophilic syndrome'' in the lungs is characterized by infiltrates of eosinophils in the pulmonary interstitium and bronchoalveolar spaces and blood eosinophilia. Atelectasis and emphysema secondary to obstruction of airways are also common findings in many parasitic pneumonias. The adult parasites are often visible grossly. The severity of the lesions relates to numbers and size of the parasites and the nature of the host reaction, which sometimes includes hypersensitivity. A common general term for all these diseases is **verminous pneumonia.**

D. viviparus is an important pulmonary nematode (lungworm) responsible for a condition in cattle referred to as verminous pneumonia or **verminous bronchitis.** Adult parasites live in the intrapulmonary bronchi of cattle, mainly in those of the caudal lobes of the lungs. Adult parasites cause severe bronchial irritation, inflammation, edema, focal atelectasis, and interstitial emphysema. Atelectasis is clearly confined to the lobules of lungs ventilated by the obstructed bronchi (dorsocaudal); interstitial emphysema (interlobular) is caused by forced expiratory movements due to obstruction of the small bronchi. In addition to inflammation of bronchial mucosa, bronchoaspiration of larvae and eggs also causes an influx of leukocytes into the bronchoalveolar space. Verminous pneumonia is most commonly seen in calves during their first summer grazing pastures used repeatedly from year to year, particularly in regions of Europe with a moist, cool climate. The parasite can overwinter on pasture even in climates as cold as Canada's, and older animals may be carriers for a considerable length of time.

The clinical signs (coughing) vary with the severity of infection, and severe cases can be confused clinically with interstitial pneumonias. Expiratory dyspnea and death can occur in heavy infections when there is massive obstruction of airways.

At necropsy, lesions appear as large, dark or gray, depressed, wedge-shaped areas of atelectasis present usually along the dorsocaudal aspect of the lungs. On the cut surface, edematous foam and mucus mixed with white, slender (up to 80 mm long) nematodes are visible in bronchi (see Fig. 3-15). In the most severe cases, massive numbers of nematodes fill the entire bronchial tree. Microscopically, parasites in bronchi are associated with excess mucus due to goblet cell hyperplasia, metaplasia of bronchial and bronchiolar epithelium, alveolar edema, hyperplasia of BALT, hyperplasia of bronchiolar smooth muscle, and a few eosinophilic granulomas around the eggs and dead larvae. These granulomas, grossly, are gray nodules (2 to 4 mm) and may be confused with those caused by tuberculosis.

A different form of bovine pneumonia, an acute allergic reaction known as **reinfection syndrome,** occurs when previously sensitized adult cattle are exposed to large numbers of larvae *(D. viviparus).* Lesions in this syndrome are those of a hypersensitivity pneumonia as previously described.

Ascaris suum is the common intestinal roundworm of pigs and cannot complete its life cycle in calves. However, the larvae can cause severe pneumonia and death within 2 weeks of housing calves in places where infected pigs were previously kept. Pigs, the natural host, can also be killed if exposed to an overwhelming larval migration. Clinical signs due to migration of larvae through the lungs include cough and expiratory dyspnea to the point of oral breathing. The lesions are a diffuse interstitial pneumonia with hemorrhagic foci, atelectasis, and interlobular edema and emphysema. Microscopically, larvae are present in bronchioles and alveoli; the latter have thickened walls and contain edema fluid and cellular exudate (including eosinophils) in the lumina.

Hydatid cysts, the intermediate stage of *Echinococcus granulosus,* a tapeworm of canidae, can be found in the lungs of sheep. Hydatid cysts are also found in cattle, pigs, goats, and horses. However, in these latter species the cysts are generally ''sterile'' and do not contain viable protoscolices. Hydatid cysts are 5 to 10 cm in diameter; they have little clinical significance but are important as a cause of zoonotic disease and a cause of economic loss due to carcass condemnation.

Aspiration pneumonias of cattle

The inhalation of regurgitated ruminal contents or iatrogenic deposition of medicines or milk into the trachea can cause a severe and often fatal **aspiration pneumonia.** Bland substances such as mineral oil may incite only a mild suppurative bronchopneumonia, whereas some ''home remedies'' or ruminal contents may be highly irritating and cause a fibrinous, necrotizing bronchiolitis and alveolitis. In some severe cases, pulmonary necrosis can be complicated by the concurrent aspiration of saprophytic organisms, causing fatal gangrenous pneumonia. Aspiration pneumonia should always be considered in animals with cleft palate or in those in which swallowing has been compromised because of disorders such as hypocalcemia (milk fever).

Pneumonias of Pigs

Porcine pneumonias are unequivocally a major component of the problems facing the contemporary swine industry. The incidence, prevalence, and severity of pneumonias in pigs are dependent on a series of complex, multifactorial interactions. Among the most commonly recognized elements linked to porcine pneumonias are host (age, genetic makeup, immune status), infectious agents (viruses, bacteria, mycoplasmas), environmental determinants (humidity, temperature, ammonia concentrations), and management practices (crowding, mixing of animals, nutrition, stress). Because of the nature of these multifactorial interactions, it will become obvious in the following paragraphs that, more often than not, a specific type of pneumonia frequently progresses to or coexists with another one.

Porcine enzootic pneumonia (mycoplasmal pneumonia of swine)

This highly contagious disease of pigs is caused by *Mycoplasma hyopneumoniae* and is characterized pathologically by suppurative bronchopneumonia (see Fig. 3-23). When its worldwide prevalence and deleterious effect on feed conversion are taken into account, this is probably the most economically significant respiratory disease of pigs. Although an infectious disease, it is very much influenced by management factors such as crowding (airspace and floor space), ventilation (air exchange rate), concentrations of noxious gases in the air (ammonia, hydrogen sulfide), relative humidity, temperature fluctuations, and mixing of stock from various sources. The etiology remained unclear for many years, and so the disease was mistakenly known as ''virus pneumonia of pigs'' on the assumption that if the agent was hard to find it must be a virus. The causative agent, *M. hyopneumoniae,* is a fastidious organism and difficult to grow; thus, the final diagnosis is frequently based on pathologic changes alone, or supported by ancillary tests directed to the detection of this mycoplasma in affected lungs by immunohistochemistry or immunofluorescence. The bronchopneumonic lesions of porcine enzootic pneumonia are, in most cases, mild to moderate, and, thus, mortality is low unless complicated with secondary pathogens such as *P. multocida, A. pyogenes, B. bronchiseptica, Haemophilus* spp., *Mycoplasma hyorhinis,* and other mycoplasmas and ureaplasmas. Although the pathogenesis of porcine enzootic pneumonia is not completely elucidated, it is known that *M. hyopneumoniae* first adheres to cilia, produces ciliostasis, and finally colonizes the respiratory system by firmly attaching to epithelial cells of the trachea and the bronchi of the cranioventral regions of the lungs. Once attached to the respiratory epithelium, it evokes an influx of neutrophils into the tracheobronchial mucosa, causes extensive loss of cilia, stimulates an intense hyperplasia of lymphocytes in the BALT, and changes the chemical composition of mucus.

Clinically, enzootic pneumonia occurs as a herd problem in two disease forms. A newly acquired infection of a previously clean herd causes disease in all age groups, resulting in acute respiratory distress and some mortality. In a chronically infected herd, the mature animals are immune, and clinical signs are usually apparent only at times of particular stress in growing pigs, such as at weaning. In such herds, coughing and reduced rate of gain are the most notable signs unless secondary bacterial infection causes severe bronchopneumonia.

The lesions are characterized initially by a bronchointerstitial pneumonia that progresses to suppurative bronchopneumonia once secondary pathogens such as *P. multocida, B. bronchiseptica,* or *A. pyogenes* are involved. In most pigs, lesions affect only portions of the cranial and accessory lobes, but, in more severely affected pigs, lesions involve 50% or more of the cranioventral portions of the lungs. The affected lungs are dark red in the early stages and have a homogeneous pale-gray (''fish flesh'') appearance in the more chronic stages of the disease. On the cut surface, exudate can easily be expressed from airways, and, depending on the stage of the lesions and secondary infections, the exudate varies from purulent to mucopurulent to mucoid. Microscopic lesions are characterized by an influx of macrophages and neutrophils into the bronchoalveolar space with marked peribronchial and peribronchiolar lymphoid hyperplasia. Accumulation of exudate can be severe enough, in some cases, to cause occlusion of airways and atelectasis of subtending lobules. The suppurative bronchopneumonia may be accompanied by a mild fibrinous pleuritis, which is often more severe if *M. hyorhinis, P. multocida,* or *Actinobacillus pleuropneumoniae* is concurrently involved. Abscesses and pleural adhesions can be long-term sequelae in chronic complicated infections.

Porcine pasteurellosis

This infectious disease complex with an unclear pathogenesis includes primary and secondary porcine bronchopneumonias (porcine pneumonic pasteurellosis) and, in some rare cases, acutely fatal septicemias. Although *P. multocida* is part of the normal nasal flora, it is also an important secondary pathogen for porcine lungs, especially when defense mechanisms have been impaired by viral or mycoplasmal infections or following stress associated with poor management practices. In contrast to responses in cows, *P. haemolytica* can cause abortion in sows, but has no important role in respiratory diseases of swine.

The most common role of *P. multocida* in porcine pneumonias is its secondary involvement in lungs with mycoplasma infection, particularly in enzootic pneumonia. Secondary infection with *P. multocida* notably modify the early and mild bronchointerstitial reaction of enzootic pneumonia into a severe suppurative bronchopneumonia with multiple abscesses and sometimes pleuritis. The other important role for *P. multocida* in porcine pneumonias is as a cause of a fulminating, cranioventral, fibrinous bronchopneumonia (pleuropneumonia) without a previous mycoplasmal infection. The nature of the lesion and the predisposing factors of poor management and concurrent viral infections, such as swine influenza, suggest circumstances common to pneumonic pasteurellosis of cattle. Pharyngitis with cervical edema, fibrinohemorrhagic polyarthritis, and focal nephritis are associated with porcine pneumonic pasteurellosis. Whether this is a separate form of pasteurellosis (septicemic) or a concurrent change to bronchopneumonia needs to be elucidated. Sequelae to porcine pneumonic pasteurellosis include fibrous pleuritis and pericarditis, pulmonary abscesses, the formation of the so-called sequestra, and, usually, death.

Porcine pleuropneumonia

This is a highly contagious, worldwide disease of pigs, caused by *Actinobacillus pleuropneumoniae (Haemophilus pleuropneumoniae),* that is characterized pathologically by a severe, often fatal, fibrinous bronchopneumonia with extensive pleuritis (pleuropneumonia). Survivors generally develop notable residual lesions and become carriers of the organisms. In the past, porcine pleuropneumonia was known as "haemophilus pleuropneumonia," because the causative bacterium was named *Haemophilus parahaemolyticus,* which was later changed to *H. pleuropneumoniae* and most recently named *A. pleuropneumoniae.* Porcine pleuropneumonia is used here for the disease but not necessarily for the pathologic changes of pleuropneumonia. Porcine pleuropneumonia is an increasingly important cause of acute and chronic pneumonias, particularly in intensively raised pigs. Transmission of *A. pleuropneumoniae* occurs by the respiratory route, and the disease can be reproduced experimentally by intranasal inoculation of the bacterium. Twelve serotypes of the organism, most of which can cause the disease, are currently identified. The pathogenesis is not yet well understood, but specific virulence factors such as capsular factors, lipopolysaccharide, hemolysins, cytotoxins, and permeability factors can damage capillaries and impair phagocytic function, resulting in vascular leakage or thrombosis and failure of clearance mechanisms.

Clinically, **porcine pleuropneumonia** can vary from a peracute form with sudden death and blood-stained froth at the nostrils and mouth to a chronic form, characterized by decreased growth rate and persistent cough. In the acute form, pigs have high fever, anorexia, lethargy, dyspnea, and coughing.

The gross lesions in the peracute and acute forms consist of a fibrinous bronchopneumonia characterized by severe consolidation with a fibrinous exudate on the pleural surface. Although all lobes can be affected, a common site is the dorsal area of the caudal lobes (Fig. 3-36). In fact, a large area of fibrinous pleuropneumonia involving the caudal lobe of a pig is considered almost pathognomonic for this disease. On the cut surface, consolidated lungs have marked dilatation of interlobular septa and irregular, but well-circumscribed areas of coagulative necrosis. Except for the distribution, pulmonary lesions of porcine pleuropneumonia are identical to those of pneumonic pasteurellosis of cattle. The microscopic lesions are also very similar to those of bovine pneumonic pasteurellosis and include areas of necrosis surrounded by a thick cluster of "streaming (oat-shaped) leukocytes," and a notable distention of the interlobular septa due to severe edema and lymph vessel thrombosis. Animals that survive the acute phase of the disease often have multiple pulmonary abscesses and large pieces of necrotic lung encapsulated by connective tissue (sequestra). These sequestra and abscesses result in a sub-

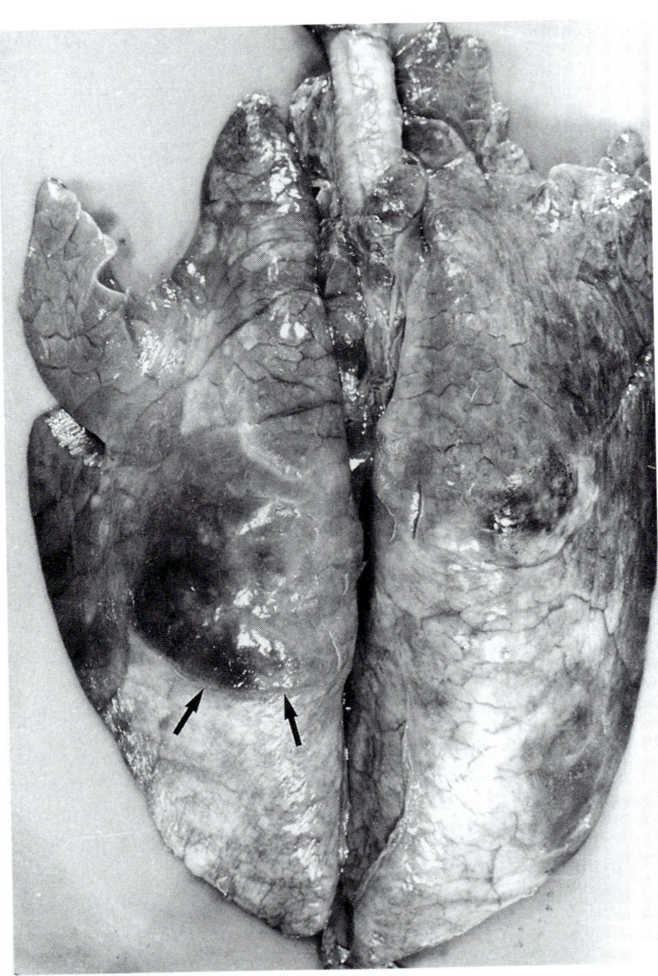

Fig. 3-36 Lungs; 4-month-old pig. Porcine pleuropneumonia *(Actinobacillus pleuropneumoniae).* Note the large focus of hemorrhagic, necrotizing fibrinous bronchopneumonia involving the dorsal aspect of the left caudal lobe *(arrows).* This dorsocaudal location is typical of porcine pleuropneumonia. *Courtesy of Western College of Veterinary Medicine.*

clinical carrier state and shedding of the organism, resulting in an occasional abortion and a high incidence of pleural adhesions at slaughter.

Haemophilus pneumonia

In addition to **polyserositis and polyarthritis (Glasser's disease),** *Haemophilus parasuis* (originally, *H. suis*) can also cause pulmonary infections characterized by a suppurative bronchopneumonia that, in some severe cases, can be fatal. The causal organism, *H. parasuis,* is usually carried in the nasopharynx of normal pigs and requires abnormal circumstances such as those following stress (weaning, cold weather) or viral infections (e.g., swine influenza) to cause pulmonary infection. Specific pathogen free (SPF) pigs seem to be particularly susceptible to Glasser's disease.

Streptococcal pneumonia

Streptococcus suis **type II,** a pathogen that produces lesions in several body systems, has been a problem in Europe for two decades and is of increasing concern in North America. It is a serious zoonosis capable of causing death by meningitis and residual deafness in survivors; butchers and pig farmers are particularly at risk. In pigs, *S. suis* type II has been associated with neonatal septicemia, meningitis, arthritis, polyserositis, myocardial necrosis, myocarditis, valvular endocarditis, abortion, and pneumonia. This organism is carried in the nasal cavity, tonsils, and mandibular lymph nodes of healthy pigs, particularly in survivors in the aftermath of an outbreak. In addition to septicemia, endocarditis, and polyserositis, infection with *S. suis* also causes a suppurative bronchopneumonia, generally in combination with *P. multocida* and *E. coli* (mixed infection). It can also produce fibrinous bronchopneumonia when the *S. suis* infection occurs in combination with *A. pleuropneumonia.*

Tuberculosis

This is an important disease in pigs, which, in many countries, including those of North America, has a much greater prevalence in pigs than in cattle or other domestic mammals. Because pigs are susceptible to *Mycobacterium avium, M. bovis,* and *M. tuberculosis,* the incidence of porcine tuberculosis in a geographic region reflects what is occurring in the poultry, cattle, and human populations. A common scenario in small mixed farming operations is the diagnosis of avian tuberculosis at the time that pigs are slaughtered, the source being ingestion of tuberculous chickens. The route of infection in pulmonary tuberculosis of pigs is most often hematogenous after oral exposure. Therefore, the gross lesions are multifocal or even miliary granulomas. Typical calcified granulomas similar to those seen in cattle are generally associated with *M. bovis* infection, while *M. avium* infection frequently causes poorly delineated, noncalcified nodules resembling neoplasms. Tuberculous lesions can be present in other tissues, such as the liver and spleen. The microscopic lesions are basically those of a tubercle, but the lesions vary with the causative species (see Bovine Tuberculosis).

Swine influenza

This disease originated in North America, and it is generally accepted that the swine disease resulted from adaptation of the **type A influenza virus,** the cause of the human influenza pandemic during World War I. Swine influenza is enzootic in the United States and occurs sporadically in Canada and Europe. The virus can be transmitted by lungworms and the common earthworm (when ingested), but influenza can also occur even when these factors are controlled. The pathogenesis of the disease is infection of epithelium throughout the respiratory tract, with the more severe outbreaks reflecting more involvement of intrapulmonary airways and secondary infection with *P. multocida, A. pyogenes,* or *Haemophilus* spp.

Clinically, a sudden onset of painful and often paroxysmal coughing is followed by respiratory distress, high fever, stiffness, and weakness or even prostration in most or all of the herd, including animals of all age groups. This often follows stressful management changes or a bout of inclement weather, particularly in the fall or winter. The outbreak subsides virtually without mortality within a week; the clinical appearance is much more alarming than the pathologic changes, unless the pigs have secondary infection with bacteria.

Grossly, a copious catarrhal to mucopurulent inflammation extends from the nasal passages to the bronchioles, the volume of mucus being sufficient to plug small airways and cause a lobular or multilobular pattern of atelectasis in the cranioventral regions of the lungs. The appearance can be quite similar grossly, though not microscopically, to that of mycoplasmal pneumonia. Fatal cases have severe pulmonary edema. Microscopically, the lesions are typical of a virus-induced, necrotizing bronchitis-bronchiolitis that, in severe cases, extends into the alveoli as a bronchointerstitial pneumonia. Exfoliated epithelial cells and neutrophils mix with mucus, and, if these changes are extensive enough, the lumen of bronchioles can be occluded by exudate. In the later stages of inflammation, neutrophils are progressively replaced by alveolar macrophages, unless the pneumonia is complicated by secondary bacterial infections. The most important effect of most outbreaks of influenza is severe weight loss, but pregnant sows may also abort or give birth to weak piglets.

Other pneumonias of pigs

Pulmonary lesions can be part of any systemic disease. Septicemias often cause petechiae and pulmonary edema, and these features may be a part of African swine fever, hog cholera, pseudorabies, and other diseases. Salmonellae, *E. coli,* and *Listeria monocytogenes* can cause severe interstitial pneumonia as part of a septicemic process in very young animals. *Salmonella choleraesuis* causes a necrotizing fibrinous pneumonia, and *S. typhisuis,* a chronic suppurative bronchopneumonia.

Several countries in Europe and North America have reported outbreaks of a new, presumably contagious disease of pigs that affects primarily the reproductive and respiratory systems. Names for this new disease rapidly proliferated, including **''mystery disease of swine,'' ''swine infertility and respiratory syndrome'' (SIRS), ''new pig disease,'' ''blue ear disease,'' ''porcine epidemic abortion and respiratory syndrome'' (PEARS).** More recently, **Porcine Reproductive and Respiratory Syndrome (PRRS)** has been recognized as the official name. Several viruses have been proposed as the etiologic agent for PRRS. The respiratory form is generally seen in young pigs and is clinically characterized by anorexia, dyspnea, cough, and, occasionally, death. On postmortem examination, pulmonary lesions vary from very mild changes to failure to collapse when the thorax is opened. Microscopically, lesions are those of an interstitial pneumonia characterized by thickening of alveolar walls due to infiltration of macrophages and a few lymphocytes and a few necrotic cells in the alveolar lumina. Unlike some other viral infections, bronchiolar epithelium appears not to be affected.

Another novel disease of uncertain etiology but referred to as **severe proliferative and necrotizing pneumonia** has been recently described in Canada. The age of affected pigs varies from 2 weeks to 4 months, and the clinical signs are those of fever and dyspnea but without noticeable cough. Depending on the stage of the disease, postmortem lesions vary from a cranioventral consolidation with mild pleuritis to a diffuse pulmonary involvement. On cut surface, affected lungs often have a ''meaty'' appearance resembling the thymus. Microscopically, there is necrotizing bronchiolitis with marked hyperplasia of type II pneumonocytes (Fig. 3-37), alveoli filled with proteinaceous eosinophilic fluid, occasional formation of hyaline membranes, and abundant alveolar macrophages, some of which appear necrotic. Although the epidemiologic attributes and type of lesions are compatible with a viral infection, a causative virus has not been confirmed. Some investigators believe that this disease is just a variant of PRRS.

Foreign body granulomatous pneumonia occurs frequently in pigs following inhalation of vegetable material, presumably from dusty (nonpelleted) feed. Lesions are clinically silent but are often mistaken for other pneumonic processes during inspection at slaughter houses. Microscopically, pulmonary changes are typical of foreign body granulomatous inflammation in which variably sized feed particles are surrounded by macrophages and neutrophils and are commonly found within multinucleated giant cells.

Parasitic pneumonias of pigs

Metastrongylus apri (elongatus), M. salmi, and *M. pudendotectus* (lungworms) of pigs occur throughout most of the world and require earthworms as intermediate hosts for

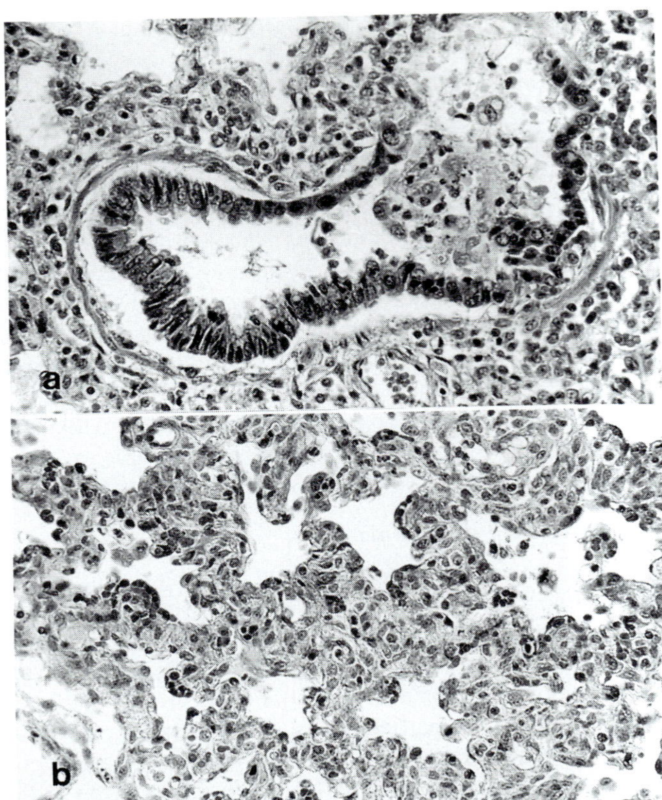

Fig. 3-37 Lung; pig. Bronchointerstitial pneumonia (unidentified virus). **A**, Focal necrosis and exfoliation of bronchiolar epithelium with discrete infiltrates of mononuclear cells in the peribronchiolar interstitium. **B**, Thickening of alveolar walls by mononuclear cells and proliferating type II pneumonocytes. H & E stain. López et al. *Can Vet J* 1993; 34:622–623.

transmission. Lungworms may transmit the virus of swine influenza. Generally, lungworm disease in swine is less severe than the disease caused by the lungworms of cattle. The importance of swine lungworms is mainly due to growth retardation of the host. Clinical signs include coughing due to the parasitic bronchitis.

The gross lesions, when noticeable, consist of small gray nodules, particularly along the ventral borders of the caudal lobes. Microscopically, the nodules are foci of peribronchial and peribronchiolar lymphoid hyperplasia. Larvae are surrounded by eosinophils, the reaction becoming granulomatous with time. The adult worms are grossly visible in bronchioles and small bronchi and cause a catarrhal inflammation with infiltration of eosinophils.

During migration through the lungs of pigs, larvae of *Ascaris suum* can cause edema, focal subpleural hemorrhages, and interstitial inflammation (Fig. 3-38). Hemorrhages also occur in the liver, and these later become the large, white ''milk spots'' seen so frequently as incidental findings at necropsy.

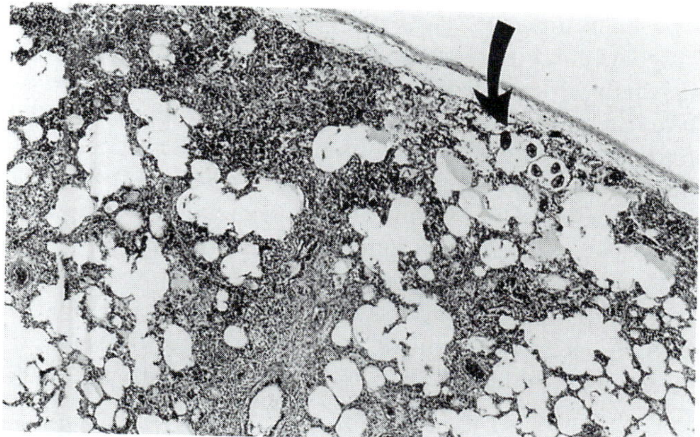

Fig. 3-38 Lung; pig. Larva migrans. Cross sections of *Ascaris suum* larvae *(arrow)* are located subpleurally and have caused focal hemorrhage and interstitial inflammation. H & E stain. *Courtesy of Western College of Veterinary Medicine.*

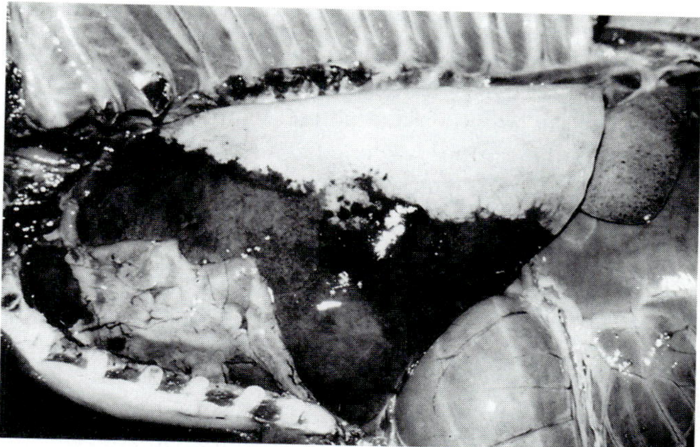

Fig. 3-39 Thoracic cavity, left lung; 3-week-old lamb. Fibrinous bronchopneumonia. Pneumonic pasteurellosis *(P. haemolytica).* The cranioventral aspects of the lungs were red, swollen, and very firm with some fibrin on the pleural surface. *Courtesy of Western College of Veterinary Medicine.*

Pneumonias of Sheep and Goats

Four major forms of *Pasteurella haemolytica* infection occur in sheep. Two are acute or chronic pulmonary infections and are referred to as **ovine pneumonic pasteurellosis** and **chronic enzootic pneumonia,** respectively; the third form is a systemic and often fulminating infection known as **septicemic pasteurellosis;** the last form is related to severe **mastitis** in ewes (blue bag). These forms of pasteurellosis are generally associated with particular biotypes and serotypes of *P. haemolytica* usually carried in the tonsils and upper respiratory tract of normal sheep.

Ovine pneumonic pasteurellosis

This is one of the most common and economically significant diseases in most areas where sheep are raised. It is caused by *P. haemolytica* biotype A and has pathogenetic features and lesions similar to that of pneumonic pasteurellosis of cattle. Colonization and infection of the lungs are encouraged by stressors such as changes in weather, handling, deworming, dipping, and by viral infections such as PI-3 virus, respiratory syncytial virus, adenovirus, and probably chlamydiae. Lesions are characterized by a severe fibrinous bronchopneumonia (lobar, cranioventral) (Fig. 3-39) with pleuritis. Subacute to chronic cases appear as a fibrinopurulent bronchopneumonia, and sequelae include abscesses and fibrous pleural adhesions.

Chronic enzootic pneumonia

In sheep, this is a multifactorial disease complex that, in contrast to ovine pneumonic pasteurellosis, causes only a mild to moderate pneumonia, and it is rarely fatal. It generally affects animals under 1 year of age. Significant costs associated with chronic enzootic pneumonia include reduction of weight gain, labor costs, veterinary fees, and slaughterhouse waste. The modifier ''chronic'' is used here to avoid any confusion with pneumonic pasteurellosis (''acute enzootic pneumonia''). It is also sometimes called *atypical pneumonia, chronic nonprogressive pneumonia, proliferative pneumonia,* or other names.

Chronic enzootic pneumonia is a clinicoepidemiologic term and does not imply a single causal agent, but a combination of infectious, environmental, and managerial factors. The list of infectious agents involved in ovine enzootic pneumonia includes PI-3, adenovirus, reovirus, and respiratory syncytial viruses, as well as chlamydiae, pasteurellae, and mycoplasmas *(M. ovipneumonia).*

In the early stages of the disease, cranioventral bronchointerstitial pneumonia causes moderate thickening of alveolar walls due to hyperplasia of type II pneumonocytes. In some cases, it may progress to suppurative bronchopneumonia when further colonization of the lungs takes place. One might expect some specific evidence pointing to the infectious agents (for example, large intranuclear inclusion bodies in epithelial cells with adenoviral infection), but such is not often the case, either because examination is seldom done at acute stages when the evidence is still present or because secondary bacterial infections mask the primary lesions. In the late stages, chronic enzootic pneumonia is characterized by atelectasis, hyperplastic bronchitis, alveolar and bronchiolar fibrosis, and severe peribronchial lymphoid hyperplasia (cuffing pneumonia).

Septicemic pasteurellosis

This is a common ovine disease caused by *P. haemolytica* biotype T in animals 5 months or older, or by the biotype A in lambs under 2 months of age. Both biotypes of *P. haemolytica* are carried in the tonsils and oropharynx of normal sheep; but, under abnormal circumstances, bacteria can invade adjacent tissues, enter the bloodstream, and cause septicemia particularly in association with stresses, such as dietary or environmental changes. Affected animals die after short illness and only rarely have clinical signs such as dullness, recumbency, and dyspnea. Gross lesions include a distinctive necrotizing pharyngitis in the tonsillar region, severe congestion and edema of the lungs, and infarcts and petechiae in various organs, but particularly of the pleura. Microscopically, the hallmark lesion is a disseminated vascular thrombosis often associated with the presence of bacterial colonies in affected tissues.

Contagious caprine pleuropneumonia

This disease in goats is the counterpart of contagious bovine pleuropneumonia in cattle; sheep do not have a corresponding disease. The etiopathogenesis and geographic distribution of contagious caprine pleuropneumonia are yet to be determined. Three mycoplasmas, namely, *M. mycoides* spp. *mycoides* large colony, *M. mycoides* spp. *capri,* and *Mycoplasma* strain *F38,* have all been associated with respiratory infections in goats; however, the classification of these mycoplasmas and their relation to specific diseases remain unsettled.

Caprine pleuropneumonia is important in Africa, the Middle East, and parts of Asia, but is also seen elsewhere; one of the etiologic agents, *M. mycoides* spp. *mycoides* large colony, is widespread in North America, yet the actual importance of this organism as cause of disease is unclear. Although it is unwise to speak in absolute terms when dealing with many aspects of biology, transmission from goats to sheep or cattle does not occur to any significant degree.

Clinically, the disease is similar to contagious bovine pleuropneumonia, with high morbidity and mortality, fever, cough, dyspnea, and increasing distress and debility. The gross lesions, particularly those caused by the *F38* strain, are similar to the bovine disease and consist of a severe fibrinous bronchopneumonia and pleuritis; however, sequestra formation in the lungs and interlobular septal distention are less obvious than in the bovine disease. Fibrinous polyarthritis, septicemia, meningitis, mastitis, peritonitis, and abortion are other lesions.

Other mycoplasma infections

The pathogenicity of other mycoplasmas such as *M. ovipneumoniae* and *M. capricolum* in sheep and goats is still being defined, and specific description of the lesions would be premature. These organisms probably cause disease only in circumstances similar to those for enzootic pneumonia, where host, infectious, and environmental factors play a complex interaction in the pathogenesis of the disease.

Maedi (maedi-visna)

This is an important slow viral disease of sheep and occurs in most countries, except Australia and New Zealand. The name means "shortness of breath" in the Icelandic language, and it is known locally as **Graaff-Reinet disease** in South Africa, **Zwoegerziekte** in the Netherlands, **la bouhite** in France, and **ovine (Montana** or **Marsh) progressive pneumonia (OPP)** in the United States. More recently, the disease has also been referred to as **lymphoid interstitial pneumonia (LIP).** Nucleic acid hybridization studies have indicated differences in the genome of the various viruses isolated from diverse parts of the world, but, for all practical purposes, the epidemiologic, clinical, and pathologic findings are indistinguishable. Goats are also considered susceptible, although this may have been confused with caprine arthritis-encephalitis.

Maedi is caused by a nononcogenic retrovirus of the lentivirus subfamily antigenically related to the retrovirus causing caprine arthritis-encephalitis. Seroepidemiologic studies indicate that infection is widespread in the sheep population, yet the clinical disease seems to be rare. The pathogenesis is incompletely understood, but it is known that transmission occurs presumably through ingestion of infected colostrum. The virus remains for long periods of time within monocytes and macrophages, and clinical signs do not develop until after a long incubation period of 2 years or more (slow virus infection). Experimentally, the incubation period can be notably reduced if lambs are inoculated intratracheally with ovine lentivirus during the perinatal period.

Maedi is clinically characterized by dyspnea and an insidious, slowly progressive emaciation despite good appetite. Death is inevitable once clinical signs are present, but may take many months.

Pulmonary lesions are a severe interstitial pneumonia, and the lungs fail to collapse when the thorax is opened. Often notable rib imprints are present on the pleural surface. The lungs are pale and mottled (Fig. 3-40) and typically heavy (2 to 3 times normal weight), and the regional lymph nodes are enlarged. Microscopically, alveolar walls are markedly thickened with distention of the perivascular spaces due to a massive infiltration of lymphocytes (Fig. 3-41). Hyperplasia of type II pneumonocytes is not a prominent feature of maedi, and secondary bacterial infections often confound the microscopic lesions of the disease. Enlargement of lymph nodes is largely due to severe lymphoid hyperplasia, primarily of B-lymphocytes.

The virus(es) can also infect many other tissues, causing encephalitis (visna), nonsuppurative arthritis with periarticular fibrosis, lymphofollicular mastitis, or vasculitis. An individual sheep can have one or a combination of these lesions (although affliction with maedi and visna concurrently is rare), or they can remain infected but disease free for life.

Pulmonary adenomatosis

This disease, also known as **ovine pulmonary carcinoma** and **jaagsiekte** (from the South African Afrikaans word for

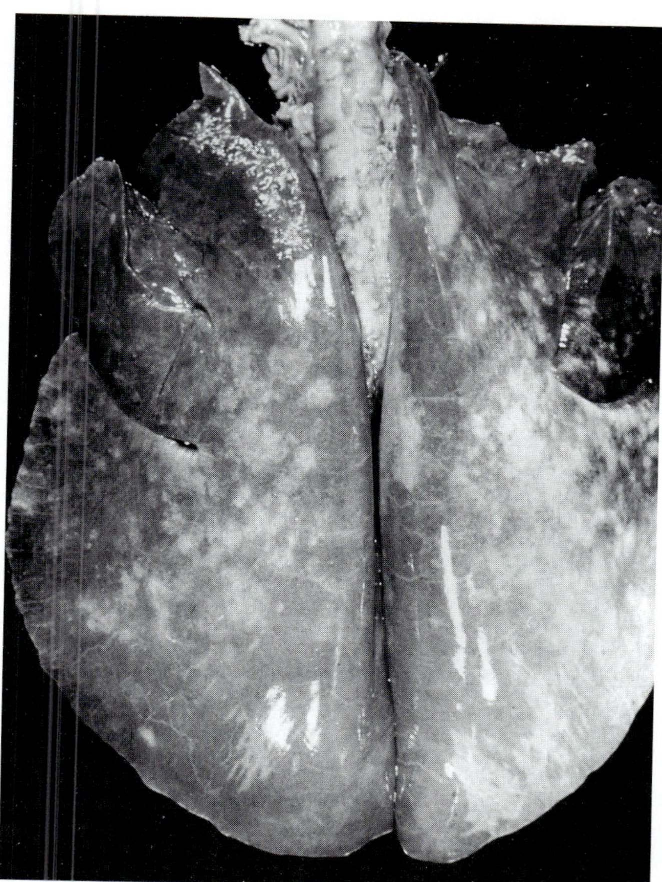

Fig. 3-40 Lungs; 7-year-old ewe. Maedi (lymphoid interstitial pneumonia, lentivirus). The lungs were extremely heavy and very firm. The interstitial pneumonia has a mottled pattern in all but the dorsocaudal areas, where it is diffuse. *Courtesy of Western College of Veterinary Medicine.*

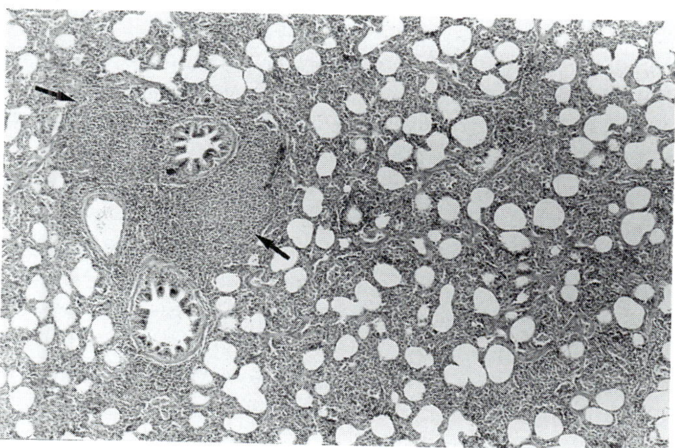

Fig. 3-41 Lung; aged ewe. Maedi (lymphoid interstitial pneumonia, lentivirus). Peribronchiolar lymphoid nodules *(arrows)* are hyperplastic, and interalveolar septa are thickened by lymphocytes and other mononuclear leukocytes. H & E stain. *Courtesy of Western College of Veterinary Medicine.*

''driving sickness''), is a highly transmissible, retroviral-induced neoplasia of the ovine lungs clinically characterized by a long incubation period (slow viral disease). It occurs in sheep around the world with the notable exception of Australia and New Zealand; its prevalence is great in Scotland and unknown, but probably low, in North America. Although a neoplastic disease, it is discussed here because the neoplasm behaves very much like a chronic pneumonia, and the putative etiology shares many epidemiologic similarities with the ovine lentivirus responsible for maedi. Pulmonary adenomatosis has been transmitted to goats experimentally but is not known to be a spontaneous disease in that species.

This disease affects mainly mature sheep but can occasionally affect young stock. Clinical signs are a gradual loss of condition, sometimes coughing, and respiratory distress, especially after exercise (such as herding or ''driving''). Appetite and temperature are normal, unless there are secondary complications. An important differentiating feature from maedi can be observed if the pelvic limbs are raised: copious, thin, mucoid fluid, presumably produced by neoplastic cells in the lungs, pours from the nostrils of some animals with pulmonary adenomatosis. Intensive husbandry probably encourages transmission through this copious nasal discharge, and may explain why the disease occurred in Iceland as a devastating epizootic disease with 5% to 80% mortality.

During the early stages of the disease, the lungs are enlarged, heavy, and wet and contain several firm, gray, variably sized nodules. In the later stages, the nodules become confluent, and large segments of both lungs are diffusely, but not symmetrically, infiltrated by neoplastic cells. On cross section, a copious mucoid secretion is in the airways. Microscopically, the nodules are composed of cuboidal or columnar epithelial cells lining airways and alveoli and forming papillary ingrowths in adenomatous (glandlike) patterns (Fig. 3-42). These cells have been identified ultrastructurally as originating from both the type II alveolar epithelial cells and the nonciliated bronchiolar epithelial (Clara) cells. Sequelae often include secondary bronchopneumonia, abscesses, and fibrous pleural adhesions; and metastases occur to tracheobronchial and mediastinal lymph nodes and to a lesser extent to other tissues such as pleura, muscle, liver, and kidneys. Death is inevitable after several months. Differential diagnosis between maedi and pulmonary adenomatosis often proves difficult, since both diseases often coexist in the same flock or in the same animal.

Caprine arthritis-encephalitis (CAE)

This is a slow viral disease of goats. It is caused by a retrovirus (lentivirus) that has a viral pathogenesis remarkably similar to that of maedi in sheep. It was first described in the United States in the 1970s, but also occurs in Canada, Europe, Australia, and probably elsewhere. There are two

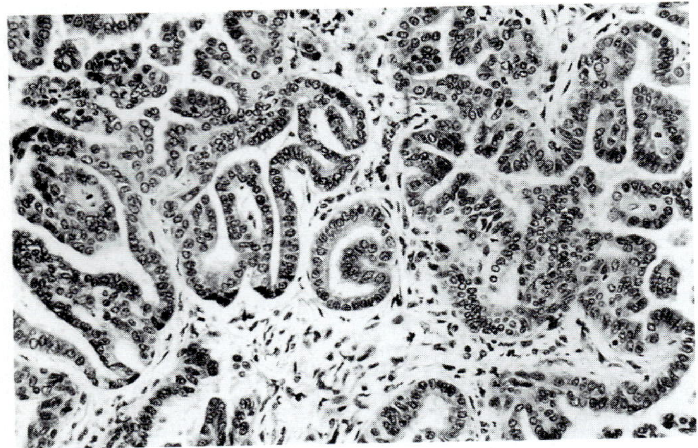

Fig. 3-42 Lung; sheep. Ovine pulmonary carcinoma (pulmonary adenomatosis, jaagsiekle). Papillary proliferation of cuboidal epithelial cells (presumed type II pneumonocytes) in a pulmonary nodule of a lamb with experimentally induced ovine pulmonary carcinoma. H & E stain. *Rosadio et al. Vet Pathol 1988; 25:475-483.*

major clinicopathologic forms: one involves the central nervous system of goat kids and young goats and is characterized by a nonsuppurative leukoencephalomyelitis; the other involves the joints of adult goats and is characterized by a chronic, nonsuppurative arthritis-synovitis. In addition, infection with CAE virus can also cause chronic interstitial pneumonia and presumably mastitis (''hard udder'').

The lentivirus of CAE is closely related to the maedi-visna virus, and, in fact, cross infection between species can be achieved experimentally. Like with maedi, infection of CAE presumably occurs during the first weeks of life when the doe transmits the virus to her offspring through infected colostrum or milk. The virus initially replicates in monocytes-macrophages; and inflammatory processes elsewhere promote recruitment of these infected macrophages, thus facilitating the viral dissemination to central nervous system, joints, lungs, and mammary glands. It can take several months before antibodies can be measured in infected goats.

Clinically, goats are active and afebrile, but progressively lose weight in spite of normal appetite. The encephalitic or arthritic signs tend to obscure the respiratory signs, which are only evident on exertion. Secondary bacterial infections are common in affected goats.

Grossly, a diffuse interstitial pneumonia tends to be most severe in the caudal lobes. The lungs are gray-pink and firm in texture with numerous, 1- to 2-mm, gray-white foci on the cut surface. The tracheobronchial lymph nodes are consistently enlarged. Microscopically, thickening of the alveolar walls is due to infiltration of lymphocytes and conspicuous hyperplasia of type II pneumonocytes. These lesions are accompanied by accumulation of proteinaceous eosinophilic material in the alveoli, which in electron micrographs has structural features of pulmonary surfactant.

Tuberculosis

This disease is uncommon in sheep and goats, but infection with *M. bovis* or *M. avium* does occur when the disease is prevalent in other species in a locality. The pulmonary form, similar to that seen in cattle, is characterized by a granulomatous pneumonia with multiple, large, caseous, calcified, and well-encapsulated granulomas scattered throughout the lungs.

Parasitic pneumonias of sheep and goats

Dictyocaulus filaria is a serious, worldwide, parasitic disease of the lungs, most commonly of lambs and goat kids, but occurring in adults as well. The life cycle and lesions are similar to those of *D. viviparus* of cattle. The clinical signs (cough, moderate dyspnea, and loss of condition) and lesions relate mainly to obstruction of the small bronchi by adult worms and exudate. As is seen in cattle with *D. viviparus,* areas of atelectasis and pneumonia are microscopically characterized by a catarrhal, eosinophilic bronchitis with peribronchial lymphoid hyperplasia, thickening of alveolar interstitium due to hyperplasia of type II pneumonocytes and focal infiltration of lymphocytes, and an alveolar exudate. Secondary bacterial pneumonia is common.

Muellerius capillaris, also called the nodular lungworm, occurs in sheep and goats in most areas of the world and is the most common lung parasite of sheep in Europe. It requires slugs or snails as intermediate hosts. Clinical signs are usually not apparent. The lesions in sheep are typically multifocal, subpleural nodules that tend to be most numerous in the dorsal areas of the caudal lobes. These nodules are soft and hemorrhagic in the early stages but, later, become gray-green and hard or even calcified. Microscopically, a focal, eosinophilic, and granulomatous reaction occurs in the subpleural alveoli where the adults, eggs, and larvae reside (Fig. 3-43).

Goats differ from sheep by having diffuse interstitial rather than focal lesions, and the reaction to the parasites seen microscopically varies from almost no lesions to a severe pneumonia with some eosinophils. Secondary effects include decreased weight gain and, possibly, secondary bacterial infections.

Protostrongylus rufescens is a worldwide parasite of sheep and goats. Infection is usually subclinical, but *P. rufescens* can be pathogenic for lambs and goat kids. It requires an intermediate snail host. The parasite lives in bronchioles and causes lobular areas of pneumonia that are not distinctly different from those caused by other lungworms.

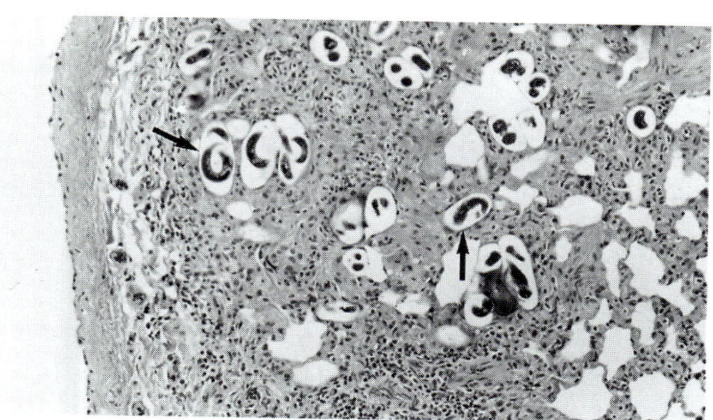

Fig. 3-43 Lung; adult ewe. Granulomatous (parasitic) pneumonia *(Muellerius capillaris).* Cross section of adults *(arrows),* larvae, and ova. H & E stain. *Courtesy of Western College of Veterinary Medicine.*

Pneumonias of Horses

Viral infections of the respiratory tract, particularly equine viral rhinopneumonitis and equine influenza, are important diseases of horses around the world. The effects of these and other respiratory viruses on the horse can be manifested in three distinct ways. First, as pure viral infections, their severity may range from mild to severe, making them a frequent interfering factor in training and performance. Second, superimposed infections by opportunists such as *P. multocida, Streptococcus* spp., *E. coli, Rhodococcus equi,* and various anaerobes can cause fibrinous or suppurative bronchopneumonias. Third, it is possible, but yet unproven, that viral infections may also predispose horses to ''airway hyperresponsiveness'' and ''chronic obstructive pulmonary disease.''

Equine viral rhinopneumonitis (EVR)

This respiratory disease of young horses is particularly important in weanlings between 4 to 8 months of age and, to a much lesser extent, in young foals and adult horses. The causative agent is an equine herpesvirus that, in addition to respiratory disease, can cause abortion in pregnant mares and neurologic diseases in horses of all ages. The taxonomy of equine herpesvirus has changed in the last few years. Currently, it is accepted that **EHV-1** and **EHV-4,** previously classified together as EHV-1 (subtypes 1 and 2), are the dominant strains responsible for respiratory disease; EHV-1 can also cause fetal infections and abortion, but EHV-4 has a low abortiogenic potential. The respiratory and abortive forms of EVR occur independently. Infection with EHV-2 and EHV-3 strains of equine herpesvirus is not clinically or pathologically associated with significant respiratory disease. Equine cytomegalovirus (EHV-2) is widely distributed in the equine population, but its role as a respiratory pathogen is still debatable. Finally, EHV-3 causes **equine coital exanthema,** a venereal disease responsible for vesicles and pustules of the vulva and penis.

The respiratory form of EVR in adult horses is mild and transient, and is seen by pathologists only when complications with secondary bacterial infections cause a fatal bronchopneumonia. Uncomplicated lesions in EVR are seen only in aborted fetuses or in foals that die within the first few days of life. They consist of focal areas of necrosis (0.5 to 2 mm) in various organs, including the liver, adrenal glands, and lungs.

Equine influenza

This contagious respiratory disease of horses has high morbidity and low mortality, and severe outbreaks occur in susceptible populations of horses. The course of the disease is generally mild and transient, and its importance is primarily due to its economic impact on the equine industry. Uncomplicated lesions in the lungs are those of a mild and self-limiting bronchointerstitial pneumonia (see Specific Diseases of the Nasal Cavity and Sinuses, Equine Diseases).

Equine viral arteritis (EVA)

This pansystemic disease of horses occurs sporadically throughout the world and is caused by a togavirus. Clinical signs are respiratory distress, fever, abortion, diarrhea, colic, and edema of the limbs and ventral abdomen. Respiratory signs are characterized by serous to mucopurulent rhinitis and conjunctivitis with palpebral edema. Like most viral respiratory infections, EVA can also predispose horses to opportunistic secondary bacterial pneumonias. Gross lesions consist of hemorrhage in most tissues, pulmonary edema, voluminous hydrothorax and hydroperitoneum, enteritis, and edema of the intestinal wall. Fibrinoid degeneration and inflammation of the walls, particularly of small muscular arteries, are the underlying microscopic lesions that explain most of the clinical and pathologic features.

African horse sickness

This vector-borne disease of horses and, to a lesser extent, other equidae is caused by an orbivirus (family Reoviridae) and is characterized by respiratory distress or cardiovascular failure. It has a high mortality rate—up to 95% in the native population of horses in Africa, the Middle East, India, Pakistan, and, most recently, in Spain. Although the virus is transmitted primarily by insects *(Culicoides)* to horses, other animals such as dogs can be infected by eating infected equine flesh. Based on clinical signs (not pathogenesis), African horse sickness is arbitrarily divided into four different forms, namely: ''pulmonary,'' ''cardiac,'' ''mixed,'' and ''mild.'' The pulmonary form is characterized by severe respiratory distress and rapid death due to massive pulmonary edema. Grossly, large amounts of froth are present in airways, lungs fail to collapse, subpleural lymph vessels appear distended, and the ventral parts of the lungs appear notably edematous. In the cardiac form, recurrent fever is detected, and heart failure results in subcutaneous and interfascial edema, most notably in the neck and supraorbital region. The mixed form is a combination of the respiratory and cardiac forms. Finally, the mild form is characterized by fever and clinical signs resembling those of equine influenza; it is in most cases, transient and followed by a complete recovery. This mild form is most frequently seen in donkeys, mules, and zebras and in horses with some degree of immunity. The pathogenesis of this disease is yet to be elucidated.

Rhodococcosis

Rhodococcus equi, formerly known as *Corynebacterium equi,* is an important cause of morbidity and mortality in foals around the world. Infection occurs in two major forms—one involves the intestine, causing ulcerative enterocolitis, and the other affects the respiratory tract, resulting in a severe and fatal bronchopneumonia. Although half of foals with pneumonia have enterocolitis, it is rare to find animals with enterocolitis alone. Occasionally, infection disseminates to lymph nodes, joints, bones, genital tract, and other organs. Because *R. equi* is present in soil and the feces of herbivores (particularly foals), it is not unusual for the disease to become enzootic on farms where the organism has been shed earlier by infected foals. Serologic evidence of infection in horses is widespread, yet clinical disease is sporadic and largely restricted to young foals or to adult horses suffering severe immunosuppression. This bacterium has been incriminated also in cases of cervical lymphadenitis in cattle and pigs and in pneumonia in immunosuppressed human beings infected with the AIDS virus.

Clinically, *R. equi* infection can be acute, with rapid death due to severe bronchopneumonia, or chronic, with depression, cough, weight loss, and respiratory distress. In either form, there may be diarrhea, arthritis, or subcutaneous "abscessation."

It is still debatable whether natural infection starts as a bronchopneumonia (aerogenous route) from which *R. equi* reaches the intestine via swallowed sputum or whether infection starts as an enteritis (oral route) with subsequent bacteremic emboli to the lungs. The results of experimental studies suggest that natural infection with this organism likely starts from inhalation. Once in the lung, *R. equi* is rapidly phagocytosed by alveolar macrophages, but defective phagosome-lysosome fusion and premature lysosomal degranulation result in bacteria survival and multiplication, eventually leading to the destruction of the macrophage. Released lysosomal enzymes and bacterial toxins are responsible for extensive caseous necrosis of the lungs and the intense recruitment of neutrophils, macrophages, and giant cells. These changes eventually lead to a pyogranulomatous pneumonia (Fig. 3-44) with abscesses and

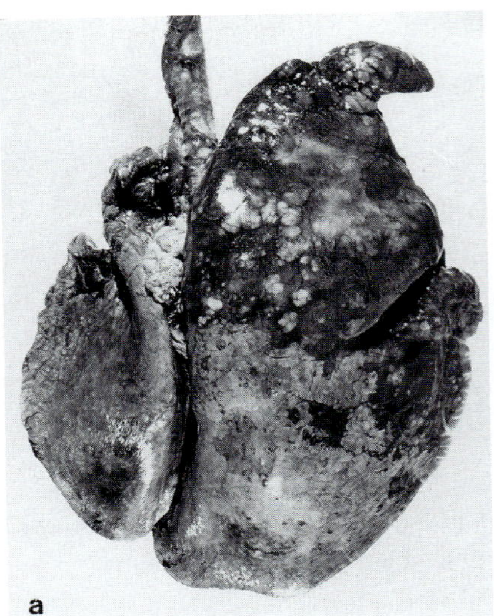

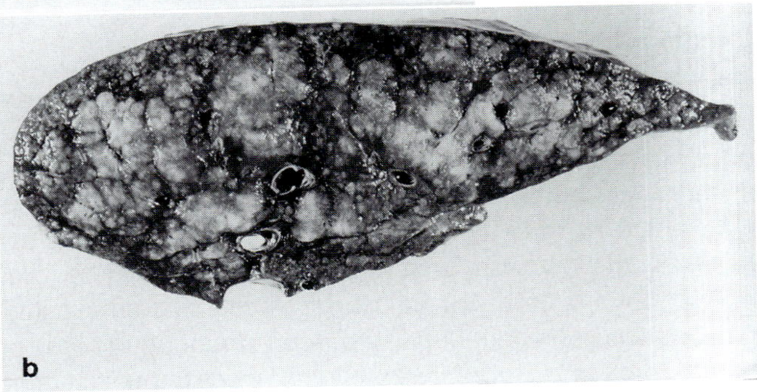

Fig. 3-44 Lungs; foal. Granulomatous pneumonia *(Rhodococcus equi).* **A**, Cranioventral consolidation of the lungs with subpleural granulomas. **B**, Cut surface. Note the large, often confluent, caseated granulomas. *Johnson et al. Vet Pathol 1983; 20:440-449.*

tracheobronchial pyogranulomatous lymphadenitis, the hallmark lesions of *R. equi* disease.

Other pneumonias of horses

Chlamydia psittaci can cause systemic infection in many species; in horses, it has been associated with keratoconjunctivitis, rhinitis, bronchopneumonia, abortion, polyarthritis, diarrhea, and hepatitis. Serologic studies suggest that infection without apparent disease may be common in horses. Horses experimentally infected with chlamydial organisms develop a mild and transient bronchointerstitial pneumonia.

Horses are susceptible to *Mycobacterium avium, M. tuberculosis,* and *M. bovis.* The intestinal tract and associated lymph nodes are usually affected, but with hematogenous dissemination, the lungs are involved (Fig. 3-45). The tubercules differ from those in ruminants and pigs, being smooth, gray, solid nodules without grossly visible caseous necrosis or calcification; they appear more like sarcomas. Microscopically, the tubercles are composed of macrophages, epithelioid cells, and multinucleated giant cells.

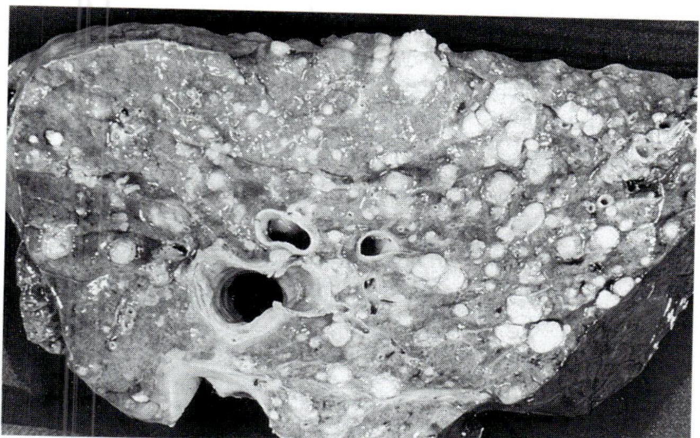

Fig. 3-45 Lung, cut surface; aged horse. Tuberculosis *(Mycobacterium avium-intracellulare).* Multifocal, granulomatous pneumonia. *Courtesy of Western College of Veterinary Medicine.*

Fibrosis increases with time, accounting in part for the sarcomatous appearance.

Adenovirus and *Pneumocystis carinii* infections occur commonly in Arabian foals with **combined immunodeficiency,** a hereditary lack of B- and T-lymphocytes. In cases of viral infection, large basophilic adenoviral inclusion bodies (Cowdry types A and B) are present in the nuclei of tracheal, bronchial, bronchiolar, alveolar, renal, and intestinal epithelia. In infections with *P. carinii,* the pulmonary lesion is an interstitial pneumonia. Characteristically, alveoli are filled with a distinctive foamy exudate that contains the organism (not visible in H & E) but easily demonstrated with silver stains such as Gomori's methenamine silver. In human beings, *P. carinii* pneumonia (pneumocystosis) is one of the most common and often fatal complications in AIDS patients.

Diffuse proliferative interstitial pneumonias of undetermined etiology have been repeatedly reported in North American horses. The gross and microscopic lesions are reminiscent of bovine pulmonary edema and emphysema in cattle. The etiology of these interstitial pneumonias in horses is not known, but toxic and viral etiologies have been proposed.

Parasitic pneumonias of horses

Parascaris equorum is a large nematode (roundworm) of the small intestine of horses; the larval stages migrate through the lungs as ascarid larvae do in pigs. It is still unclear whether migration of *P. equorum* larvae can cause significant pulmonary lesions under natural conditions. Experimentally, migration of larvae results in coughing, anorexia, and weight loss. Small necrotic foci and petechiae occur in the liver, hepatic and tracheobronchial lymph nodes, and lungs. These changes are also apparent microscopically, but eosinophils are also prominent as part of a focal, granulomatous, interstitial pneumonia associated with the larvae. Eosinophilic bronchitis and bronchiolitis also occur.

Dictyocaulus arnfieldi is not a very pathogenic nematode, but should be considered if there are signs of coughing in horses that are pastured together with donkeys. Donkeys are considered the natural hosts and can tolerate large numbers of parasites without ill effects. *D. arnfieldi* does not usually become patent in horses, so examination of fecal samples is not useful. The lesion is an eosinophilic bronchitis similar to the less acute infestations seen in cattle and sheep with their *Dictyocaulus* species.

Pneumonias of Dogs

In general, inflammatory diseases of the lungs are less of a problem in dogs than in food-producing species. Of the infectious causes, two account for most cases: infectious tracheobronchitis (kennel cough), which was discussed previously, and canine distemper. Uremia and paraquat toxicity are perhaps the two most notable noninfectious causes of pulmonary disease in dogs.

Canine distemper

This is an important and ubiquitous infectious disease of dogs, other canidae, and mustelidae around the world. It is caused by a paramyxovirus that is antigenically related to the human measles and rinderpest viruses. Distemper virus invades through the upper respiratory tract, proliferates in all lymphoid tissues, becomes viremic, and, in dogs with an inadequate antibody response, infects nearly all body tissues (pantropic), particularly the epithelial cells. This virus can target the lungs either directly as a viral pneumonia or by its immunosuppressive effects rendering the lungs susceptible to secondary infections. Clinical signs may consist of biphasic fever, diarrhea, vomiting, weight loss, mucopurulent oculonasal discharge, coughing, respiratory distress, and possible loss of vision. Weeks later, hyperkeratosis of foot pads (''hard pad'') and nose are observed, along with nervous signs including ataxia, paralysis, convulsions, or residual myoclonus (muscle twitches, chorea, ''tics'').

Gross lesions in the acute stages may include serous to catarrhal to mucopurulent nasopharyngitis. The lungs are edematous, have a diffuse interstitial pneumonia, and appear somewhat mottled because of variations in cellularity. Secondary infection with bacteria, including mycoplasmas, is common, resulting in suppurative bronchopneumonia. The thymus may be small relative to the age of the animal. Microscopically, eosinophilic inclusions are present in the epithelium of many tissues, in the nuclei or cytoplasm or in both. They appear early in the bronchiolar epithelium, but are most prominent in the epithelium of the stomach, renal pelvis, and urinary bladder, making these tissues good choices for diagnostic examination. The suppurative secondary pneumonias may obscure evidence of the viral infection such as inclusion bodies.

Distemper virus also has a tendency to affect developing tooth buds, causing enamel hypoplasia in dogs that recover from infection. Of all distemper lesions, demyelinating encephalomyelitis, which develops late, is the most devastating (see Diseases of the Nervous System). Sequelae to distemper include the nervous and pneumonic complications mentioned previously and such various systemic infections as toxoplasmosis.

Canine adenovirus type 2 (CAV-2) infection

This is a common and contagious disease of the respiratory tract of dogs, causing mild fever, oculonasal discharge, and coughing. Pulmonary lesions are initially those of a bronchointerstitial pneumonia, with necrosis and exfoliation of bronchiolar and alveolar epithelium and the presence of large, basophilic intranuclear viral inclusions. A few days later, the lesions change into a proliferation of type II pneumonocytes and hyperplastic bronchitis and bronchiolitis. The disease is sometimes associated with the infectious tracheobronchitis complex (kennel cough) and occasionally can coexist with distemper. It is clinically mild unless complicated with a secondary bacterial infection.

Canine herpesvirus 1

This viral infection can cause fatal generalized disease in puppies, and it is probably part of the variety of factors that result in the "fading puppy syndrome." It may also cause necrotizing rhinotracheitis and secondary bronchopneumonia in older animals.

Bacterial pneumonias

Dogs generally have bacterial pneumonias when the pulmonary defense mechanisms have been impaired. *P. multocida, Streptococcus* spp., *E. coli, Klebsiella pneumonia,* and *B. bronchiseptica* can be involved in pneumonia secondary to distemper or after aspiration of gastric contents. *S. zooepidemicus* also causes acute and fatal hemorrhagic pleuropneumonia with hemorrhagic pleural effusion in dogs. It is generally a consequence of generalized septic embolism affecting lungs, liver, brain, and lymph nodes, but, often, the primary source of the infection cannot be determined. The role of **mycoplasmas** in canine pneumonia is still unclear.

Tuberculosis is uncommon in dogs, but dogs are susceptible to the human *(M. tuberculosis),* bovine *(M. bovis),* and avian *(M. avium)* strains and, therefore, the incidence in dogs reflects the incidence of these bacteria in their environment. The clinicopathologic manifestation is pulmonary after inhalation or alimentary after oral exposure. The gross pulmonary lesions are focal, firm nodules, often in the caudal lobes, and, as in the horse, they appear like neoplasms (sarcomas) rather than calcified or caseous. Diffuse granulomatous pleuritis with copious serofibrinous and sanguineous effusion is common.

Mycotic pneumonias

These are serious diseases seen commonly in animals in some areas. There are two main types: those caused by opportunistic fungi and those caused by a group of fungi associated with systemic "deep" mycoses. All these fungi affect human beings and most domestic animals but are probably not transmitted between species.

Opportunistic fungi, such as *Aspergillus fumigatus,* are important in birds, but in domestic animals they mainly affect immunosuppressed animals or those on prolonged antibiotic therapy. The pulmonary lesion is a focal, nodular, pyogranulomatous or granulomatous pneumonia. Microscopically, the fungal hyphae are apparent, and there are usually necrosis, vasculitis, and the expected components of granulomas.

Systemic (deep) mycoses are caused by *Blastomyces dermatitidis, Histoplasma capsulatum, Coccidioides immitis,* and *Cryptococcus neoformans.* Blastomycosis mainly affects dogs and is discussed here, whereas cryptococcosis is discussed in the section Pneumonias of Cats. In contrast to other fungi such as *Aspergillus* sp., organisms of the systemic mycosis group are all primary pathogens of human beings and animals and, thus, do not necessarily require a preceding immunosuppression in order to cause disease.

Blastomycosis occurs in many countries of the American continent, Africa, and the Middle East and occasionally in Europe. In the United States, it is most prevalent in the Atlantic, St. Lawrence, and Ohio-Mississippi River Valley states as compared with the Mountain-Pacific region. In addition, sport (outdoor and hunting) dogs appear to have an increased risk of developing infection. *B. dermatitidis* is a dimorphic fungus (mycelia-yeast) seen mainly in young dogs and occasionally in cats. This fungus is present in the soil, and inhalation of spores is considered the principal route of infection. Clinical signs can reflect involvement of virtually any body tissue; pulmonary effects include cough, decreased exercise tolerance, and terminal respiratory distress. Pulmonary involvement is characterized by a granulomatous pneumonia, generally with multiple firm nodules (pyogranulomas) scattered throughout the lungs (Fig. 3-32). Microscopically, nodules are granulomas with a connective tissue stroma containing numerous macrophages (epithelioid cells), some neutrophils, multinucleated giant cells, and thick-walled yeasts (Fig. 3-46). Yeasts are 5 to 25 μm in diameter and are much better visualized when tissue sections are stained with PAS or with silver stains. Nodules can also be present in other tissues, chiefly lymph nodes, skin, spleen, liver, kidneys, and eyes.

Coccidioidomycosis (San Joaquin Valley Fever), caused by the dimorphic fungus *Coccidioides immitis,* occurs mainly in animals living in arid regions of the southwestern United States and Central and South America. It is a primary respiratory tract (aerogenous) infection seen com-

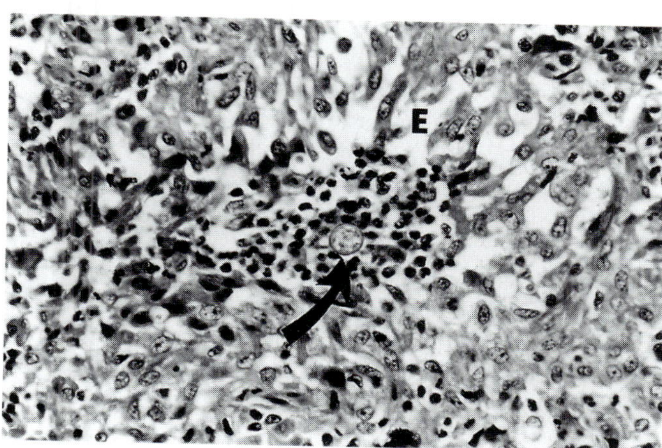

Fig. 3-46 Lung, histologic section; 2-year-old dog. Blastomycosis *(Blastomyces dermatitidis)*. Granulomatous pneumonia. A fungal yeast *(arrow)* is surrounded by neutrophils, which are in turn surrounded by a layer of epithelioid cells *(E)*. H & E stain. *Courtesy of Western College of Veterinary Medicine.*

monly at slaughter in clinically normal feedlot cattle and only becomes systemic in dogs. In dogs, the signs relate to the chance location of lesions, so there can be respiratory distress, lameness, or cutaneous lesions, among others. Again, the lesions are focal granulomas or pyogranulomas that can have suppurative or caseated centers. The organisms are present in affected tissues as small spores or large spherules (10 to 80 μm).

Histoplasmosis is a systemic infection that results from inhalation of another dimorphic fungus, *H. capsulatum*. The geographic distribution of histoplasmosis in North America is similar to that of blastomycosis, that is, more prevalent in the Mississippi–Ohio–St. Lawrence valleys. Bat and bird droppings appear to promote its growth and survival in the soil of enzootic areas. Histoplasmosis occurs in young dogs and, to a lesser extent, in cats. Pulmonary histoplasmosis is grossly characterized by variably sized, firm, well-encapsulated granulomas, and, sometimes, more diffuse involvement of the lungs. Microscopically, granulomatous tissue typically has many macrophages filled with small (1 to 3 μm) yeasts, best demonstrated with PAS or Gomori-methenamine-silver stains. Similar nodules can be present in other tissues, chiefly lymph nodes, spleen, intestines, and liver.

Toxic pneumonias

Paraquat, a herbicide widely used in gardening and agriculture, can cause severe and often fatal pulmonary lesions in dogs, human beings, and other species. Following ingestion or inhalation (airborne), paraquat metabolites promote local release of free radicals, which cause extensive injury to the air-blood barrier, presumably through lipid-peroxidation of type I pneumonocytes. Soon after poisoning, the lungs are heavy, edematous, and hemorrhagic, with bullae of emphysema and pneumomediastinum. The lungs of animals that survive acute paraquat toxicosis become pale and fail to collapse when the thorax is opened. Microscopic findings in the acute and subacute phases include necrosis of type I pneumonocytes, edema, hemorrhages, and proliferation of type II alveolar cells. In the chronic stages (4 to 8 weeks later), the lesions are characterized by severe interstitial and intraalveolar fibrosis.

Uremic pneumonopathy (pneumonitis) is one of the many nonrenal lesions seen in dogs with chronic uremia. Lesions are characterized by a combination of pulmonary edema and calcification of smooth muscle, which in some severe cases, extends into the alveolar walls. When lesions are severe, the lungs fail to collapse when the thorax is opened and have a "gritty" texture due to severe calcification. Since this is not primarily an inflammatory lesion, the term pneumonitis should be avoided.

Parasitic pneumonias of dogs

Toxoplasmosis is a worldwide disease caused by the protozoal parasite *Toxoplasma gondii.* Cats and other felidae are the definitive host where the mature parasite divides sexually in the intestinal mucosa. Mammals, including human beings, can become intermediate hosts following accidental ingestion of fertile oocysts shed in cat feces. In most instances, the parasite infects many cells but does not cause clinical disease. Toxoplasmosis is often preceded by immunosuppression, such as that caused by canine distemper virus. Pulmonary toxoplasmosis is characterized by a severe, focal necrotizing interstitial pneumonia with notable proliferation of type II pneumonocytes, especially in cats. Lesions in other organs include focal necrotizing hepatitis, encephalitis, splenitis, myositis, and retinitis. The parasites appear microscopically as small (3 to 6 μm) basophilic bodies that can be found free in affected tissues or within the cytoplasm of many epithelial cells and macrophages.

Pneumocystis carinii has also been reported as a sporadic cause of chronic interstitial pneumonia in dogs with a compromised immune system (see Equine Pneumonias).

Filaroides hirthi, a lungworm of the alveoli and bronchioles of dogs, has long been known as a cause of mild subclinical infection in large colonies of beagle dogs in the United States. However, it can on occasion cause severe and even fatal disease in individual pets. Clinical signs may include coughing and terminal respiratory distress in such cases. Grossly, the lesions are multifocal subpleural nodules, often with a green hue due to eosinophils, scattered throughout the lungs. Microscopically, these nodules are eosinophilic granulomas associated with larvae or dead worms, as little reaction develops to the live adults.

Crenosoma vulpis is a lungworm seen occasionally in dogs with access to the intermediate hosts, slugs and snails.

The adults live in small bronchi and bronchioles, causing eosinophilic, catarrhal bronchitis-bronchiolitis manifested grossly as gray areas of inflammation and atelectasis in the caudal lobes.

Paragonimus kellicotti in North America and *P. westermanii* in Asia are asymptomatic fluke infections in fish-eating species; cats and dogs acquire it in North America by eating crayfish. Gross lesions include pleural hemorrhages when the metacercariae migrate into the lungs. Later, multifocal eosinophilic pleuritis and cysts up to 7 mm long, containing pairs of adult flukes, are found along with eosinophilic granulomas around clusters of eggs. Pneumothorax can occur if a cyst that communicates with an airway ruptures to the pleural surface.

Angiostrongylus vasorum and *Dirofilaria immitis* are parasites of the vascular system. They can cause chronic arteritis leading to pulmonary hypertension and, eventually, congestive right cardiac failure. Recently, pleural lesions of focal hemorrhage, fibrosis, and diffuse hemosiderosis have been described.

Pneumonias of Cats

Although upper respiratory infections are common and important in cats, pneumonias are uncommon except when there is immunosuppression. Viral infections such as *feline rhinotracheitis* and *calicivirus* may cause lesions in the lungs, but, unless there is secondary invasion by bacteria, they do not usually pose a problem. Pleural effusions are significant in cats.

Feline pneumonitis

This mild, subclinical bronchointerstitial pneumonia is caused by *Chlamydia psittaci (felis)*. The term feline pneumonitis is a misnomer since infections with chlamydia cause a severe conjunctivitis and rhinitis (see Nasal Cavity and Sinuses) and only a mild pneumonia. The elucidation of the importance of feline viral rhinotracheitis and feline calicivirus has probably removed most of the confusion amid which chlamydia had taken on an artificially inflated importance.

Bacterial pneumonias

Bacteria from the nasal flora such as *Pasteurella multocida* and *Pasteurella*-like organisms are occasionally associated with secondary bronchopneumonias in cats. *P. multocida* also causes otitis media and meningitis, but its role as a respiratory pathogen is mainly associated with pyothorax. Mycoplasmas are often isolated, but are not established as primary pathogens in feline pneumonias.

Cats are susceptible to the bacteria of the three main types of **tuberculosis,** but *Mycobacterium bovis* is the most frequent cause. The usual route of infection is oral, through infected milk, so the lesions are mainly in the alimentary tract. The gross appearance of tuberculous nodules is similar to that of neoplasms, so they must be differentiated from pulmonary neoplasms (e.g., lymphosarcomas).

Mycotic Pneumonias

Cryptococcosis *(Cryptococcus neoformans)* is a systemic mycosis akin to those discussed under the section on Mycotic Pneumonias under Pneumonias of Dogs. It occurs worldwide in all species, but is diagnosed most frequently in cats. Animals that are compromised immunologically, such as by feline leukemia virus infection, malnutrition, or corticosteroid treatment, are most susceptible.

Lesions can occur in nearly any tissue, resulting in a wide variety of clinical signs. However, granulomatous rhinitis, sinusitis, pulmonary involvement, ulcerative skin lesions, meningitis, and encephalitis are common. The pulmonary lesion is a multifocal granulomatous pneumonia and, as with those occurring in other internal organs, has the appearance of small, gelatinous, white foci. The gelatinous appearance is due to the wide mucus capsule around the yeast (4 to 10 μm).

Endogenous lipid pneumonia

This is an obscure, subclinical pulmonary disease of cats and occasionally of dogs, which is unrelated to aspiration of foreign material. Although the pathogenesis is not understood, it is presumed that lipids from pulmonary surfactant and from degenerated cells accumulate within alveolar macrophages. The gross lesions are multifocal, white, firm nodules scattered throughout the lungs. Microscopically, the alveoli are filled with foamy macrophages accompanied by interstitial infiltration of lymphocytes and plasma cells, fibrosis, and alveolar epithelialization. Endogenous lipid pneumonia should not be confused with accidental aspiration of oil (exogenous lipid pneumonia).

Aspiration pneumonias

This is common in cats given mineral oil (exogenous lipid pneumonia) by their owners in attempts to remove hairballs, or as a result of vomiting.

Parasitic pneumonias

Aelurostrongylus abstrusus, known as ''feline lungworm,'' is a parasite that occurs wherever the necessary slug and snail intermediate hosts are found. It can cause chronic respiratory disease with coughing and weight loss and, sometimes, severe dyspnea and death, particularly if there are secondary bacterial infections. The gross lesions are multifocal subpleural nodules up to 1 cm in diameter throughout the lungs. On incision, these nodules contain eggs, larvae, and turbid, viscous exudate. Microscopically, the parasites and their eggs and larvae are in the bronchioles and alveoli where they cause catarrhal bronchiolitis, hyperplasia of submucosal glands, granulomatous alveolitis, and fibromuscular hyperplasia. Pyothorax is an occasional sequela.

Toxoplasma gondii and *Paragonimus kellicotti* can also affect cats (see Parasitic Pneumonias under Pneumonias of Dogs).

Fetal and Perinatal Pneumonias

Pneumonia is one of the most frequent lesions found in fetuses submitted for postmortem examination, particularly in foals and food-producing animals. Because of autolysis, lack of inflation, and lungs being at various stages of development, lesions are often missed or misdiagnosed. In the nonaerated fetal lung, the bronchoalveolar spaces are filled with a viscous, locally produced fluid known as "lung fluid" or "lung liquid." This fluid normally moves along the tracheobronchial tree, reaching the oropharynx and, finally, the amniotic fluid. At the time of birth, this fluid is rapidly reabsorbed from the lungs by the pulmonary lymph vessels.

Aspiration of amniotic fluid contaminated with meconium and bacteria is the most common route by which pathogens reach the fetal lungs. This form of pneumonia is associated with intrauterine hypoxia and acidosis that cause the fetus to relax the anal sphincter, release meconium into the amniotic fluid, and, in the terminal stages, inspire deeply with open glottis, resulting in the aspiration of contaminated fluid. Gross lesions are only occasionally seen, but microscopic changes are similar to those of a bronchopneumonia. Microscopically, bronchoalveolar spaces contain variable numbers of neutrophils, macrophages, and pieces of meconium that appear as bright yellow material because of the bile content. In contrast to postnatal bronchopneumonia, lesions in fetuses are not restricted to the cranioventral aspects of the lungs, but involve all pulmonary lobes.

In cattle, *Brucella abortus* and *Actinomyces pyogenes (Corynebacterium pyogenes)* are two of the most common bacteria isolated from the lungs of aborted fetuses. These organisms are usually present in large numbers in the amniotic fluid of cows with bacterial placentitis. Aspiration of contaminated amniotic fluid carries the organisms into the fetal lungs, causing a suppurative bronchopneumonia characterized by severe necrosis and cellular exudation into bronchi, bronchioles, and alveoli. Microscopically, leukocytes, bacteria, necrotic debris, and occasional pieces of meconium are present in the bronchoalveolar spaces. *Aspergillus* spp. (mycotic abortion) and *Ureaplasma diversum* are sporadically associated with placentitis and pneumonia in aborted calves.

In addition to aspiration of bacteria, pathogens can also reach the lungs via fetal blood and cause interstitial pneumonia. Listeriosis *(Listeria monocytogenes)*, salmonellosis (*Salmonella* spp.), and chlamydiosis *(Chlamydia psittaci)* are the best known examples of blood-borne diseases causing fetal pneumonia in farm animals. Gross lesions in the lungs are generally undetected, but microscopic lesions include focal necrotizing interstitial pneumonia, as well as focal necrosis in the liver, spleen, or brain. Fetal bronchointerstitial pneumonia occurs also in some viral abortions, such as those caused by infectious bovine rhinotracheitis virus and PI-3 virus in cattle and equine viral rhinopneumonitis virus in horses. Fetal pneumonias in dogs and cats are infrequently described, perhaps because aborted puppies and kittens are rarely submitted for postmortem examination.

Neonatal pneumonias and septicemias

These are rather common in newborn animals lacking passive immunity (failure of passive transfer) because of the lack of ingestion or absorption of maternal colostrum. In addition to septicemic states and associated interstitial pneumonia, farm animals suffering with hypogammaglobulinemia can also develop bronchopneumonia by inhalation of secondary bacterial pathogens such as *Streptococcus* spp. in calves, foals, and lambs, and *E. coli* and streptococci in pigs.

"Meconium aspiration syndrome"

This important but preventable condition in human babies originates when amniotic fluid contaminated with meconium is aspirated during labor. The pathogenesis is basically the same as in fetal bronchopneumonia and abortion, except that in this syndrome aspiration of amniotic fluid takes place during delivery and babies are born alive. This syndrome is well known in human babies, but the occurrence and significance in animals remain largely unknown. Although pulmonary lesions in affected children and animal neonates are only mild and transient, this syndrome can be life threatening since it is always accompanied by severe acidosis. In the most severe cases, focal (patchy) atelectasis can be observed grossly (see Fig. 3-13). Microscopically, keratin exfoliated from skin into the amniotic fluid and meconium are present in bronchoalveolar spaces accompanied by a mild alveolitis.

Neoplasms of the Lungs

Malignant pulmonary neoplasms in animals are relatively rare. The nomenclature of pulmonary neoplasms in domestic animals is not universal, and, as a consequence, a multiplicity of names and synonyms occur in the veterinary literature. The most common types of pulmonary neoplasms described in domestic mammals are given in Table 3-5.

Primary neoplasms of the lungs arise from cells normally present in the pulmonary tissue and can be epithelial or mesenchymal, although the latter are rare. Primary benign neoplasms of the lungs, such as **pulmonary adenomas,** are highly unusual in domestic animals. Most primary neoplasms are malignant and appear as solitary masses of variable size that, with time, can metastasize to other areas of the lungs and to distal organs.

It is often difficult to determine the precise topographic origin of a neoplasm within the lungs, for instance, whether it originates in the conductive system **(bronchogenic carcinoma),** transitional system **(bronchiolar carcinoma),** exchange system **(alveolar carcinoma),** or bronchial glands **(bronchial gland carcinoma).** However, according to the literature, pulmonary carcinomas in animals seem to arise

Table 3-5. Classification of pulmonary neoplasms

Primary
Epithelial origin
Benign
- Bronchial papilloma
- Bronchial gland adenoma
- Bronchiolar-alveolar adenoma

Malignant
- Bronchogenic carcinoma
  - Squamous cell (epidermoid) carcinoma
  - Adenocarcinoma
  - Adenosquamous carcinoma
  - Anaplastic (undifferentiated) carcinoma
    - Small cell
    - Large cell
- Bronchiolar-alveolar carcinoma
- Alveolar carcinoma
- Bronchial gland carcinoma
- Carcinoid tumor (neuroendocrine)

Mesenchymal origin
- Benign, e.g., hemangioma; granular cell tumor (myoblastoma) of horses
- Malignant, e.g., hemangiosarcoma

Secondary = metastatic
Any malignant tumor metastatic from another body location, e.g., osteogenic sarcoma in dogs, uterine carcinoma in cows, malignant melanoma in horses

generally from the bronchiolar-alveolar region (Clara cells or type II pneumonocytes), in contrast to those in human beings, which are mostly bronchogenic. Because of histologic architecture, many malignant epithelial neoplasms are frequently classified as **pulmonary adenocarcinomas** irrespective of their cell of origin.

Dogs and cats are the species most frequently affected with primary pulmonary neoplasms, largely carcinomas and generally in animals 6 years of age or older (Fig. 3-47). Pulmonary carcinomas in other domestic animals are less common, possibly because fewer are allowed to live a natural life span. These neoplasms can be invasive or expansive, color and texture varying, but often have areas of necrosis and hemorrhage, resulting in a ''craterous'' or ''umbilicate'' appearance.

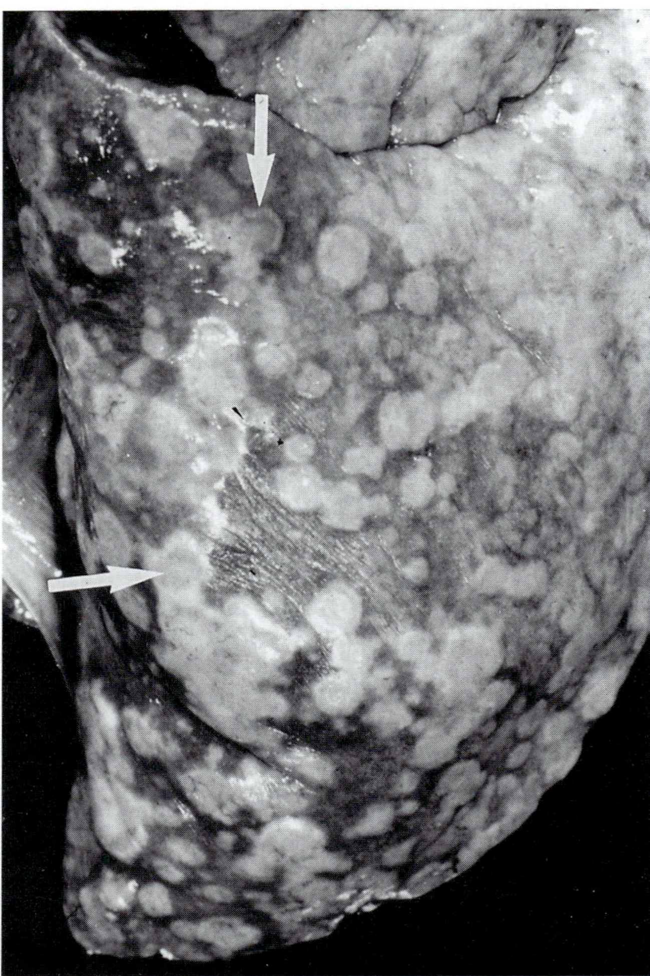

Fig. 3-47 Lungs, right caudal lobe; 12-year-old dog. Pulmonary adenocarcinoma. Metastases are present widely within the lung but not beyond. Some of the tumorous nodules are ''umbilicated'' *(arrows)* due to central necrosis. *Courtesy of Western College of Veterinary Medicine.*

Ovine pulmonary carcinoma (pulmonary adenomatosis)

This disease is common in some areas of the world (see Pneumonia of Sheep).

Carcinoid of the lungs

This neoplasm, presumably arising from neuroendocrine cells, is occasionally seen in dogs as multiple, large, firm masses closely associated with the main bronchi.

Secondary neoplasms of the lungs

These are all malignant by definition because they are the result of metastasis to the lungs from malignant neoplasms elsewhere. They too can be of epithelial or mesenchymal origin. Common sources include **mammary** and **thyroid carcinomas** in cats, **uterine carcinoma** in cows, **hemangiosarcoma** (Fig. 3-48), **osteogenic sarcoma,** and **malignant melanoma** in dogs, and **malignant lymphoma** in dogs and pigs. Secondary neoplasms are relatively common in comparison to primary ones, but even at that metastasis is an inefficient process with millions of embolic cells per day slipping through without fixing at a site. Secondary pulmonary neoplasms are usually multiple, of variable size, and, according to distribution, can be nodular (''cannonball''), diffuse, or radiating. The appearance of metastatic neoplasms differs according to the type of neoplasm. For instance, dark cystic nodules containing blood are indicative of hemangiosarcoma; dark solid nodules, of melanoma; and hard solid nodules with bone spicules, of osteogenic sarcoma.

Proper diagnoses of pulmonary neoplasia require his-

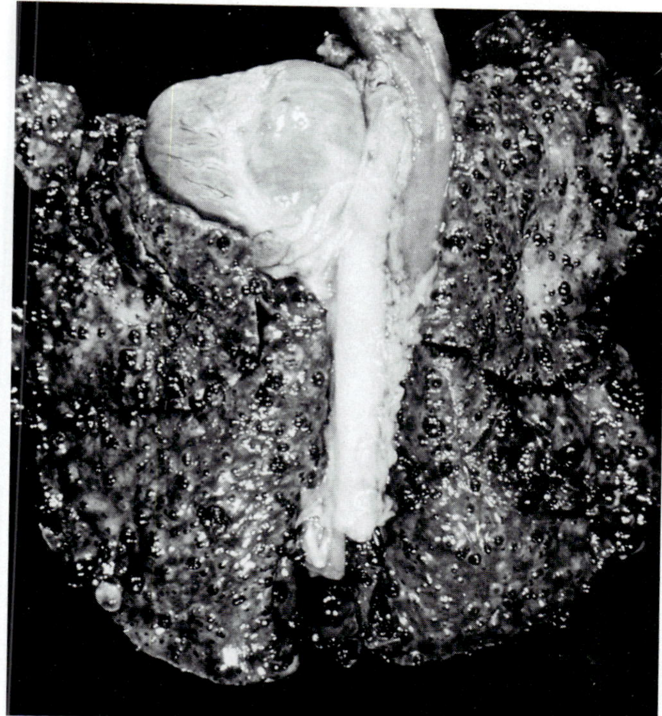

Fig. 3-48 Lungs; 9-year-old boxer dog. The animal collapsed suddenly and died of hemothorax. Metastatic hemangiosarcoma. Note the numerous, blood-filled, cystic nodules. The primary site was the right atrium. *Courtesy of Western College of Veterinary Medicine.*

tory, clinical signs, radiographs, and gross and microscopic examination with routine and special stains. Identification of a specific lineage of neoplastic cells is difficult and often requires special techniques, such as electron microscopy, by which distinctive cellular components may be seen (melanosomes in melanoma, lamellar phospholipid bodies in alveolar type II epithelial cells), and immunocytochemistry by which particular cellular structures or cell types are identified with immunologically specific markers.

Clinically, the signs vary with the degree of invasiveness, the amount of parenchyma involved, and locations of metastases. Signs may be vague, such as cough, lethargy, anorexia, weight loss, and, perhaps, dyspnea. In addition, paraneoplastic syndromes have also been associated with pulmonary neoplasia, particularly in human beings and dogs. The occurrence of these syndromes, such as hypercalcemia, endocrinopathies, and pulmonary hypertrophic osteoarthropathy (see Skeletal System), cannot be explained by the simple physical presence of the neoplasm alone.

DISEASES OF THE PLEURA AND THORACIC CAVITY

The thoracic wall, diaphragm, and mediastinum are lined by the parietal pleura, which reflects at the hilum and continues as the visceral pleura, covering the entire surfaces of the lungs. The space between these two pleurae is only minimal and, under normal conditions, contains only traces of clear fluid with a few exfoliated cells. Volumetric, biochemical, and cytologic changes in this fluid are routinely used in veterinary diagnostics. Sampling of this fluid is accomplished by thoracocentesis, a simple surgical procedure in which a needle passed into the thoracic cavity permits the retrieval of pleural effusions.

Anomalies

Congenital defects are rare. **Cysts** within the mediastinum of dogs can be large enough to compromise pulmonary function. Anomalies of the thoracic duct may cause some of the cases of chylothorax.

Degenerative Disturbances

Pleural calcification

This disorder is commonly found in dogs with chronic uremia. Lesions appear as linear white streaks in parietal pleura, mainly over the intercostal muscles of the cranial part of the thoracic cavity. The lesions are not functionally significant but indicate a severe underlying renal problem. **Vitamin D toxicity (hypervitaminosis D)** can cause a similar pleural lesion (Fig. 3-49).

Pneumothorax

This disorder is the presence of air in the thoracic cavity where there should normally be negative pressure to facilitate inspiration. Human beings have a complete and strong mediastinum so that pneumothorax is generally unilateral and, thus, not a serious problem. In dogs, the barrier is variable but, in general, less complete, so often some communication exists between left and right sides. However, processes can be unilateral if appropriately walled off by fibrinous exudate or other lesions.

Causes of pneumothorax include accidental (penetrating

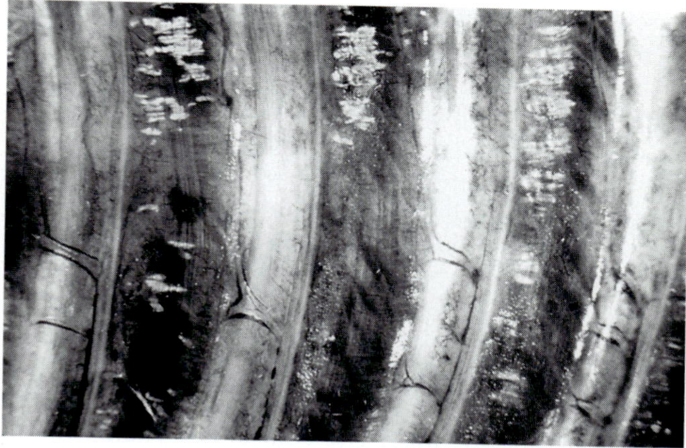

Fig. 3-49 Rib cage; 5-year-old male dog. Hypervitaminosis D. Foci of mineralization in the intercostal pleura caused by excessive vitamin D in the diet. Identical lesion occurs in dogs with uremia. *Courtesy of Western College of Veterinary Medicine.*

wound) or iatrogenic trauma (biopsy of the lung) and spontaneous rupture of emphysematous bullae or parasitic cysts that communicate with airways (*Paragonimus* spp.). Clinical signs include respiratory distress, and the lesion is simply a collapsed, atelectatic lung. The air is readily reabsorbed from the cavity if the source of air is sealed.

Circulatory Disturbances

Pleural effusion

This general term is used to describe accumulation of fluid (transudate, exudate, blood, lymph) in the thoracic cavity. When this fluid is serous, clear, and odorless, and fails to coagulate when exposed to air, the condition is referred to as **hydrothorax.** Causes of hydrothorax are the same as those involved in edema formation in other organs: increased hydrostatic pressure (heart failure), decreased oncotic pressure (hypoproteinemia, as in liver disease), alterations in vascular permeability (ANTU toxicity), or obstruction of lymph drainage (neoplasia). In cases where the leakage is corrected, fluid is rapidly reabsorbed, but, when leakage becomes chronic, persistent irritation of the serosal surface by transudate results in mesothelial hyperplasia and fibrosis with concurrent thickening of the pleura.

In severe cases, the amount of fluid present in the thoracic cavity can be considerable. For instance, a medium-sized dog can have 2 L of fluid, and a cow may accumulate 25 L or more. Excessive fluid in the thorax causes compressive atelectasis and respiratory distress. Hydrothorax is most commonly seen in cattle with right heart failure or cor pulmonale, dogs with congestive heart failure or nephrotic syndrome, pigs with mulberry heart disease, and horses with African horse sickness.

Hemothorax

Blood in the thoracic cavity is called hemothorax, but the term may be used for exudates with a sanguineous component. Causes include rupture of a major blood vessel as a result of severe trauma (e.g., hit by car), erosion of a vascular wall by malignant cells or inflammation (e.g., aoartitis caused by *Spirocerca lupi*), or ruptured aneurysms. It also can result from clotting defects (coagulopathies such as that in warfarin toxicity), disseminated intravascular coagulation, and bone marrow suppression. It is generally acute and fatal. On gross examination, the thoracic cavity is filled with blood, and the lungs are partially or completely atelectatic (Fig. 3-50).

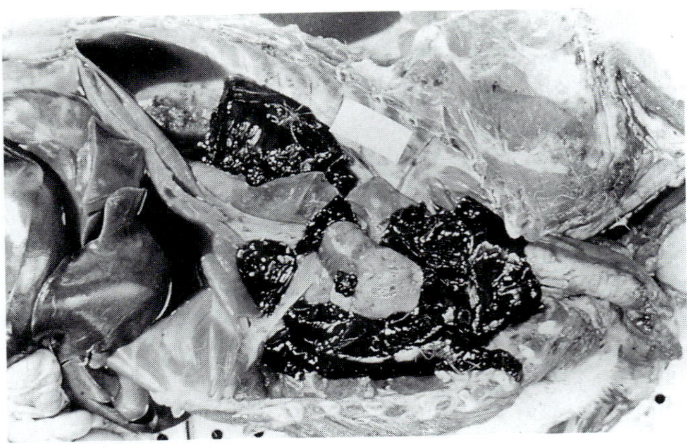

Fig. 3-50 Thoracic cavity; dog. Hemothorax. A large ruptured aneurysm of the thoracic aorta caused sudden death. Aortic aneurysms are associated with migration of *Spirocerca lupi* larvae.

Chylothorax

The accumulation of chylous fluid (lymph rich in triglycerides) in the thoracic cavity (Fig. 3-51) is due to rupture of major lymph vessels, chiefly the thoracic duct and the right lymphatic duct. The clinical and pathologic effects of chylothorax are similar to those of the other pleural effusions. Causes of lymph leakage include neoplasia (the most common cause in human beings but a distant second to idiopathic cases in dogs), trauma, congenital lymph vessel anomalies, and iatrogenic rupture of thoracic duct during surgery. The source of the leakage of the chyle is rarely found at necropsy.

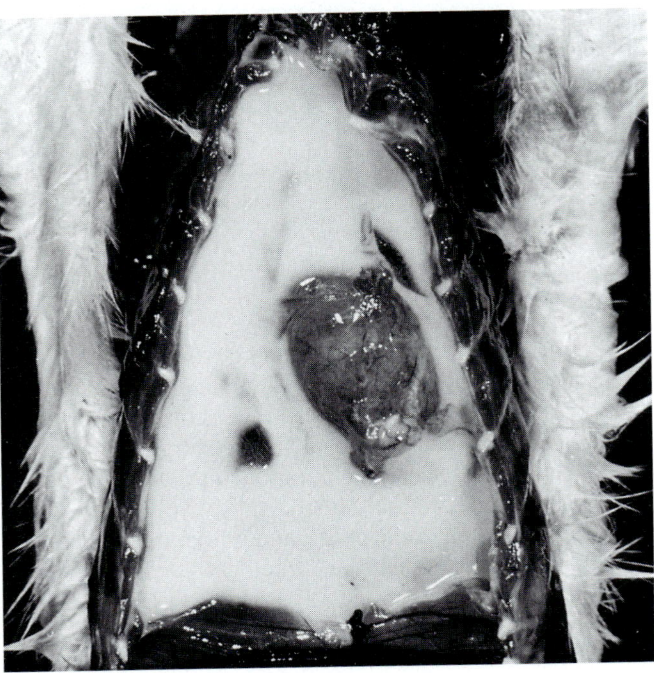

Fig. 3-51 Thoracic cavity; cat. Chylothorax (etiology unknown). Lymph (chyle) fills the thoracic cavity. *Courtesy of Western College of Veterinary Medicine.*

Inflammation

Pleuritis or pleurisy

Inflammation of the visceral or parietal pleurae is called pleuritis and, according to the type of exudate, can be fibrinous, suppurative, granulomatous, hemorrhagic, or a combination of exudates. When suppurative pleuritis results in purulent exudate in the cavity, the lesion is called **pyothorax** or **thoracic empyema** (Fig. 3-52). Clinically, pleuritis causes considerable pain, and, in addition, empyema can result in severe toxemia. **Pleural adhesions** and **fibrosis** are the most common sequelae to chronic pleuritis and can notably interfere with pulmonary expansion.

Pleuritis can occur as part of pneumonia, particularly in fibrinous bronchopneumonias (pleuropneumonia), or it can occur alone, without notable pulmonary involvement. Bovine and ovine pneumonic pasteurellosis and porcine and bovine pleuropneumonia are good examples of pleuritis associated with fibrinous bronchopneumonias. Polyserositis in pigs and pleural empyema, particularly in cats and horses, are examples of pleural inflammation in which involvement of the lungs may not accompany the pleurisy. Pleuritis is most frequently caused by bacteria, which can reach the pleural surface hematogenously, as in bacteremias with polyserositis. Examples of hematogenous pleuritis and polyserositis include *Haemophilus parasuis* (Glasser's disease) *Streptococcus suis* type II, and some strains of *P. multocida* in pigs, *S. equi* in horses, *E. coli* in calves, and *Mycoplasma* spp. and *Haemophilus* spp. in sheep and goats. Implantation of bacterial pathogens onto the pleural surface can also occur by extension from a septic process, such as a puncture wound of the thoracic wall, and traumatic reticulopericarditis or ruptured pulmonary abscesses *(A. pyogenes)* in cattle.

In dogs and cats, bacterial species (such as *Nocardia, Actinomyces,* and *Bacteroides*) can cause **pyogranulomatous pleuritis** characterized by accumulation of blood-stained pus (''tomato soup'') in the thoracic cavity. This exudate usually contains yellowish flecks called ''sulfur granules'' (Fig. 3-53), although these may not occur in nocardial empyema in cats. Many bacteria can be present in pyothorax of dogs and cats, alone or as mixed infections, such as *E. coli, A. pyogenes, P. multocida,* and *Fusobacterium necrophorum.* The pathogenesis of pleural empyema in cats is still debatable, but bite wounds or penetration of foreign material (migrating grass awns) are likely involved.

Cats with the noneffusive (''dry'') form of **feline infectious peritonitis** frequently have focal, pyogranulomatous pleuritis, in contrast to those with the ''wet'' or ''effusive'' form, in which thoracic involvement is primarily that of a pleural effusion.

Pleuritis is also an important problem in horses. *Nocardia asteroides* and *N. brasiliensis* can cause fibrinopurulent pneumonia and pyothorax with characteristic sulfur granules. Although *Mycoplasma felis* can be isolated from the respiratory tract of normal horses, it is also isolated from horses with pleuritis and pleural effusion, particularly during the early stages of infection.

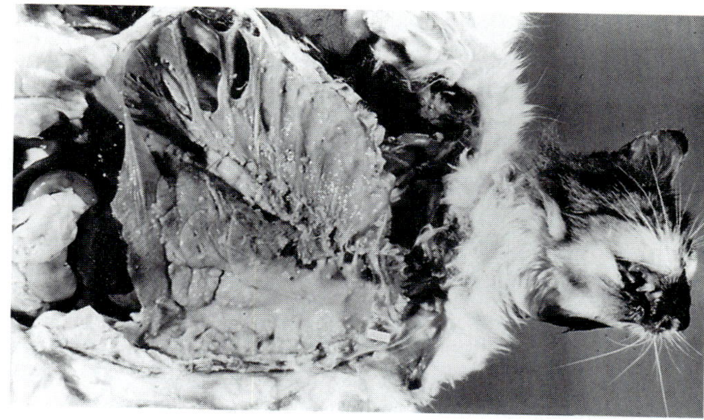

Fig. 3-52 Right thoracic cavity; cat. Pyothorax *(Pasteurella multocida).* Large amounts of purulent exudate have caused thickening of visceral and parietal pleurae.

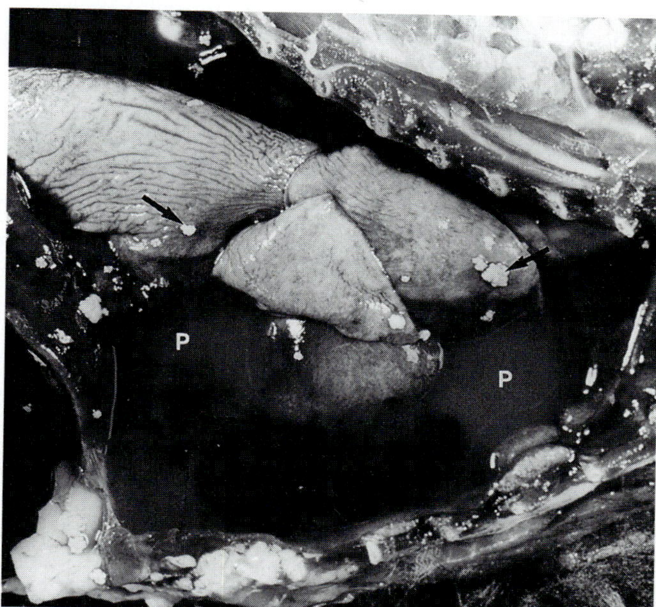

Fig. 3-53 Right thorax and lung; cat. Nocardiosis *(Nocardia asteroides).* Note flecks of exudate (''sulfur granules'') *(arrows),* fibrinopurulent pleuritis, and mild pyothorax (*P*). *Courtesy Dr. M.D. McGavin.*

Neoplasms

The pleural surface of the lung is often involved in neoplasms that have metastasized from other organs to the pulmonary parenchyma. Mesothelioma is the only primary neoplasm of the pleura.

Mesothelioma

This rare neoplasm of the thoracic and peritoneal mesothelium of human beings and most domestic animals is seen most commonly in calves, in which it can be congenital. In human beings, it has long been associated with asbestos exposure (asbestos mining, ship building), where with other factors, such as cigarette smoking, it is probably a cocarcinogen; no association between mesothelioma and asbestos has been made convincingly in domestic animals. In animals, there may be pleural effusion with resulting respiratory distress, cough, and weight loss.

Grossly, mesothelioma appears as multiple, discrete nodules or arborescent, spreading growths on the pleural surface. Microscopically, either the mesothelial covering cells or the supporting tissues can be the predominant malignant component, so the neoplasm can appear microscopically as a carcinoma or as a fibrosarcoma. Although considered malignant, mesothelioma rarely metastasizes.

Acknowledgments

This chapter is based on the one by Dr. William Yates (Agriculture Canada) published in the first edition of *Special Veterinary Pathology*. For his past contribution and his assistance I sincerely thank him. I also thank Shelley Ebbett and Tom MacDonald for photographic assistance and Glenda Clements for illustrations; Eileen Kinch, Sharon Martin and Kathleen Wilson for preparation of the manuscript; all pathologists at the Atlantic Veterinary College for providing case material; Dr. Manuel Chirino, Western College of Veterinary Medicine; Dr. Donald McGavin, University of Tennessee; and Dr. William Stokoe, Atlantic Veterinary College for critically reviewing the text. Finally, I thank Dr. Reginald G. Thomson, former Dean of the Atlantic Veterinary College for years of advice.

Suggested Readings

Beech J. Equine Respiratory Disorders. Philadelphia: Lea & Febiger, 1991.

Blood DC, Radostits OM. Veterinary Medicine: A Textbook of the Diseases of Cattle, Sheep, Pigs, Goats and Horses. 8th ed. London: Bailliere Tindall, 1994.

Breeze RG, Pirie HM, Dawson CO, Selman IE, Wiseman A. The pathology of respiratory diseases of adult cattle in Britain. Folia Vet Latina 1975; 5:95-128.

Castleman WL, Sorkness RL, Lemanske RF, McAllister PK. Viral bronchiolotis during early life induces increased numbers of bronchiolar mast cells and airway hyperresponsiveness. Am J Pathol 1990; 137:821-831.

Cutlip RC, Lehmkuhl HD, Schmerr MJF, Brogden KA. Ovine progressive pneumonia (maedi-visna) in sheep. Vet Microbiol 1988; 17:237-250.

Dungworth DL. Interstitial pulmonary disease. Adv Vet Sci Comp Med 1982; 26:173-200.

Dungworth DL. The respiratory system. In: Jubb KVF, Kennedy PC, Palmer N, eds. Pathology of Domestic Animals. 3rd ed. Vol 2. Toronto: Academic Press, 1993:539.

Dungworth DL, Schwartz LW. The reaction of lung to injury. In: Philippson AT, Hall LW, eds. Pritchard WR, Scientified Foundations of Veterinary Medicine. London: William Heinemann Medical Book LTD, 1980.

Ettinger SJ, ed. Textbook of Veterinary Internal Medicine: Diseases of the Dog and Cat. 3rd ed. Toronto: WB Saunders, 1989.

Fossum TW, Jacobs RM. Chylothorax in 34 dogs. J Am Vet Med Assoc 1986; 188:1315-1318.

Gail DB, Lenfant CJM. Cells of the lung: Biology and clinical implications. Am Rev Respir Dis 1983; 127:366-387.

Goyal SM. Porcine reproductive and respiratory syndrome. J Vet Diagn Invest 1993; 5:656-664.

Green GM, Jakab GJ, Low RB, Davis GS. Defense mechanisms of the respiratory membrane. Am Rev Respir Dis 1977; 115:479-514.

Griffiths IR. The pathogenesis of equine laryngeal hemiplegia. Equine Vet J 1991; 23:75-76.

Gyles CL, Thoen CO, eds. Pathogenesis of bacterial infections in animals. 2nd ed. Ames: Iowa State University Press, 1993.

Jakab GJ. Viral-bacterial interactions in pulmonary infection. Adv Vet Sci Comp Med 1982; 26:155-171.

Johnson JA, Prescott JF, Markham RJF. The pathology of experimental *Corynebacterium equi* infection in foals following intrabronchial challenge. Vet Pathol 1983; 20:440-449.

Jones GE. Mycoplasmas of sheep and goats: A synopsis. Vet Rec 1983; 113:619-620.

Mehlhaff CJ, Mooney S. Primary pulmonary neoplasia in the dog and cat. Vet Clin North Am Small Anim Pract 1985; 15:1061-1068.

Moulton JE. Tumors of the respiratory system. In: Moulton JE, ed. Tumors in Domestic Animals. 3rd ed. Berkeley: University of California Press, 1990:308.

Norris AM, Laing EJ. Diseases of the nose and sinuses. Vet Clin North Am Small Anim Pract 1985; 15:865-890.

Powell DG. Viral respiratory disease of the horse. Vet Clin North Am Equine Pract 1991; 7:27-52.

Robinson NE. Some functional sequences of species differences in lung anatomy. Adv Vet Sci Comp Med 1982; 26:1-33.

Rosadio RH, Lairmore MD, Russell HI, DeMartini JC. Retrovirus-associated ovine pulmonary carcinoma (sheep pulmonary adenomatosis) and lymphoid interstitial pneumoia. I. Lesion development and age susceptibility. Vet Pathol 1988; 25:475-483.

Sanford SE, Tilker AME. *Streptococcus suis* type II–associated diseases in swine: Observations of one-year study. J Am Vet Med Assoc 1982; 181:673-676.

Sibille Y, Reynolds HY. Macrophages and polymorphonuclear neutrophils in lung defense and injury. Am Rev Respir Dis 1990; 141:471-501.

Slauson DO. The mediation of pulmonary inflammatory injury. Adv Vet Sci Comp Med 1982; 26:99-153.

Slauson DO, Cooper BJ. Mechanisms of Disease: A Textbook of Comparative General Pathology. 2nd ed. Baltimore: Williams & Wilkins, 1990.

Sweeney CR. Exercise-induced pulmonary hemorrhage. Vet Clin North Am Equine Pract 1991; 7:93-103.

Timotey JF, Gillispie JH, Scott FW, Barlough JE. Hagan and Bruner's Microbiology and Infectious Diseases of Domestic Animals. 8th ed. Ithaca: Cornell University Press, 1988.

Yates WDG. A review of infectious bovine rhinotracheitis, shipping fever pneumonia, and viral-bacterial synergism in respiratory disease of cattle. Can J Comp Med 1982; 46:225-263.

Zink MC, Yager JA, Myers JD. Pathogenesis of caprine arthritis encephalitis virus. Am J Pathol 1990; 136:843-954.

CHAPTER

4

Pathology of the Cardiovascular System

JOHN F. VAN VLEET
VICTOR J. FERRANS

HEART

Introduction

Normal morphology

The heart is a conical, muscular organ that in mammals and birds has evolved to form a four-chambered pump with four valves. During early fetal development, the heart is converted from an elongated muscular tube into a C-shaped structure by a process termed looping. Subsequently, septation occurs to produce right and left atrial and ventricular chambers and separation of the common truncus arteriosus into the aorta and pulmonary artery. The heart lies within a fibroelastic sac, the pericardium, that normally contains a small amount of clear, serous fluid. The heart is interposed as a pump into the vascular system, with the right side supplying the pulmonary circulation and the left side the systemic circulation.

The wall of the heart is composed of three layers: the epicardium, the myocardium, and the endocardium. The epicardium, the outermost layer of the heart, is formed by the visceral pericardium, which is continuous at the cardiac base with the parietal pericardium, the fibrous pericardium. The entire surface of the pericardial cavity is covered by mesothelium. The subepicardial layer is attached to the myocardium; it contains a thin layer of fibrous connective tissue; variable, but generally abundant, amounts (in well-nourished animals) of adipose tissue; as well as numerous blood vessels, lymphatic vessels, and nerves (Fig. 4-1).

The myocardium is the prominent muscular layer of the heart. It is composed of cardiac muscle cells (myocytes) arranged in overlapping spiral patterns. These sheets of cells are anchored to the fibrous skeleton of the heart that surrounds the atrioventricular valves and the origins of the aorta and pulmonary artery. The myocardial thickness is related to the pressures present in each chamber; the atria are thin and the ventricles are thicker. The thickness of the left ventricular free wall is approximately threefold greater than that of the right ventricle when measured in a transverse section across the middle of the ventricles, because the pressures are greater in the systemic circulation than in the pulmonary circuit.

The endocardium is the innermost layer of the heart and lines the chambers and extends over projecting structures such as the valves, chordae tendineae, and papillary mus-

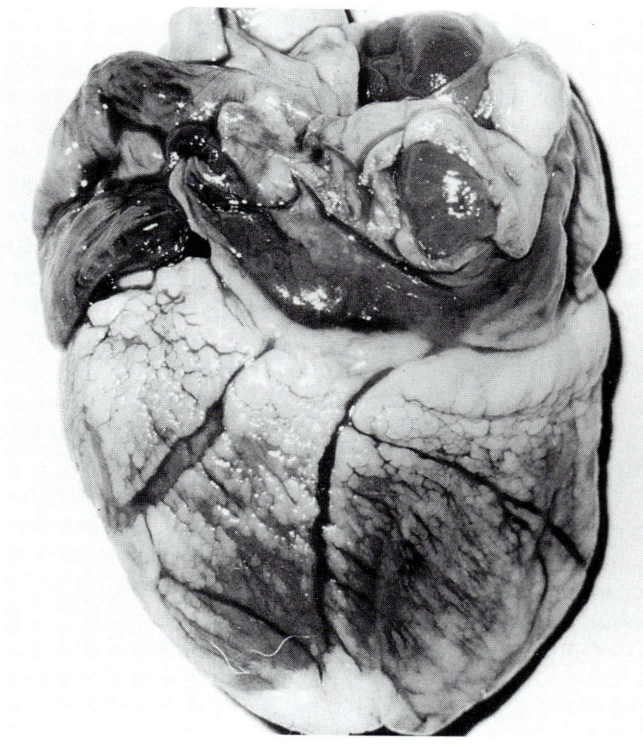

Fig. 4-1 Normal heart; rabbit. Abundant white subepicardial deposits of adipose tissue are present in the ventricular epicardium.

cles. The endocardium of the atria is thicker than that lining the ventricles and normally appears white at gross examination. The surface of the endocardium is lined by endothelium lying on a thin layer of connective tissue; the subendocardial layer contains blood vessels, nerves, and connective tissue. Purkinje fibers are distributed throughout the ventricles in the subendocardium.

The arterial supply to the heart is the left and right coronary arteries, which arise from the aorta at the sinuses of Valsalva behind the left and right cusps of the aortic valves. The arteries radiate over the heart in the subepicardium and give off perforating intramyocardial arteries that supply a rich capillary bed throughout the myocardium. Extensive anastomoses occur between the capillaries that tend to run parallel to the elongated cardiac muscle cells. The ratio of capillaries to muscle cells is approximately 1:1; a fact evident when the fibers are viewed in cross section.

The cardiac conduction system is infrequently examined in animals. Components include (1) the sinoatrial node at the junction of the cranial vena cava and the right atrium, (2) the atrioventricular node and bundle located beneath the septal leaflet of the tricuspid valve and traversing the lower atrial septum onto the upper portion of the muscular ventricular septum, and (3) the right and left bundle branches that descend on each side of the muscular ventricular septum and eventually ramify over the ventricles as the Purkinje fiber network.

Normal features in animal hearts may occasionally be misinterpreted as lesions. The epicardial lymph vessels, especially in cattle, may appear as prominent white streaks that might be interpreted as areas of necrosis. The septal cusp of the tricuspid valve in dogs is normally rather tightly attached to the ventricular septum. In young ruminants, the ductus arteriosus and foramen ovale may be probe-patent, but, unless the openings are large, there was probably no significant shunting of blood during life. The overall shape of normal hearts may vary from the elongated conical profile in the horse to the somewhat rounded shape of the dog. Cardiac weights vary greatly among species, from pigs having relatively small hearts (approximately 0.3% of body weight) to dogs having relatively large hearts (from 0.75% of body weight in nonathletic breeds to 1.25% in athletic breeds).

Postmortem alterations in hearts must be recognized and correctly interpreted. Rigor mortis occurs in myocardium much as in skeletal muscles and produces contracted, rigid ventricular walls, which empties the more powerful left ventricle. Postmortem blood clotting produces red (''currant jelly'') clots in the atria, right ventricle, and large vessels at the base of the heart. Occasionally, pale ''chicken fat'' clots that are poor in erythrocytes form in animals with severe anemia or after prolonged agonal periods. Horses more often have pale clots due to a rapid sedimentation rate. Postmortem inhibition of hemoglobin will produce diffuse red staining of the endocardium and epicardium and simulate the appearance of hemorrhage.

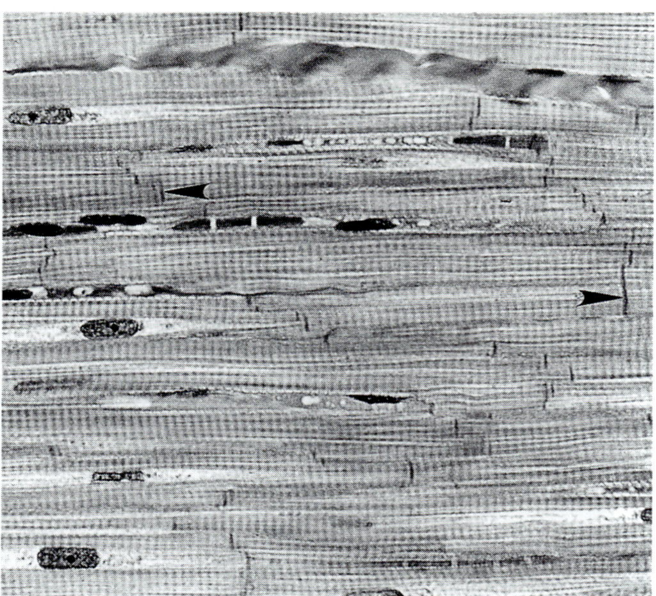

Fig. 4-2 Normal left ventricular myocardium; dog. The longitudinally sectioned myocytes show prominent cross-striations and several intercalated discs *(arrowheads).* Toluidine-blue stained, plastic-embedded section. ×425.

Other potentially misleading findings at necropsy of young dogs and horses include diffuse or patchy myocardial pallor that subsequently fails to correlate with any detectable microscopic alterations. Also, the intracardiac injection of euthanasia solution and other substances can cause hemopericardium and myocardial discoloration at the site of solution deposition.

Cardiac muscle cells are surrounded by interstitial components including blood vessels, lymphatics, nerves, connective tissue cells such as fibroblasts, histiocytes, mast cells, pericytes, and primitive mesenchymal cells and extracellular elements of connective tissue, including collagen fibrils, elastic fibers, connective tissue microfibrils, and acid mucopolysaccharides. Cardiac muscle cells can be divided into two populations: the working myocytes and the specialized fibers of the conduction system. The basic design of the working myocyte is a cross-striated fiber of an irregular cylindrical shape that measures 60 to 100 μm in length and 10 to 20 μm in diameter (Fig. 4-2). Myocytes in young animals are smaller and have small amounts of sarcoplasm. Atrial myocytes are smaller than ventricular myocytes. Adjacent myocytes are joined end-to-end by specialized junctions known as intercalated discs and, less frequently, by side-to-side connections termed lateral junctions. Myocytes have centrally located, elongated nuclei. Multinucleated fibers with nuclei arranged in central rows are frequently seen in growing swine (Fig. 4-3). In old animals, large polyploid nuclei are common. The cytoplasm (sarcoplasm) of myocytes is largely occupied by the contractile proteins that are highly organized into sarco-

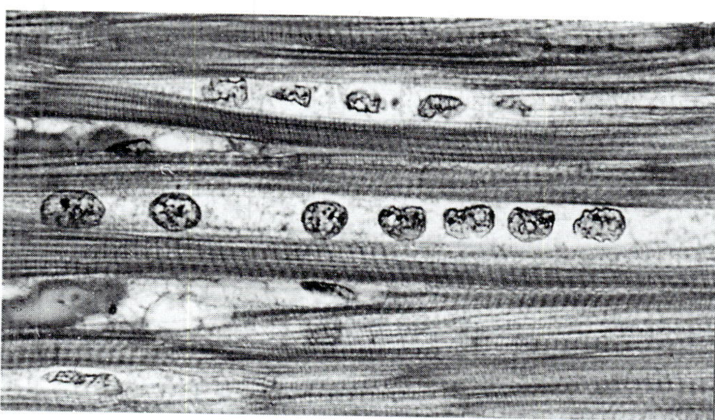

Fig. 4-3 Left ventricular myocardium; normal young pig. Multinucleated myocytes are present. Toluidine-blue stained, plastic-embedded section. ×375.

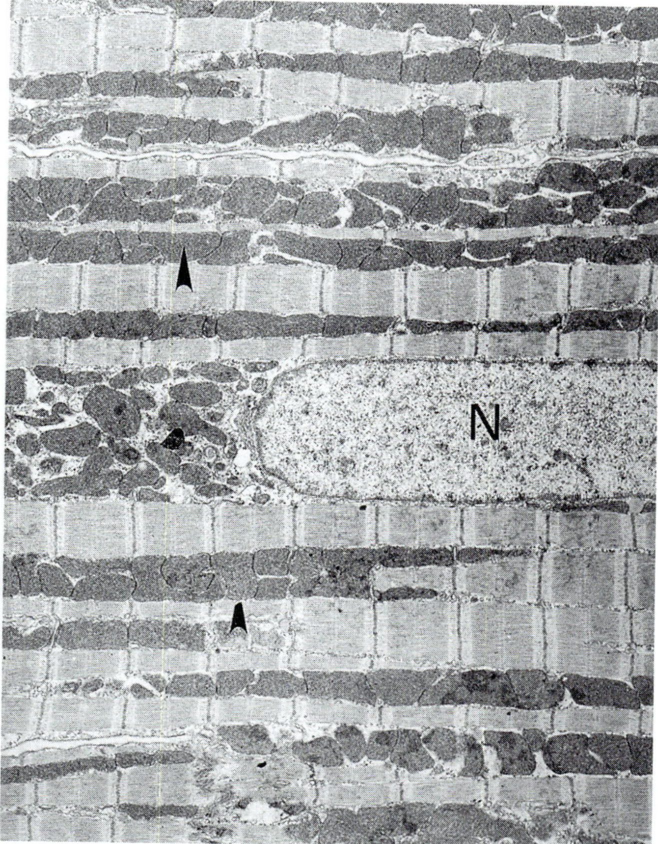

Fig. 4-4 Transmission electron micrograph. Heart, longitudinally sectioned left ventricular myocytes; normal rat. Numerous dense mitochondria *(arrowheads)* lie between myofibrils which have prominent bands. *N*, nucleus. ×8250.

meres. Myofibrils are formed by end-to-end attachment of many sarcomeres. The cross-striated or banded appearance of myocytes is the result of sarcomere organization into A bands containing myosin in the form of "thick" filaments (12 to 16 nm in diameter), I bands containing actin in the form of "thin" filaments (5 to 8 nm in diameter), and dense

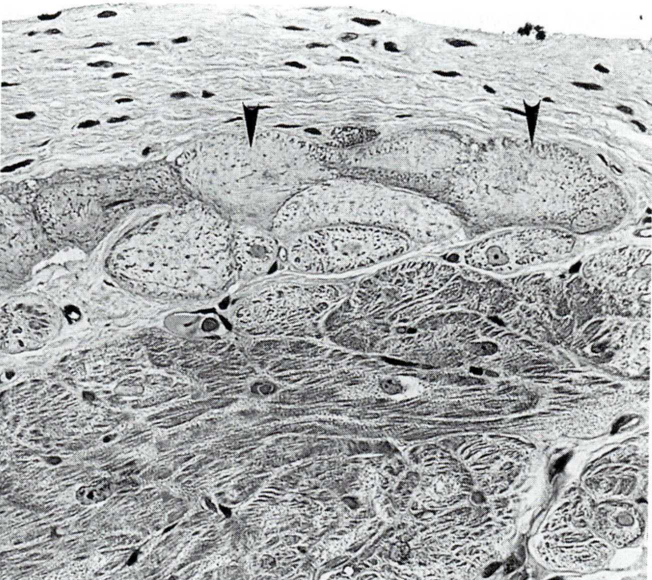

Fig. 4-5 Inner left ventricular wall; normal pig. Note fibrous endocardium *(top),* several large pale Purkinje fibers *(arrowheads),* and underlying contractile myocytes. Toluidine-blue stained, plastic-embedded section. ×530.

Z bands at the ends of sarcomeres. Thick and thin filaments interdigitate and provide the basis for the sliding mechanism of muscle contraction. Myocytes are surrounded by the sarcolemma, which consists of the plasma membrane and the covering basal lamina (external lamina). Other important components of cardiac muscle cells are generally only apparent by electron microscopy and include abundant mitochondria, a highly organized network of intracellular tubules termed the sarcoplasmic reticulum, cylindrical invaginations of the plasma membrane called T tubules, ribosomes, cytoskeletal filaments, glycogen particles, lipid droplets, Golgi complexes, atrial granules, lysosomes, and residual bodies (Fig. 4-4).

The cardiac muscle cells of the specialized conduction tissues, including the sinoatrial node, atrioventricular node, atrioventricular bundle (bundle of His), and bundle branches, have marked variability in morphology at different sites and among animal species, but generally differ from working myocytes by appearing as thin fibers surrounded by abundant fibrous connective tissue stroma and containing only small amounts of contractile material. The Purkinje fibers are distinguished by their large diameters (in large mammals) and abundant pale eosinophilic sarcoplasm rich in glycogen and containing few myofibrils (Fig. 4-5).

Reaction to injury

Cardiac muscle cells respond to injury by a limited spectrum of reactions. Reversible morphologic alterations include cellular growth disturbances that lead to atrophy or hypertrophy (Fig. 4-6). Various sublethal injuries or de-

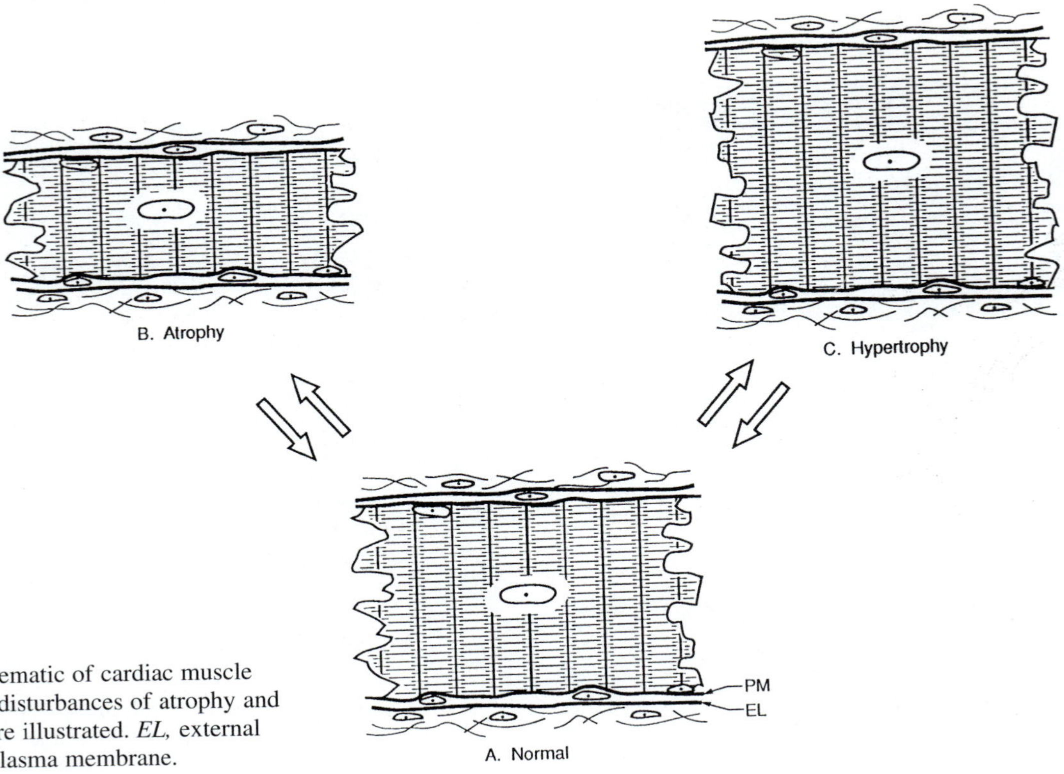

B. Atrophy

C. Hypertrophy

PM

EL

A. Normal

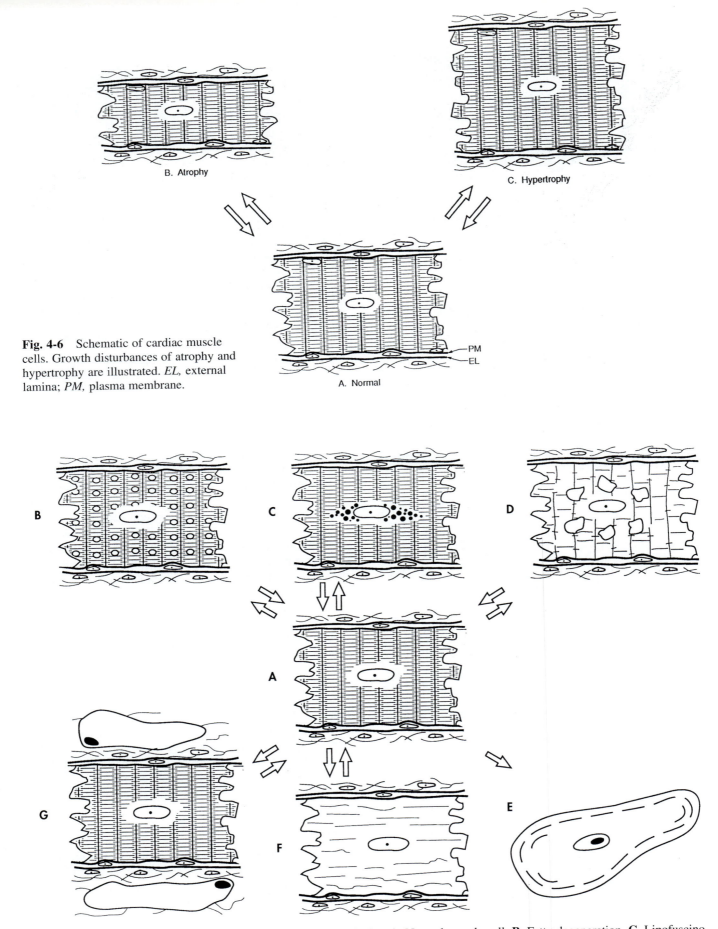

Fig. 4-6 Schematic of cardiac muscle cells. Growth disturbances of atrophy and hypertrophy are illustrated. *EL,* external lamina; *PM,* plasma membrane.

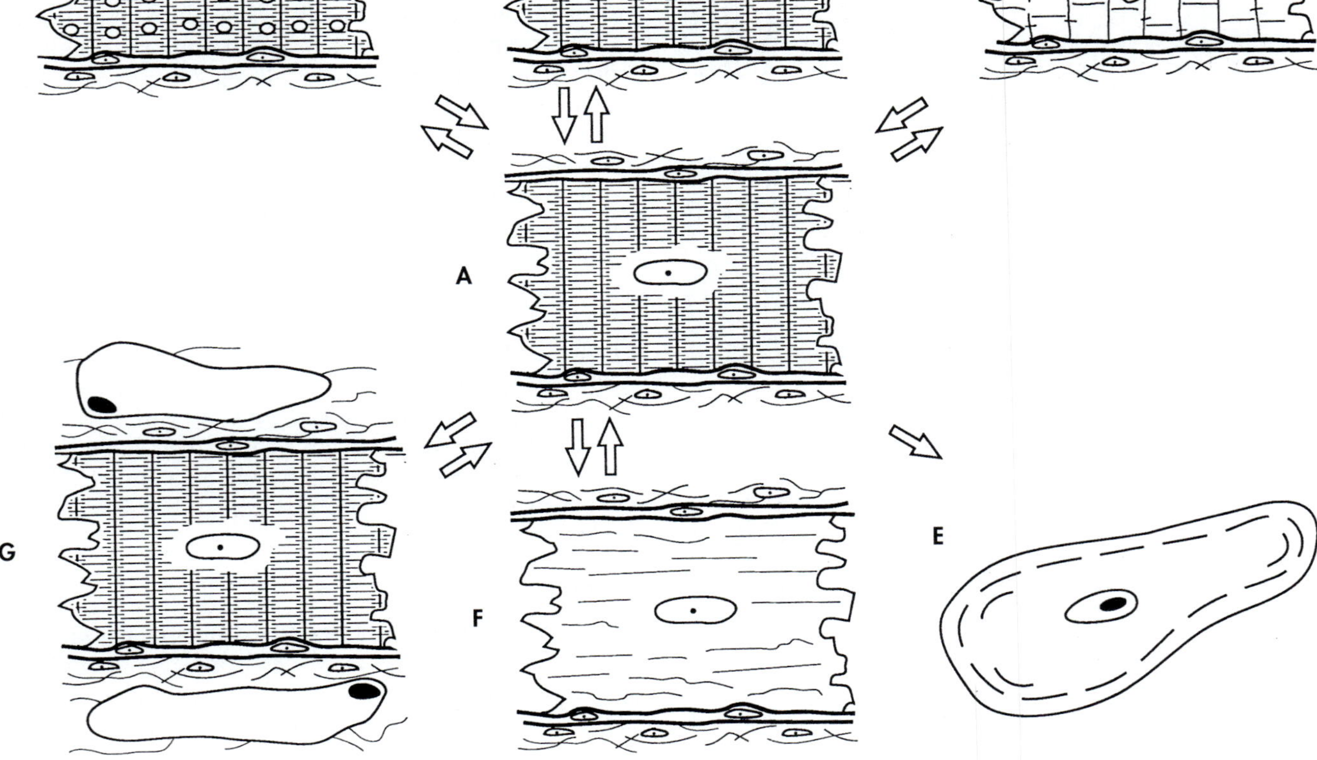

Fig. 4-7 Schematic of various cardiac muscle cell sublethal injuries. **A**, Normal muscle cell. **B**, Fatty degeneration. **C**, Lipofuscinosis. **D**, Vacuolar degeneration. **F**, Myocytolysis. Also illustrated is fatty infiltration of interstitium, **G**, and neoplastic transformation of myocytes, **E**.

generations such as fatty degeneration, lipofuscinosis, vacuolar degeneration, and myocytolysis result in distinctive myocyte alterations (Fig. 4-7). Lethal injury to myocytes results in necrosis (Fig. 4-8).

Necrosis of cardiac muscle cells is generally followed by leukocytic invasion and phagocytosis of sarcoplasmic debris. The end result is persistence of sarcolemmal "tubes" of basal lamina surrounded by condensed interstitial stroma and vessels. In some lesions with severe disruption of the myocardium, the residual effects will be fibroblastic proliferation and collagen deposition to form scar tissue. Regeneration of cardiac muscle cells generally does not occur. Evidence suggests that the continual contraction of intact cardiac muscle cells impairs the opportunity for regeneration of necrotic cells. Rarely, in very young animals and especially in avian hearts, a limited amount of myocyte regeneration will take place. Hyperplasia of myocytes is a normal component of cardiac growth in the first several months of life, but, then, proliferation ceases and then growth is the result of hypertrophy of myocytes until normal cell sizes are reached.

Diagnostic specificity of histopathologic study of the myocardium is substantially limited and only rarely can an etiologic diagnosis be made from the morphologic alterations. This limitation results because the range of pathologic reactions is limited and many damaging agents produce similar lesions. Myocardial necrosis may be confused with myocardial inflammation with secondary necrosis as both lesions have substantial leukocytic infiltration. Animals that die peracutely from cardiac failure may lack detectable microscopic alterations. Hearts with long-standing myocardial damage will have foci of fibrosis, regardless of the cause. Correlation between the severity of clinical cardiac disease and the severity of myocardial injury may be poor—a small lesion in a critical site such as a major portion of the conduction system can be fatal, but a widespread myocardial lesion, such as in myocarditis, may be asymptomatic.

Cardiac pathophysiology

Normal cardiac function results in maintenance of adequate blood flow to the peripheral tissues to provide delivery of oxygen and nutrients, removal of carbon dioxide and

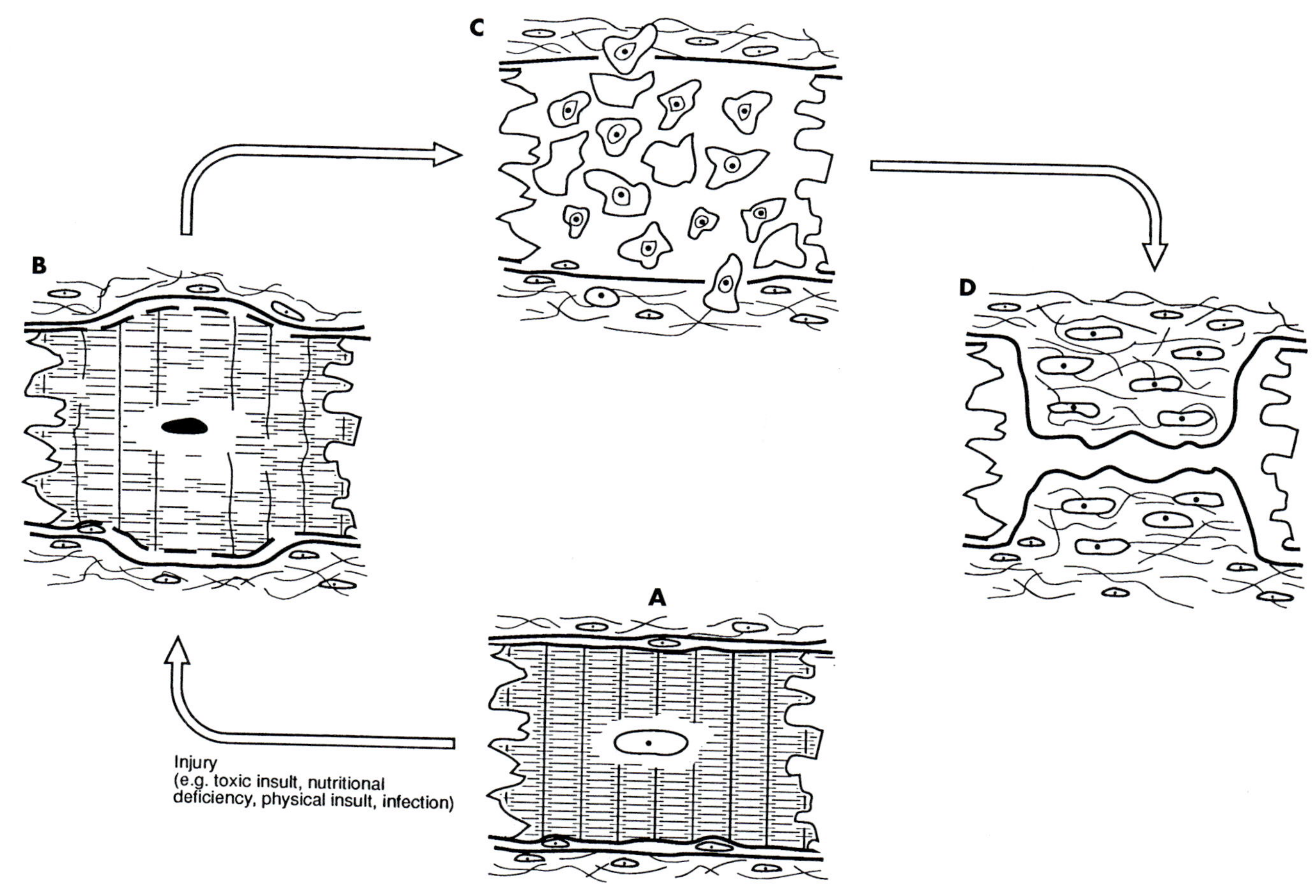

Fig. 4-8 Schematic of the sequential events in myocardial necrosis. **A,** Various injuries lead to **B,** hyaline necrosis of myocyte, **C.** Resolution follows with macrophagic invasion, **D,** and subsequent healing with fibrosis, rather than by regeneration.

other metabolic products, distribution of hormones and other cell regulators, and maintenance of adequate thermoregulation and urine output. The normal heart has a three- to fivefold functional reserve capacity that eventually will be lost with cardiac disease and, subsequently, result in impaired function. A variety of compensatory mechanisms operate in normal and diseased hearts in an attempt to meet both the short-term and long-term demands for adequate cardiac output. These mechanisms include cardiac dilatation, myocardial hypertrophy, increase in heart rate, increase in peripheral resistance, increase in blood volume, and redistribution of blood flow. These compensatory mechanisms may allow maintenance of adequate cardiac output for some time in animals with rather severe cardiac disease that may have compromised cardiac function from loss of myocardial contractility, sustained pressure overload, or sustained volume overload.

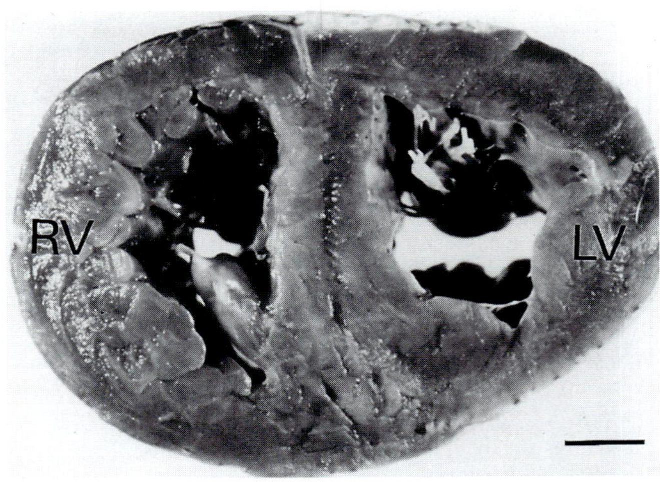

Fig. 4-10 Heart, right ventricular myocardium; dog. Hypertrophy, tetralogy of Fallot. Note similar thickness of the right *(RV)* and left *(LV)* ventricular walls. Bar = 1 cm.

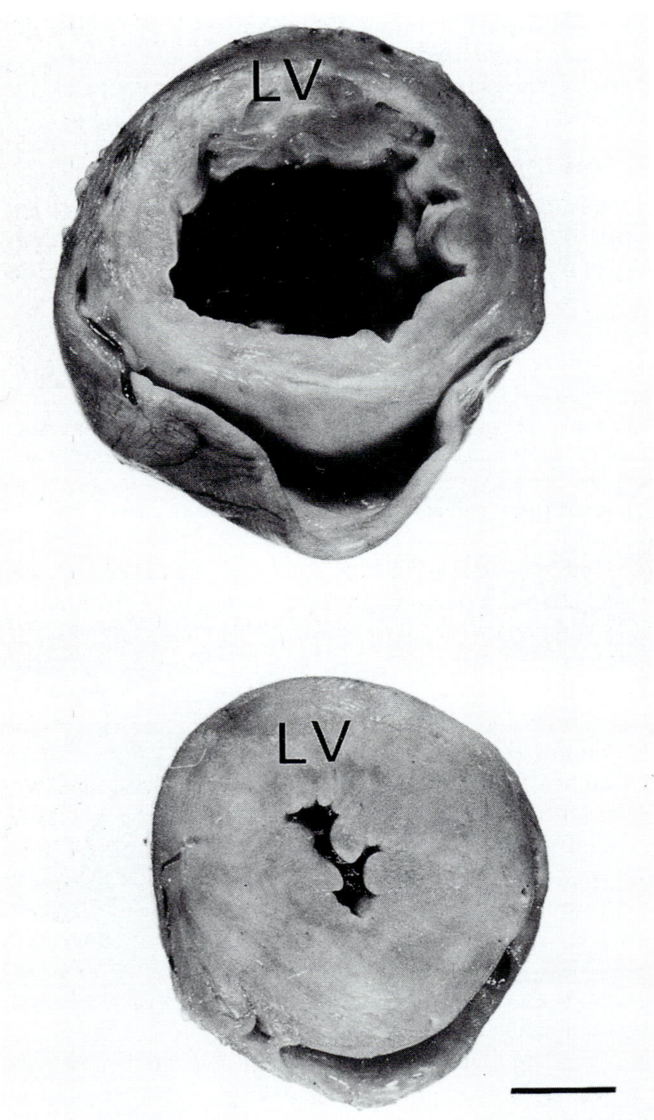

Fig. 4-9 Heart, transected ventricles; turkey poult. Cardiac dilatation, ''round heart disease.'' Note dilated ventricular chambers with thin walls in affected heart *(top)* as compared with those of adjacent normal heart *(bottom). LV,* left ventricular free wall. Bar = 1 cm.

Cardiac dilatation may occur as a terminal lesion in many cardiac diseases (Fig. 4-9). As a compensatory response to achieve increased cardiac output, dilatation allows stretching of cardiac muscle cells to increase contractile force according to the Frank-Starling phenomenon and increased stroke volume is the result. However, stretching beyond certain limits will result in decreased contractile strength.

Myocardial hypertrophy is an important long-term compensatory response of the heart to maintain adequate cardiac output in the face of increased pressure or volume overload (see Myocardial Diseases p. 189) (Fig. 4-10).

Syndromes of cardiac failure or decompensation (Table 4-1)

Cardiac syncope, an acute expression of cardiac disease, is characterized clinically by collapse, loss of consciousness, and extreme change in heart rate and blood pressure, and with or without demonstrable organic lesions. Syncope may develop with massive myocardial necrosis, ventricular fibrillation, heart block, arrhythmias, and reflex cardiac inhibition (e.g., that associated with high intestinal blockage).

Congestive heart failure usually develops slowly from gradual loss of cardiac pumping efficiency associated with

Table 4-1. Experimental models of heart failure*

Experimental technique	Species
Pressure loading	
Pulmonary artery banding	Rat, dog, pig, sheep, pony
Aortic constriction	Rat, rabbit, dog, sheep
Supravalvar aortic constriction	Dog
Aortic valve stenosis	Rabbit, dog
Pulmonary valve stenosis	Dog
Experimental hypertension	Rat, dog
Volume loading	
Fluid overload	Baboon
Aorta-to-vena cava fistula	Rat, dog
Aortic valve incompetence	Rat, rabbit
Atrial septal defect	Cat
Myocardial infarction	
Sustained atrial pacing	Dog
Coronary ligation	Dog, pig
Controlled occlusion-subclavian-to-carotid shunt	Dog
Coronary embolism	Dog, calf, pig
Thrombus generation	Dog
Chronic hypoxia	Rat
Cardiomyopathy and other conditions	
Left ventricular dacron patch	Dog
Spontaneous cardiomyopathy	Hamster, mouse, cow, rat, turkey, cat, dog
Barbiturate overdosage	Dog
Furazolidone cardiomyopathy	Turkey, duckling
Adriamycin cardiomyopathy	Rat, dog, mouse, pig
Isoprenaline	Rat
Noradrenaline	Dog
Amphetamine	Rat
Cobalt chloride	Rat, pig
Vitamin E deficiency	Rat, mouse, calf, lamb
Alcohol intoxication	Rat
Coxsackie viral myocarditis	Mouse
Viral encephalomyocarditis	Mouse

*Modified from Smith HJ, Nuttal A. Cardiovasc Res 1985; 19:181.

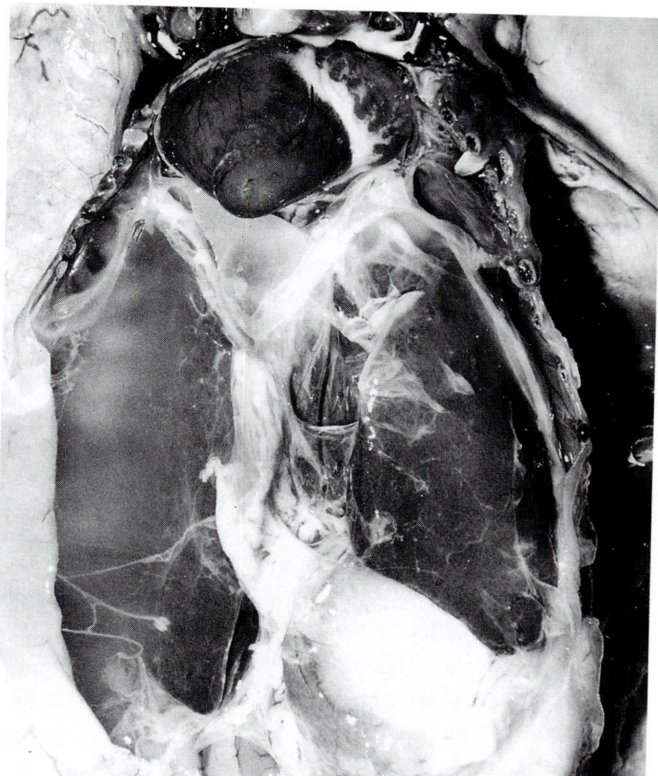

Fig. 4-11 Heart, liver; duckling. Congestive heart failure, furazolidone cardiotoxicity. Note prominent accumulations of serous fluid in the abdomen and fibrin deposits over the liver. The heart *(top)* is dilated.

either pressure or volume overload or myocardial damage (Fig. 4-11). Pathogenetically, congestive heart failure is initiated by development of cardiac disease (myocardial, valvular, congenital, etc.) or increased work load associated with pulmonary, renal, or vascular disease leading to loss of cardiac reserve and development of decreased blood flow to peripheral tissues (forward failure) and accumulation of blood behind the failing chamber (backward failure). Reduced renal blood flow creates hypoxia in the kidneys and increases renin release from the juxtaglomerular apparatus, resulting in stimulation of aldosterone release from the adrenal cortex; sodium and water retention result from the action of aldosterone on the kidneys; and increased plasma volume follows, as does accumulation of edema fluid (mainly in body cavities). Hypoxia also stimulates the marrow to increase erythropoiesis, and, subsequently, polycythemia develops. The increased viscosity of polycythemic blood and the hypervolemia from aldosterone-induced water retention place further work load on the failing heart, and a vicious cycle of cardiac decompensation is initiated which will lead to death from cardiac failure unless therapeutic intervention occurs. Some compensation for increased work load is possible by cardiac dilatation, hypertrophy, and increased heart rate.

Left heart failure is manifested by pulmonary congestion and edema. The most common causes are (1) myocardial contractility loss associated with myocarditis, myocardial necrosis, or cardiomyopathy; (2) dysfunction of the mitral or aortic valves; and (3) several congenital heart diseases.

Chronic right heart failure results in hepatic congestion (''nutmeg liver'') and more severe sodium and water retention than seen with left heart failure. Edema is evident predominantly as ventral subcutaneous edema in horses and ruminants, ascites in dogs, and hydrothorax in cats. Causes of right-sided failure include (1) pulmonary hypertension, (2) cardiomyopathy, and (3) disease of the tricuspid and pulmonary valves.

Diagnostic procedures

The array of diagnostic tools available to the veterinarian to evaluate changes in cases of cardiac disease has grown dramatically in the past decade as many procedures have been adapted from use in human patients. Procedures include physical examination, radiography, electrocardiology, echocardiography, angiocardiography, and cardiac catheterization. Cardiac damage may be detected by increased activity of serum enzymes and isoenzymes, such as creatine phosphokinase, lactate dehydrogenase, and aspartate aminotransferase, that are specifically released from injured cardiac muscle cells. In research studies of cardiac diseases in animals, endomyocardial biopsies have been used to assess the microscopic and ultrastructural alterations during the course of the disease.

Congenital Anomalies

The complex events involved in the embryologic development of the heart and great vessels allow substantial opportunities for the development of congenital anomalies. The functional significance of these anomalies varies widely. Animals with the most extreme defects will be unable to survive in utero, and those with the mildest lesions may have no clinical signs of disease throughout their lives. However, the group of defects with intermediate severity are most likely to be presented to a veterinarian because of gradually developing signs of cardiac failure, including poor exercise tolerance, cyanosis, and stunted body growth. The most frequently observed cardiovascular anomalies in domestic animals are listed in Box 4-1.

The etiologies of congenital cardiovascular anomalies are varied. Most animal species have a low background frequency of spontaneous cardiac malformations. In many species, especially in dogs, these defects are heritable and may be attributed to either single or multiple gene effects. Under experimental conditions, at least, cardiovascular congenital defects may be elicited by exposure of pregnant dams to various chemicals and drugs, physical agents, or nutritional deficiencies and toxicities. Implicated chemical compounds include thalidomide, ethanol, salicylates, griseofulvin, and cortisone. Prenatal exposure to x-irradiation or fetal hypoxia may induce defects. Maternal nutritional deficiencies of vitamin A, pantothenic acid, riboflavin, or zinc and feeding excesses of vitamin A, retinoic acid, or copper may result in newborn with cardiovascular anomalies.

Box 4-1 MOST COMMON CARDIOVASCULAR ANOMALIES IN SEVERAL DOMESTIC ANIMAL SPECIES

Dog
Patent ductus arteriosus, pulmonic stenosis, subaortic stenosis, persistent right aortic arch

Cat
Endocardial cushion defects, mitral malformation

Cow
Atrial septal defect, ventricular septal defect, transposition of aorta and pulmonary artery, valvular hematomas

Pig
Subaortic stenosis, endocardial cushion defect

Anomalies from failure of closure of fetal cardiovascular shunts

Patent ductus arteriosus is a frequent anomaly in poodle, collie, and Pomeranian dogs (Fig. 4-12). In poodles, it is an inherited lesion. This vascular channel between the pulmonary artery and aorta allows blood to bypass the lungs during fetal life and is normally converted to the solid ligamentum arteriosum postnatally, but remains patent with this anomaly. Generally, blood will shunt from left to right ventricle with resulting pulmonary hypertension.

An **atrial septal defect** may represent failure of closure of the foramen ovale, a fetal interatrial septal shunt that allows blood to bypass the lungs of the fetus, or it may be the result of true septal defects from faulty development of the septum (Fig. 4-13).

A **ventricular septal defect** indicates failure of complete development of the ventricular septum and will allow shunting of blood between the ventricular cavities (Fig. 4-14). The defect occurs in many species and develops more commonly in the upper, membranous portion of the septum rather than in the lower, muscular septum.

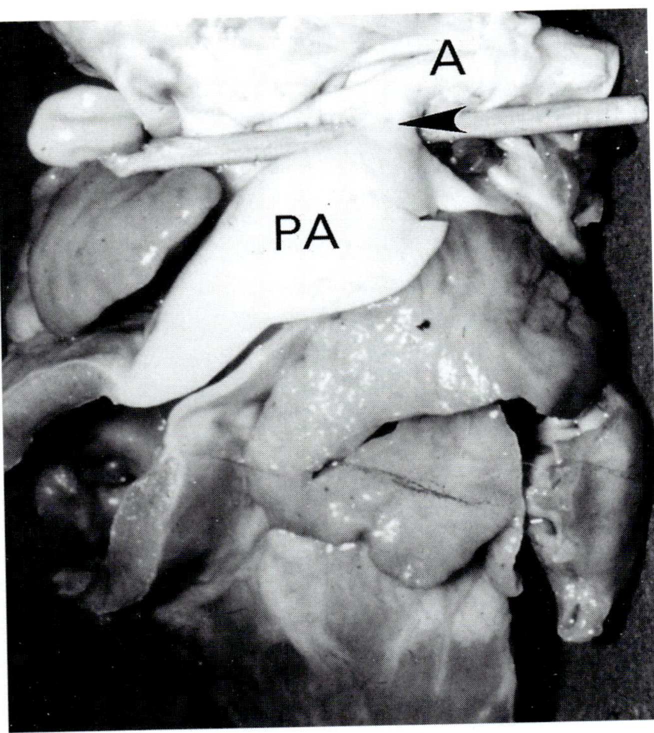

Fig. 4-12 Heart; pig. Patent ductus arteriosus. Note the prominent ductus *(arrowhead)* between the pulmonary artery *(PA)* and aorta *(A)*.

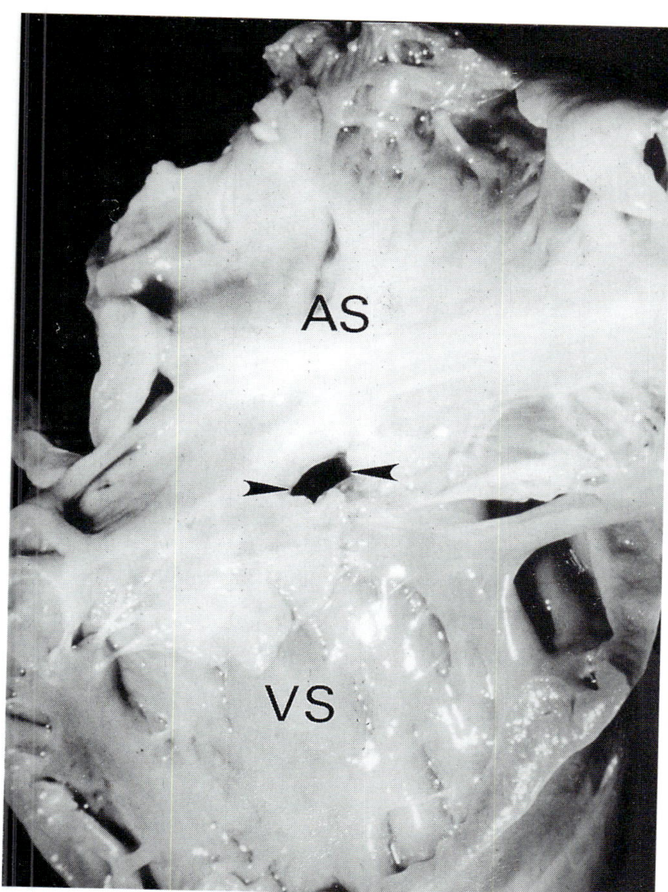

Fig. 4-13 Heart, opened right side; pig. Atrial septal defect. There is a prominent opening *(arrowheads)* low in the atrial septum *(AS)*. *VS,* ventricular septum.

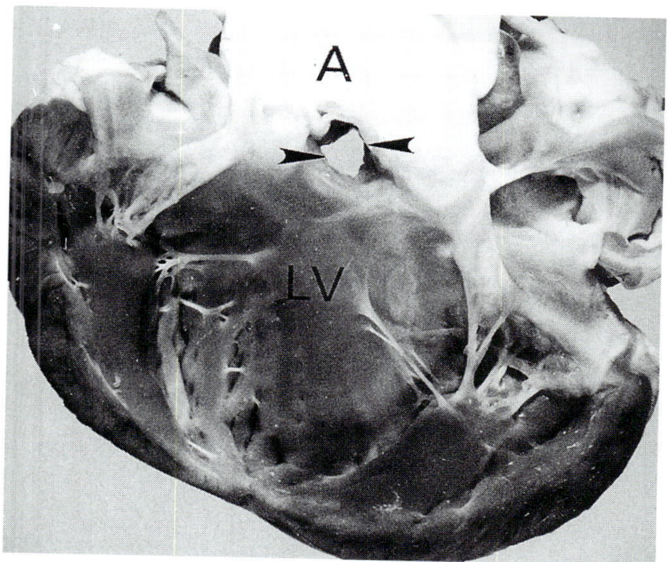

Fig. 4-14 Heart, left side; dog. Ventricular septal defect. Note the large opening in the basal portion of the septum *(arrowheads)*. *LV,* left ventricle; *A,* aorta.

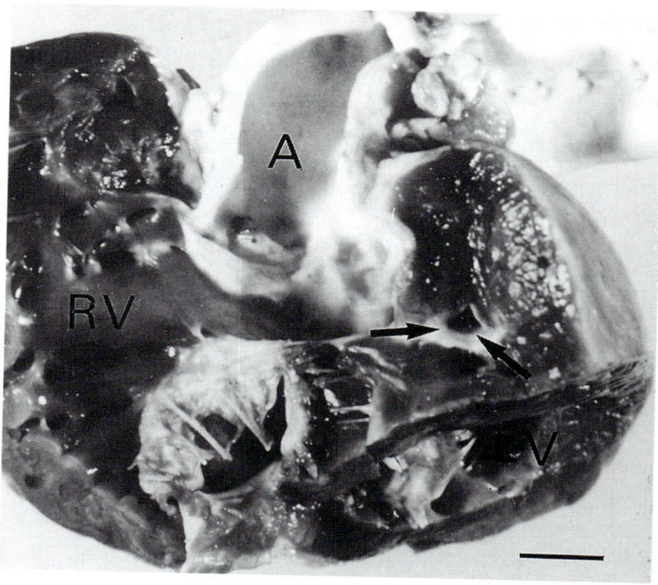

Fig. 4-15 Heart, dissected; dog. Tetralogy of Fallot. This large basal ventricular septal defect has an overlying, straddling aorta (*A*) and severe pulmonic stenosis *(arrowheads)* with massive right ventricular hypertrophy. *RV,* right ventricle; *LV,* left ventricle. Bar = 1 cm.

The **tetralogy of Fallot** is a complicated cardiac anomaly with four lesions (Fig. 4-15). The three primary defects are a ventricular septal defect located high in the septum, pulmonic stenosis (see below), and dextroposition of the aorta (see below). The fourth defect, which develops secondarily, is hypertrophy of the right ventricular myocardium. This complex anomaly is inherited in Keeshond dogs; it often is associated with cyanosis and is one of the most common cardiac anomalies of human beings (so-called blue babies). By genetic and pathologic studies in Keeshond dogs, the basic defect has been determined to be hypoplasia and malpositioning of the conotruncal septum. Wide variability in the development of lesions occurs from case to case.

Anomalies from failure of normal valvular development

Pulmonic stenosis has been recognized as a frequent anomaly in dogs and is inherited in beagles, English bulldogs, and Chihuahuas (Fig. 4-16). Several types of valvular lesions have been described and include formation of a band of fibrous and/or muscular tissue proximal to the valve (subvalvular stenosis) or malformation of the valve (valvular stenosis), with a small central orifice in a dome of thickened valvular tissue. Marked concentric hypertrophy of the right ventricle will develop from the resulting pressure overload.

Subaortic stenosis is a frequent cardiac anomaly of swine and dogs; it apparently is inherited in Newfoundland, boxer, and German shepherd dogs (Fig. 4-17). The stenosis is produced by the presence of a thick zone of

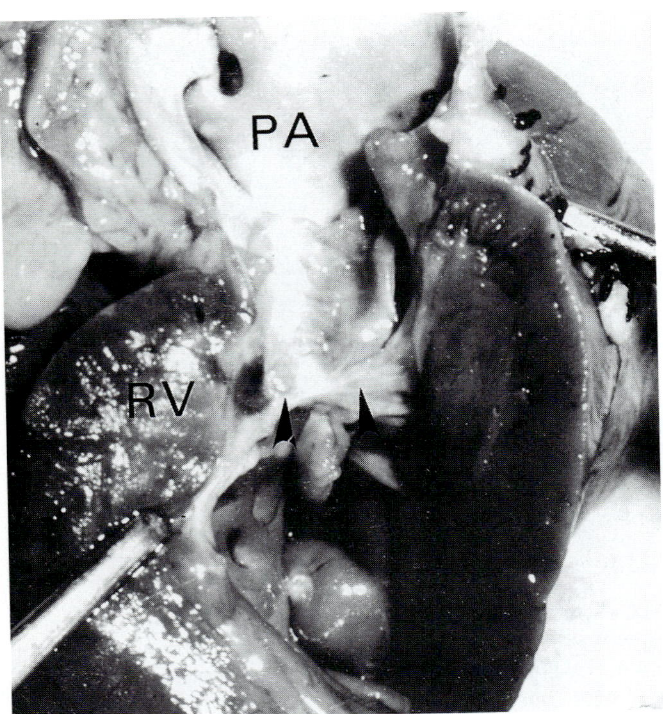

Fig. 4-16 Heart; dog. Pulmonic stenosis. Note the prominent right ventricular *(RV)* hypertrophy and white, thick mass of fibrous connective tissue *(arrowheads)* lining the outflow tract beneath the pulmonary valve. The pulmonary artery *(PA)* is dilated above the stenotic valve.

endocardial fibrous tissue that encircles the left ventricular outflow tract below the valve. Microscopically, the altered endocardial tissue may contain proliferated mesenchymal cells, mucinous ground substance, and foci of cartilaginous metaplasia. Other cardiac lesions develop secondarily to the altered left ventricular outflow, and these include left ventricular concentric hypertrophy, disseminated foci of myocardial necrosis and fibrosis in the inner left ventricular wall, and thickening of the walls of intramyocardial arteries.

Valvular hematomas (hematocysts) are frequently observed on the atrioventricular valves of young ruminants (Fig. 4-18). These lesions, which generally regress spontaneously by several months of age and do not produce any functional abnormalities, are bulging, blood-filled cysts, several millimeters in diameter, on the margins of the atrioventricular valves.

Other valvular developmental anomalies include **endocardial cushion defects** (persistent atrioventricular canal) in pigs and cats, **mitral malformation** in cats, and **tricuspid dysplasia** in cats.

Anomalies from malpositioning of great vessels

Persistent right aortic arch occurs in dogs; German shepherd and Irish setter dogs are predisposed (Fig. 4-19).

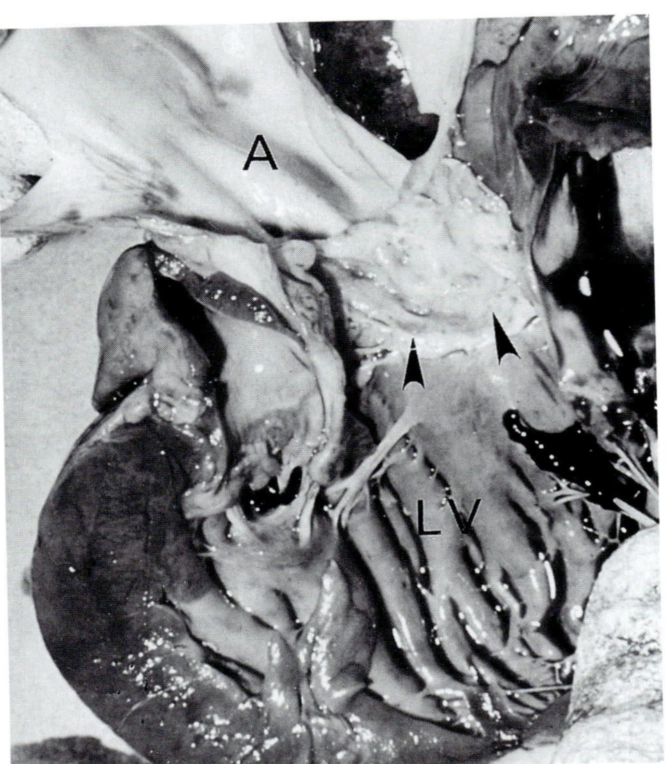

Fig. 4-17 Heart, opened left side; dog. Subaortic stenosis. A thick, white, broad band of fibrous connective tissue *(arrowheads)* lies along the left ventricular outflow tract below the aortic valve (*A*, aorta). Left ventricular hypertrophy is evident by the thick wall and prominent muscular trabeculae. *LV,* left ventricle.

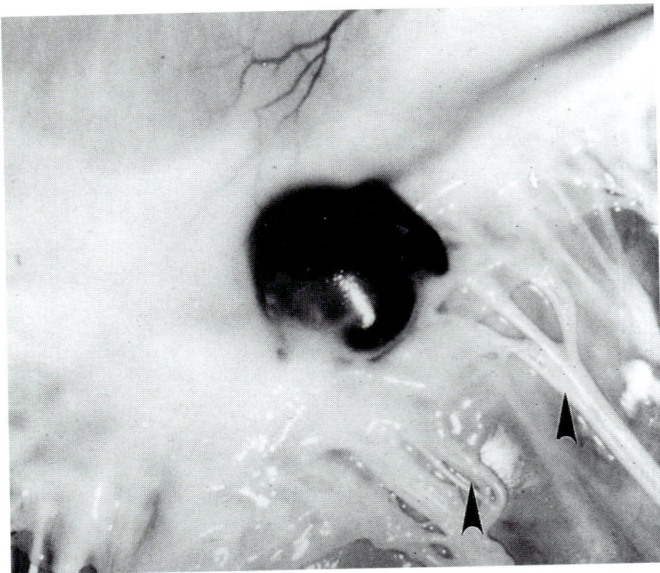

Fig. 4-18 Heart, opened left side; calf. Valvular hematoma. A dark, blood-filled cyst is on a cusp of the mitral valve. Chordae tendinae *(arrowheads)* are present.

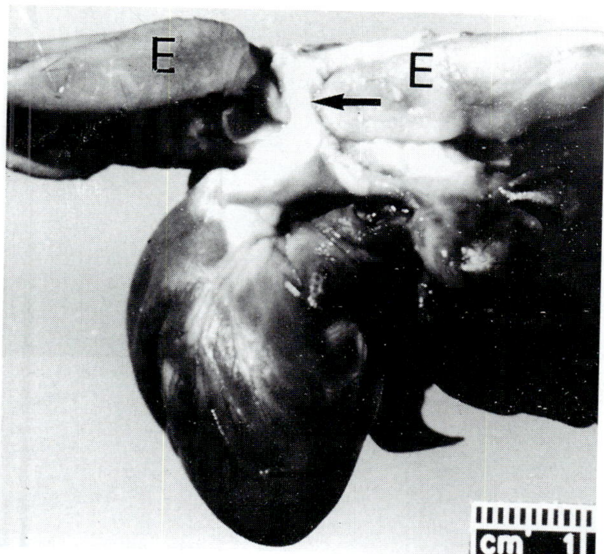

Fig. 4-19 Heart, esophagus; dog. Persistent right aortic arch. Vascular ring *(arrowheads)* overlies the esophagus (*E*), which is dilated proximally, and the trachea.

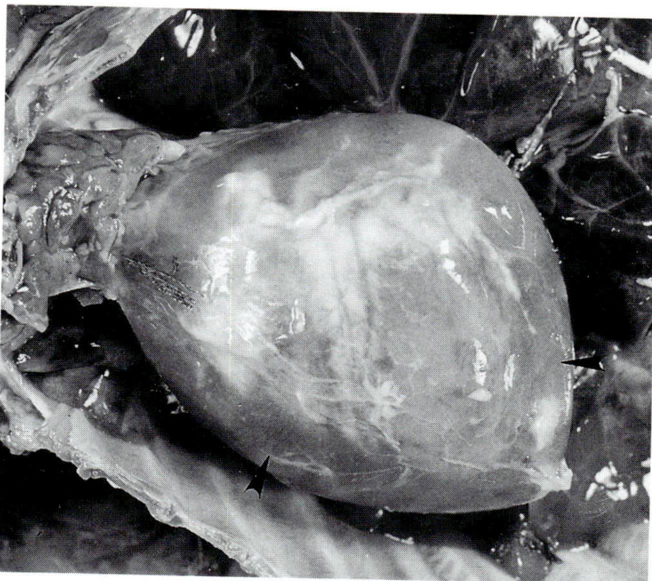

Fig. 4-20 Pericardial sac (opened), rib cage *(bottom)*, hydropericardium; pig. "Mulberry heart disease." The thin-walled pericardial sac *(arrowheads)* is distended by serous fluid that has a few clumps of fibrin.

This defect arises because the right fourth aortic arch, rather than the left, develops and ascends on the right side of the midline and results in the ligamentum arteriosum forming a vascular ring over the esophagus and trachea. This arrangement will eventually result in esophageal obstruction and proximal dilatation (megaesophagus) as the animal matures and consumes solid feed.

Transposition of the aorta and pulmonary artery are severe anomalies that occur as several types.

Other cardiac anomalies

Ectopia cordis is the congenital development of the heart at an abnormal site outside of the thoracic cavity. In cattle, cases in healthy adult animals have been described where the heart was located in the caudoventral neck area.

Endocardial fibroelastosis in animals has been best recognized as a primary cardiac defect in Burmese cats. The heritable disease leads to prominent, white, thickened endocardium, especially of the left ventricle, from proliferation of fibroelastic tissue.

Pericardial Diseases

Noninflammatory fluid accumulations in the pericardial sac

Hydropericardium is the accumulation of clear to light yellow, watery, serous fluid in the pericardial sac, which becomes distended. In cases associated with vascular injury, such as "mulberry heart disease" or dietary microangiopathy of swine, a few fibrin strands are present, and the fluid may clot following exposure to air (Fig. 4-20). The exposed pericardial surfaces are smooth and glistening in cases with sudden onset, but, in long-standing cases, the epicardium may become opaque from mild fibrous thickening and may appear roughened and granular from villous proliferation, especially over the atria and great vessels.

Hydropericardium occurs in those diseases that have generalized edema. Thus, ascites and hydrothorax often occur concurrently with hydropericardium. Congestive heart failure is an important mechanism of hydropericardium and is usually due to primary myocardial, valvular, congenital, or neoplastic diseases. Common specific diseases include dilated cardiomyopathy of dogs and cats and "ascites syndrome" of poultry. Hydropericardium may also accompany pulmonary hypertension (e.g., "brisket disease" or "high altitude disease" of cattle), renal failure, and hypoproteinemia from various chronic debilitating diseases. Hydropericardium may also occur in various systemic diseases with vascular injury such as "mulberry heart disease" and septicemia in swine, "heartwater" (*Cowdria ruminantium* infection) in small ruminants, African horse sickness, and bovine ephemeral fever.

Hydropericardium of rapid onset leads to development of cardiac tamponade or compression, which interfere with cardiac filling (especially of the atria) and venous return to the heart. In cases with slow development, stretching of the pericardium allows accumulation of large volumes of fluid without tamponade. Hydropericardium may be reversible if the underlying initiating cause is removed, but many cases are associated with progressive cardiac diseases, and death is the outcome.

Hemorrhagic pericardial effusion of unknown etiology is seen in dogs. Similar effusions may occur in dogs with cardiac hemangiosarcomas and heart base tumors, common cardiac neoplasms in this species.

Hemopericardium is accumulation of whole blood in the pericardial sac. Death often occurs suddenly from cardiac tamponade. Bleeding may be the result of spontaneous atrial rupture in dogs or rupture of the intrapericardial aorta in horses or be a complication of intracardiac injections.

Metabolic alterations

Serous atrophy of fat is readily detected by the gray gelatinous appearance of epicardial fat deposits (Fig. 4-21). Microscopically, lipocytes are atrophic, and edema involves interstitial tissues. Healthy animals normally have abundant white to yellow epicardial fat deposits, especially along the atrioventricular junction. Serous atrophy of epicardial fat occurs rapidly from mobilization of fat following anorexia, starvation, or cachexia.

Epicardial mineralization (cardiac calcinosis) is a striking lesion of certain inbred strains of mice (Fig. 4-22). The inherited disorder may lead to formation of white, firm, mineralized plaques, especially over the right ventricular epicardium. The lesion, arising by dystrophic calcification, does not tend to cause cardiac dysfunction.

Urate deposits in the pericardium may occur in birds and snakes with visceral gout. The affected serosal surface appears thickened and white, as though covered by plaster of Paris.

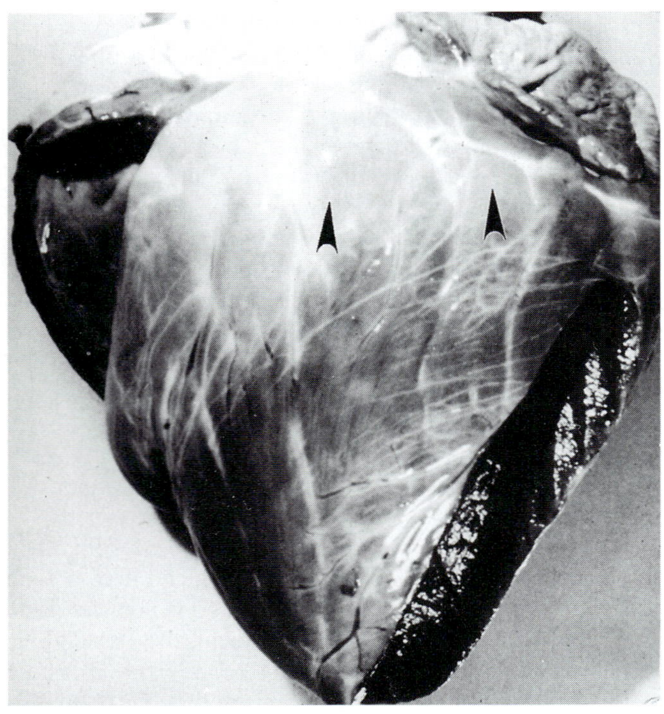

Fig. 4-21 Heart, myocardium; cow. Serous atrophy of fat and brown atrophy of myocardium. The epicardial fat deposits appear gray and gelatinous *(arrowheads),* and the incised myocardium is dark brown due to deposits of lipofuscin in myocytes.

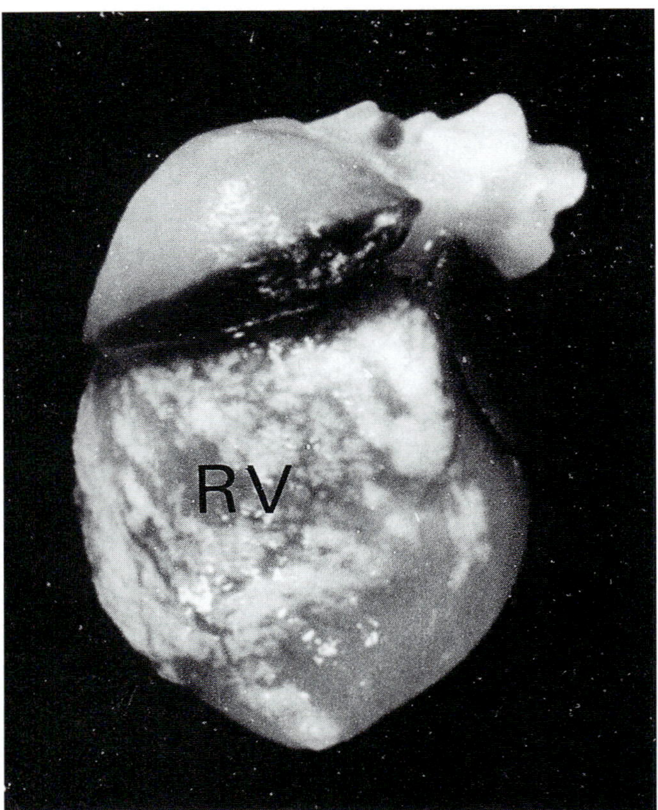

Fig. 4-22 Heart, right ventricle; mouse. Epicardial calcification. Note the prominent white mineralized deposits over the right ventricle *(RV).*

Inflammation

Fibrinous pericarditis, the most common type of pericardial inflammation in animals, is usually the result of hematogenous infection. Specific diseases with this lesion include, cows—pasteurellosis, blackleg, coliform septicemias, and sporadic bovine encephalomyelitis; pigs—Glasser's disease, streptococcal infections, pasteurellosis, enzootic mycoplasmal pneumonia, and salmonellosis; horses—streptococcal infections; birds—psittacosis. Grossly, the pericardial surfaces are covered by variable amounts of yellow fibrin deposits that result in adherence between the parietal and visceral layers. When the pericardial sac is laid open at necropsy, these attachments are torn away (so-called bread-and-butter heart) (Fig. 4-23). Microscopically, an eosinophilic layer of fibrin with admixed neutrophils lies over the congested pericardium.

The outcome of fibrinous pericarditis varies. Early death is frequent because many of these lesions result from in-

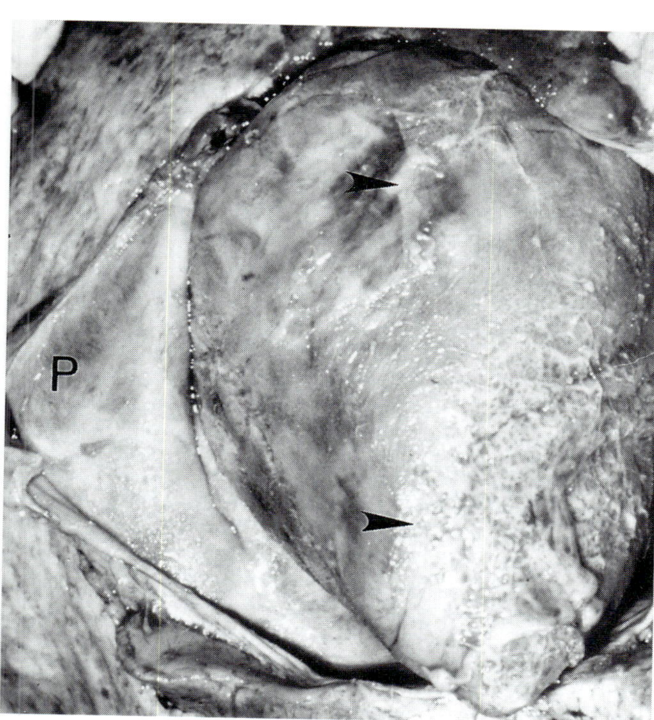

Fig. 4-23 Heart, epicardium; horse. Fibrinous pericarditis. The epicardium is covered by a thick, yellow layer of fibrin *(arrowheads). P*, reflected pericardium.

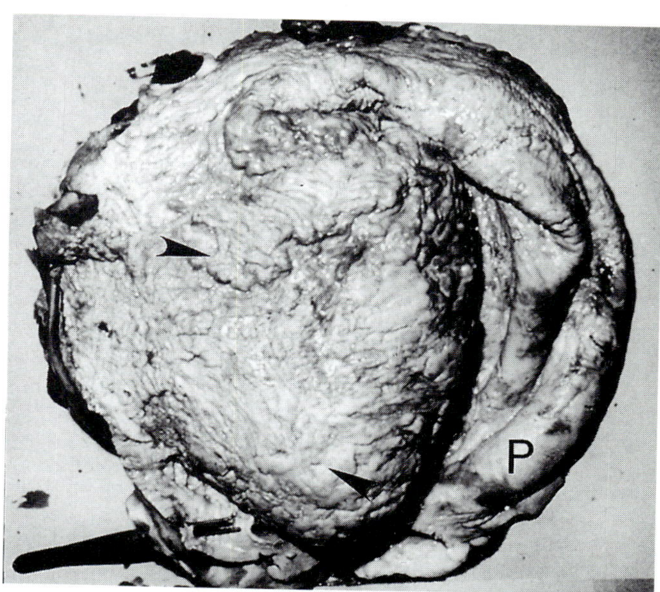

Fig. 4-24 Heart, pericardium; cow. Suppurative pericarditis, traumatic reticuloperitonitis (''hardware disease''). The exposed pericardial surface is markedly thickened by fibrous connective tissue and is covered by shaggy, white masses of fibrinopurulent exudate *(arrowheads). P*, reflected pericardium.

fection by highly virulent bacteria and concurrent septicemia. Survival is prolonged in some cases with formation of fibrous adhesions between the pericardial surfaces from fibrous organization of the exudate.

Suppurative pericarditis is seen mainly in cattle as a complication of traumatic reticuloperitonitis (''hardware disease''). Foreign bodies, such as nails or pieces of wire that accumulate in the reticulum, may occasionally penetrate the abomasum, diaphragm, and adjacent pericardial sac and introduce infection. Affected cattle may survive for weeks to months until death ensues from congestive heart failure and septicemia. Grossly, the pericardial surfaces are markedly thickened by white, often rough, shaggy-appearing masses of fibrous connective tissue with an accumulation of white to gray, thick, foul-smelling, purulent exudate in the pericardial sac (Fig. 4-24).

Constrictive pericarditis is a chronic inflammatory lesion of the pericardium accompanied by extensive fibrous proliferation and eventual formation of fibrous adhesions across the pericardial space. Severe lesions may result in obliteration of the pericardial sac and constriction of the heart by fibrous tissue to the point of interference with cardiac filling. Compensatory myocardial hypertrophy may result in diminished chamber volumes and further contribute to the eventual development of congestive cardiac failure.

Endocardial Diseases

Degeneration

Endocardial mineralization and **endocardial fibrosis** may be single lesions or occur together. Mineralization occurs with vitamin D toxicosis and from intoxication by calcinogenic plants that contain vitamin D analogs *(Cestrum diurnum, Tristetum flavescens, Solanum malacoxylon, Solanum torvum).* These plant-induced syndromes of cattle have been called by various names in various areas of the world, including ''Manchester wasting disease'' in Jamaica, ''enzootic calcinosis'' in Europe, ''naahelu disease'' in Hawaii, ''enteque seco'' in Argentina and ''espichamento'' in Brazil. Multiple, large, white, rough, firm plaques from mineralization of fibroelastic tissue are present in the endocardium and on the intima of large elastic arteries. Fibrosis, with or without mineralization, may occur in chronically dilated hearts, in debilitated cattle with Johne's disease (Fig. 4-25), in dogs with healed lesions of left atrial ulcerative endocarditis associated with a prior uremic episode, and in so-called jet lesions produced in response to trauma by refluxed blood in valvular insufficiencies.

Valvular endocardiosis is an important age-related cardiac disease of old dogs. Other names for this disease include valvular fibrosis and myxomatous or mucoid valvular degeneration. This disease, the most common cause of congestive heart failure in old dogs, may also have genetic influences as males of certain breeds are most frequently affected. Lesions are most frequent on the mitral valve, less common on the tricuspid, and infrequent on the

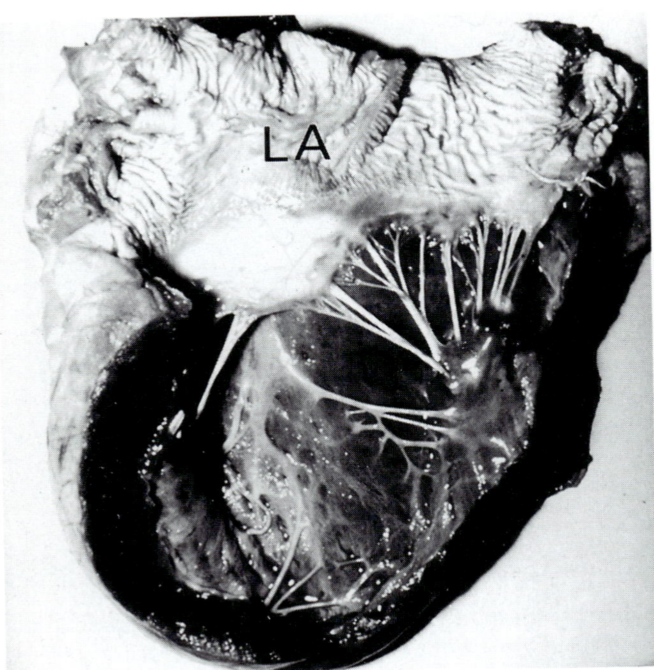

Fig. 4-25 Heart, left atrial endocardium; cow. Endocardial mineralization, Johne's disease. The left atrial *(LA)* endocardium is white, thick, and wrinkled.

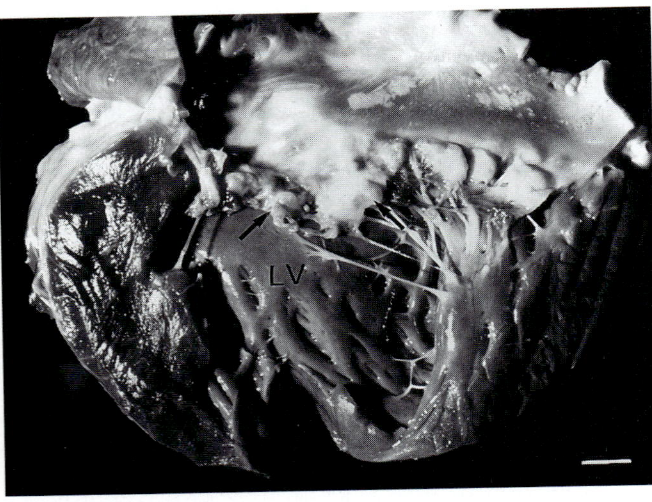

Fig. 4-26 Heart, left ventricle; dog. Valvular endocardiosis. The affected cusps of the mitral valve are thickened by white, smooth, fibrotic nodules *(arrowheads)*. *LV,* left ventricle. Bar = 1 cm. *Courtesy Dr. M.D. McGavin.*

aortic and pulmonary valves. Affected valves are shortened and thick, either diffusely or nodular, and appear smooth rather than rough, as is usual in cases of valvular endocarditis (Fig. 4-26). These lesions result in valvular insufficiency with subsequent atrial dilatation and ''jet lesions.'' Other complications include occasional rupture of the chordae tendineae and occasional splitting or rupture of the left atrial wall. Microscopically, the thickened valves have markedly increased fibroblastic proliferation and deposition of acid mucopolysaccharides. Frequent accompanying myocardial alterations include arteriosclerosis of intramyocardial arteries and multifocal myocardial necrosis and fibrosis.

Circulatory disturbances

Atrial thrombosis is a frequent finding in aged Syrian hamsters and in certain strains of mice and may be present in the failing hearts of dogs and cats with idiopathic cardiomyopathies. In affected hamsters and mice, the atria are swollen, firm, mottled and contain gray to tan, laminated masses of fibrin. Fibroblastic organization occurs rapidly in the thrombi. Etiologic factors include aging and genetic and dietary influences. Susceptible strains fed a thrombogenic diet (high fat, low protein, and hypolipotropic) have a high incidence of atrial thrombosis.

Inflammation

Endocarditis is usually the result of bacterial infections, except for lesions produced by migrating *Strongylus vulgaris* larvae in horses and an occasional instance of mycotic infection. The lesions are generally very large by the time of death and are present on the valves (valvular endocarditis), although some lesions may extend to the adjacent wall (mural endocarditis). Grossly, the affected valves have large, adhering, friable, yellow to gray masses termed ''vegetations'' that may largely occlude the valvular orifice (Fig. 4-27). In chronic lesions, the fibrin deposits are organized by fibrous connective tissue to produce irregular nodular masses termed ''verrucae'' (wartlike lesions). Microscopically, the lesion consists of accumulated layers of fibrin and numerous embedded bacterial colonies underlain by a zone of infiltrated leukocytes and granulation tissue (Fig. 4-28). Relative frequency of valvular involvement with endocarditis in animals is mitral > aortic > tricuspid > pulmonary.

The pathogenesis of endocarditis is complicated and frequently incompletely understood. Affected animals generally have preexisting extracardiac infections that have resulted in one or more bouts of bacteremia. Focal endothelial disruption on the surface of the normally avascular valves allows bacterial adherence and proliferation and initiation of the inflammatory reaction with subsequent deposition of masses of fibrin. Agents frequently recovered from the lesions are *Actinomyces pyogenes* in cattle and *Streptococcus* spp. and *Erysipelothrix rhusiopathiae* in pigs. Death is the result of cardiac failure from valvular dysfunction along with the effects of bacteremia. Some cases will have septic embolization of various organs such as the heart and kidneys.

Ulcerative endocarditis of the left atrium is a distinctive lesion associated with acute renal insufficiency in dogs. Grossly, after healing of the initial ulceration, the area is replaced by raised, white plaques of fibrous and mineralized tissue.

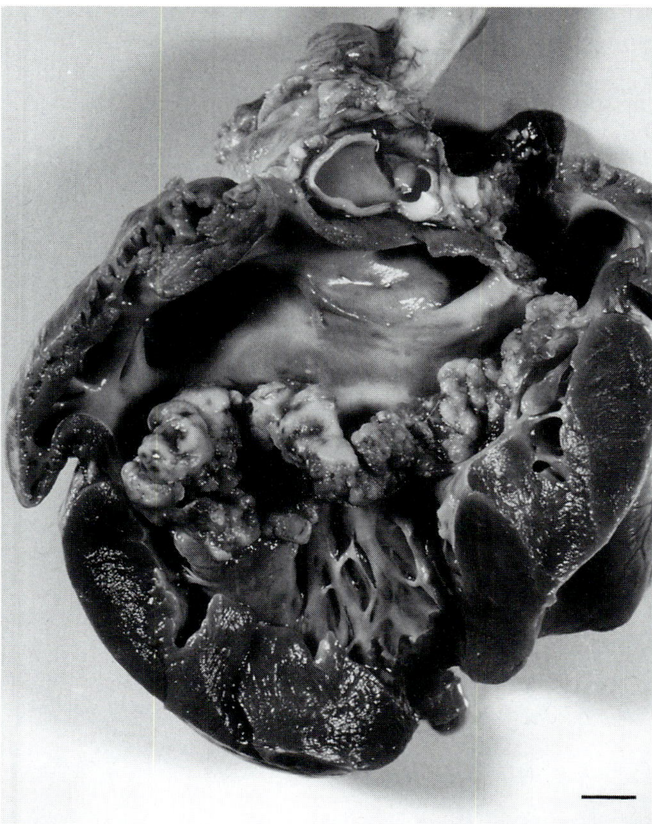

Fig. 4-27 Heart, mitral valve; pig. Vegetative valvular endocarditis, streptococcal infection. Multiple, large, raised, friable, yellowish-red thrombotic masses are attached to the affected mitral valve. Bar = 1 cm. *Courtesy Dr. M.D. McGavin.*

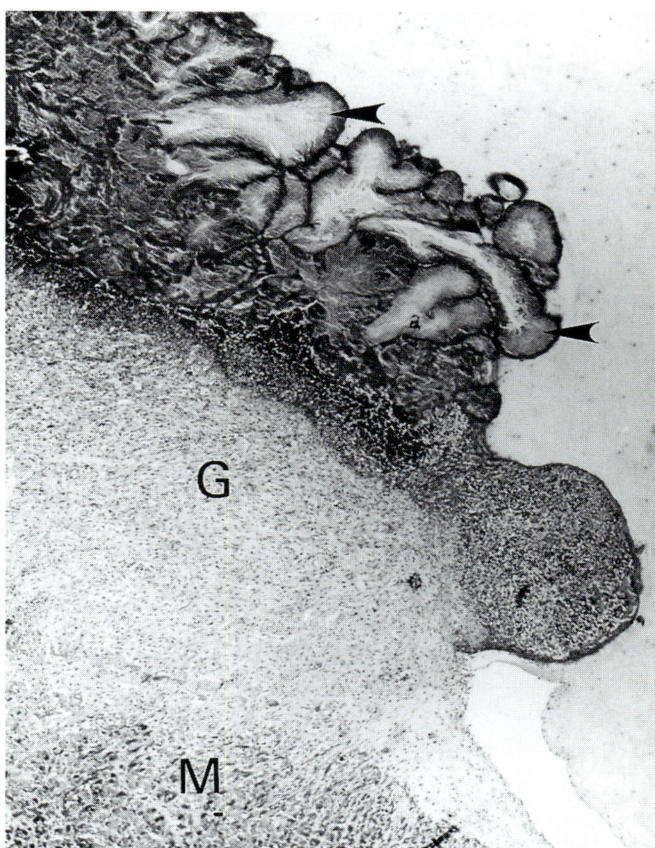

Fig. 4-28 Heart, section of endocardium and myocardium from the affected valve cusp; pig. Vegetative valvular endocarditis. Note abundant masses of bacterial colonies *(arrowheads)* overlying a zone of inflammatory cells and granulation tissue (*G*). *M*, myocardium. Hematoxylin-eosin (H & E) stain. ×105.

Myocardial Diseases

Growth disturbances

Hypertrophy of the myocardium represents an increase in muscle mass associated with increased size of cardiac muscle cells. Hypertrophy is generally secondary and is the result of a compensatory response to increased work load; it is usually reversible upon removal of the cause. However, primary hypertrophy also occurs, as in cats and dogs with idiopathic hypertrophic cardiomyopathy (see below), and is not reversible. Two anatomic forms of hypertrophy are recognized. **Eccentric hypertrophy** results in an enlarged cardiac chamber with walls of normal to somewhat decreased thickness and is produced by lesions with increased blood volume load, such as valvular insufficiencies and septal defects. **Concentric hypertrophy** is characterized by small cardiac chambers with thick walls and results from lesions with increased pressure load, such as valvular stenosis, systemic hypertension, and pulmonary disease. Cats with hyperthyroidism may have cardiac hypertrophy mediated by enhanced production of myocardial contractile proteins under the influence of excess concentration of circulating thyroid hormones. The hypertrophy is reversible upon return to euthyroidism.

Three stages of myocardial hypertrophy are recognizable: (1) initiation, (2) stable hyperfunction, and (3) deterioration of function associated with degeneration of hypertrophied myocytes. Microscopically, myocyte hypertrophy is seen as enlarged fibers with large nuclei.

Diseases that may result in right ventricular hypertrophy include dirofilariasis (Fig. 4-29) and congenital pulmonic stenosis in dogs, ''brisket disease'' (''high altitude disease'') in cattle, and chronic alveolar emphysema (''heaves'') in horses. Cattle maintained under the hypoxic conditions that exist at altitudes over 7000 feet above sea level develop pulmonary hypertension and subsequent right heart failure with subcutaneous edema, chronic passive congestion of the liver (''nutmeg liver''), and right ventricular hypertrophy. Exposure to certain poisonous plants (*Oxytropis* spp. and *Astragalus* spp.) may increase the severity of the disease.

Left ventricular hypertrophy occurs in dogs with congenital subaortic stenosis. Biventricular hypertrophy may occur with hypertrophic cardiomyopathy and various congenital cardiac anomalies. Eccentric hypertrophy may develop in the late stages of diseases that cause concentric hypertrophy.

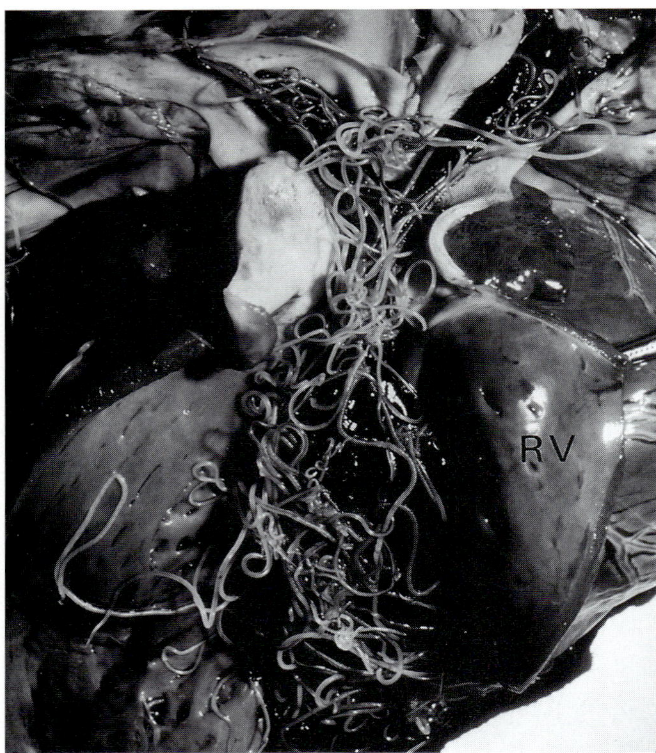

Fig. 4-29 Heart, opened; dog. Dirofilariasis. Multiple, adult *Dirofilaria immitus* are embedded in clotted blood in the right ventricle *(RV),* and pulmonary artery. *Courtesy Dr. M.D. McCracken.*

Infiltration

Fatty infiltration is the presence of increased numbers of lipocytes interposed between myocardial fibers. The lesion is associated with obesity and abundant epicardial deposits of adipose tissue.

Degeneration

Fatty degeneration (fatty change) is the accumulation of abundant lipid droplets in the sarcoplasm of myocytes. Grossly, the myocardium will be pale and flabby. Microscopically, affected myocytes have numerous variably sized spherical droplets that appear as empty vacuoles in paraffin sections, but stain positively for lipids with lipid-soluble stains in frozen sections. This lesion may occur with systemic disorders such as severe anemia, toxemia, and copper deficiency, but is less often seen in the heart than in the liver and kidneys.

Hydropic degeneration, a distinctive microscopic alteration in cardiac muscle cells, is associated with chronic administration of anthracyclines, a group of antineoplastic drugs. Affected fibers have extensive sarcoplasmic vacuolization that is initiated by distention of elements of sarcoplasmic reticulum and, eventually, ends in lysis of contractile material (Figs. 4-30 and 4-31).

Lipofuscinosis (brown atrophy) of the myocardium occurs in aged animals and in animals with severe cachexia,

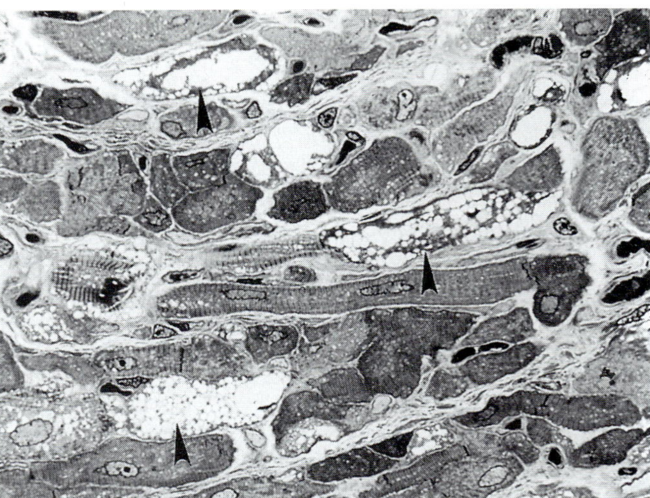

Fig. 4-30 Heart, section of myocardium; dog. Myocardial vacuolar degeneration, chronic doxorubicin cardiotoxicity. The affected myocytes have prominent sarcoplasmic vacuolation *(arrowhead).* Plastic-embedded, toluidine-blue stained section. ×425.

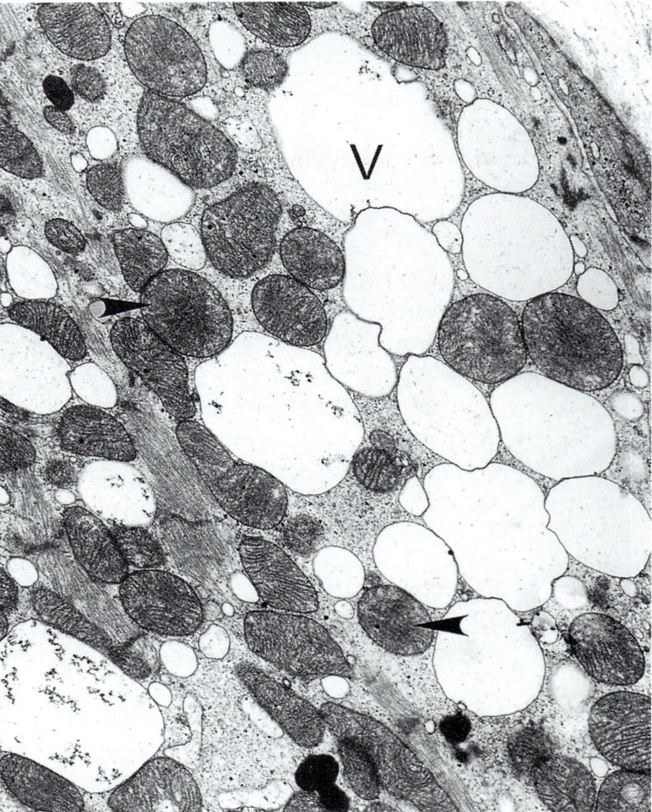

Fig. 4-31 Transmission electron micrograph. Heart, section of myocardium; dog. Chronic doxorubicin cardiotoxicity. The prominent sarcoplasmic vacuolation (*V*) is produced by distention of elements of sarcoplasmic reticulum. Even though the myofibrils have extensive lysis, mitochondria *(arrowheads)* are intact. ×14,400.

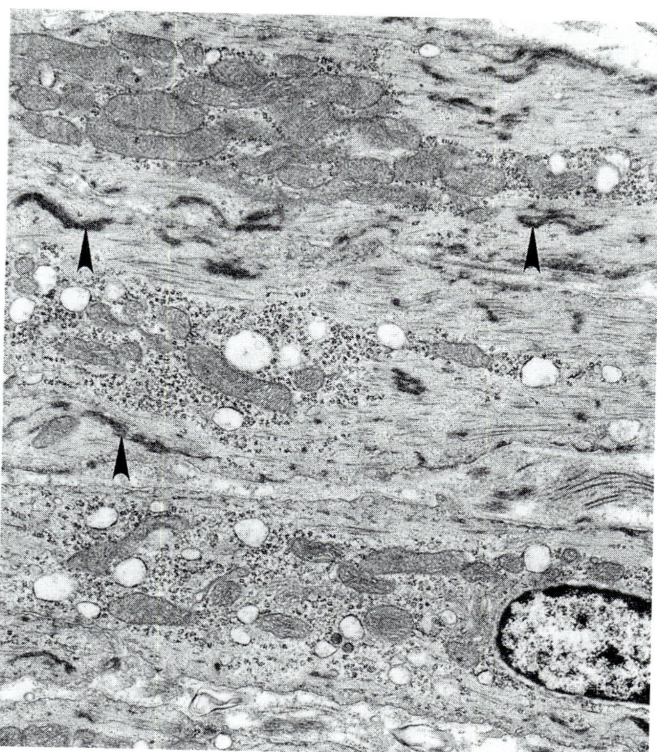

Fig. 4-32 Transmission electron micrograph. Heart, ventricular myocardium; duckling. Myofibrillar lysis, furazolidone cardiotoxicity. Affected myocytes have extensive dissolution of myofibrils with scattered free myofilaments and dense clumps of Z-band material *(arrowheads)*. Other organelles appear normal. ×12,350.

Box 4-2 CAUSES OF MYOCARDIAL NECROSIS IN ANIMALS

Nutritional deficiencies
Selenium–vitamin E, potassium, copper, thiamine, magnesium, protein, choline

Toxicities
Cobalt, catecholamines (isoproterenol, epinephrine, norepinephrine, salbutamol, terbutaline, ephedrine), histamine, vasodilator antihypertensives (minoxidil, hydralazine, diazoxide), methylxanthines (theobromine, theophylline, caffeine), ionophores (monensin, lasalocid, salinomycin, narasin), vitamin D and calcinogenic plants *(Cestrum diurnum, Trisetum flavescens, Solanum malacoxylon, Solanum torvum)*, other poisonous plants (*Acacia georginae, Gastrolobium* spp., *Oxylobium* spp., *Dichapetalum cymosum, Pachystigma pygmaeum, Pachystigma thamnus, Pavetta harborii, Pavetta schumaniana, Fadogia monticola, Cassia occidentalis, Cassia obtusifolia, Karwinskia humboldtiana, Vicia villosa, Trigonella foenum-graceum, Palicourea marcgravii*), blister beetles (Epicauta), high-erucic-acid rapeseed oil, brominated vegetable oils, rancid fat, gossypol, chloroquine, T-2 mycotoxin, papain, paraphenylenediamine, allylamine, plasmocid, oxygen, emetine, uremia

Physical injuries and shock
Central nervous system lesions and trauma, stress, overexertion, electrical defibrillation, acceleration stress, hemorrhagic shock

but it also has been described as a hereditary lesion in healthy Ayrshire cattle (see Fig. 4-21). Affected hearts appear brown and microscopically have clusters of yellow-brown granules at the nuclear poles of myocytes. These granules represent intralysosomal accumulation of membranous and amorphous debris (residual bodies).

Myofibrillar degeneration (myocytolysis) represents a distinctive sublethal injury of cardiac muscle cells. Affected fibers have pale eosinophilic sarcoplasm and lack cross striations. Ultrastructurally, myofibrils have variable extent of dissolution (myofibrillar lysis). This lesion has been described in furazolidone cardiotoxicity in birds (Fig. 4-32) and potassium deficiency in rats.

Necrosis and mineralization

Myocardial necrosis may result from a number of causes, including nutritional deficiencies, chemical and plant toxins, ischemia, metabolic disorders, and physical injuries (Box 4-2). From this large list of causes of myocardial injury, some of the most frequently observed current examples are ionophore toxicity in horses and ruminants, vitamin E–selenium deficiency in the young of all species, anthracycline toxicity in dogs, and gossypol toxicosis in swine. In various localized areas throughout the world, numerous deaths in ruminants may result from consumption of poisonous plants such as *Acacia georginae* and *Dichapetalum cymosum.*

Cardiotoxicity has emerged as a significant clinical entity in veterinary medicine in recent years with the growing use of antineoplastic drugs in small animal practice and the widespread use of growth promotants in ruminants. The mechanisms of cardiotoxicities include (1) exaggerated pharmacologic action of cardiovascular drugs, (2) exposure to myocardial depressants, (3) direct injury of cardiac muscle cells by chemicals, and (4) of hypersensitivity reactions.

Grossly, affected areas appear pale initially, and these may progress to prominent yellow to white, dry areas made gritty by dystrophic mineralization (Figs. 4-33 to 4-35). The lesions may be focal, multifocal, or diffuse. The most frequent sites of focal lesions are the left ventricular papillary muscles and the subendocardial myocardium, especially when such lesions are related to transient reduction of vascular perfusion. These lesions may be overlooked at necropsy unless multiple incisions are made in the ventricular myocardium. In diseases with diffuse cardiac necrosis, such as so-called white muscle disease of calves and lambs with selenium–vitamin E deficiency, the pale lesions may

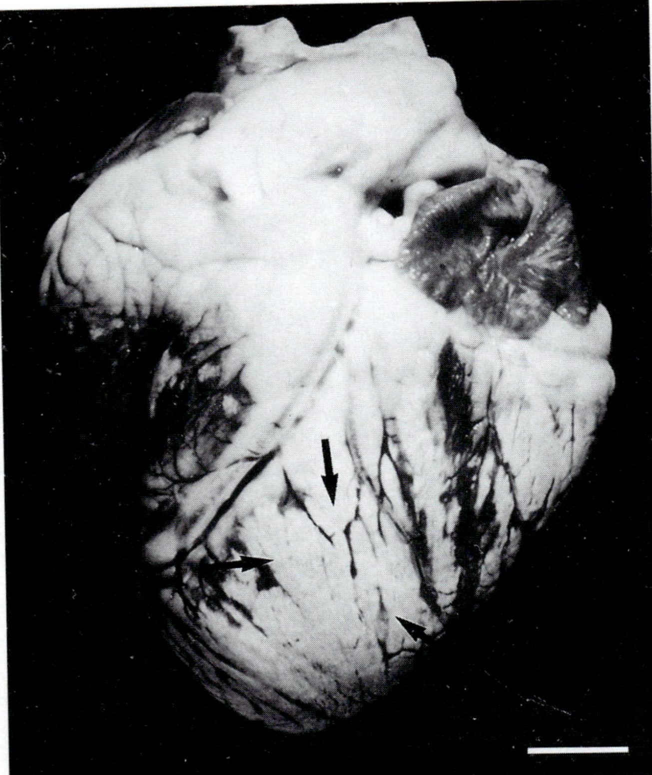

Fig. 4-33 Heart, left ventricular myocardium; calf. Myocardial necrosis, selenium–vitamin E deficiency. Note prominent white chalky areas of necrosis with mineralization *(arrows)*. Bar = 2 cm.

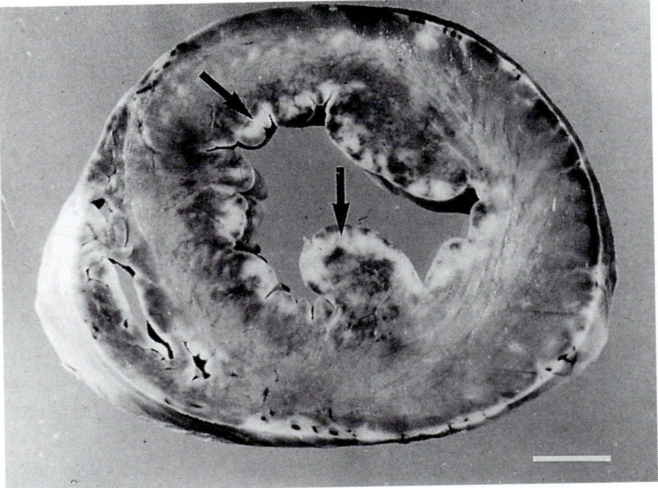

Fig. 4-34 Heart, transected ventricles; dog. Myocardial necrosis and hemorrhage. Prominent pale and red affected areas are concentrated in the subendocardium *(arrows)* and subepicardium. Bar = 1 cm.

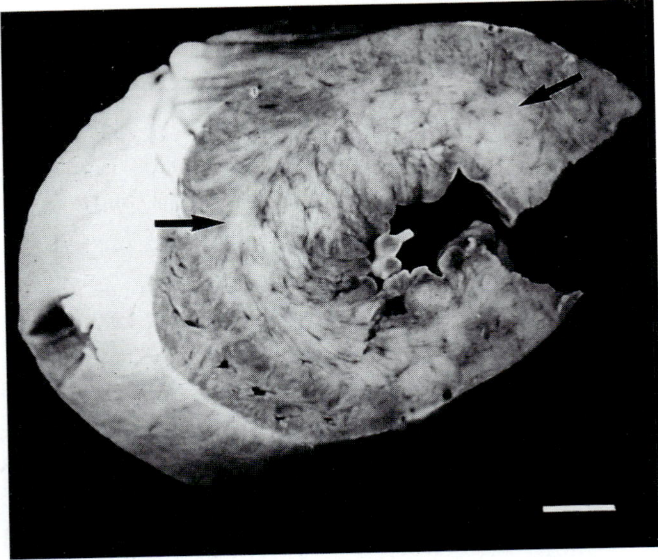

Fig. 4-35 Heart, ventricular myocardium; calf. Myocardial necrosis, acute monensin toxicosis. Note the pale, mottled, necrotic areas *(arrows)* distributed throughout the cross-sectioned ventricular myocardium. Bar = 1 cm.

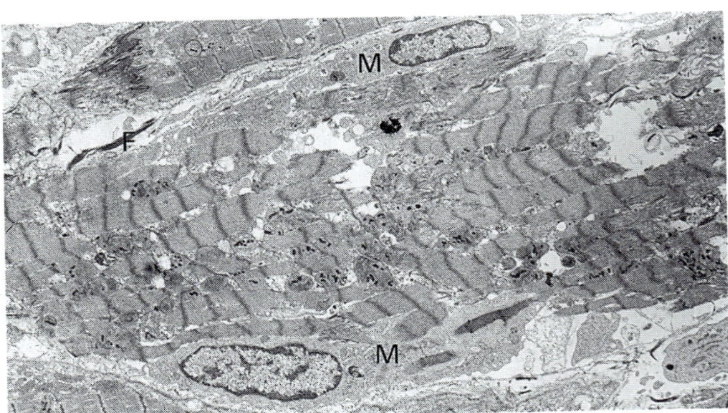

Fig. 4-36 Transmission electron micrograph. Heart, necrotic myocyte, longitudinal section; calf. Myocardial necrosis, monensin toxicosis. The necrotic myocyte *(center)* has disrupted myofibrils, damaged mitochondria with matrical densities, and several invading macrophages (*M*). *F*, fibrin. ×6000.

be readily observed on the epicardial and endocardial surfaces.

Microscopically, fibers in areas of recent necrosis often appear swollen and hypereosinophilic (hyaline necrosis). Striations are indistinct, and nuclei are pyknotic. Necrotic fibers often have scattered basophilic granules that represent mitochondrial accumulation of calcium salts, which can be confirmed by electron microscopy (Fig. 4-36). A second pattern of necrosis may be observed when affected myocytes have a ''shredded'' appearance from hypercontraction and formation of multiple transversely oriented bars of disrupted contractile material (often termed contraction band necrosis). A third pattern is seen in necrotic myocytes in large areas of ischemic necrosis (infarcts). These myocytes have features of coagulation necrosis, and have relaxed rather than hypercontracted contractile elements.

Within 24 to 48 hours after injury, necrotic areas will be infiltrated by inflammatory cells, mainly macrophages and a few neutrophils; these phagocytose and lyse the necrotic cellular debris (Fig. 4-37). In early stages of resolution of necrosis, it may be difficult to distinguish the lesions from those produced by some types of myocarditis (see below).

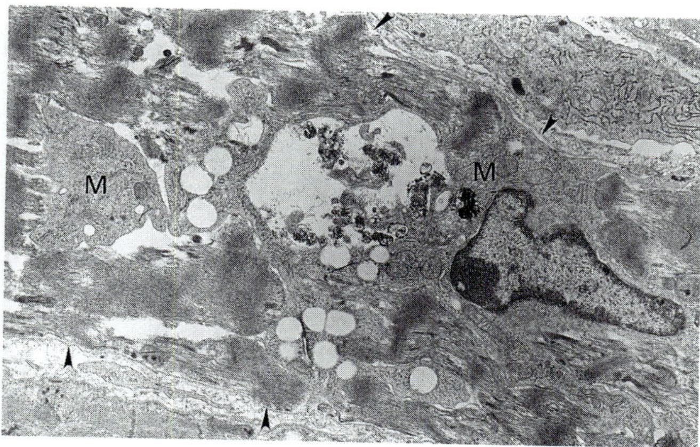

Fig. 4-37 Transmission electron micrograph. Heart, section of myocardium; calf. Myocardial necrosis, monensin toxicosis. Necrotic myocyte has disrupted contractile material invaded by a macrophage (*M*). The basal lamina of the necrotic myocyte is marked by arrowheads. ×6000.

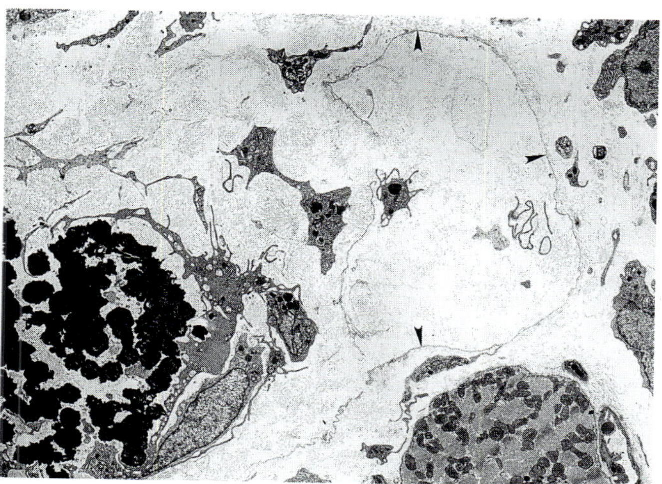

Fig. 4-38 Transmission electron micrograph. Heart, section of myocardium; mouse. Myocardial necrosis and calcification, cardiac calcinosis. Necrotic myocyte *(lower left)* has dark granular masses of calcified debris and several invading macrophages. Another necrotic myocyte *(right center)* is outlined by a shell of external lamina *(arrowheads)*. Numerous macrophages are scattered in the interstitium. ×3000.

Later, when the necrosis has resolved somewhat, lesions will consist of persistent stromal tissues (interstitial fibroblasts and collagen and capillaries) and empty "tubes" of basal laminae of necrotic myocytes (Fig. 4-38). The healing phase is further characterized by proliferation of connective tissue cells (fibroblasts and capillary endothelial cells) and by deposition of connective tissue (collagen and elastic tissue and acid mucopolysaccharides). Grossly, these areas with resolution of myocardial necrosis will appear as white scars.

The outcome of myocardial necrosis will vary depending on the extent of the damage. First, many animals will die acutely from cardiac failure if the myocardial damage is extensive. Second, early deaths from necrosis-related arrhythmias may also occur when cardiac conduction is disrupted. Third, some cases may eventually develop cardiac decompensation and die with cardiac dilatation and scarring and lesions of chronic congestive failure. A number of hearts with minimal damage will have only microscopically detectable myocardial lesions when death eventually occurs from other diseases.

Myocardial mineralization may be a prominent feature in several diseases, such as hereditary calcinosis in mice, cardiomyopathy in hamsters, vitamin E–selenium deficiency in sheep and cattle, vitamin D toxicity in several species, calcinogenic plant toxicosis in cattle ("Manchester wasting disease"), and spontaneous myocardial calcification in aged rats and guinea pigs.

Cardiomyopathies

Primary and **secondary cardiomyopathies** (Box 4-3) represent important generalized myocardial diseases of either idiopathic or known causation. The primary or idio-

Box 4-3 CARDIOMYOPATHIES IN ANIMALS

Primary cardiomyopathies (idiopathic)

Hypertrophic: cat, dog, rat, pig
Dilated (congestive): cat, dog, hamster, turkey, pig, cow
Restrictive: cat

Secondary cardiomyopathies (specific heart muscle diseases)

Heritable (known or suspected): hereditary cardiomyopathy of hamsters, mice, rats, turkeys, and cattle; x-linked muscular dystrophy of dogs; glycogenoses
Nutritional deficiencies: see list in Box 4-2; other examples include taurine deficiency in cats and foxes
Toxic: see list in Box 4-2; other examples include anthracycline toxicity, furazolidone toxicity, NaCl toxicity
Physical injuries and shock: see list in Box 4-2
Endocrine disorders: hypothyroidism, hyperthyroidism, glucocorticoid excess, functional pheochromocytomas, diabetes mellitus
Infections: see list in Box 4-4

pathic cardiomyopathies result in progressive cardiac disease. These diseases affect cats and dogs and resemble similar diseases of human beings. These diseases are divided into three morphologic types: hypertrophic, dilated, and restrictive cardiomyopathies.

Hypertrophic cardiomyopathy occurs frequently in cats, especially in middle-aged males, and is seen infrequently in dogs, usually affecting males of large breeds. Cats usually are presented with congestive heart failure, and approximately half will have posterior paresis from concurrent thromboembolism of the caudal abdominal aorta ("saddle thrombosis"). Some dogs die suddenly and unexpectedly as the first clinical expression of the disease. In both cats and dogs, the affected hearts are enlarged with prominent hypertrophy of the left ventricle and ventricular septum. The left ventricular cavity is small, and the left atrium is dilated. In occasional cases, the ventricular septum is disproportionately hypertrophied in relation to the remainder of the myocardium. Microscopically, the myocardium may have prominent disarray or disorganization of myocytes with interweaving rather than parallel arrangement of fibers (Fig. 4-39). Interstitial fibrosis and various degenerative alterations in myocytes also may be present.

Dilated or **congestive cardiomyopathy** is an important cause of congestive heart failure in cats and dogs. Many affected cats have low tissue concentrations of taurine, and supplementation with taurine has reversed the cardiac failure syndrome. Foxes with taurine depletion also develop cardiac failure.

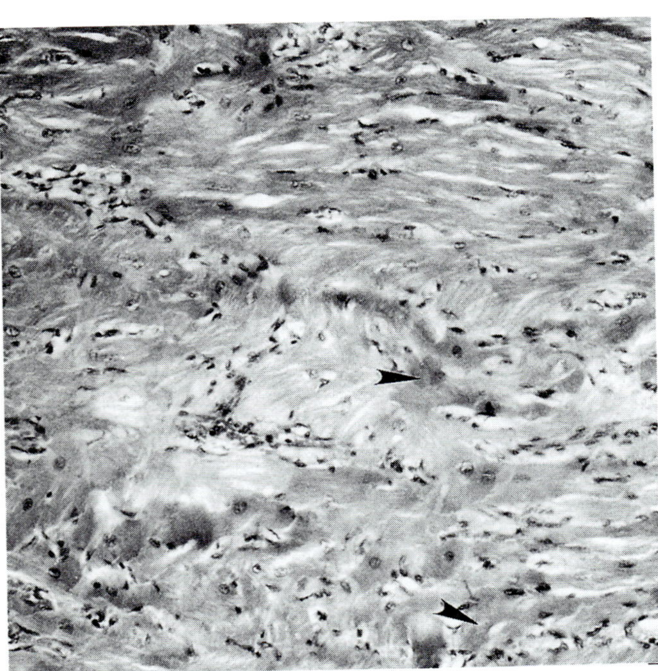

Fig. 4-39 Heart, section of the ventricular myocardium; cat. Hypertrophic cardiomyopathy. Large hypertrophied myocytes with interweaving patterns are indicated by the arrowheads. H & E stain. ×105.

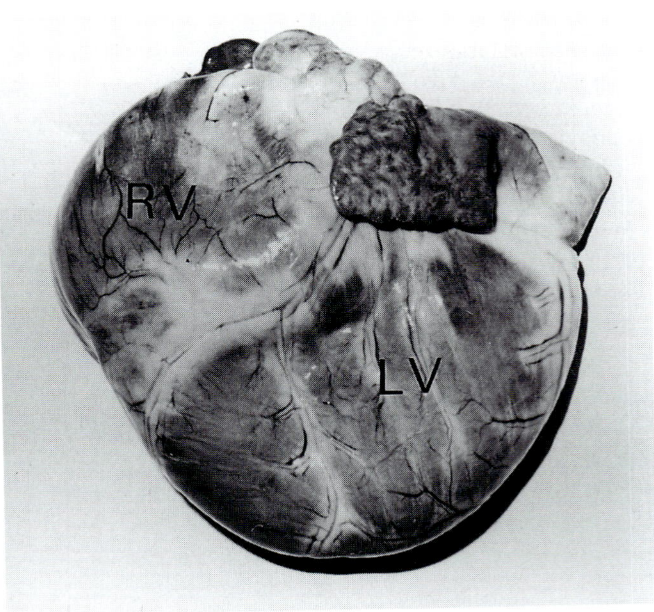

Fig. 4-40 Heart, left ventricle *(LV)* and right ventricle *(RV)*; dog. Dilated (congestive) cardiomyopathy. Biventricular dilatation has given the heart a rounded profile.

Affected cats often are middle-aged males and affected dogs often are males of large breeds, such as Doberman pinscher, Great Dane, and boxer dogs. Cats may develop aortic thromboembolism. At necropsy, lesions of congestive heart failure are present, and the hearts appear rounded from biventricular dilatation (Fig. 4-40). The dilated cardiac chambers often have diffusely white, thickened endocardial tissue. Microscopic and ultrastructural alterations are nonspecific, may be either mild or absent, and include interstitial fibrosis and myocyte degenerative changes.

Restrictive cardiomyopathy occurs infrequently. It is found in cats as one of two types of endocardial lesions that result in impaired ventricular filling. In one type, the left ventricular endocardium has diffuse marked fibrosis. The other type results from numerous anomalous moderator bands that traverse the left ventricular cavity. Other examples of restrictive cardiomyopathy in animals include endocardial fibrosis in certain strains of aged rats and congenital endocardial fibroelastosis in Burmese cats.

Secondary cardiomyopathies (also termed specific heart muscle diseases) are those generalized myocardial diseases of known causation. Box 4-2 lists examples (many are discussed either above under Degeneration and Necrosis of the Myocardium or below under Myocarditis).

Circulatory disturbances

Hemorrhage is a frequent lesion of the epicardium, endocardium, and myocardium. The hemorrhages vary from

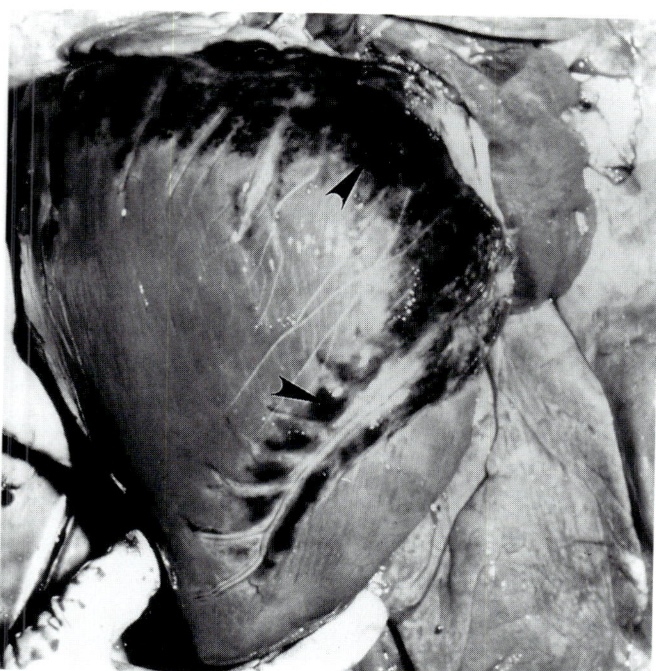

Fig. 4-41 Heart, epicardial surface; horse. Epicardial hemorrhage. A dark sheet of suffusive hemorrhage *(arrowheads)* extends along coronary vessels and atrioventricular groove.

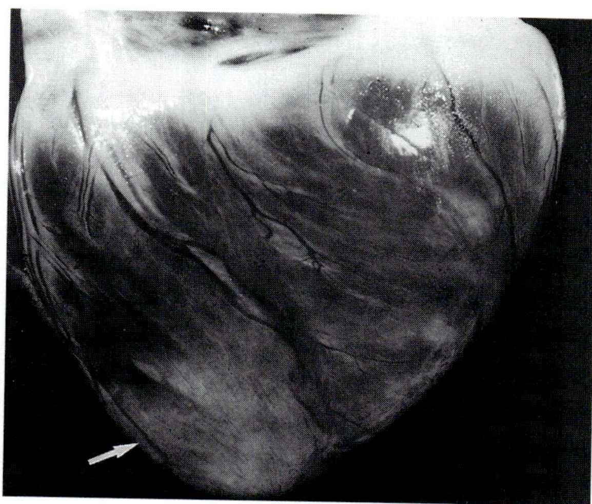

Fig. 4-42 Heart, left and right ventricles; dog. Myocardial infarction. Pale, necrotic, circumscribed area *(arrowhead)* are present in the ventricular wall. *Courtesy Dr. C.S. Patton.*

petechial to ecchymotic to suffusive in extent. Animals dying from septicemia, anoxia, or electrocution often have prominent epicardial and endocardial hemorrhages (Fig. 4-41). Horses dying of any cause usually have agonal hemorrhages on the epicardial and endocardial surfaces. A distinctive example of a specific disease with cardiac hemorrhage is so-called mulberry heart disease, associated with selenium–vitamin E deficiency in growing swine. In these pigs, hydropericardium accompanies severe myocardial hemorrhage that results in a red, mottled (mulberry-like) appearance of the heart.

Thrombosis or **embolism** of the coronary arteries may result in **myocardial infarction** (Fig. 4-42) and cardiac failure. However, these lesions are much less common in animals than in human beings. Affected animals generally have one of several types of coronary arterial disease, including atherosclerosis, arteriosclerosis, or periarteritis. In atherosclerosis associated with hypothyroidism (discussed below), severe lesions are present in extramural coronary arteries of dogs, but this only rarely leads to thrombosis and myocardial infarction. In contrast, severe arteriosclerosis of intramural cardiac arteries in aged dogs may cause small disseminated myocardial infarcts. Often affected dogs also have valvular endocardiosis.

Septic emboli may be disseminated into the coronary circulation from fragments of infective material derived from lesions of vegetative valvular endocarditis of the mitral or aortic valves. These infective emboli may initiate disseminated lesions of suppurative myocarditis that may evolve into multiple myocardial abscesses.

Inflammation

Myocarditis generally is the result of hematogenous infection of the myocardium and may occur with various systemic diseases. Infrequently, myocarditis is the primary lesion in affected animals and responsible for their death. A wide range of types of inflammation is provoked by the spectrum of infectious agents that produce myocarditis and includes suppurative, necrotizing, hemorrhagic, lymphocytic, and eosinophilic responses. **Suppurative myocarditis** results from the myocardial localization of pyogenic bacteria, which often originate from left-sided lesions of vegetative valvular endocarditis. Pale disseminated lesions are present grossly. Neutrophilic infiltration and myocyte necrosis form abscesses that may be confirmed microscopically. **Necrotizing myocarditis** is a frequent lesion of toxoplasmosis, a common disease of cats and dogs. **Hemorrhagic myocarditis** may also occur together with the hemorrhagic inflammation typically found in skeletal muscle of cattle with blackleg *(Clostridium chauvoei)*. **Lymphocytic myocarditis** is usually a lesion of viral infections and is well illustrated by the lesions of parvoviral myocarditis of puppies. Affected dogs die suddenly and unexpectedly with generalized lesions of acute congestive heart failure, but lack evidence of the enteric lesions that are the primary site of viral damage in approximately 95% of clinical cases. The heart is pale and flabby and has disseminated interstitial lymphocytic infiltration, scattered myocytes with large, basophilic, intranuclear viral inclusion bodies, and, in later lesions, fibrosis is present (Fig. 4-43).

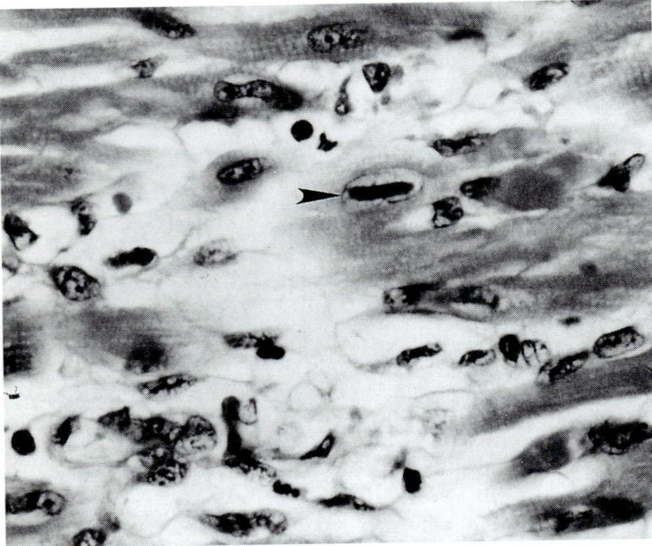

Fig. 4-43 Heart, section of myocardium; dog. Myocarditis, parvovirus infection. Note intranuclear inclusion body in a myocyte *(arrowhead)*. H & E stain. ×425.

Box 4-4 DISEASES THAT CAUSE MYOCARDITIS IN ANIMALS

Viral
Canine parvovirus, encephalomyocarditis, foot and mouth disease, pseudorabies, canine distemper, cytomegalovirus, Newcastle disease, avian encephalomyelitis, Eastern and Western equine encephalomyelitis

Bacterial
Blackleg *(Clostridium chauvoei)*, listeriosis *(Listeria monocytogenes)*, Tyzzer's disease *(Bacillus piliformis)*, necrobacillosis *(Fusobacterium necrophorum)*, tuberculosis (*Mycobacterium* sp.), caseous lymphadenitis *(Corynebacterium pseudotuberculosis)*, disseminated infections by *Actinobacillus equuli, Staphylococcus* sp., *Corynebacterium kutscheri, Pseudomonas aeruginosa,* and *Diplococcus pneumoniae*

Protozoan
Toxoplasmosis *(Toxoplasma gondii)*, sarcosporidiosis (*Sarcocystis* sp.), encephalitozoonosis *(Encephalitozoon cuniculi)*, trypanosomiasis (Chagas' disease [*Trypanosoma cruzi*])

Parasitic
Cysticercosis *(Cysticercus cellulosae)*, trichinosis (*Trichinella* sp.)

Idiopathic
Eosinophilic myocarditis

Eosinophilic myocarditis may accompany various parasitic infections, such as sarcocytosis. Box 4-4 summarizes the various infectious diseases that cause myocarditis in animals.

The pathogenesis and expected outcome of cases of myocarditis remain an important area of research because of the importance of this lesion in cardiac failure in human beings. The sequellae to myocarditis may be (1) complete resolution of lesions, (2) scattered residual myocardial scars, or (3) progressive myocardial damage with acute or, in some cases, chronic cardiac failure as secondary dilated (congestive) cardiomyopathy. In experimental studies of myocarditis induced by infection with Coxsackie B virus in mice, the severity of myocarditis was influenced by the virulence of the virus and was enhanced by various host factors such as young age, male sex, pregnancy, poor nutrition, whole-body ionizing radiation, cold environmental temperatures, alcohol ingestion, exercise, cortisone administration, and mouse strain. Much of the myocardial damage in Coxsackie B virus infection is induced by immunologic reactions rather than by direct viral injury, and T-lymphocytes are involved.

Conduction System Diseases

Conduction system disorders have been described mainly in dogs and horses, probably because clinical cardiologic evaluations are done most frequently in these species. Few pathologic evaluations of the tissues of the conduction system have been reported. Specific diseases presumably inherited in dogs include (1) sudden death in Doberman pinscher dogs associated with focal degeneration of the bundle of His; (2) syncope in pug dogs with lesions of the bundle of His; (3) intermittent sinus arrest in deaf dalamatian dogs, presumably associated with lesions in the sinus node; and (4) sinoatrial syncope (sick sinus syndrome) in miniature schnauzers. Other arrhythmias in dogs and horses are atrial fibrillation and heart block. Dogs with atrial fibrillation usually have short survival times and have atrial dilatation with mitral insufficiency, but horses may have prolonged survival and evidence of atrial fibrosis at necropsy. Heart block of first degree (incomplete), second degree (incomplete with dropped beats), and third degree (complete) have been associated with various myocardial lesions, such as areas of scar formation in horses and dogs. However, some investigators consider second-degree heart block in horses to be a normal phenomenon.

Neoplastic Diseases

Various primary and secondary neoplasms may develop either in or near the heart. The primary neoplasms include rhabdomyoma, rhabdomyosarcoma, schwannoma, and hemangiosarcoma. **Rhabdomyomas** and **rhabdomyosarcomas** are rare in animals and form gray nodules in the myocardium that often project into the cardiac chambers. **Congenital rhabdomyomatosis**, non-neoplastic hamartoma, in swine and guinea pigs is characterized by multi-

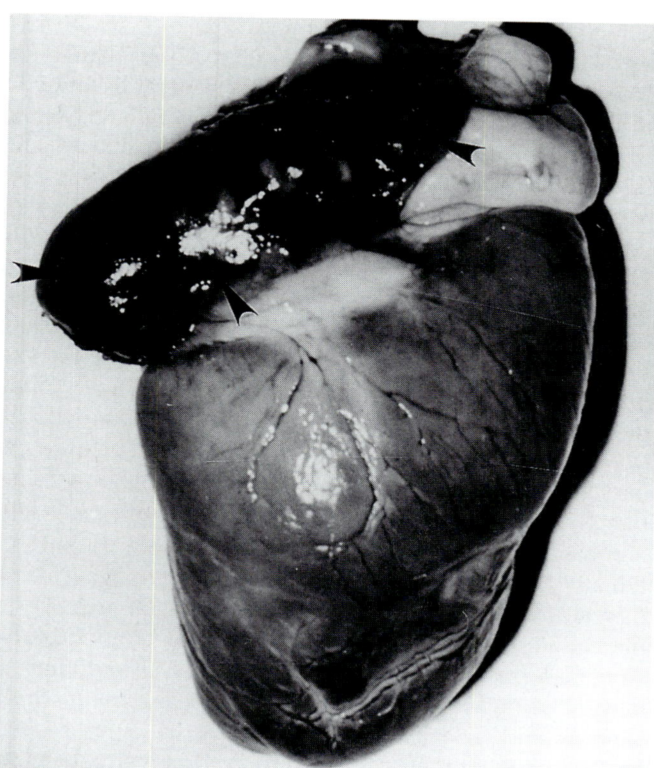

Fig. 4-44 Heart, right atrium; dog. Hemangiosarcoma. The atrium is enlarged by the dark red neoplastic mass *(arrowheads).*

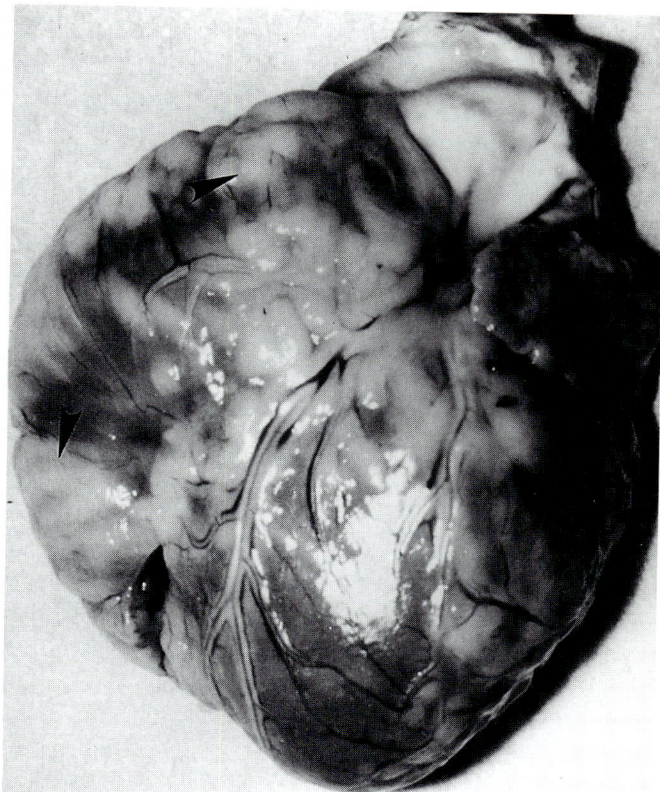

Fig. 4-45 Heart, myocardium; dog. Lymphosarcoma. Neoplastic infiltration of the ventricular myocardium is evident by the numerous white areas *(arrowheads).*

ple, pale, poorly circumscribed areas scattered in the myocardium composed of large glycogen-laden myocytes. **Schwannomas** may involve cardiac nerves in cattle and appear as single or multiple white nodules along the epicardial nerves.

Cardiac **hemangiosarcomas** are important neoplasms of dogs and may arise in the heart (primary) or represent metastatic lesions (secondary) from other sites, such as the spleen. This neoplasm is usually seen in the right atrium and occasionally may involve the right ventricle. Grossly, protruding red to red-black blood-containing masses are located on the epicardial surface. These may rupture and produce fatal hemopericardium and cardiac tamponade (Fig. 4-44). Microscopically, the neoplasms are composed of scattered, elongated, plump neoplastic endothelial cells that may or may not be arranged to form vascular spaces containing blood. Pulmonary metastases are frequent.

Malignant lymphoma (lymphosarcoma) often causes lesions in the hearts of affected cattle, and these may be severe enough to cause death from cardiac failure. The neoplastic invasion may be diffuse or nodular and involve the myocardium and pericardium. Lymphomatous tissue may appear as white masses that resemble deposits of fat (Fig. 4-45). Microscopically, infiltration by neoplastic lymphocytes is extensive in the myocardium (Fig. 4-46). Various

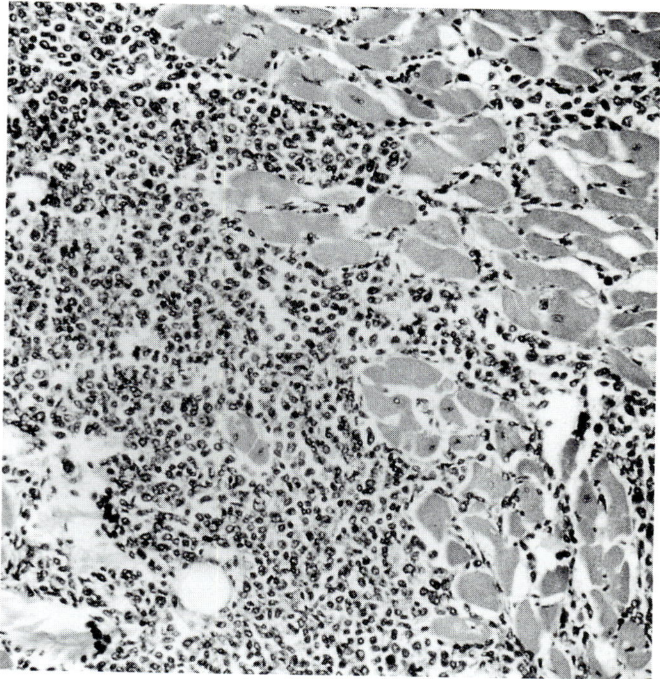

Fig. 4-46 Heart, section of myocardium; cow. Lymphosarcoma. Neoplastic lymphocytes have extensively infiltrated the ventricular myocardium. H & E stain. ×265.

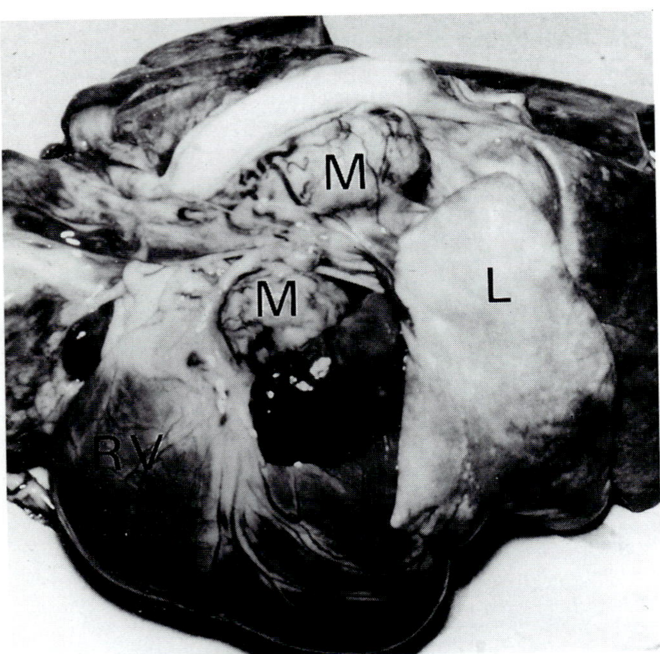

Fig. 4-47 Heart, lung (*L*); dog. Heart base tumor (aortic body tumor, chemodectoma). Multiple tumor masses (*M*) surround the large vessels at the base of the heart.

other generalized neoplasms may occasionally produce metastatic lesions in the heart.

Chemodectomas (heart base tumors) are primary neoplasms of extracardiac tissues in dogs, but arise at the base of the heart and may produce vascular obstruction and cardiac failure. The usual neoplasm arising in this location is the **aortic body tumor** or chemodectoma (paraganglioma), but, occasionally, neoplasms in this location arise from ectopic thyroid or parathyroid tissue. The aortic body is a chemoreceptor organ, as is the carotid body, and either structure may become neoplastic. Aortic body tumors may become large, white, firm masses that surround and compress the great vessels and atria (Fig. 4-47). Brachycephalic dog breeds are most frequently affected. Microscopically, the neoplastic polyhedral cells with vacuolated cytoplasm are supported by an abundant, fine connective tissue stroma.

VESSELS

Introduction

Normal morphology

The vascular system is subdivided into **arterial, capillary, venous,** and **lymph segments.** The arteries are classified into three types—elastic arteries, muscular arteries, and arterioles. The venous vessels are termed venules and veins. The lymph vasculature includes lymph capillaries and lymph vessels. Interposed between the arterial and venous segments are the capillary beds. A vascular segment termed the **microcirculation** includes arterioles, capillaries, and venules and serves as the major area of exchange between the circulating blood and the peripheral tissues.

The overall design of the blood and lymph vessels is similar, except that luminal diameter, wall thickness, and the presence of other anatomic features such as valves vary between the different segments. The luminal surface of all vessels is lined by longitudinally aligned endothelial cells lying over a basal lamina. Vessel walls are divided into three layers or tunics: intima, media and adventitia. However, some or all of the layers may be deleted or thinned in some segments of the vascular system, depending on the intravascular pressures. The large **elastic arteries,** such as the aorta, have (1) an intimal layer composed of endothelium and subendothelial connective tissue, (2) a very thick tunica media composed of fenestrated elastic laminae with interposed smooth muscle cells and ground substance and bordered internally by the internal elastic lamina and externally by the external elastic lamina, and (3) an outer tunica adventitia layer composed of collagen and elastic fibers and connective tissue cells with penetrating blood vessels, termed the vasa vasorum, supplying nutrients to the adventitia and the outer half of the media. In **muscular arteries** and **arterioles,** the tunica media is composed largely of smooth muscle cells arranged in a circumferential pattern. Arterioles are the smallest arterial channels and are generally recognizable as vessels of less than 100 μm in diameter and surrounded by one to three layers of smooth muscle cells.

Capillaries are 5 to 10 μm in diameter and may have endothelium of one of three types: (1) continuous, (2) fenestrated (as in the endocrine glands), and (3) porous (as in renal glomeruli). The endothelium rests on an external lamina surrounded by pericytes. Lesions in endothelium may not be evident by light microscopy and require electron microscopy for characterization.

Veins have thin walls in relation to their luminal size when compared with arteries, in which blood pressures are greater. The adventitia is the thickest layer. Valves are present to prevent retrograde blood flow (i.e., away from the heart).

Lymph capillaries lack basal laminae. **Large lymph vessels** are similar to veins; have large lumina, thin walls, and intimal valves; but will contain lymph. In contrast, veins contain blood.

Reactions to injury

The response of vessels to injury involves a complex interaction among the cellular and noncellular elements of the vessel wall and the cellular and noncellular elements of the blood. The cells of vessels key to these reactions are endothelial cells and smooth muscle cells. Endothelial cells are metabolically active and provide a thromboresistant monolayer at the interface of blood constituents and the vessel wall. Key functions of endothelial cells include prostacyclin production, macromolecular transport, and recruitment of inflammatory cells. Injury of endothelial cells will result in movement of plasma proteins into the subendothelium. Necrosis of endothelium will expose subendothelial collagen and elicit thrombus formation. Endothelial cells at the margin of denuded areas proliferate and reendothelialize the damaged area. The arterial intima has regional differences in the uptake of macromolecules as well as other unique structural and functional features that result in lesion-prone areas of the vasculature.

The other major vascular cellular component involved in reaction to injury is the smooth muscle cell. These cells have a number of important functions, including production of extracellular components such as collagen, elastin, and proteoglycans; maintainance of vascular tone; blood monocyte recruitment; lipoprotein metabolism; production of bioactive lipids such as prostaglandins; and formation of oxygen free radicals. These functions are regulated by a wide variety of biochemical mediators, such as various growth factors, cytokines, and inflammatory mediators.

Postmortem alterations

After death, usually after 12 to 24 hours, erythrocytes lyse and the resultant **imbibition of hemoglobin** will produce red discoloration of the normally white intimal surface of blood vessels. Postmortem clotting must be differentiated from thrombosis. **Postmortem clots,** found in veins and large elastic arteries as red "currant jelly" type or, occasionally, as pale "chicken fat" type, are readily removed by traction or gentle flushing at necropsy in contrast to thrombi, which are adherent. Muscular arteries undergo **postmortem contraction** due to rigor mortis and, microscopically, will appear devoid of blood, and their internal elastic lamina has a scalloped appearance in cross sections.

Arterial Diseases

Aneurysms and ruptures

An **aneurysm** is a localized dilatation or outpouching of a thinned and weakened portion of a vessel. Usually arteries are affected, especially large elastic arteries, but the lesion can also affect veins. Known causes include copper deficiency in pigs, as copper is needed for normal elastic tissue development, and infection with *Spirocera lupi,* but most cases are idiopathic. **Dissecting aneurysms** are infrequent but may be seen in birds and result from intimal disruption and entry of blood into the media to dissect along the wall (Fig. 4-48). Aneurysms are subject to rupture with rapid fatal consequences as rather large arteries are usually involved.

Arterial ruptures may follow severe trauma or occur as spontaneous lesions. Horses are susceptible to sudden rupture of the ascending aorta associated with marked exertion. Death ensues rapidly from cardiac tamponade as the tear is within the region of the aorta covered by the pericardium. In horses, rupture of the carotid artery into the guttural pouch with subsequent epistaxis is a complication of deep mycotic infection of the guttural pouch. Aortic rupture, with or without dissection, is an important cause of death in male turkeys.

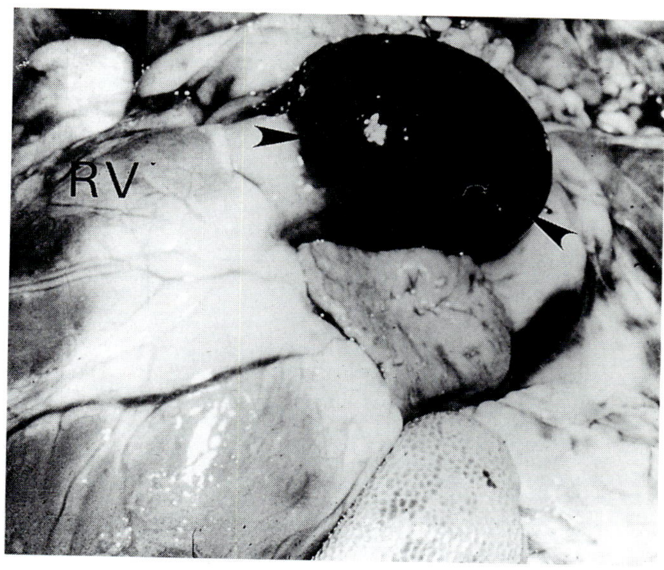

Fig. 4-48 Heart, pulmonary artery, right ventricle (*RV*); pig. Dissecting aneurysm, copper deficiency. The dark, blood-filled, bulging segment of the artery wall *(arrowheads)* has resulted from disruption of elastic fibers.

Growth disturbances

Arterial hypertrophy is a response to sustained increases in pressure or volume loads. Affected vessels are generally muscular arteries, and the increased wall thickness is predominantly due to hypertrophy (and, to some degree, hyperplasia) of smooth muscle cells of the tunica media. Muscular pulmonary arteries of cats are frequently affected, and the condition has been associated with infection by several parasites, including *Aelurostrongylus abstrusus* (the lungworm of cats), *Toxocara* sp., and *Dirofilaria immitis* (Fig. 4-49). However, the lesions often occur in the absence of parasitic infections. No clinical disease is associated with the lesion in cats. Similar hypertrophy of muscular pulmonary arteries occurs in cattle with pulmonary hypertension associated with exposure to high altitudes (so-called high-altitude disease or "brisket disease"). (See Myocardial Hypertrophy p. 180 and Myocardial Diseases p. 189.) Also, animals with cardiovascular anomalies that result in left-to-right shunting of blood and resulting pulmonary hypertension will have hypertrophy of the muscular pulmonary arteries. Uterine arteries in pregnant animals also hypertrophy.

Degeneration and necrosis

Generalized vascular degenerative diseases in animals are classified into three principal groups. Arteriosclerosis

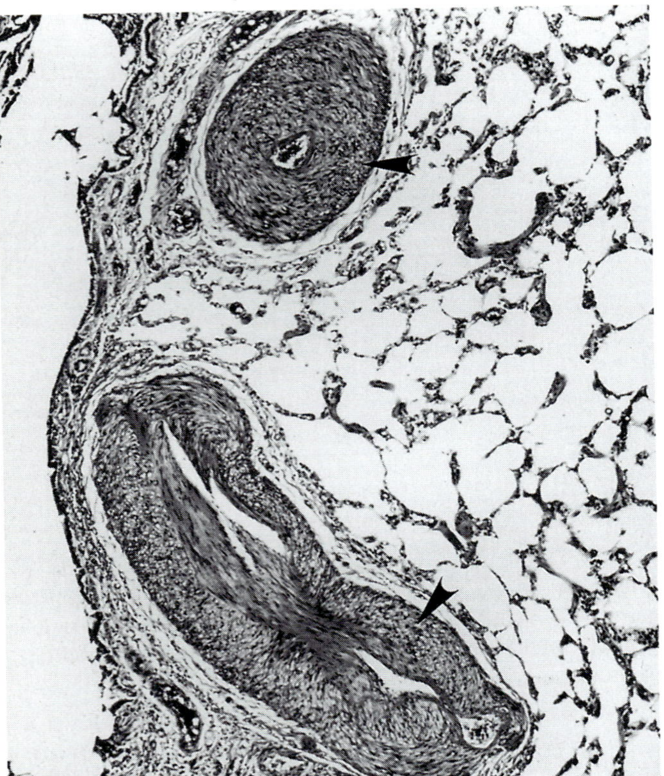

Fig. 4-49 Lung, small pulmonary arteries; cat. Medial hypertrophy. Proliferation of smooth muscle cells *(arrowheads)* has resulted in marked thickening of the media. Note luminal narrowing. H & E stain. ×50.

is characterized by intimal fibrosis of large elastic arteries, and atherosclerosis by intimal and medial lipid deposits in elastic and muscular arteries. Medial calcification has characteristic mineralization of the walls of elastic and muscular arteries.

Arteriosclerosis is an age-related disease that is frequent in many animal species but rarely causes clinical signs. The disease develops as chronic degenerative and proliferative responses in the arterial wall and results in loss of elasticity (''hardening of the arteries'') and luminal narrowing. The abdominal aorta is most frequently affected, with lesions often localized around the orifice of arterial branches, but other elastic arteries and peripheral large muscular vessels may also be involved. Etiologic factors in the development of arteriosclerotic lesions are not well defined, but the significant role of hemodynamic influences is suggested by the frequent involvement of arterial branch sites where blood flow is turbulent. Grossly, the lesions are seen as slightly raised, firm, white plaques. Microscopically, the intima is thickened by accumulations of mucopolysaccharides with subsequent proliferation of medial smooth muscle cells and fibrous tissue infiltration into the intima and splitting and fragmentation of the internal elastic lamina.

Atherosclerosis is the vascular disease of greatest importance in human beings, but occurs only infrequently in animals and rarely leads to clinical disease, such as results from infarction of the heart or brain. The principal alteration is accumulation of extensive deposits (atheroma) of lipid, fibrous tissue, and calcium in vessel walls, with eventual luminal narrowing. Many experimental studies have established that species such as the pig, rabbit, and chicken are susceptible to the experimental disease produced by feeding high-cholesterol diets, but the dog, cat, cow, goat, and rat are resistant. Lesions of the naturally occurring disease may be detected in aged swine and birds, and in dogs with hypothyroidism that develop hypercholesterolemia. Vessels of the heart, mesentery, and kidneys are prominently thickened, firm, and yellow-white (Fig. 4-50). Microscopically, lipid globules accumulate in the cytoplasm of smooth muscle cells and macrophages, often termed ''foam cells,'' in the media and intima (Fig. 4-51). Necrosis and fibrosis may develop in the arterial lesions.

Arterial medial calcification is a frequent lesion in animals and may involve both elastic and muscular arteries that often have concurrent endocardial mineralization. The

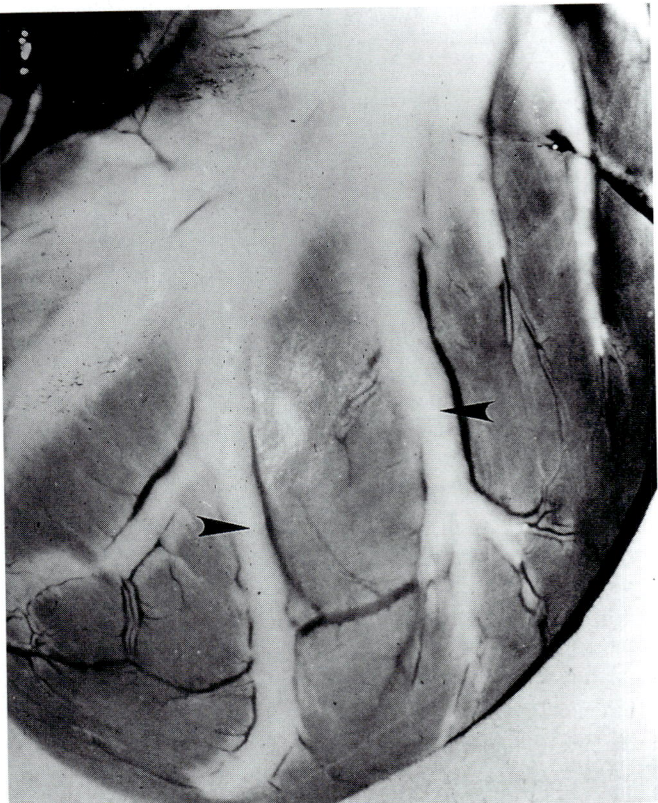

Fig. 4-50 Heart, left ventricle; dog. Coronary atherosclerosis, hypothyroidism. The affected epicardial arteries appear as prominent, white, cordlike structures *(arrowheads)*.

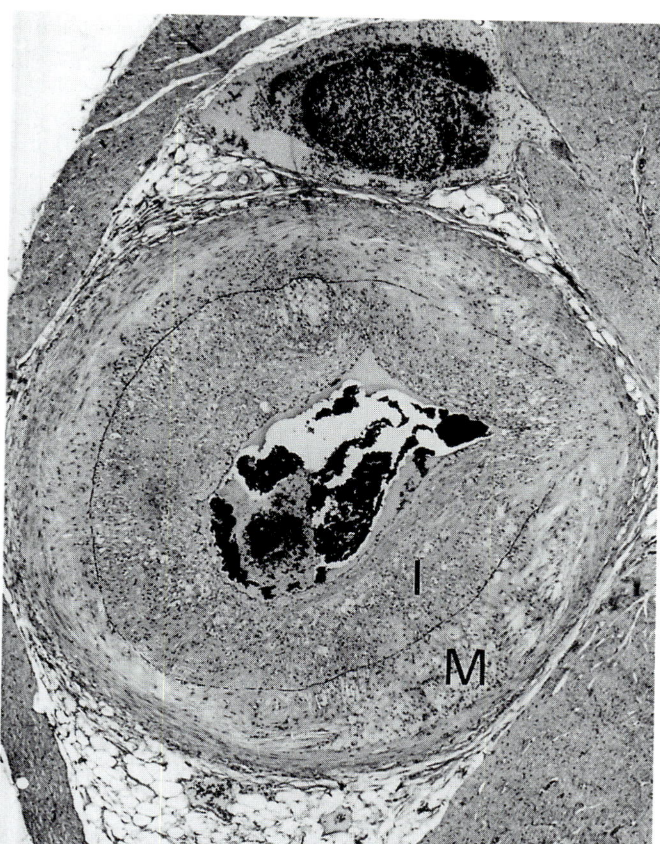

Fig. 4-51 Heart, cross section of affected epicardial artery; dog. Coronary atherosclerosis. Note extensive accumulation of lipid in "foam cells" throughout the thickened intimal (*I*) and medial (*M*) layers. H & E stain. ×25.

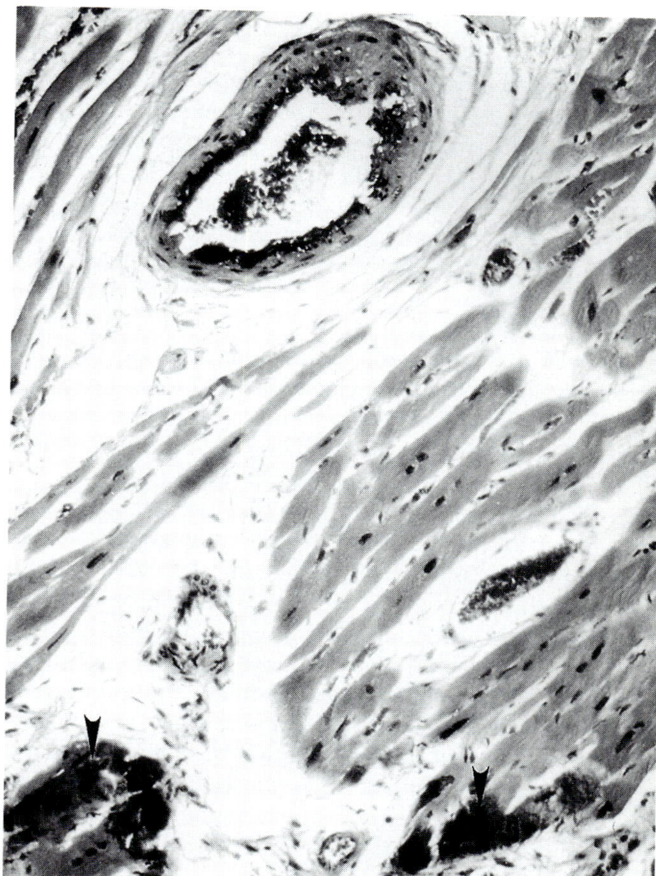

Fig. 4-52 Heart, section of myocardium; pig. Arterial and myocardial calcification, vitamin D toxicosis. Dark, basophilic masses of calcium deposits are present in the arterial intima and media *(top)* and in scattered necrotic myocytes *(arrowheads at bottom)*. H & E stain. ×105.

etiologies for arterial calcification include calcinogenic plant toxicosis, vitamin D toxicosis, renal insufficiency, and severe debilitation, as seen in cattle with Johne's disease. The disease occurs spontaneously in rabbits and in aged guinea pigs and rats with chronic renal disease. Affected arteries such as the aorta have an unique appearance. They appear grossly as solid, dense, pipelike structures or as raised, white, solid intimal plaques. Microscopically, prominent basophilic granular mineral deposits are either present on elastic fibers of the media of elastic arteries or may form a complete ring of mineralization in the medial musculature of muscular arteries (Fig. 4-52). **Siderocalinosis** (so-called iron rings) is a finding in the cerebral arteries of aged horses where both iron and calcium salts are deposited in the vessel walls. Lesions in the surrounding brain tissue are generally absent, and, thus, these vascular lesions are incidental.

Arterial intimal calcification (intimal bodies) are distinctive findings in small muscular arteries and arterioles of horses. These lesions represent small mineralized masses within the subendothelium and have no deleterious effect.

Hyaline degeneration, fibrinoid necrosis, and **amyloidosis** are vascular lesions of small muscular arteries and arterioles and occur in all animal species. These lesions are generally not detected grossly, but, in some diseases with fibrinoid necrosis, grossly apparent hemorrhages or edema is seen in affected organs. The microscopic feature shared by these lesions is the formation of a homogeneous eosinophilic zone in the vessel wall. Application of special stains will allow differentiation of the three lesions based on (1) specific staining of amyloid deposits by such stains as Congo red and methyl violet; (2) positive staining of fibrinoid deposits by the periodic acid–Schiff method; and (3) absence of staining of hyaline deposits by these several stains. Vascular amyloidosis and hyaline degeneration often are observed in small muscular arteries of the myocardium and spleen of old dogs. Lesions of the intramyocardial arteries may be accompanied by small foci of myocardial infarction.

Fibrinoid necrosis of arteries is associated with endothelial damage and is characterized by entry and accumulation of serum proteins and fibrin polymerization in the wall. This forms an intensely eosinophilic collar that obliterates the cellular detail. This lesion may be a feature of many acute degenerative and inflammatory diseases of small arteries and arterioles. The lesion is particularly frequent in swine and is an important diagnostic feature in cases of selenium–vitamin E deficiency (heart), edema disease (gastric submucosa), cerebrospinal angiopathy, and organic mercury toxicosis (meninges). Fibrinoid necrosis is seen frequently in dogs with uremia and also may be seen with hypertension, although this is a rather uncommon finding in animals as compared to human beings.

In swine with selenium–vitamin E deficiency, the lesions may occur as cardiac hemorrhage (''mulberry heart disease'') and as massive hemorrhagic hepatic necrosis (hepatosis dietetica). With either form of the disease, widespread vascular lesions may be present as fibrinoid necrosis of small muscular arteries and arterioles with accompanying evidence of microvascular damage as fibrin thrombi of capillaries, especially in the myocardium (Fig. 4-53). This complex of vascular lesions has been termed dietary microangiopathy. Similar capillary lesions with endothelial damage and occlusion by fibrin thrombi are seen in the cerebellum of vitamin E–deficient chicks with ischemia-induced encephalomalacia and in the skin and skeletal muscles of selenium–vitamin E–deficient chicks with exudative diathesis.

Cerebrospinal angiopathy in swine is a disease characterized clinically by sporadic cases with signs of nervous system disease. Vascular lesions, which include fibrinoid necrosis, are present consistently in arteries of the central nervous system. Similar vascular lesions occur in the gastric submucosa of pigs with edema disease, a form of colibacillosis, and many researchers believe that cerebrospinal angiopathy represents a subacute form of edema disease.

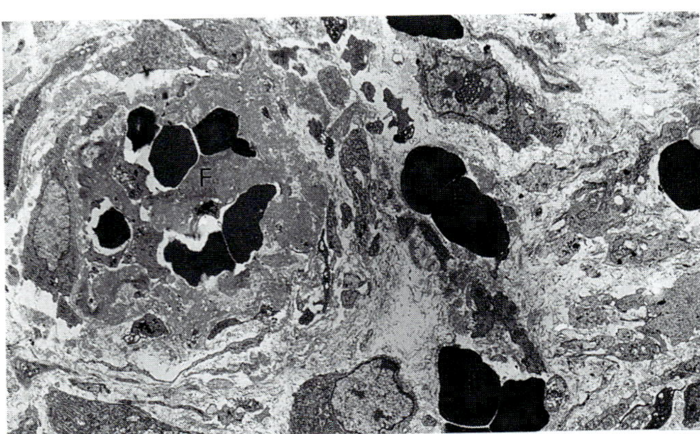

Fig. 4-53 Transmission electron micrograph. Heart, section of myocardium; pig. Fibrinoid necrosis, ''mulberry heart disease,'' selenium–vitamin E deficiency. The affected arteriole *(left)* has intraluminal masses of fibrin (*F*) and entrapped erythrocytes. Fibrin masses are also present in the vessel wall, and the adjacent interstitium has edema and hemorrhage. Note scattered erythrocytes (*E*). ×3500.

Thrombosis and embolism

Thrombosis represents the product of intravascular coagulation or clotting during life. Predisposing factors to thrombosis include (1) endothelial damage, (2) altered blood flow, and (3) hypercoagulative states. Endothelial damage can be a feature of many arterial diseases. It is frequently present in arteritis, but is uncommon with most of the degenerative arterial diseases other than fibrinoid necrosis. Alterations in blood flow may occur with vascular or cardiac valvular lesions that cause turbulence; stasis of blood flow can accompany congestive cardiac failure and cardiovascular collapse, as occurs in systemic shock. Hypercoagulative states may exist in dogs with amyloidosis and some types of renal disease.

Frequently observed examples of arterial thrombosis in animals include caudal aortic thromboemboli in cats and dogs with primary cardiomyopathy (Fig. 4-54), thrombosis

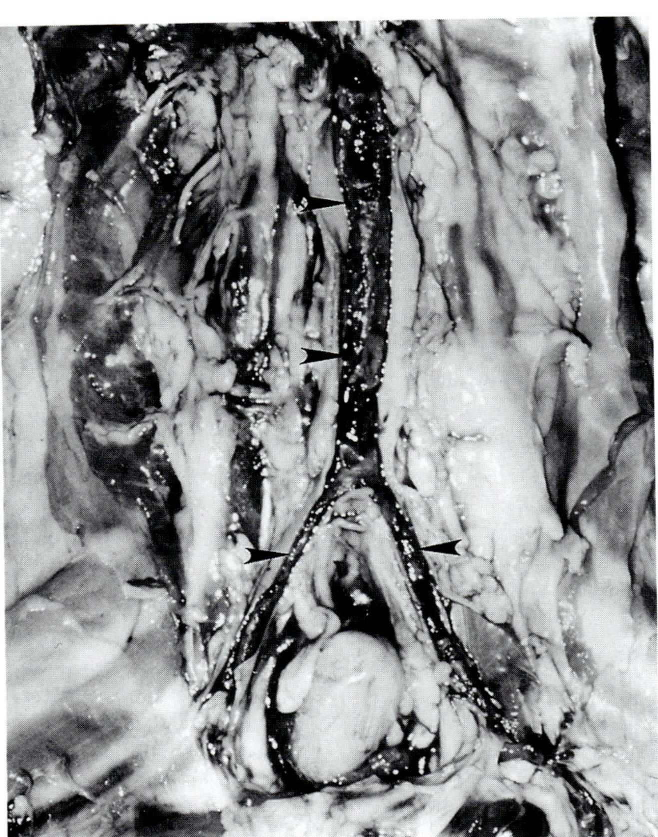

Fig. 4-54 Aorta and iliac arteries; dog. Aortic thrombosis. Dark-red, friable masses of fibrin thrombus occlude the caudal abdominal aorta and iliac arteries *(arrowheads)*.

of mesenteric and intestinal arteries in horses with strongylosis, thrombosis of the pulmonary arteries in dogs with dirofilariasis, and aorto-iliac thrombosis in horses. In these diseases, because large arteries may be affected, ischemia in the peripheral tissues results unless adequate collateral circulation exists. Recently formed mural thrombi appear as yellow, firm masses of fibrin adhered focally to the arterial intima. Fibroblastic proliferation and organization develop within days in the thrombi.

Disseminated intravascular coagulation, initiated by a variety of causes, results in formation of widespread clotting within arterioles and blood capillaries. This clotting phenomenon is largely due to (1) endothelial damage with exposure of subendothelial collagen and subsequent platelet aggregation and (2) intravascular activation of the coagulation process. Diseases that may be accompanied by disseminated intravascular coagulation include bacterial endotoxemias, certain viral infections such as feline infectious peritonitis and infectious canine hepatitis, dirofilariasis, certain neoplastic diseases, shock, hemolysis, and extensive tissue necrosis, such as occurs in animals with burns. Extensive clotting results in depletion of coagulation factors (termed consumption coagulopathy) and in widespread hemorrhages. Hemorrhagic lesions produced by this mechanism include hemorrhagic renal cortical necrosis (Shwartzman-like reaction) or hemorrhagic adrenal gland necrosis in cases of septicemia. Microscopically, organs in cases of disseminated intravascular coagulation will have numerous fibrin thrombi in arterioles and capillaries (Fig. 4-55). Fibrinolysis, an intravascular enzymatic process to lyse clots, may continue to be active following death of the animal and could lead to failure to observe fibrin thrombi in autolyzed tissue.

Embolism is the occlusion of arteries by lodgment of foreign materials, such as disrupted fragments of thrombi, neoplastic cells, and bacteria. Thromboemboli originating from thrombotic lesions may be either bland (sterile) or septic. Septic emboli most often originate from lesions of vegetative endocarditis, with right-sided lesions being disseminated into the lungs and left-sided lesions being found in sites such as the myocardium, kidneys, and spleen. Other types of emboli include air bubbles or hair fragments forced into the circulation during intravenous injections, release of fat into the vasculature from fractures, release of fragments of dead intravascular parasites such as *Dirofilaria immitis* into the pulmonary circulation of carnivores following administration of adulticidal drugs, and introduction of fragments of fibrocartilage into spinal arteries of dogs and other species from disruption of degenerated intervertebral disc material.

Inflammation

Arteritis may occur as a feature of many infections and immune-mediated diseases (Box 4-5). Often, all types of vessels are affected rather than only arteries, and then vas-

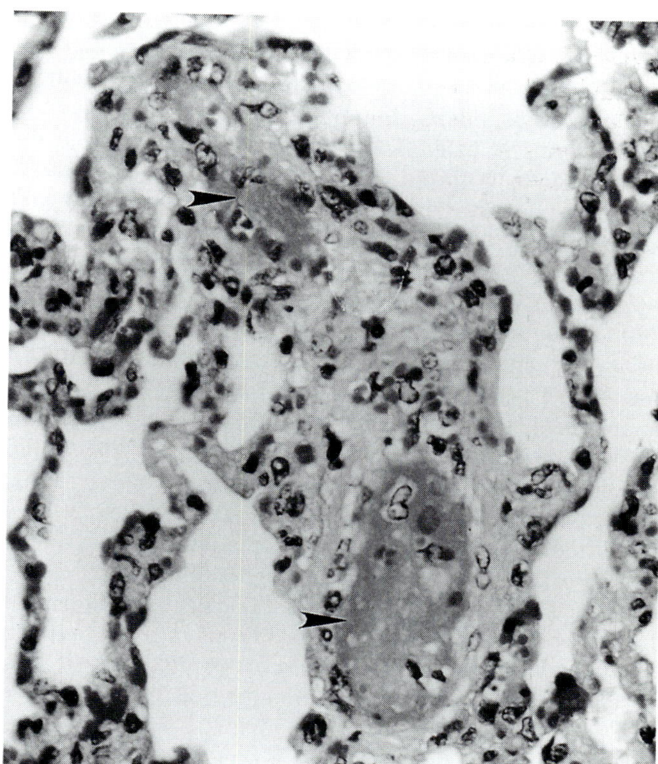

Fig. 4-55 Lung; horse. Fibrin thrombi, disseminated intravascular coagulation. Multiple fibrin thrombi *(arrowheads)* occlude pulmonary vessels. H & E stain. ×265.

Box 4-5 DISEASES THAT CAUSE VASCULITIS IN ANIMALS

Viral
Equine viral arteritis, malignant catarrhal fever, hog cholera, feline infectious peritonitis, bluetongue, African swine fever

Bacterial
Salmonellosis, erysipelas *(Erysipelothrix rhusiopathiae), Hemophilus somnus* infections

Mycotic
Phycomycosis, aspergillosis

Parasitic
Equine strongylosis *(Strongylus vulgaris),* dirofilariasis *(Dirofilaria immitis),* spirocercosis *(Spirocerca lupi),* onchocerciasis, elaeophoriasis *(Elaphora schneideri),* filariasis in primates, aelurostrongylosis, angiostrongylosis

Immune-mediated
Canine systemic lupus erythematosus, Aleutian disease, polyarteritis nodosa, lymphocytic choriomeningitis, drug-induced hypersensitivity (?)

culitis or angiitis is the term applied to the lesions. In inflamed vessels, leukocytes will be present within and surrounding the walls and damage to the vessel wall will be evident as fibrin deposition or necrosis of endothelial and smooth muscle cells. These vascular alterations may be accompanied by thrombosis and the attending complications of ischemic injury or infarction in the circulatory field as seen in the ''diamond skin'' lesions of cutaneous infarction in porcine erysipelas caused by infection with *Erysipelothrix rhusiopathiae* (Fig. 4-56).

Arteritis and vasculitis may develop from endothelial injury by either infectious agents or immune-mediated mechanisms or may be established by local extension of suppurative and necrotizing inflammatory processes into adjacent vessel walls. Equine viral arteritis is a systemic viral infection with a tropism for vascular endothelial cells. The walls of affected small muscular arteries have lesions of fibrinoid necrosis, extensive edema, and leukocytic infiltration. Grossly, the vascular injury is reflected by severe edema of the intestinal wall and mesentery accompanied by marked accumulation of serous fluids in body cavities.

Arteritis is a prominent feature of several parasitic diseases. In dirofilariasis (heartworm infection), maturation of adult parasites occurs in the pulmonary arteries and right side of the heart of dogs. The pulmonary arteries containing parasites initially have an eosinophilic infiltration of the intima (termed endarteritis), with subsequent development of an irregular fibromuscular proliferation of the intima that can be observed grossly as a rough granular or shaggy appearance of the luminal surface (Fig. 4-57). Live or dead parasites may be present within these vascular lesions, and thromboembolism and pulmonary infarction may occur. Infection of horses by *Strongylus vulgaris* is very common. Development of the parasite includes migration through the intestinal arteries, with the most severe lesions generally found in the cranial mesenteric artery. The affected vessel is enlarged, and the wall is firm and fibrotic. The intimal surface often has adhering thrombotic masses admixed with larvae. Microscopically, the altered vessel has extensive infiltration of inflammatory cells and proliferation of fibroblasts throughout the wall. Thromboembolism frequently occurs, but the abundant collateral circulation

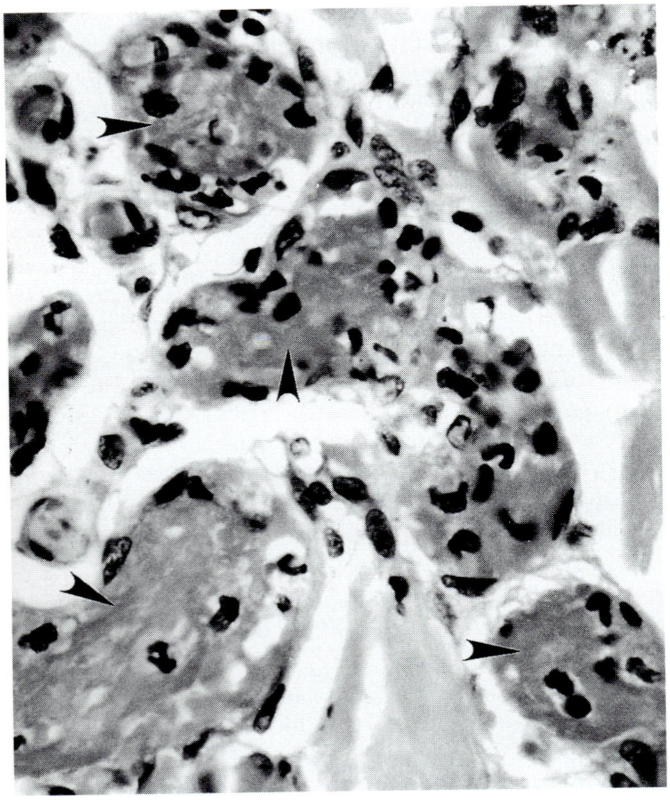

Fig. 4-56 Skin; pig. Arteritis, erysipelas. The dermal vessels *(arrowheads)* contain masses of fibrin and have numerous invading leukocytes scattered throughout the walls. H & E stain. ×425.

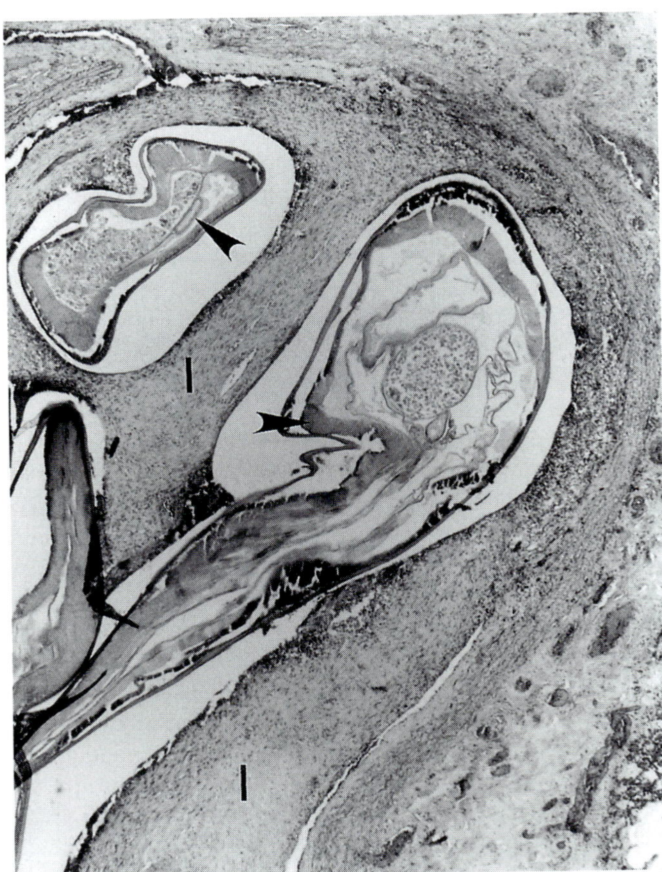

Fig. 4-57 Pulmonary artery; dog. Chronic proliferative verminous arteritis, dirofilariasis. Multiple, dead adult *Dirofilaria immitis (arrowheads)* are in the lumen, with surrounding marked fibrous intimal proliferation (*I*). H & E stain. ×25.

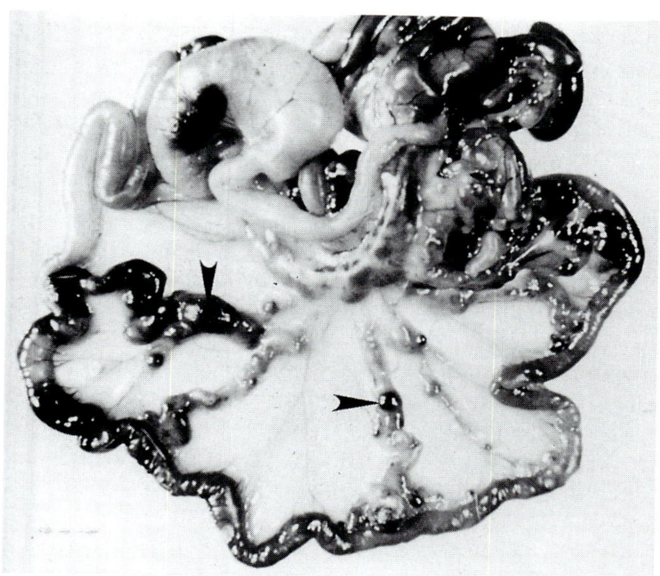

Fig. 4-58 Mesenteric arteries; rat. Polyarteritis nodosa. The affected segments of the arteries appear in the mesentery as thick, red, hemorrhagic, tortuous structures *(arrowheads).*

to the equine intestinal tract makes intestinal infarction an unusual event.

Polyarteritis is a disease that occurs sporadically in many animal species and is an important disease of aged rats. Several reports have described the occurrence of polyarteritis (idiopathic necrotizing arteritis) involving the coronary and meningeal arteries in colonies of beagle dogs (''canine pain syndrome''). The lesions are usually attributed to an immune-mediated vascular injury. Medium-sized muscular arteries are selectively involved and appear thick and tortuous, have associated focal hemorrhage, and develop aneurysms and thrombosis (Fig. 4-58). Microscopically, the early lesions include fibrinoid necrosis and leukocytic invasion of the intima and media. In chronic lesions, inflammatory cells and fibrosis involve all layers of the vascular wall.

Neoplastic diseases

Neoplasms arising from vascular endothelial cells may develop in many different organs. **Hemangiomas** are benign neoplasms often found in the skin of dogs. These red, blood-filled masses are well circumscribed. The malignant neoplasm, the **hemangiosarcoma,** occurs frequently in the spleen and the right side of the heart of dogs. This neoplasm is also generally a red mass, but, microscopically, the neoplastic cells are pleomorphic and do not form distinct vascular spaces. Another neoplasm of vascular origin is the **hemangiopericytoma** of the canine skin. The distinctive microscopic feature is a laminated arrangement of elongated, plump neoplastic pericytes around small blood vessels.

Venous Diseases

Congenital anomalies

Portocaval shunts occur in dogs and, because blood bypasses the liver, may result in signs of nervous system disease associated with failure of hepatic degradation of nitrogenous products such as ammonia. This nervous syndrome is termed hepatic encephalopathy. Specifically, the shunts may represent retained fetal vascular structures, as in persistent ductus venosus, or arise from prominent dilatation of various portosystemic shunts that normally are quite small vessels.

Dilatation

Venous dilatation from weakened vascular walls is termed a **varicosity** (localized involvement) or **phlebectasia** (generalized alteration). Although a frequent lesion in the superficial veins of the legs in women, it is rather uncommon in animals. The pampiniform plexus in the spermatic cord in aged rams and bulls may be affected.

Inflammation

Phlebitis is a common vascular lesion and is often complicated by thrombosis. The vascular lesion may arise from (1) systemic infections, (2) local extension of infection, and (3) faulty intravenous injection procedure. Systemic infections with phlebitis as a lesion include salmonellosis in several species and feline infectious peritonitis. In pigs with various septicemias, the gastric fundic mucosa is often severely congested and hemorrhagic because of venous endothelial damage and thrombosis. Severe local infections, as in metritis or hepatitis, may extend into the walls of adjacent veins and produce phlebitis, with or without thrombosis. Intravenous injections of irritant solutions, failure to inject solutions into the lumen, or intimal trauma produced by indwelling venous catheters will result in vascular damage and create an opportunity for localization and proliferation of infectious agents and development of phlebitis. Cases of phlebitis complicated by thrombosis will have the additional risk of septic embolism and development of additional lesions such as endocarditis and pulmonary abscesses.

Omphalophlebitis (''navel ill'') is inflammation of the umbilical vein and often occurs in farm animals due to bacterial contamination of the umbilicus immediately following parturition. Other lesions that often evolve in affected neonates include septicemia, suppurative polyarthritis, hepatic abscesses, and umbilical abscesses.

Cats with feline infectious peritonitis often develop phlebitis in various abdominal organs. This lesion appears to result from deposition of immune complexes and subsequent evolution of the inflammatory reaction in affected vessels. Occasionally, in some cattle with hepatic abscesses, infection will extend into the adjacent large hepatic veins and result in formation of a septic thrombus (usually a mural thrombus) in the caudal vena cava. Sometimes, focal devitalization of the wall of the vena cava occurs, and rupture of the abscess releases the contents into the lumen, producing sudden death of the affected animal.

Several parasitic diseases important in tropical regions of the world are characterized by presence of parasites in the lumina of veins. These diseases include schistosomiasis (blood fluke infection) and infection of cats in South America by *Gurltia paralysans.* Affected cats have spinal cord damage from thrombophlebitis in the lumbar veins, associated with the presence of adult parasites in affected vessels. In schistosomiasis, adult parasites are present in the mesenteric and portal veins, and the resulting phlebitis is characterized by intimal proliferation and thrombosis.

Lymph Vessel Diseases

Congenital anomalies

Hereditary lymphedema has been described in dogs, Ayrshire calves, and pigs. Affected animals have prominent subcutaneous edema that, in calves, often causes severe swelling of the tips of the ears. Interference with lymph drainage results from defective development of the lymph vessels. The affected vessels may be aplastic or hypoplastic.

Dilatation and rupture

Lymphangiectasis is dilatation of lymph vessels. One cause is obstruction of lymph drainage by invading masses of malignant neoplasms. Another example is intestinal lymphangiectasis, an important disease of dogs in which there is a protein-losing enteropathy. Lacteals in the intestinal villi are prominently dilated, and lymph vessels throughout the wall of the bowel and the mesentery are distended. The role of lymph vessel obstruction in the pathogenesis of this disease is still unclear. Many diseases with severe acute inflammatory alterations accompanied by vascular damage, as with the pulmonary lesions of bovine pasteurellosis, will have prominent dilatation of the lymph vessels.

Rupture of the thoracic duct, either as a result of trauma or from spontaneous disruption, has been associated with development of chylothorax in dogs and cats. However, many cases of chylothorax occur without injury to the thoracic duct.

Inflammation

Lymphangitis is a feature of many diseases (Box 4-6). The affected vessels are often located in the distal limbs as thick, cordlike structures. Lymphedema may be present. Nodular suppurative lesions may ulcerate and discharge pus onto the surface of the skin. In Johne's disease, the mesenteric lymph vessels are often prominent and have evidence of extension of the enteric infection as granulomatous lymphangitis (Fig. 4-59).

Box 4-6 DISEASES THAT CAUSE LYMPHANGITIS IN ANIMALS

Bacterial
Porcine anthrax *(Bacillus anthracis),* Johne's disease *(Mycobacterium paratuberculosis),* tuberculosis (*Mycobacterium* spp.), actinobacillosis *(Actinobacillus lignieresii),* glanders ("farcy") *(Pseudomonas mallei),* cutaneous streptothricosis *(Dermatophilus congolensis),* bovine farcy, ulcerative lymphangitis of horses, sporadic lymphangitis of horses

Mycotic
Epizootic lymphangitis of horses *(Histoplasma farciminosum),* sporotrichosis *(Sporothrix schenckii)*

Parasitic
Brugia spp. infection of dogs and cats

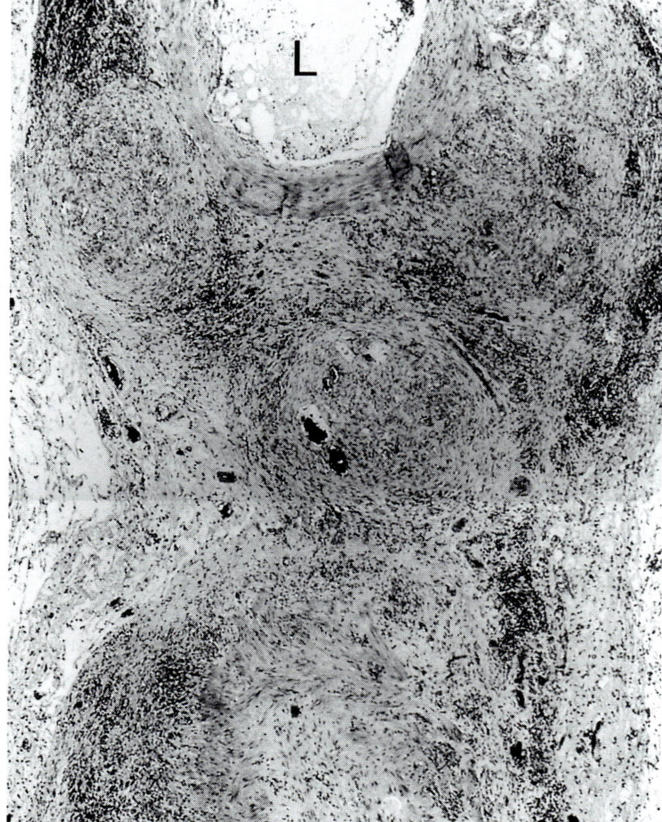

Fig. 4-59 Mesenteric lymph vessel; cow. Granulomatous lymphangitis, Johne's disease. The vessel wall is markedly thickened by infiltration of mononuclear leukocytes and proliferation of fibrous connective tissue. *L,* lumen. H & E stain. ×25.

Neoplastic diseases

Lymphangioma represents a rare benign neoplasm composed of lymph channels. The lymphangiosarcoma occurs more often than the benign neoplasm. Vascular spaces contain lymph rather than the blood seen in hemangiomas. Lymph vessels are frequently invaded by primary carcinomas, and this is a common route of metastasis.

Suggested Readings

Allen A. The cardiotoxicity of chemotherapeutic drugs. Semin Oncol 1992; 19:529-542.

Ayers KM, Jones SR. The cardiovascular system. In: Benirschke K, Garner FM, Jones TC, eds. Pathology of Laboratory Animals. Vol I. New York: Springer-Verlag, 1978, 1-69.

Balazs T, ed. Cardiac Toxicology. Vols I, II, III. Boca Raton, Fl: CRC Press, 1981.

Bishop SP. Cardiovascular system. In Andrews ET, Ward BC, Altman NH, eds. Spontaneous Animal Models of Human Disease. Vol I. New York: Academic Press, 1979:39-79.

Bristow MR. Drug-Induced Heart Disease. New York: Elsevier/North Holland Biomedical Press, 1980.

Buchanan JW. Chronic valvular disease (endocardiosis) in dogs. Adv Vet Sci Comp Med 1977; 21:75-104.

Combs AG, Acosta D. Toxic mechanisms of the heart: A review. Toxicol Pathol 1990; 18:583-596.

Czarnecki CM. Animal models of drug-induced cardiomyopathy. Comp Biochem Physiol 1984; 79C:9-14.

Easley JR. Necrotizing vasculitis: An overview. J Am Anim Hosp Assoc 1979; 15:207-211.

Ferrans VJ. Overview of morphologic reactions of the heart to toxic injury. In: Balazs T, ed. Cardiac Toxicology. Boca Raton, Fl: CRC Press, 1981:83-109.

Gibbs C, Gaskell CJ, Darke PGG, Wotton PR. Idiopathic pericardial hemorrhage in dogs: A review of fourteen cases. J Small Anim Pract 1982; 23:483-500.

Harpster NK. Cardiovascular diseases of the domestic cat. Adv Vet Sci Comp Med 1977; 21:39-74.

Hayes TJ, Roberts GKS, Halliwell WH. An idiopathic febrile necrotizing arteritis syndrome in the dog: Beagle pain syndrome. Toxicol Pathol 1989; 17:129-137.

Holman RL. Acute necrotizing arteritis, aortitis, and auriculitis following uranium nitrate injury in dogs with altered plasma proteins. Am J Pathol 1941; 17:359-381.

Jonsson L. Coronary arterial lesions and myocardial infarcts in the dog: A pathologic and microangiographic study. Acta Vet Scand 1972; 38(Suppl):1-80.

Kellerman TS, Coetzer JAW, Naudé TW. Heart. In: Plant Poisonings and Mycotoxicoses of Livestock in Southern Africa. Capetown, South Africa: Oxford University Press, 1988:83-130.

King JM, Roth L, Haschek WM. Myocardial necrosis secondary to neural lesions in domestic animals. J Am Vet Med Assoc 1982; 180:144-148.

Liu S-K, Hsu FS, Lee RCT. An Atlas of Cardiovascular Pathology. Taiwan: Pig Research Institute of Taiwan and the Animal Medical Center, 1989:1-371.

Liu S-K, Peterson ME, Fox PR. Hypertrophic cardiomyopathy and hyperthyroidism in the cat. J Am Vet Med Assoc 1984; 185:52-57.

Luginbuhl H, Detweiler D. Cardiovascular lesions in dogs. Ann NY Acad Sci 1965; 127:517-540.

Luginbuhl H, Rossi GL, Ratcliffe HL, Muller R. Comparative atherosclerosis. Adv Vet Sci Comp Med 1977; 21:421-448.

Newsholme SJ. Reaction patterns in myocardium in response to injury. J S Afr Vet Assoc 1982; 53:52-59.

Patterson DF. Congenital defects of the cardiovascular system of dogs: Studies in comparative cardiology. Adv Vet Sci Comp Med 1976; 20:1-35.

Pion PD, Kittleson MD, Rogers QR, Morris JG. Myocardial failure in cats associated with low plasma taurine: A reversible cardiomyopathy. Science 1987; 237:764-768.

Reichenbach DD, et al. Myofibrillar degeneration: A response of the myocardial cell to injury. Arch Pathol 1968; 85:189-199.

Riddell C. Cardiovascular system. In: Avian Histopathology. Lawrence, Kans: Allen Press, 1987:31-36.

Robinson WF, Huxtable CR, Pass DA. Canine parvoviral myocarditis: A morphologic description of the natural disease. Vet Pathol 1980; 17:282-293.

Robinson WF, Maxie MG. The cardiovascular system. In: Jubb KVF, Kennedy PC, Palmer N, eds. Pathology of Domestic Animals. Vol. 3, 4th ed. New York: Academic Press, 1993:1-100.

Smith HJ, Nuttall A. Experimental models of heart failure. Cardiovasc Res 1985; 19:181-186.

Szabo KT. Heart and cardiovascular system. In: Congenital malformations in laboratory and farm animals. New York: Academic Press, 1989:216-226.

Tanigawa G, Jarcho JA, Kass S, Solomon SD, Vosberg H, Seidman JG, Seidman CE. A molecular basis for familial hypertrophic cardiomyopathy: An α/β cardiac myosin heavy chain hybrid gene. Cell 1990; 62:991-998.

Van Stee EW, ed. Cardiovascular Toxicology. New York: Raven Press, 1982.

Van Vleet JF, Amstutz HE, Weirich WE, Rebar AH, Ferrans VJ. Clinical, clinicopathologic and pathologic alterations in acute monensin toxicosis in cattle. Am J Vet Res 1983; 44:2133-2144.

Van Vleet JF, Ferrans VJ. Clinical and pathologic features of chronic adriamycin toxicosis in rabbits. Am J Vet Res 1980; 41:1462-1469.

Van Vleet JF, Ferrans VJ. Congestive cardiomyopathy induced in ducklings fed graded amounts of furazolidone. Am J Vet Res 1983; 44:76-85.

Van Vleet JF, Ferrans VJ. Myocardial disease of animals. Am J Pathol 1986; 124:98-178.

Van Vleet JF, Ferrans VJ, Herman E. Cardiovascular and skeletal muscular systems. In: Haschek WM, Rousseaux CG, eds. Handbook of Toxicologic Pathology. New York: Academic Press, 1991:539-624.

Van Vleet, JF, Ferrans VJ, Weirich WE. Cardiac disease induced by chronic adriamycin administration in dogs and an evaluation of vitamin E and selenium as cardioprotectants. Am J Pathol 1980; 99:13-42.

Van Vleet JF, Ferrans VJ, Weirich WE. Pathologic alterations in congestive cardiomyopathy of dogs. Am J Vet Res 1981; 42:416-424.

Van Vleet JF, Ferrans VJ, Weirich WE. Pathologic alterations in hypertrophic and congestive cardiomyopathy of cats. Am J Vet Res 1980; 41:2037-2048.

Van Vleet JF, Rebar AH, Ferrans VJ. Acute cobalt and isoproterenol cardiotoxicity in swine: Protection by selenium-vitamin E supplementation and potentiation by stress-susceptible phenotype. Am J Vet Res 1977; 38:991-1002.

Vracko R, Cunningham D, Frederickson RG, Thorning D. Basal lamina of rat myocardium: Its fate after death of cardiac myocytes. Lab Invest 1988; 58:77-87.

Vracko R, Throning D, Frederickson RG, Cunningham D. Myocytic reactions at the borders of injured and healing rat myocardium. Lab Invest 1988; 59:104-114.

Woodruff JF. Viral myocarditis. Am J Pathol 1980; 101:427-484.

CHAPTER

5

The Urinary System

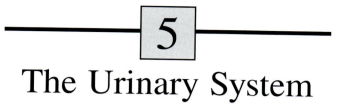

ANTHONY W. CONFER
ROGER J. PANCIERA

GENERAL RESPONSE TO INJURY

The urinary system is composed of kidneys, ureters, urinary bladder, and urethra. Injury to or obstruction of any component that significantly decreases or blocks renal function can result in major systemic effects, including azotemia; uremia; plasma protein loss; water, electrolyte, and acid/base imbalances; hyperparathyroidism and osteodystrophy; and retention of drugs. The functional unit of the kidney is the nephron. Each nephron contains a glomerulus, proximal convoluted tubule, loop of Henle, distal convoluted tubule, collecting duct, and a closely associated blood-vascular system. Because the nephron is a functional unit, destruction of any component of that unit results in damage to other components and in diminished function of the entire nephron.

Primary glomerular damage often occurs as a result of deposition of immune complexes, thrombosis, embolism, or direct viral or bacterial infection of glomerular components. Such insults are reflected morphologically by necrosis or proliferation of cells or membranes of the glomerulus or by infiltration with leukocytes and functionally by reduced vascular perfusion or by leakage of large quantities of proteins and other macromolecules into the glomerular filtrate. Continued or severe injury causes chronic lesions characterized by atrophy and fibrosis of the tuft and secondary atrophy of renal tubules. Similar chronic glomerular lesions occur secondarily to chronic loss of tubular function or reduced blood flow to the glomerulus.

Tubules respond to injury by cellular degeneration, necrosis, and atrophy. Tubular disease may occur as a result of tubular epithelial damage from infection, direct toxic damage, or ischemia. When nephrons are lost due to injury, remaining tubules have the capacity to undergo compensatory hypertrophy, which can maintain overall renal function. In many instances of necrosis, particularly in response to toxins, tubular epithelium can regenerate and restore function. Severe insult and loss of tubular basement membranes result in loss of tubular segments, failure of functional repair, and permanent loss of function of the entire nephron. Tubules may atrophy due to reduced oxygen tension, interstitial fibrosis, or tubular obstruction or secondary to diminished glomerular perfusion and function.

The renal interstitium is significantly involved in renal disease in ascending urinary tract infections (pyelonephritis), systemically derived infections of tubules and interstitium, and secondary to injury of tubules or glomeruli. Common acute lesions of the interstitium include edema, hemorrhage, and inflammation characterized by neutrophil infiltration. As lesions become subacute to chronic, neutrophils become less prominent, and, in several diseases, infiltrates of macrophages, lymphocytes, and plasma cells predominate. With chronic injury to or atrophy of nephrons, fibrosis of the interstitium is prominent, resulting in marked reduction in nephron function.

Diseases of the lower urinary tract may result from infection, obstruction, intoxication, congenital defects, physical trauma, or neoplasia. The initial sequence of events after insult to the lower urinary tract is erosion/ulceration of the transitional epithelium, neutrophilic infiltrates in the lamina propria, hemorrhage, and edema. With time, complete healing may occur. Chronic insults result in hyperplasia or metaplasia of transitional epithelium, lymphocytes, and plasma cell infiltrates; fibrosis of the lamina propria; and hypertrophy of smooth muscle.

THE KIDNEYS

Normal Structure and Function

Gross anatomy

Mammalian kidneys are complex, paired organs that lie in the retroperitoneum adjacent to the lumbar vertebrae. In domestic animals, only bovine kidneys have external lobation. Kidneys are covered by a fibrous capsule that normally may be easily removed from the renal surface. The renal parenchyma is divided into a cortex and a medulla. The cortex/medulla ratio is usually approximately 1:2 or 1:3 in domestic animals. The ratio varies among species;

for example, those adapted to the desert have a far wider medulla and, thus, a lower cortex/medulla ratio. That ratio may also be altered in disease states. The medulla can be generally subdivided into an outer zone, that portion of the medulla closer to the cortex, and an inner zone, that portion that is closer to the pelvis. Normally, the cortex is radially striated and dark red-brown except in mature cats, in which the cortex is often yellow because of the lipid content of tubular epithelial cells. The renal medulla is pale gray and has a single renal papilla in cats; a fused, crestlike papilla (renal medullary crest) in dogs, sheep, and horses; and multiple renal papillae in swine and cattle.

Organization and functions of the kidneys

The functional unit of the kidneys is the nephron, which includes the glomerulus and a tubular system with convoluted and straight tubules that become collecting ducts (Fig. 5-1). The glomerulus is a complex, convoluted tuft of capillaries held together by a supporting structure of cells in a glycoprotein matrix, the mesangium. The capillary tuft is covered by the visceral epithelial cells and contained within a membranous "cap," called Bowman's capsule, which is lined by parietal epithelial cells. Blood perfusing the glomerulus is the source of the glomerular filtrate. This ultrafiltrate of plasma, which contains water, salts, ions, glucose, and albumin, passes between visceral epithelial cells into Bowman's space and then into the proximal convoluted tubule. This tubule is lined by columnar epithelial cells that have a microvillous border, which greatly increases their absorptive surface. A major function of the proximal tubules is to reabsorb sodium, albumin, glucose, and water, and to reclaim bicarbonate. The proximal tubule is continuous with the loop of Henle, which is closely associated with the capillary network referred to as the vasa recta. The loop of Henle, via a countercurrent mechanism, absorbs Na^+ and Cl^- ions, producing a hypotonic filtrate that flows into the next portion of the nephron, the distal convoluted tubule. There, water is reabsorbed from the tubule into the interstitium because of a solute concentration gradient and by the effects of antidiuretic hormone. The filtrate is further concentrated in the collecting ducts by water reabsorption into the medullary interstitium by a urea gradient. Thus, the final excretory product, urine, is formed.

Renal function can be summarized into the following five basic components:

1. Formation of urine for the purpose of elimination of metabolic wastes.
2. Acid-base regulation, predominantly through reclamation of bicarbonate from the glomerular filtrate.
3. The conservation of water through reabsorption by the proximal convoluted tubules, the countercurrent mechanism of the loop of Henle, antidiuretic hormone activity in the distal tubules, and the urea gradient in the medulla. The tubular system normally reabsorbs approximately 99% of the water of the glomerular filtrate.
4. The maintenance of normal extracellular potassium ion concentration through passive reabsorption in the proximal tubules and tubular secretion in the distal tubules under the influence of aldosterone.
5. Endocrine function through three hormonal axes (erythropoietin, renin-angiotensin, and vitamin D). Erythropoietin produced in the kidneys in response to reduced oxygen tension stimulates bone marrow to produce erythrocytes. Renin, produced by cells in the juxtaglomerular apparatus, stimulates the production of the angiotensins that constrict afferent arterioles,

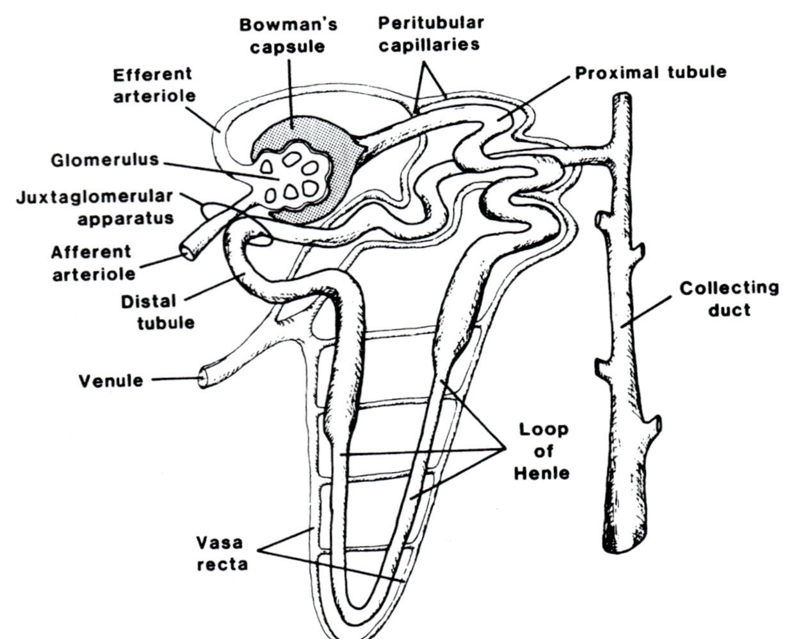

Fig. 5-1 Kidney, normal. The diagram depicts the organization of the normal nephron.

maintain renal blood pressure, and stimulate aldosterone secretion from the adrenal glands, thus increasing sodium reabsorption. Vitamin D is converted in the kidneys to its most active form [1,25-dihydroxycholecalciferol (calcitriol)]. This compound facilitates calcium absorption by the intestine (see Endocrine System).

Thus, renal malfunction may result in deficiency of one or more of these basic functions.

Renal Failure

Renal functional capacity can be impaired such that kidneys fail to carry out their normal metabolic and endocrine functions. Renal function can be reduced by prerenal factors, such as reduced renal blood flow, circulatory collapse, obstruction of vascular supply to the kidneys, shock, or severe hypovolemia. Renal function can be impaired by renal disease or by postrenal causes, such as obstruction of urine outflow through the lower urinary tract. Impairment of renal function results in the retention of those constituents of plasma that are normally removed by the kidneys. Assays of plasma or serum concentrations of urea and creatinine, nitrogenous waste products of protein catabolism, are routinely used as indices of diminished renal function. The intravascular elevation of these nitrogenous waste products is referred to as **azotemia.** Renal failure can result in intravascular accumulation of other metabolic wastes, such as guanidines, phenolic acids, and large-molecular-weight alcohols (example: myoinositol); in reduced blood pH (metabolic acidosis); in alterations in plasma ion concentrations, particularly potassium, calcium, and phosphate; and in hypertension. The result of renal failure is a toxicosis called **uremia.** Uremia is a syndrome associated with multisystemic clinical signs and lesions.

Table 5-1. Nonrenal lesions of uremia

Lesion	Mechanism
Pulmonary edema	Increased vascular permeability
Fibrinous pericarditis	Increased vascular permeability
Ulcerative and hemorrhagic gastritis	Ammonia secretion and vascular necrosis
Ulcerative and necrotic stomatitis	Ammonia secretion in saliva and vascular necrosis
Atrial and aortic thrombosis	Endothelial and subendothelial damage
Hypoplastic anemia	Increased erythrocyte fragility and lack of erythropoietin production
Soft-tissue mineralization (stomach, lungs, pleura, kidneys)	Altered calcium-phosphorus metabolism
Fibrous osteodystrophy	Altered calcium-phosphorus metabolism
Parathyroid hyperplasia	Altered calcium-phosphorus metabolism

Animals that die of renal failure usually do so because of the cardiotoxicity of elevated serum potassium, metabolic acidosis, and pulmonary edema. Nonrenal lesions of uremia recognizable clinically and at necropsy are often present in animals and are useful indicators of renal disease (Table 5-1). The severity of nonrenal lesions of uremia is dependent on the length of time that the animal has survived in the uremic state. Therefore, in acute renal failure, few, if any, nonrenal lesions occur, whereas in chronic renal failure many lesions may be seen. Many of the lesions can be attributed either to endothelial degeneration and necrosis resulting in thrombosis and infarction or to the excretion of high concentrations of ammonia in the saliva and gastric juice. Lesions of uremia include ulcerative and necrotic stomatitis characterized by a brown, foul-smelling, mucoid material adherent to the eroded and ulcerated lingual and oral mucosae (Fig. 5-2). Ulcers are most commonly present on the underside of the tongue. Ulcerative and hemorrhagic lesions often occur in the stomachs of dogs and cats and the colon of horses and cattle (Fig. 5-3). Large areas of mucosa are often edematous and dark red due to hemorrhage. The gastrointestinal contents may be

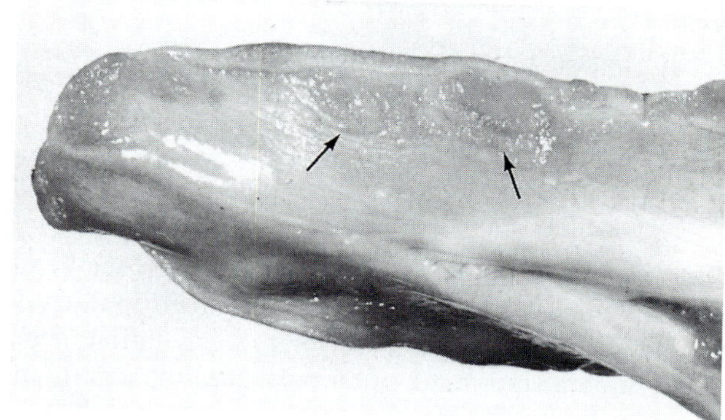

Fig. 5-2 Tongue; dog. Ulcerative glossitis. Uremia-induced ulcers *(arrows)* are on the ventral surface of the tongue.

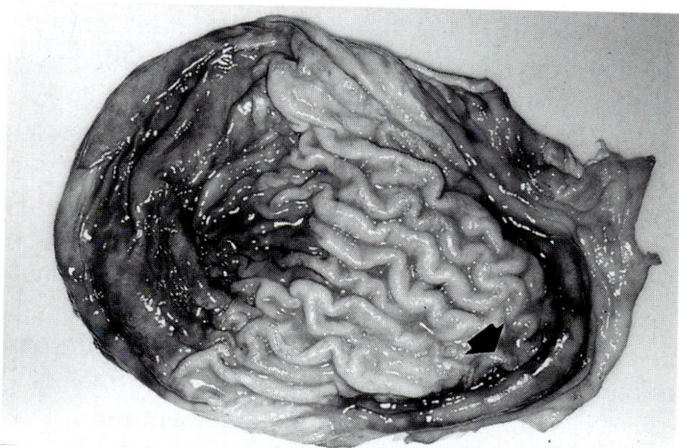

Fig. 5-3 Stomach; dog. Uremic gastritis. Due to uremia, the stomach wall is hemorrhagic and contains bloody mucus. Note the edematous mucosal thickening *(arrowhead).*

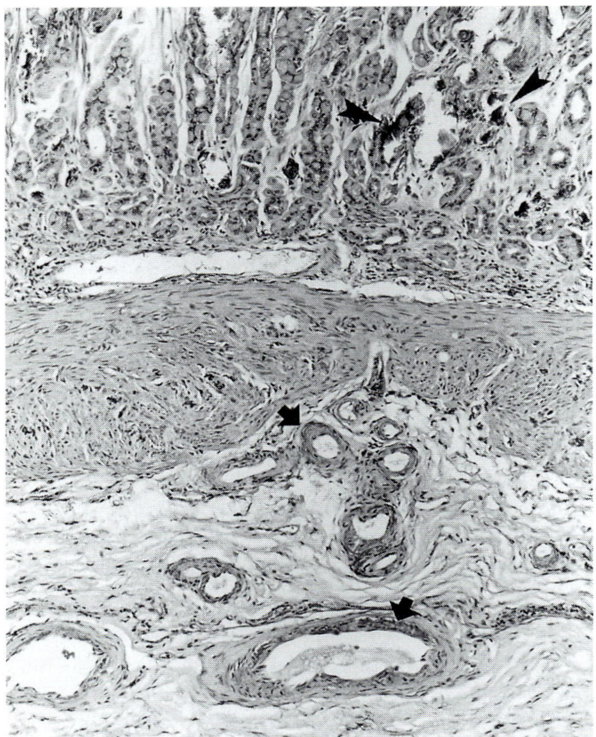

Fig. 5-4 Stomach. Uremic gastritis. Submucosal vessels are thickened, hyalinized, and mineralized *(arrows)*. The mucosa has multifocal mineralization of gastric glands *(arrowheads)*. Hematoxylin-eosin (H & E) stain.

bloody and have the odor of ammonia. Microscopically, coagulative necrosis, hemorrhage, and a neutrophilic infiltrate occur in the mucosa. Arteriolar degeneration, necrosis, and mineralization are often present in the gastric mucosa and submucosa (Fig. 5-4).

Increased vascular permeability in uremia occasionally results in a fibrinous pericarditis, characterized by fine granular fibrin deposits on the epicardium (visceral pericardium), and diffuse pulmonary edema. In the lungs, alveoli contain fibrin-rich fluid and often a mild infiltrate of macrophages and neutrophils. This lesion is called **uremic pneumonitis (uremic pneumonopathy).**

In the uremic animal, focal subendothelial degeneration can occur in the left atrial endocardium and, less frequently, on the endothelial surface of the proximal aorta and pulmonary trunk. These arterial lesions, called **mucoarteritis,** appear as finely granular, roughened plaques. Large thrombi may develop at these sites because of the predisposition to thrombosis, due to loss of antithrombin III in the urine, in dogs with protein-losing lesions of glomeruli. Chronic renal failure often results in reduced production of erythropoietin causing nonregenerative anemia. Increased erythrocytic fragility also contributes to the anemia. Most animals in renal failure have hyperphosphatemia and normocalcemia or hypocalcemia. Alterations in calcium-phosphorous metabolism in the uremic animal result from a complex set of events. When the glomerular filtration rate is reduced to less than 25% of normal, hyperphosphatemia results. This results in reduced ionized calcium in the blood, which stimulates parathyroid hormone secretion, causing calcium and phosphate reabsorption from bone through osteocytic osteolysis. These changes in calcium-phosphorous metabolism are made more severe by the reduced ability of the diseased kidney to hydroxylate 25-hydroxycholecalciferol to the more active 1,25-dihydroxycholecalciferol (calcitriol), resulting in decreased intestinal absorption of calcium. Calcitriol production is further inhibited by hyperphosphatemia. With time, these events lead to parathyroid hyperplasia (renal secondary hyperparathyroidism), fibrous osteodystrophy (renal osteodystrophy), and soft tissue calcification. Hyperparathyroidism is thought to perpetuate and enhance renal disease by stimulating nephrocalcinosis, the process by which renal tubular epithelium is damaged by an increase in intracellular calcium with its precipitation in mitochrondria.

Soft tissue calcification associated with uremia occurs in numerous sites and represents both dystrophic and metastatic calcification. The stomach wall may be gritty when cut, due to calcification of the inner and middle layers of the mucosa as well as the submucosal arterioles. Necrotic arterioles throughout the body are particularly susceptible to calcification during uremia. A characteristic lesion, particularly in dogs, is calcification of the subpleural connective tissue of the intercostal spaces (Fig. 5-5). These lesions are white-gray, granular pleural thickenings with a horizontal ''ladderlike'' arrangement. The intercostal muscles are only superficially calcified. Patchy or diffuse pulmonary calcification results in failure of the lungs to collapse, areas of paleness, mild to moderate firmness, and crunchi-

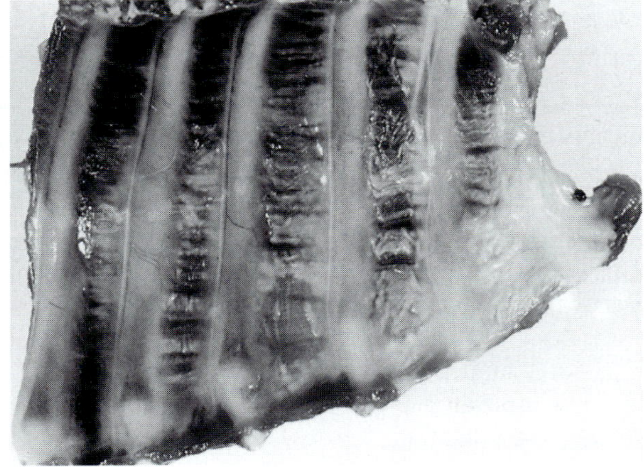

Fig. 5-5 Thoracic cavity, parietal pleura; dog. Intercostal mineralization. Transversally oriented streaks of mineralization are present in the subpleural intercostal connective tissue due to chronic uremia.

ness, and occurs occasionally in conjunction with the lesions of uremic pneumonitis. Microscopically, the interalveolar septa are calcified and may focally rupture, causing small emphysematous bullae. Although usually not visible at necropsy, calcification occurs in the kidneys. The kidneys may be gritty when cut, due to calcification of tubular basement membranes, Bowman's capsules, and necrotic tubular epithelium, especially in the medulla and inner cortex.

Necropsy Examination of the Kidneys

Examination of the kidneys should include assessment of their position relative to vertebrae and abdominal viscera, size relative to normal (approximately 2.5 to 3 vertebrae in length), color, contour, topographic features, turgidity, thickness, and degree of adherence of the capsule. The capsule should always be completely stripped from the kidneys so that the surface can be examined to evaluate the distribution of cortical lesions. This is particularly important for localizing small lesions. Kidneys should be incised longitudinally and the cut surfaces examined. Lesions visible on the surface should be evaluated on cut surface to assess whether they are superficial or extend deeply into the underlying parenchyma. On cut surface, the thickness of the cortex relative to normal and relative to the medulla should be assessed as well as bulging of the parenchyma to evaluate renal swelling, the color and moistness of the cortex and medulla, and the distinctness and intensity of cortical and medullary striations. Diminution or effacement of the striations is often a key observation in the gross recognition of degenerative and inflammatory lesions in the kidneys. The renal papillae (crests) should be examined, particularly for evidence of erosion or necrosis. Dilatation, inflammation, calculosis, and other lesions of the renal pelvis and its extensions should be noted.

Developmental Abnormalities

Renal aplasia, hypoplasia, and dysplasia

Renal **aplasia (agenesis)** is failure of development of one or both kidneys such that there is no recognizable renal tissue. In these cases, the ureter may be present or absent. If present, the cranial extremity of the ureter begins as a blind pouch. Unilateral aplasia is compatible with life, provided the other kidney is normal. Unilateral aplasia may be unnoticed during life and recognized only at necropsy. Bilateral aplasia, obviously incompatible with life, occurs sporadically. There may be a familial tendency in Doberman pinscher and beagle dogs.

Renal **hypoplasia** designates incomplete development of the kidney such that there are fewer nephrons, lobules, and calyces at birth. Hypoplasia can be unilateral or bilateral; it occurs rarely and is difficult to diagnose. Two rigid criteria have been suggested as being required before a diagnosis of renal hypoplasia can be established in human beings. These are: "in the absence of acquired disease, reduction in size of one kidney by more than 50 percent or in total renal mass by more than one-third . . ." and, more important, "a markedly reduced number of reniculi [renal lobules] and calyces." The latter criterion is likely to be useful only when evaluating the kidneys of cattle or pigs, which have renal lobular and calyceal structures analogous to those in human beings. These anatomic divisions are fused in most animal species. In cattle and pigs, the number of renal papillae in the hypoplastic kidney is reduced compared with the number in a normal kidney. Occasionally, bovine kidneys have reduced numbers of external lobules. These kidneys are not hypoplastic but are microscopically and functionally normal, and the reduction of numbers merely represents fusion of external lobules. Renal hypoplasia has been documented as an inherited disease of purebred or crossbred Large White pigs in New Zealand and has been recently described in foals of various breeds. In hypoplastic kidneys from pigs and foals, a marked reduction in the number of glomeruli was observed. In foals, for example, 5 to 12 glomeruli were present per low power field in affected kidneys compared with 30 to 35 glomeruli per low power field for normal kidneys from adults. The shrunken, pitted kidneys in young animals, particularly dogs, are often diagnosed as hypoplastic. However, most of these cases represent renal fibrosis (due to renal disease developing at an early age), progressive juvenile nephropathy, or dysplasia.

Renal **dysplasia** is an abnormality of altered structural organization resulting from abnormal differentiation with presence of structures not representative of normal nephrogenesis. Microscopically, five primary features of dysplasia are described. These include asynchronous differentiation of nephrons, persistence of mesenchyme such that the interstitial connective tissue has a myxomatous appearance, the persistence of metanephric ducts, atypical (adenomatoid) tubular epithelium, and the presence of cartilaginous or osseous tissues. Interstitial fibrosis, renal cysts, and a few enlarged hypercellular glomeruli (compensatory hypertrophy) are seen secondarily to the primary dysplastic lesions. Renal dysplasia occurs infrequently and, like renal hypoplasia, must be differentiated from renal fibrosis and from progressive juvenile nephropathy. Dysplastic lesions may be unilateral or bilateral and can involve much of the kidneys or occur as only focal lesions. Dysplastic kidneys may be small and/or misshapen. The number of nephrons, lobules, and calyces is normal. Bilateral renal dysplasia characterized by persistent mesenchyme and atypical tubular development has been described in foals. Cystic renal dysplasia has been described in sheep and is inherited as an autosomal dominant trait.

Progressive juvenile nephropathy (familial renal disease) of Lhaso apso and Shih Tzu dogs, and perhaps other breeds, may be a dysplasia. Asynchronous differentiation is often seen and, to a lesser extent, several other lesions of dysplasia. However, until these hereditary lesions of dogs are better characterized, it is probably best to retain the diagnosis of progressive juvenile nephropathy (see Chronic Renal Diseases).

Ectopic and fused kidneys

Ectopic kidneys are misplaced from their normal sublumbar location by abnormal migration during fetal development. These occur most frequently in pigs and dogs and usually involve only one kidney. Ectopic locations often include the pelvic cavity or inguinal region. Although ectopic kidneys are usually structurally and functionally normal, malposition of the ureter predisposes them to obstruction and secondary hydronephrosis.

Fused (horseshoe) kidneys result from the fusion of the cranial or caudal poles of the kidneys during nephrogenesis. This results in the appearance of one large kidney with two ureters. The histologic structure and function of fused kidneys are usually normal.

Renal cysts

Congenital renal cysts can accompany renal dysplasia or can occur as primary entities. Kidneys may contain single or multiple cysts that cause no alteration in renal function and are, therefore, incidental findings. Such renal cysts are common in pigs and calves.

Cysts may arise anywhere along the nephron and be located in either cortex or medulla. Cysts range from those barely visible to those several centimeters in diameter; are usually spherical, thin walled, and lined by flattened epithelium; and contain clear, watery fluid. When viewed from the renal surface, the cyst wall is pale gray, smooth, and translucent. **Polycystic** kidneys contain many cysts that involve numerous nephrons, such that the kidney may have a ''Swiss cheese'' appearance (Fig. 5-6). As cysts enlarge, they compress adjacent parenchyma. When kidneys are polycystic, renal function may be compromised. Congenital polycystic kidneys occur sporadically in many species but may be inherited as an autosomal dominant lesion in pigs and lambs and may be inherited along with cystic biliary disease in cairn terrier dogs. The lesion is also seen in families of Persian cats. A polycystic renal disease with cysts arising from glomeruli has been described in collie puppies.

The pathogenesis of renal cysts is not entirely understood. It was once thought that congenital cysts arose from failure of nephrons and collecting ducts to unite; however, this theory has not been substantiated. Cysts appear to derive from normal or noncystic segments of the nephron, including Bowman's space, renal tubules, and collecting ducts. Results of experimental studies with chemicals indicate that genetic predisposition is not a requirement for renal cyst formation. Three mechanisms of renal cyst formation are now considered plausible. First, obstruction of nephrons may cause elevated luminal pressure and secondary dilatation. Second, defective tubular basement membranes allow saccular dilatation of tubules. Third, focal tubular epithelial hyperplasia with production of new basement membranes causes development of enlarged, dilated tubules.

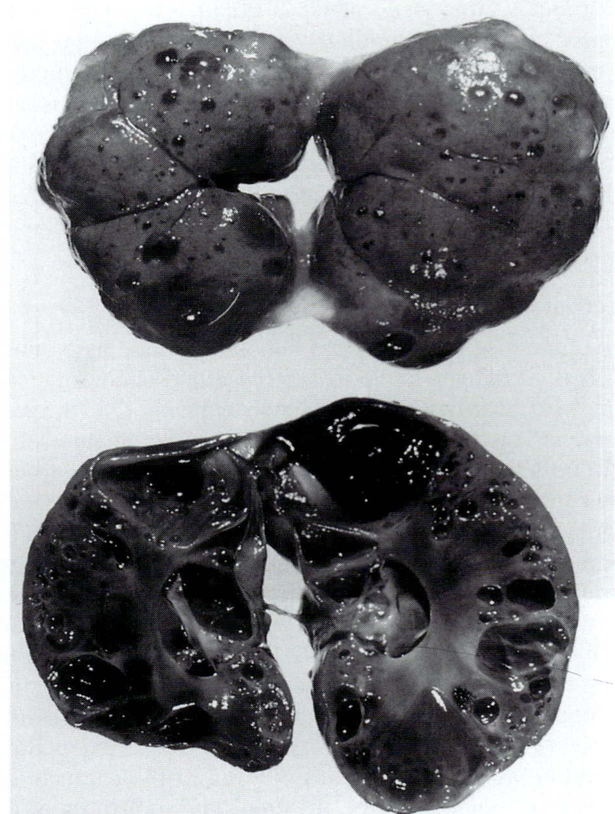

Fig. 5-6 Kidney; cat. Polycystic disease. Numerous cortical and medullary renal cysts are present. One cyst contains a blood clot.

Acquired renal cysts may occur as a result of renal interstitial fibrosis (see Chronic Renal Diseases) or of other renal diseases that cause intratubular obstruction. These cysts are usually very small (1 to 2 mm) and occur primarily in the cortex.

Inherited abnormalities in renal tubular function

Inherited abnormalities of tubular metabolism, in transport, or in reabsorption of glucose, amino acids, ions, and proteins have been described in dogs. These are not associated with consistent morphologic changes in the kidneys. The excretion of large quantities of cystine in the urine **(cystinuria)** is a sex-linked inherited disease seen occasionally in purebred or mongrel male dogs. It is of importance because it predisposes affected dogs to calculus formation and obstruction of the lower urinary tract. Primary renal **glucosuria,** an inherited disorder in Norwegian elkhounds and found sporadically in other dogs, occurs when the capacity of tubular epithelial cells to reabsorb glucose is significantly reduced. Glucosuria predisposes dogs to infections of the lower urinary tract and urinary bladder emphysema. An hereditary generalized defect in tubular reabsorption similar to the **Fanconi syndrome** in human beings has been described in basenji dogs. This disease is characterized by aminoaciduria, glucosuria, proteinuria, and increased phosphaturia and is often associated with progressive renal insufficiency.

Circulatory Disturbances

Hyperemia/congestion

As in other organs, renal **hyperemia** and **congestion** may be physiologic, active, passive, or hypostatic. Hyperemic kidneys are darker red than normal, may be perceptibly swollen, and ooze blood on a cut surface. At necropsy, unilateral renal hypostatic congestion is present in animals that have died in lateral recumbency.

Hemorrhage

Renal cortical hemorrhages occur in association with many septicemic diseases and result from vasculitis or vascular necrosis. Petechiae are commonly seen on the surface and throughout the cortex of kidneys from pigs that died of such septicemias as hog cholera (swine fever), African swine fever, erysipelas, streptococcal infections, or salmonellosis (Fig. 5-7). Renal cortical ecchymotic hemorrhages associated with multifocal tubular and vascular necrosis are salient and diagnostically important lesions of herpesvirus septicemia of neonatal puppies (Fig. 5-8).

Large intrarenal or subcapsular hemorrhages may occur in association with direct trauma, bleeding disorders such as hemophilia, and disseminated intravascular coagulation.

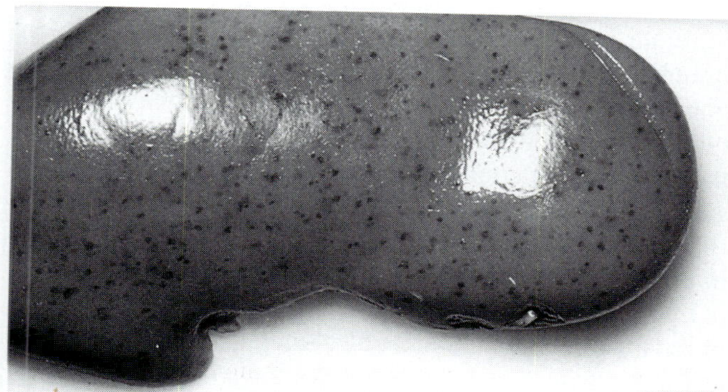

Fig. 5-7 Kidney; pig. Renal hemorrhages. Cortical petechial hemorrhages are randomly scattered throughout the kidney. This kidney is from a pig with a septicemic illness (in this case, hog cholera [swine fever]). Bar = 5 mm.

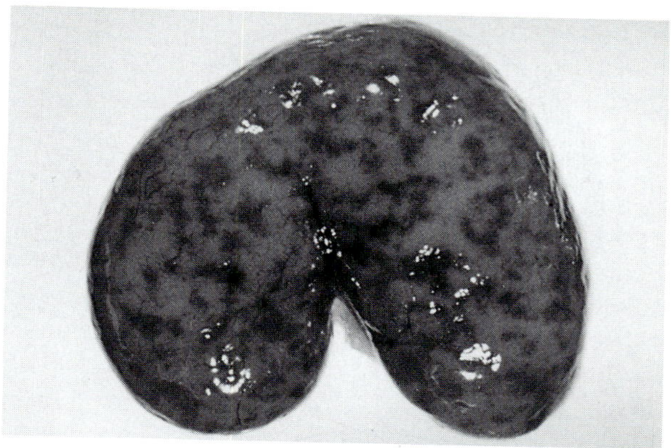

Fig. 5-8 Kidney; dog. Renal hemorrhages. Characteristic cortical petechial and ecchymotic hemorrhages from a puppy with herpesvirus canis septicemia.

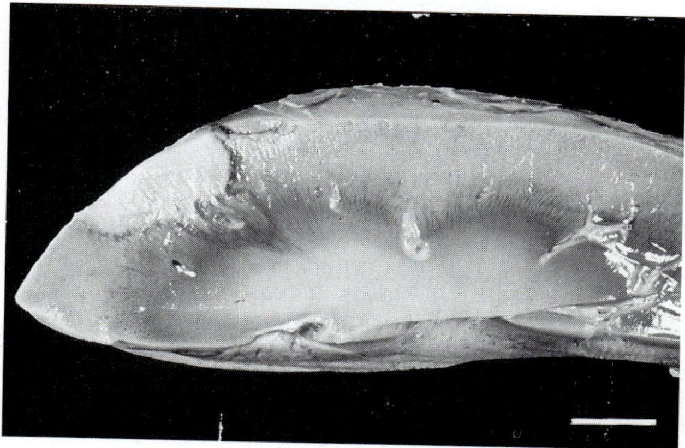

Fig. 5-9 Kidney; horse. Acute infarct. The renal cortex contains a pale, wedge-shaped renal infarct. Bar = 1 cm.

Infarction

Renal **infarcts** are areas of coagulative necrosis that result from the ischemia of vascular occlusion and are usually due to thrombosis or aseptic emboli. Grossly, renal infarcts appear red or pale, depending on several factors including the interval after vascular occlusion and whether arteries or veins are occluded (Fig. 5-9). Occlusion of arteries results in infarcts that are initially hemorrhagic and turn pale yellow-gray within 2 to 3 days due to lysis of erythrocytes and leaching of hemoglobin (Fig. 5-10). Pale infarcts have a central area of coagulative necrosis and are usually surrounded by a zone of congestion and hemorrhage along with a pale margin due to a zone of leukocytes (Fig. 5-11). Infarcts are often wedge-shaped, with the base against the cortical surface and the apex pointing toward the medulla, conforming to the distribution of the obstructed vessel(s). That appearance, however, may not be apparent when infarcts are extremely large or confluent.

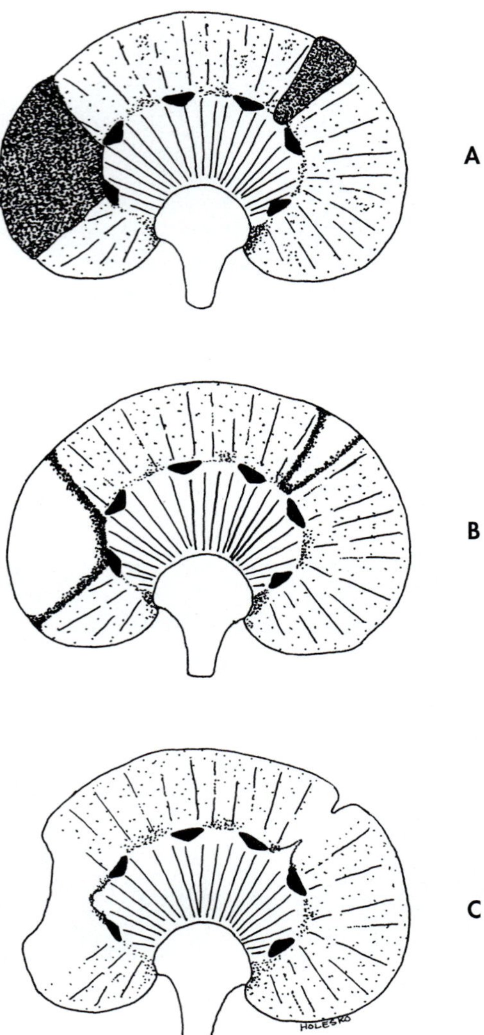

Fig. 5-10 Kidney. Renal infarcts. The normal progression of renal infarcts is outlined. **A**, **B**, Acute renal infarcts. Initially, renal infarcts are swollen and hemorrhagic. In 2 to 3 days, infarcts become pale, surrounded by a zone of hyperemia and hemorrhage. **C**, Chronic infarcts are pale, shrunken, and fibrotic, resulting in distortion of the renal contour.

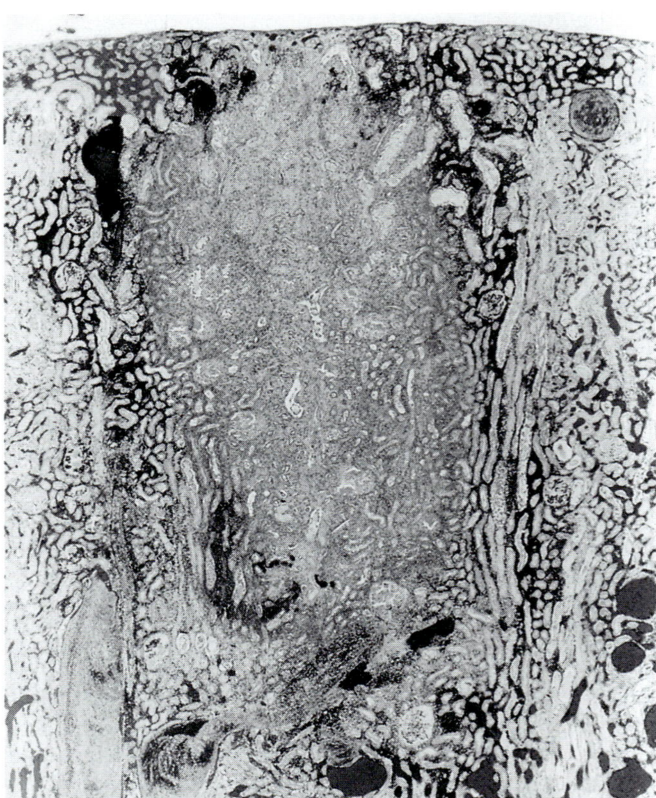

Fig. 5-11 Kidney, cortex. Acute infarct. The renal cortex contains an acute infarct with a central zone of coagulation necrosis surrounded by a zone of hyperemia and hemorrhage. H & E stain.

Infarcts can involve the cortex only or the cortex and medulla, depending on the size of the occluded vessel and the site of obstruction. For example, thrombosis of an arcuate artery, which supplies both cortex and medulla, would result in coagulative necrosis of a segment of both the cortex and medulla. Thrombosis of a cortical interlobular artery would result in an infarct of the cortex only. Although less common, infarcts due to venous occlusion are seen occasionally, and their hemorrhagic appearance is more prolonged than that of infarcts resulting from arterial occlusion because the former have continued arterial blood flow to the area.

Microscopically, in acute renal infarcts, all structures in the central zone of the infarct are necrotic. At the periphery of the infarct, only the proximal tubules may be affected, due to their high metabolic rate. The glomeruli may be spared. Along the margin of the necrotic zone, the limited infiltrate consists of neutrophils, macrophages, and a few lymphocytes. Associated capillaries are markedly engorged with blood. Healing of the infarcted area occurs by lysis and phagocytosis of the necrotic tissue and replacement by fibrous connective tissue, leaving a discrete, linear, fibrotic scar (Fig. 5-12). Various causes of renal scarring and differentiation of scarred lesions will be discussed in the section on Chronic Renal Disease.

Endocardial thrombosis frequently results in embolism of renal vessels due to the high percentage of cardiac output (20% to 25%) that goes to the kidneys. Therefore, renal infarcts resulting from thromboemboli are commonly present in cats with left atrial thrombosis associated with cardiomyopathy or in any animal species with endocarditis involving the left heart. In rare cases, emboli may be large enough to occlude the renal artery, causing infarction of

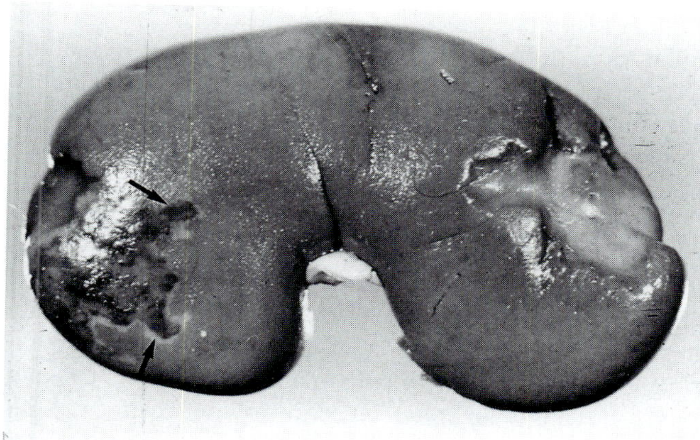

Fig. 5-12 Kidney; dog. Multiple renal infarcts. The depressed foci represent healing (scarred) stages of infarction. An acute infarct is at the lower left *(arrows)*. *Courtesy Dr. L. Roth.*

the entire kidney. More commonly, emboli obstruct many smaller vessels, causing multiple small infarcts in the kidneys. In general, renal infarction may occur due to thrombosis associated with a generalized vascular disease such as polyarteritis or arteriosclerosis or with cardiovascular collapse and shock. Renal infarcts may occur rarely in horses due to emboli arising from thrombosed cranial mesenteric arteries associated with migrating larvae of *Strongylus vulgaris.* Thrombosis of pulmonary, coronary, splenic, or renal arteries and resultant infarction are common in dogs with renal amyloidosis due primarily to loss through the urine of plasma anticoagulants such as antithrombin III. Endotoxin-mediated arterial or capillary thrombosis is a common cause of infarction in association with gram-negative sepsis or endotoxic shock.

Septic emboli, particularly those from valvular endocarditis, can cause renal infarcts as well. Septic infarcts are initially hemorrhagic but eventually become abscesses.

Renal cortical necrosis

This lesion results from the widespread thrombosis that occurs in the glomerular capillaries, interlobular arteries, and afferent arterioles in disseminated intravascular coagulation. This lesion is not to be confused with ischemic acute tubular necrosis discussed under the section on Tubular Necrosis. Partial or complete renal cortical necrosis is usually a bilateral lesion that occurs in all animal species, especially in association with gram-negative septicemias or endotoxemias, and is related to endotoxin-induced endothelial damage, activation of the clotting mechanism, and widespread capillary thrombosis. The lesion may be experimentally induced in animals by two endotoxin injections 24 hours apart and is a manifestation of the generalized Shwartzman reaction.

The resulting microthrombosis of vessels throughout the renal cortex results in widespread ischemia and large and small areas of hypoxic coagulation necrosis and hemorrhage. The renal cortex may be diffusely pale with a zone of hyperemia separating the necrotic cortex from the viable medulla, or, more often, the cortex is a mosaic of large, irregular hemorrhagic areas, resembling hemorrhagic infarcts interspersed with large yellow-gray areas resembling pale infarcts. The necrotic tissue may involve the full width of the cortex or only the outer portion (Fig. 5-13). Thrombi are demonstrable in interlobular and afferent arterioles and glomerular capillaries (Fig. 5-14). Special stains are useful in identifying microthrombi in histologic sections.

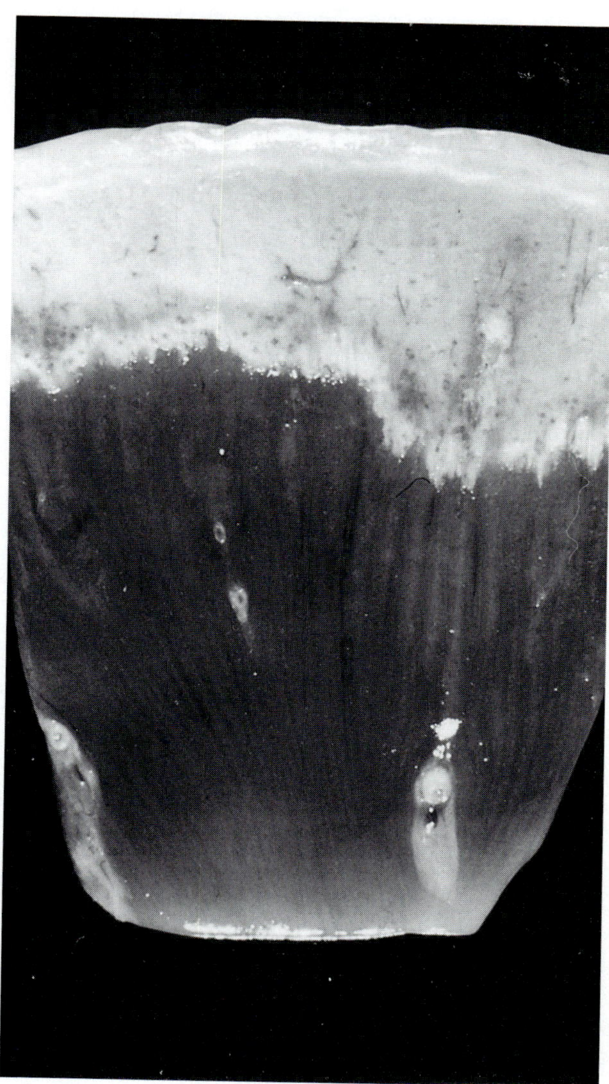

Fig. 5-13 Kidney; horse. Bilateral renal cortical necrosis. Virtually the entire renal cortex is necrotic. The lesion was bilateral and diffuse and due to widespread capillary thrombosis. *Courtesy Dr. J. Long.*

Papillary (Medullary Crest) Necrosis

Necrosis of the renal papillae or their anatomic counterpart, the medullary crest, is a response of the inner medulla to ischemia. Papillary necrosis occurs as a primary lesion or in association with other renal lesions. The inner medulla, including the papillae, normally is less well perfused with blood than are other zones of the kidneys. Because of this limited blood flow, any lesion or process that further reduces medullary blood flow may cause ischemic necrosis (infarction) of the papillae. Thus, papillary necrosis can be seen secondary to scarring of the outer medulla, medullary amyloidosis, pyelitis, or renal pelvic calculi or with the increased intrapelvic pressure that occurs with obstruction of the lower urinary tract.

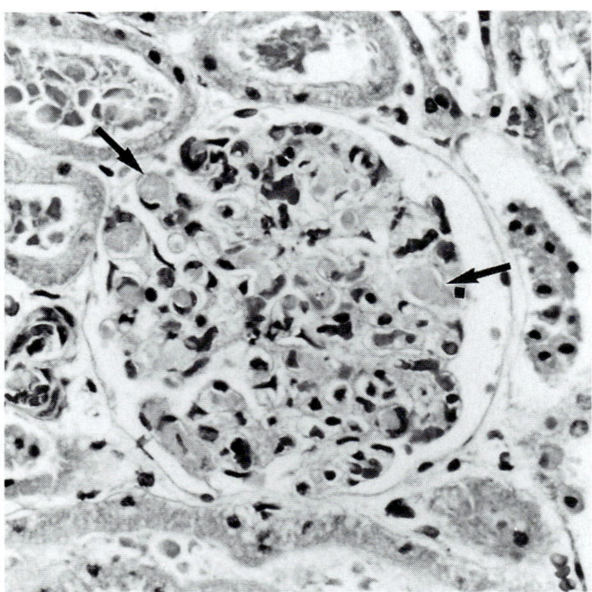

Fig. 5-14 Kidney, cortex; dog. Glomerular capillary thrombosis. Capillaries are dilated with microthrombi *(arrows)* due to disseminated intravascular coagulation. Cortical tubules are undergoing pyknosis and karyolysis. H & E stain.

Papillary necrosis also occurs as a primary disease in animals treated with nonsteroidal antiinflammatory-analgesic drugs and is analogous to **analgesic nephropathy** in human beings. The primary disease occurs quite frequently in horses treated for prolonged periods with phenylbutazone or banamine. It is of potential importance in dogs and cats following accidental ingestion of or treatment with ibuprofen, aspirin, or acetaminophen at excessive dosages. Some of these drugs inhibit prostaglandin biosynthesis, and, because prostaglandins are important for the maintenance of normal blood flow in the vasa recta, these compounds can reduce blood flow and cause ischemic necrosis of the papillae. In addition to its inhibition of prostaglandin biosynthesis, acetaminophen also causes direct oxidative damage to medullary tubular epithelium after covalent binding to the cells, further enhancing necrosis of the renal papillae.

Papillary necrosis is usually an incidental finding at necropsy, but rarely may lead to progressive renal failure. Typical lesions are discolored areas of necrotic inner medulla sharply delineated from the surviving medullary tissue (Fig. 5-15). The necrotic tissue may be yellow-gray, green, or pink stained; friable or plastic; attached, detached, or absent, leaving a roughened, attenuated, ulcerated papilla, depending on the stage/duration of the lesion (Fig. 5-16). Sloughed necrotic medullary tissue may form a nidus for precipitation of minerals, resulting in formation of pelvic or ureteral calculi.

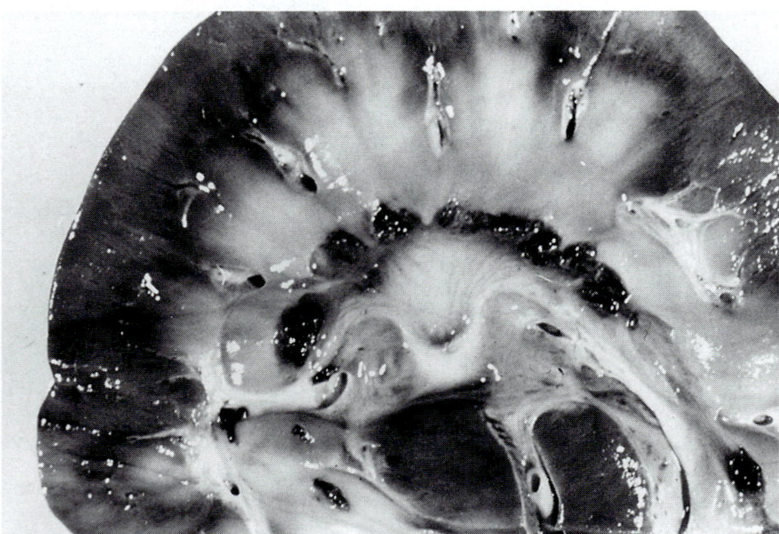

Fig. 5-15 Kidney; horse. Papillary (medullary crest) necrosis. Acute coagulation necrosis of the inner medulla resulted from chronic administration of a nonsteroidal antiinflammatory drug. *Courtesy Dr. L. Roth.*

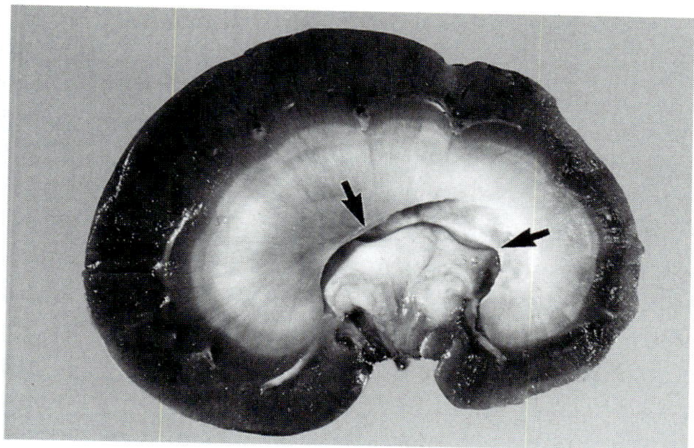

Fig. 5-16 Kidney; dog. Chronic papillary (medullary crest) necrosis. The medullary crest is irregularly attenuated *(arrows)*, and there is scarring and contraction of the overlying cortex and medulla.

Tubular Necrosis

General considerations

Acute tubular necrosis, often referred to as **nephrosis,** is the result of an ischemic or a toxic insult to the renal tubular epithelial cells. Tubular epithelial cells respond to prolonged ischemia or to nephrotoxins by undergoing degeneration, followed by necrosis and desquamation of the cells. The proximal convoluted tubular epithelium is most susceptible to ischemia or toxic injury due to its high metabolic rate. Animals that have severe tubular necrosis often have signs of uremia. Characteristically associated with uremia of tubular necrosis origin is a decrease in urine production **(oliguria)** or absence of urine production **(anuria).** Acute tubular necrosis induces oliguria by one of several mechanisms. These include the leakage of urine from damaged tubules across disrupted basement membranes into the renal interstitium or intratubular obstruction due to loss of necrotic epithelium. In addition, because of activation of the renin-angiotensin system, particularly affecting outer cortical nephrons, glomerular blood flow and filtration are decreased, resulting in reduced formation of urine.

At necropsy, the recognition of acute tubular necrosis is often difficult. Nevertheless, the kidneys are swollen; the capsular surface is smooth and pale and has a slightly translucent appearance. The cut surface is usually pale and excessively moist; striations may be muted, or they may be accentuated by radially oriented, opaque, white streaks. The medulla may be pale or congested. The microscopic appearance of kidneys with acute tubular necrosis can be variable, depending on the severity of the insult, the duration of exposure to the insult, and the length of time between insult and death. Tubular epithelium may be swollen, the microvilli lost, and the cytoplasm vacuolated or granular and intensely eosinophilic, indicative of coagulation necrosis. In such tubules, the nuclear changes are pyknosis, karyorrhexis, or karyolysis. Necrotic tubular epithelium is desquamated, resulting in dilated, markedly hypocellular tubules that may contain necrotic cellular debris and hyalinized or granular casts (Figs. 5-17 and 5-18).

If the insult is removed and the tubular basement membranes remain intact, tubular epithelial regeneration occurs with restitution of renal function. Recent evidence indicates that epidermal growth factor secreted by distal convoluted tubules mediates the tubular repair process. In an experimental model system of tubular necrosis caused by the nephrotoxin mercuric chloride, morphologic evidence of regeneration of proximal convoluted tubules is seen within 3 days after a toxic insult. Microscopically, basement membranes are partially covered with flattened and elongated to low cuboidal cells that stain more basophilic than normal due to the increased concentrations of cytoplasmic ribosomes and rough endoplasmic reticulum producing protein for repair. Nuclei are hyperchromatic, and mitotic figures are seen. Normal-appearing tubular epithelium became prominent between 7 and 14 days after toxin exposure. Normal renal structure without residual evidence of tubular damage is restored between 21 and 56 days after exposure to the nephrotoxin. Similar time frames for tubular regeneration have been described in human patients naturally exposed to inorganic mercury.

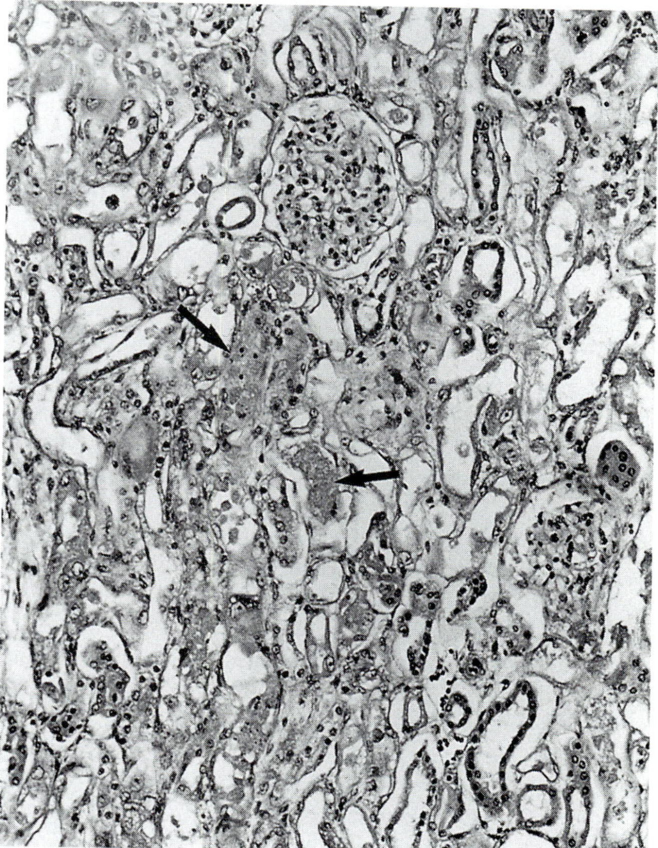

Fig. 5-17 Kidney. Acute tubular necrosis. The lesion is characterized by epithelial coagulation necrosis *(arrows)*, dilated hypocellular tubules, and intratubular nuclear and proteinaceous debris. H & E stain.

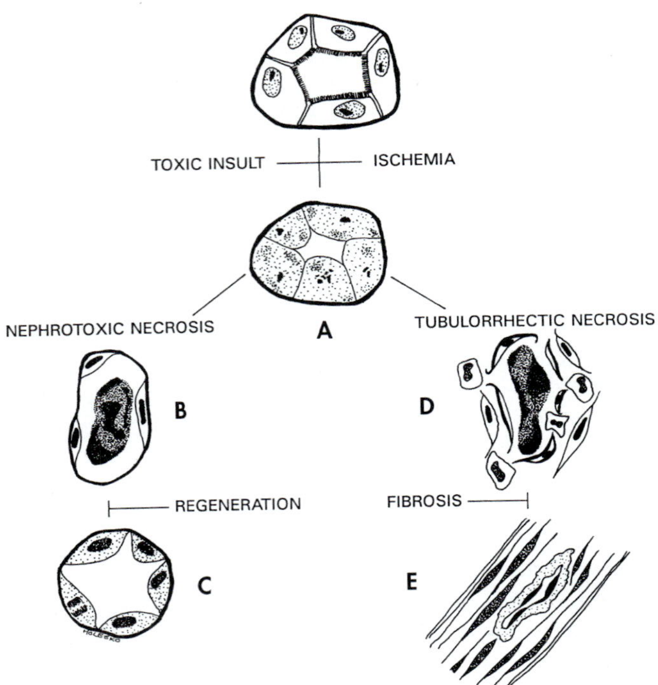

Fig. 5-18 Kidney, proximal tubules. Acute tubular necrosis. Acute tubular necrosis results from a nephrotoxin or ischemia. **A**, Both insults cause acute necrosis characterized by cellular swelling, pyknosis, karyorrhexis, and karyolysis. **B**, Subsequent to nephrotoxic necrosis, there is sloughing of necrotic epithelium into the tubular lumina and the basement membranes remain intact allowing, **C**, regeneration to occur. **D**, Ischemia may result in tubulorrhectic necrosis. Necrotic epithelium sloughs into the tubular lumen, the basement membrane is disrupted, macrophages infiltrate, and fibroblasts proliferate. **E**, Fibrosis with tubular atrophy results.

Causes of acute tubular necrosis

As stated earlier, acute tubular necrosis occurs by two general mechanisms: ischemic and nephrotoxic. Numerous causes of markedly reduced renal perfusion may lead to **ischemic tubular necrosis.** Severe hypotension, associated with shock, results in preglomerular vasoconstriction and reduced glomerular filtration, resulting in renal ischemia and ischemic tubular necrosis. Complete ischemia for longer than 2 hours usually results in tubular necrosis. Cell death results from decreased ATP production, increased membrane permeability, calcium ion influx, phospholipase activation, and generation of oxygen radicals. Thus, mitochondrial respiration is disrupted, and further cell membrane damage occurs. Initially, tubular necrosis is randomly distributed in nephrons, but the proximal convoluted tubules are most severely affected. Prolonged ischemia can result in necrosis of epithelium throughout the cortex and, to a lesser extent, the medulla. Glomeruli often remain morphologically normal even when ischemia is prolonged. One characteristic of ischemic tubular necrosis is that disruption of the tubular basement membranes can occur, a process referred to as **tubulorrhectic necrosis** (see Fig. 5-18). Tubular repair in such kidneys is imperfect because regenerating epithelial cells have lost their normal scaffolding, and tubular atrophy and interstitial fibrosis are the results. Gross and microscopic lesions resemble those described in the section on Tubular Necrosis.

A frequent set of events leading to ischemic tubular necrosis occurs in hypoperfused kidneys complicated by hemoglobinuria or myoglobinuria. Hemoglobinuria accompanies episodes of severe intravascular hemolysis and hemoglobinemia, as in chronic copper toxicity in sheep, leptospirosis or babesiosis in cattle, red maple toxicity in horses, and babesiosis or autoimmune hemolytic anemia in dogs. Myoglobinuria accompanies acute rhabdomyolysis, as in azoturia of horses, capture myopathy in exotic or wild animals, or severe trauma. In these disease states, elevated serum concentrations of hemoglobin or myoglobin pass into the glomerular filtrate and accumulate in renal tubules, causing **hemoglobinuric** or **myoglobinuric nephrosis.** Hemoglobin and myoglobin are not nephrotoxic themselves, in that intravenous infusions of these compounds into healthy animals produce no recognizable lesions. However, stromal components of erythrocytes may be toxic, and hemoglobin may enhance the tubular necrosis associated with ischemia. The renal cortices of animals with severe hemoglobinuria or myoglobinuria are diffusely stained red-brown to blue-black and often have intratubular heme casts that appear as red-black stippling on the external surface and continue into the cortex as radially oriented, dark red streaks. The medulla may be stained dark red or contain red streaks (Fig. 5-19). Microscopically, tubular lumina contain an abundance of orange-red, granular, refractile material, the characteristic appearance of a heme compound (Fig. 5-20). Cellular swelling and pigmentation of tubular epithelial cells may be seen in association with

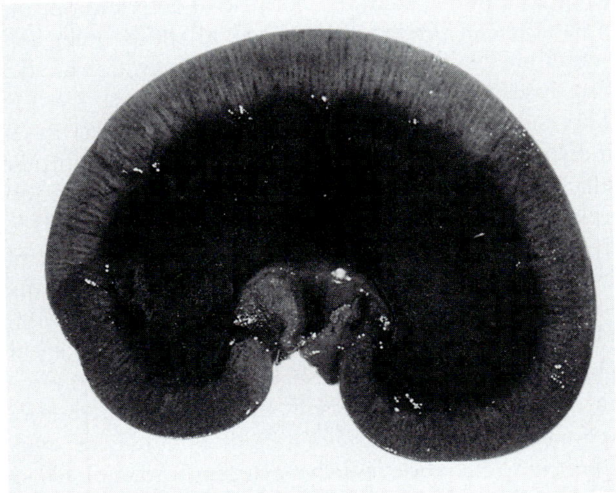

Fig. 5-19 Kidney; dog. Hemoglobinuric nephrosis. Diffuse hemoglobin staining of the medulla is present due to a severe intravascular hemolytic crisis.

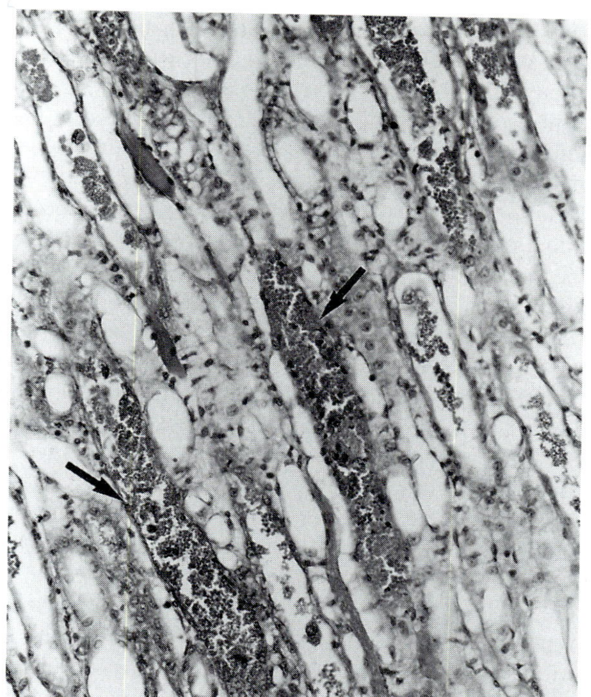

Fig. 5-20 Kidney; cow. Myoglobinuric nephrosis. Heme casts *(arrows)* are present in dilated medullary tubules as a result of acute severe rhabdomyolysis. H & E stain.

Box 5-1 COMMON NEPHROTOXINS OF DOMESTIC ANIMALS

Heavy metals
Mercury
Lead
Arsenic
Cadmium
Bismuth

Antibacterial/antifungal agents
Aminoglycosides
- gentamicin
- neomycin
- kanamycin
- streptomycin
- tobramycin
- amikacin

Tetracyclines
Amphotericin B
Monensin

Mycotoxins
Ochratoxin A
Citrinin

Plants
Pigweed *(Amaranthus retroflexus)*
Oaks (*Quercus* sp.)
Isotropis sp.
Yellow wood tree *(Terminalia oblongata)*

Oxalates
Ethylene glycol (antifreeze)
Halogeton *(Halogeton glomeratus)*
Greasewood *(Sarcobatus vermiculatus)*
Rhubarb *(Rheum rhaponticum)*
Sorrel, dock (*Rumex* sp.)

Vitamin D
Vitamin D supplements
Calciferol-containing rodenticides
Cestrum diurnum
Solanum sp.
Trisetum sp.

Antineoplastic compounds
Cisplatin

increased serum concentrations of bilirubin, especially due to obstructive jaundice. The term **cholemic nephrosis** has been applied to this lesion; however, its significance is doubtful. Acute tubular necrosis, when seen in association with severe bilirubinemia, the so-called **hepatorenal syndrome,** is probably not due to bile acid or bilirubin retention per se, but to prerenal causes such as constriction of renal vessels.

Nephrotoxic tubular necrosis may be caused by various classes of naturally occurring or synthetic compounds (Box 5-1). Gross and microscopic lesions resemble those described in the section on Tubular Necrosis. Nephrotoxins, however, usually do not damage the tubular basement membranes. One group of nephrotoxins includes the heavy metals, such as inorganic mercury, inorganic arsenic, lead, cadmium, and thallium. Common sources of heavy metals include herbicides (arsenics), old paint, batteries, automobile components (lead), impure petroleum distillates, and other environmental contaminants. Acute tubular necrosis results from cell membrane or mitochondrial damage induced by these toxins and is often related to interaction of metals with protein sulfhydryl groups. In mercury toxicosis, mercury concentrates in the rough endoplasmic reticulum and causes early tubular changes, including loss of brush borders and dispersion of ribosomes followed by mitochondrial swelling and cellular death. The specific metal involved in toxic tubular injury cannot be identified by the renal lesions except in lead toxicity, in which epithelial

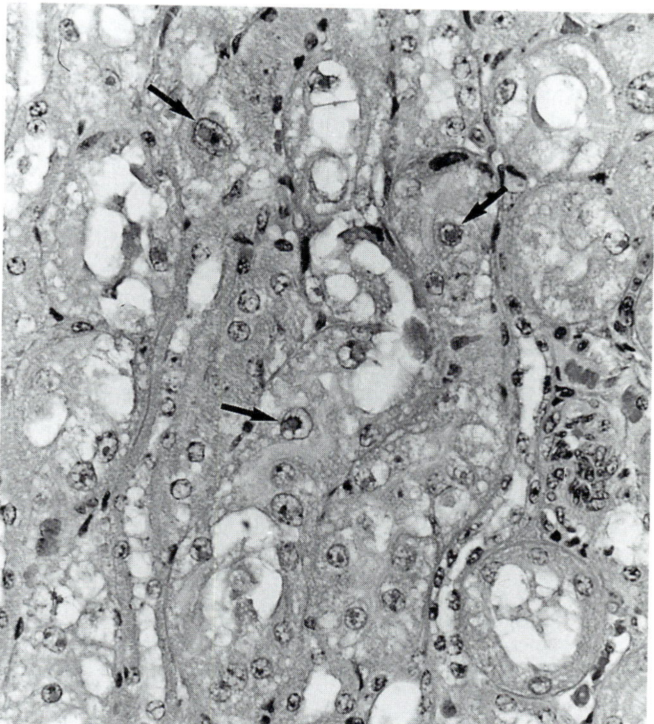

Fig. 5-21 Kidney, cortex; rat. Lead nephrosis. Acid-fast intranuclear inclusion bodies *(arrows)* are present in convoluted tubular epithelium as a result of lead intoxication. Acid-fast stain.

cells of affected tubules may contain acid-fast intranuclear inclusions formed by lead-protein complexes (Fig. 5-21). Acute nephrosis has occurred in sheep after exposure to natural gas condensate, a complex mixture of hydrocarbon compounds. The mechanism of nephrotoxicity was not identified but was not associated with heavy metal contaminants.

Certain pharmaceutic agents are nephrotoxic and cause acute tubular necrosis when administered at excessive dosages. Cisplatin, a platinum-containing cancer chemotherapeutic agent, causes tubular necrosis by direct tubular damage and by reducing renal blood flow. Aminoglycoside antimicrobials such as gentamicin, neomycin, kanamycin, tobramycin, amikacin, and streptomycin are nephrotoxic. Variations in susceptibility of animal species to the nephrotoxic effects of these drugs are related to differences in susceptibility of tubules and/or the rate of excretion/inactivation of the drug among species. Tubular toxicity due to gentamicin occurs with some frequency because of its common use in veterinary medicine. Several aminoglycosides alter tubular cell membrane transport by inhibition of sodium-potassium-ATPase, resulting in an intracellular influx of hydrogen and sodium ions and water. Acute cellular swelling, mitochondrial swelling, and cell death result. Another mechanism of action, particularly with gentamicin, is inhibition of phospholipase activity with the accumulation of phospholipids intracellularly. This results in ultrastructural alterations in lysosomes, with the formation of cytosegresomes, lysosomal leakage, and cellular death. Amphotericin B, an antifungal polyene antibiotic, is nephrotoxic through direct disruption of the cellular membrane by interfering with normal cholesterol-lipid interactions, causing potassium ion loss, intracellular hydrogen ion accumulation, and acute cellular swelling and necrosis. These changes are not confined to overdosage of the drug but can occur with the recommended therapeutic dosage. Use of some of these drugs necessitates continued monitoring of renal function. Sulfonamide-induced tubular necrosis, a common entity in years past, now occurs infrequently because the presently used sulfonamides have greater solubility than those used in the past. Sulfonamides produce tubular necrosis most readily in dehydrated animals. Crystals form in tubules, and necrosis occurs due to local toxicity and mechanical effects. Fine, granular, yellow, crystalline deposits may be seen grossly in the medullary tubules of affected animals but are dissolved during normal fixation and histologic processing of tissue. Monensin is an ionophore antibiotic used as a feed additive to control coccidiosis and stimulate weight gains in poultry and cattle. Horses are particularly susceptible to toxicosis with monensin, and, although striated muscle necrosis is the major effect of toxicosis, renal tubular degeneration and/or necrosis may also occur.

Among the naturally occurring nephrotoxins are ochratoxins and citrinin, mycotoxins produced by *Aspergillus* sp. and *Penicillium* sp. Ochratoxin A is nephrotoxic for monogastric animals, particularly pigs, and has been associated with tubular degeneration and necrosis, with subsequent diffuse renal fibrosis, after long-term ingestion.

Acute tubular necrosis can result from ingestion of nephrotoxic plants. Several species of pigweed, particularly *Amaranthus retroflexus,* cause acute tubular necrosis and perirenal edema in pigs and cattle. The toxic principle has not been identified. Ruminants can develop tubular necrosis after ingestion of leaves, buds, or acorns from oak trees and shrubs (*Quercus* sp.). The toxic substances are metabolites of tannins; however, the mechanism of tubular damage is unknown. Acutely affected cattle often have swollen, pale kidneys that occasionally have cortical petechiae (Fig. 5-22). Perirenal edema is a common lesion, and the body cavities may contain excessive, clear, edema fluid. The kidneys in chronic cases become fibrotic and, thus, are pale, are reduced in size, and have finely pitted or dimpled surfaces and thinned, pale cortices.

Ingestion of antifreeze is a common cause of acute tubular necrosis in dogs and cats. Ethylene glycol, the major constituent of antifreeze, is readily absorbed from the gastrointestinal tract, and a small percentage is oxidized by alcohol dehydrogenase in the liver to the toxic metabolites glycolaldehyde, glycolic acid, glyoxylate, and oxalate. Ethylene glycol and its toxic metabolic products are filtered by the glomeruli. Acute tubular necrosis results from direct interaction of these toxic metabolites, especially glycolic acid, with tubular epithelium. Of particular significance is that calcium oxalate precipitates as crystals in renal tubular lumina. These crystals cause intrarenal obstruction and de-

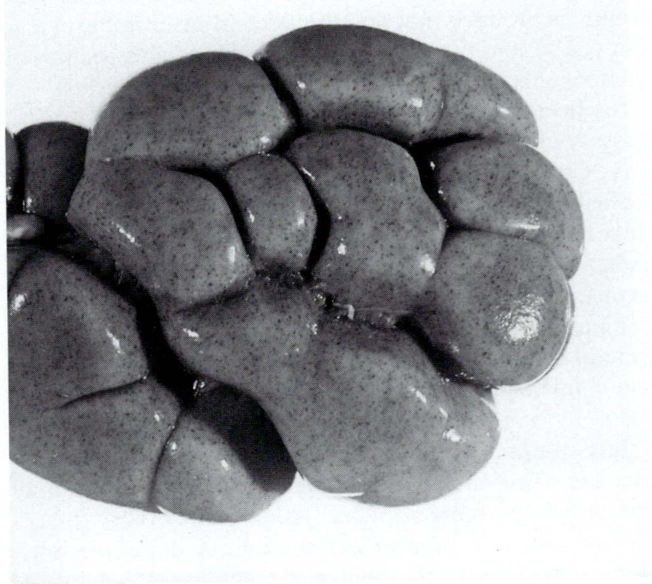

Fig. 5-22 Kidney; calf. Oak nephrosis. Acute tubular necrosis is associated with oak toxicity. The kidney is pale, swollen, and moist and has pinpoint hemorrhages throughout the cortex.

generation and necrosis of tubular epithelium. The microscopic identification using polarized light of large numbers of these birefringent crystals in renal tubules is virtually pathognomonic for ethylene glycol toxicity in dogs and cats.

Oxalate-induced tubular necrosis also occurs in sheep and cattle after ingestion of toxic quantities of oxalates that accumulate in plants of several genera (Fig. 5-23). After absorption from the intestine, calcium oxalates form and precipitate in vessels and in renal tubules where they cause obstruction and epithelial cell necrosis. Illness in oxalate poisoning may occur due not only to renal damage but also to neuromuscular dysfunction that occurs as a result of the hypocalcemia resulting from chelation of serum calcium by oxalates. Recently, oxalate-induced nephrosis was described in Tibetan spaniel dogs with an inherited hyperoxaluria.

Nephrosis occurs in dogs or cats receiving prolonged, excessive vitamin D supplementation (vitamin D intoxication [**vitamin D nephropathy**]) or by accidental ingestion of calciferol-containing rodenticides. In livestock, prolonged ingestion of plants such as *Cestrum diurnum* in the southern United States or *Solanum* sp. or *Trisetum* sp. abroad, each of which has vitamin D–like biologic activity, can also cause nephrosis. Ingestion of excessive vitamin D induces hypercalcemia. Subsequently, tubular necrosis is the consequence of renal ischemia resulting from vasoconstriction and of nephrotoxicity resulting from tubular absorption of calcium, causing mitochondrial calcification and cellular death. Tubular basement membranes are also calcified. Lesions depend on time postexposure for rodenticides or time of continued exposure to vitamin D. In acute cases, the kidneys have a smooth capsular surface. Microscopically, tubular epithelium is necrotic or atrophic, with a few calcific deposits in tubules randomly scattered throughout the cortex. In more chronic cases, the surface of the kidney is finely granular. White, chalky calcific deposits may be seen within the cortex. Interstitial fibrosis, tubular dilatation and atrophy, glomerular atrophy, and extensive calcification are seen microscopically.

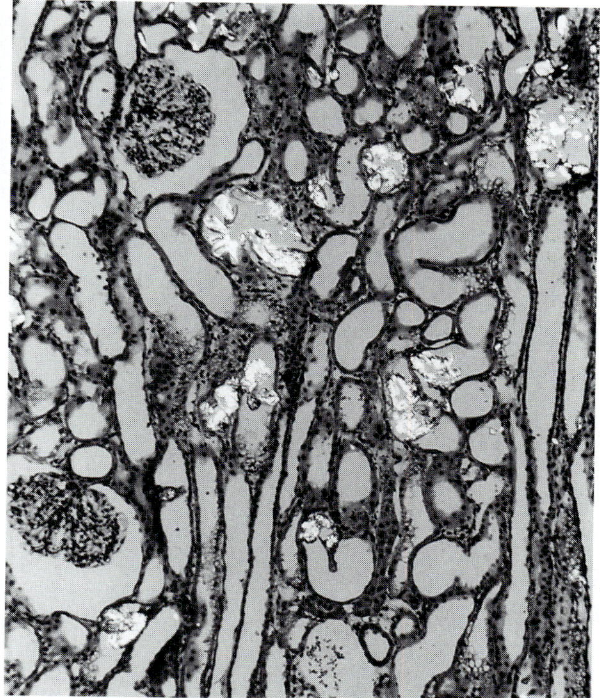

Fig. 5-23 Kidney, cortex; sheep. Oxalate nephrosis. Tubular dilatation and tubular necrosis are severe. Numerous tubules contain birefringent calcium oxalate crystals (photographed with polarized light). H & E stain.

Incidental lesions of renal tubules

Pigment can be present in the renal tubules. In dogs, microscopic granules of hemosiderin are frequent incidental findings in the cytoplasm of cells of proximal convoluted tubules. The origin of this pigment is most likely from degradation of hemoglobin resorbed from the glomerular filtrate by tubular epithelium. However, a history of concurrent lesions of a prior hemolytic crisis is often lacking. The kidneys usually appear normal grossly. Fine, golden granules of lipofuscin (''wear and tear pigment'') can accumulate in the renal convoluted tubules of aged cattle, often associated with striated muscle **lipofuscinosis.** Grossly, the renal cortex may have streaks of brown discoloration, but renal function is not affected. **Cloisonné kidneys** occur in goats and have diffuse, intense, black or brown discoloration of the cortex (Fig. 5-24). The medulla is spared. The lesion is the result of tubular membrane thickening due to deposits of ferritin and hemosiderin. Although this lesion is striking, it is not associated with abnormal renal function. Incidental tubular changes also occur. In the neuronal lysosomal storage diseases, feline sphingomyelinosis, and ovine GM_1 gangliosidosis, vacuolation of renal tubular epithelium is seen. In dogs, intranuclear eosinophilic crystalline inclusions may occur in re-

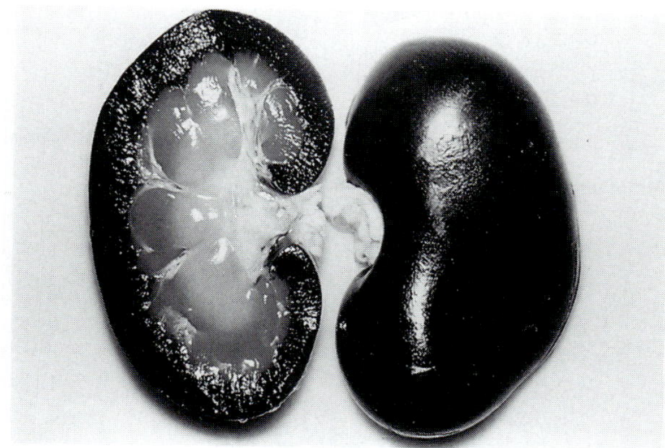

Fig. 5-24 Kidney; goat. Cloisonné kidney. The cortex is diffusely black pigmented; the medulla is unaffected.

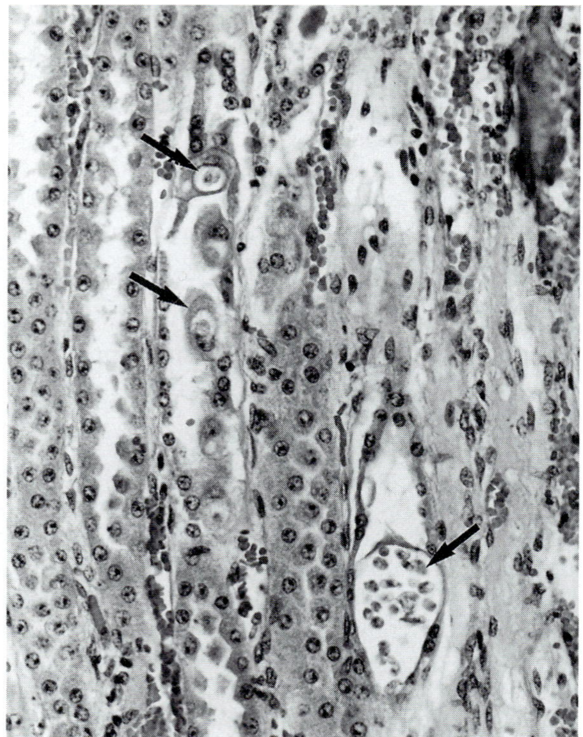

Fig. 5-25 Kidney, medulla; horse. *Klossiella equi* infection. Tubular epithelium containing various developmental stages of *K. equi (arrows).* H & E stain.

nal tubular epithelium. These can be round or rectangular and often greatly distort the nuclei.

Klossiella equi is a sporozoan parasite of the horse. Various stages of schizony can be found microscopically in proximal convoluted tubular epithelium and, to a lesser extent, in glomerular endothelium (Fig. 5-25). Stages of sporogony are present in the loop of Henle. Tubules with coccidial forms occur multifocally and, usually, produce no gross lesions or alterations of renal function. Occasionally, however, *K. equi* has been associated with lesions of mild tubular necrosis and interstitial nephritis.

Glomerular Diseases

General considerations

Glomeruli are complex capillary tufts whose main function is to form a filtrate of plasma that, in its passage through a multifunctional tubular system, is excreted into the lower urinary tract as urine. The glomerular capillaries are supported on a basement membrane and are held in their tufted arrangement by the mesangium, a glycoprotein matrix that is formed and maintained by myofibroblasts called mesangial cells (Fig. 5-26). The mesangium also contains macrophages that phagocytose particles that enter the mesangium. The capillaries are lined by a fenestrated endothelium, and their outer surface is covered by visceral epithelial cells (podocytes) whose processes (foot processes) interdigitate such as to have epithelial slit pores between them. The endothelium, basement membrane, and slit pores constitute the glomerular filtration barrier that

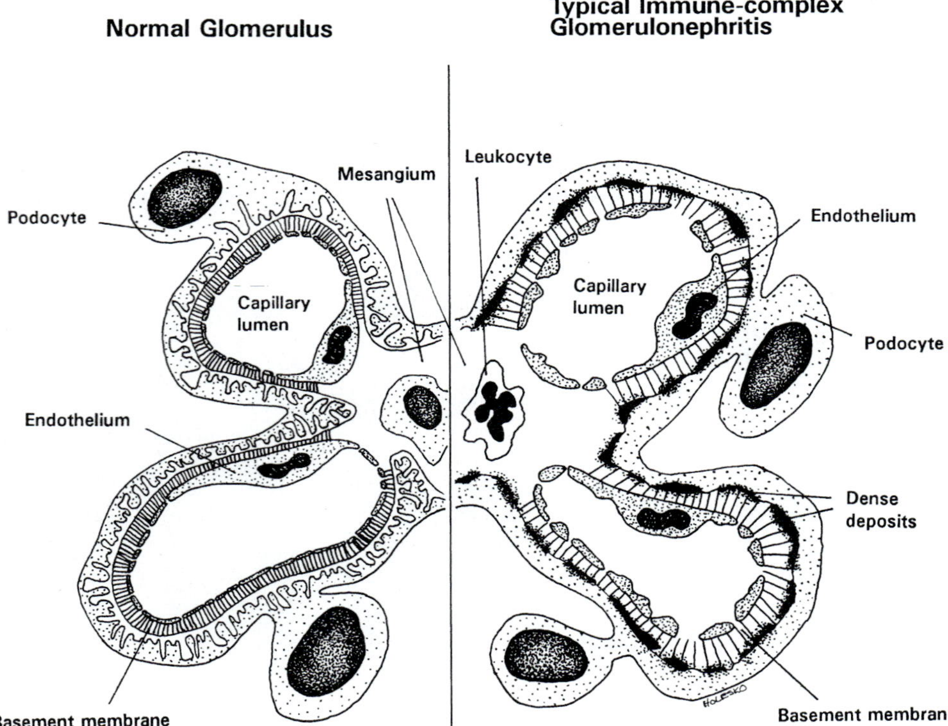

Fig. 5-26 Kidney, glomerulus. Normal glomerulus and immune complex glomerulonephritis. *Left,* A normal glomerulus; *right,* a glomerulus with immune complex glomerulonephritis. Typically, immune complex glomerulonephritis is characterized by fusion of visceral epithelial (podocyte) foot processes, thickening of the capillary basement membranes, leukocyte infiltrates, hypertrophy of endothelium, and dense granular deposits of immune complexes associated with the basement membrane.

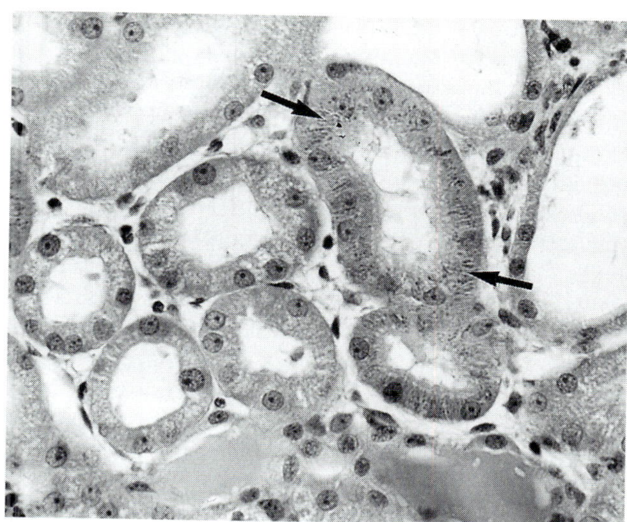

Fig. 5-27 Kidney, cortex; dog. Intratubular protein. Due to glomerulonephritis and increased protein in the glomerular filtrate, intracytoplasmic hyalin droplets are present in proximal tubular epithelium *(arrows)*. Other tubules contain intraluminal proteinaceous material. H & E stain.

selectively filters molecules based on size (<70,000 daltons), electrical charge, and capillary pressure.

Damage to the glomerular filtration barrier can result in renal disease with a variety of clinical manifestations. A major expression of glomerular disease is the leakage of various low-molecular-weight (small molecule size) proteins into the glomerular filtrate and into urine. Renal diseases that result in **proteinuria** are called **protein-losing nephropathies.** A large quantity of plasma protein, particularly albumin, filters through the damaged glomerular filtration barrier and overloads the protein reabsorption capabilities of the proximal convoluted tubules to such an extent that protein appears in the urine. In such diseases, the proximal tubules often have microscopic eosinophilic intracytoplasmic bodies, referred to as **hyaline droplets,** that represent accumulations of pinocytized intracytoplasmic protein (Fig. 5-27). Microscopically, tubular lumina are often dilated and filled with proteinaceous material as well. Prolonged, severe renal protein loss results in hypoproteinemia, reduced plasma colloid osmotic (oncotic) pressure, and loss of antithrombin III. Protein-losing nephropathy is one of several causes of severe hypoproteinemia and the resulting generalized edema, ascites, and pleural effusion called the **nephrotic syndrome.**

Viral glomerulitis

Glomerular lesions occur in acute systemic viral diseases such as acute infectious canine hepatitis, septicemic cytomegalovirus infection (inclusion body rhinitis) in neonatal pigs, equine arteritis virus infection, hog cholera, and Newcastle disease in birds. The lesions are mild and usually transient, resulting from viral replication in capillary endothelium. Transient proteinuria may occur. Viral-induced intranuclear inclusions are present in endothelium during viremia with infectious canine hepatitis and cytomegalovirus infections. In the other diseases, viral antigens may be demonstrated in endothelium, epithelium, or mesangial cells by immunofluorescence. Endothelial hypertrophy, a thickened and edematous mesangium, hemorrhage, and individual cell necrosis may be present as well. However, those lesions are best demonstrated in electron micrographs. In addition to these lesions, infectious canine hepatitis virus is associated with a transient immune complex glomerulonephritis (see Immune-Mediated Glomerulonephritis).

Suppurative glomerulitis (embolic nephritis)

Acute **suppurative glomerulitis,** which is also called embolic nephritis, is the result of a bacteremia, whereby bacteria become lodged in glomeruli and, to a lesser extent, in interstitial capillaries and cause the formation of multiple foci of inflammation randomly scattered throughout the renal cortex (Fig. 5-28). Microscopically, glomerular capillaries contain numerous bacterial colonies. Necrosis and extensive infiltration with neutrophils often result in obliteration of the glomeruli. Glomerular or interstitial hemorrhage may occur as well. This lesion occurs commonly in actinobacillosis of foals caused by *Actinobacillus equuli.* Foals with actinobacillosis die within a few days after birth and have small abscesses in many visceral organs and a fibrinopurulent polysynovitis. Suppurative glomerulitis also occurs in other animal species due to bacteremia with any of several bacterial species. In pigs, *Erysipelothrix* sp., *Streptococcus* sp., and *Antinomyces* sp. (*Corynebacterium* sp.) are frequently isolated from this lesion.

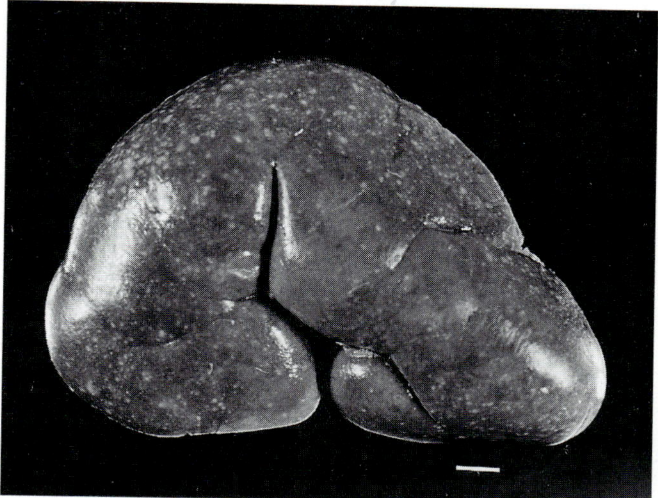

Fig. 5-28 Kidney; horse. Suppurative glomerulitis (embolic nephritis). Multiple, small abscesses are randomly scattered throughout the cortex as a result of *Actinobacillus equuli* septicemia. Bar = 1 cm.

Immune-mediated glomerulonephritis

Glomerulonephritis results most often from immune-mediated mechanisms, most notably involving antibodies to glomerular basement membranes or the deposition of soluble immune complexes within the glomeruli. Diagnosis of an immune-mediated glomerulonephritis is confirmed by demonstrating immunoglobulin (Ig) and complement components, usually C3, in the glomeruli by immunofluorescent or immunohistochemical techniques.

Antibodies to basement membrane bind to glomerular basement membranes **(antibasement membrane disease)** and result in damage to the glomerulus through fixation of complement and resulting leukocyte infiltration. This mechanism of glomerulonephritis has been well documented in human beings and lower primates but only rarely in other species. To confirm the diagnosis of antibasement membrane disease, Ig and C3 must be demonstrated within glomeruli, and antibodies must be eluted from the kidneys and bind to normal glomerular basement membranes of the appropriate species.

Immune complex glomerulonephritis occurs in association with persistent infections or other diseases that characteristically have a prolonged antigenemia. In domestic animals, immune complex glomerulonephritis occurs most commonly in dogs and cats and is associated with specific viral infections such as feline leukemia virus or feline infectious peritonitis virus, bacterial infections such as pyometra, chronic parasitism such as dirofilariasis, autoimmune diseases such as systemic lupus erythematosus, or neoplasia (Box 5-2). However, as in the well-documented disease, feline progressive membranous glomerulonephritis, the specific cause of immune complex glomerulonephritis may not be identifiable.

Box 5-2 DISEASES IN WHICH IMMUNE COMPLEX GLOMERULONEPHRITIS MAY OCCUR

Dogs	Infectious canine hepatitis Bacterial endometritis (pyometra) Dirofilariasis Leishmaniasis Ehrlichiosis Borreliosis (Lyme disease) Chronic inflammatory skin disease Systemic lupus erythematosus Polyarteritis Autoimmune hemolytic anemia Neoplasia Hereditary C3 deficiency
Cats	Feline leukemia virus infection Feline infectious peritonitis Progressive polyarteritis Neoplasia Progressive membranous glomerulonephritis
Horses	Equine infectious anemia *Streptococcus* sp.
Cattle	Bovine virus diarrhea Trypanosomiasis
Pigs	Hog cholera African swine fever
Sheep	Hereditary hypocomplementemia in Finnish Landrace lambs

Immune complex glomerulonephritis is initiated by the formation of soluble immune complexes (antigen-antibody complexes) in the presence of antigen-antibody equivalency or slight antigen excess in the plasma. These complexes are selectively deposited in the glomerular capillaries, stimulating complement fixation with formation of C3a, C5a, and C567, which are chemotactic for neutrophils. During early stages, infiltrating neutrophils damage the basement membrane through release of hydrolytic enzymes; later, monocytes infiltrate into the glomeruli and are responsible for continuing damage to the glomeruli.

Many specific factors determine the extent of deposition of soluble immune complexes in the glomerular capillary walls. These include persistence of appropriate quantities of immune complexes in the circulation, local vascular permeability, the size and molecular charge of the soluble complexes, and the strength of the bond between the antigen and antibody (avidity). The most damaging complexes are small or intermediate, whereas large complexes are removed from the circulation through phagocytosis by the mononuclear-phagocyte system in the liver and spleen. An increase in local vascular permeability is necessary for complexes to leave the microcirculation and deposit in the glomerulus. This usually occurs via vasoactive amine release from platelets, basophils, and/or mast cells. Release of vasoactive amines can occur from mast cells or basophils by the interaction of the immune complexes with antigen-specific IgE on the surface of these cells, by stimulation of the mast cells or basophils by cationic proteins from neutrophils, or by the anaphylatoxin activity of C3a and C5a. Platelet activation factor is released from immune complex–stimulated mast cells, basophils, or macrophages and causes platelets to release vasoactive amines as well. Localization of the complexes within the basement membrane or in subepithelial locations depends on their molecular charge and avidity. Within the capillary wall, soluble immune complexes can then become greatly enlarged due to interactions with free antibodies, free antigens, complement components, or other immune complexes.

Once immune complexes are deposited in the glomerular capillary basement membranes, a series of events ensue that lead to glomerular lesions and altered permeability. Activation of the complement cascade results in the generation of chemotactic factors that attract neutrophils to glomeruli. Neutrophils release proteinases, arachidonic acid metabolites (such as thromboxane), and oxygen-derived free radicals, causing degradation of glomerular basement membranes. The release of biologically active molecules from glomerular mesangial cells, monocytes, and macrophages adds to the glomerular injury.

Glomerular injury may occur in the absence of neutrophil infiltration through aggregation of platelets and activation of Hageman factor, causing fibrin thrombi and glomerular ischemia. Furthermore, glomerular cell damage can result directly from terminal membrane attack complex of the activated complement cascade. Finally, if exposure of the glomerulus to immune complexes is short-lived, as in a transient infection such as infectious canine hepatitis, immune complexes will be phagocytosed by macrophages or mesangial cells and removed, and glomerular lesions and clinical signs will resolve. Conversely, continual exposure of glomeruli to soluble immune complexes, such as with persistent viral infections, can result in progressive glomerular injury, severe lesions, and disease.

Ultrastructurally, immune complexes either in the glomerular basement membrane or in a subepithelial location appear as electron-dense bodies (Figs. 5-26 and 5-29). Complexes that are poorly soluble, fairly large, or of high avidity rather than localizing in capillaries often enter the mesangium, where they may be phagocytosed by macrophages, and are detectable ultrastructurally as dense, granular deposits. Other ultrastructural changes commonly seen are fusion of podocytic foot processes and infiltrates of neutrophils and monocytes.

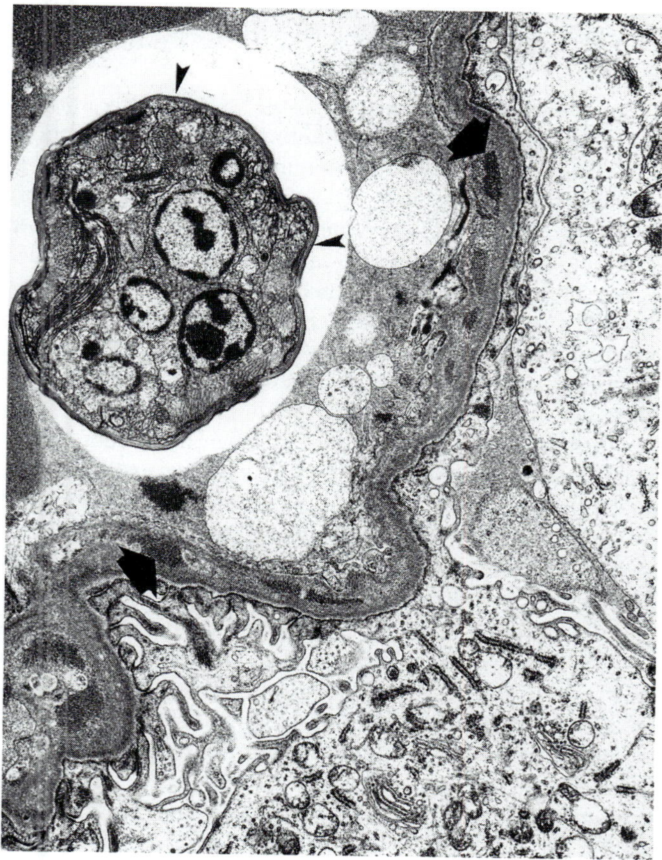

Fig. 5-29 Kidney, glomerulus; dog. Immune complex glomerulonephritis. Electron photomicrograph of a glomerulus with immune complex deposits due to dirofilariasis. A heartworm microfilaria is present in the capillary lumen *(arrowheads)*. The basement membrane is irregularly thickened and contains granular, electron-dense deposits *(arrows)*. The podocytic foot processes are fused. *Courtesy Dr. N. Cheville.*

A tentative diagnosis of immune complex glomerulonephritis can be made by demonstration of Ig and C3 in glomerular tufts. In dogs, IgG is the most common Ig isotype demonstrated in glomerulonephritis; however, combinations of IgG, IgM, and IgA may occur in the glomeruli in some dogs. Recently, IgA was the only Ig demonstrated in three dogs with immune complex glomerulonephritis. Both Ig and C3 are usually seen in a granular (''lumpy-bumpy'') pattern under immunofluorescent or immunohistochemical techniques (Fig. 5-30); however, occasionally the deposits are in a linear distribution, conforming to basement membranes. The diagnosis of immune complex glomerulonephritis can be confirmed only by ruling out anti-basement membrane disease after demonstrating that the antibodies eluted from glomeruli do not bind to normal glomeruli. Once a diagnosis of immune complex glomerulonephritis is confirmed, it would be ideal to identify the causative antigen present in immune complexes. This is done by eluting antibodies from diseased glomeruli and attempting to identify their specificity for suspected antigens. For example, antibodies eluted from the glomeruli of dogs with severe heartworm disease and its associated glomerulonephritis bind to several *Dirofilaria immitis* antigens, including the wall of adult worms, parasitic uterine fluid, and microfilariae. In cases of immune complex glomerulonephritis, however, the specific causative antigen usually escapes determination. This is the case in sheep, in which subclinical lesions of immune complex glomerulonephritis are often present.

Gross lesions of acute immune complex glomerulone-

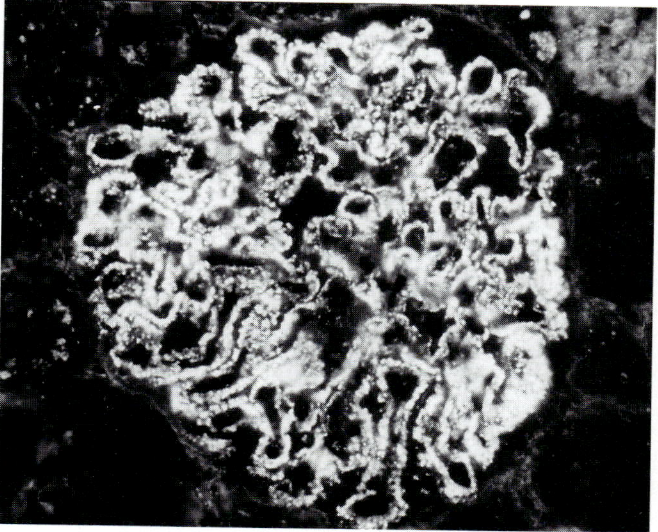

Fig. 5-30 Kidney, glomerulus; dog. Immune complex glomerulonephritis. Intraglomerular immunoglobulin deposits demonstrated by immunofluorescence. Note the granular (''lumpy-bumpy'') pattern of fluorescence. *Courtesy Dr. R. Lewis.*

phritis are usually subtle. The kidneys are often swollen, have a smooth capsular surface, are normal color or pale, and have glomeruli that are visible as pinpoint red dots on the cut surface of the cortex. The glomeruli of horses are usually visible, so this criterion cannot be used in that species. If lesions do not resolve but become subacute to chronic, the renal cortex becomes somewhat shrunken, with a generalized fine granularity of the capsular surface. On cut surface, the cortex may be thinned, and glomeruli may appear as pale gray dots. With time, more intense scarring may develop throughout the cortex (see Renal Fibrosis).

Microscopically, immune complex glomerulonephritis has one of several anatomic forms. Although various classifications of glomerulonephritis exist, the following simple classification is well understood among veterinary pathologists. Lesions in the glomeruli may be described as the following:

Proliferative when there is increased cellularity in the glomerular tufts due to a proliferation of glomerular cells and an influx of leukocytes involving both the capillary loops and the mesangium (Fig. 5-31).

Membranous when diffuse capillary basement membrane thickening is the predominant change (Fig. 5-32). This is the most common form of immune complex glomerulonephritis in cats,

Membranoproliferative (mesangiocapillary, mesangioproliferative) when both hypercellularity and capillary basement membrane thickening are present. This is the most common form of immune complex glomerulonephritis in the dog.

Several other changes usually accompany the lesions discussed above. These include adhesions between the glomerular tuft and Bowman's capsule, hypertrophy and hyperplasia of the parietal epithelium, fibrinous thrombi in glomerular capillaries, and tubular dilatation with homogenous proteinaceous fluid. An increase in mesangial matrix often accompanies these changes. If the damage is mild and the cause is removed, glomeruli may heal without obvious or with minimal residual lesions. However, if the lesion is severe and prolonged, subacute to chronic glomerular changes develop. Bowman's capsule can become thickened and hyalinized. Proliferation of parietal epithelium, an influx of monocytes, and deposition of fibrin can result in the formation of a semicircular, hypercellular, intraglomerular lesion known as a **glomerular crescent** (Fig. 5-33). Fibrosis can develop in the glomerular crescent, and when Bowman's capsule ruptures, glomerular fibrosis may become continuous with interstitial fibrosis. Accompanying chronic glomerulonephritis are interstitial and periglomerular fibrosis and foci of interstitial lymphocytes and plasma cells (see Renal Fibrosis). Finally, glomeruli shrink and, with an increase in fibrous connective tissue and mesangial matrix and obliteration of glomerular capillaries, become hyalinized (Fig. 5-34). These glomeruli are hypocellular and essentially nonfunctional. This process is referred to as **glomerulosclerosis.** It should be noted that glomerulosclerosis is not only the end stage of glomerulonephritis but can result from any chronic insult that results in loss of glomerular or nephron function. Numerous factors are associated with and accelerate glomerulosclerosis, including unrestricted protein in the diet, increased glomerular capillary pressure in functional glomeruli in the chronic diseased kidney, and cytokines and platelet-derived growth factors. Glomerulosclerosis is sometimes seen in animals

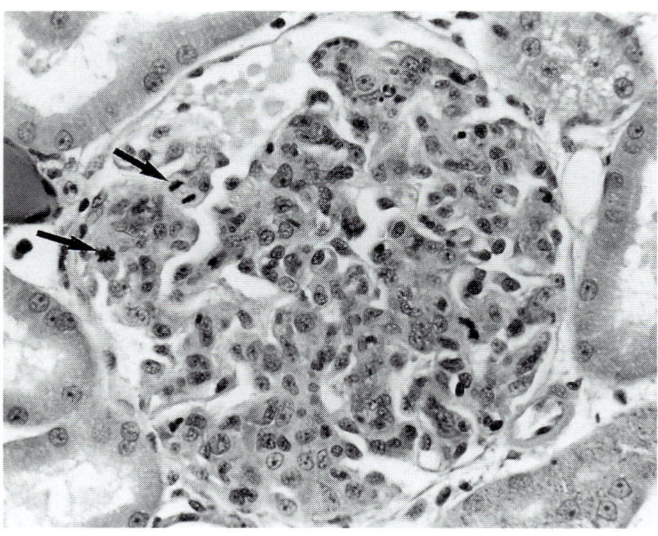

Fig. 5-31 Kidney, glomerulus; dog. Proliferative glomerulonephritis. The lesion is characterized by hypercellularity of a glomerulus. There are mitotically active epithelial cells *(arrows).* H & E stain.

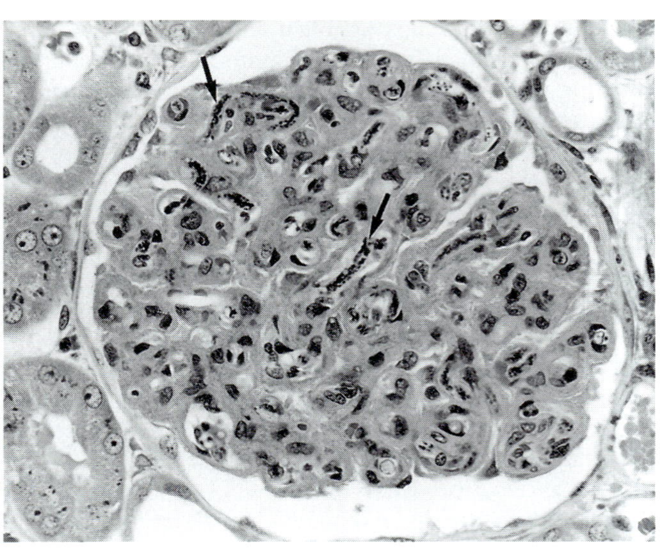

Fig. 5-32 Kidney, glomerulus; dog. Membranous glomerulonephritis. The lesion is associated with dirofilariasis and is characterized by generalized hyalin thickening of glomerular capillary basement membranes. Note also microfilaria within vessel lumina *(arrows).* H & E stain.

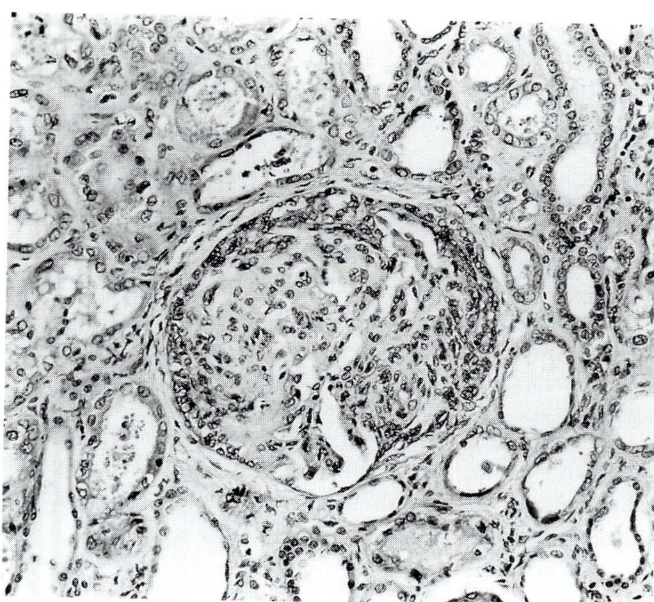

Fig. 5-33 Kidney, glomerulus; chimpanzee. Chronic glomerulonephritis. A glomerular crescent is associated with chronic proliferative glomerulonephritis. H & E stain.

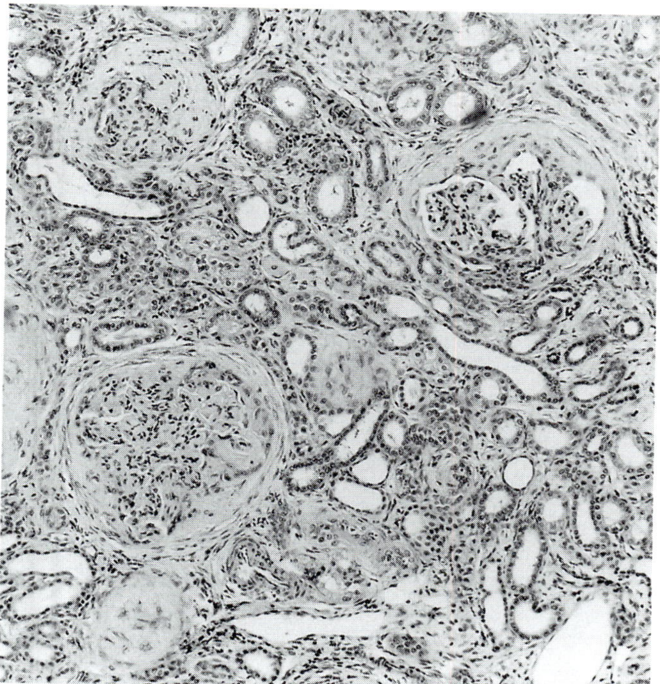

Fig. 5-34 Kidney, glomerulus; dog. Glomerulosclerosis. Chronic glomerulonephritis is characterized by various stages of shrinkage, hyalinization, and fibrosis of the glomerular tufts and periglomerular and interstitial fibrosis. H & E stain.

with diabetes mellitus in which diffuse or nodular eosinophilic glycoprotein material (hyaline) is deposited in the glomerular mesangium.

Amyloidosis

Amyloid, an insoluble fibrillar protein with a β-pleated sheet conformation, is produced after limited proteolysis of several soluble amyloidogenic proteins. Amyloid deposits in patients with plasma cell myelomas or other B-lymphocyte dyscrasias (called AL amyloidosis) are composed of fragments of the light chains of immunoglobulins. In domestic animals, spontaneously occurring amyloidosis is usually an example of what is called reactive amyloidosis (AA amyloidosis). This form of the disease is often associated with chronic inflammatory stimuli and diseases, and amyloid deposits are composed of fragments of a serum acute-phase reactant protein called serum amyloid-associated (AA) protein. Amyloid fibrils from either source are deposited in tissues along with a glycoprotein called amyloid P-component.

Glomeruli are the most common renal site for deposition of amyloid, although the medullary interstitium is a common site for deposition in cats. Renal amyloidosis may occur in association with other diseases, particularly chronic inflammatory or neoplastic diseases. Idiopathic renal amyloidosis, that is, amyloidosis in which an associated disease process is not recognized, often occurs in dogs and cats. However, the underlying pathogenic mechanisms of that form of renal amyloidosis are not known. An hereditary predisposition for amyloidosis has been found in Abyssinian cats and Chinese Shar Pei dogs. A familial tendency is suspected in beagle dogs. In cattle, renal amyloidosis is nearly always secondary to chronic systemic infectious disease. Glomerular amyloidosis is a protein-losing nephropathy that results in marked proteinuria and uremia. It can, like immune complex glomerulonephritis, result in the nephrotic syndrome. Medullary amyloidosis is usually asymptomatic unless it leads to papillary necrosis (see Circulatory Disturbances).

Kidneys affected with glomerular amyloidosis are often enlarged and pale, with a smooth to finely granular capsular surface. Amyloid-laden glomeruli may be visible as fine tan dots on the capsular and cut surfaces. The cortex may have a finely granular appearance. Treatment of kidneys with an iodine solution, such as Lugol's, may result in brown staining of glomeruli, which become purple when exposed to dilute sulfuric acid (Fig. 5-35). Long-standing glomerular amyloidosis and consequent diminished renal vascular perfusion can lead to renal tubular atrophy, degeneration, and diffuse fibrosis. Medullary amyloidosis is usually not grossly recognizable.

Microscopically, amyloid is deposited in the mesangium and subendothelial locations. Amyloid is acellular and may accumulate in foci within glomerular tufts; thus, a portion of the normal glomerular architecture is replaced by eosinophilic, homogeneous to slightly fibrillar material (Fig. 5-

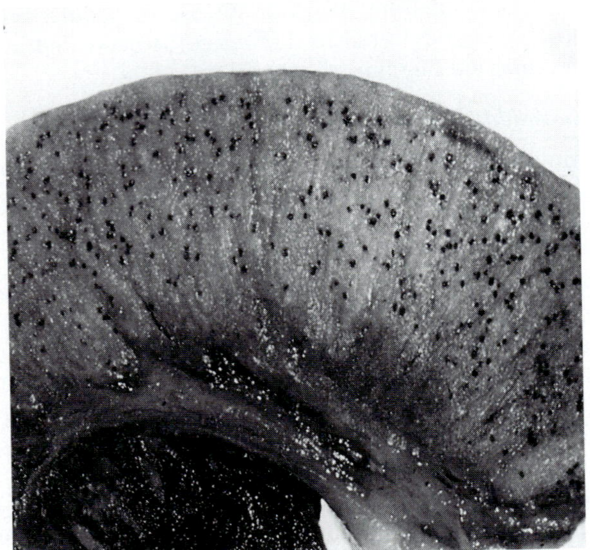

Fig. 5-35 Kidney; dog. Amyloidosis. The cut surface of a kidney is stained with iodine/acid to demonstrate amyloid-infiltrated glomeruli.

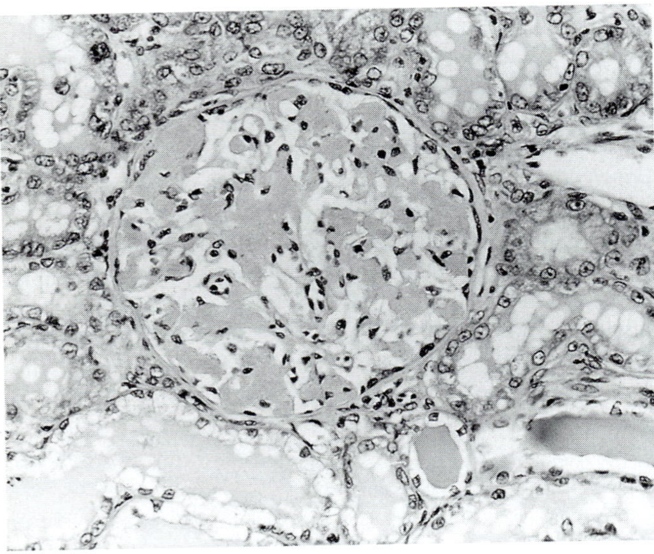

Fig. 5-36 Kidney, glomerulus; dog. Amyloidosis. Amyloid is seen as pale, hyalinized deposits within the glomerular tuft. Note also the dense proteinaceous material in tubular lumina. H & E stain.

36). When amyloidosis involves the entire glomerular tuft, the glomerulus is enlarged, capillary lumina become obliterated, and the tuft may appear as a large, hypocellular, eosinophilic hyaline sphere. Amyloid may be present in renal tubular basement membranes as well, resulting in hyalinized thickening of the membranes. Tubules in kidneys with glomerular amyloidosis are usually markedly dilated and contain proteinaceous material. Amyloid is confirmed microscopically by staining with Congo red stain. Such stained sections will have green birefringence or dichroism when viewed with polarized light. Loss of Congo Red staining after treatment of a section with potassium permanganate suggests the presence of amyloid of acute-phase reactant protein origin.

Miscellaneous glomerular lesions

Glomerular lipidosis, characterized by small aggregates of lipid-laden, foamy macrophages in glomerular tufts, is an occasional incidental finding in dogs. A similar but more extensive glomerular lipidosis has been described in cats with inherited hyperlipoproteinemia, a generalized disease characterized by hyperchylomicronemia, atherosclerosis, and xanthogranulomas in numerous parenchymatous organs, including the kidneys (see Granulomatous Nephritis). Microscopically, glomeruli contain foamy macrophages, characteristic of glomerular lipidosis, as well as thickened mesangium and Bowman's capsule.

An idiopathic renal glomerular and cutaneous vasculopathy occurs in greyhound dogs. Affected greyhound dogs have multifocal, cutaneous, erythematous, ulcerated lesions and distal limb edema. Variable systemic signs of uremia often accompany the cutaneous lesions. Thrombocytopenia is frequently seen. At necropsy, kidneys from affected dogs are swollen and congested, with small, cortical petechiae. Microscopically, numerous glomeruli have segmental or diffuse fibrinous thrombi, hemorrhage, and necrosis (Fig. 5-37). Afferent arterioles at the glomerular vascular pole have fibrin deposition and vascular necrosis. The cause of this disease is unknown, but renal lesions are similar to those seen in disseminated intravascular coagulation, thrombotic thrombocytopenic purpura, and hemolytic-anemia syndrome in human beings.

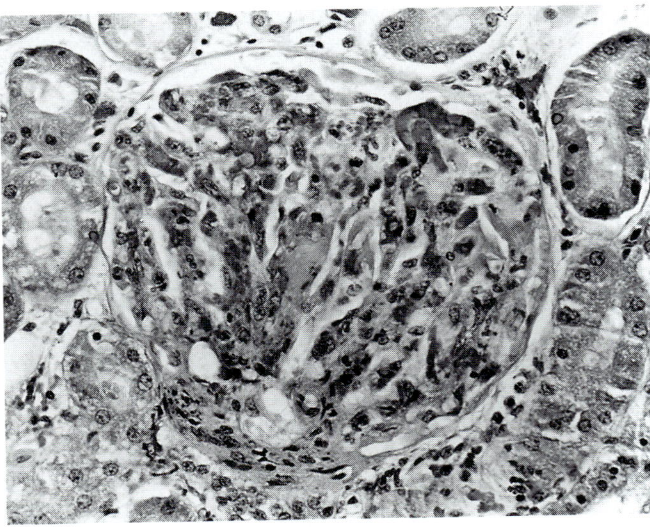

Fig. 5-37 Kidney, glomerulus; dog. Glomerular vasculopathy. Necrosis of glomerular vascular pole and extensive glomerular capillary thrombosis are present, which is typical of the idiopathic glomerular and cutaneous vasculopathy syndrome in greyhound dogs. H & E stain.

Tubulointerstitial Disease

Interstitial nephritis

Aggregates of inflammatory cells may be present in the renal interstitium in various systemic infectious diseases of domestic animals. In many of these diseases, the inflammatory cell infiltrates are visible only microscopically, are not associated with renal failure, and are generally inconsequential (examples are canine erhlichiosis and equine infectious anemia). In other diseases, interstitial inflammatory responses are more severe and grossly visible, are associated with renal failure, and have traditionally been called **interstitial nephritis.** More recently, the term **tubulointerstitial nephritis** has been used to acknowledge that changes in tubules are often present and may actually be the primary process. Interstitial nephritis can be acute, subacute, or chronic, and it is traditionally associated with a lymphoplasmacytic infiltrate. Chronic interstitial nephritis is associated with renal fibrosis (see Renal Fibrosis).

Interstitial nephritis is the result of bacterial and viral septicemias, whereby these infectious agents infect the kidney tubules and incite an inflammatory response in the interstitium (Box 5-3). The actual pathogenesis of these lesions is often unknown. The best understood causes of interstitial nephritis in domestic animals are serovars of *Leptospira interrogans.* Serovars *canicola* and *icterohemorrhagiae* are the most common cause of canine leptospirosis, whereas serovar *pomona* is the most common cause of the lesion in pigs. Other serovars such as *grippotyphosa* and *bratislava* have also been associated with renal leptospirosis in several species.

The pathogenesis of leptospirosis will be discussed as an example of a bacterial acute interstitial nephritis. Following exposure to the bacterium, leptospiremia occurs and organisms localize in the renal interstitial capillaries, migrate through vascular endothelium, persist in the interstitial spaces, and immigrate via the lateral intercellular junctions to reach tubular lumina. Within tubules, leptospires are associated with epithelial microvilli and within phagosomes of the epithelium of the proximal and distal convoluted tubules. Tubular epithelial cells undergo degeneration and necrosis due either to direct toxic effects of the leptospires or to the accompanying interstitial inflammatory reaction. Although neutrophils may be present in tubular lumina, the predominant lesion is in the interstitium, which becomes infiltrated with monocytes, macrophages, lymphocytes, and plasma cells. In affected dogs, interstitial plasma cells secrete *Leptospira*-specific antibodies. However, the role of those antibodies in pathogenesis or resolution of the lesion is not known. *Escherichia coli* septicemia in calves can result in interstitial nephritis. The pathogenesis is most likely similar to that of leptospirosis.

Another well-documented mechanism for the production of interstitial nephritis is exemplified by the immune response to infectious canine hepatitis virus infection in dogs. During the viremic phase of the disease, virus initially localizes in the glomeruli (viral glomerulitis), producing a transient immune complex glomerulonephritis. As the dog recovers from the acute phase of the disease and with onset of the systemic immune response, virus disappears from the glomeruli only to reappear in tubular epithelial cells where it may persist for weeks and months and causes tubular epithelial necrosis by a viral-induced cytolysis. Tubular necrosis is followed by a lymphocytic and plasmacytic interstitial nephritis. Basophilic intranuclear inclusions typical of infectious canine hepatitis virus are present in infected epithelium.

Deposition of immune complexes in or interactions between antibasement membrane antibodies and tubular basement membranes can initiate immune-mediated tubulointerstitial disease in human beings and laboratory animals. Depositions of Ig and complement have rarely been identified in renal tubular basement membranes in domestic animals. At present, immune-mediated mechanisms are questionable as causes of interstitial nephritis in domestic animals.

Gross lesions of interstitial nephritis discussed herein can be classified as acute or subacute; descriptions of chronic interstitial nephritis are discussed in the section on Renal Fibrosis. The distribution of lesions can be diffuse, as in canine leptospirosis, or multifocal, as in **"white spotted kidneys"** of calves due to *E. coli* septicemia, infectious canine hepatitis, malignant catarrhal fever, or porcine leptospirosis (Figs. 5-38 and 5-39). In diffuse interstitial nephritis, kidneys may be swollen and pale, with a random gray mottling seen from the capsular surface. The cut surface may bulge; gray infiltrates of varying size obscure the normally radially striated cortical architecture. The infiltrates are manifested as coalescing gray foci, particularly obvious in the inner cortex. Focal interstitial nephritis is less severe and composed of more discrete gray areas in the cortex and, sometimes, the outer medulla.

Microscopically, aggregates of lymphocytes, plasma cells, and monocytes and a few neutrophils are randomly scattered or intensely localized throughout the interstitium

Box 5-3 CAUSES OF INTERSTITIAL NEPHRITIS

Dogs	*Leptospira interrogans* serovar *canicola*
	Leptospira interrogans serovar *icterohemorrhagiae* (and other serovars)
	Infectious canine hepatitis virus, recovery phase
Cattle	*Escherichia coli,* "white spotted kidney"
	Malignant catarrhal fever virus
	Theileria parva
Pigs	*Leptospira interrogans* serovar *pomona*
Sheep	Sheeppox

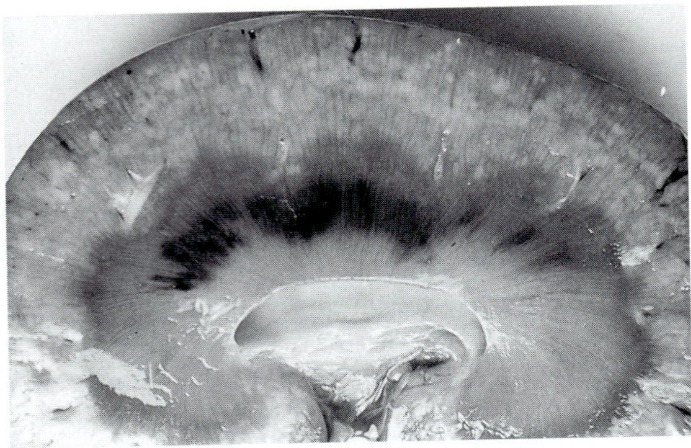

Fig. 5-38 Kidney; dog. Interstitial nephritis. Pale foci of inflammatory cellular infiltrate are in the cortex, concentrated near the corticomedullary junction. These lesions are typical for subacute leptospirosis. Note there is a zone of medullary hemorrhage.

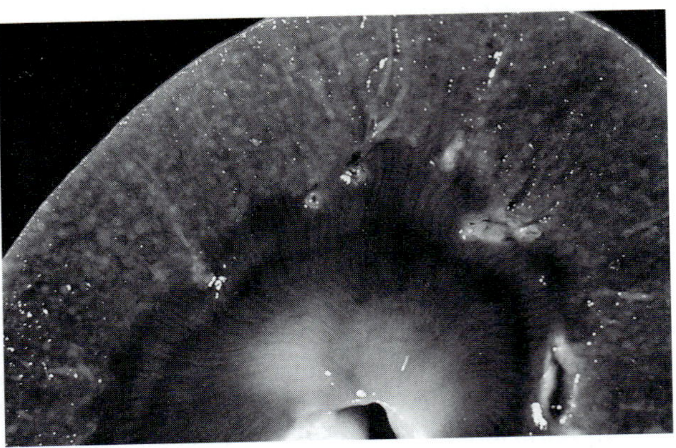

Fig. 5-39 Kidney; gaur. Interstitial nephritis. The cortex has multiple, pale, discrete interstitial inflammatory cell infiltrates throughout due to malignant catarrhal fever virus infection. Note that the cortical striations are effaced.

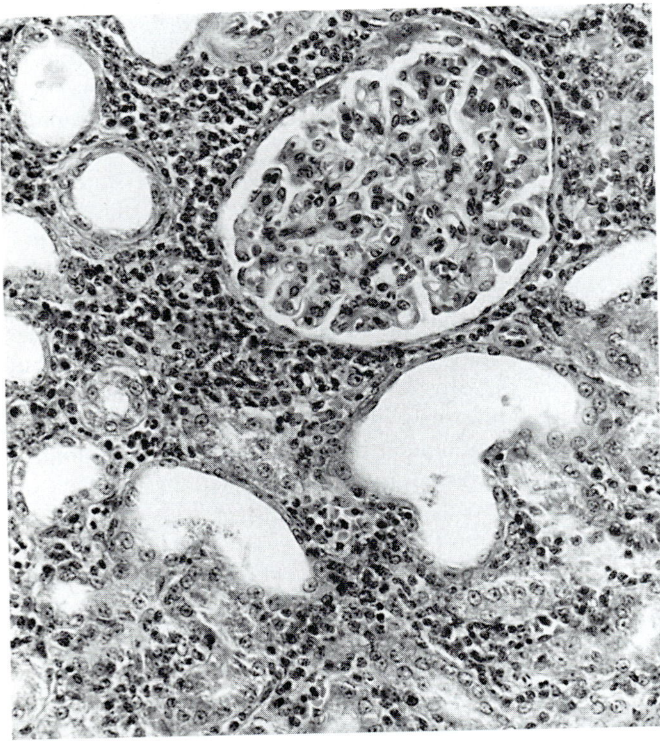

Fig. 5-40 Kidney, cortex; dog. Interstitial nephritis. There are extensive lymphoplasmacytic infiltrates in the cortical interstitium due to leptospirosis. Note the normal glomerulus. H & E stain.

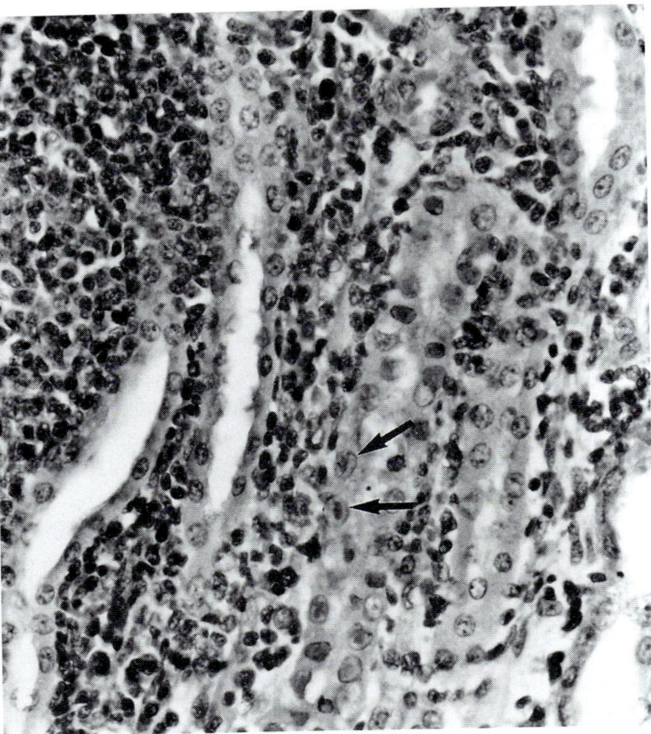

Fig. 5-41 Kidney; medulla; dog. Interstitial nephritis. Lesion is typical for the convalescent phase of infectious canine hepatitis. There is an intense lymphoplasmacytic interstitial infiltrate. Renal tubular epithelial cells contain intranuclear inclusion bodies *(arrows)*. H & E stain.

(Figs. 5-40 and 5-41). The interstitium may be edematous. The epithelium of tubules within intensely inflamed areas has alterations of degeneration and necrosis.

Granulomatous nephritis

Granulomatous nephritis is a manifestation of tubulointerstitial disease that usually accompanies chronic systemic diseases characterized by multiple granuloma formation in various organs. In domestic animals, granulomatous nephritis may be associated with a variety of infectious agents, including viruses, bacteria, fungi, and parasites. Common to each, however, is the formation of grossly visible granulomas randomly scattered throughout the kidneys, but especially in the cortex.

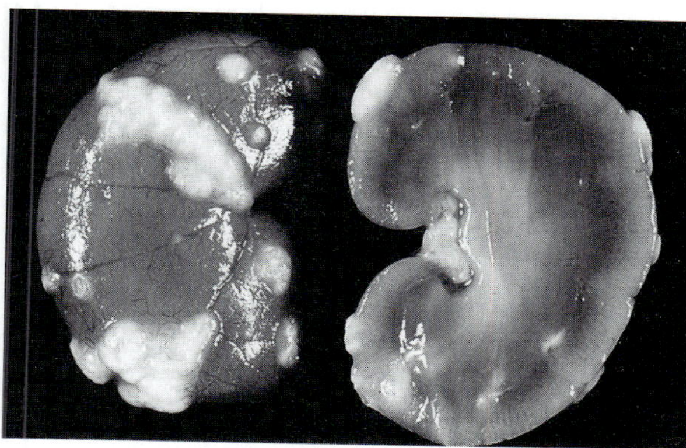

Fig. 5-42 Kidney; cat. Granulomatous nephritis. Lesions are typical for the noneffusive form of feline infectious peritonitis. There are multifocal, coalescing granulomas that extend into the cortical parenchyma. *Courtesy Dr. D.Y. Cho.*

Cats with **feline infectious peritonitis,** particularly the noneffusive (dry) form, often have a multifocal pyogranulomatous nephritis characterized grossly by multiple, large, irregular, pale gray cortical foci that are firm and granular on cut surface (Fig. 5-42). These lesions are somewhat circumscribed and bulge from the capsular surface such that they may be misinterpreted as neoplastic infiltrates. Microscopically, extensive accumulations of macrophages are interspersed with lymphocytes, plasma cells, and neutrophils (pyogranuloma). The pathogenesis of this lesion is thought to be related to cell-mediated hypersensitivity (type IV) to the feline infectious peritonitis virus.

Lymphoplasmacytic to granulomatous nephritis occurs in puppies with systemic *Encephalitozoon cuniculi* infection. Marked interstitial aggregates of lymphocytes, plasma cells, and macrophages are present in the cortex and medulla. Cats with inherited hyperlipoproteinemia have xanthogranulomas in various organs, including the kidneys. These lesions are characterized by foamy, lipid-laden macrophages, lymphocytes, plasma cells, and fibrosis interspersed with lenticular spaces typical of cholesterol deposits (cholesterol clefts). The authors have seen similar renal xanthogranulomas in dogs with hypothyroidism and severe atherosclerosis.

Granulomatous nephritis may also be caused by a variety of granuloma-inducing infectious agents, including fungi such as *Aspergillus* sp., Phycomycetes, or *Histoplasma capsulatum;* algae such as *Prototheca* sp.; and higher bacteria such as *Mycobacterium* sp. *M. tuberculosis* may be a cause of granulomatous nephritis, particularly in cattle. Small, gray-white, granulomatous foci (2 to 5 mm) may be present, randomly scattered throughout the kidneys of animals with generalized miliary tuberculosis. A coarse, nodular, renal tuberculosis occurs also. Kidneys are permeated with large granulomas, up to 10 cm in diameter. These foci are dry and granular and may have calcified, caseous centers. Microscopically, lesions are characterized by central foci of necrosis surrounded by epithelioid macrophages and giant cells that contain acid-fast bacteria.

Migratory *Toxocara canis* larvae can induce small, gray to white granulomas (2 to 3 mm) randomly scattered throughout the subcapsular renal cortex of dogs (Fig. 5-43). Such lesions are probably due to cell-mediated im-

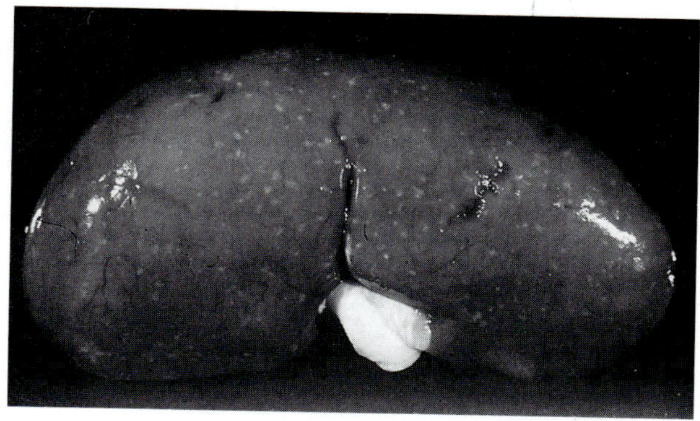

Fig. 5-43 Kidney; dog. Granulomatous nephritis. Widespread multifocal, small, discrete granulomatous foci in the renal cortex are due to extensive ascarid larval migration.

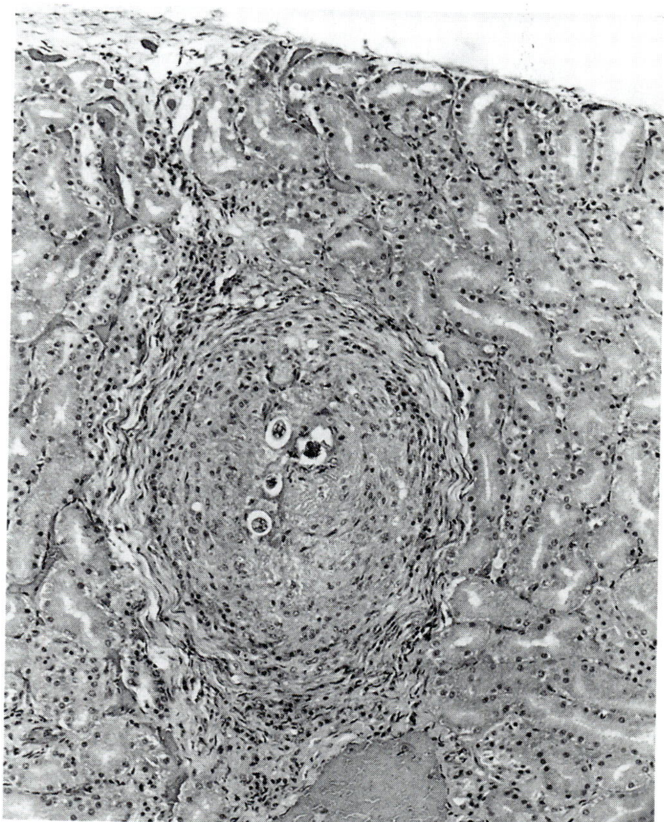

Fig. 5-44 Kidney; cortex; dog. Granulomatous nephritis. A mature granuloma contains ascarid larvae. The center contains epithelioid cells and is surrounded by concentrically arranged fibrous connective tissue and inflammatory cells. H & E stain.

mune responses to the larvae and are composed of aggregates of macrophages, lymphocytes, and eosinophils surrounded by fibroblasts within concentrically arranged fibrous connective tissue (Fig. 5-44). In recently acquired lesions, nematode larvae can often be seen in the center of these lesions. Following death, the larvae become fragmented and are absorbed. Lesions heal by fibrosis, leaving a few fine, pitted foci on the capsular surface.

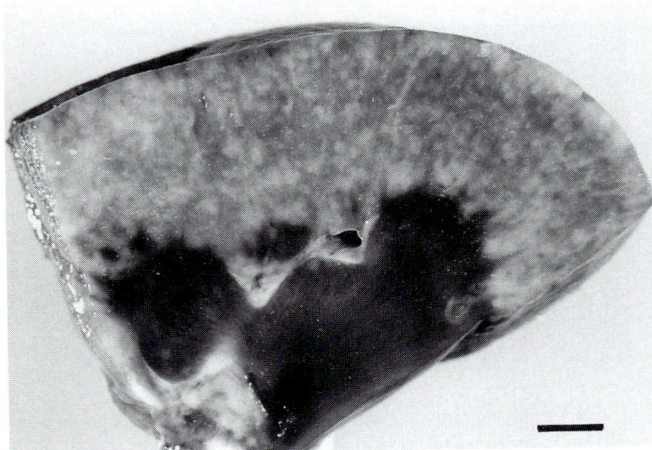

Fig. 5-45 Kidney; cow. Granulomatous nephritis. Cortical striations are obliterated by coalescing granulomatous foci associated with hairy vetch toxicosis. Bar = 1 cm.

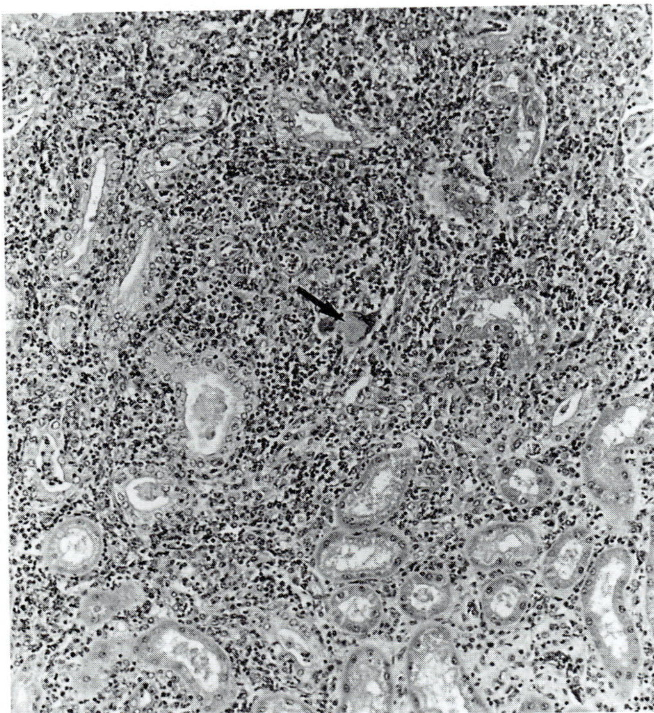

Fig. 5-46 Kidney; cortex; cow. Granulomatous nephritis. Lesions associated with hairy vetch toxicosis are characterized by a mixed inflammatory cell infiltrate with renal tubular atrophy and replacement. Note the multinucleated giant cell *(arrow)*. H & E stain.

In cattle, granulomatous nephritis is part of the multisystemic granulomatous disease associated with hairy vetch *(Vicia villosa)* toxicosis. Lesions are characterized by multifocal and coalescing infiltrates of monocytes, lymphocytes, plasma cells, eosinophils, and multinucleated giant cells (Figs. 5-45 and 5-46).

Pyelonephritis

While **pyelitis** refers to inflammation of the renal pelvis, **pyelonephritis** is inflammation of both the renal pelvis and renal parenchyma and is an excellent example of suppurative tubulointerstitial disease. Each usually originates as an extension of bacterial infection of the lower urinary tract (see Lower Urinary Tract) that ascends the ureters to the kidneys and establishes infections in the pelvis and inner medulla. Rarely, pyelonephritis may result from descending bacterial infections, bacterial contamination of the kidneys having arisen hematogenously, e.g., embolic nephritis. Ascending infection, however, is by far the most common cause of pyelonephritis.

The pathogenesis of ascending pyelonephritis depends on the abnormal reflux of bacterial-contaminated urine from the lower tract to the renal pelvis and collecting tubules **(vesicoureteral reflux).** Normally, there is little vesicoureteral reflux during micturition. Vesicoureteral reflux occurs more readily when there is increased pressure within the urinary bladder, as with urethral obstruction. In addition, bacterial infection of the lower urinary tract can enhance vesicoureteral reflux by several mechanisms. When the bladder wall is inflamed (cystitis), the normal competency of the vesicoureteral valve may be compromised, allowing greater freedom for urine reflux. Cystitis and urethritis, associated with narrowing of the urethra, or obstruction by urinary calculi, may cause increased intracystic pressure and enhanced reflux. Endotoxin liberated from gram-negative bacterial infections of the ureter and bladder can inhibit normal ureteral peristalsis, increasing reflux.

Bacteria that colonize the pelvis can easily infect the inner medulla. The medulla is highly susceptible to bacterial infection because of its poor blood supply (see Papillary Necrosis); its high interstitial osmolality, which inhibits neutrophil function; and its high ammonia concentration, which inhibits complement activation. Thus, bacteria can randomly infect and ascend collecting ducts, cause tubular epithelial necrosis and hemorrhage, and stimulate an inflammatory response. Bacterial infection can progressively ascend within both tubules and interstitium until the inflammatory lesions (tubulointerstitial inflammation) extend from pelvis to capsule.

Because most occurrences of pyelonephritis are ascending infections and because females are more susceptible to lower urinary tract infection, pyelonephritis occurs more frequently in females than males. *E. coli* (particularly alpha hemolysin–producing strains), *Proteus* sp., *Klebsiella* sp., *Staphylococcus* sp., *Streptococcus* sp., and *Pseudomonas aeruginosa* are common causes of lower urinary tract infection and pyelonephritis in all species. *Corynebacterium renale* and *Eubacterium suis (C. suis)* are specifically pathogenic for the lower urinary tract of cattle and swine, respectively, and are common causes of pyelonephritis.

Pyelonephritis is recognized by the existence of an acute or chronic pyelitis and an associated inflammation of the renal parenchyma. The pelvic and ureteral mucous membranes may be acutely inflamed, thickened, reddened, roughened or granular, and coated with a thin exudate or may be markedly dilated and contain purulent exudate (Fig. 5-47). The medullary crest (papilla) is often ulcerated and necrotic. Renal involvement is marked by irregular, radially oriented, red or gray streaks involving the medulla, extending toward and often reaching the renal surface (Fig. 5-48). The distribution of lesions in the kidneys is somewhat unique as aggregates of inflamed foci distributed over the renal capsular surface and cut surface, but separated from each other by areas of normal renal parenchyma (Fig. 5-49). Inflammatory foci are often most severe at the renal poles. The renal lesions of advanced chronic pyelonephritis include most of the elements of acute inflammation de-

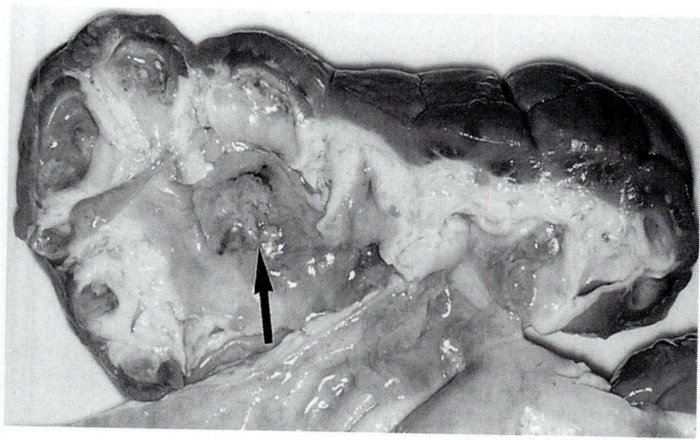

Fig. 5-47 Kidney; cow. Pyelonephritis. There are ureteral and pelvic dilatation, pelvic exudate *(arrow),* and cortical and medullary atrophy.

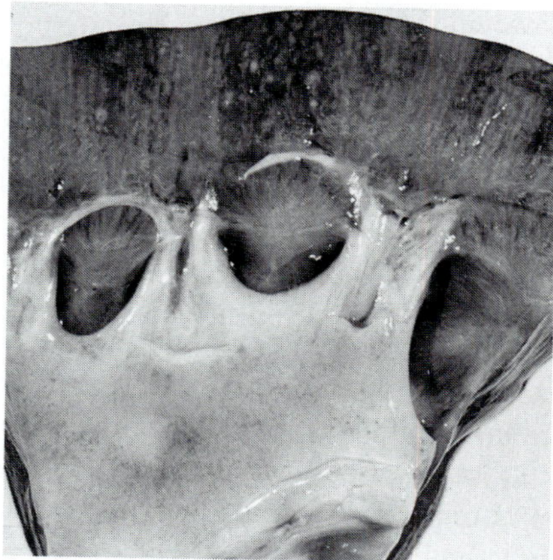

Fig. 5-48 Kidney; sow. Pyelonephritis. The pelvic mucosa is hyperemic, the calyces are dilated, the papillae are attenuated, and there are radiating zones of hyperemia and purulent foci in the cortex.

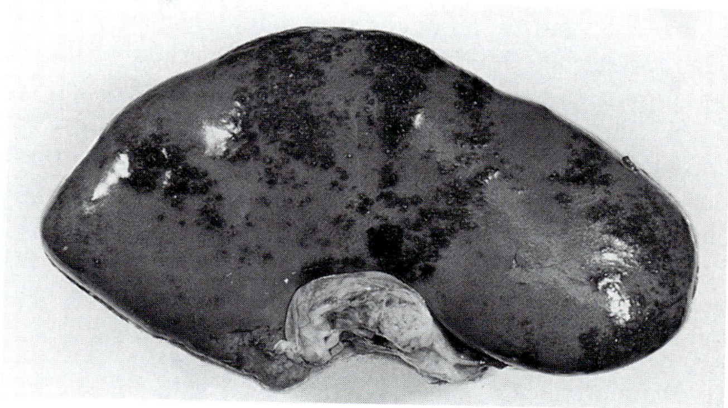

Fig. 5-49 Kidney; sow. Pyelonephritis. There are irregularly distributed patches of hyperemia and purulent foci in the subcapsular cortex. The irregular and patchy distribution is a frequent feature of ascending pyelonephritis.

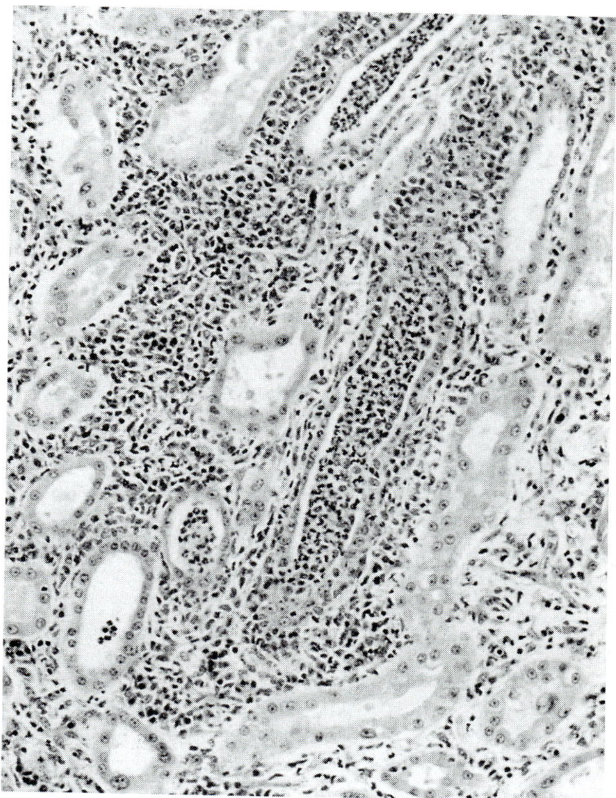

Fig. 5-50 Kidney; cow. Pyelonephritis. There is both intratubular and interstitial inflammation. Tubules contain dense neutrophil aggregates. H & E stain.

scribed above as well as extensive necrosis with destruction of the medulla and fibrosis with patchy scarring of the outer medulla and cortex. Pyelonephritis may be unilateral. Occasionally, inflammation extends through the surface of the kidneys to produce extensive subcapsular inflammation and localized peritonitis.

Microscopically, the most severe lesions are in the inner medulla. The transitional epithelium is usually focally or diffusely necrotic and desquamated. Necrotic debris, fibrin, neutrophils, and bacterial colonies may be adherent to the denuded surface. Medullary tubules are markedly dilated, and lumina contain neutrophils and bacterial colonies (Fig. 5-50). The tubular epithelium is focally necrotic. An intense neutrophilic infiltrate present in the renal interstitium may be accompanied by marked interstitial hemorrhages and edema. Coagulative necrosis of the inner medulla may be severe if vascular obstruction has occurred. Similar tubular and interstitial lesions, although less severe, extend radially into the cortical tubules and interstitium.

Hydronephrosis

Hydronephrosis refers to dilatation of the renal pelvis due to obstruction of urine outflow and is associated with increased pelvic pressure, dilatation of the pelvis, and progressive renal parenchymal atrophy. Hydronephrosis occurs in all domestic animals. Obstruction leading to hydronephrosis may occasionally be caused by congenital malformation of the ureter, vesicoureteral junction, or urethra, but the more common causes of hydronephrosis are ureteral or urethral blockage due to urinary tract calculi (see Lower Urinary Tract), chronic inflammation, or neoplasia of the ureter or bladder. Congenitally malpositioned kidneys may result in a kinking of the ureter and obstruction. Hydronephrosis may be unilateral or bilateral. When hydronephrosis is unilateral, renal cystic enlargement may become extensive before the lesion is recognized. When the destructive lesion is bilateral and complete, death due to uremia may occur before cystic enlargement becomes extensive. However, if the obstructive process causes partial or intermittent blockage, bilateral hydronephrosis can become marked.

The increased intratubular pressure following ureteral obstruction results in renal tubular dilatation. Glomeruli remain functional, but much of the glomerular filtrate diffuses into the interstitium, where it is initially removed via lymph vessels and veins. As intrapelvic pressure increases, the interstitial vessels collapse, and renal blood flow is reduced, accompanied by ischemia, tubular atrophy and necrosis, and interstitial fibrosis. The glomeruli maintain a relatively normal morphologic appearance for a prolonged period but eventually become atrophic and sclerotic.

Early lesions of hydronephrosis are dilated pelvis and calyces with blunting of the renal crest/papillae (Fig. 5-51). With progressive pelvic dilatation, the kidney silhouette enlarges and becomes rounder than normal, with progressive thinning of the cortex and medulla (Fig. 5-52). Interstitial vascular obstruction may occur, resulting in cortical ischemia, possibly infarction, and necrosis. In its most advanced form, the hydronephrotic kidney is a thin-walled (2 to 3 mm thick), fluid-filled sac caused by pelvic dilatation and degeneration, severe atrophy, and fibrosis of the renal parenchyma. This sac is lined by transitional epithelium, which is spared during lesion development.

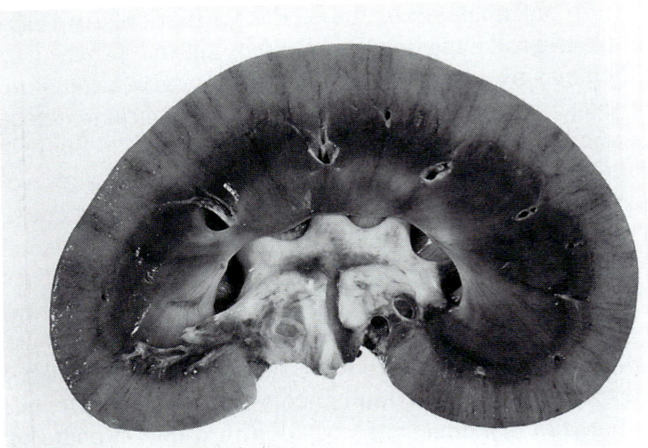

Fig. 5-51 Kidney; sheep. Hydronephrosis. Both the pelvis and calyces are dilated, typical of early hydronephrosis.

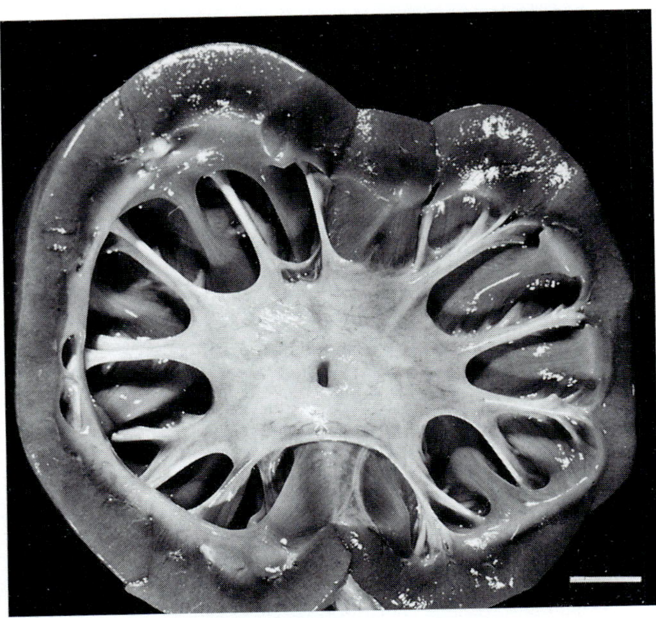

Fig. 5-52 Kidney; dog. Hydronephrosis. Advanced hydronephrosis is characterized by marked pelvic and calyceal dilatation and medullary atrophy. The ureter is dilated also. Bar = 1 cm.

Occasionally, a severely hydronephrotic kidney becomes bacterially contaminated, such that the thin-walled sac becomes filled with pus instead of urine. This lesion is referred to as **pyonephrosis** and is probably the result of descending pyelonephritis.

Renal Nematodes

The giant kidney worm of dogs *(Dioctophyma renale)* is seen infrequently in dogs in temperate and cold countries worldwide. It is endemic in Canada and in northern regions of the United States. Because of a prolonged and complex life cycle, this nematode is seen only in dogs 2 years old or older. The adult nematode, which may be up to 100 cm long, inhabits the renal pelvis, where it causes severe hemorrhagic or purulent pyelitis and ureteral obstruction. The renal parenchyma may be destroyed, causing the kidney to be transformed into a cyst that contains the nematode and purulent exudate.

In North America, the swine kidney worm *(Stephanurus dentatus)* is found most often in adult swine in southern regions of the United States. The parasite is also a problem in other countries with warm climates. Adult worms normally encyst in perirenal fat; however, cysts that contain the nematode may be found in the kidneys. Peripelvic cysts often communicate with the renal pelvis or ureter, and there may be localized fibrosis and chronic granulation tissue surrounding the parasite.

Capillaria plica and *Capillaria feliscati* have been identified infrequently in dogs and cats worldwide. Typically, these nematodes are attached to the renal pelvis, ureter, or urinary bladder of animals of various ages. Microscopic inflammatory cell infiltrates and focal hemorrhages are associated with sites of attachment.

Chronic Renal Diseases

Renal fibrosis (scarring)

Renal fibrosis can occur as a primary event, but, more frequently, it occurs as a chronic manifestation of the healing phase of a preexisting renal lesion. It occurs following primary inflammation of glomeruli, tubules, or interstitial tissue or following severe degeneration or necrosis of renal tubules. The severity of renal fibrosis usually parallels the intensity of the antecedent renal disease. Renal fibrosis and chronic renal disease are the most frequently recognized renal pathologic processes in mature or aging domestic animals, particularly dogs and cats. When renal fibrosis and accompanying loss of nephrons are severe, they can be manifested in the live animal as renal failure and uremia. One of the most common expressions of this chronic disease state is the inability of an animal to concentrate urine, resulting in frequent urination **(polyuria)** of a dilute urine **(isosthenuria).** Polyuria is accompanied by dehydration and intense water drinking **(polydipsia).** Hypoplastic anemia occurs as well, due to failure of the kidney to synthesize and secrete erythropoietin.

Fibrotic kidneys are pale, shrunken, and firm, with excessive adhesion of the capsule to the underlying cortex. Without careful attention to the pattern of fibrosis, such kidneys may be indiscriminately evaluated as representing **chronic interstitial nephritis, end-stage kidney,** or **nephrosclerosis.** However, fibrosis generally follows a pattern characteristic of the antecedent lesion; it may be diffuse and finely stippled, diffuse or multifocal and coarse, or patchy. For example, fibrosis often is initiated by circulatory disturbances predicated upon compromise of blood flow through glomerular capillaries in glomerulonephritides and amyloidosis. Thus, because most primary glomerular lesions involve glomeruli diffusely throughout the renal cortex, the distribution of fibrosis secondary to glomerular disease is diffuse, finely stippled, and primarily cortical; and because all components of the nephron are interdependent, glomerular fibrosis and loss of function ultimately result in secondary atrophy of cortical and medullary tubules and degrees of fibrosis in the adjoining interstitial connective tissue.

Diffuse fibrosis with a finely stippled pattern may also occur subsequent to widespread necrosis of renal tubular epithelium (acute tubular necrosis) (Fig. 5-53). In oak poisoning, severe tubular necrosis with destruction of the tubular basement membrane, leakage of tubular contents, and failure of epithelial cell regeneration may occur as a prelude to fibrosis.

Coarser patterns of renal fibrosis occur when the antecedent lesion is less evenly distributed in the kidney. Fibrosis secondary to the tubulointerstitial inflammation of pyelonephritis follows the pattern of the acute disease and results in irregularly distributed, patchy scarring, often deeply depressed on the renal surface with linear areas of fibrosis extending through both the cortex and medulla to

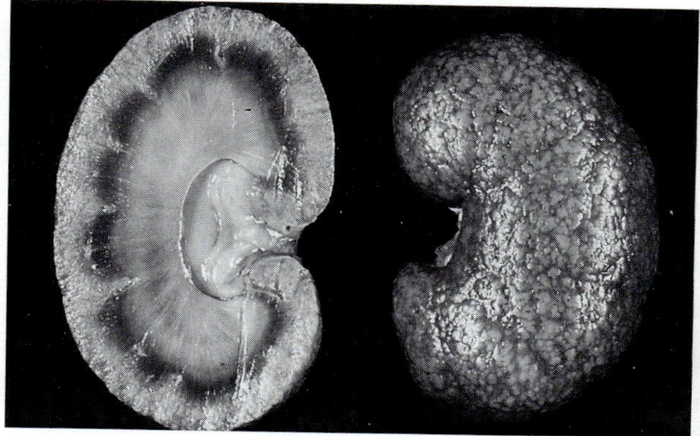

Fig. 5-53 Kidney; dog. Fibrosis. Diffuse interstitial fibrosis is present as a finely stippled pattern characterized by fine pitting on the surface and a thin, granular cortex on cut surface. *Courtesy Dr. D.Y. Cho.*

the pelvis (Fig. 5-54). Like the acute lesion, fibrosis frequently has a polar distribution. The scarring that follows embolic or thrombotic vascular obstruction and infarction is related to the size of the ischemic area caused by vascular compromise (Fig. 5-55). Obstruction of relatively large vessels causes large, deeply depressed scars that involve primarily the cortex but can extend into the medulla, whereas obstruction of smaller vessels heals as small-diameter pits in the renal surface with an accompanying pale, linear scar on the cut surface. A coarser pattern of diffuse renal fibrosis occurs in chronic interstitial nephritis and certain progressive juvenile nephropathies of dogs. Both cortex and medulla are "equivalently" fibrotic, cortical striations are severely distorted or effaced, and multiple cysts are common.

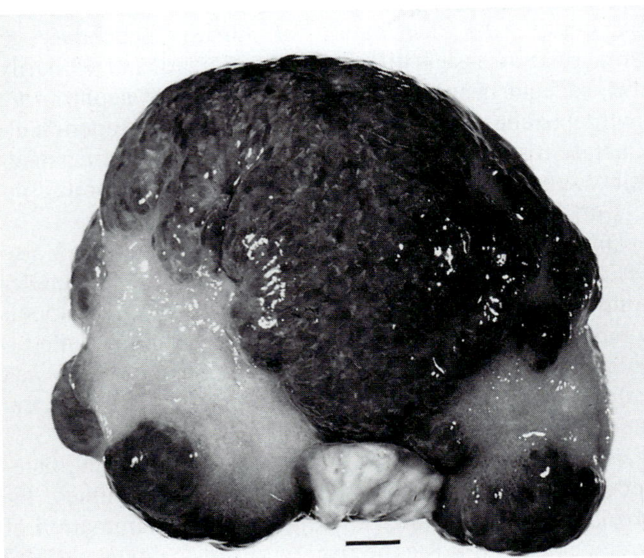

Fig. 5-54 Kidney; dog. Fibrosis. There are large patches of advanced cortical scarring at the poles and a finely stippled pattern of fibrosis in the remaining kidney. This pattern suggests previous pyelonephritis. Bar = 1 cm.

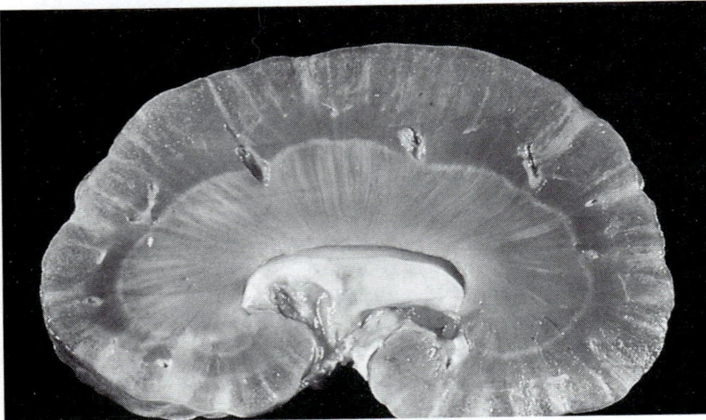

Fig. 5-55 Kidney; dog. Fibrosis. There are multiple radial-oriented scars randomly involving the renal cortex, a pattern that suggests previous vascular obstruction.

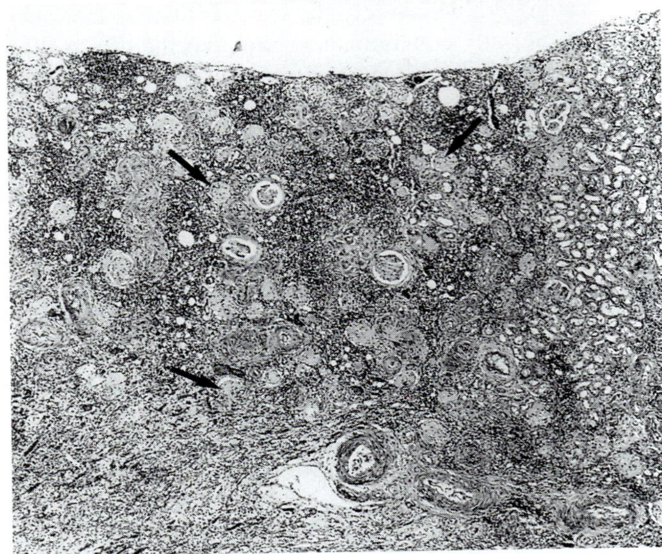

Fig. 5-56 Kidney; cortex; dog. Fibrosis. The lesion is characterized by interstitial fibrosis, tubular atrophy, and interstitial inflammatory cell infiltration. Note the depressed capsular surface due to scarring and the shrunken sclerotic glomeruli *(arrows)*. H & E stain.

Microscopically, renal fibrosis is characterized by an increase in interstitial connective tissue and by atrophy and disappearance of associated renal tubules. Atrophic tubules have a reduced diameter, have a thickened, hyalinized basement membrane, and are lined by flattened epithelium. The interstitium usually has foci of lymphocytes and plasma cells randomly scattered throughout, giving rise to the often-used diagnosis of chronic interstitial nephritis (Fig. 5-56). Multiple cysts can be present throughout the cortex and medulla. These acquired cysts are lined by flattened epithelial cells and are the result of dilated Bowman's capsules, with associated atrophic glomerular tufts or dilated, sequestered tubular segments that became isolated by connective tissue (Fig. 5-57). Glomerulosclerosis is commonly present, particularly in areas of intense interstitial fibrosis. Calcification of vessels, tubular basement membranes, Bowman's capsule, and degenerate tubular epithelium is common in fibrotic kidneys due to alterations in calcium-phosphorous metabolism associated with chronic renal failure.

Progressive juvenile nephropathy

The development of severe bilateral renal fibrosis has been described in young dogs of several breeds and has been designated progressive juvenile nephropathy or familial (hereditary) renal disease (Box 5-4). A familial-tendency has been demonstrated in many dogs, but the

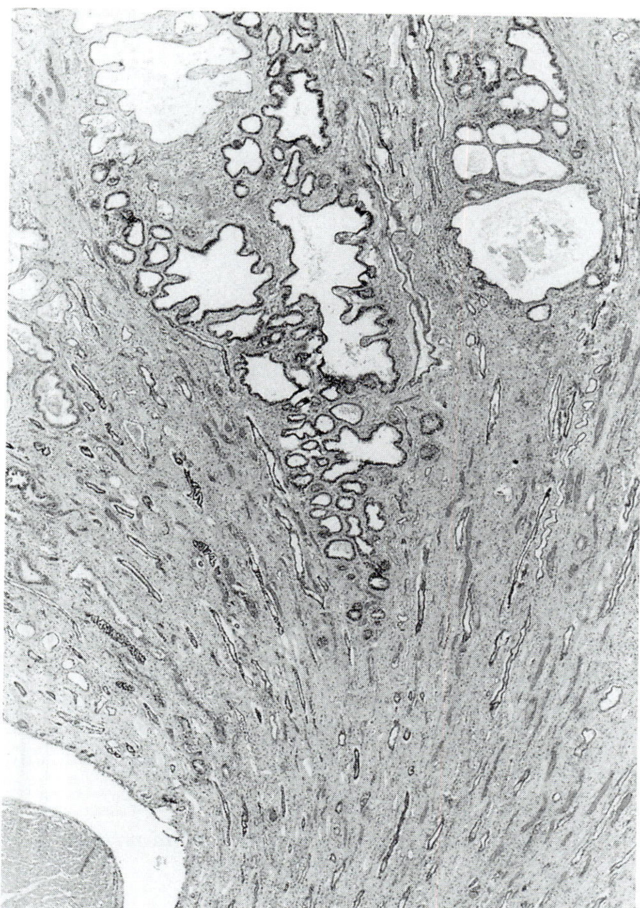

Fig. 5-57 Kidney; dog. Fibrosis. The lesion is characterized by renal interstitial fibrosis with dilated tubules and acquired renal cysts. H & E stain.

Box 5-4 BREEDS OF DOGS WITH PROGRESSIVE JUVENILE NEPHROPATHY

Cocker spaniels	Standard poodles
Norwegian elkhounds	Alaskan malamutes
Samoyeds	Miniature schnauzers
Doberman pinschers	German shepherds
Lhaso apsos	Keeshounds
Shih tzus	Chow chows
Soft-coated wheaten terriers	

mode of inheritance has been determined only in Samoyed dogs and is sex-linked. The disease in shih tzu dogs appears to have a simple autosomal recessive inheritance. Although variations exist in microscopic and gross lesions as well as in the pathogenesis of progressive nephropathy among the different breeds, a typical case is usually seen in a dog 4 months to 2 years old that has signs of polyuria, polydipsia, and uremia. The clinical presentation and gross lesions are identical to those of chronic renal disease in mature or aging dogs.

In the Doberman pinscher dog, the primary lesion is a glomerulopathy that microscopically is a membranoproliferative glomerulonephritis. Subsequently, the lesions are extensive periglomerular fibrosis, tubular atrophy, and cystic dilatation of Bowman's capsule and renal tubules. In affected Samoyed dogs, multilamellar splitting of the glomerular basement membrane is due to abnormalities in basement membrane collagen. These lesions progress to severe glomerulosclerosis. A tubular disorder resulting in periglomerular and interstitial fibrosis, tubular atrophy, and glomerulosclerosis without indication of primary glomerular disease has been observed in Norwegian elkhound dogs. In Lhaso apso, shih tzu, Wheaten terrier, and standard poodle dogs, renal dysplasia has been hypothesized. Small, shrunken, fetal-like glomeruli composed of small cells with dense nuclei, minimal mesangial tissue, and nonpatent capillaries may be seen interspersed with normal, sclerotic, or compensatorily hypertrophied glomeruli. Other lesions include marked interstitial fibrosis and tubular dilatation. Most of these lesions have minimal inflammatory cell infiltrates. Thus, progressive juvenile nephropathy is a syndrome, the lesions of which are the result of any of several chronic pathologic processes.

Gross renal lesions of progressive juvenile nephropathy are variable among affected breeds and among affected dogs within a breed. Generally, kidneys are markedly shrunken, pale, and firm. The surface may be diffusely pitted and have a fine stippled pattern, particularly in those dogs where glomerular disease is the primary event; or the surface may have patchy areas of deep cortical scarring. On cut surface, the cortex is thin and has linear scars. The medulla is usually diffusely fibrotic. Small, variably sized cysts often occur in the cortex and medulla.

Neoplasia

The prevalence of primary renal neoplasms in domestic animals is less than 1% of the total neoplasms reported. They are usually unilateral and can be of epithelial, mesenchymal, or embryonal origin.

Renal adenomas

These neoplasms are rare, are incidental findings at necropsy, and usually appear as a small, solitary, well-circumscribed mass in the cortex. Microscopically, adenomas are composed of solid sheets, tubules, or papillary proliferations of cuboidal epithelial cells that are uniform in size and have granular eosinophilic cytoplasm and small, round to oval nuclei. Mitotic figures, necrosis, and fibrosis are rarely seen.

Renal carcinomas

These are the most common primary renal neoplasms and occur most frequently in older dogs. The neoplasms

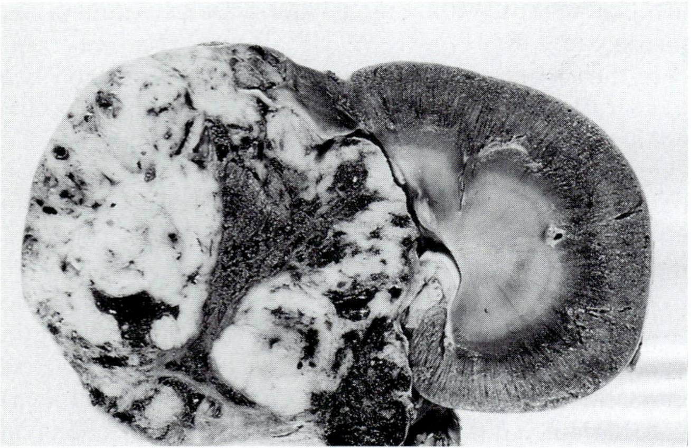

Fig. 5-58 Kidney; dog. Renal carcinoma. The neoplasm has infiltrated and replaced one half of the kidney. *Lucke VM, Kelly DF, Vet Pathol 13: 264–276, 1976.*

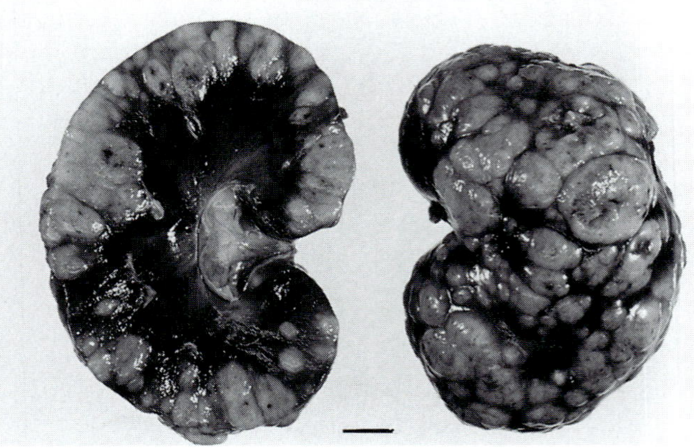

Fig. 5-59 Kidney; dog. Metastatic neoplasm. Multiple pale, neoplastic nodules are randomly scattered throughout the kidneys as a result of disseminated mast cell tumors. Bar = 1 cm.

are usually large (up to 20 cm in diameter), spherical to oval, and firm. They often are pale yellow and have dark areas of hemorrhage and necrosis and foci of cystic degeneration. The masses usually occupy and obliterate one pole of a kidney and grow by expansion, compressing the adjacent renal tissue (Fig. 5-58). Metastasis to the lungs is frequent. In German shepherd dogs, a variant of the typical renal carcinoma has been seen in conjunction with nodular dermatofibrosis. The lesions are hereditary and consist of multifocal, bilateral, renal cystadenocarcinomas. Neoplastic cells occur in solid sheets, tubules, or papillary patterns. Cells vary in shape from cuboidal to columnar to polyhedral, vary in size, and may have clear or granular eosinophilic cytoplasm. Nuclei range from small, round, granular, and uniform to large, oval, vesicular, and pleomorphic. Mitotic figures are numerous. These neoplasms have a moderate fibrovascular stroma.

Nephroblastomas (embryonal nephroma, Wilm's tumor)

These are common renal neoplasms of pigs and chickens and are usually recognized at slaughter or necropsy. They occur in cattle and dogs as well, but less frequently. These neoplasms are of embryonal origin, arising from the metanephric blastema, and, thus, occur in young animals. It is speculated that neoplasms result from malignant transformation during normal nephrogenesis or from neoplastic transformation of nests of embryonic tissue that persist in the postnatal kidney. At necropsy, nephroblastomas may be solitary or multiple masses that often reach a great size and in which renal tissue may be difficult to recognize. They usually are soft to rubbery, gray with foci of hemorrhage, and lobulated on cut surface. Because nephroblastomas arise from primitive pluripotential tissue, microscopic features vary but are morphologically similar to the developmental stages of embryonic kidneys. Characteristically, primitive, loose myxomatous mesenchymal tissue predominates. Interspersed in this tissue are primitive tubules lined by elongated, deeply staining cells and structures that resemble primitive glomeruli. Nests of cells resembling the metanephric blastema may be present. Nephroblastomas may also contain such mesenchymal components as cartilage, bone, skeletal muscle, and adipose tissue.

Transitional cell neoplasms, sarcomas, and metastatic tumors

These neoplasms may arise in the renal pelvis and lower urinary tract and can obstruct urinary outflow. Such carcinomas may invade the kidneys. The morphologic features of transitional cell neoplasms will be discussed under the section on The Lower Urinary Tract. Occasionally, **fibromas, fibrosarcomas,** or **hemangiosarcomas** arise in the kidneys. Metastatic neoplasms, both carcinomas and sarcomas, occur in the kidneys and are characteristically composed of randomly scattered, multiple nodules, usually involving both kidneys (Fig. 5-59). Renal **lymphosarcoma** occurs with some frequency in cattle and cats, particularly as part of generalized or multicentric lymphosarcoma. The lesions appear as single or multiple, homogeneous, gray-white nodules or as diffuse lymphomatous infiltrates that uniformly enlarge the affected kidney.

THE LOWER URINARY TRACT

General Considerations

The lower urinary tract consists of the ureters, urinary bladder, and urethra. The renal pelvis, ureters, and urinary bladder are lined by transitional epithelium, whereas the urethra is lined by transitional epithelium cranially and stratified squamous epithelium caudally. As in other mucous membranes, the lamina propria contains small lymphoid follicles that, on occasion, may be large enough to be seen grossly as discrete, circular, white foci (2 to 4 mm) in the mucosa. The vesicoureteral valve, created by the oblique passage of the ureter through the wall of the urinary bladder, is an important structure as it normally prevents reflux of bladder urine into the ureter and pelvis. At death, the urinary bladder may constrict, such that the normal bladder wall appears thick at necropsy. The normal mucosa of the lower urinary tract should be smooth and glistening. Urine should be clear, except in horses, where, due to the normal presence of mucus or fine crystals, it is cloudy.

Developmental Anomalies

Ureteral aplasia (agenesis)

This lesion is rare, but may occur by itself or in association with renal aplasia. Ectopic ureters are found most frequently in dogs; certain breeds, especially the Siberian husky dog, are at greater risk. The involved ureter empties into the urethra, vagina, neck of the bladder, vas deferens, or prostate. Ectopic ureters are more subject to obstruction or infection, thus they predispose animals to pyelitis and pyelonephritis. Occasionally, anomalies of the lower urinary tract mucosa are such that transitional epithelium is focally replaced by skin or alimentary tract mucosa.

Patent urachus

The most common malformation of the urinary bladder is **patent (pervious) urachus.** This develops when the fetal urachus fails to close and, therefore, forms a direct channel between the bladder's apex and the umbilicus. Foals are affected most often and have dribbling of urine at the umbilicus. Affected animals have increased susceptibility to bacterial infections of the urinary bladder. Failure of the urachal remnant and the umbilical arteries and vein to involute is a very frequent manifestation of ''neonatal'' omphalitis. Although unusual, urachal patency may occur under that circumstance as well. Patent urachus has also been reported secondary to congenital urethral obstruction. Increased bladder pressure due to the obstruction forces urine out the urachus.

Occasionally, during urachal closure, the mucosa closes, but closure of the bladder musculature is incomplete. When this occurs, a **bladder diverticulum** (outpouching) of the apex of the bladder can develop. Urine stasis may occur in the diverticulum, predisposing the animal to cystitis or urinary calculi.

Urolithiasis

Urinary calculi (uroliths)

These are concretions formed in the urinary tract and are usually composed of salts of inorganic or organic acids or other materials, such as cystine or xanthine. Struvite (ammoniomagnesium phosphate hexahydrate), carbonate, silica, urate, cystine, xanthine, or benzocoumarin (''clover stone'') calculi have been seen in domestic animals. Calculi can be found in the renal pelvis, ureter, or any portion of the lower urinary tract. Calculi vary in size and shape. Renal pelvic calculi classically have a ''staghorn'' appearance because they take the shape of the renal calyces (Fig. 5-60). These calculi predispose to pyelitis and pyelonephritis. Bladder calculi can be single or multiple, vary in size (2 mm to 10 cm), and sometimes are composed of a fine, sandlike material that may appear as cloudy urine (Fig. 5-61). Calculi may have smooth or rough surfaces; they may be white, yellow, or brown, depending on their

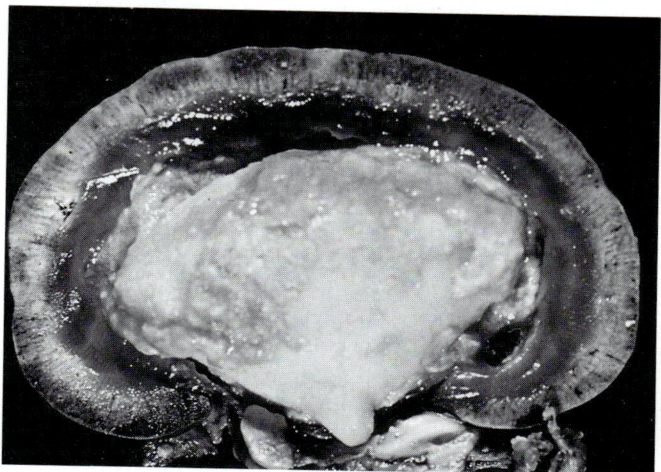

Fig. 5-60 Kidney; dog. Urolithiasis. A calculus is filling and distending the renal pelvis and causing extensive erosion and attenuation of the medulla. The apex of the calculus conforms to the ureteral opening.

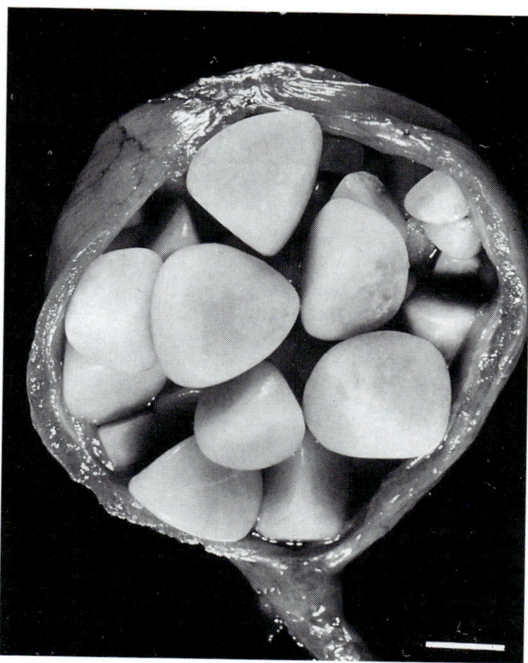

Fig. 5-61 Urinary bladder; dog. Urolithiasis. Multiple smooth calculi are present in the urinary bladder. The bladder wall is diffusely thickened (scale in centimeters). Bar = 1 cm.

composition. Urolithiasis causes urinary obstruction or traumatic injury to the bladder mucosa. These changes are manifested as difficult or painful urination **(stranguria, dysuria)** and/or hematuria.

Both males and females are subject to urolithiasis, but calculi cause urinary obstruction more commonly in males because of the narrow urethral diameter and longer urethra of males. When obstruction or dysuria occurs in females, calculi are usually large and located in the renal pelvis or urinary bladder. In males, dysuria may result from large calculi, but urinary tract obstruction with uremia most commonly occurs because of obstruction of the urethra with small calculi. The most common sites of lodgment of urethral calculi in bulls are at the ischial arch and the proximal end of the sigmoid flexure; in rams and wethers, the urethral process (vermiform appendage) is the most common site (Fig. 5-62), and in dogs, it is the base of the os penis. In cats, fine struvite crystals (sand) in a rubberlike protein matrix fill the entire urethra and are typical for the condition called feline urologic syndrome. Urethral calculi are least commonly seen in horses and swine.

Calculi form due to precipitation of salts in urine, usually in association with an organic (protein) matrix. A number of factors predispose the lower urinary tract to calculus formation. Urine pH is important to the development of calculi, in that some salts precipitate more readily at acid pH (oxalates) and others more readily at alkaline pH (struvite and carbonate). Bacterial infections predispose to urolithiasis (particularly struvite calculi in dogs) because bacterial colonies, exfoliated epithelium, or leukocytes can serve as the nidus around which precipitation of the mineral constituents occurs. A cell-associated herpesvirus has been one of many factors that predispose cats to struvite urolithiasis.

Nutritional and dietary factors have been associated with the formation of urinary calculi. In sheep, diets rich in phosphate, such as milo or sorghum products, predispose to struvite urolithiasis. In cats, dry commercial food rich in magnesium is another predisposing factor for the feline urologic syndrome. Ingestion of oxalate-accumulating plants predisposes to oxalate urolithiasis. Vitamin A deficiency may predispose to urolithiasis by the development of metaplastic changes in the transitional epithelium. Dehydration, as occurs when water intake is limited, can precipitate or aggravate calculus formation by allowing a supersaturated state of mineral constituents in the concentrated urine. Supersaturation may be unstable and predispose animals to spontaneous precipitation. Ingestion of estrogens, such as after consumption of subterranean clover, as well as implantation or injection of estrogens can predispose sheep to so-called clover stones (benzocoumarin) or carbonate calculi.

Hereditary defects that result in urinary excretion of xanthine **(xanthinuria)** or cystine **(cystinuria)** can cause urinary calculi of the appropriate compound (see Inherited Abnormalities in Renal Tubular Function). Urate calculi form most commonly in Dalmatian dogs due to their high urinary excretion of uric acid.

At necropsy, animals that die of urinary obstruction have greatly distended, turgid or ruptured urinary bladders and often dilated ureters and renal pelves. The urinary bladder wall is thin and often diffusely hemorrhagic (Fig. 5-63). When urine is released from the urinary bladder, the wall is flaccid, the mucosa is often ulcerated, and the urine may contain clotted blood. Mucosal ulceration, localized lamina propria hemorrhage, and necrosis are usually present in the ureter, urinary bladder, or urethra adjacent to an obstructive calculus. The urinary bladder may rupture antemortem, whereby there is clotted blood and fibrin at the site of rupture and possibly an acute, localized, chemically induced peritonitis.

Microscopically, inflammation and hemorrhage are present in the lower urinary tract. Lesions are most severe in

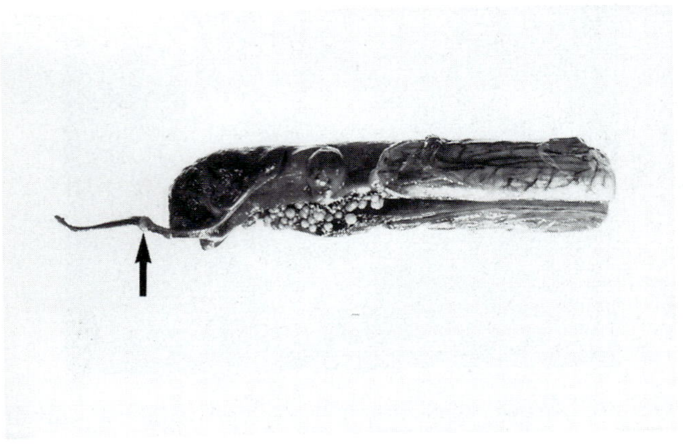

Fig. 5-62 Penis; lamb. Urolithiasis. Multiple calculi are in the penile urethra and in the urethral process *(arrow)*.

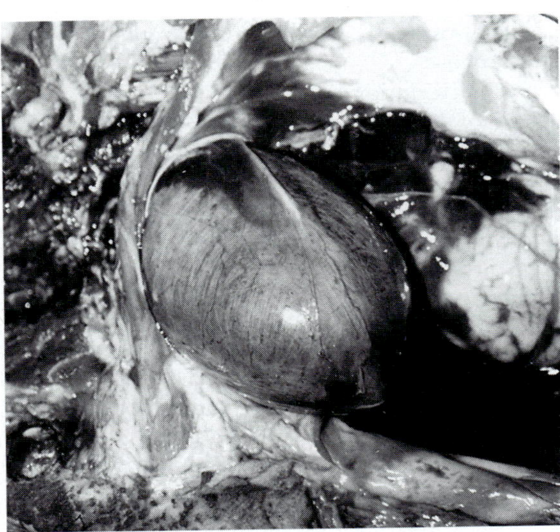

Fig. 5-63 Urinary bladder; lamb. Urolithiasis. The bladder is overdistended and turgid due to urethral obstruction. Note hemorrhages at the neck and apex of the bladder.

cases where obstruction has been complete. The mucosa is usually ulcerated, and areas of transitional epithelial cell hyperplasia may have numerous goblet cells. The lamina propria is usually infiltrated with pleocellular inflammatory exudates; neutrophils are associated with foci of ulceration, whereas lymphocytes and plasma cells may infiltrate perivascularly or more uniformly throughout the lamina propria. Hemorrhage is transmural and often causes wide separation of smooth muscle bundles. Degeneration and necrosis of smooth muscle occur in severe cases.

Inflammatory Diseases

Inflammation of the bladder **(cystitis)** is common in domestic animals. Because inflammation of the ureter **(ureteritis)** or urethra **(urethritis)** in the absence of cystitis is rare, this discussion will concentrate on cystitis. Cystitis can result from several chemical causes. Active metabolites of cyclophosphamide, a drug used to treat neoplastic and immune-mediated diseases of dogs and cats, can cause a sterile hemorrhagic cystitis. Cantharidin toxicosis in horses results from ingestion of blister beetles (*Epicauta* sp.) in alfalfa hay, and necrotic and hemorrhagic cystitis is a common finding. Chronic ingestion of bracken fern *(Pteridium aquilinum)* by cattle can result in the syndrome enzootic hematuria, which can be manifested as acute bladder hemorrhage, chronic cystitis, or bladder neoplasia. In cats, a cell-associated herpesvirus has been associated with mild cystitis. However, cystitis most commonly is associated with bacterial infection of the mucosa. Bacterial cystitis is more common in females because their relatively short urethra provides a lesser barrier to ascending infections than the longer, narrow-diameter male urethra. The bacterial species most commonly associated with cystitis are *Escherichia coli* (alpha hemolysin–producing strains), *Proteus* sp., *Corynebacterium renale, Eubacterium suis (Corynebacterium suis), Klebsiella* sp., streptococci, and staphylococci.

Except for the distal urethra, the lower urinary tract is normally free of bacteria. Sterility of the urinary bladder is maintained by normal repeated voiding of urine and by the antibacterial properties of urine. Antibacterial properties are attributable to the acidic urine of carnivores; secretory IgA; secreted mucin, which inhibits bacterial adhesion; high concentrations of urea and organic acids; and high urine osmolality. Cystitis occurs when bacteria overcome normal defense mechanisms and attach to or invade (colonize) the urinary bladder mucosa. Several factors can enhance colonization and predispose animals to cystitis. Colonization is more likely for strains of bacteria that express molecules on their surfaces that enhance adhesion, e.g., the P and type 1 fimbriae of certain strains of *E. coli.* Retention of urine due to obstruction or neurogenic causes related to spinal cord diseases often leads to cystitis. Trauma to the urinary bladder mucosa due to calculi, faulty catheterization, and parturition causes erosion and hemorrhage and can predispose to bacteria invasion of the lamina propria. Hydrolysis of urea by urease-producing bacteria, such as *C. renale* and *Eubacterium suis,* releases excessive ammonia, which can damage the mucosa. Bacterial growth can be enhanced when glucosuria is present. Urinary bladder emphysema may occur in conjunction with glucosuria-associated cystitis due to fermentation of glucose by certain bacterial species. Compromise of the host immune system, as with feline immunodeficiency virus infection, can result in increased susceptibility to bacterial cystitis. Other bacterial virulence factors, such as the *E. coli* hemolysin, enhance pathogenicity and help bacteria overcome antibacterial factors.

Once bacteria gain access to the lamina propria, lesions include vascular damage and inflammation. Acute cystitis is often hemorrhagic, fibrinopurulent, necrotizing, or ulcerative. However, in each case, components of several of these processes are present. The urinary bladder wall may be thickened due to edema and an inflammatory cell infiltrate, and diffusely or focally hemorrhagic. Hemorrhage is most common when obstruction is concurrently present. Urine may be cloudy, flocculent, foul smelling, ammoniacal, and often red-tinged. The mucosa may have nonreflectant foci of erosion or ulceration, patches or sheets of adherent exudate and necrotic debris, or adherent blood clots (Fig. 5-64). Microscopically, acute cystitis is characterized by epithelial denudation with bacterial colonies present on the surface. The lamina propria is intensely

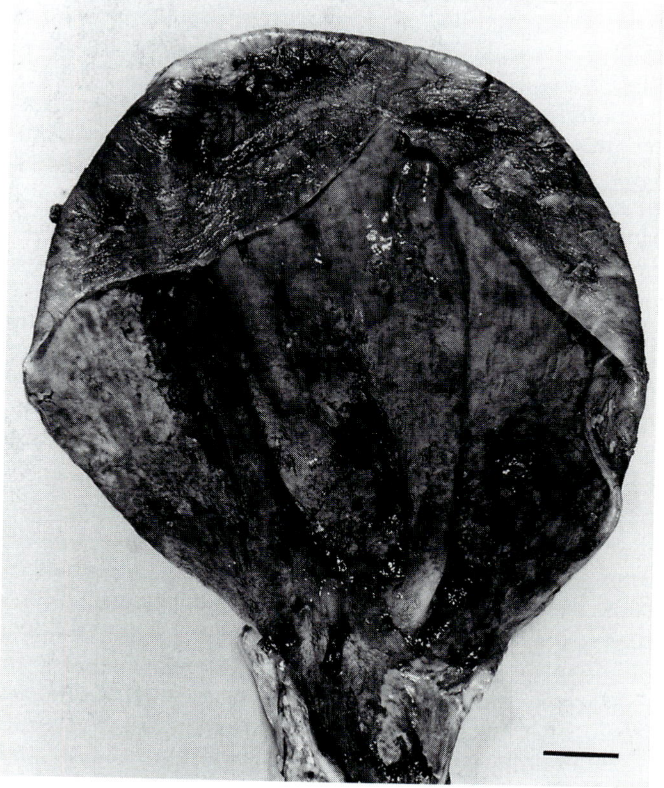

Fig. 5-64 Urinary bladder; calf. Acute cystitis. Patchy areas of ulceration are interspersed with inflamed mucosa. Bar = 3 cm.

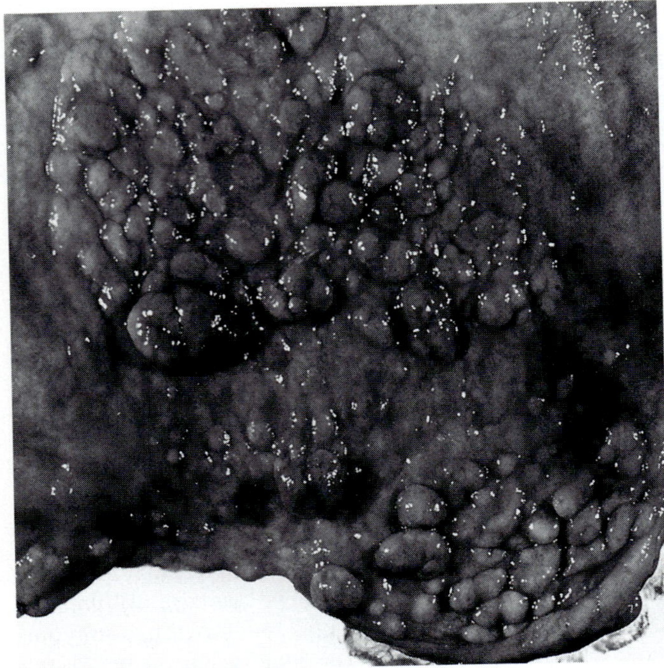

Fig. 5-65 Urinary bladder; dog. Chronic cystitis. Multiple polypoid proliferations are seen from the mucosal surface.

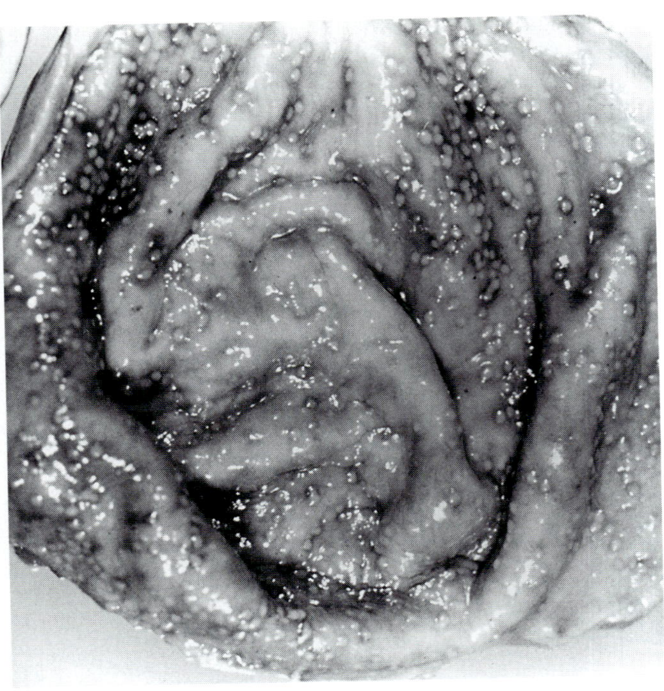

Fig. 5-66 Urinary bladder; dog. Chronic cystitis. The lesion is characterized by multiple follicular lymphoid proliferations. *Courtesy Dr. L. Roth.*

edematous and has a diffuse neutrophilic infiltrate. Superficial hyperemia and hemorrhage are usually present. A mild perivascular leukocytic infiltrate may occur in the muscularis.

Chronic cystitis may occur in any of several forms. Often, the lesions are a diffusely thickened, hyperplastic mucosa with goblet cell hyperplasia and a chronic lymphoplasmacytic infiltrate and fibrosis in the lamina propria. Hyperplasia of the muscularis may be present. This is particularly common when cystitis is associated with chronic urolithiasis. Several specific anatomic forms of chronic cystitis may occur. Chronic **polypoid cystitis** is a form found especially in dogs. The mucosa contains single or multiple, nodular mucosal masses (Fig. 5-65) composed of fibrous connective tissue and infiltrated with neutrophils and mononuclear leukocytes. The masses may be broad-based or pedunculated, ulcerated or covered by hyperplastic epithelium with goblet cell metaplasia. Chronic cystitis may also take the form of disseminated nodular, submucosal lymphoid, proliferations (2 to 4 mm in diameter), such that the mucosa has a cobblestone appearance **(follicular cystitis)** (Fig. 5-66). These white-gray, lymphoid foci are often surrounded by a zone of hyperemia.

Mycotic cystitis is occasionally seen when opportunistic fungi, such as *Candida albicans* or *Aspergillus* sp., colonize the urinary bladder mucosa. Such infections usually occur secondary to chronic bacterial cystitis, especially when animals are immunosuppressed or subjected to prolonged antibiotic therapy. The urinary bladder is usually ulcerated, with proliferation of underlying lamina propria and generalized thickening of the wall due to extensive inflammation, edema, and fibrosis.

Neoplasms

Neoplasms of the lower urinary tract occur predominantly in the urinary bladder. They are observed most frequently in dogs, occasionally in cats, and rarely in other species. Lower urinary tract neoplasms occupy space and often cause mucosal ulceration, resulting in clinical signs of dysuria, hematuria, or obstruction. Urinary bladder neoplasms constitute less than 1% of the total of canine neoplasms. Most occur in old dogs; there is no sex predisposition. Many chemicals, including intermediate components of aniline dyes, aromatic hydrocarbons, and tryptophan metabolites, have been found experimentally or epidemiologically to induce urinary bladder neoplasms. Bracken fern *(Pteridium aquilinum)* contains quercetin, a carcinogen; cattle grazing bracken fern develop various neoplasms of the urinary bladder.

Epithelial neoplasms are most common and are classified as **transitional cell papillomas, transitional cell carcinomas, squamous cell carcinomas, adenocarcinomas,** and **undifferentiated carcinomas.** Papillomas have a papilliferous or pedunculated appearance. Microscopically, papillary structures are covered by well-differentiated transitional epithelium. Carcinomas are focal, raised nodules or diffuse thickenings of the urinary bladder wall. Transitional cell carcinomas are composed of anaplastic transitional epithelium. They are observed most commonly in the trigone area of the urinary bladder. Neoplastic transitional cells cover the mucosal surface in irregular layers and readily invade the lamina propria in the form of solid nests and acini (Fig. 5-67). Squamous cell carcinomas, adenocarcinomas, and undifferentiated carcinomas most likely arise from transitional epithelium. In the bitch, carcinomas are often multicentric in origin, developing not only in the urinary bladder but also in the urothelium of ureters, urethra, and renal pelvis and often extend to the vagina and vestibule. Metastasis of urinary bladder carcinomas is most often to the regional lymph nodes.

Mesenchymal tumors, including **fibromas/fibrosarcomas, leiomyomas/leiomyosarcomas, rhabdomyosarcomas, lymphosarcomas,** and **hemangiomas/hemangiosarcomas,** occur in the lower tract. Leiomyomas are the most common and appear as solitary or multiple, circumscribed, firm, pale masses in the urinary bladder wall. They have the macroscopic consistency and microscopic appearance of normal smooth muscle. Fibromas arise from lamina propria connective tissue and project into the bladder lumen as solitary nodules. Primary fibrosarcomas, leiomyosarcomas, and vascular neoplasms are rare. Lymphosarcoma occasionally infiltrates the wall, not only of the urinary bladder but also of the ureters and renal pelves of cattle with lymphosarcoma. Rhabdomyosarcomas are rare but occur in young dogs (less than 18 months old), suggesting an embryonal origin. These masses are described as **botryoid** (grapelike) because they are large, fungating masses (4 to 18 cm in diameter) that protrude into the lumen. They infiltrate the urinary bladder wall and may metastasize. Microscopically, the neoplasms are composed of sheets of fusiform cells interspersed with pleomorphic cells. Microscopic demonstration of longitudinal and cross-striations typical of skeletal muscle or immunohistochemical demonstration of the intermediate filament desmin are needed to confirm the diagnosis of rhabdomyosarcoma.

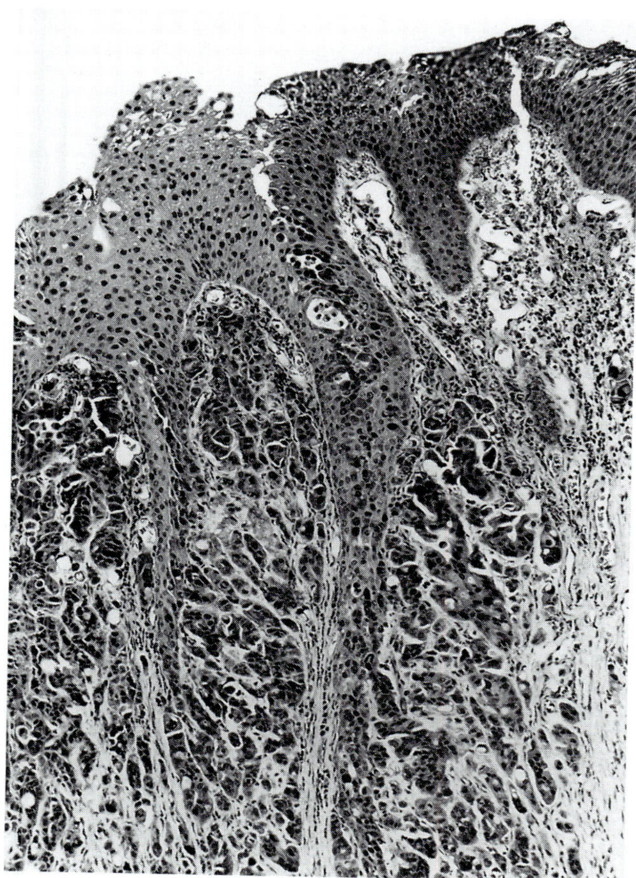

Fig. 5-67 Urinary bladder; dog. Transitional cell carcinoma. There is neoplastic transformation of superficial epithelium and infiltration of the lamina propria with neoplastic cells. H & E stain.

Enzootic hematuria is a disease of cattle caused by prolonged ingestion of bracken fern *(Pteridium aquilinum).* The urinary bladder lesion is initially one of hemorrhagic cystitis resulting in marked persistent hematuria, hence the name enzootic hematuria. The mucosa is hemorrhagic, with marked capillary congestion and ectasia. With time, epithelial (papillomas or carcinomas), mesenchymal (fibromas, hemangiomas, and their malignant counterparts), or mixed epithelial-mesenchymal neoplasms develop in association with the primary lesions of chronic cystitis. These neoplasms usually ulcerate the mucosa and bleed freely into the lumen.

Suggested Readings

Breitschwerdt EB. Nephrology and Urology, Contemporary Issues in Small Animal Practice. Vol. 4. New York: Churchill Livingstone, 1986.

Center SA, Smith CA, Wilkinson E, Erb HB, Lewis RM. Clinicopathologic, renal immunofluorescent, and light microscopic features of glomerulonephritis in the dog: 41 cases (1975-1985). J Am Vet Med Assoc 1987; 190:81-90.

Cotran RS, Kumar V, Robbins SL. Robbins' Pathologic Basis of Disease. 4th ed. Philadelphia: Saunders, 1989:1011-1098.

DiBartola SP, Rutgers HC, Zack PM, Tarr MJ. Clinicopathologic findings associated with chronic renal disease in cats: 74 cases (1973-1984). J Am Vet Med Assoc 1987; 190:1196-1202.

DiBartola SP, Tarr MJ, Parker AT, Powers JD, Pultz JA. Clinicopathologic findings in dogs with renal amyloidosis: 59 cases (1976-1986). J Am Vet Med Assoc 1989; 195:358-364.

Divers TJ. Diseases of the renal system. In Smith BP, ed. Large Animal Internal Medicine. St. Louis: Mosby, 1990:872-900.

Divers TJ, Crowell, WA, Duncan JR, Whitlock RH. Acute renal disorders in cattle: A retrospective study of 22 cases. J Am Vet Med Assoc 1982; 181:694-699.

Grauer GF. Glomerulonephritis. Semin Vet Med Surg (Small Anim) 1992; 7:187-197.

Lulich JP, Osborne CA, O'Brien TD, Polzin DJ. Feline renal failure: Questions, answers, questions. Compendium. 1992; 14:127-153.

Maxie GM. The urinary system. In Jubb KVF, Kennedy PC, Palmer N, eds. Pathology of Domestic Animals. Vol. 2. 4th ed. San Diego: Academic, 1993:447-538.

Nagode LA, Chew DJ. Nephrocalcinosis caused by hyperparathyroidism in progression of renal failure: Treatment with calcitriol. Semin Vet Med Surg (Small Anim) 1992; 7:202-220.

Picut CA, Lewis RM. Comparative pathology of canine hereditary nephropathies: An interpretive review. Vet Res Commun 1987; 11:561-581.

Rebhun WC, Dill SG, Perdrizet JA, Hatfield CE. Pyelonephritis in cows: 15 cases (1982-1986). J Am Vet Med Assoc 1989; 194:953-955.

Tisher CC, Brenner BM. Renal Pathology with Clinical and Functional Correlations. Vols. 1 & 2. Philadelphia: Lippincott, 1989.

CHAPTER

6 Endocrine System

CHARLES C. CAPEN

Endocrine glands are collections of specialized cells that synthesize, store, and release their secretions directly into the bloodstream. They are sensing and signaling devices located in the extracellular fluid compartment and are capable of responding to changes in the internal and external environments to coordinate a multiplicity of activities that maintain homeostasis.

Endocrine cells that produce polypeptide hormones have a well-developed, rough endoplasmic reticulum that assembles hormone and a prominent Golgi apparatus that packages hormone into granules for intracellular storage and transport. Secretory granules are unique to polypeptide hormone- and catecholamine-secreting endocrine cells and provide a mechanism for intracellular storage of substantial amounts of preformed active hormone. When the cell receives a signal for hormone secretion, secretory granules are directed to the periphery of the endocrine cell, probably by the contraction of microfilaments.

Steroid hormone–secreting cells are characterized by large cytoplasmic lipid bodies that contain cholesterol and other precursor molecules. The lipid bodies are in close proximity to an extensive tubular network of smooth endoplasmic reticulum and large mitochondria that contain hydroxylase and dehydrogenase enzyme systems. These enzyme systems function to attach various side chains to the basic steroid nucleus. Steroid-producing cells lack secretory granules and do not store significant amounts of preformed hormone. They are dependent on continued biosynthesis to maintain the normal secretory rate of a particular hormone.

PATHOGENIC MECHANISMS OF ENDOCRINE DISEASES

Many diseases of the endocrine system are characterized by dramatic functional disturbances and characteristic clinicopathologic alterations affecting one or several body systems. The affected animal may be presented because of changes that primarily involve the skin (hair loss caused by hypothyroidism), nervous system (seizures caused by hyperinsulinism), urinary system (polyuria caused by diabetes mellitus, diabetes insipidus, or hyperadrenocorticism), or skeletal system (fractures induced by hyperparathyroidism).

Primary Hypofunction of an Endocrine Gland

Hormone secretion is subnormal because of extensive destruction of secretory cells by a disease process, the failure of an endocrine gland to develop properly, or the result of a specific biochemical defect in the synthetic pathway of a hormone. In animals, immune-mediated injury causes hypofunction of several endocrine glands, including the parathyroid glands, adrenal cortex, and thyroid gland. Thyroiditis caused by this mechanism is characterized by marked infiltration of lymphocytes and plasmacytes and deposition of electron-dense immune complexes along the follicular basement membranes, with progressive destruction of secretory parenchyma.

Failure of development also results in primary hypofunction of an endocrine gland. The classic example of this mechanism is the failure of oropharyngeal ectoderm to differentiate completely into tropic hormone-secreting cells of the adenohypophysis in dogs, resulting in pituitary dwarfism.

Secondary Hypofunction of an Endocrine Gland

In this mechanism a destructive lesion in one organ, such as the pituitary gland, interferes with the secretion of a tropic hormone. This results in hypofunction of the target endocrine gland. Large, endocrinologically inactive pituitary neoplasms in adult dogs, cats, and other animal species may interfere with the secretion of multiple pituitary tropic hormones and may result in clinically detectable hypofunction of the adrenal cortex (Fig. 6-1), follicular cells of the thyroid gland, and gonads.

Primary Hyperfunction of an Endocrine Gland

This is one of the most important pathologic mechanisms of endocrine disease in animals. A lesion, often a neoplasm derived from endocrine cells, synthesizes and secretes a hormone at an autonomous rate in excess of the body's ability to utilize and to degrade, thereby resulting in a syndrome of hormone excess. Examples are summarized in Table 6-1. These include hyperfunction of parathyroid chief cells, thyroid C (parafollicular) cells, beta cells of the pancreatic islets, secretory cells of the adrenal medulla, and follicular cells of the thyroid gland.

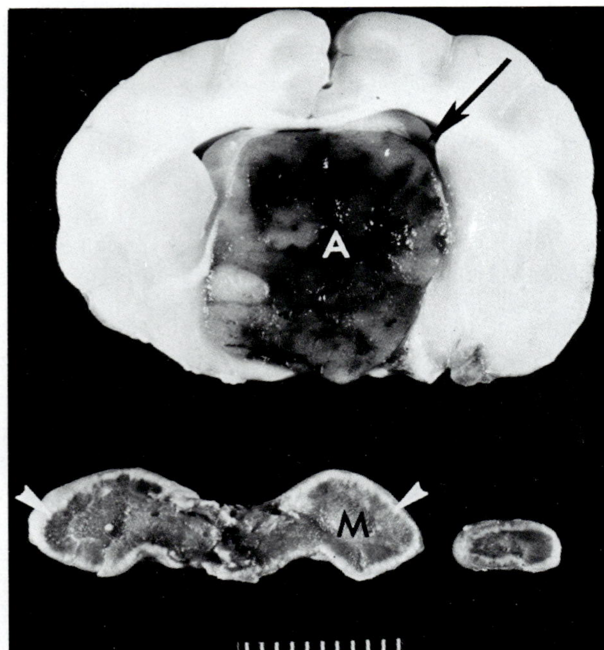

Fig. 6-1 Pituitary gland; dog. Secondary hypofunction of an endocrine gland. A large nonfunctional chromophobe adenoma (*A*) has completely incorporated and destroyed the adenohypophysis and hypothalamus, thereby interrupting the secretion of thyrotropin, adrenocorticotropin, and other pituitary tropic hormones, and extended into the thalamus *(arrow)*. This resulted in severe tropic atrophy of the adrenal cortex *(white arrowheads)*, especially the ACTH-dependent zonae fasciculata and reticularis, and a relatively more prominent medulla (*M*). Bar = 1 cm.

Secondary Hyperfunction of an Endocrine Gland

In this mechanism of endocrine disease, a lesion in one organ (e.g., adenohypophysis) secretes an excess of a tropic hormone that leads to long-term stimulation and hypersecretion of a hormone by a target organ. The classic example in animals is the adrenocorticotropic hormone (ACTH)–secreting neoplasm derived from pituitary corticotrophs in dogs (Fig. 6-2).

Hypersecretion of Hormones or Hormone-like Factors by Nonendocrine Neoplasms

The hypersecretion by nonendocrine neoplasms of hormones or "hormonelike factors" that are similar chemically and/or biologically to the native hormone has recently been recognized in animals and human beings. Most of these substances are peptides. Steroids and iodothyronines do not appear to be secreted by nonendocrine neoplasms.

A classic example in animals is the adenocarcinoma derived from apocrine glands of the anal sac in dogs. This neoplasm produces parathyroid hormone–related protein (PTHrP) that stimulates calcium mobilization in bone, kidneys, and intestine. The resulting accelerated mobilization of calcium leads to the development of persistent hypercalcemia, even though the animal's parathyroid glands are smaller than normal and composed of inactive and atrophic chief cells.

Endocrine Dysfunction Due to Failure of Target Cell Response

This response has been appreciated more recently, coincident with our more complete understanding of mechanisms of hormone action. Steroid and iodothyronine hormones penetrate the cell membrane, bind to cytosolic receptors, and are transported to the nucleus, where they interact with the genetic information in the cell to increase new protein synthesis. Polypeptide and catecholamine hormones bind to receptors on the surface of target cells and activate a membrane-bound enzyme that generates an intracellular messenger (cAMP) that elicits the physiologic response.

Failure of target cells to respond to hormone may be due

Table 6-1. Examples of primary hyperfunction of endocrine glands

Example	Hormone secreted in excess	Animal most frequently affected	Principal lesion or functional disturbance
Chief cell adenoma or carcinoma	Parathyroid hormone	Dog	Generalized osteitis fibrosa
Thyroid C cell adenoma or carcinoma	Calcitonin	Bull	Osteosclerosis
Beta cell adenoma or carcinoma	Insulin	Dog	Hypoglycemia
Sertoli cell tumor (testis)	Estrogens	Dog (male)	Feminization
Pheochromocytoma	Norepinephrine, epinephrine	Dog	Hypertension, hyperglycemia
Thyroid follicular cell adenoma or carcinoma	Thyroxine, triiodothyronine	Cat	Increased metabolic rate, weight loss, hyperactivity
Adrenal cortical adenoma or carcinoma (zona fasciculata)	Cortisol	Dog	Cushing's syndrome

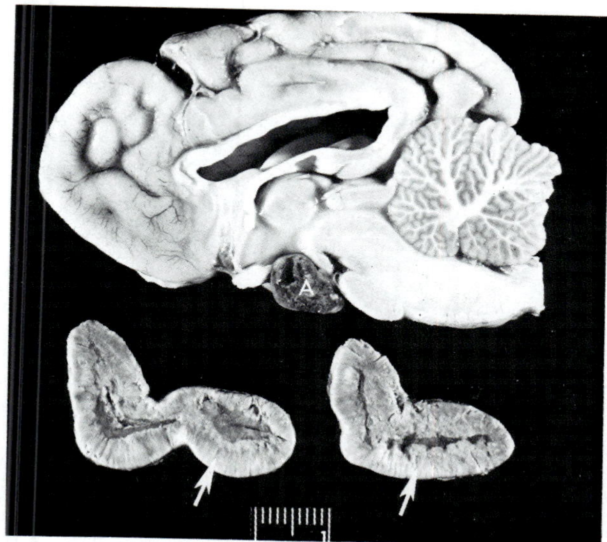

Fig. 6-2 Pituitary gland and adrenal glands; dog. Secondary hyperfunction of an endocrine organ. Corticotroph (ACTH-secreting) chromophobe adenoma (*A*) in the pituitary gland and bilateral enlargement of the adrenal glands. The long-term secretion of ACTH has resulted in hypertrophy and hyperplasia of secretory cells of the zone fasciculata and reticularis in the adrenal cortex *(white arrows)* and an excessive secretion of cortisol. Bar = 1 cm.

to lack of adenylate cyclase in the cell membrane or to an alteration in hormone receptors on the cell surface. Certain forms of insulin resistance associated with obesity in animals and human beings result from a decrease in the number of receptors on the surface of target cells.

Endocrine Hyperactivity Secondary to Diseases of Other Organs

The best characterized example of this response is the hyperparathyroidism that develops secondary to chronic renal failure or nutritional imbalance. In the renal form, early retention of phosphorus and subsequent progressive destruction of cells in the proximal convoluted tubules interfere with the metabolic activation of vitamin D by 1-hydroxylase in the kidneys. This is the rate-limiting step in the metabolic activation of vitamin D that is tightly controlled by multiple factors. The impaired intestinal absorption of calcium results in the development of progressive hypocalcemia, which leads to long-term parathyroid stimulation and subsequent generalized demineralization of the skeleton.

Failure of Fetal Endocrine Function

Subnormal function of the fetal endocrine system, especially in ruminants, may disrupt normal fetal development and result in prolonged gestation. In Guernsey and Jersey cattle, there is a genetically determined failure of adenohypophysis development, although the neurohypophysis develops normally. This results in a lack of fetal pituitary tropic hormone secretion during the last trimester and hypoplasia of target endocrine organs, namely, the adrenal cortex, gonads, and follicular cells of the thyroid glands. Fetal development is normal up to approximately 7 months' gestation, but fetal growth subsequently ceases, irrespective of how long the viable fetus is retained in the uterus.

Prolongation of the gestation period occurs in sheep after ewes consume the plant *Veratrum californicum* early in gestation. Toxins in the plant cause extensive malformations of the central nervous system (CNS) and hypothalamus in the lamb. Although the adenohypophysis is present, it lacks the necessary fine control derived from the releasing hormones of the hypothalamus and is unable to secrete normal amounts of tropic hormones (adrenocorticotropin). Target endocrine organs in the fetus are hypoplastic, and the adrenal cortex fails to differentiate completely into the three distinctive zones that secrete corticosteroid hormones.

V. californicum contains potent steroidal alkaloids that inhibit neural tube development when ingested by the ewe between the 9th and 14th day of gestation. Cyclopia and extensive CNS malformations are found in lambs. Arhinencephalia and lack of development of nasal bones accompany the formation of a proboscis-like structure. The lambs retained in the uterus beyond the normal gestation interval continue to grow.

The concepts that have emerged from the study of these two valuable experiments of nature are (1) that in certain animals, fetal hormones are necessary for final growth and development of the fetus; and (2) that in these species, normal parturition at term requires an intact fetal hypothalamic-adenohypophyseal-adrenocortical system working in concert with trophoblasts of the placenta.

Although the presence or absence of functional adenohypophyseal tissue determines whether the fetus continues to grow in utero, the pathogenesis of prolongation of the gestational interval is similar in these two examples. Subnormal development of the fetal adrenal cortex in calves and lambs results in an inadequate secretion of cortisol and a failure of induction of 17-hydroxylase in the placenta that converts precursor molecules, such as progesterone, to estrogen. This results in maintenance of the dam's circulating progesterone at near-midgestation concentrations and a lack of the marked increase in estrogens that normally occurs at term and that results in parturition. The estrogen surge stimulates a synthesis of prostaglandins in the uterus. The local accumulation of prostaglandins results in the smooth muscle contractions and biochemical changes in collagen along the birth canal that normally permit delivery of the fetus.

Endocrine Dysfunction Resulting from Abnormal Degradation of Hormone

In these diseases, secretion of hormone by an endocrine gland is normal, but concentrations in the blood are elevated persistently, since a decreased rate of degradation simulates a state of hypersecretion. The syndrome of feminization in human beings due to hyperestrogenism, associated with cirrhosis and decreased hepatic degradation of estrogens, is a classic example of this pathogenic mechanism.

Chronic renal disease in animals may be associated with subnormal, normal, or elevated blood concentrations of calcium. In animals with hypercalcemia and renal failure, the parathyroid glands are often atrophic and composed of inactive chief cells. The hypercalcemia associated with certain forms of renal disease may be related, in part, to diminished renal degradation of parathyroid hormone as well as to decreased urinary excretion of calcium by diseased kidneys. Biologically active parathyroid hormone is normally degraded in the kidneys either by peptidase on the surface of tubular cells or by lysosomal enzymes after uptake of the hormone from the glomerular filtrate.

Iatrogenic Syndromes of Hormone Excess

The administration of hormone, either directly or indirectly, influences the activity of target cells and results in clinical disturbances. The prolonged daily administration of high doses of potent preparations of adrenal corticosteroids in the symptomatic treatment of various diseases will reproduce most of the functional disturbances associated with cortisol excess, including muscle weakness, marked hair loss, and deposition of calcium in the skin. The elevated blood concentrations of exogenous cortisol result in marked tropic atrophy of the adrenal cortex, particularly the ACTH-dependent zona fasciculata and zona reticularis (Fig. 6-3).

The administration of certain progestogens to dogs will indirectly result in a syndrome of hormone excess. For example, the injection of medroxyprogesterone acetate for

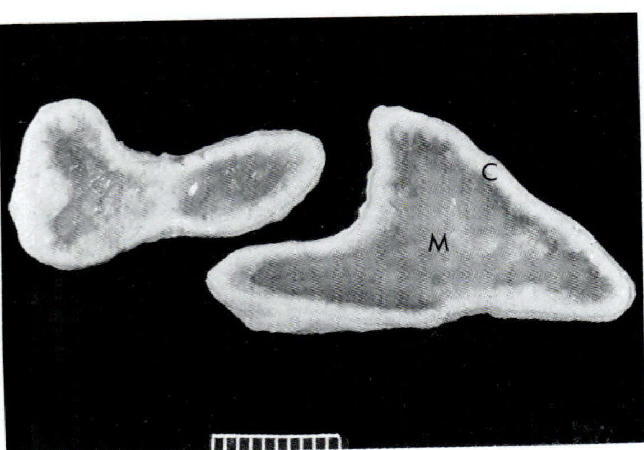

Fig. 6-3 Adrenal glands; dog. Iatrogenic syndrome of hormone excess. Hyperadrenocorticism caused by long-term administration of exogenous corticosteroids has resulted in marked tropic atrophy of the ACTH-dependent zona fasciculata and zona reticularis of the adrenal cortex (*C*). The adrenal medulla (*M*) occupies a relatively greater percentage of the atrophic adrenal gland than of a normal adrenal. Bar = 1 cm.

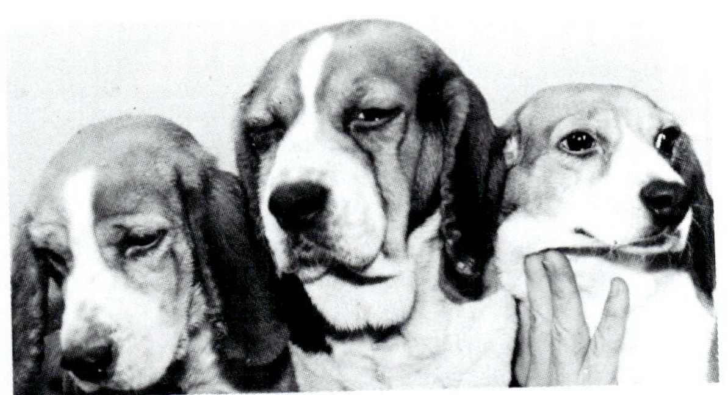

Fig. 6-4 Iatrogenic acromegaly; beagle dog, *center* (compared with unaffected littermates, *left* and *right*). Note the coarseness of the facial features and the marked thickening and folding of the skin of the face. These characteristics are the result of the protein anabolic effects of pituitary somatotropin that has been stimulated by the exogenous administration of medroxyprogesterone acetate. *Courtesy Dr. P. Concannon.*

the prevention of estrus in dogs stimulates an increased secretion of growth hormone by pituitary somatotrophs, resulting in acromegaly. The excessive skin folds (Fig. 6-4), expansion of interdigital spaces, and abdominal enlargement in dogs with iatrogenic acromegaly are related to the protein anabolic effects of growth hormone on connective tissues.

PITUITARY GLAND (HYPOPHYSIS)

The **adenohypophysis** consists of three portions: the pars distalis, pars tuberalis, and pars intermedia (Fig. 6-5). In many animal species, the adenohypophysis completely surrounds the pars nervosa of the neurohypophyseal system. The pars distalis is the largest portion and contains the different populations of endocrine cells that secrete the pituitary tropic hormones. The secretory cells are surrounded by abundant capillaries (Fig. 6-6).

The pars tuberalis consists of dorsal projections of cells along the infundibular stalk. It functions primarily as a scaffold for the capillary network of the hypophyseal portal system in its course from the median eminence to the pars distalis. The pars intermedia forms the junction between the pars distalis and pars nervosa. It lines the residual lumen of Rathke's pouch and often contains two populations of cells. In the dog, one of these cell types synthesizes and secretes ACTH.

A specific population of endocrine cells is present in the pars distalis (and in the pars intermedia of dogs for ACTH) that synthesizes and secretes each of the pituitary tropic hormones. Secretory cells in the adenohypophysis are classified as acidophils, basophils, or chromophobes, based on reaction of their secretory granules with pH-dependent histochemical stains. Based upon specific immunocytochemical staining, acidophils are further subclassified functionally into somatotrophs that secrete growth hormone (GH; somatotropin) and luteotrophs that secrete luteotropic hormone (LTH; prolactin). Their granules contain hormones

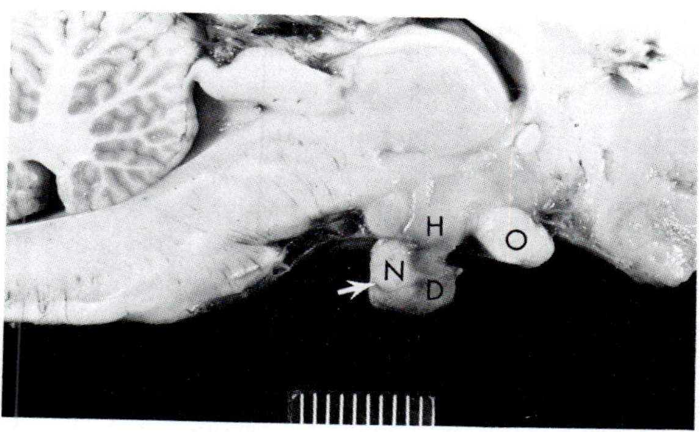

Fig. 6-5 Pituitary gland; normal dog. Longitudinal section of the pituitary region illustrating the close relationship to the optic chiasm (*O*), hypothalamus (*H*), and overlying brain. The pars distalis (*D*) forms a major part of the adenohypophysis and completely surrounds the pars nervosa (*N*). The residual lumen of Rathke's pouch *(white arrow)* separates the pars distalis and pars nervosa and is lined by the pars intermedia. Bar = 1 cm.

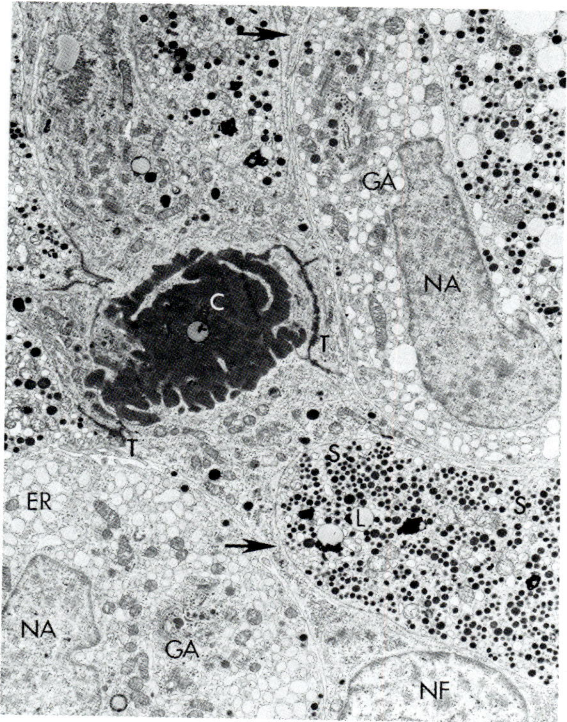

Fig. 6-6 Pituitary gland, pars distalis; normal dog. Follicular cells *(NF)* in the pars distalis form a framework and extend cytoplasmic processes *(arrows)* around extracellular accumulations of colloid (*C*). Adjacent follicular cells are joined by prominent terminal bars (*T*). Acidophils in the storage phase of the secretory cycle contain numerous large, uniformly electron-dense secretory granules (*S*), scattered lipofuscin (*L*) bodies, but a small amount of endoplasmic reticulum *(ER)* and a small Golgi apparatus. Hypertrophied acidophils *(NA)* have few mature secretory granules but many distended profiles of endoplasmic reticulum *(ER)* and large Golgi apparatuses *(GA)* associated with prosecretory granules in the process of formation. ×7500.

that are simple proteins. Basophils include both gonadotrophs that secrete luteinizing hormone (LH) and follicle-stimulating hormone (FSH) and thyrotrophs that secrete thyrotropic hormone (thyroid-stimulating hormone [TSH]). Chromophobes are pituitary cells that by light microscopy do not have obvious cytoplasmic secretory granules. They include the pituitary cells concerned with the synthesis of ACTH and melanocyte-stimulating hormone (MSH) in some species, nonsecretory follicular (stellate) cells (Fig. 6-6), degranulated chromophils (acidophils and basophils) in the actively synthesizing phase of the secretory cycle, and undifferentiated stem cells of the adenohypophysis.

Each type of endocrine cells in the adenohypophysis appears to be under the control of a corresponding releasing hormone (''factor'') from the hypothalamus. These releasing hormones are small peptides synthesized by neurosecretion in neurons of the hypothalamus. They are transported by axonal processes to the median eminence, where they are released into capillaries and conveyed by the hypophyseal portal system to specific endocrine cells in the adenohypophysis. Each hormone stimulates the rapid release of secretory granules containing a specific, preformed tropic hormone.

The **neurohypophysis** has three anatomic subdivisions. The pars nervosa (posterior lobe) represents the distal component of the neurohypophyseal system. It is composed of numerous capillaries that are supported by modified glial cells (pituicytes). The capillaries in the pars nervosa are termination sites for the nonmyelinated axonal processes of neurosecretory neurons in the hypothalamus. Secretion granules that contain the neurohypophyseal hormones, i.e., oxytocin and antidiuretic hormone, are synthesized in hypothalamic neurons but are released into the bloodstream in the pars nervosa. The infundibular stalk joins the pars nervosa to the overlying hypothalamus and is composed of axonal processes from neurosecretory neurons.

Neurosecretory neurons in the hypothalamus receive neural input from higher centers, resulting in hormonal secretion. Antidiuretic hormone (ADH or vasopressin) and oxytocin are nonapeptides synthesized by neurons situated in either the supraoptic or paraventricular nuclei of the hypothalamus. ADH and its corresponding neurophysin appear to be synthesized as part of a common, larger, biosynthetic precursor molecule, **propressophysin.** The hormones are packaged with a corresponding binding protein (i.e., neurophysin) into membrane-limited neurosecretory granules and transported to the pars nervosa by axonal processes of the neurosecretory neurons. These axons terminate on fenestrated capillaries in the pars nervosa and release ADH or oxytocin into the circulation.

Developmental Disturbances of Adenohypophysis

Pituitary cyst

Pituitary dwarfism in dogs usually is associated with a failure of the oropharyngeal ectoderm of Rathke's pouch

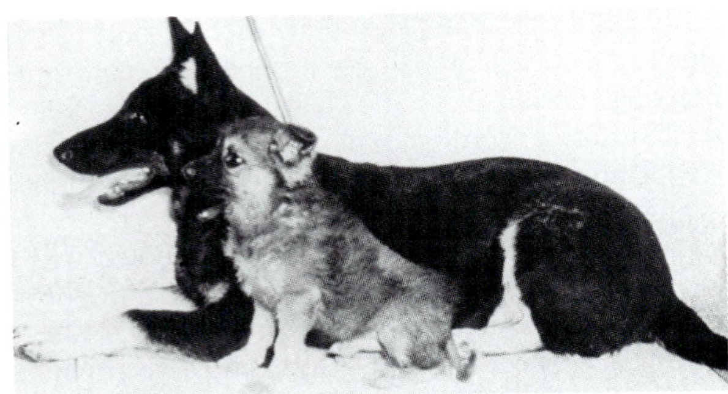

Fig. 6-7 Panhypopituitarism (''pituitary dwarfism''); 5-month-old German shepherd dog. The unaffected littermate weighed 27.3 kg while the dwarf puppy weighed only 4 kg. The pituitary dwarf has retained the puppy hair coat. *Courtesy Dr. J. E. Alexander and Can Vet J.*

to differentiate into tropic hormone–secreting cells of the pars distalis. This results in a progressively enlarging, multiloculated cyst in the sella turcica and an absence of the adenohypophysis.

Juvenile panhypopituitarism occurs most frequently in German shepherd dogs, but it has been reported in Spitz, toy pinscher, and Carelian Bear dogs. The dwarf pups appear normal from birth to about 2 months of age. Then, the slower growth, retention of puppy hair coat, and lack of primary guard hairs gradually become evident (Fig. 6-7). A bilaterally symmetrical alopecia develops gradually and often progresses to complete alopecia, except for the head and tufts of hair on the legs. There is progressive hyperpigmentation of the skin until it is uniformly brown-black over most of the body. Adult German shepherd dogs with panhypopituitarism vary in size from as small as 2 kg to nearly half normal size, apparently depending upon whether the failure of formation of the adenohypophysis is nearly or only partially complete.

The mode of inheritance is a simple autosomal recessive. The activity of somatomedin (a nonspecies-specific, cartilage growth–promoting peptide whose production in the liver and plasma activity is controlled by somatotropin) is low in dwarf dogs. Intermediate somatomedin activity is present in the phenotypically normal ancestors suspected to be heterozygous carriers. Assays for somatomedin provide an indirect measurement of circulating growth hormone activity in dogs with suspected pituitary dwarfism.

NEOPLASMS OF ADENOHYPOPHYSIS

Adenomas of Pars Intermedia

Adenomas derived from cells of the pars intermedia are the most common type of pituitary neoplasm in horses, the second most common type in dogs, and rare in other species. Adenomas develop in older horses, more frequently in females. Nonbrachycephalic breeds of dogs have adenomas of the pars intermedia more often than brachycephalic breeds.

In dogs, adenomas of the pars intermedia result in only a moderate enlargement of the pituitary gland. The pars distalis is readily identifiable and sharply demarcated from the anterior margin of the neoplasm, usually by an incomplete layer of condensed stroma. The neoplasm may extend across the residual hypophyseal lumen and result in compression atrophy, but it usually does not invade the pars distalis. The posterior lobe is incorporated within the neoplasm, but the infundibular stalk is intact.

Endocrinologically active (ACTH-secreting) adenomas of the pars intermedia in dogs have prominent groups of corticotrophs, with an abundant eosinophilic cytoplasm with more widely scattered follicles. Adenomas of the pars intermedia in dogs are either functionally inactive and associated with varying degrees of hypopituitarism and diabetes insipidus or endocrinologically active and secrete excessive ACTH, leading to bilateral adrenal cortical hyperplasia and a syndrome of cortisol excess.

In horses, adenomas of the pars intermedia often are large neoplasms that extend out of the sella turcica and severely compress the overlying hypothalamus. The adenomas are yellow to white and multinodular and incorporate the pars nervosa. When the neoplasm is incised, the pars distalis usually can be identified as a compressed subcapsular rim of tissue on the anterior margin. A sharp line of demarcation remains between the neoplasm and the compressed pars distalis.

The neoplastic cells arranged in cords and nests along the capillaries and connective tissue septa are large and cylindrical, spindle-shaped or polyhedral, with an oval, hyperchromatic nucleus. The pattern is often reminiscent of that of the prominent pars intermedia of normal horses. More cuboidal neoplastic cells occasionally form follicular structures that contain dense, eosinophilic colloid (Fig. 6-8). The clinical syndrome associated with neoplasms of the pars intermedia in horses is characterized by polyuria, polydipsia, ravenous appetite, muscle weakness, somnolence, intermittent hyperpyrexia, and generalized hyperhidrosis. The affected horses often develop a striking hypertrichosis (''hirsutism'') because of failure to seasonally shed hair. The hair over most of the trunk and extremities is long (up to 10 to 12 cm), abnormally thick, wavy, and often matted (Fig. 6-9).

Horses with larger neoplasms may have hyperglycemia (insulin-resistant) and glycosuria, probably the result of a down-regulation of insulin receptors on target cells induced by the chronic excessive intake of feed and hyperinsulinemia. The disturbances in carbohydrate metabolism, ravenous appetite, hypertrichosis, and hyperhidrosis are considered to be primarily a reflection of deranged hypothalamic function, caused by compression of the overlying hypothalamus by the large pituitary neoplasms. The hypothalamus is the primary center for homeostatic regulation of body temperature, appetite, and cyclic shedding of hair.

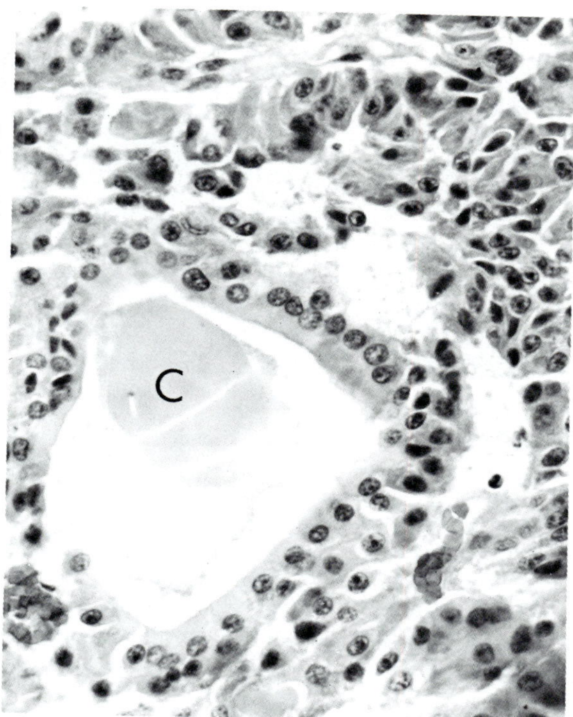

Fig. 6-8 Pituitary glands, pars intermedia; horse. Adenoma. The follicle is lined by cuboidal cells and contains colloid (*C*). ×450.

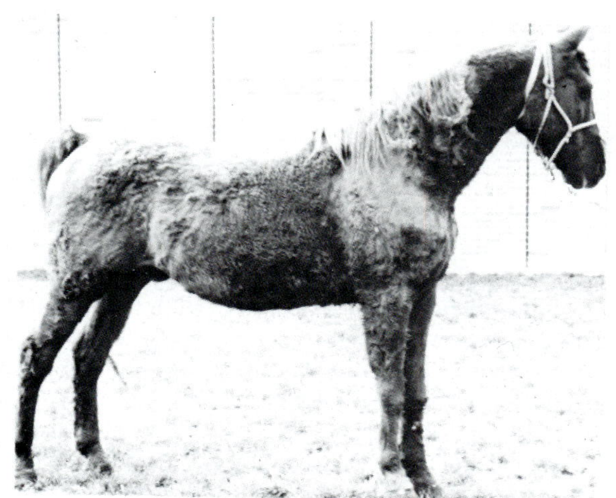

Fig. 6-9 Hirsutism is the result of a failure to shed due to an adenoma of the pars intermedia.

ACTH-secreting (Corticotroph) Adenoma

Functional (endocrinologically active) neoplasms arising in the pituitary gland most likely are derived from corticotroph (ACTH-secreting) cells in either the pars distalis or the pars intermedia of dogs. They cause a clinical syndrome of cortisol excess (Cushing's disease). These neoplasms are encountered most frequently in dogs, particularly in adult to aged boxers, Boston terriers, and dachshunds.

The pituitary gland is consistently enlarged (see Fig. 6-2); however, neither the occurrence nor the severity of functional disturbances appears to be directly related to the size of the neoplasm. In the dog, the diaphragma sellae is incomplete; therefore, the line of least resistance favors dorsal expansion of the gradually enlarging pituitary mass and invagination into the infundibular cavity, dilatation of the infundibular recess and the third ventricle, with eventual compression or replacement of the hypothalamus, and possible extension of the neoplasm into the thalamus (see Fig. 6-1).

Bilateral enlargement of the adrenal glands occurs in dogs with functional corticotroph adenomas (see Fig. 6-2). This enlargement is due to increased cortical parenchyma, primarily in the zona fasciculata and zona reticularis. Nodules of yellow-orange cortical tissue often are found outside the capsule as well as extending down into and compressing the adrenal medulla.

Pituitary corticotroph adenomas are composed of well-differentiated, large or small, chromophobic cells supported by fine connective tissue septa. The cytoplasm of the neoplastic cells usually is devoid of secretory granules, but stains immunocytochemically for ACTH and MSH. Hormone-containing secretory granules can be demonstrated by electron microscopy in functional corticotroph adenomas of dogs.

Endocrinologically Inactive Chromophobe Adenoma

Nonfunctional pituitary neoplasms occur in dogs, cats, laboratory rodents, and parakeets but are uncommon in other species. Although chromophobe adenomas appear to be endocrinologically inactive, they may result in significant functional disturbances and clinical signs by virtue of compression atrophy of adjacent portions of the pituitary gland and dorsal extension into the overlying brain (Fig. 6-10). They result in clinical disturbances as the result of either a lack of secretion of pituitary tropic hormones and diminished target organ function (e.g., adrenal cortex; see Fig. 6-1) or dysfunction of the CNS. Affected animals often have decreased spontaneous activity, have incoordination and other disturbances of balance, are weak, and may collapse with exercise. In chronically affected animals, blindness with dilated and fixed pupils is due to compression and disruption of the optic nerves by dorsal extension of the pituitary neoplasms (Fig. 6-10). Endocrinologically inactive pituitary adenomas often attain considerable size before they cause obvious signs or kill the animal (see Figs. 6-1 and 6-10). Clinical signs associated with nonfunctional pituitary adenomas and hypopituitarism are not specific and can be confused with other disorders of the CNS, such as brain neoplasms and encephalitis, or with chronic renal disease. There is no effect on body stature associated with compression of the

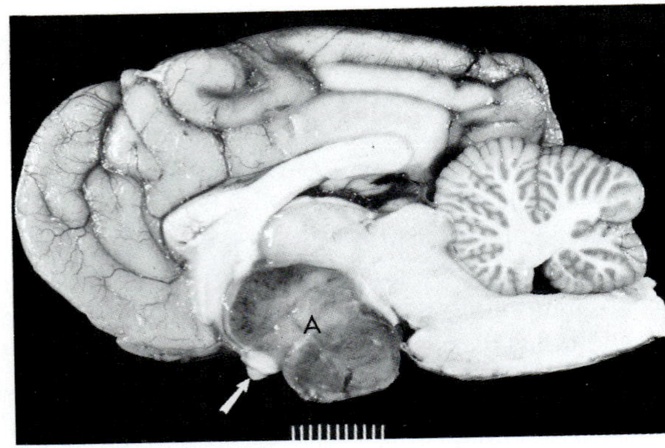

Fig. 6-10 Pituitary gland; dog. Adenoma. A large pituitary adenoma (*A*) extends dorsally out of the sella turcica into the overlying brain. The optic chiasm *(white arrow)* is severely compressed. The adenohypophysis, neurohypophysis, and hypothalamus have been invaded and destroyed by the neoplasm. Bar = 1 cm.

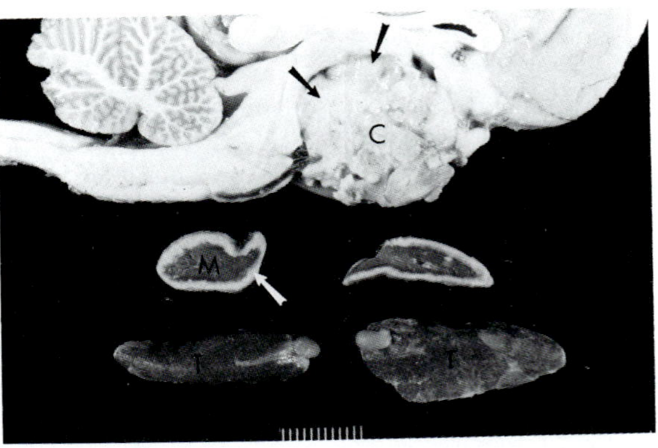

Fig. 6-11 Pituitary area, adrenal glands, thyroid glands; dog. Craniopharyngioma. The tumor has extended dorsally through the hypothalamus and compressed the thalamus *(black arrows)*. The tumor has also destroyed the adenohypophysis and neurohypophysis, resulting in severe tropic atrophy of the adrenal cortex *(white arrow)*. The adrenal glands consist predominantly of medulla (*M*) surrounded by a thin rim of cortex (capsule plus zona glomerulosa). Although the thyroid follicular cells are atrophic, the overall gland (*T*) size is within normal limits due to colloid involution of the follicles. Bar = 1 cm.

pars distalis and interference with growth hormone secretion, because these neoplasms usually arise in adult-aged animals that have already completed their growth. However, the atrophy of the skin and loss of muscle mass may be related, in part, to a lack of the protein anabolic effects of growth hormone. Interference in the secretion of pituitary tropic hormones often leads to reduced basal metabolic rate due to diminished TSH secretion and hypoglycemia from tropic atrophy of the adrenal cortex (see Fig. 6-1).

Craniopharyngioma

Craniopharyngioma is a benign tumor that is derived from epithelial remnants of the oropharyngeal ectoderm of the craniopharyngeal duct (Rathke's pouch). It often occurs in animals younger than those with other types of pituitary neoplasms and is present in either a suprasellar or infrasellar location. One cause of panhypopituitarism and dwarfism in young dogs, craniopharyngioma is due to a subnormal secretion of somatotropin and other tropic hormones beginning at an early age, before closure of the growth plates.

Craniopharyngiomas often are large and grow along the ventral aspect of the brain, where they can surround several cranial nerves. In addition, they extend dorsally into the hypothalamus and thalamus (Fig. 6-11). The resulting clinical signs often are a combination of (1) lack of secretion of pituitary tropic hormones, resulting in tropic atrophy and subnormal function of the adrenal cortex and thyroid, atrophy of the gonads, and failure to attain somatic maturation due to a lack of secretion of growth hormone; (2) disturbances in water metabolism (polyuria, polydipsia, and low urine specific gravity and osmolality) from an interference in the release and synthesis of ADH by the large tumor; (3) deficits in cranial nerve function; and (4) CNS dysfunction due to extension into the overlying brain. Microscopically, craniopharyngiomas have alternating solid and cystic areas. The solid areas are composed of nests of epithelial cells (cuboidal, columnar, or squamous) with focal areas of mineralization. The cystic spaces are lined by either columnar or squamous cells and contain keratin debris and colloid.

Pituitary Carcinoma

Pituitary carcinomas are uncommon compared with adenomas but have been seen in older dogs and cows. They usually are endocrinologically inactive but may result in significant functional disturbances by destruction of the pars distalis and neurohypophyseal system, leading to panhypopituitarism and diabetes insipidus. Carcinomas are large and extensively invade the overlying brain, along the ventral aspect of the skull, and the sphenoid bone of the sella turcica, causing osteolysis. Metastases may occur to regional lymph nodes or to distant sites, such as the spleen or liver. Carcinomas are highly cellular and often have large areas of hemorrhage and necrosis. Giant cells, nuclear pleomorphism, and mitotic figures are encountered more frequently than in adenomas.

DISORDERS OF NEUROHYPOPHYSIS

Diabetes Insipidus

Diabetes insipidus results when inadequate ADH is produced or target cells in the kidneys lack the biochemical pathways necessary to respond to the secretion of normal or elevated circulating concentrations of hormone. The hypophyseal form of diabetes insipidus results from compression and destruction of the pars nervosa, infundibular stalk, or supraoptic nucleus in the hypothalamus. The disruption of ADH synthesis or secretion in hypophyseal diabetes insipidus occurs as the result of large pituitary neoplasms, a dorsally expanding cyst, or inflammatory granuloma or by traumatic injury to the skull with hemorrhage and glial proliferation in the neurohypophyseal tissues. Compression or disruption of the posterior lobe, infundibular stalk, and hypothalamus by neoplastic cells interrupts the nonmyelinated axons that transport ADH from its site of production, primarily in the supraoptic nucleus of the hypothalamus, to the site of release in the capillary plexus of the pars nervosa.

Animals with diabetes insipidus excrete large volumes of hypotonic urine, which in turn obliges them to drink equally large amounts of water to prevent dehydration and hyperosmolality of body fluids. Urine osmolality is decreased below normal plasma osmolality (approximately 300 mOsm/kg) in both hypophyseal and nephrogenic forms of diabetes insipidus. In response to water deprivation, urine osmolality remains below that of plasma in both forms of diabetes insipidus, in contrast to increased osmolality observed in normal animals. The elevation of urine osmolality above that of plasma in response to exogenous ADH in hypophyseal but not in nephrogenic diabetes insipidus is useful in the differential diagnosis.

ADRENAL CORTEX

Structure and Function

The adrenal glands of mammals consist of two distinct parts that differ not only in morphology and function but also in embryologic origin. Because of their close structural relationships, the outer cortex and inner medulla of the adrenal glands usually have been considered as parts of one organ. The adrenal cortex develops from cells of the coelomic epithelium that are of mesodermal origin. The chromaffin tissue and sympathetic ganglion cells of the adrenal medulla are derived from ectoderm of the neural crest.

The adrenal cortex of normal dogs is firm, yellow, and of nearly uniform thickness. The soft, brown medulla is surrounded by the cortex. In normal dogs, the cortical/medulla ratio is approximately 2:1. The adrenal glands are richly vascularized, and a sinusoidal network about the cell columns of the adrenal cortex empties into the venous tree at the periphery of the medulla.

The adrenal cortex microscopically and functionally is subdivided into three layers or zones, although the demarcation between zones often is not distinct. The zona glomerulosa (multiformis) (outer zone) is composed of columns of cells adjacent to the capsule that have a sigmoid or arclike arrangement. It represents about 10% to 15% of the cortex and is responsible for the secretion of mineralocorticoid hormones. The secretory cells of the zona fasciculata are arranged in long, anastomosing cords separated by numerous small capillaries. This middle zone, which comprises about 65% to 70% of the cortex, is composed of cells that contain abundant cytoplasmic lipid and are responsible for the secretion of the glucocorticoid hormones. The zona reticularis (inner zone) accounts for the remainder of the cortex. The secretory cells, arranged in small groups surrounded by capillaries, are responsible for the secretion of sex steroids.

Mineralocorticoids are adrenal steroids that have their principal effects on ion transport by epithelial cells, which results in loss of potassium and conservation of sodium. The most potent and important naturally occurring mineralocorticoid is aldosterone. The enzymatically controlled electrolyte "pumps" in epithelial cells of the renal tubule, and sweat glands respond to mineralocorticoids by conserving sodium and chloride and by excreting potassium. In the distal convoluted tubule of the mammalian nephron, a cation-exchange mechanism is responsible for the resorption of sodium from the glomerular filtrate and secretion of potassium into the lumen. These reactions are accelerated by mineralocorticoids but still proceed, although at a much slower rate, in their absence (Fig. 6-12). A lack of secretion of mineralocorticoids (such as in the Addison's-like disease of dogs) may result in a lethal retention of potassium and loss of sodium (see Fig. 6-12).

Cortisol and lesser amounts of corticosterone are the most important naturally occurring glucocorticoid hormones secreted by the adrenal glands in many animal species. In general, the actions of glucocorticoids on carbohydrate, protein, and lipid metabolism result in a sparing of glucose and a tendency to hyperglycemia and increased glucose production. In addition, glucocorticoids decrease lipogenesis and increase lipolysis in adipose tissue, which results in release of glycerol and free fatty acids.

ACTION OF ALDOSTERONE*
ON RENAL TUBULE

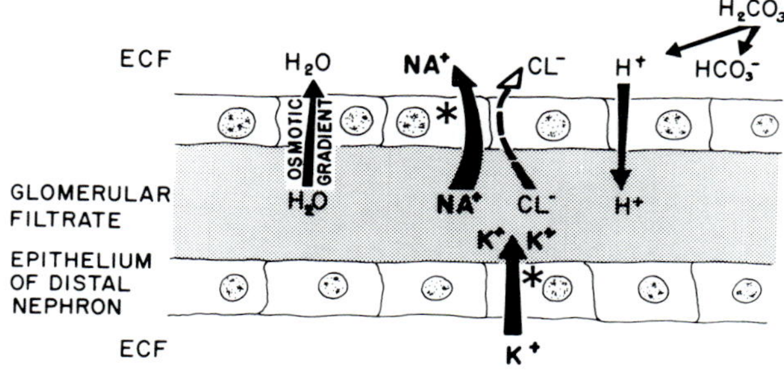

Fig. 6-12 Aldosterone secreted by the zona glomerulosa of the adrenal cortex acts on the distal portions of the nephron to increase tubular excretion of potassium and increase resorption of sodium (and, secondarily, chloride). The resulting osmotic gradient facilitates movement of water from the glomerular filtrate into the extracellular fluid.

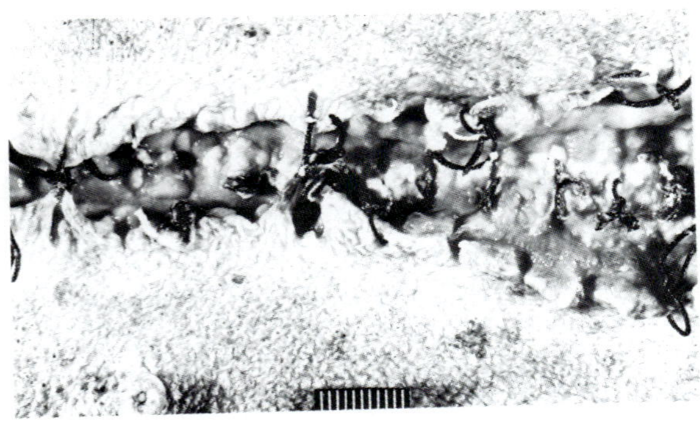

Fig. 6-13 Skin; dog. Dehiscence of surgical wound. Wounds heal slowly in dogs with cortisol excess because of an inhibition of fibroblastic proliferation.

Glucocorticoids also function to suppress both inflammatory and immunologic responses and, thereby, reduce the associated necrosis and fibroplasia. However, under the influence of elevated concentrations of glucocorticoids, an animal has reduced resistance to a number of bacterial, viral, and fungal diseases. Glucocorticoids may impair the immunologic response at any stage from the initial interaction and processing of antigens by cells of the macrophage-monocyte system through the induction and proliferation of immunocompetent lymphocytes and subsequent antibody production. Inhibition by glucocorticoids of a number of functions of lymphoid cells forms part of the basis for suppression of the immunologic response.

Glucocorticoids exert a profound negative effect on wound healing. Dogs with hypercortisolism may have wound dehiscence (Fig. 6-13). The basic mechanism involved is an inhibition of fibroblast proliferation and collagen synthesis, leading to a decrease in scar tissue formation.

Progesterone, estrogens, and androgens are sex hormones synthesized by secretory cells of the zona reticularis of the adrenal cortex. An excessive secretion of adrenal sex steroids may occur infrequently, associated with a neoplasm arising in the zona reticularis. The clinical manifestations of virilism, precocious sexual development, or feminization depend upon which steroid is secreted in excess, the sex of the patient, and the age of onset.

Developmental Disturbances

Hypoplasia of the adrenal cortex is seen in association with maldevelopment of the hypophysis associated with anencephaly, in some cases of cyclopia, and in hypophyseal aplasia. The adrenal cortices are small, but the adrenal medulla is normal.

Degenerative and Inflammatory Lesions

Calcification of the adrenal glands

Extensive deposits of calcium salts occur frequently in the adrenal glands of adult cats. The cause is unknown. The calcium deposits, although often bilateral and extensive, usually are not associated with clinical signs. A few dogs with extensive calcification and degeneration of the adrenal glands may die suddenly after relatively minor stress. Extensively calcified adrenal glands are coarsely nodular, firm, and mottled, with multiple, yellow-white, gritty foci throughout the cortex. Some have large areas of necrosis, with calcium deposition adjacent to areas of nodular regenerative hyperplasia. These hypertropic cortical cells have abundant lipid in their expanded cytoplasmic area and appear to be able to maintain near-normal blood cortisol concentrations in response to an apparent increased secretion of ACTH.

Amyloid

Amyloid deposition in the adrenal glands occurs in all species and usually involves only the cortex. The affected adrenal cortices often are widened, and the amyloid deposits may be grossly visible as translucent areas. Amyloid deposition begins around the sinusoids in the inner portions of the zona fasciculata and often is largely confined to this zone. Signs of adrenal cortical insufficiency usually are not observed.

Adrenalitis

Infectious and parasitic agents frequently localize in the adrenal gland and elicit varying degrees of inflammation and necrosis. Focal inflammations usually are suppurative, arising in the course of bacterial septicemias. The adrenal capsule provides an effective barrier against direct invasion by inflammatory reactions in adjacent tissue. Granulomatous adrenalitis due to *Histoplasma capsulatum, Coccidioides immitis,* or *Cryptococcus neoformans* occasionally occurs in dogs and cats. Multiple, distinct granulomas with central areas of necrosis and mineralization may destroy nearly the entire adrenal cortex. *Toxoplasma gondii* produces necrosis, with an infiltration of histiocytes, in the adrenal cortex of many species of animals. There is good experimental evidence to suggest that the high local concentration of antiinflammatory steroids in the adrenal cortex (e.g., cortisol and corticosterone) suppresses local cell-mediated immunity and permits the progressive growth of certain fungi (e.g., *H. capsulatum, Coccidioides immitus*). protozoa (e.g., *Babesia darlingi, B. jellisoni,* or *T. gondii*), and bacteria (e.g., *Mycobacterium tuberculosis*).

Hyperplasia and Neoplasia of Adrenal Cortex

Accessory adrenal tissue

Accessory cortical nodules are common in the adrenal glands of adult to aged animals and are found in the capsule, cortex, and medulla. Many of these nodules arise either as evaginations of the cortex into the capsule and surrounding periadrenal fat or as invaginations of the cortex into the medulla.

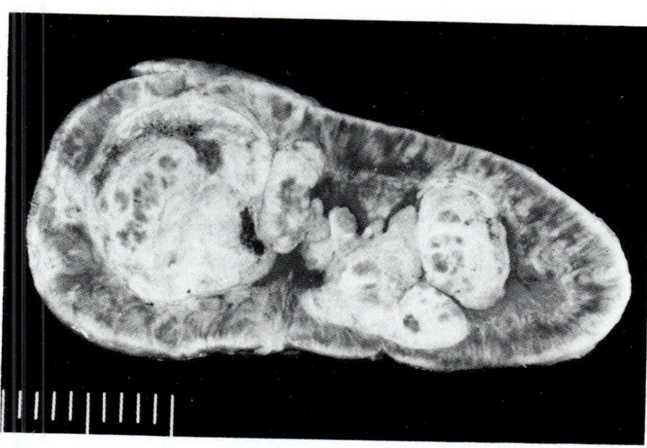

Fig. 6-14 Adrenal gland; dog. Nodular adrenal cortical hyperplasia. Multiple discrete nodules of cortical hyperplasia extend into the medulla. Bar = 1 cm.

Hyperplasia

Nodular hyperplasia also is common in the adrenal cortex as well-defined spherical nodules in the cortex or attached to the capsule (Fig. 6-14). Hyperplastic nodules are usually multiple, bilateral, and yellow and may involve any of the three zones of the cortex. Histologically, the nodules near the capsule resemble zona glomerulosa (multiformis) and sometimes have areas that resemble zona fasciculata. The lipid content in these hyperplastic nodules is not depleted in circumstances that reduce the amount of lipid in the remainder of the cortex. Hyperplastic cortical nodules are most common in older horses, dogs, and cats. Nodular hyperplasia of the zona reticularis has been seen in animals with functional disturbances, suggesting androgen excess (e.g., greater muscle mass, well-developed crest, hypertrophy of clitoris, and involution of mammary gland).

Diffuse cortical hyperplasia results in a uniform, usually bilateral, enlargement of the adrenal cortices. Marked hypertrophy and hyperplasia of cells of the zona fasciculata and zona reticularis occur in response to an autonomous hypersecretion of ACTH by a corticotropic adenoma of the pituitary gland (see Fig. 6-2). The hyperplastic cells of the zona fasciculata are vacuolated due to their lipid content. Cells of the outer zona glomerulosa (multiformis) may be compressed by the expanded inner two zones. Nodular hyperplasia can be present in a diffusely hyperplastic cortex.

Cortical adenomas

Adenomas of the adrenal cortex occur most frequently in older dogs and sporadically in horses, cattle, and sheep. Castrated male goats have a greater incidence of cortical adenomas than intact males. Although usually incidental findings at necropsy, the neoplasms occasionally are endocrinologically active. Cortical adenomas are well demarcated, usually single nodules in one adrenal gland. Larger cortical adenomas are yellow to red, distort the gland, compress the adjacent cortical parenchyma, and are partially or completely encapsulated. Cortical adenomas often develop in an adrenal gland with multiple nodules of hyperplasia, and adenomas may be difficult to differentiate grossly from the nodules of hyperplasia. However, nodular hyperplasia consists of multiple small foci, usually in both adrenals with no evidence of encapsulation, and often is associated with extracapsular nodules of hyperplastic cortical tissue. Cortical adenomas are composed of well-differentiated cells that resemble secretory cells of the normal zona fasciculata or zona reticularis. The abundant cytoplasm of neoplastic cells is lightly eosinophilic, often vacuolated, and filled with lipid droplets. Adenomas are partially or completely surrounded by a fibrous connective tissue capsule of varying thickness and a rim of compressed cortical parenchyma.

Cortical carcinomas

Adrenal cortical carcinomas occur less frequently than adenomas and have been reported most often in cattle and older dogs but infrequently in other species. Carcinomas develop in adult to older individuals with no apparent breed or sex prevalence. Adrenal carcinomas are larger than adenomas and are more likely to be bilateral. In dogs, they are composed of a variegated, yellow-red, friable tissue and may invade extensively into surrounding tissues and into the caudal vena cava, resulting in thrombus formation. Carcinomas attain considerable size in cattle (up to 10 cm or more in diameter) and have multiple areas of calcification or ossification.

Carcinomas are composed of more highly pleomorphic secretory cells than are adenomas and are subdivided by a usually fine fibrovascular stroma. The affected adrenal gland usually is completely obliterated by the carcinoma. The pattern of growth varies among neoplasms and within the same carcinoma and includes trabeculae, lobules, or nests of neoplastic cells. Neoplastic cells usually are large and polyhedral, with prominent nucleoli and densely eosinophilic or vacuolated cytoplasm.

Carcinomas and adenomas of the adrenal cortex in dogs occasionally are functional and secrete excessive amounts of cortisol. The clinical picture of adrenal cortical carcinomas may be complicated by compression of adjacent organs if the neoplasm is large; by invasion into the aorta or caudal vena cava, leading to intraabdominal hemorrhage; and by metastases to distant sites (e.g., liver, kidneys, mesenteric lymph nodes, and lungs). Functional cortical adenomas and carcinomas are associated with severe atrophy of the contralateral adrenal cortex because of negative feedback inhibition of the pituitary ACTH secretion by the elevated blood cortisol concentrations. The atrophic cortex consists primarily of the adrenal capsule and zona glomerulosa (multiformis) (Fig. 6-15). Atrophy may be present also in the remnants of the adrenal cortex compressed by functional adenomas. The adrenal medulla ap-

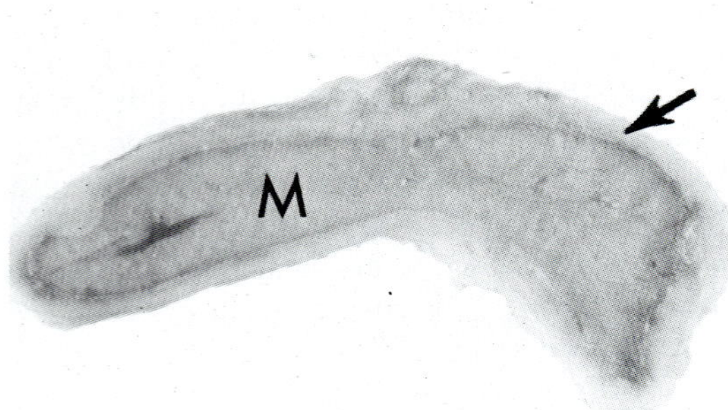

Fig. 6-15 Adrenal gland; dog. Cortical atrophy. The adrenal cortex is markedly thin *(arrow)* due to severe tropic atrophy and consists of the zona glomerulosa and a thickened fibrous capsule. The adrenal medulla (*M*) is relatively more prominent due to the tropic atrophy of the cortex.

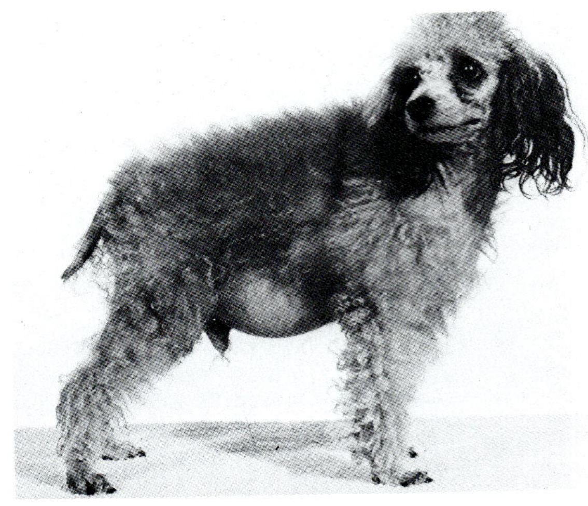

Fig. 6-16 Poodle. Cushing's-like disease of hypercortisolism due to idiopathic adrenal cortical hyperplasia. Muscle asthenia is evident from the pendulous abdomen, and there is alopecia of the abdomen, ventral cervical region, and tail.

pears more prominent because of the lack of cortical tissue (see Fig. 6-15).

Hypercortisolism (Cushing's Disease or Syndrome)

The clinical manifestations and lesions associated with the syndrome of hyperadrenocorticism primarily result from chronic overproduction of cortisol by hyperactive adrenal cortices. Affected dogs develop a spectrum of functional disturbances and lesions from the combined glyconeogenic, lipolytic, protein catabolic, and antiinflammatory effects of the glucocorticoid hormones on many organs. The disease is insidious and slowly progressive. Cortisol excess is one of the most common endocrinopathies in adult and aged dogs, but occurs infrequently in other domestic animals.

The increase in circulating cortisol concentrations in dogs with hyperadrenocorticism may result from one of several different pathogenetic mechanisms. The most common cause is a functional corticotroph (ACTH-secreting) adenoma of the pituitary gland, which causes bilateral adrenal cortical hypertrophy and hyperplasia (see Fig. 6-2). The cortex of both adrenal glands is widened considerably owing to diffuse and nodular hyperplasia, primarily in the zona fasciculata. Functional adrenal neoplasms are an infrequent (10% to 15% of cases) cause of the Cushing's-like syndrome of cortisol excess in the dog. Many of the clinical signs and lesions of the naturally occurring hyperadrenocorticism can be induced by long-term, daily administration of large doses of corticosteroids, as used for the treatment of other diseases. To accurately separate the different pathogenetic mechanisms responsible for cortisol excess, plasma cortisol concentrations must be evaluated with the animal in the basal state and after dexamethasone (high or low dose) suppression and ACTH stimulation.

Functional disturbances and lesions of cortisol excess

The appetite and intake of food often are increased as a direct result of either the hypercortisolism or the involvement of hypothalamic appetite centers by a large pituitary neoplasm. The muscles of the extremities and abdomen are weakened and atrophied. The loss in tone of the muscles of the abdomen and abaxial skeleton results in gradual abdominal enlargement (Fig. 6-16), lordosis, muscle trembling, and a straight-legged, skeletal-braced posture assumed in order to support the body's weight. Hepatomegaly due to increased fat and glycogen deposition may contribute to the development of the distended, often pendulous, abdomen. The muscular asthenia and wasting are the result of increased catabolism of structural proteins combined with diminished protein synthesis under the influence of long-term cortisol excess. Skin lesions occur frequently in dogs with hyperadrenocorticism. The initial changes in the skin often are observed over points of wear (e.g., neck, flanks, behind the ears, and over bony prominences). These changes spread in a bilaterally symmetric pattern to involve a significant percentage of the body surface. Skin lesions caused by excessive cortisol include atrophy of the epidermis and pilosebaceous apparatus, combined with loss of collagen and elastin in the dermis and subcutis. Cutaneous calcification is a characteristic lesion in dogs with hypercortisolism (approximately 30% to 40%). Numerous calcium crystals are deposited along collagen and elastin fibers in the dermis and may protrude through the atrophic and thinned epidermis. These calcium deposits occur in dogs with normal blood calcium and phosphorus concentrations. This manifestation of hypercortisolism most likely is related to the glyconeogenic and protein catabolic action of cortisol, resulting in the rearrangement of the molecular structure of proteins such as collagen and elastin, and the formation of an organic matrix that attracts and binds calcium. Severe calcification also occurs in other tissues, and the lungs are most frequently affected. However, active skeletal muscles and the wall of the stomach also may have extensive areas of calcification.

Hypoadrenocorticism (Addison's Disease)

Chronic adrenocortical insufficiency was the first recognized endocrine disease. Dogs with hypoadrenocorticism have bilateral adrenocortical atrophy involving all layers of the adrenal cortex. Production of all three classes of corticosteroids (mineralocorticoids, glucocorticoids, and adrenal sex steroids) is deficient. The adrenal cortex is reduced to one tenth or less of its normal thickness and consists primarily of the adrenal capsule (Fig. 6-17). Thus, the adrenal medulla becomes relatively more prominent and, along with the capsule, makes up the bulk of the remaining adrenal tissues.

The precise pathogenesis of idiopathic adrenocortical atrophy is unknown, but the lesion may be immune-mediated. Early in the disease, multiple foci of lymphocytes and plasma cells are interspersed between the adrenal sinusoids and groups of fibroblasts. The entire three zones of the cortex are nearly absent in dogs that die from untreated hypoadrenocorticism. The capsule is thickened due to collapse of the adrenal cortex and fibroblastic proliferation. Pituitary gland lesions have not been observed in dogs with idiopathic adrenal cortical atrophy in which all three zones of the adrenal cortex are atrophic, including the zona glomerulosa (multiformis) that is not under ACTH control. By comparison, atrophy of the adrenal cortex secondary to a destructive pituitary gland lesion that decreases ACTH secretion is characterized by severe atrophy only of the inner two cortical zones. The zona glomerulosa remains intact (see Fig. 6-1), and these animals do not have electrolyte abnormalities since the secretion of aldosterone remains within normal limits.

Chronic adrenal insufficiency is recognized as a distinct and common endocrinopathy of dogs. Idiopathic adrenocortical insufficiency occurs more frequently in young adult dogs and may have an immune-mediated pathogenesis. The synthesis and secretion of mineralocorticoids are reduced, resulting in marked alterations of serum potassium, sodium, and chloride concentrations. Less potassium is excreted by the kidneys (hypokaluria), resulting in a severe hyperkalemia. Less sodium and chloride are reabsorbed from renal tubules, leading to varying degrees of hypernatruria and hyperchloruria and a corresponding decline in blood concentrations of these ions. The severe hyperkalemia frequently produces marked cardiovascular disturbances. A pronounced bradycardia develops in some dogs (heart rate of 50 or fewer beats per minute) and does not change with exercise, predisposing to weakness or circulatory collapse after minimal exertion.

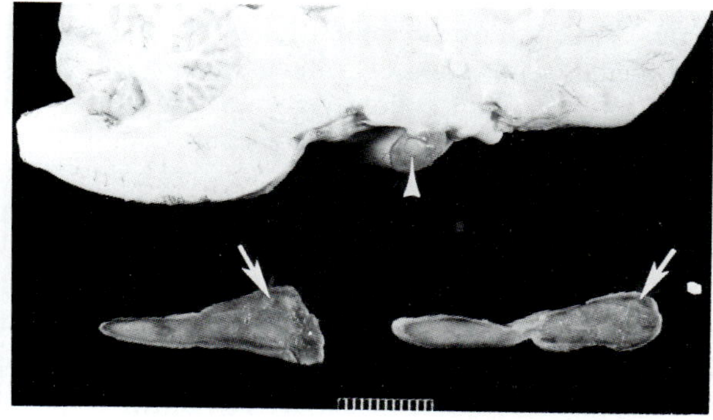

Fig. 6-17 Adrenal glands; dog. Cortical atrophy. Bilateral atrophy of all three cortical layers *(white arrows)* is characteristic of hypoadrenocorticism. The pituitary gland *(white arrowhead)* was grossly normal with histologic evidence of corticotropic hyperplasia. Bar = 1 cm.

A decreased production of glucocorticoids results in several characteristic functional disturbances of hypoadrenocorticism. The failure of gluconeogenesis and increased sensitivity to insulin contribute to the development of moderate hypoglycemia. Hyperpigmentation of the skin occurs in some dogs with long-standing adrenocortical insufficiency and is a common finding in Addison's disease of human beings. This change results from a lack of negative feedback on the pituitary gland and increased release of ACTH (and possibly MSH). The plasma cortisol concentrations in dogs with hypoadrenocorticism are low and range from 0.1 to 1.5 μg/dl. Due to the severe atrophy of the adrenal cortex, little or no increase in blood cortisol concentrations results from the administration of ACTH.

ADRENAL MEDULLA

The adrenal medulla is derived from neuroectoderm of the neural crest and produces catecholamine hormones. The main biosynthetic pathway for catecholamines in mammals starts with tyrosine, which is converted first to 1-dihydroxyphenylalanine (Dopa) by tyrosine hydroxylase. Dopa is then decarboxylated to 3,4-dihydroxyphenylethylamine (dopamine) by 3,4-amino acid decarboxylase, which subsequently undergoes beta-hydroxylation (by dopamine beta-oxidase) to norepinephrine. In mammals, the medulla is completely surrounded by the adrenal cortex, and venous blood from the cortex bathes the medullary cells. This blood contains the highest concentration of corticosteroids of any fluid in the body. This close anatomic association between the adrenal cortex and medulla in mammals is not fortuitous because the N-methylating enzyme (phenylethanolamine-N-methyl transferase) that converts norepinephrine to epinephrine is corticosteroid hormone–dependent.

Proliferative Lesions

Adrenal medullary hyperplasia

Diffuse or nodular adrenal medullary hyperplasia appears to precede the development of pheochromocytoma in bulls and human beings with C cell neoplasms of the thyroid gland. The proliferated chromaffin cells are nonencapsulated but compress the surrounding adrenal cortex.

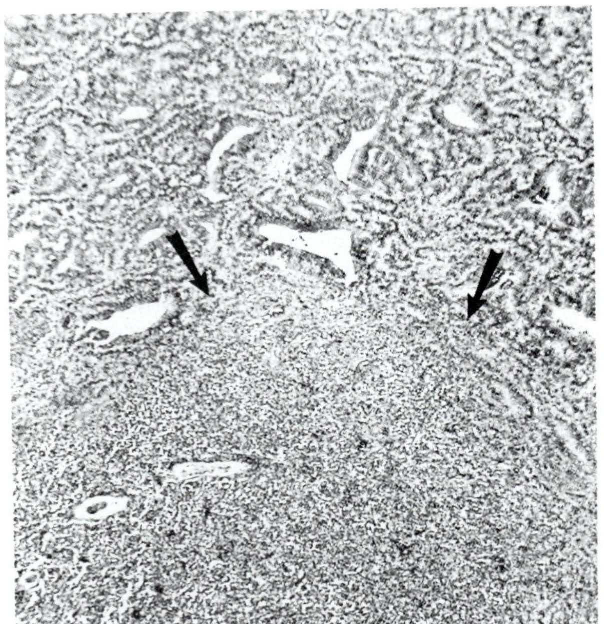

Fig. 6-18 Adrenal medulla; bull. Bilateral diffuse hyperplasia of adrenal medulla in a bull with a concomitant C cell carcinoma of the thyroid gland. The expanded adrenal medulla *(bottom)* compresses the surrounding adrenal cortex *(arrow)*. Bar = 1 cm. *Yarrington JT, Capen CC. Vet Pathol 1981; 18:316-325.*

The hyperplastic cells are round to oval and have a lightly basophilic cytoplasm. Some bulls with prominent diffuse medullary hyperplasia often have a few small nodules of proliferated medullary cells (Fig. 6-18). Medullary hyperplasia is diagnosed on the basis of these criteria: an increased adrenal weight, a decrease in corticomedullary ratio due to an increase in the size and number of medullary cells, and the presence of numerous mitotic figures in the adrenal medulla.

Neoplasms

Neuroblastomas and ganglioneuromas

Neuroblastomas usually occur in young animals, arising from primitive neuroectodermal cells and forming a large intraabdominal mass. Ganglioneuromas are usually small neoplasms that have well-differentiated, multipolar ganglion cells and neurofibrils. Neuroblastomas are composed of small neoplastic cells that have a hyperchromatic nucleus and a scant amount of cytoplasm and, thus, resemble lymphocytes. They tend to aggregate about vessels to form pseudorosettes. Neurofibrils or unmyelinated nerve fibers can be demonstrated in neuroblastomas.

Ganglioneuromas are benign neoplasms composed of multipolar ganglion cells and neurofibrils and have a prominent fibrous connective tissue stroma. The surrounding adrenal cortex may be severely compressed. Occasionally, neoplastic cells in medullary neoplasms may differentiate into two cell lines, resulting in pheochromocytoma and ganglioneuroma in the same adrenal gland.

Pheochromocytoma

Pheochromocytomas are the most common neoplasms in the adrenal medulla of animals, occurring most often in cattle and dogs and infrequently in other species. In bulls and human beings, pheochromocytomas develop concurrently with calcitonin-secreting C cell neoplasms of the thyroid gland. Malignant pheochromocytomas invade through the capsule of an adrenal gland and into adjacent structures (e.g., caudal vena cava) or metastasize to distant sites (e.g., liver, regional lymph nodes, or lungs).

Pheochromocytomas are unilateral or bilateral neoplasms of chromaffin cells located in the adrenal glands of animals. Pheochromocytomas often are large (10 cm or more in diameter) and replace most of the affected adrenal gland. Smaller neoplasms are completely surrounded by a thin, compressed rim of adrenal cortex. Large pheochromocytomas are multilobular and are variegated and light brown to yellow-red, due to areas of hemorrhage and necrosis.

Neoplastic cells in pheochromocytomas vary from small, round to polyhedral cells to large pleomorphic cells with multiple hyperchromatic nuclei. The cytoplasm is lightly eosinophilic, finely granular, and often indistinct. Pheochromocytomas are composed of either epinephrine- or norepinephrine-secreting cells or both.

THYROID GLAND

Thyroid Follicular Cells

The thyroid gland in most animal species is located as two lobes on the lateral surfaces of the trachea. In pigs, the main lobe of the thyroid gland is on the midline in the ventral cervical region with dorsolateral projections from each side. In dogs, the right lobe of the thyroid gland is situated slightly cranial to the left lobe and almost touches the caudal aspect of the larynx.

The thyroid gland is the largest of the endocrine organs that function exclusively as an endocrine gland. The basic histologic structure of the thyroid gland is unique for endocrine glands, consisting of follicles of varying size (20 to 250 μ) that contain colloid produced by the follicular cells. The follicular cells are cuboidal to columnar, and their secretory pole is directed toward the lumen of the follicles. An extensive network of interfollicular and intrafollicular capillaries provides the follicular cells with an abundant blood supply. Follicular cells have extensive profiles of rough endoplasmic reticulum and a large Golgi apparatus for the synthesis and packaging of substantial amounts of protein that are then transported into the follicular lumen. The interface between the luminal side of follicular cells and the colloid is modified by numerous microvilli (Fig. 6-19).

The synthesis of thyroid hormones is unique among

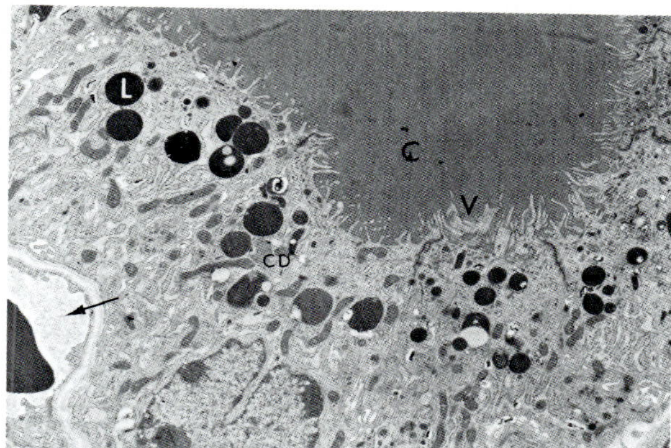

Fig. 6-19 Thyroid gland; normal dog. Thyroid follicular cells with long microvilli (*V*) that extend into the colloid (*C*) in follicular lumen. Numerous lysosomes (*L*) and colloid droplets *(CD)* are present in the apical portion of the follicular cells. An interfollicular capillary *(arrow)* is present at the base of the follicle.

those of the endocrine glands because the final assembly of hormone occurs extracellularly within the follicular lumen. Follicular cells trap essential raw materials, such as iodide from plasma, transport them rapidly against a concentration gradient to the lumen, and, here, the iodine is oxidized by a peroxidase in the microvilli to iodine (I_2) (Fig. 6-20). The assembly of thyroid hormones within the follicular lumen is made possible by a unique protein (thyroglobulin). Thyroglobulin is a high-molecular-weight (600,000 to 750,000 daltons) glycoprotein synthesized in successive subunits on the ribosomes of the endoplasmic reticulum in follicular cells. The constituent amino acids (tyrosine and others) and carbohydrates (i.e., mannose, fructose, galactose) are derived from the circulation. Recently synthesized thyroglobulin (17S) leaving the Golgi apparatus is packaged into apical vesicles and extruded into the follicular lumen (Fig. 6-20). The amino acid tyrosine, an essential component of thyroid hormones, is incorporated in the molecular structure of thyroglobulin. Iodine is bound to tyrosyl residues in thyroglobulin at the apical surface of follicular cells to form, successively, monoiodotyrosine (MIT) and diiodotyrosine (DIT). The resulting MIT and DIT combine to form the two biologically active iodothyronines (thyroxine [T_4], triiodothyronine [T_3]) secreted by the thyroid gland.

The secretion of thyroid hormones into the bloodstream from luminal colloid is initiated by elongation of microvilli and formation of pseudopodia on follicular cells. These elongated cytoplasmic projections are increased by pituitary thyrotropin, extend into the follicular lumen, and indiscriminatingly phagocytose adjacent colloid. Colloid droplets within follicular cells fuse with numerous lysosomes. T_3 and T_4 are released from the thyroglobulin molecule, diffuse from the follicular cell, and enter adjacent

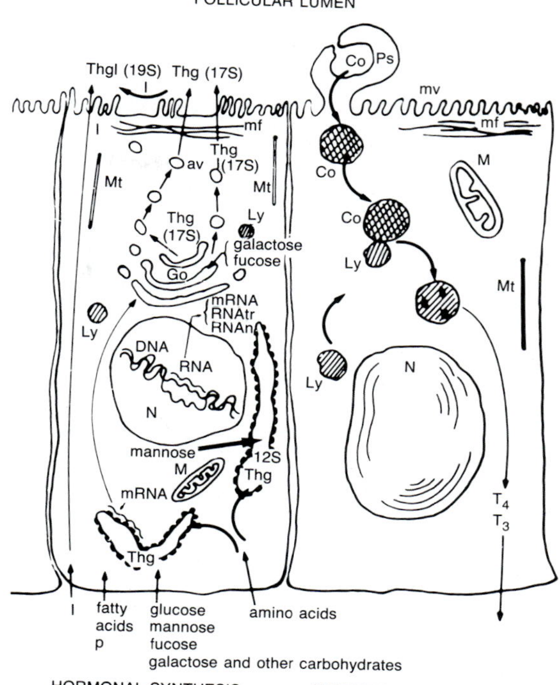

Fig. 6-20 Thyroid follicular cells illustrating two-way traffic of materials from capillaries into the follicular lumen. Raw materials, such as iodine, are concentrated by follicular cells and rapidly transported into the lumen (*left side* of the drawing). Amino acids (tyrosine and others) and sugars are assembled by follicular cells into thyroglobulin, packaged into apical vesicles *(av)* and released into the lumen. The iodination of tyrosyl residues with the thyroglobulin molecule to form thyroid hormones occurs within the follicular lumen. Elongation of microvilli and endocytosis of colloid by follicular cells occur in response to TTH stimulation (*right side* of drawing). The intracellular colloid droplets *(Co)* fuse with lysosomal bodies *(Ly),* active thyroid hormone is enzymatically cleaved from thyroglobulin, and free T_4 and T_3 are released into the circulation. *Bastenie PA, Ermans AM, Bonnyns M, Neve P, Delespesse G. Lymphocytic thyroiditis as an autoimmune disease. In: Good RA, Day SB, Yunis JJ, eds. Molecular Pathology. Springfield, Ill.: Charles C Thomas, 1975.*

capillaries. Negative feedback control of thyroid hormone secretion is accomplished by the coordinated response to circulating concentrations of T_4 and T_3 by the adenohypophysis and certain hypothalamic nuclei.

Thyrotropin (TTH or TSH) is conveyed to thyroid follicular cells where it binds to the basilar aspect of the cell, activates adenylate cyclase, and increases the rate of biochemical reactions concerned with the biosynthesis and secretion of thyroidal hormones. If the secretion of TTH is sustained (hours or days), thyroid follicular cells become more columnar and follicular lumina become smaller due to increased endocytosis of colloid (Fig. 6-21). Numerous PAS-positive colloid droplets are present in the luminal aspect of the hypertrophied follicular cells. The converse

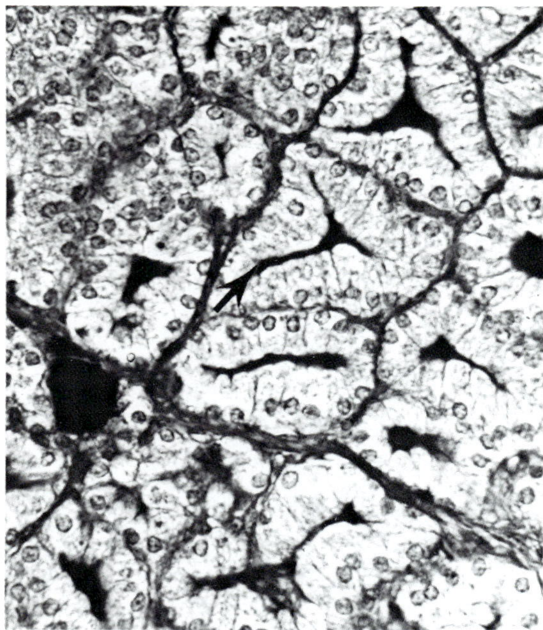

Fig. 6-21 Thyroid gland; dog. Hyperplasia. Follicular cells 8 hours post-TSH stimulation are columnar, and many follicles are nearly depleted of colloid and are partially collapsed *(arrow).*

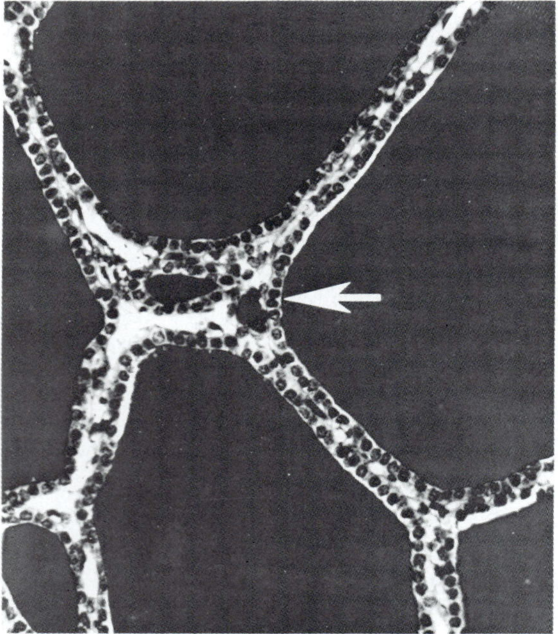

Fig. 6-22 Thyroid gland; dog. Atrophy. Thyroid follicular cells after long-term administration of exogenous thyroxine *(arrow)* are cuboidal. Thyroid follicles are distended with dense colloid.

of what has been just described occurs in response to an increase in circulating thyroid hormone (T_4 and T_3) and a corresponding decrease in circulating pituitary TTH. Thyroid follicles become enlarged and distended with colloid due to decreased TTH-mediated endocytosis of colloid. Follicular cells lining the involuted follicles are low cuboidal, and there are few endocytotic vacuoles at the interface between the colloid and follicular cells (Fig. 6-22).

T_4 and T_3, once released into the circulation, act on many different target cells in the body. The overall functions of T_4 and T_3 are similar, although much of the biologic activity appears to be the result of monodeiodination to 3,5,3′-triiodothyronine (T_3) prior to interacting with target cells. Under certain conditions (protein starvation, the neonatal period, hepatic and renal disease, febrile illness, etc.), T_4 is preferentially monodeiodinated to 3,3′,5′-triiodothyronine (''reverse T_3''). Since ''reverse'' T_3 produced by target cells is biologically inactive, monodeiodination to form reverse T_3 provides a mechanism to attenuate the overall metabolic effects of thyroid hormones. The subcellular mechanism of action of thyroid hormones resembles that of steroids in that free hormone enters target cells and binds to cytosol-binding proteins and nuclear receptors.

Developmental Disturbances

Accessory thyroid tissue

The thyroid gland originates embryologically as a thickened plate of epithelium in the floor of the pharynx. Because it is intimately related to the aortic sac in its development, this leads to the frequent occurrence of accessory thyroid tissue, which is usually in the mediastinum, particularly in adult dogs, but may be located anywhere from the base of the tongue to the diaphragm. About 50% of adult dogs have nodules of accessory thyroid tissue embedded in the fat around the base of the heart and origin of the aorta. The follicular structure and function are the same as those of the main thyroid lobes. Attempts to induce hypothyroidism in the dog by surgical thyroidectomy are not successful because the accessory thyroids readily respond to the prompt increase in endogenous TTH secretion and can undergo sufficient hyperplasia to sustain adequate hormone production. This accessory thyroid tissue may undergo neoplastic transformation.

Thyroglossal duct cysts

Thyroglossal duct cysts develop most frequently in dogs and pigs and occasionally in other animals by a persistence of portions of the midline embryologic primordia of the thyroid gland, which migrates caudally from the floor of the primitive pharynx to form the postnatal thyroid lobes. These cysts are present in the ventral aspect of the cervical region in dogs as fluctuant masses. They may rupture and form a fistulous tract to the exterior. Their lining epithelium consists of multiple layers of follicular cells in which are occasionally colloid-containing follicles that may undergo neoplastic transformation and give rise to papillary carcinomas.

Degenerative and Inflammatory Lesions

Idiopathic follicular atrophy ("collapse")

In follicular atrophy, there is a progressive loss of follicular epithelium and replacement by adipose connective tissue with a minimal inflammatory response. The gland usually is smaller and lighter in color than normal. The early lesion in dogs with mild clinical signs of hypothyroidism appears to be confined to one part of the thyroid gland. This affected part contains small follicles, lined by tall columnar follicular cells and often containing little colloid. A more advanced form of follicular atrophy is present in dogs with clinical hypothyroidism and low blood concentrations of thyroidal hormones. These thyroid glands are composed predominantly of adipose connective tissue with only a few clusters of small follicles containing vacuolated colloid. The thyroid gland, markedly reduced in size, consists primarily of small follicles and individual follicular cells containing PAS-positive colloid within a microfollicle in the cytoplasm. The mild increase of connective tissue in the interstitium results from condensation of the stroma.

Lymphocytic (immune-mediated) thyroiditis

Lymphocytic thyroiditis in dogs, obese strains of chickens, nonhuman primates, and Buffalo rats closely resembles Hashimoto's disease in human beings. Although the exact pathogenetic mechanism in the dog is not completely established, evidence suggests a polygenic pattern of inheritance similar to that observed in human beings. The immunologic basis of the development of chronic lymphocytic thyroiditis in both human beings and dogs appears to be through production of autoantibodies directed against thyroglobulin, a microsomal antigen, and a second colloid antigen. The fact that thyroglobulin autoantibodies have been found in 48% of pet dogs with hypothyroidism may be related to the cause of thyroiditis. Laboratory beagle dogs with naturally occurring lymphocytic thyroiditis also have circulating thyroidal autoantibodies, but the focal thyroiditis usually is not associated with clinical signs of hypothyroidism.

Microscopic alterations consist of multifocal to diffuse infiltrates of lymphocytes, plasma cells, macrophages, and, sometimes, lymphoid nodules. Thyroid follicles are small and lined by columnar epithelial cells; lymphocytes, macrophages, and degenerate follicular cells are often present in vacuolated colloid (Fig. 6-23). Thyroid C cells are present as small nests or nodules between follicles and often are more prominent than those in normal dogs. Some remaining follicular cells may be transformed into large oxyphilic cells with densely eosinophilic granular cytoplasm.

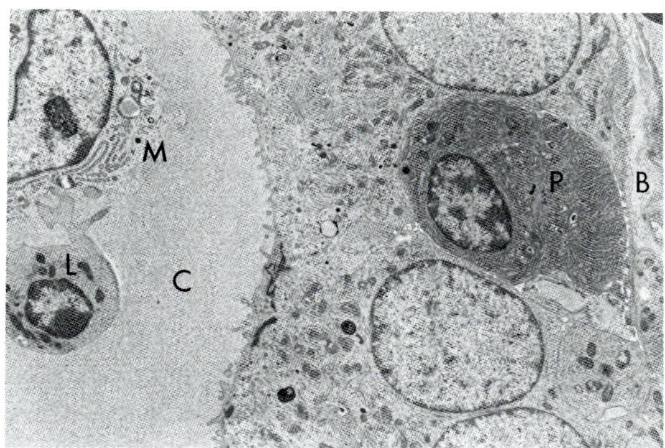

Fig. 6-23 Lymphocytic thyroiditis in a dog with severe hypothyroidism. A lymphocyte (*L*) and macrophage (*M*) are present in the colloid (*C*) of a thyroid follicle. A plasma cell (*P*) within the follicular basement membrane (*B*) is infiltrating between thyroid follicular cells. *Gosselin SJ, Capen CC, Martin SL, Krakowka S. Vet Immunol Immunopathol 1982; 3:185-201.*

Goiter

Hyperplasia of thyroid follicular cells ("goiter")

Nonneoplastic and noninflammatory enlargement of the thyroid gland develops in all domestic mammals, birds, and other submammalian vertebrates. Certain forms of thyroid hyperplasia, especially nodular, may be difficult to differentiate from adenomas. The major pathogenic mechanisms responsible for the development of thyroid hyperplasia include iodine-deficient diets, goitrogenic compounds that interfere with thyroxinogenesis, excess dietary iodide, and genetically determined defects in the enzymes responsible for biosynthesis of thyroidal hormones. All these result in inadequate thyroxine synthesis and decreased blood concentrations of T_4 and T_3. This is detected by the hypothalamus and pituitary gland, stimulating an increase in the secretion of TTH, which results in hypertrophy and hyperplasia of follicular cells.

Diffuse hyperplastic and colloid goiter

Dietary iodine deficiency that resulted in diffuse thyroid hyperplasia was common in many areas of the world before the widespread addition of iodized salt to animal diets. Iodine-deficient goiter still occurs worldwide in domestic animals, but cases are sporadic and few animals are affected. Marginally, iodine-deficient diets that contain goitrogenic compounds may cause severe thyroid follicular cell hyperplasia and goiter. These substances include thiouracil, sulfonamides, anions of the Hofmeister series, and a number of plants from the family *Brassicacceae.* Offspring of females fed iodine-deficient diets are more likely to develop severe thyroidal follicular cell hyperplasia and have clinical signs of hypothyroidism. Both lateral lobes of the thyroid gland are uniformly enlarged in young animals due to diffuse hypertrophy and hyperplasia of follicular cells (Fig. 6-21). The enlargements may be extensive and result in palpable or visible swellings in the cranial cervical area. The affected lobes are firm and dark red because an extensive interfollicular capillary network develops under the influence of long-term TTH stimulation.

Colloid goiter represents the involutionary phase of diffuse hyperplastic goiter in young adult and adult animals. The markedly hyperplastic follicular cells continue to produce colloid, but endocytosis of colloid is decreased due to diminished pituitary TTH concentrations in response to the return of blood T_4 and T_3 to normal. Both thyroid lobes are diffusely enlarged but are more translucent and lighter in color than in hyperplastic goiter. These differences in macroscopic appearances are the result of less vascularity in colloid goiter and development of macrofollicles distended with colloid.

Colloid goiter may develop either after sufficient amounts of iodide have been added to the diet or after the requirements for thyroid hormones have diminished in an older animal. Blood T_4 and T_3 concentrations return toward normal, and the secretion of TTH by the pituitary gland is correspondingly decreased. Follicles are progressively distended (Fig. 6-22) with densely eosinophilic colloid due to diminished TTH-induced endocytosis. The follicular cells lining the macrofollicles are flattened and atrophic. The interface between the colloid and luminal surface of the follicular cells is smooth and lacks the characteristic endocytotic vacuoles of actively secreting follicular cells. Some involuted follicles in colloid goiter have remnants of the papillary projections of follicular cells extending into their lumina.

The changes in diffuse hyperplastic and colloid goiters are consistent throughout the diffusely enlarged thyroid lobes. Follicles are irregular in size and shape in hyperplastic goiter because they contain varying amounts of colloid that is lightly eosinophilic and vacuolated. Some follicles collapse from the lack of colloid. Their lining epithelial cells are columnar and have a deeply eosinophilic cytoplasm and small hyperchromatic nuclei that often are situated in the basilar portion of the cell. The follicles are lined by single or multiple layers of hyperplastic follicular cells that, in some follicles, may form papillary projections into the lumen (Fig. 6-24). Similar proliferative changes are present in ectopic thyroid tissue in the neck and mediastinum.

Although seemingly paradoxic, an excess of iodide in the diet also can result in thyroid hyperplasia in animals and human beings. Foals of mares fed dry seaweed containing excessive iodide may develop thyroid hyperplasia and clinically evident goiter. The thyroid glands of the young are exposed to greater blood iodide concentrations than are those of the dam because iodide is concentrated first by the placenta and then by the mammary gland. High blood iodide interferes with one or more steps of thyroidal hormone synthesis and secretion, leading to lowered blood T_4 and T_3 concentrations and a compensatory increase in pituitary TTH secretion. Excess iodine appears to particularly block the release of T_3 and T_4 by interfering with proteolysis of colloid by lysosomes.

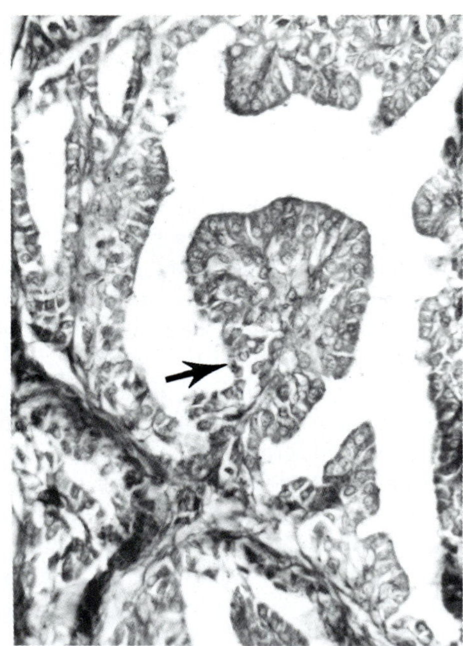

Fig. 6-24 Thyroid gland, dog. Hyperplastic goiter. Papillary projections *(arrow)* extend into follicular lumina. The partial collapse of follicles is due to increased endocytosis of colloid.

Multifocal nodular hyperplasia

Nodular hyperplasia (''goiter'') in thyroid glands of old horses, cats, and dogs appears as multiple, white to tan nodules of varying sizes (Fig. 6-25). The affected lobes often are moderately enlarged and irregular in contour. Multifocal nodular goiter in most animals (except cats) is endocrinologically inactive and is an incidental lesion at necropsy. However, functional thyroid adenomas often develop in a thyroid gland of aged cats with hyperthyroidism and multinodular hyperplasia of follicular cells. In contrast to thyroid adenomas, the areas of nodular hyperplasia are not encapsulated and result in minimal compression of adjacent parenchyma. Thus, nodular goiter consists of multiple foci of hyperplastic follicular cells that are sharply demarcated but not encapsulated from the adjacent thyroid tissue.

The microscopic appearance of multinodular goiter often is variable. Some hyperplastic cells form small follicles with little or no colloid. Other nodules are composed of larger, irregularly shaped follicles lined by one or more layers of columnar cells that form papillary projections into the lumen. Some of the follicles have undergone colloid involution and are filled with densely eosinophilic colloid.

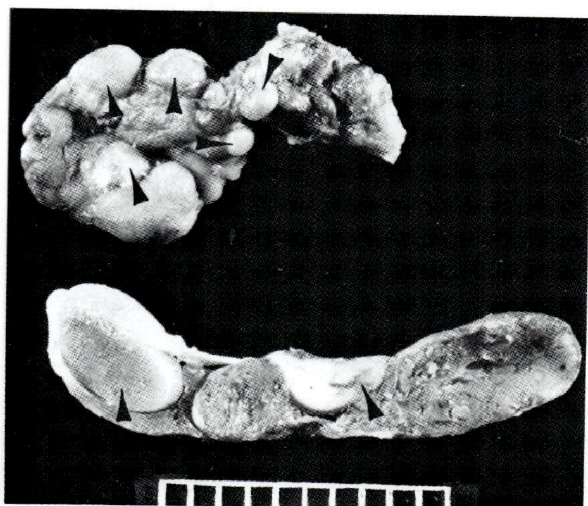

Fig. 6-25 Thyroid glands; cat. Hyperplasia, hyperthyroidism. Multinodular follicular cell hyperplasia *(arrowheads)* involves both thyroid lobes.

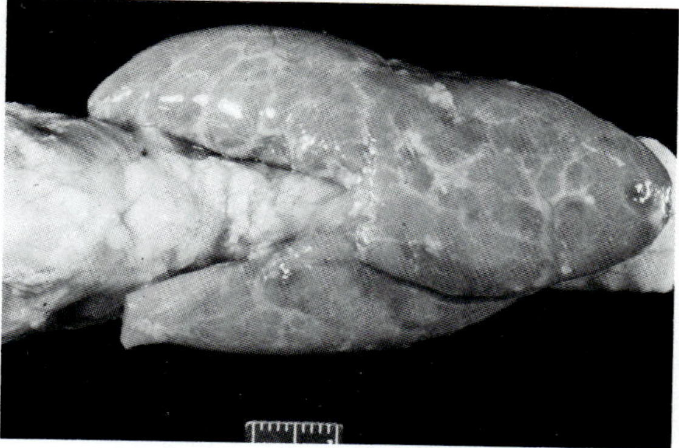

Fig. 6-26 Thyroid gland; lamb. Congenital dyshormonogenetic goiter. The symmetrically enlarged thyroid (*T*) lobes are fused on the midline beneath the larynx (*L*) and trachea.

These changes appear to be the result of alternating periods of hyperplasia and colloid involution in the thyroid glands of aged animals.

Congenital dyshormonogenetic goiter

Congenital dyshormonogenetic goiter in sheep (Corriedale, Dorset Horn, Merino, and Romney breeds), Afrikander cattle, and Saanen dwarf goats is inherited as an autosomal recessive gene. The subnormal growth rate; absence of normal wool development or a rough, sparse hair coat; subcutaneous myxedematous swellings; weakness; and sluggish behavior suggest that the affected young are clinically hypothyroid. Most lambs with congenital goiter either die shortly after birth or are highly sensitive to the effects of adverse environmental conditions, particularly cold.

Thyroid lobes are symmetrically enlarged at birth due to an intense, diffuse hyperplasia of follicular cells (Fig. 6-26). Thyroid follicles are lined by tall columnar cells but often are collapsed because of lack of colloid resulting from the marked endocytotic activity. The tall columnar follicular cells lining thyroid follicles have extensively dilated profiles of rough endoplasmic reticulum and large mitochondria, but there are relatively few dense granules associated with the Golgi apparatus and few apical vesicles near the luminal plasma membrane. Numerous long microvilli extend into the follicular lumen.

Although thyroidal uptake and turnover of ^{131}I are greatly increased compared with euthyroid controls, circulating T_4 and T_3 concentrations are consistently low. The lack of a defect in the iodide transport mechanism and organification or dehalogenation, plus an absence of normal 19S thyroglobulin in goitrous thyroids and only minute amounts of thyroglobulin-related antigens (0.01% of normal), suggest an impairment in thyroglobulin biosynthesis. A closely related or similar defect appears to operate in congenital goiter of sheep, cattle, and goats.

Neoplasms of the Thyroid Gland

Follicular cell adenoma

Adenomas usually are white to tan, small, solid nodules that are well demarcated from the adjacent thyroid parenchyma. The affected thyroid lobe is only moderately enlarged and distorted; usually only a single adenoma is present in a thyroid lobe. A distinct, white, fibrous connective tissue capsule of variable thickness separates the adenoma from the compressed parenchyma. Some thyroid adenomas are composed of thin-walled cysts filled with a yellow to red fluid. Their external surfaces are smooth and covered by an extensive network of blood vessels. Small masses of neoplastic tissue remain in the wall and form rugose projections into the cyst. Adenomas are classified into follicular and papillary types, and follicular types are more common.

Follicular cell carcinoma

In dogs, thyroid carcinomas occur more often than adenomas, but, in cats, adenomas are more common. Boxer dogs develop thyroidal carcinomas more frequently than any other breed, but beagle and golden retriever dogs have a significant risk for the development of thyroid carcinoma. In dogs, about 60% of thyroid carcinomas are detectable clinically by palpation as a firm mass in the neck and by evidence of respiratory distress. Carcinomas become fixed in position by extensive local invasion of adjacent structures, whereas adenomas (which do not invade) are freely movable under the skin. Neoplasms of thyroid origin also may occur in accessory thyroidal tissue located anywhere from the base of the tongue to the cranial mediastinum.

Thyroid carcinomas often grow rapidly and invade adjacent structures, such as the trachea, esophagus, and larynx. The earliest and most frequent site of metastasis is to the lungs because thyroid carcinomas early in the course of development invade branches of the thyroid vein. The retropharyngeal and caudal cervical lymph nodes are infrequent sites of metastasis.

Hyperthyroidism

Proliferative lesions that secrete excess thyroidal hormones are common in the thyroid glands of adult and aged cats. Follicular cell adenomas, which often develop in a thyroid gland with multinodular hyperplasia, are encountered more commonly than thyroid carcinomas. In aged cats, a syndrome of hyperthyroidism associated with multinodular hyperplasia, adenomas, or carcinomas derived from follicular cells of the thyroid is being recognized more frequently. Follicles in the rim of thyroid tissue around a functional adenoma are markedly enlarged and distended by an accumulation of colloid. The follicular cells are low cuboidal and atrophic with little evidence of endocytotic activity in response to the elevated concentrations of thyroid hormones. In cats with solitary adenomas, the opposite thyroid lobe should be carefully evaluated for evidence of nodular hyperplasia or ''microadenomas.'' These small areas of multinodular hyperplasia of follicular cells may cause recurrence of hyperthyroidism several months to a year or more after surgical removal of the functional adenoma.

Hyperthyroidism in cats also occurs in association with bilateral multinodular (''adenomatous'') hyperplasia. These multiple areas of thyroidal cell hyperplasia usually cause only slight enlargement of the affected lobe(s) (see Fig. 6-25). In contrast to adenomas, the areas of nodular hyperplasia are not encapsulated and the adjacent thyroid tissue is not compressed. Microscopically, hyperplastic nodules are composed of irregularly shaped, colloid-filled follicles lined by cuboidal follicular cells. These multiple nodules of follicular cell hyperplasia may coalesce to form macroscopically observable thyroidal cell adenomas.

Thyroid neoplasms in the dog may secrete sufficient thyroidal hormones to produce mild clinical signs of hyperthyroidism, including weight loss, polyphagia, weakness and fatigue, intolerance to heat, and nervousness. However, because the efficient enterohepatic excretory mechanism for T_4 and T_3 is difficult to overload, clinical hyperthyroidism in dogs with functional thyroidal cell neoplasms is infrequent.

Hypothyroidism

Hypothyroidism is a well-recognized and clinically important disease in dogs but is encountered only occasionally in other animals. Although the disease may occur in many adult purebred and mixed breed dogs, certain breeds (golden retriever, Doberman pinscher, dachshund, Shetland sheepdog, Irish setter, miniature schnauzer, cocker spaniel, and Airedale) have been reported to be more commonly affected. Hypothyroidism in dogs usually is the result of primary lesions in the thyroid gland, particularly idiopathic follicular collapse and lymphocytic thyroiditis. Less common causes of hypothyroidism include bilateral nonfunctional thyroidal cell neoplasms and severe iodine-deficient goiter. Hypothyroidism secondary to long-standing pituitary gland or hypothalamic lesions that prevent the release of either TTH or thyrotropin-releasing hormone (TRH) is encountered infrequently in the dog. In these cases, the thyroid gland is moderately reduced in size and composed of colloid-distended follicles lined by flattened follicular cells.

Many functional disturbances associated with hypothyroidism are due to a reduction in basal metabolic rate. A gain in body weight without an associated change in appetite occurs in some hypothyroid dogs. There is thinning of the hair coat and, often, a bilaterally symmetrical alopecia. Areas affected initially by hair loss are those receiving frictional wear, such as the tail and cervical area.

Hyperkeratosis is a consistent finding in hypothyroidism and results in an increased scaliness of the skin. It may become severe and occur as circular scaling patches suggestive of seborrhea. Microscopically, the skin has striking hyperkeratosis (Fig. 6-27) that involves the external root sheath, resulting in follicular keratosis. Hyperpigmentation, especially in such localized areas of alopecia as the dorsal aspect of the nose and distal portion of the tail, occurs in many dogs with hypothyroidism. Myxedema may develop, the result of accumulation of mucin (neutral and acid mucopolysaccharides combined with protein) in the dermis and subcutis. These substances bind considerable amounts of water, which produces marked thickening of the skin. Microscopically, mucin appears as granular or fibrillar material in H & E–stained sections.

Abnormalities in reproduction include lack of libido, reduction in sperm count, and abnormal or absent estrus cycles and reduced conception rates. The spermatogenic ep-

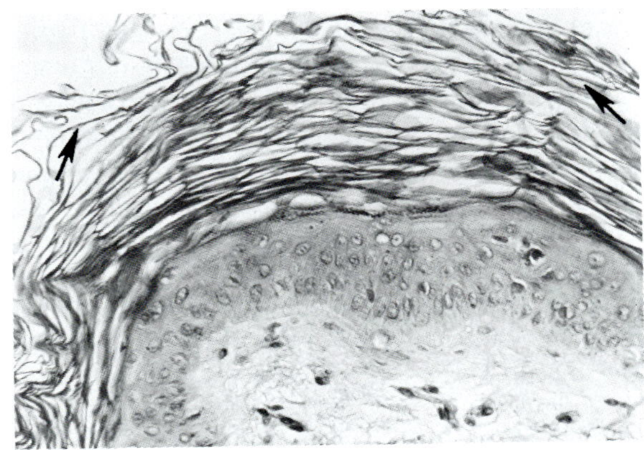

Fig. 6-27 Skin; dog. Hypothyroidism. Hyperkeratosis *(arrows)* involves the skin.

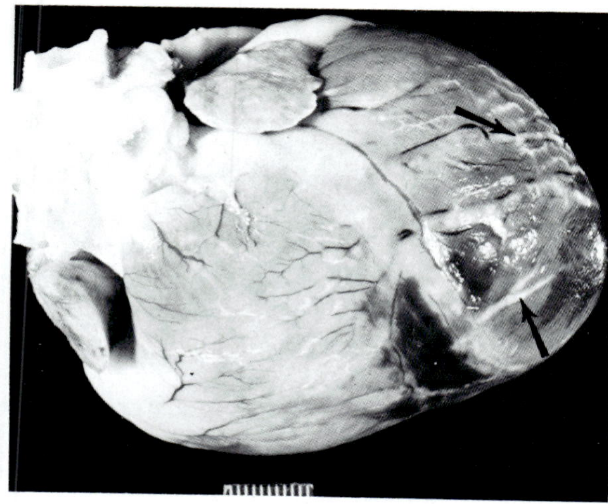

Fig. 6-28 Heart; dog with marked hyperlipidemia associated with severe primary hypothyroidism. Note coronary atherosclerosis *(arrows)* with areas of ischemic necrosis and hemorrhage of myocardium (*H*). Bar = 1 cm.

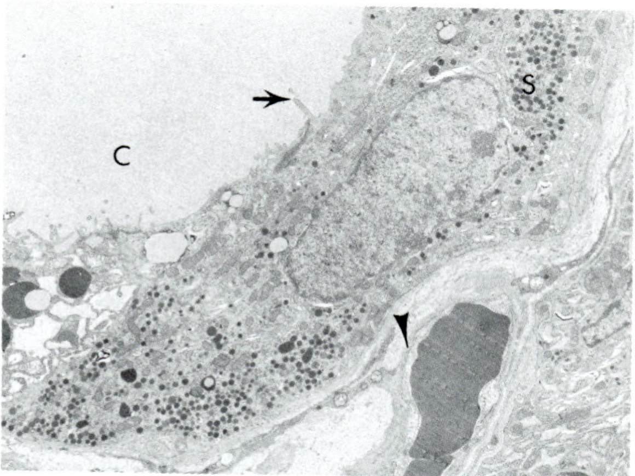

Fig. 6-29 Thyroid gland; normal dog. Thyroid C (parafollicular) cell with numerous secretory granules (*S*) and moderate development of Golgi apparatuses and rough endoplasmic reticulum. Microvilli from follicular cells *(arrow)* extend into the colloid of the follicular lumen (*C*). The secretory polarity of the C cell is directed toward an interfollicular capillary *(arrowhead)* with fenestrae.

ithelium in the testes is often markedly atrophic in chronic hypothyroidism.

Hypothyroidism in dogs is accompanied by low circulating thyroidal hormone concentrations and decreased ^{131}I uptake by the thyroid gland. In dogs with hypothyroidism, the T_4 concentration is usually below 0.8 μg/dl (normal: 1.5 to 3.4 μg/dl) and that of T_3 is below 50 ng/dl (normal: 48 to 150 ng/dl). In the euthyroid dog, the T_4 concentrations will at least double, 8 hours after intravenous or intramuscular injection of TTH. In dogs with hypothyroidism, the T_4 concentrations do not change significantly after injection of TTH.

The serum cholesterol concentration is elevated significantly (300 to 900 mg/dl) in many hypothyroid dogs. The marked hypercholesterolemia in long-standing and severe hypothyroidism results in a variety of secondary lesions, including atherosclerosis, hepatomegaly, glomerular and corneal lipidosis. Atherosclerosis of coronary (Fig. 6-28) and cerebral vessels may develop in dogs with severe hypothyroidism and long-standing hyperlipidemia.

Thyroid C (Parafollicular) Cells

Calcitonin is secreted by a second endocrine cell population, C (parafollicular) cells, in the mammalian thyroid gland. These cells are situated either within the follicular wall between follicular cells (Fig. 6-29) or as small groups of cells between follicles. C cells do not border the follicular colloid directly, and their secretory pole is oriented toward the interfollicular capillaries. The distinctive feature of C cells is the presence of numerous small, membrane-limited secretory granules in their cytoplasm (Fig. 6-29). Immunocytochemical techniques have localized the calcitonin activity of C cells to these secretory granules.

Calcitonin is a polypeptide hormone, and concentration of calcium ions in plasma and extracellular fluids is the principal physiologic stimulus for the secretion of calcitonin by C cells. The rate of secretion of calcitonin is increased greatly in response to elevations in blood calcium concentration.

C cells store substantial amounts of calcitonin in their cytoplasm, and in response to hypercalcemia the hormone is discharged rapidly from C cells into interfollicular capillaries. Hyperplasia of C cells occurs in response to long-term hypercalcemia. When the blood calcium concentration is reduced, the stimulus for calcitonin secretion is diminished, and numerous secretory granules accumulate in the cytoplasm of C cells (Fig. 6-30). Calcitonin exerts its function by interacting with target cells located primarily in bones and kidneys. The actions of parathyroid hormone and calcitonin are antagonistic to bone resorption but synergistic to decreasing the renal tubular reabsorption of phosphorus.

Thyroid C (ultimobranchial) cell neoplasms

Neoplasms derived from C cells of the thyroid gland are most frequently encountered in adult to aged bulls (but not in cows fed similar diets), certain strains of laboratory rats, and adult to aged horses, but infrequently in other species. A high percentage of aged bulls fed calcium-rich diets develop C cell neoplasms (30%) or hyperplasia of C cells and ultimobranchial derivatives (15% to 20%). The incidence of C cell neoplasms increases with advancing age in bulls and may be associated with the development of increased vertebral density. The syndrome of C cells neoplasms in bulls shares many similarities with that of medullary thy-

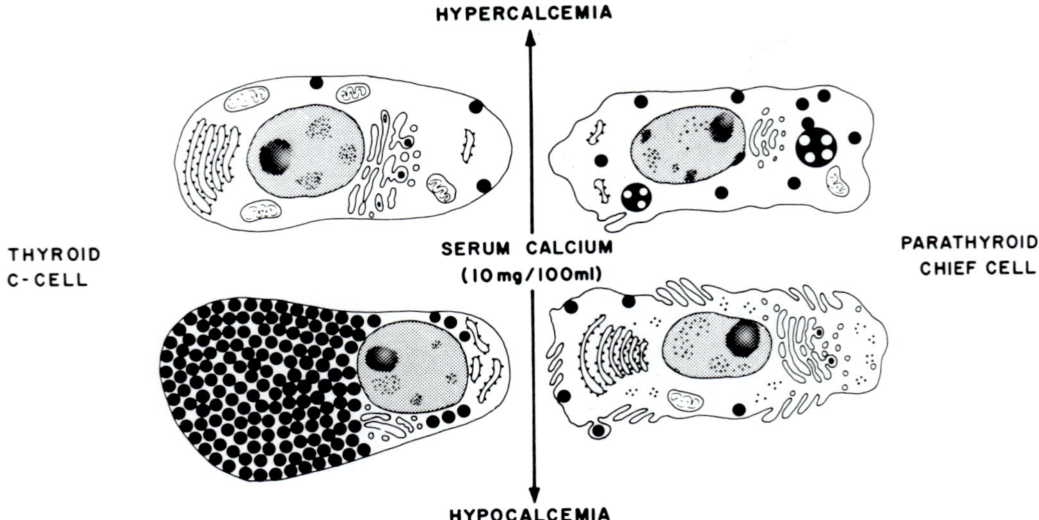

Fig. 6-30 Response of thyroid C cells and parathyroid chief cells to hypercalcemia and hypocalcemia. C cells accumulate secretory granules in response to hypocalcemia, whereas chief cells are nearly degranulated but have an increased development of synthetic and secretory organelles. In response to hypercalcemia, C cells are degranulated, and parathyroid chief cells are predominantly in the inactive stage of the secretory cycle.

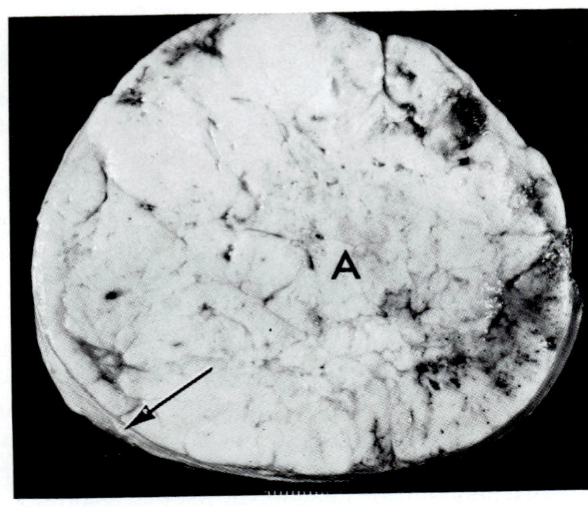

Fig. 6-31 Thyroid gland; horse. Adenoma. The adenoma (*A*) is confined by the thyroid capsule, and a rim of compressed thyroid *(arrow)* is present at the periphery of the mass. Bar = 1 cm.

roid carcinoma in human beings. Multiple endocrine neoplasms, especially bilateral pheochromocytomas and occasionally pituitary adenomas, may also be present in bulls and human beings with C cell neoplasms. A diffuse or nodular hyperplasia in the adrenal medulla precedes the development of pheochromocytoma.

Adenomas. C cell adenomas occur as discrete, single or multiple, gray to tan nodules in one or both thyroid lobes. Adenomas are smaller (approximately 1 to 3 cm in diameter) than carcinomas and are separated from the adjacent compressed thyroid parenchyma by a thin, fibrous connective tissue capsule. Larger C cell adenomas replace most of the thyroid lobe, but a rim of dark, brown-red thyroid often is present on one side (Fig. 6-31). Microscopically, a thyroid C cell adenoma is a discrete, expansive mass of cells larger than a colloid-distended follicle. The adenoma is well circumscribed or partially encapsulated, and adjacent follicles are compressed to varying degrees. The neoplastic C cells are well differentiated and have abundant to clear, lightly eosinophilic cytoplasm.

Carcinomas. Thyroid C cell carcinomas result in extensive multinodular enlargements of one or both thyroid lobes and may replace the entire thyroid gland. Thyroid C cell neoplasms in bulls, other animal species, and human beings are firm, and, in some areas, the stroma consists of dense bands of fibrous connective tissue. Multiple metastases that occur in cranial cervical lymph nodes are usually large (Fig. 6-32) and have areas of necrosis and hemorrhage. Pulmonary metastases appear as discrete tan nodules and occur infrequently. C cell carcinomas are composed of neoplastic cells that are more pleomorphic than cells of C cell adenomas. The carcinomatous cells are poorly differentiated, polyhedral to spindle-shaped, with lightly eosinophilic, finely granular, indistinct cytoplasm. Both adenomas and carcinomas have deposits of amyloid.

The etiology of C cell neoplasms is unknown, but the chronic stimulation of C cells by high concentrations of calcium absorbed from the digestive tract may be responsible for their high incidence. A significant decline in the incidence of C cell neoplasms occurs when the high cal-

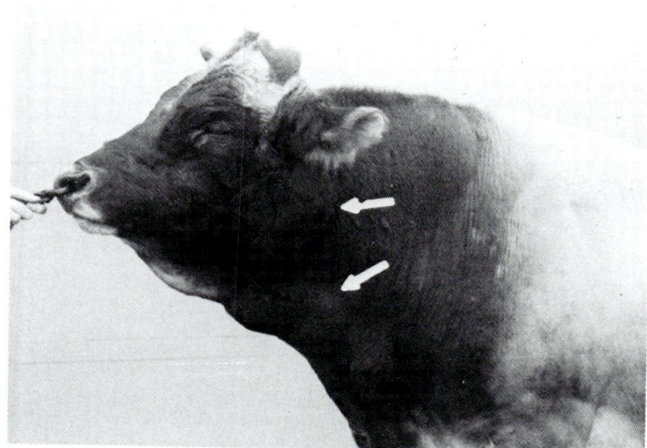

Fig. 6-32 Jersey bull. C cell carcinoma with multiple metastases to anterior cervical lymph nodes. Note the swellings in the neck as a result of the metastases.

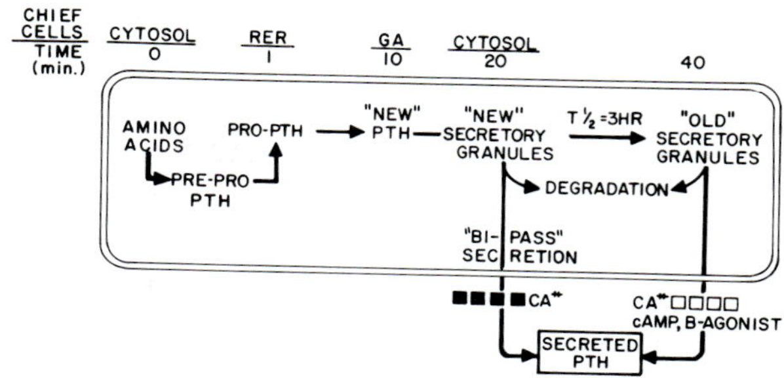

Fig. 6-33 Bypass secretion of PTH in response to increased demand signaled by decreased blood calcium ion concentration. Recently synthesized and progressed active PTH (1-84) may be released directly and not enter the storage pool of mature (''old'') secretory granules in the cytoplasm of chief cells. PTH from the storage pool can be mobilized by cAMP and β-agonists (such as epinephrine, norepinephrine, and isoproterenol), as well as by lowered blood calcium ion, whereas secretion from the pool of recently synthesized PTH can be stimulated only by a decreased calcium ion concentration. *RER,* rough endoplasmic reticulum; *GA,* Golgi apparatus.

cium intake of bulls is reduced. Cows fed similar rations rarely develop proliferative lesions of C cells because of the high physiologic requirements of pregnancy and lactation for calcium.

PARATHYROID GLANDS

Parathyroid glands in most animal species consist of two pairs of glands situated in the cranial cervical region. In the dog and cat, both the external and internal parathyroids are located close to the thyroid gland. Other animal species, such as the pig, have only a single pair of parathyroids cranial to the thyroid gland, embedded either in the thymus in young animals or in adipose connective tissue in adult animals. In cattle and sheep, the larger external parathyroid gland is located a considerable distance cranial to the thyroid gland in the loose connective tissue along the common carotid artery. The smaller internal parathyroid glands are situated on the dorsal and medial surface of the thyroid gland. In horses, the larger (''lower'') parathyroid gland in horses is located a considerable distance from the thyroid in the caudal cervical region near the bifurcation of the bicarotid trunk at the level of the first rib, while the smaller (''upper'') parathyroid is situated near the thyroid gland.

The parathyroid glands contain a single type of secretory cell responsible for the elaboration of one hormone. The parathyroids of animals and human beings are composed predominantly of chief cells in different stages of secretory activity and, in certain species, in transition to oxyphilic cells. Oxyphilic cells increase in number with advancing age and often form nodules in parathyroids of aged animals. They are larger than chief cells, and their abundant cytoplasm is filled with numerous large, often bizarre-shaped mitochondria.

Biologically active parathyroid hormone (PTH) secreted by chief cells is a straight-chain polypeptide consisting of 84 amino acid residues with a molecular weight of approximately 9,500. Secretory cells in the parathyroid glands of most animals store relatively small amounts of preformed hormone but are capable of responding to minor fluctuations in calcium ion concentration by rapidly altering the rate of hormonal secretion and, more slowly, by altering the rate of hormonal synthesis (Fig. 6-33). In contrast to most endocrine organs, which are under complex control, the parathyroid glands have a unique feedback control system based primarily on the concentration of calcium (and, to a lesser extent, of magnesium) ion in blood. Calcium ion concentration controls not only the rate of biosynthesis and secretion of parathyroid hormone but also other metabolic and intracellular degradative processes within chief cells. Increased calcium ion concentration in extracellular fluids rapidly inhibits the uptake of amino acids by chief cells, synthesis of proPTH and conversion to PTH, and secretion of stored PTH (Fig. 6-33).

PTH is the principal hormone involved in the minute-to-minute, fine regulation of blood calcium concentration in mammals. It does this by directly influencing the function of target cells located primarily in bone and kidneys and indirectly acting in the intestine to maintain plasma calcium concentration sufficient to ensure the optimal functioning of a wide variety of body cells. The overall action of PTH on bone is to mobilize calcium from skeletal reserves into extracellular fluids (Fig. 6-34). The response of bone to PTH is the result of increasing the activity of existing osteoclasts and osteocytes present in bone.

PTH has a rapid (within 5 to 10 minutes) and direct effect on renal tubular function, leading to decreased reabsorption of phosphate and phosphaturia. The site of ac-

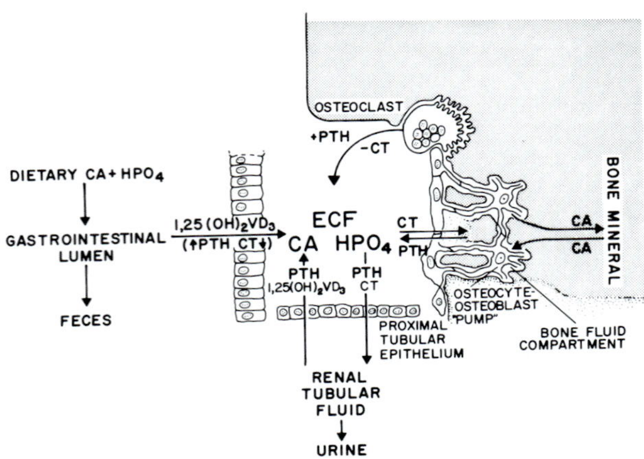

Fig. 6-34 Interrelation of PTH, calcitonin, and 1,25-$(OH)_2D_3$ in hormonal regulation of calcium and phosphorus in extracellular fluids.

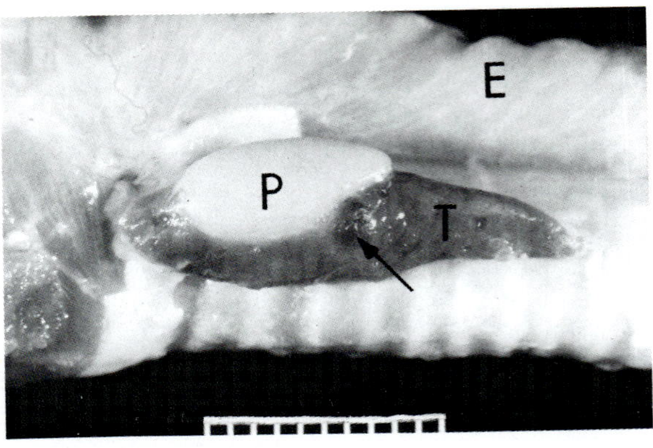

Fig. 6-35 Parathyroid gland; dog. Parathyroid cyst. The parathyroid cyst *(arrow)* was formed from the persistent and distended embryonic duct (*E*) that connects parathyroid-thymic primordia in the III and IV pharyngeal pouches (Kürsteiner's cyst). *T*, thyroid gland. Hyperplastic parathyroids (*P*) from a dog with chronic renal failure. Bar = 1 cm.

tion where PTH blocks tubular reabsorption of phosphate has been localized to the proximal tubule. Also, the ability of PTH to enhance the renal absorption of calcium is of considerable importance in the maintenance of calcium homeostasis. This effect of PTH upon tubular reabsorption of calcium appears to be due to a direct action on the distal convoluted tubule. Calcitonin and PTH, acting in concert, provide a dual negative feedback control mechanism to maintain within narrow limits the concentration of calcium in extracellular fluids.

The third major hormone involved in the regulation of calcium metabolism and skeletal remodeling is cholecalciferol or vitamin D_3 (Fig. 6-34). Cholecalciferol is ingested in small amounts in the diet and can be synthesized in the epidermis by the action of ultraviolet light on precursor molecules (e.g., 7-dehydrocholesterol) through a pre–vitamin D_3 intermediate form. The active metabolites of vitamin D increase the absorption of calcium and phosphorus from the intestine and, thereby, maintain adequate concentrations of these electrolytes in the extracellular fluids required for the appropriate mineralization of bone matrix. From a functional point of view, vitamin D brings about the retention of sufficient mineral ions to ensure mineralization of bone matrix, whereas PTH maintains the proper ratio of calcium to phosphorus in extracellular fluids. The major target tissue for 1,25-dihydroxycholecalciferol [1,25-$(OH)_2VD_3$] is the mucosa of the small intestine, where the vitamin increases the active transcellular transport of calcium (proximal small intestine) and phosphorus (distal small intestine).

Developmental Disturbances

Parathyroid cysts

Small cysts within the parenchyma of the parathyroid or in the immediate vicinity of the glands occur frequently in dogs but only occasionally in other animal species (Fig. 6-35). Parathyroid cysts are usually multiloculated, are lined by a cuboidal to columnar (often ciliated) epithelium, and contain a densely eosinophilic proteinic material. Parathyroid cysts (Kürsteiner's cysts) appear to develop from persistent and dilated remnants of the duct that connects the parathyroid and thymic primordia during embryonic development. Parathyroid cysts are distinct from midline cysts derived from remnants of the thyroglossal duct. The latter are lined by multilayered thyroidogenic epithelium that often has colloid-containing follicles and are usually located near the midline, from the base of the tongue to the mediastinum.

Degenerative Lesions of Parathyroid Chief Cells

Multinucleated syncytial cells

Parathyroid glands of dogs and rats may develop a unique multinucleated syncytial giant cell, which appears to form by the fusion of the cytoplasm of adjacent chief cells. These cells are often more numerous near the periphery of the parathyroid gland, but considerable numbers can be present in the more central portions. The number of syncytial cells varies considerably between parathyroids in the same animal and may equal half the parenchyma of the gland. Their cytoplasm is densely eosinophilic and homogeneous, and their plasma membrane is often indistinct. The nuclei are smaller, more hyperchromatic, and more oval than those of adjacent chief cells.

Inflammatory Lesions and Hypoparathyroidism

Lymphocytic parathyroiditis and hypoparathyroidism

In hypoparathyroidism, either the parathyroid glands secrete subnormal amounts of PTH or the hormone secreted is unable to interact with target cells. Hypoparathyroidism has been recognized in dogs—particularly in smaller breeds, such as schnauzers and terriers—but infrequently in other animal species. Idiopathic hypoparathyroidism in adult dogs is usually associated with diffuse lymphocytic parathyroiditis and is characterized by extensive degeneration of chief cells and replacement fibrosis. Early lesions are infiltrates of lymphocytes and plasma cells and nodular hyperplasia of remaining chief cells. Later, the parathyroid gland is completely replaced by lymphocytes, fibroblasts, and neocapillaries, with only an occasional viable chief cell remaining (Fig. 6-36). Lymphocytic parathyroiditis may develop by an immune-mediated mechanism, since a similar lymphocytic infiltration and destruction of secretory parenchyma has been produced in dogs by injection of emulsions of parathyroid gland in adjuvant. Other infrequent causes of hypoparathyroidism include invasion and destruction of parathyroid glands by primary or metastatic neoplasms in the cranial cervical region and tropic atrophy of parathyroid glands associated with long-term hypercalcemia. Also, the parathyroid glands may be damaged or inadvertently removed during thyroid surgery.

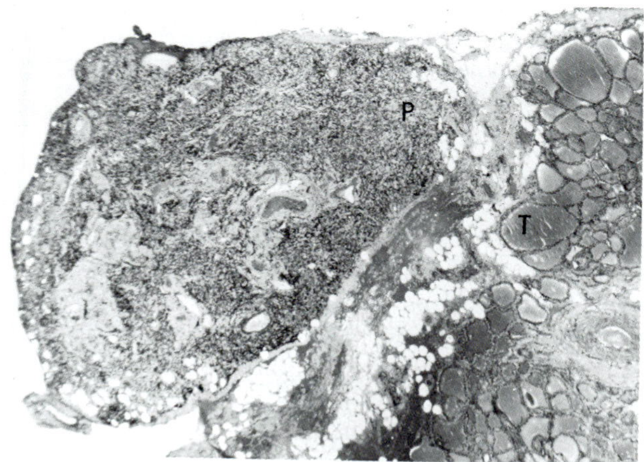

Fig. 6-36 Parathyroid gland, dog. Diffuse lymphocytic parathyroiditis (*P*). The external parathyroid gland has been completely replaced by lymphocytes, plasma cells, fibroblasts, and neocapillaries. *T*, thyroid gland. ×16.

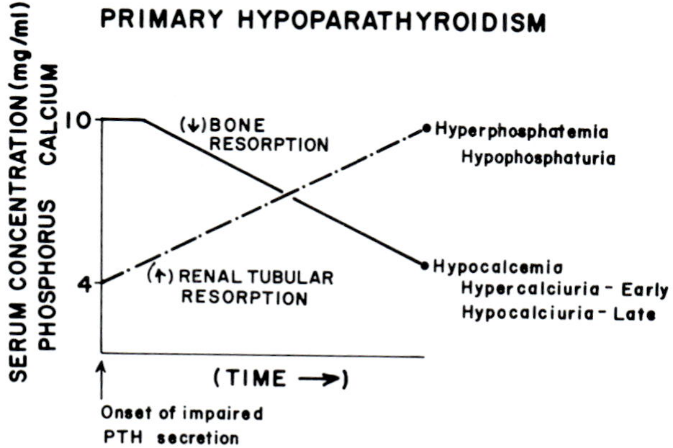

Fig. 6-37 Alterations in serum and phosphorus in response to an inadequate secretion of PTH. A progressive increase in serum phosphorus and a marked decline in the levels of serum calcium have resulted in increased neuromuscular excitability and tetany.

The functional disturbances and clinical manifestations of hypoparathyroidism are primarily the result of increased neuromuscular excitability and tetany. Because of the lack of PTH, bone resorption is decreased, and blood calcium concentrations diminish progressively to 4 to 6 mg/100 ml (Fig. 6-37). Affected animals are restless, nervous, ataxic, and weak and have intermittent tremors of separate muscle groups. Tremors may progress to generalized tetany and convulsive seizures. Concurrently, blood phosphorus concentrations are elevated because of increased renal tubular reabsorption.

Hyperplasia of Chief Cells

Hyperparathyroidism secondary to nutritional imbalances

Nutritional hyperparathyroidism occurs commonly in cats, dogs, certain nonhuman primates, horses, domestic and captive birds, and reptiles. The increased secretion of PTH is a compensatory mechanism induced by nutritional imbalances. Such imbalances occur with diets low in calcium, diets with excess phosphorus but with normal or low calcium, and diets with inadequate amounts of vitamin D_3 fed to New World primates housed indoors. The significant result is hypocalcemia, which stimulates the parathyroid glands. An elevated blood phosphorus concentration may contribute indirectly to parathyroid stimulation by decreasing the blood calcium concentration.

In response to the diet-induced hypocalcemia, chief cells undergo hypertrophy and, eventually, hyperplasia with increased lightly eosinophilic or vacuolated cytoplasm. The organelles concerned with protein synthesis and packaging of secretory products are well developed, and many chief cells stimulated chemically by 5 to 14 weeks of hypocalcemia may accumulate glycogen.

The most frequent nutritional imbalance causing hyperparathyroidism in horses is the ingestion of excessive amounts of phosphorus. Hyperphosphatemia stimulates the parathyroid gland indirectly by lowering the blood calcium concentration. These horses usually have been fed grain-rich diets with below-average-quality roughage. Evidence of high phosphorus intake may be difficult to establish as the excess phosphorus may have been in the form of a bran supplement to the grain ration. The diet is usually palatable and nutritious, except for the excessive phosphorous and marginal or deficient calcium content. A diet deficient in calcium fails to supply the daily requirement, and hypocalcemia develops, even though a greater proportion of ingested calcium is absorbed. Because in horses, changes in concentrations of urinary calcium and phosphorus are more consistent, they are more useful in the clinical diagnosis of nutritional secondary hyperparthyroidism than changes in blood concentrations of these minerals. The increased secretion of PTH acts on normal kidneys to markedly increase urinary phosphorus excretion, but to decrease calcium loss in the urine.

Hyperparathyroidism secondary to renal disease

Hyperparathyroidism as a complication of chronic renal failure is characterized by excessive production of PTH in response to chronic hypocalcemia. When the renal disease is severe enough to reduce the glomerular filtration rate, phosphorus is retained, and hyperphosphatemia develops. The increased blood phosphorus concentration contributes to parathyroid stimulation by lowering blood calcium concentration. Chronic renal disease impairs the production of 1,25-$(OH)_2VD_3$ by the kidneys and, thereby, diminishes intestinal calcium transport and increases mobilization of calcium from the skeleton. All four parathyroid glands undergo marked chief cell hyperplasia, and the bones have varying degrees of generalized fibrous osteodystrophy.

Hypocalcemia associated with parturition: Acute parathyroid stimulation

Parturient paresis in dairy cattle is a complex metabolic disease characterized by the development of severe hypocalcemia and hypophosphatemia near the time of parturition and the initiation of lactation. The serum calcium concentration falls to less than 50% of normal in spite of an increased secretion of PTH. Bone resorption remains low, and few osteoclasts are present on bone surfaces. Biochemical and ultrastructural studies indicate that the parathyroid glands are capable of responding to the acute hypocalcemia by increased development of cellular organelles for hormonal synthesis and by the increased secretion of PTH.

The composition of the diet fed to dairy cows is a significant factor in the pathogenesis of parturient hypocalcemia. High-calcium diets have been incriminated in significantly increasing the incidence of the disease. Conversely, low-calcium diets or diets supplemented with pharmacologic doses of vitamin D reduce the incidence of parturient hypocalcemia. Calcium homeostasis in pregnant cows fed a high-calcium diet appears to be maintained principally by intestinal calcium absorption (Fig. 6-38). This greater reliance on intestinal absorption rather than on PTH-stimulated bone resorption probably is a significant factor in the more frequent development of profound hypocalcemia near parturition in cows fed high-calcium prepartal diets.

An increased secretion of calcitonin, prepartum, in cows that develop parturient hypocalcemia (''milk fever''), especially those fed high-calcium diets, may be one factor that contributes to the inability of increased PTH concentrations to mobilize calcium rapidly from skeletal reserves

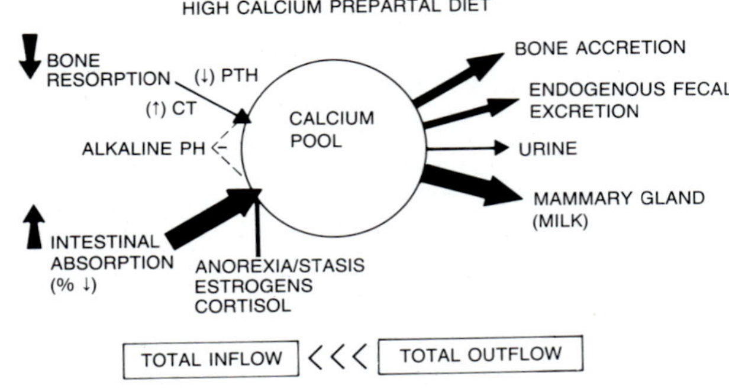

Fig. 6-38 Calcium homeostasis in cows fed a high-calcium prepartal diet. The calcium homeostasis is primarily dependent upon intestinal calcium absorption. The rate of bone resorption is low, and parathyroid glands are inactive. Anorexia and gastrointestinal stasis, which often occur near parturition, interrupt the major inflow into the extracellular fluid calcium pool. Outflow of calcium with the onset of lactation exceeds the rate of inflow into the calcium pool, and the cows develop a progressive hypocalcemia and paresis.

and maintain blood calcium concentrations during the critical period near parturition. The thyroid's content of calcitonin is reduced, many C cells are degranulated, and plasma concentrations of calcitonin often are increased in cows prior to the development of profound hypocalcemia.

Neoplasms of Chief Cells: Primary Hyperparathyroidism

Adenomas and carcinomas of parathyroid glands often secrete PTH far in excess of normal, resulting in a syndrome of primary hyperparathyroidism. A prolonged increased secretion of PTH accelerates osteolytic and osteoclastic bone resorption. Mineral removed from the skeleton at an accelerated rate is replaced by immature fibrous connective tissue. The lesions of fibrous osteodystrophy are generalized throughout the skeleton, but are accentuated in local areas.

Adenomas of parathyroid glands are encountered in older animals, particularly in dogs and infrequently in certain strains of rats. Parathyroid gland carcinomas are rare in animals. Chief cell adenomas usually cause considerable enlargement of a single parathyroid gland. Grossly, these are light brown to red and are located either in the cervical region adjacent to the thyroid gland or, infrequently, within the thoracic cavity near the base of the heart. Parathyroid adenomas are encapsulated and sharply demarcated from the adjacent thyroid gland.

Parathyroid gland adenomas are composed of closely packed, small groups of chief cells enclosed by delicate connective tissue septa that have many capillaries (Fig. 6-39). The chief cells are round to polyhedral and have lightly eosinophilic cytoplasm. The expanded cytoplasm of neoplastic chief cells contains few electron-dense secretory

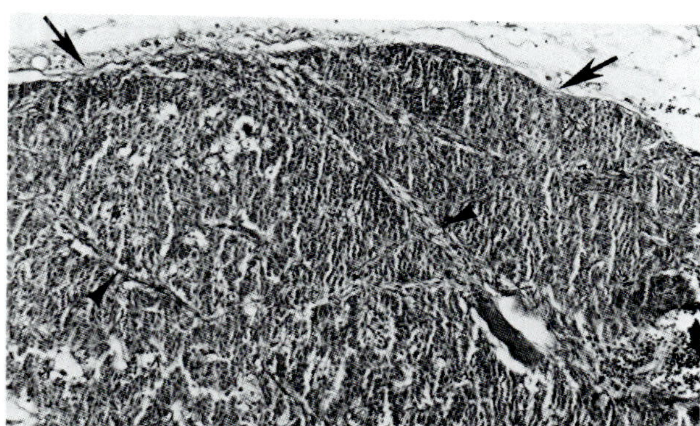

Fig. 6-39 Parathyroid gland; dog. Adenoma. Closely packed chief cells are formed into small groups by fine fibrous septa containing capillaries *(arrowheads)*. A thin capsule of fibrous connective tissue *(arrows)* surrounds the neoplasm. Hematoxylin-eosin (H & E) stain; ×125.

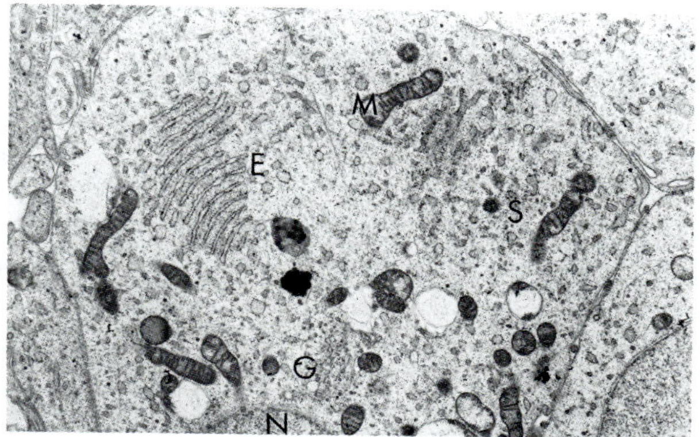

Fig. 6-40 Parathyroid gland; dog. Adenoma. Active chief cells have large lamellar arrays of rough endoplasmic reticulum (*E*), prominent Golgi apparatus (*G*), and large mitochondria (*M*) but few secretory granules (*S*). *N*, nucleus of chief cell. ×7100.

granules and prominent arrays of endoplasmic reticulum and Golgi complexes (Fig. 6-40).

The functional disturbances observed with endocrinologically active chief cell neoplasms are primarily the result of a weakening of bones by excessive resorption of calcium. Cortical bone is thinned due to increased resorption by osteoclasts stimulated by the autonomous secretion of PTH (Fig. 6-41). Lameness due to fractures of long bones may occur after relatively minor physical trauma. Compression fractures of vertebral bodies can exert pressure on the spinal cord and nerves, resulting in motor or sensory dysfunction or both. Facial hyperostosis due to extensive osteoblastic proliferation and deposition of poorly mineralized osteoid and loosening or loss of teeth from alveolar sockets has been observed in dogs with primary hyperparathyroidism. Hypercalcemia results in anorexia, vomiting, constipation, depression, polyuria, polydipsia, and generalized muscular weakness due to decreased neuromuscular excitability.

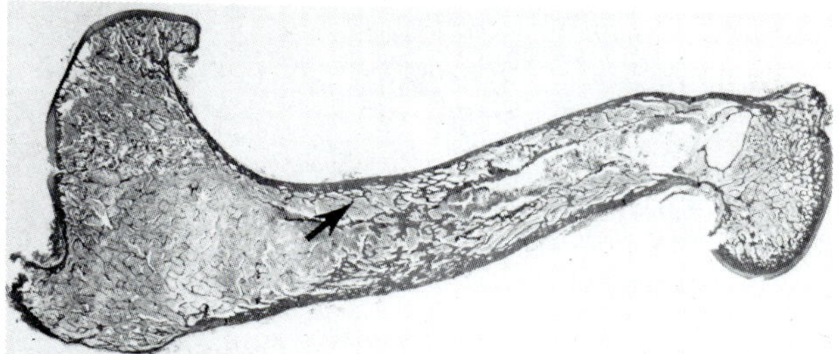

Fig. 6-41 Humerus; dog. Primary hyperparathyroidism. Severe thinning of cortical bone and large resorptive cavities *(arrow)* results from localized resorption of bone by osteoclasts.

The most important and practical laboratory test to aid in the diagnosis of primary hyperparathyroidism is quantification of the total blood calcium concentration. Dogs with primary hyperparathyroidism have greatly elevated blood calcium concentrations (12 to 20 mg/100 ml or above). The blood phosphorus concentration is low (4 mg/100 ml or less) or in the low-normal range because of inhibition of renal tubular reabsorption of phosphorus by the autonomous secretion of PTH. The urinary excretion of calcium and phosphorus is increased and may predispose to the development of nephrocalcinosis and urolithiasis.

Humoral Hypercalcemia of Malignancy: Pseudohyperparathyroidism

Humoral hypercalcemia of malignancy (HHM) is a metabolic disorder in which PTH-related peptides or other bone-resorbing substances are secreted in excessive amounts by malignant neoplasms of non–parathyroid gland origin. Criteria for the diagnosis of HHM include (1) persistent hypercalcemia and hypophosphatemia, (2) absence of radiographic or pathologic evidence of metastases in bone, (3) atrophy of parathyroid glands and thyroid C cell hyperplasia, (4) remission of hypercalcemia when the neoplasm is destroyed or excised, (5) demonstration of immunologically or biologically active bone-resorbing substances in the neoplasm, and (6) exacerbation of hypercalcemia if the neoplasm recurs following therapy. Dogs and human beings develop hypercalcemia and hypophosphatemia with several different types of malignant neoplasms, but metastases to bone and functional lesions of the parathyroid glands are absent. The persistent hypercalcemia is the result of the combined effects of humoral factors on the calcium homeostasis of bone, kidneys, and intestine.

A syndrome of HHM in aged, primarily female dogs with anal sac apocrine gland adenocarcinomas has been characterized. The dogs have persistent hypercalcemia (range: 11.4 to 24 mg/dl; mean: 16.2 mg/dl) and, often, hypophosphatemia that returns to normal following surgi-

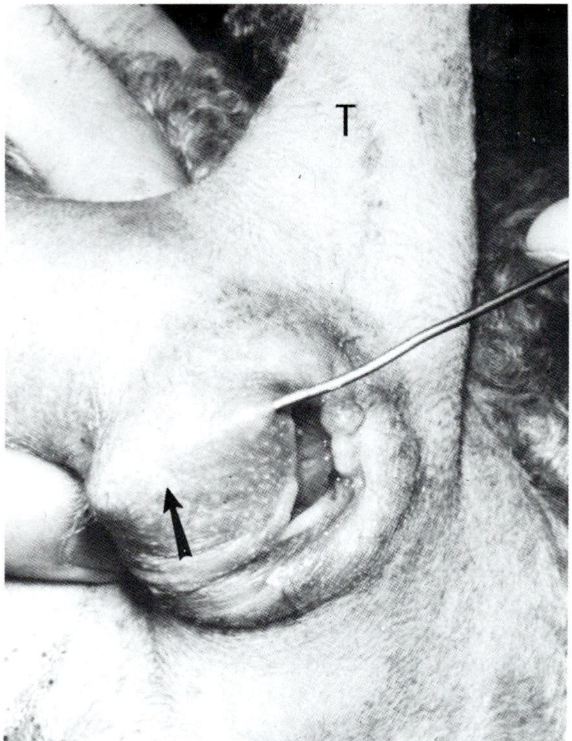

Fig. 6-42 Perirectal region; dog. Small adenocarcinoma *(arrow)* derived from apocrine glands of the anal sac enlarges the region and protrudes as a nodular lesion. *T*, tail.

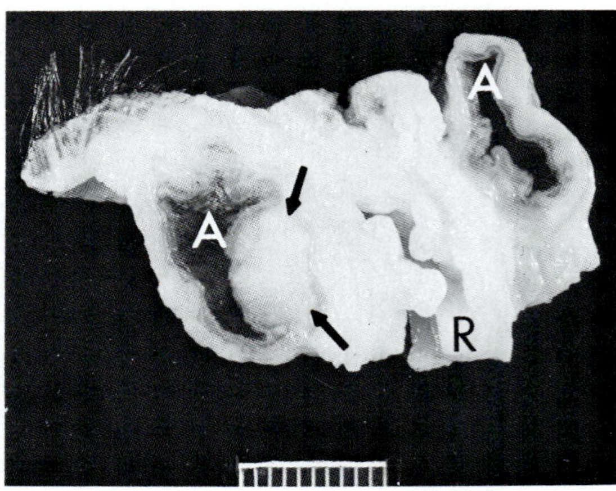

Fig. 6-43 Perineum (transverse section); dog. Adenocarcinoma. A neoplasm derived from apocrine glands of the anal sac is present as a 1-cm diameter nodule *(arrows)* arising in the wall of the left anal sac and protruding into its lumen. Anal sacs (*A*) are present on both sides of the rectum (*R*). Bar = 1 cm. *Meuten DJ, Cooper BJ, Capen CC, et al. Vet Pathol 1981; 18:454-471.*

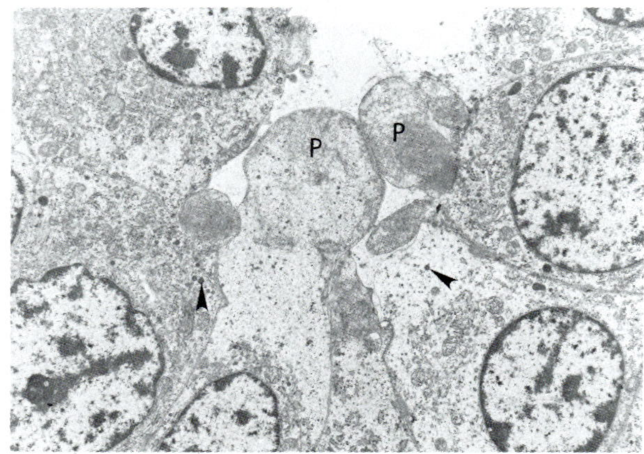

Fig. 6-44 Anal sac; dog. Adenocarcinoma. Projections (*P*) of apical cytoplasm extend into the lumen of acinus. Small membrane-limited secretory granules *(arrowheads)* are present in the cytoplasm. *Meuten DJ, Capen CC, Kociba GJ, Chew DJ. Am J Pathol 1982; 107:167-175.*

cal excision of the neoplasm. The hypercalcemia persists following removal of the parathyroid glands, suggesting that the factor produced by neoplastic cells does not stimulate an increased secretion of PTH. Increased circulating concentrations of PTH-related protein (PTHrP) have been observed in these dogs. Most neoplasms are histopathologically malignant, and most have metastasized to iliac and sublumbar lymph nodes. Clinical signs include generalized muscular weakness, anorexia, vomiting, bradycardia, depression, polyuria, and polydipsia. These signs are primarily the result of severe hypercalcemia.

Anal sac apocrine adenocarcinomas develop as a firm mass, usually unilateral, ventrolateral to the anus, close to the anal sac but not attached to the overlying skin (Fig. 6-42). The neoplasm arises in the wall of the anal sac and projects as a variably sized mass into its lumen (Fig. 6-43).

This unique adenocarcinoma forms glandular acini and projections of apical cytoplasm that extend into the lumen (Fig. 6-44) and is histologically distinct from the more common perianal (circumanal) gland tumor. The majority of neoplasms are histologically bimorphic and contain glandular and solid areas. The solid pattern is characterized by sheets, microlobules, and packets separated by a thin, fibrovascular stroma. Pseudorosettes are common in solid areas adjacent to small blood vessels.

The parathyroid glands are small and difficult to locate or not visible macroscopically. Atrophic parathyroid glands in dogs with HHM are characterized by narrow cords of inactive chief cells with an abundant fibrous connective tissue stroma and widened perivascular spaces. The parathyroid glands respond to the persistent cancer-associated hypercalcemia by tropic atrophy. Thyroid C cells, in response to the persistent elevation in the blood calcium concentration, undergo either diffuse or nodular hyperplasia.

Renal calcification has been detected microscopically in

approximately 90% of dogs with HHM associated with anal sac apocrine gland adenocarcinomas, particularly when the calcium × phosphorus product is 50 or greater. Tubular calcification is most pronounced near the corticomedullary junction but also is present in cortical and deep medullary tubules, Bowman's capsule, and the glomerular tuft. Calcification also occurs in the gastric fundic mucosa and endocardium.

Hypercalcemia Associated with Lymphosarcoma

Lymphosarcoma is the most common neoplasm associated with hypercalcemia in dogs and cats. Estimates of the prevalence of hypercalcemia in dogs with lymphosarcoma vary from 10% to 40%. Peripheral lymph node enlargement may or may not be present, but usually cranial mediastinal or visceral nodes are involved. The hypercalcemia may be in response to the production of humoral substances by neoplastic cells, physical disruption of trabecular bone by lymphosarcoma in bone marrow, or both mechanisms. Serum immunoreactive PTH concentrations have been subnormal, and plasma prostaglandin E_2 concentrations did not differ from those of controls. Circulating concentrations of PTHrP are increased when compared with those of controls and normocalcemic dogs with lymphosarcoma. PTHrP concentration decreased following medical or surgical treatment of the lymphosarcoma.

PANCREATIC ISLETS

The endocrine function of the pancreas is performed by small groups of cells ("islets of Langerhans") that are completely surrounded by acinar (exocrine) cells that produce digestive enzymes (Fig. 6-45). During embryonic development of the pancreas, a close relationship exists between the endocrine and exocrine portions. Evidence suggests that islet, acinar, and ductal cells arise from a common multipotential precursor cell. In early embryonic development, the endocrine cells are integrated within the exocrine matrix of the pancreatic bud. They subsequently accumulate in nonvascularized clusters and later become isolated from the exocrine tissue and independently vascularized.

The pancreatic islets of normal animals contain multiple types of cells. Beta cells, the predominant secretory cells, function in the biosynthesis of insulin. The glucagon-secreting alpha cells are less numerous. The different cell types of the endocrine pancreas can be differentiated by immunohistochemical techniques (Fig. 6-45) and by electron microscopy (Fig. 6-46). Alpha, beta, and delta cells have well-developed cytoplasmic organelles that synthesize polypeptide hormones. The rough endoplasmic reticulum and Golgi apparatus are prominent, and numerous secretory ("storage") granules are present in the cytoplasm. Each type of endocrine cell in the pancreatic islets has distinctive secretory granules with characteristics that aid in their identification (Fig. 6-46).

The major physiologic stimulus for the release of insulin from beta cells is glucose. The plasma membrane of beta cells has specific receptors that bind glucose; as a result, the adenylate cyclase system in the plasma membrane is activated, leading to formation of cAMP from ATP in the presence of magnesium ion. An appropriate concentration of calcium ion in extracellular fluids is required for induction of insulin release from beta cells.

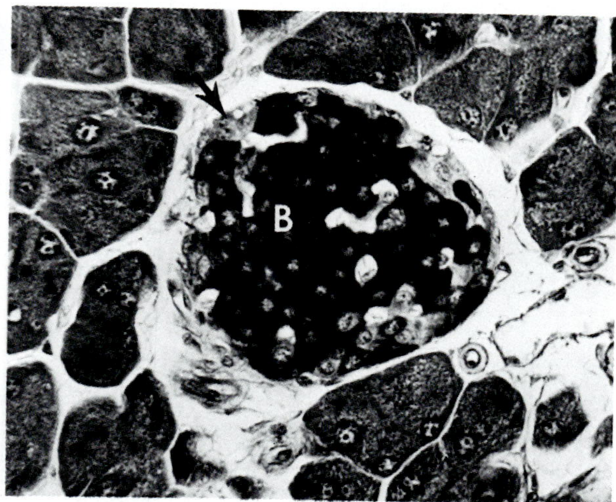

Fig. 6-45 Pancreatic islet; dog. Normal. Gomori's aldehyde fuchsin stains the centrally located beta cells (*B*) surrounded by a thin rim of poorly staining alpha and delta cells *(arrows)* at the periphery. The islets are surrounded by the exocrine pancreas (*P*).

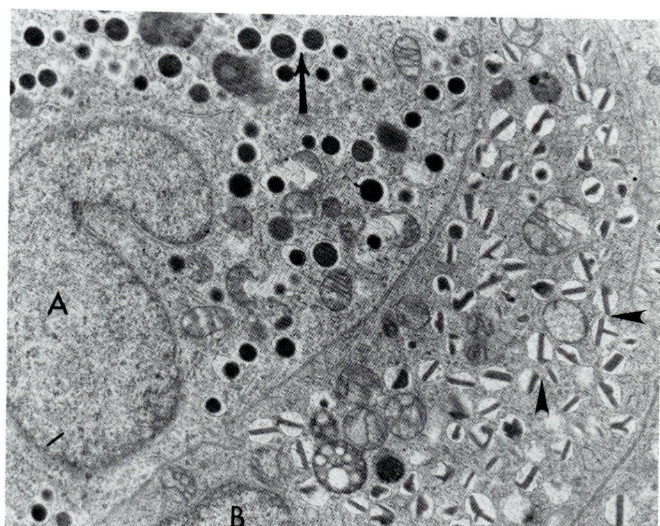

Fig. 6-46 Pancreatic islet; normal dog. Differences in secretion granules between beta (*B*) and alpha (*A*) cells; the internal cores of secretion granules in beta cells *(arrowheads)* are bar- or Y-shaped, with a prominent space between the limiting membrane and internal core. Secretion granules of the glucagon-secreting alpha cell have an electron-dense, circular, internal core with a narrow submembranous space *(arrow)*.

Insulin is a powerful hormone with broad biologic influences and affects either directly or indirectly the structure and function of every organ in the body. Tissues and cells especially responsive to insulin include skeletal and cardiac muscle, adipose tissue, fibroblasts, liver, leukocytes, mammary glands, cartilage, bone, skin, aorta, pituitary gland, and peripheral nerves. The main function of insulin is to stimulate anabolic reactions involving carbohydrates, fats, proteins, and nucleic acids. It catalyzes the formation of macromolecules used in cell structure, energy stores, and regulation of many cell functions. Liver, adipose cells, and muscle are three principal target sites for the action in insulin. In general, insulin increases the transfer of glucose and certain other monosaccharides, some amino acids and fatty acids, and potassium and magnesium ions across the plasma membrane of target cells; enhances glucose oxidation and glycogenesis; and stimulates lipogenesis and the formation of ATP, DNA, and RNA. Insulin also decreases the rate of lipolysis, proteolysis, ketogenesis, and gluconeogenesis.

Glucagon secreted in response to a reduction in blood glucose concentration is a hormone that stimulates energy release from target cells. It mobilizes stores of energy-yielding nutrients by increasing glycogenolysis, gluconeogenesis, and lipolysis, thereby increasing the blood concentration of glucose. At physiologic concentrations, glucagon increases both hepatic glycogenolysis and gluconeogenesis. Insulin and glucagon act in concert to maintain the concentration of glucose in extracellular fluids within relatively narrow limits. A "glucose sensor" in the pancreatic islets controls the relative mixture of these two biologic antagonists secreted from the beta and alpha cells of the islets. Glucagon controls the influx of glucose into the extracellular space from the liver, and insulin controls efflux of glucose from the extracellular space into such insulin-sensitive tissues as fat, muscle, and liver.

Hypofunction: Diabetes Mellitus

Diabetes mellitus is a metabolic disorder that results from diminished availability of insulin for normal function of many cells of the body. In some cases, increased concentrations of glucagon contribute to development of the persistent hyperglycemia. Insulin unavailability may be due to degenerative changes in beta cells of the pancreatic islets, reduced effectiveness of the hormone due to the formation of antiinsulin antibodies or inactive complexes, immune-mediated islet cytotoxicity, and inappropriate secretion of hormones by neoplasms in other endocrine organs.

With a reported incidence of 1:200, diabetes mellitus is a common endocrinopathy in dogs. Most cases of spontaneous diabetes occur in mature dogs, and in females approximately twice as often as males. There appears to be an increased incidence of diabetes mellitus in certain small breeds of dogs, such as miniature poodle, dachshund, and terrier, but nearly all breeds of dogs can be affected.

The pathogenic mechanisms of diabetes mellitus responsible for the diminished available insulin are multiple. Destruction of islets secondary to severe pancreatitis or selective degeneration of islet cells is the usual cause. In dogs, the pancreatic islets are often destroyed secondary to an inflammatory disease of the exocrine pancreas. Chronic relapsing pancreatitis with progressive loss of both exocrine and endocrine cells and replacement by fibrous connective tissue is a frequent cause of diabetes mellitus. In these dogs, the pancreas becomes firm and multinodular and often has scattered areas of hemorrhage and necrosis (Fig. 6-47). Later in the course of the disease, all that remains of the pancreas may be a thin fibrous band or nodule near the duodenum and stomach (Fig. 6-48). Selective destruction of islet cells by infiltration of islets with amyloid, glycogen, and collagen is a less frequent cause of diabetes mellitus in dogs than in cats. In other cases, beta cells are decreased and have vacuolated cytoplasm; in long-standing cases, the islets are difficult to find.

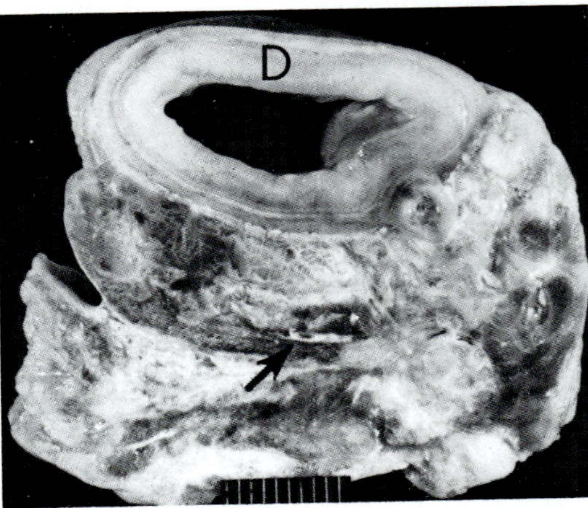

Fig. 6-47 Pancreas; dog. Chronic relapsing pancreatitis. The pancreas is multinodular and firm with areas of hemorrhage *(arrow)* and necrosis. *D*, duodenum. Bar = 1 cm.

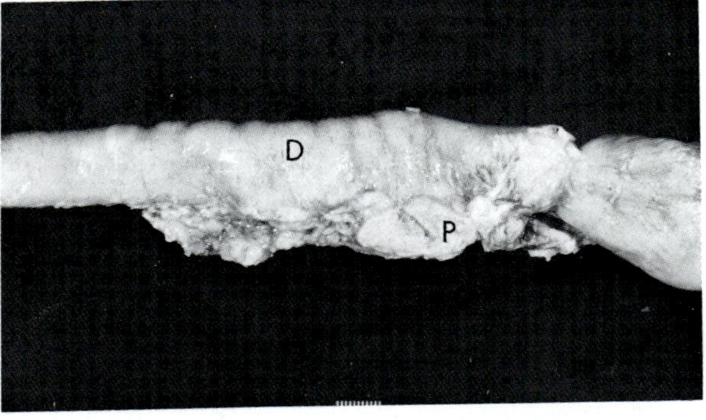

Fig. 6-48 Pancreas; dog. Chronic pancreatitis. The parenchyma of the pancreas (*P*) is nearly replaced by fibrous connective tissue in "end-stage" pancreatitis. *D*, duodenum.

Development of diabetes mellitus in young dogs may be associated with idiopathic atrophy of the pancreas, acute pancreatitis with necrosis and hemorrhage, and aplasia of pancreatic islets. The overall size of the pancreas with idiopathic atrophy is reduced to a third or less of normal. Hypoplasia of pancreatic islets has caused diabetes mellitus in young dogs (2 to 3 months of age). The islets are absent, but the pancreatic acini and ducts are present and functional.

Cats with diabetes mellitus usually have specific degenerative lesions localized selectively in the islets of Langerhans, whereas the remainder of the pancreas appears normal. The selective deposition of amyloid in islets, resulting in degenerative changes in alpha and beta cells, is the most common pancreatic lesion in cats with diabetes; however, scattered amyloid deposits occur in the pancreatic islets of many cats without diabetes mellitus. Another common islet lesion in cats with diabetes mellitus is hydropic (vacuolar) degeneration of the beta and alpha cells (Fig. 6-49). The cytoplasm of beta cells is expanded by massive accumulation of glycogen particles (Fig. 6-50). Vacuolar degeneration with glycogen accumulation in cats appears to develop in beta cells in response to long-term overstimulation (''exhaustion'') because of insulin resistance.

The onset of diabetes is insidious, and the clinical course is often chronic. In dogs, the signs most often associated with diabetes mellitus include polydipsia, polyuria, increased feed consumption, weight loss, bilateral cataracts, and weakness. The disturbances in water metabolism have a primarily osmotic basis. In dogs with persistent hyperglycemia and glycosuria, the renal tubular epithelium is unable to concentrate the urine effectively against the osmotic attraction of glucose in the glomerular filtrate.

Animals with diabetes have diminished resistance to bacterial or fungal infections and often develop chronic or recurrent infections, such as suppurative cystitis, prostatitis, bronchopneumonia, and dermatitis. This increased susceptibility to infection in patients with poorly controlled diabetes may be related in part to impaired chemotactic, phagocytic, and microbicidal functions and adherence of polymorphonuclear leukocytes. The impaired microbicidal function may have a metabolic basis, the result of diminished cellular energy production from glucose. These defects in leukocyte function are at least partially corrected by appropriate treatment of the diabetes. Radiographic evidence of emphysematous cystitis is strongly suggestive of diabetes mellitus. Infections of the urinary bladder with glucose-fermenting organisms, such as *Proteus* sp., *Aerobacter aerogenous,* and *Escherichia coli,* result in gas formation in the wall and lumen. Emphysema also may develop in the gallbladder wall in dogs with diabetes.

Hepatomegaly, due to fatty degeneration and cirrhosis, may occur. Lipids accumulate in the liver as the result of increased fat mobilization, and hepatocytes, injured by ketonemia, have decreased utilization of fats. Individual hepatocytes are greatly enlarged by multiple droplets of neutral lipid (Fig. 6-51). If the accumulation of lipid is extensive and long-standing, nutritional cirrhosis may develop. The liver remains enlarged, and its surface becomes coarsely nodular because of extensive remodeling of hepatic parenchyma (Fig. 6-52). Degenerated hepatocytes are replaced by regenerative nodules and interlobular fibrosis. Icterus and bilirubinuria often accompany severe cirrhosis.

Cataracts often develop in dogs with poorly controlled diabetes mellitus. They are stellate (''asteroidal'') (Fig. 6-53) and initially appear along the suture lines of lenticular

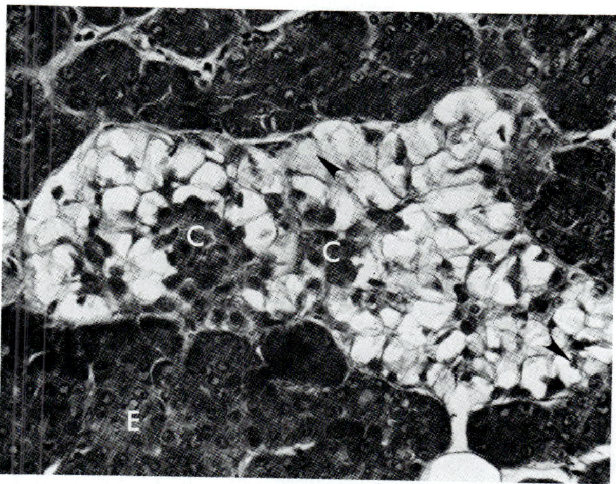

Fig. 6-49 Pancreas; islet, cat. Hydropic (''vacuolar'') degeneration. Discrete vacuoles *(arrowheads)* are present in the cytoplasm of beta cells. A few viable secretory cells remain adjacent to several capillaries (*C*). *E*, exocrine pancreas. ×315.

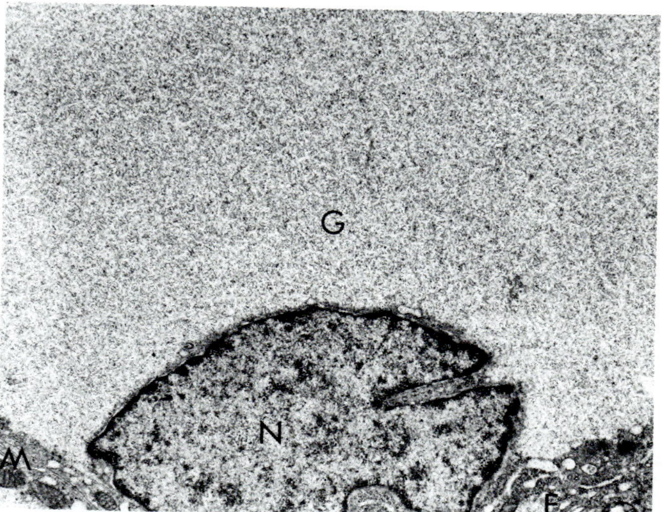

Fig. 6-50 Pancreas, islet; cat. Glycogen accumulation in beta cell. The nucleus (*N*) and secretory organelles are displaced to the periphery of the beta cell by the accumulation of glycogen (*G*) particles. ×4000.

fibers. Their formation is related to the unique sorbitol pathway by which glucose is metabolized in the lens. Glucose is first converted to sorbitol by the enzyme aldose reductase and, subsequently, to fructose by sorbitol dehydrogenase. These sugar alcohols accumulate within the lens and result in an intracellular accumulation of solute and hypertonicity. The initial structural change in the lens consists of swelling and hydropic degeneration of lenticular fibers, and, in long-standing cases, the majority of lenticular fibers are affected. In the later phases, macromolecular aggregation or precipitation of normally translucent lenticular proteins by disruption of lenticular fibers and formation of interfibrillar clefts occurs. This results in the diffuse, often bilateral, opacity of the lens observed in animals with chronic diabetes mellitus.

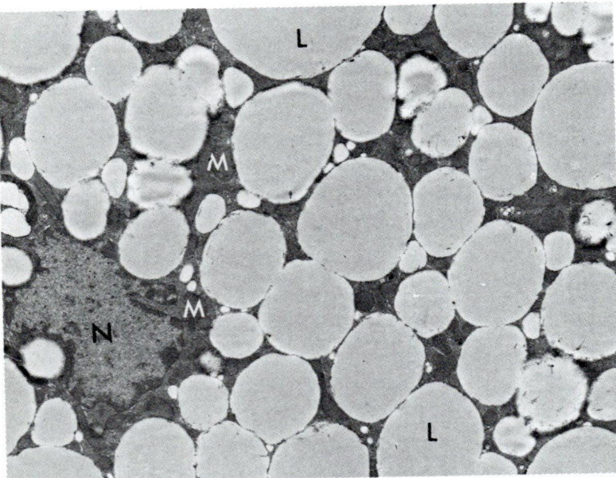

Fig. 6-51 Liver; dog. Fatty degeneration. The cytoplasm contains multiple large lipid droplets (*L*) that have displaced the nucleus (*N*) peripherally and compressed cytoplasmic organelles such as mitochondria (*M*). ×6600.

Other extrapancreatic lesions of diabetes mellitus, such as chronic renal disease, blindness, and gangrene, are the result of microangiopathy characterized by thickening of the capillary basement membrane. Dogs with long-standing, poorly controlled, spontaneous diabetes mellitus may develop nodular or diffuse glomerulosclerosis characterized by PAS-positive fibrillar deposits of glycoprotein that sometimes form spherical nodules in the glomerular capillary tufts. Other renal lesions include accumulation of glycogen within cells of Henle's loop (intracytoplasmic) and distal convoluted tubule (intranuclear) (Fig. 6-54).

Complete expression of the complex metabolic disturbances in diabetes mellitus appears to be the result of a bihormonal abnormality. Although a relative or absolute deficiency of insulin action in response to a rising extracellular glucose concentration has been long recognized as the *sine qua non* of diabetes mellitus, the importance of an absolute or relative increase of glucagon secretion in most forms of the disease has been appreciated only recently. Hyperglucagonemia in patients with diabetes may be the result of increased secretion of pancreatic glucagon, of enteroglucagon, or of both. Increased blood glucagon con-

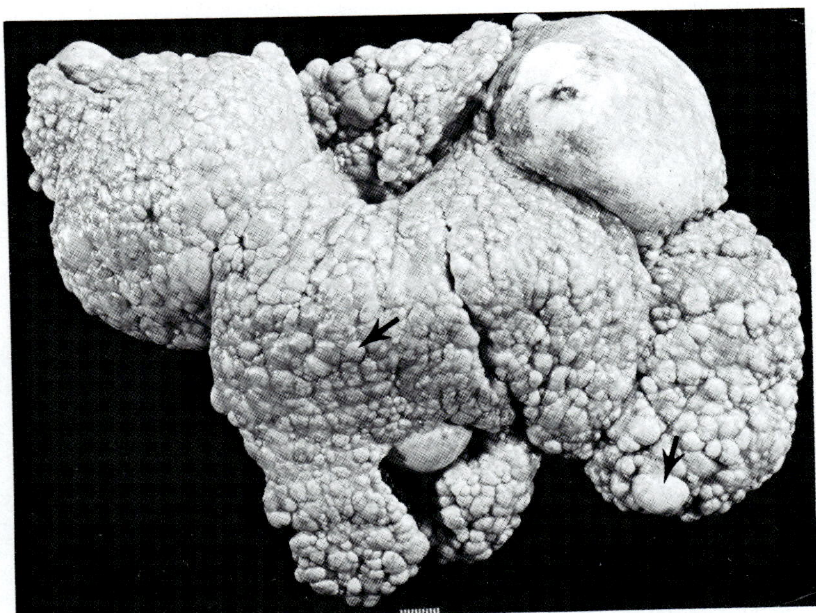

Fig. 6-52 Liver; dog. Cirrhosis. All lobes of the liver were considerably enlarged and firm and had a coarsely nodular surface. The nodules *(arrows)* represent areas of regenerative hyperplasia of hepatocytes.

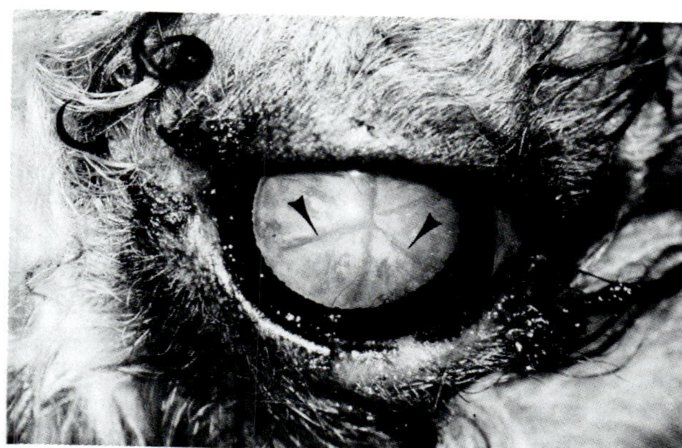

Fig. 6-53 Eyeball, lens; dog. Diabetes mellitus. Early stellate cataract *(arrowheads)* along the sutures of the lens.

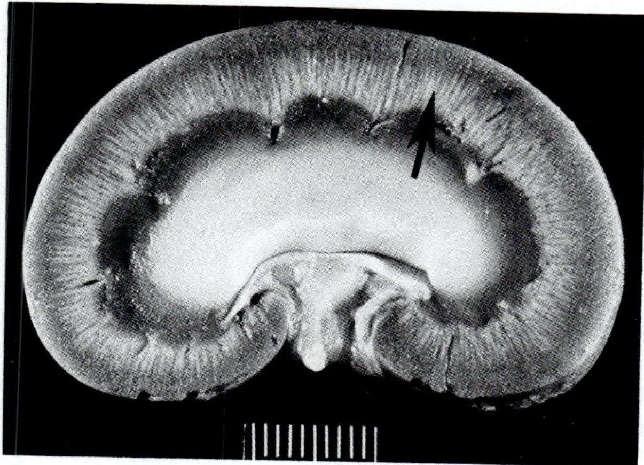

Fig. 6-54 Kidney, dog. Glycogen ''nephrosis,'' diabetes mellitus. The radially arranged light areas in the inner cortex of the kidney *(arrow)* represent prominent tubules with an abnormal accumulation of glycogen.

tributes to the severe endogenous hyperglycemia by mobilizing hepatic stores of glucose and to the development of ketoacidosis by increasing the oxidation of fatty acids by the liver. The major glucoregulatory consequence of insulin deficiency is reduction of movement of glucose into insulin-sensitive tissues (e.g., liver, fat, and muscle), with a corresponding increase in hepatic glucose production, resulting in marked endogenous hyperglycemia. Two abnormalities in alpha cell function have been described in severe diabetes: (1) loss of the glucose-sensing capacity, resulting in increased glucagon secretion associated with an increasing blood glucose concentration; and (2) an exaggerated response to stimulation with arginine or alanine.

Hyperfunction of Pancreatic Islets

Beta cell (insulin-secreting) neoplasms

The most frequently occurring neoplasms arising in pancreatic islets are adenomas and carcinomas derived from beta cells. These neoplasms often are endocrinologically active and produce dramatic functional disturbances. Other pancreatic neoplasms appear to be derived from multipotential ductal epithelial cells, which differentiate into one of the several other cell types of the pancreatic islets. Beta cell neoplasms are seen most frequently in dogs 5 to 12 years of age (mean: 9 years). These neoplasms also occur in older cattle and may be associated with periodic convulsive seizures.

Adenomas of the beta cells of the pancreatic islets (''insulinomas'') usually appear as a single yellow to dark red, spherical, small (1 to 3 cm) nodule. They are of a consistency similar to or slightly firmer than that of the surrounding pancreas. Adenomas occur singly or occasionally as multiple nodules in the same or different lobes of the pancreas. A thin layer of fibrous connective tissue separates the adenoma from the adjacent parenchyma (Fig. 6-55).

In dogs, carcinomas of the pancreatic islets are more common than adenomas and are more common in the duodenal (right) lobe of the pancreas. Carcinomas of the pancreatic islets can be differentiated from adenomas by their larger size, multilobular appearance, extensive invasion of adjacent parenchyma and lymph vessels, and metastases to extrapancreatic sites, such as regional lymph nodes, liver, mesentery, and omentum.

Islet cell adenomas are sharply delineated and surrounded by a thin capsule of fibrous connective tissue (Fig. 6-55). Small nests of acinar epithelial cells may be present throughout the neoplasm, particularly at the periphery. Numerous connective tissue septa containing small capillaries radiate from the capsule into the neoplasm, subdividing it into small lobules or packets. The neoplastic cells are well differentiated, vary from round to polyhedral, have a lightly eosinophilic and finely granular cytoplasm, and have indistinct cellular membranes.

Islet cell carcinomas are consistently larger than ade-

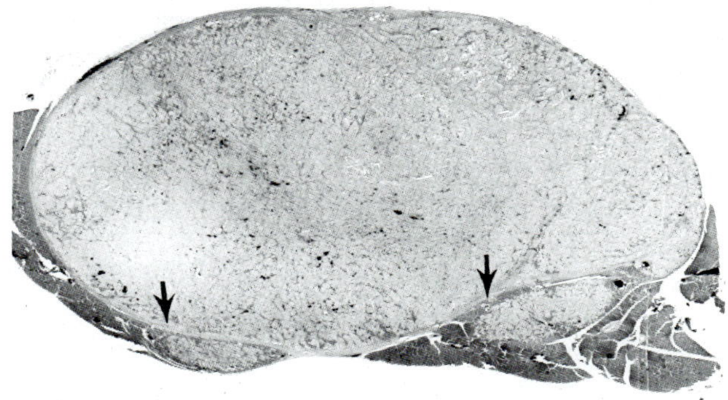

Fig. 6-55 Pancreas, islet; dog. Beta cell adenoma. The thin fibrous capsule around the adenoma may be incomplete at several points *(arrows)* where there is intermingling of islet and acinar epithelial cells.

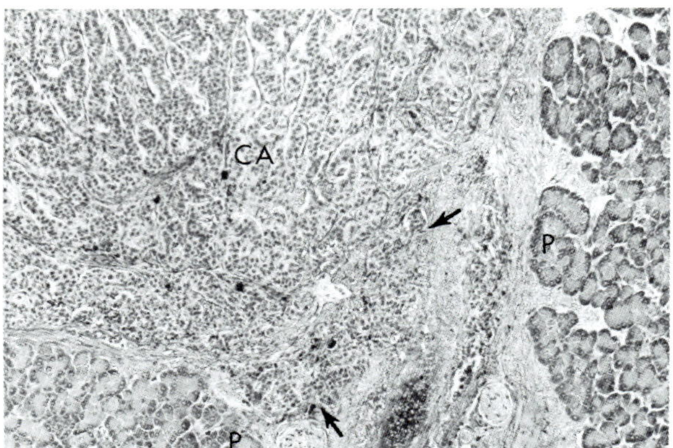

Fig. 6-56 Pancreas, islet; dog. Beta cell carcinoma. Neuroendocrine packeting of neoplastic cells (*CA*) and invasion of carcinoma through the fibrous capsule *(arrows)* into adjacent exocrine pancreas.

nomas, are multilobular, and invade into and through the fibrous capsule of the adjacent pancreas (Fig. 6-56). The dense bands of fibrous tissue that course through the neoplasm give rise to fine connective tissue septa containing capillaries that subdivide the neoplasm into small cords or lobules. The well-differentiated neoplastic cells in islet cell carcinomas are closely packed but may be less uniform in size and shape than cells of adenomas. They are round to polyhedral and have a granular eosinophilic cytoplasm. Mitotic figures are not numerous. Cells composing functional islet cells neoplasms in dogs have ultrastructural, histochemical, and immunocytochemical characteristics of beta cells. The neoplastic beta cells are electron-dense because of the numerous cytoplasmic organelles.

The clinical alterations observed with functional beta cell neoplasms are the result of excessive insulin secretion and the development of severe hypoglycemia. The clinical signs are reflective of hypoglycemia and are not specific for the hyperinsulinism produced by beta cell neoplasms. Initial signs include weakness, fatigue after vigorous exercise, generalized muscular twitching and weakness, ataxia, mental confusion, and changes of temperament. These dogs are easily agitated and have intermittent periods of excitability and restlessness. Periodic convulsive seizures of the tonic-clonic type occur later in the disease and increase progressively in frequency and intensity.

The predominance of clinical signs relating to the CNS demonstrates the primary dependence of the brain on the metabolism of glucose for energy. The failure to recognize that dogs with functional islet cell neoplasms may be presented with clinical signs suggesting primary disease of the nervous system has frequently prolonged the misdiagnoses of idiopathic epilepsy, brain neoplasm, or other organic neurologic disease. Repeated episodes of prolonged and severe hypoglycemia result in neuronal death and permanent neurologic disability with terminal coma, and, eventually, death.

Non–beta (gastrin-secreting) islet cell neoplasms

Gastrin-secreting, non–beta islet cell neoplasms of the pancreas have been reported in human beings, dogs, and cats. The hypersecretion of gastrin in human beings results in the well-documented Zollinger-Ellison syndrome, consisting of hypersecretion of gastric acid and recurrent peptic ulceration in the GI tract. Non–beta islet cell neoplasms derived from ectopic APUD (**a**mine **p**recursor **u**ptake **d**ecarboxylation) cells in the pancreas produce an excess of gastrin, which normally is secreted by cells of the antral and duodenal mucosa. The incidence of gastrin-secreting pancreatic neoplasms in dogs and cats is uncertain, but it appears to be uncommon compared with that of insulin-secreting beta cell neoplasms. The comparatively few cases studied in the dog and cat have had clinical signs of anorexia, vomiting of blood-tinged material, intermittent diarrhea, progressive weight loss, and dehydration. The prominent functional disturbances result from multiple ulcerations of the gastrointestinal mucosa, the result of gastrin hypersecretion.

Animals with Zollinger-Ellison–like syndrome have had single or multiple variably sized neoplasms in the pancreas. The neoplasms are firm and have increased amounts of fibrous connective tissue and partial encapsulation, but the neoplasm usually extends into the surrounding pancreas.

The basic histologic patterns of pancreatic islet cell neoplasms in animals are similar, irrespective of whether they are secreting insulin or gastrin. Three histologic patterns of non–beta islet cell neoplasms are recognized in dogs: the ribbon or trabecular pattern; solid nests of cells with a delicate, highly vascularized stroma; and an acinar pattern with arrangement of cuboidal neoplastic cells around a central lumen. The stroma may be prominent and hyalinized in some gastrin-secreting neoplasms.

Gastrin-secreting islet cell neoplasms in dogs invade locally into the adjacent parenchyma and often metastasize to regional lymph nodes and liver. These dogs have either single or multiple ulcerations in the gastric and/or duodenal mucosa and free blood in their lumina.

CHEMORECEPTOR ORGANS

Chemoreceptor organs are sensitive barometers of changes in blood carbon dioxide content, pH, and oxygen tension, thereby aiding in the regulation of respiration and circulation. Carotid and aortic bodies can initiate an increase in the depth and rate of respiration and minute volume by way of parasympathetic nerves and an increased heart rate and elevated arterial blood pressure by way of the sympathetic nervous system. The bodies are composed of parenchymal (chemoreceptor) cells and stellate (sustentacular) cells. Nerve endings with synaptic vesicles as well as nerve fibers occur in close association with the chemoreceptor cells. Chemoreceptor tissue is present at several sites in the body, including the carotid body, aortic bodies, nodose ganglion of the vagus nerve, ciliary ganglion in the orbit, pancreas, bodies on the internal jugular vein below the middle ear, and glomus jugular along the recurrent branch of the glossopharyngeal nerve.

Although chemoreceptor tissue appears to be widely distributed in the body, neoplasms develop principally in the aortic and carotid bodies of animals, and, aortic body chemodectomas are more frequent than those of the carotid body. The reverse is true for human beings. These neoplasms develop primarily in dogs and rarely in cats and cattle. Brachycephalic breeds of dogs, such as the boxer and Boston terrier, are highly predisposed.

Neoplasms

Neoplasms of aortic body

Aortic body neoplasms appear most frequently as single masses or as multiple nodules within the pericardial sac near the base of the heart. They vary considerably in size (from 0.5 to 12.5 cm), with carcinomas, in general, being larger than adenomas. Solitary, small adenomas either are attached to the adventitia of the pulmonary artery and ascending aorta or are embedded in the adipose connective tissue between these major vessels. They have a smooth external surface and, on cross section, are white and mottled with red to brown areas. Larger adenomas are multilobular and may indent the atria or displace the trachea and partially surround the major arterial trunks at the base of the heart. In dogs, aortic body carcinomas occur less frequently than adenomas. Carcinomas may infiltrate the wall of the pulmonary artery to form papillary projections into the lumen or invade through the wall of the atria into the lumen (Fig. 6-57). Although neoplastic cells often invade blood vessels, metastases to the lungs and liver occur infrequently in dogs with aortic body carcinomas.

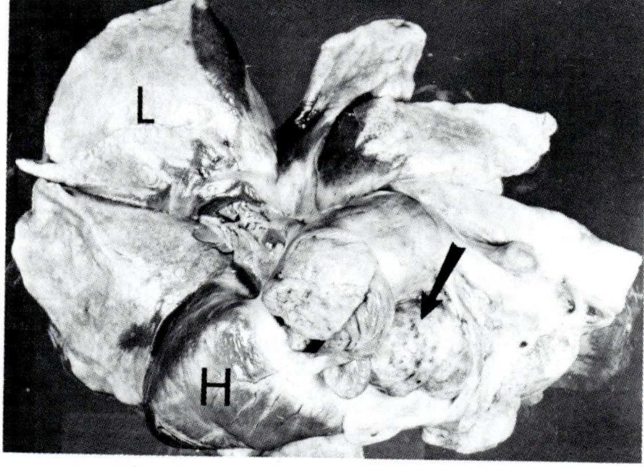

Fig. 6-57 Aortic body; dog. Carcinoma. Multiple nodules *(arrow)* are at the base of the heart *(H)*. *L*, diaphragmatic lobe of lung.

Neoplasms of the aortic bodies in animals are not functional (i.e., they do not secrete excess hormone into the circulation), but, as space-occupying lesions, they may produce a variety of functional disturbances. Due to pressure on the atria, vena cava, or both, larger aortic body adenomas and carcinomas may cause manifestations of cardiac decompensation. More aortic body neoplasms than carotid body neoplasms are benign. Aortic body carcinomas may invade locally into the atria, pericardium, and adjacent large, thin-walled vessels.

Neoplasms of carotid body

Carotid body neoplasms arise near the bifurcation of the common carotid artery in the cranial cervical area. They are usually unilateral, rarely bilateral, slow-growing masses. Adenomas vary from approximately 1 to 4 cm in diameter, are well encapsulated, and have a smooth external surface. The bifurcation of the carotid artery is incorporated in the mass, and neoplastic cells are firmly adherent to the tunica adventitia. Adenomas are firm and white, with scattered areas of hemorrhage, and are extremely vascular.

Carotid body carcinomas are larger, more coarsely multinodular than adenomas, invade the capsule, and penetrate into the walls of adjacent blood and lymph vessels. The external jugular vein and some cranial nerves may be incorporated into the neoplasm. Metastases of carotid body carcinomas occur in approximately 30% of cases and have been found in the lungs, tracheobronchial and mediastinal lymph nodes, liver, pancreas, and kidneys. Multicentric neoplastic transformation of chemoreceptor tissue occurs frequently in brachycephalic breeds of dogs.

The microscopic features of chemoreceptor neoplasms (''chemodectomas'') are essentially similar whether they are derived from either the carotid or aortic body. The neoplasm is subdivided into lobules by prominent branching trabeculae of connective tissue that originate from the fibrous capsule and are further subdivided into smaller nests by fine septa that contain collagenous and reticulin fibers and small capillaries. Neoplastic cells are commonly aligned along and around small capillaries; are discrete, round to polyhedral, and closely packed; and have lightly eosinophilic, finely granular, and often vacuolated cytoplasm.

Although the etiology of carotid and aortic body neoplasms is unknown, a genetic predisposition aggravated by chronic hypoxia may account for the greater risk of development in certain brachycephalic breeds, such as the boxer and Boston terrier dogs. Carotid bodies of several mammalian species, including dogs, have developed hyperplastic foci when the animals are subjected to the chronic hyp-

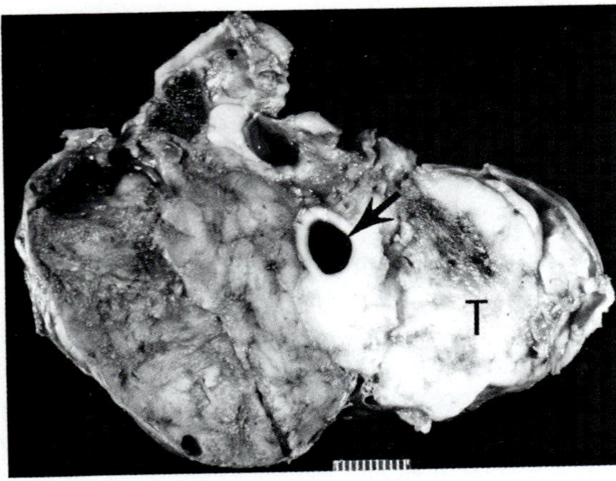

Fig. 6-58 Ectopic thyroid tissue; dog. Adenocarcinoma. Neoplastic tissue (*T*) surrounds the trachea *(arrow)* and other structures in the cranial mediastinum.

oxia of high altitude. Human beings living at high altitudes have 10 times the frequency of chemodectomas as those residing at sea level.

Heart-base neoplasms derived from ectopic thyroid

Adenomas and carcinomas derived from ectopic thyroid tissue account for approximately 5% to 10% of ''heart-base'' neoplasms in dogs. They often compress or invade structures in the cranial mediastinum near the base of the heart (Fig. 6-58). Areas of ectopic thyroid neoplasms with a compact cellular (solid) pattern of arrangement are difficult to distinguish histologically from aortic body tumors. Cells of ectopic thyroid neoplasms generally are smaller than those of aortic body neoplasms and have more hyperchromatic nuclei and an eosinophilic cytoplasm. Thyroidal neoplasms of follicular cells are not consistently subdivided into small packets by fine strands of connective tissue. Giant cells are infrequent in ectopic thyroid neoplasms, and the stroma is not prominent. Usually, primitive follicular structures or colloid-containing follicles can be demonstrated in ectopic thyroid neoplasms but not in aortic body neoplasms.

Suggested Readings

General considerations

Aurbach GD. Inherited disorders of hormone resistance. In: Desnick RJ et al., eds. Animal Models of Inherited Metabolic Diseases. New York: Alan R. Liss, 1982. Binns W, James LF, Shupe JL, Evertte G. A congenital cyclopian-type malformation in lambs induced by maternal ingestion of a range plant, *Veratrum californicum.* Am J Vet Res 1963; 24:1164-1175.

Chan L, O'Malley BW. Mechanism of action of the sex steroid hormones. N Engl J Med 1976; 294:1322-1328.

Cox RI. The endocrinologic changes of gestation and parturition in the sheep. In: Brandly CA et al., eds. Advances in Veterinary Science and Comparative Medicine. Vol. 19. New York: Academic Press, 1975.

Gosselin SJ, Capen CC, Krakowka S, Martin SL. Lymphocytic thyroiditis in dogs: Induction with local graft-versus-host reaction. Am J Vet Res 1981; 42:1856-1864.

Gosselin SJ, Capen CC, Martin SL. Histopathologic and ultrastructural evaluation of thyroid lesions associated with hypothyroidism in dogs. Vet Pathol 1981; 18:299-309.

Gosselin SJ, Capen CC, Martin SL, Krakowka S. Autoimmune lymphocytic thyroiditis in dogs. Vet Immunol Immunopath 1982; 3:185-201.

Holzworth J, Theran P, Carpenter JF, Harpster NK, Todoroff RJ. Hyperthyroidism in the cat: Ten cases. J Am Vet Med Assoc 1980; 176:345-353.

Kennedy PC, Kendrick JW, Stormont C. Adenohypophyseal aplasia, an inherited defect associated with abnormal gestation in Guernsey cattle. Cornell Vet 1957; 47:160-178.

Leav I, Schiller AL, Rijnberg A, Legg MA, de Kinderen PJ. Adenomas and carcinomas of the canine and feline thyroid. Am J Pathol 1976; 83:61-122.

Meuten DJ, Capen CC, Kociba GJ, Chew DJ. Ultrastructural evaluation of an adenocarcinoma derived from apocrine glands of the anal sac associated with hypercalcemia in dogs. Am J Pathol 1982; 107:167-175.

Pammenter M, Albrecht C, Kiebenberg vdW, van Jaarsveld P. Afrikander cattle congenital goiter: Characteristics of its morphology and iodoprotein pattern. Endocrinology 1978; 102:954-965.

Roth J. Polypeptide hormone receptors. In: Membrane Receptors for Viruses, Antigens and Antibodies, Polypeptide Hormones, and Small Molecules. New York: Raven Press, 1976.

van Herle AJ, Vassart G, Dunmont JE. Control of thyroglobulin synthesis and secretion. N Engl J Med 1979; 301:239-249.

van Voorthuizen WF, Dinsort C, Flavell RA, de Vijlder JJM, Vassart G. Abnormal cellular localization of thyroglobulin mRNA associated with hereditary congenital goiter and thyroglobulin deficiency. Proc Natl Acad Sci U S A 1978; 75:74-78.

Vogelgesand G, Harmeyer J, vonGrabe C. Measurements of intestinal calcium uptake in pigs with vitamin D-dependent rickets. In: Nuclear Techniques in Animal Production and Health. Vienna: Proc Joint JAEA/FAO, 1976.

Pituitary gland

Capen CC. Tumors of the endocrine glands. In: Moulton JE, ed. Tumors in Domestic Animals. 3rd ed. Berkeley/Los Angeles: University of California Press, 1990.

Capen CC, Koestner A. Functional chromophobe adenomas of the canine adenohypophysis: An ultrastructural evaluation of a neoplasm of pituitary corticotrophs. Vet Pathol 1967; 4:326-347.

Capen CC, Martin SL. Animal model: Hyperadrenocorticism (Cushing's-like syndrome and disease in dogs). Am J Pathol 1975; 81:459-462.

Capen CC, Martin SL, Koestner A. Neoplasms in the adenohypophysis of dogs: A clinical and pathologic study. Vet Pathol 1967; 4:301-325.

Muller GH. Pituitary dwarfism: Cutaneous manifestations of an endocrine disorder. Vet Clin North Am 1979; 9:41-48.

Richards MA. Polydipsia in the dog: The differential diagnosis of polyuric syndromes in the dog. J Small Anim Pract 1970; 10:651-667.

Adrenal cortex

Anderson MP, Capen CC. Diseases of the endocrine system. In: Benirschke K et al., eds., Pathology of Laboratory Animals. Vol. 1. Chap. 6. New York: Springer-Verlag, 1978; 423-508.

Hullinger RL. Adrenal cortex of the dog (*Canis familiaris*): Histomorphological changes during growth, maturity, and aging. Zbl Vet Med C Anat Histol Embryol 1978; 7:1-27.

Mulnix JA. Hypoadrenocorticism in the dog. J Am Anim Hosp Assoc 1971; 7:220-241.

Peterson ME, Gilbertson SR, Drucker WD. Plasma cortisol response to exogenous ACTH in 22 dogs with hyperadrenocorticism caused by adrenocortical neoplasia. J Am Vet Med Assoc 1982; 180:542-544.

Schaer M, Chen CL. A clinical survey of 48 dogs with adrenocortical hypofunction. J Am Anim Hosp Assoc 1983; 19:443-452.

Adrenal medulla

Howard EB, Nielsen SW. Pheochromocytomas associated with hypertensive lesions in dogs. J Am Vet Med Assoc 1965; 147:245-252.

Sponenberg DP, McEntee K. Pheochromocytomas and ultimobranchial (C-cell) neoplasms in the bull: Evidence of autosomal dominant inheritance in the Guernsey breed. Vet Pathol 1983; 20:396-400.

Yarrington JT, Capen CC. Ultrastructural and biochemical evaluation of adrenal medullary hyperplasia and pheochromocytoma in aged bulls. Vet Pathol 1981; 18:316-325.

Thyroid follicular cells

Bastenie PA, Ermans AM, Bonnyns M, Neve P, Delespesse G. Lymphocytic thyroiditis as an autoimmune disease. In: Good RA, Day SB, Yunis JJ, eds. Molecular Pathology. Springfield, Ill.: Charles C Thomas, 1975.

Gosselin SJ, Capen CC, Martin SL. Histopathologic and ultrastructural evaluation of thyroid lesions associated with hypothyroidism in dogs. Vet Pathol 1981; 18:299-309.

Gosselin SJ, Capen CC, Martin SL, Krakowka S. Autoimmune lymphocytic thyroiditis in dogs. Vet Immunol Immunopathol 1982; 3:185-201.

Gosselin SJ, Martin SL, Capen CC, Targowski SP. Biochemical and immunological investigations of hypothyroidism in dogs. Can J Comp Med 1980; 44:158-168.

Holzworth J, Theran P, Carpenter JL, Harpster NK, Rodoroff RJ. Hyperthyroidism in the cat: Ten cases. J Am Vet Med Assoc 1980; 176:345-353.

Leav I, Schiller AI, Rijnberk A, Legg MA, der Kinderen PJ. Adenomas and carcinomas of the canine and feline thyroid. Am J Pathol 1976; 83:61-94.

Martin SL, Capen CC. Hypothyroidism and the skin. In: Muller GH, ed. Veterinary Clinics of North America: Symposium on Skin and Internal Disease. Vol. 9. Philadelphia: Saunders, 1979: 29-40.

Peterson ME. Diagnosis and treatment of feline hyperthyroidism. In: van Marthens E, ed. Proceedings 6th Kal Kan Symposium for Treatment of Small Animal Disease, Veterinary Learning Systems, 1983; 63-66.

Rojko JL, Hoover EA, Martin SL. Histopathologic interpretation of cutaneous biopsies from dogs with various dermatologic disorders. Vet Pathol 1978; 579-589.

Thyroid C cells

Black HE, Capen CC, Young DM. Ultimobranchial thyroid neoplasms in bulls: A syndrome resembling medullary thyroid carcinoma in man. Cancer 1973; 32:865-878.

Capen CC. Metabolic bone and disease calcium regulating hormones. In: Newton CD, Nunamaker DM, eds. Textbook of Small Animal Orthopaedics. Philadelphia: Lippincott, 1985; 673-722.

Zarrin K. Naturally-occurring parafollicular cell carcinoma of the thyroid in dogs: A histological and ultrastructural study. Vet Pathol 1977; 14:556-566.

Parathyroid gland

Black HE, Capen CC, Yarrington JT, Rowland GN. Effect of a high calcium prepartal diet on calcium homeostatic mechanisms in thyroid glands, bone, and intestine of cows. Lab Invest 1973; 29:437-448.

Capen CC. Functional and fine structural relationships of parathyroid glands. Adv Vet Sci Comp Med 1975; 19:249-286.

Capen CC, Cole CR, Hibbs JW. Influences of vitamin D on calcium metabolism and the parathyroid glands of cattle. Federation Proceedings 1968; 27:142-152.

Capen CC, Young DM. The ultrastructure of the parathyroid glands and thyroid parafollicular cells of cows with parturient paresis and hypocalcemia. Lab Invest 1967; 17:717-737.

Heath H, Weller RE, Mundy GR. Canine lymphosarcoma: A model for study of the hypercalcemia of cancer. Calcif Tissue Int 1980; 30:127-133.

Hunt RD, Garcia FG, Hegsted DM. A comparison of vitamin D_2 and D_3 in New World primates. I. Production and regression of osteodystrophia fibrosa. Lab Anim Care 1967; 16:222-234.

Krook L, Barrett RB. Simian bone disease—a secondary hyperparathyroidism. Cornell Vet 1962; 52:459-492.

Meuten DJ, Capen CC, Kociba GJ, Cooper BJ. Hypercalcemia of malignancy: Hypercalcemia associated with an adenocarcinoma of the apocrine glands of the anal sac. Am J Pathol 1982; 108:366-370.

Meuten DJ, Capen CC, Thompson KG, Serge GV. Syncytial cells in canine parathyroid glands. Vet Pathol 1984; 21:463-468.

Meuten DJ, Kociba GJ, Capen CC, Chew DJ, Segre GV, Levin L, Tashjian AJ Jr, Voelkel EF, Nagode LA. Hypercalcemia in dogs with lymphosarcoma: Biochemical, ultrastructural and histomorphometric investigations. Lab Invest 1983; 49:553-562.

Meuten DJ, Segre GV, Capen CC, Kociba GJ, Voelkel EF, Levine L, Tashjian AH Jr, Chew DJ, Nagode LA. Hypercalcemia in dogs with adenocarcinoma derived from apocrine glands of anal sac: Biochemical and histomorphometric investigations. Lab Invest 1983; 48:428-435.

Strewler GJ, Nissenson RA. Nonparathyroid hypercalcemia. Adv Intern Med 1987; 32:235-258.

Pancreatic islets

Capen CC, Martin SL. Hyperinsulinism in dogs with neoplasia of the pancreatic islets: A clinical, pathologic, and ultrastructural study. Pathol Vet 1969; 6:309-341.

Happé RP, van der Gaag I, Lamers CBHW, van Toorenburg J, Renfeld JF, Larsson LI. Zollinger-Ellison syndrome in three dogs. Vet Pathol 1980; 17:177-186.

Johnson KH, Osborne CA, Barnes DM. Intracellular substance with some amyloid staining affinities in pancreatic acinar cells of a cat with amyloidosis. Pathol Vet 1970; 7:153-162.

Meier H. Diabetes mellitus in animals. Diabetes 1960; 9:485-489.

Chemoreceptor organs

Bloom F. Structure and histogenesis of tumors of the aortic bodies in dogs with a consideration of the morphology of the aortic and carotid bodies. Arch Pathol 1943; 36:1-12.

Cheville NF. Ultrastructure of canine carotid body and aortic body tumors: Comparison with tissues of thyroid and parathyroid origin. Vet Pathol 1972; 9:166-189.

Edwards C, Heath D, Harris P, Castillo Y, Kruger H, Arias-Stella J. The carotid body in animals at high altitude. J Pathol 1971; 104:231-238.

Johnson KH. Aortic body tumors in the dog. J Am Vet Med Assoc 1968; 152:154-160.

CHAPTER

7 Hemopoietic System

GENE P. SEARCY

Structure and Function

The blood, bone marrow, spleen, and lymph nodes and other lymphoid tissues comprise the hemopoietic system. The bone marrow, spleen, and lymph nodes share certain basic anatomic features. For example, specialized fibroblast-like reticular cells extend long, filamentous processes that provide a scaffolding arrangement to support populations of cells. In addition to physical support, these cells also provide a microenvironment that attracts the appropriate circulating cells and enables them to multiply and/or differentiate into cells of a particular lineage. Within the reticular networks of these organs are thin-walled sinuses that control movement of cells and large molecules into and out of the lymph. These sinuses are located between arterioles and venules in the bone marrow and spleen, but enclose lymph within lymph nodes. Macrophages, derived from monocytes, are found in most of these reticular cell networks, where they perform a wide variety of functions. They, collectively, are part of the monocyte-macrophage or mononuclear phagocyte system.

The **bone marrow** maintains an embryonic function throughout life because it must constantly renew cells of the blood. It is particularly efficient at entrapping and nurturing pluripotential stem cells. In the 1950s, it was reported that bone marrow–derived cells injected into irradiated mice formed splenic colonies. These colonies contained varying numbers of erythrocytic, granulocytic, megakaryocytic, and undifferentiated cells. It was eventually established that each of these colonies arose from a single stem cell capable of renewal and differentiation. Similar findings were confirmed in other animals and in human beings. By the use of chromosomal markers, it was confirmed that lymphoid stem cells arose from a more pluripotent stem cell that was also the origin of other hemopoietic cells (myeloid stem cells) (Fig. 7-1). Techniques that facilitate growth of hemopoietic cells in liquid culture have enabled investigators to study humoral mediators that control differentiation and maturation of blood cells. A compartment of stem cells committed to erythropoiesis was recognized and further subdivided into burst-forming

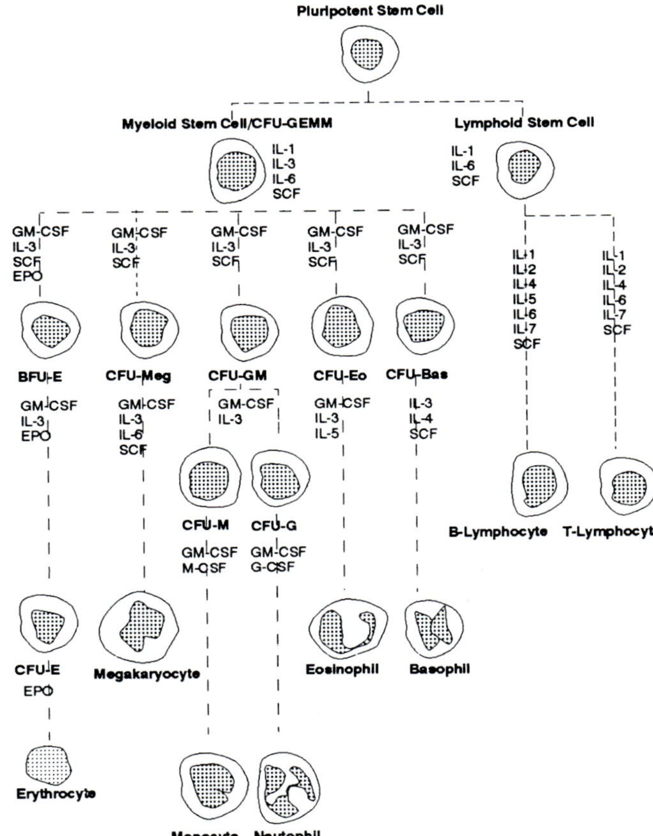

Fig. 7-1 Model of hemopoiesis. *CFU-GEMM,* colony-forming unit–granulocyte, erythroid, macrophage, megakaryocyte; *BFU-E,* burst-forming unit–erythroid; *CFU-E,* colony-forming unit–erythroid; *CFU-Meg,* colony-forming unit–megakaryocyte; *CFU-GM,* colony-forming unit–granulocyte-macrophage; *CFU-G,* colony-forming unit–granulocyte; *CFU-M,* colony-forming unit–monocyte; *CFU-Eo,* colony-forming unit–eosinophil; *CFU-Bas,* colony-forming unit–basophil; *GM-CSF,* granulocyte-macrophage colony-stimulating factor; *M-CSF,* macrophage colony-stimulating factor; *G-CSF,* granulocyte colony-stimulating factor; *SCF,* stem cell factor; *EPO,* Erythropoietin; *IL,* interleukin. *Modified from Chart of Hematopoeisis, Immunex Corporation, Seattle, Wash.*

units–erythroid (BFU-E) and colony-forming units–erythroid (CFU-E). The former is under control of interleukin 1 (IL-1) and erythropoietin, whereas CFU-E proliferation occurs in response to erythropoietin. In a similar manner, the stem cells that give rise to granulocytes and monocytes are known as colony-forming units–granulocyte-monocyte (CFU-GM) (Fig. 7-1). These are under the control of several mediators called colony-stimulating activities (CSA) or factors (CSF). Megakaryocyte-committed colonies (CFU-Meg) arise from stem cells also under control of specific mediators. It can now be appreciated that hematalogy results following bone marrow injury will vary, depending upon the stage of differentiation of the affected stem cells. For example, the diversity of bone marrow and blood disorders in feline leukemia virus–infected cats results from variation in the viral disturbance of hemopoietic cells.

Significant insight into diseases of the hemopoietic system may be gained by simply submitting blood for hematologic examination. Indeed, a complete hemogram is frequently of greater value than the necropsy in understanding disease mechanisms of the hemopoietic system. Learning to evaluate blood smears is a valuable addition to the information gained from the physical examination of an animal. Lymph node and bone marrow aspirates are also frequently indicated when studying disorders of the hemopoietic system.

Responses of System

Like other organs, the blood-forming organs, lymph nodes, and spleen may undergo atrophy, hyperplasia, hypertrophy, and neoplasia. Atrophy of the bone marrow hemopoietic cell population follows certain types of injury and results in failure of erythropoiesis (causing anemia), granulopoiesis (causing neutropenia), and thrombopoiesis (causing thrombocytopenia). Occasionally, injury to pluripotent stem cells results in complete failure of hemopoiesis and occurrence of pancytopenia. Splenic atrophy is uncommon, occurring in older animals, and is usually of little consequence. Infections with certain viruses and exposure to certain toxins as well as malnutrition can cause thymic and lymph node atrophy and impaired immune functions.

Hypertrophy of bone marrow is most unlikely in animals since hemopoietic tissue is enclosed by bone. (In children with congenital hemolytic anemias, some flat bones may become enlarged owing to years of erythroid hyperplasia.) Hypertrophy of the spleen can occur when the red pulp is engorged with erythrocytes, in which case the organ is compressable and blood oozes from the cut surface. Hyperplasia of the splenic lymphocyte or macrophage populations also results in hypertrophy; when this occurs, the spleen is firm and fleshy when incised. Lymph node enlargement secondary to cellular proliferation or hyperplasia occurs in response to inflammation and antigenic stimulation. Hypertrophy of superficial lymph nodes is usually confined to one node receiving lymph from a localized area of injury or inflammation. Generalized lymph node hypertrophy (lymphoid hyperplasia) is uncommon and occurs with systemic infections of some duration.

Hyperplasia of bone marrow hemopoietic tissue occurs following prolonged hemorrhage or hemolysis and bacterial infections. Hemopoietic tissue expands and replaces adipocytes; yellow marrow becomes red, beginning along the endosteum. Extramedullary hemopoiesis in organs such as the liver and spleen frequently accompanies hyperplasia of the bone marrow.

The hemopoietic system in some species, such as the cat, has a significant incidence of neoplasia. Although not universally practiced, the foundational terminology for neoplastic diseases as taught in general pathology can be applied to the hemopoietic system and will be used in this chapter. Sarcomas of bone marrow can be derived from erythrocytic, granulocytic, megakaryocytic, lymphocytic, and plasma cell populations. In cats infected with feline leukemia virus, a combination of erythrocytic and granulocytic sarcomas can occasionally occur. Sarcomas of bone marrow are unique in pathology because they may release neoplastic cells into the blood. It follows that identification of the sarcoma can be made by identifying the leukemic cells in blood smears. Frequently, however, bone marrow aspiration is required to identify the sarcoma; veterinarians should be capable of obtaining these samples. Lymphosarcomas arise in any organ but, as would be expected, frequently cause lymph node enlargement. Superficial lymph node aspirates for cytology and biopsies for histopathologic evaluation usually allow differentiation of lymphosarcoma from either lymphadenitis or lymphoid hyperplasia.

ERYTHROCYTE DISORDERS

Erythrocytosis (Polycythemia)

Erythrocytosis is an increase in erythrocyte numbers, hemoglobin concentration, and packed cell volume of blood; it may be classified as relative or absolute.

Relative erythrocytosis

Relative erythrocytosis is the result of dehydration or hemoconcentration, in which extracellular fluid imbalance leads to reduction of the plasma compartment. Although the packed cell volume, hemoglobin concentration, and erythrocyte numbers are increased, the total erythrocyte mass is normal. Plasma proteins are affected by shifts in fluid volume in the same manner as erythrocytes. Estimation of the packed cell volume and plasma protein provides some estimation of the degree of dehydration.

Absolute erythrocytosis

Absolute erythrocytosis is an actual increase in erythrocyte numbers. It can be further classified as primary or secondary erythrocytosis. Primary erythrocytosis is the proliferation of marrow erythroid precursors that are no

Table 7-1. Hematology of a 4-month-old Holstein calf with congenital vascular anomalies and constriction of the pulmonary artery

Hemogram	Patient values	Reference values
WBC × 10^9/L	7.9	4.0-12.0
RBC × 10^9/L	13.2	5.0-10.0
Hemoglobin g/L	261	80-150
PCV L/L	0.78	0.24-0.46
MCV fL	58	40-60
MCH pg	15	11-17
MCHC g/L	320	300-360
Platelets × 10^9/L	950	200-800
Neutrophils × 10^9/L	3.6	0.6-4.0
Lymphocytes × 10^9/L	3.80	1.5-5.5
Monocytes × 10^9/L	0.48	0.025-0.84
Protein g/L	68	68-78

WBC, white blood count; *RBC,* red blood count; *PCV,* packed cell volume; *MCV,* mean corpuscular volume; *MCH,* mean corpuscular hemoglobin; *MCHC,* mean corpuscular hemoglobin concentration.

longer influenced by erythropoietin; this form of erythrocytosis may represent the escape of a clone of such cells from normal control mechanisms. Although the disease is uncommon, it has been described in young to middle-aged dogs and in cats. Packed cell volumes in dogs have ranged from 0.65 to 0.82 L per liter (65% to 82%).

Secondary erythrocytosis results from excessive production of erythropoietin. Commonly caused by hypoxia, it probably occurs to a mild degree in older dogs with cardiac or pulmonary disease. Occasionally, marked hypoxic erythrocytosis can result from congenital anomalous transposition of major vessels in which a significant percentage of erythrocytes bypass the pulmonary circulation (Table 7-1). Erythrocytosis due to inappropriate hormonal stimulation of erythropoiesis in the absence of hypoxia occurs as a paraneoplastic syndrome. Although rare, this syndrome has been reported in dogs with renal and extrarenal neoplasms.

The clinical signs of absolute erythrocytosis include cyanotic oral mucous membranes (which can be pronounced) and marked depression. The increased viscosity of the blood causes impaired blood flow, induces cyanosis, and causes a tendency for thrombosis. Necropsy findings include marked generalized congestion, thrombosis of major vessels, and hyperplasia of bone marrow.

Anemia

Mechanisms of anemia

Anemia is the reduction of erythrocyte numbers for an animal of a particular age, species, breed, and geographic location. Erythrocyte numbers decrease in neonatal animals following ingestion of colostrum; this decrease continues during the period of rapid body growth. The age at which erythrocyte numbers begin to increase, as well as the age at which adult numbers are reached, varies among species. In dogs, adult values are usually reached between 4 to 6 months of age; in horses, this occurs at approximately 1 year of age. In most species, erythrocytes are larger at birth, and mean corpuscular volumes (MCVs) decline as fetal erythrocytes are replaced. It is important that these factors be considered when assessing hemograms in young animals. Factors such as malnutrition and parasitism will delay the age at which adult erythrocyte numbers are reached. Breed influences erythrocyte numbers in both horses and dogs. Draft horses have lower erythrocyte numbers than those of racing breeds. Some breeds of dogs such as greyhounds and whippets have higher erythrocyte numbers than most other breeds. Animals residing at higher altitudes have higher erythrocyte counts. When assessing hemograms from animals, these factors must be taken into consideration and assessment made as to what the erythrocyte values might have been for that animal prior to the current illness, even though reference to normal values may not indicate anemia.

Anemia is a significant indicator of underlying disease and should be investigated in a routine, logical manner. The initial decision is whether the anemia is regenerative or nonregenerative, based on the presence or absence of indicators of compensatory erythropoiesis. Regenerative anemias result from hemorrhage or hemolysis, which is followed by stimulation of the bone marrow with release of immature erythrocytes. A blood film contains large, immature erythrocytes that vary in size (anisocytosis). The immature erythrocytes stain blue, and polychromasia is a most useful indicator of increased erythropoiesis. Additional morphologic indicators of rapid erythropoiesis include metarubricytes and rubricytes and, in ruminants, basophilic stippling (Table 7-2). Incubation of blood with supravital stains (such as new methylene blue) results in precipitation of residual RNA as blue strands in immature cells called reticulocytes (Fig. 7-2). Enumeration of reticulocytes in 1000 erythrocytes provides the most precise estimate of erythropoietic rate. The absolute number of reticulocytes is estimated by multiplying the percentage of reticulocytes by the erythrocyte count. A reticulocyte count of greater than 60 × 10^2 L per liter (60,000/mm^3) in cats and dogs is consistent with regenerative anemia. Special precautions are necessary when enumerating reticulocytes in cats because of the occurrence of punctate reticulocytes, as well as aggregate reticulocytes similar to those of dogs. As the name implies, punctate erythrocytes contain noncoalescing blue dots. The aggregate forms are representative of immature erythrocytes, whereas the punctate forms are descendants of the aggregate type. The latter may persist for several days and indicate earlier responsive erythropoiesis. Reticulocytes appear in the blood within 2 to 3 days after hemorrhage or hemolysis. Animals with hemolytic anemias usually have evidence of compensatory erythropoiesis on initial examination, but animals presented because of hemorrhage may not. Evaluation of anemia in horses is complicated because the horse does not

Table 7-2. Nomenclature of erythrocyte shapes and associated diseases

Term	Description	Disease association
Disocyte	Normal bioconcave disc Degree of central pallor varies with species	None
Macrocyte	Large erythrocyte	Release of immature cells in response to blood loss Congenital in some poodle dogs
Polychromasia	Diffuse blue erythrocytes on Wright's-Giemsa stains	Release of immature cells in response to blood loss
Reticulocyte	Erythrocyte containing precipitated strands of RNA with supravital stains	Release of immature cells in response to blood loss
Nuclear remnant	Small, single, black-staining, round inclusion in various locations within erythrocyte	Response to blood loss; splenic malfunction
Basophilic stippling	Punctate precipitate in cytoplasm	Response to blood loss in ruminants; lead poisoning
Microcyte	Small erythrocyte	Iron deficiency
Hypochromia	Erythrocyte with thin rim of pale peripheral hemoglobin and large amount of central pallor	Iron deficiency
Leptocyte	Thin erythrocyte with increased central pallor and dense peripheral hemoglobin	Chronic diseases; liver diseases
Codocytes (target cells)	Leptocytes with a dense, round, central concentration of hemoglobin	Chronic diseases; liver diseases
Spherocyte	Small, dense erythrocyte lacking central pallor and therefore only recognizable in those species whose erythrocytes normally have central pallor, e.g., dogs	Immune-mediated hemolysis; senescent erythrocytes; accompany poikilocytosis
Spheroechinocyte	Spiculated spherocyte Short, spiny projections around periphery	Absorption of erythrocytes from body cavities
Poikilocyte	Nonspecific term for abnormally shaped erythrocyte	See more specific terms
Acanthocyte	Erythrocyte with projections of variable length at variable intervals around the cell	Splenic disease; hemangiosarcomas
Shizocyte	Small, irregular erythrocyte fragment that may have two or three pointed extremities	Intravascular coagulation; vasculitis
Eccentrocyte	Hemoglobin displaced to one side of cell	Hemolytic anemias induced by chemicals
Keratocyte	Half-moon shape with spicules	Intravascular coagulation
Dacrocyte	Teardrop cell	Myelofibrosis

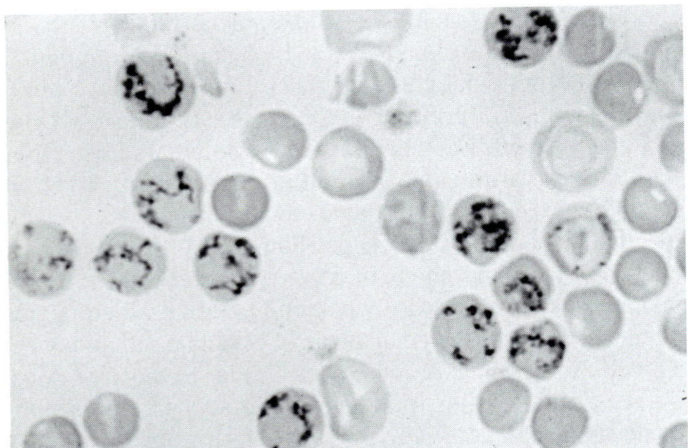

Fig. 7-2 Blood smear; dog. Reticulocytes. New methylene blue stain.

release reticulocytes from the bone marrow. Intense erythrogenesis in horses may increase the MCV and red cell distribution width (RDW); however, examination of bone marrow aspirates may also be necessary to assess erythropoietic rate.

Regenerative anemias

After establishing that an anemia is regenerative (e.g., the result of erythrocyte loss), it is necessary to differentiate between hemorrhage and hemolysis. Such differentiation is often difficult; a good history and thorough examination of the animal are required to detect occult hemorrhage, e.g., bleeding into body cavities and large muscle masses. Blood films of animals with lymph return of erythrocytes into the bloodstream following bleeding into body cavities will have spheroidal, spiculated erythrocytes known as spherochinocytes. Significant bleeding at the free gingival margin of dogs with thrombocytopenia may go undetected because of constant swallowing. Commercial tablets for detection of hemoglobin in feces are extremely sensitive and will detect the hemoglobin present in meat ingested by carnivores. It may be necessary to place animals in which gastrointestinal bleeding is suspected on cereal diets before testing their feces for occult blood. Routine urinalysis will detect bleeding into the urinary tract; samples obtained during urination are preferred because samples obtained by cystocentesis from dogs and cats frequently contain erythrocytes.

When hemorrhage has occurred within the previous 36

to 48 hours, hypoproteinemia is concurrent with the anemia; as fluid enters the vascular compartment to maintain blood pressure, the dilution that results in anemia also causes hypoproteinemia. In species with a storage spleen, such as the horse, splenic contraction initially compensates for erythrocyte loss, but dilution of plasma proteins begins within minutes.

Detection of hemolysis may also be difficult. Icteric mucous membranes and bilirubin and hemoglobin in plasma and urine indicate hemolysis. Because dogs are able to conjugate and excrete large amounts of bilirubin rapidly, they only have products of hemolysis in the blood after a hemolytic crisis. Bilirubinuria is a more constant finding. Blood films may have erythrocyte alterations suggestive of hemolysis, such as spherocytes in the canine immune-mediated hemolytic anemias. The reticulocyte response following hemolysis due to erythrophagocytosis is usually greater than that following hemorrhage owing to the efficient salvage of iron from hemoglobin and release of cytokines from activated macrophages.

Hemorrhagic anemias

An important consequence of chronic hemorrhage is the exhaustion of iron stores, which results in impaired erythropoiesis. This can occur in parasitic diseases such as bovine pediculosis, severe flea infestations of puppies and kittens, and hookworms in puppies. Chronic immune-mediated thrombocytopenia in dogs and gastrointestinal neoplasms in older animals may also cause iron deficiency owing to chronic hemorrhage. Bleeding intestinal carcinomas and lymphosarcomas in dogs deserve special emphasis; these neoplasms should be considered immediately when the hemogram has features suggestive of iron deficiency.

Hemolytic anemias

The most significant hemolytic anemias in animals are extrinsic abnormalities, acquired as a result of erythrocyte injury. Inherited hemolytic anemias result from an intracellular defect confined to a single protein. The severity of the anemia will vary, depending on the abnormal protein and the location of the abnormality within the molecule. These anemias in animals can result from abnormalities in heme synthesis, membrane skeletal proteins, and glycolytic enzymes.

Two congenital abnormalities of heme synthesis occur in cattle. **Congenital erythropoietic porphyria** occurs in Holstein and Shorthorn cattle and is characterized by red-brown discoloration of teeth and bones due to accumulation of porphyrins. Because of the circulation of the photodynamic porphyrins in blood, these animals have lesions of photosensitization of the nonpigmented skin and hemolytic anemia. All affected tissues, including nucleated erythrocytes, fluoresce with ultraviolet light. The premature destruction of developing and mature erythrocytes is caused by the accumulation of excess porphyrins. Bovine **erythropoietic protoporphyria** is an inherited disorder of heme synthetase, a terminal enzyme of the heme synthetic pathway, resulting in the accumulation of protoporphyrins in tissues and erythrocytes. It is confined to Limousin or Limousin-cross cattle. Photosensitivity is the only clinical manifestation of the disease; there is no discoloration of teeth and bones or anemia. A congenital porphyria described in Siamese and domestic short-haired cats resembles congenital erythropoeitic porphyria in cattle. These cats have brown teeth, lesions of photosensitization, and hemolytic anemia.

Two inherited glycolytic enzyme abnormalities have been described in dogs. **Pyruvate kinase deficiency** in Basenji, beagle, and West Highland white terrier dogs results in severe hemolytic anemia with marked reticulocytosis. This distal block in the Embden-Meyerhof pathway results in inadequate synthesis of adenosine triphosphate (ATP), which shortens the life span of erythrocytes (Fig. 7-3). Many of these animals develop myelofibrosis and die because of interference with the rapid compensatory erythropoiesis. **Phosphofructokinase deficiency** has been described in English springer spaniel and American cocker spaniel dogs (Fig. 7-3). The hemolytic anemia is less severe in comparison with that observed in cases of pyruvate kinase deficiency. The erythrocytes are sensitive to changes in pH and are more susceptible to hemolysis during periods of exercise, when panting results in alkalosis.

Most hemolytic anemias in animals are extravascular and caused by partial or complete phagocytosis of erythrocytes by macrophages of the mononuclear phagocyte system. The concept of partial phagocytosis is important. Here, the erythrocyte loses a portion of its membrane and has a decreased surface area relative to its volume. This disc-to-sphere transformation with loss of deformability places the cell at risk. Erythrocytes must be extremely pliable in order to traverse the splenic red pulp and sinusoidal walls (Fig. 7-4); spherocytes, therefore, tend to be retained in the spleen, with risk of further injury and phagocytosis. Erythrocyte-macrophage interaction with spherocyte formation is important for the destruction of aged erythrocytes. It is now apparent that this interaction is significantly mediated by antibody fixation to erythrocyte membrane proteins, which become exposed as the cells age. Following erythrophagocytosis, the enzymes of macrophages dissolve the erythrocytes, and hemoglobin is degraded, releasing bilirubin and iron from the porphyrin part of the molecule. The iron is efficiently returned to the bone marrow for utilization by developing erythrocytes.

Erythrocyte lysis occurring intravascularly releases hemoglobin in the plasma where it binds to haptoglobin, its principal transport protein. The hemoglobin-haptoglobin complex is then removed by hepatocytes, and the hemoglobin is degraded. Hemoglobinemia and hemoglobinuria, important indicators of intravascular hemolysis, are detectable only when the haptoglobin binding capacity is exceeded.

Infectious agents that cause hemolytic anemia include

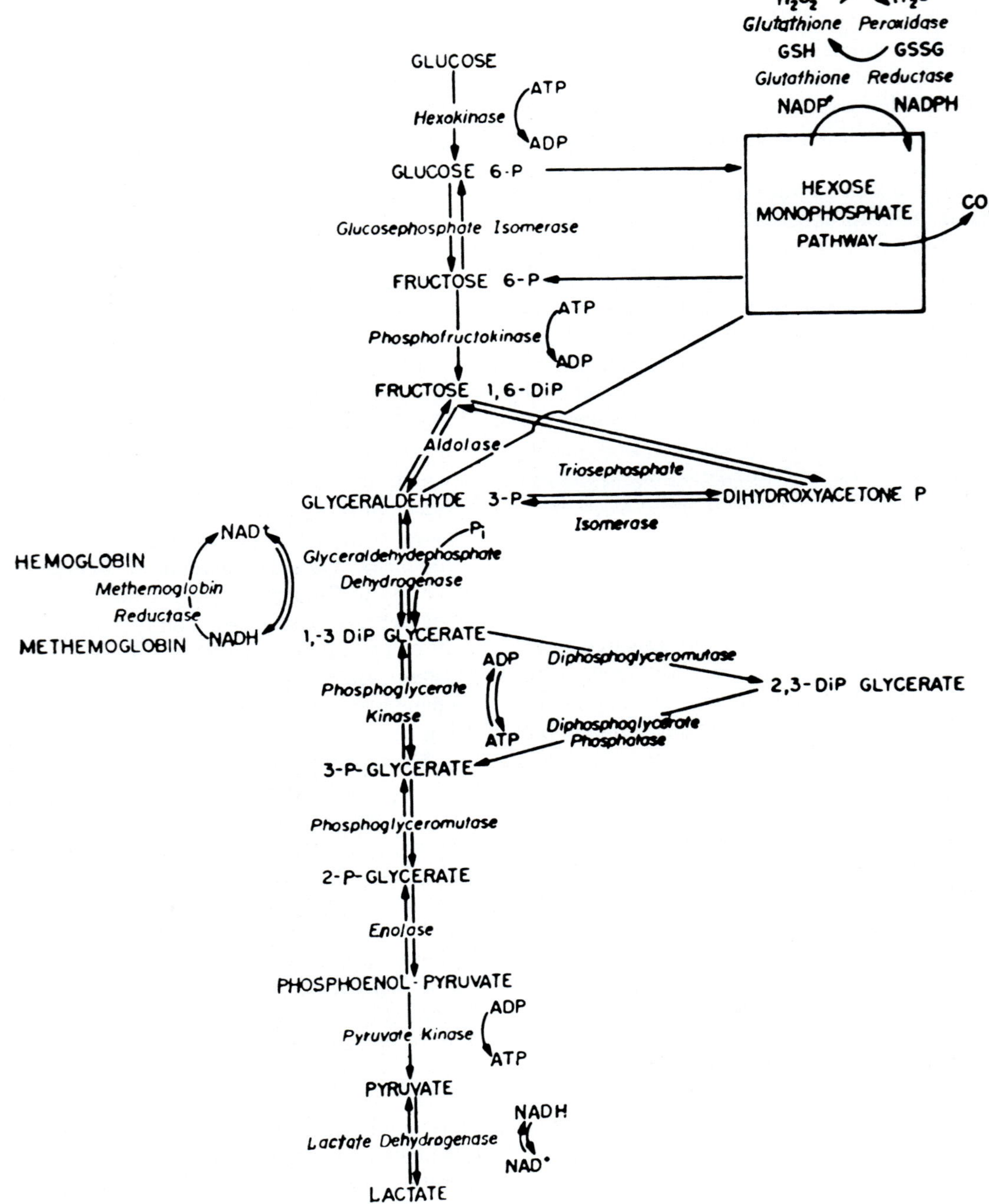

Fig. 7-3 Glucose metabolism of the erythrocyte. *From Beutler E. Energy metabolism and maintenance of erythrocytes. In: Williams WJ, Beutler E, Erslev AJ, Lichtman MA, eds. Hematology. 4th ed. New York: McGraw-Hill, 1990: 356.*

viruses, bacteria, rickettsiae, protozoa, and blood parasites. Mechanisms of erythrocyte destruction by some of these agents may involve fixation of antibody to the erythrocytic membrane, with subsequent phagocytosis by macrophages.

Equine infectious anemia is a disease of horses, mules, and donkeys caused by an arthropod-borne retrovirus. Horses may die of anemia during the initial viremia or may recover to undergo subsequent episodes of viremia and anemia. The virus replicates in macrophages and possibly other cells, which eventually release large amounts of virus. Each subsequent hemolytic crisis is caused by a new antigenic variant of the virus. Hemolysis is assumed to be immune-mediated; C3 complement is present on erythrocytes, presumably following adsorption of virus and antibody fixation and complement activation leading to erythrophagocytosis. Later in the course of the disease,

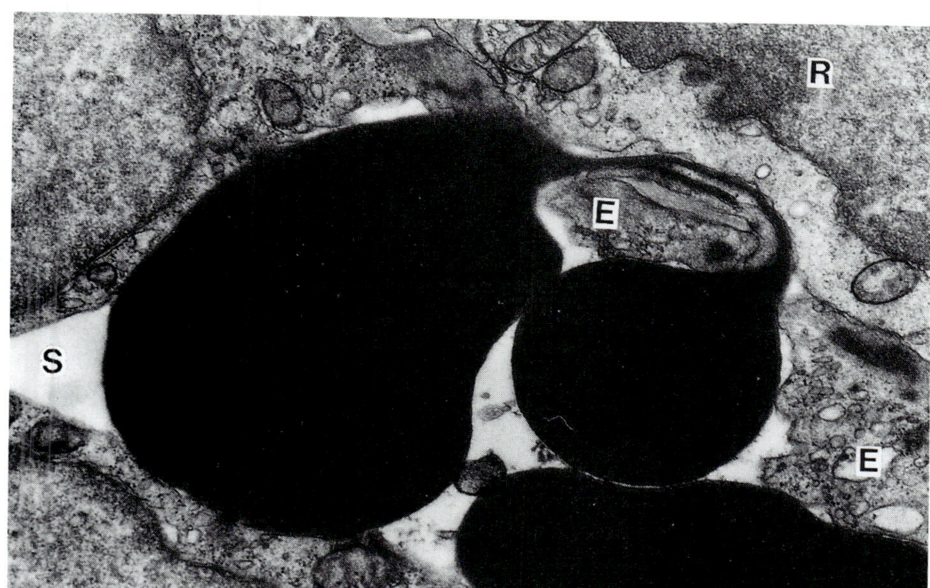

Fig. 7-4 Electron micrograph. Spleen; rabbit. The deformability of an erythrocyte is shown as it passes through two apertures of basement membrane. Two globular portions of the erythrocyte are in a sinus (*S*). An attenuated connecting portion lies deep in the basement membrane. *E*, endothelial cells; *R*, reticular cell. *From Burke JS, Simon GT. Am J Pathol 1970; 58:127-155.*

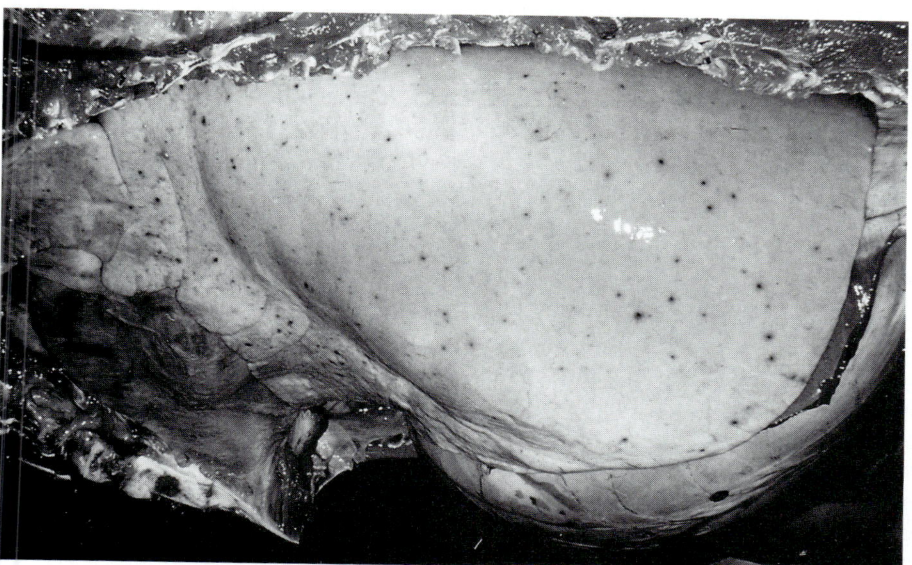

Fig. 7-5 Lung; horse. Equine infectious anemia. Focal hemorrhages are visible beneath the visceral pleura.

compensatory erythropoiesis is inhibited, presumably by mechanisms responsible for anemias of chronic inflammation.

During the viremic phase, horses with equine infectious anemia are markedly depressed and have fever, icterus, dependent pitting edema, and pallor of mucous membranes. Petechiae are frequently present on the ventral surface of the tongue and on conjunctivae. Hemograms taken during periods of anemia have severely depressed erythrocyte numbers and packed cell volumes (PCVs) as low as 0.10 L per liter (10%). There is usually bilirubinemia. The only indication of compensatory erythropoiesis may be an increased MCV and RDW. The accompanying leukopenia has components of neutropenia and a marginal lymphopenia. Monocyte numbers are increased, and, occasionally, they contain erythrocytes. Thrombocytopenia is evident within 1 or 2 days of viral inoculation, but the mechanism is unclear. Bone marrow aspirates have marked erythroid hyperplasia. Megakaryocyte numbers are not increased, suggesting that the thrombocytopenia may, in part, be due to impaired thrombopoiesis. As the disease progresses, the erythropoietic rate declines, and hemosiderin-laden macrophages and plasma cells accumulate. Confirmatory diagnosis of equine infectious anemia is by an agar-gel immunodiffusion test, in which a precipitin line develops in the presence of serum antibody to tissue culture–derived antigen.

Animals dying during hemolytic crises have icterus, anemia, and widespread hemorrhages. In more chronic cases, emaciated animals have serous atrophy of fat. The spleen and liver are enlarged, dark, and turgid, and these and other organs have superficial hemorrhages (Fig. 7-5). Petechiae are evident beneath the renal capsule and throughout the cortex and medulla. The bone marrow is strikingly red as the adipose tissue is replaced by hemopoietic tissue; the extent of replacement is reflective of the duration of the anemia.

Leptospirosis is a disease of domestic animals, rodents, and human beings caused by *Leptospira* sp. The spirochetes are subdivided into serogroups, which are further subdivided into serovars. The organisms are ubiquitous, occurring throughout the world under appropriate environmental conditions. They remain viable for some time in water but are susceptible to drying, shifts in pH, and changes in temperature. Leptospires are best studied by dark-field microscopy of fluids, in which they are visible as delicate, motile spirilla.

Leptospires are not highly host specific; thus, several serovars may cause disease in several different species. There is considerable overlap in clinical signs, laboratory results, and lesions in the diseases caused by different serovars in different animals. Infection occurs by the percutaneous route and via conjunctival mucous membranes followed by shedding of organisms in secretions and excretions, particularly urine. Animals become bacteremic, and, then, the organisms localize in the kidneys, liver, and pregnant uterus. During the bacteremic phase, animals may become icteric because of hemolysis and hepatic injury. In cattle, sheep, and horses, the icterus is mainly due to intravascular hemolysis caused by a hemolysin. Later, erythrocyte injury is mediated by antibody with continuing intravascular hemolysis.

The spirochetes, *L. icterohemorrhagia* and *L. canicola,* localized in hepatocytes of dogs can result in acute hepatic injury, increased activity of hepatic enzymes, and hyperbilirubinemia. Following this phase of the disease, the organisms localize in the kidneys. Leptospires in the kidneys cause a focal to diffuse interstitial nephritis, initially characterized by hyperemia, edema, and endothelial cell swelling and, later, by accumulation of lymphocytes and plasma cells. Although renal injury may be severe, death from renal failure is not common, occurring most often in dogs as a result of *L. canicola* infection. Those animals that survive may have organisms in their urine for years. Localization of leptospires in the pregnant uterus results in abortion, the most costly result of the disease in ruminants and swine.

Laboratory diagnosis of leptospirosis requires that precautions be taken to protect human beings from infection and to optimize isolation of such a fragile organism. The simplest procedure for diagnosis is demonstration of a rising titer in acute and convalescent serums. Demonstration of the organisms by dark-field microscopy of fluids and tissue emulsions at necropsy requires that the tissues be fresh. Inoculation of laboratory animals, followed by examination of fluids and tissue emulsions, increases the likelihood of diagnosis by microscopic visualization and cultural isolation of the organisms.

The most prominent lesions in ruminants dying of acute leptospirosis are the results of intravascular hemolysis and include anemia, icterus, pulmonary edema, and a pale, friable, bile-stained liver. The kidneys are swollen and dark because of hemoglobin staining. Later in the course of the disease, the kidneys have pale foci caused by interstitial cell infiltrates. Hemorrhages are numerous and widespread.

Dogs dying of acute leptospirosis have widespread hemorrhages and focal hepatic necrosis. The kidneys most consistently have lesions and, in the acute disease, are swollen and have subcapsular and cortical ecchymotic hemorrhages. Later in the disease, the kidneys become shrunken, with adherent capsules and varying degrees of cortical fibrosis.

Babesioses are tick-borne diseases caused by protozoa of the genus *Babesia.* They occur in all domestic animals, principally in warmer climates suitable for the tick vectors. The organisms can cause an acute syndrome characterized by hemolytic anemia, a chronic syndrome associated with anemia and weight loss, and a carrier state. Young cattle are resistant to *Babesia* infections. Infection in dogs occurs in pups. The speciation of *Babesia* is difficult because of incomplete knowledge of many of the isolates; however, *B. bigemina, B. bovis, B. divergens,* and *B. major* occur in cattle; *B. caballi* and *B. equi* occur in horses; *B. canis* and *B. gibsoni* occur in dogs; and *B. foliata, B. motasi,* and *B. ovis* occur in sheep.

Babesia produce acute disease by two principal mechanisms, hemolysis and circulatory disturbances. *Babesia* invade erythrocytes and cause intravascular and extravascular hemolysis. The precise mechanisms of intravascular hemolysis are unclear but are assumed to be directly attributable to the organism, because correlation exists between the parasitemia and the degree of anemia, hemoglobinemia, and hemoglobinuria. Phagocytosis of parasitized erythrocytes may be enhanced by antibody in the later stages of disease, as some *Babesia*-infected animals have positive direct antiglobulin tests and lowered complement levels.

B. bovis and *B. canis,* in addition to causing hemolysis, initiate events resulting in circulatory shock. The organisms activate plasma vasodilatory agents, such as kallikrein and bradykinin, resulting in sludging of blood in the microvasculature.

The wide variety of clinical signs of babesiosis is due to variations in pathogenicity of the organisms and susceptibility of the animals. The organisms usually appear in erythrocytes within 8 to 16 days following vector-transmitted infection; this appearance is accompanied by fever. Animals become listless, dehydrated, and weak with hemoglobinuria and icterus. Subcutaneous edema of the lower abdomen and thorax is detected in horses. *B. bovis* infections in cattle and *B. canis* infections in dogs result in nervous signs such as mania, recumbency with paddling of limbs, and coma, most likely due to circulatory disturbances caused by blockage or partial blockage of cerebral capillaries and resultant cerebral ischemia. If animals recover from the acute form of babesiosis, they have variable, unpredictable relapses, and some dogs experience chronic disease characterized by unthriftiness and weight loss.

Laboratory findings in animals with acute babesiosis are those of anemia with intense erythrogenesis and organisms visible in erythrocytes. Infected erythrocytes are large and tend to congregate in the feather edge of blood films. In vivo–infected erythrocytes accumulate in capillaries; therefore, blood films prepared from capillary blood, as from an ear or tail incision, are useful for finding the round to pyriform organisms (Fig. 7-6). The number of organisms per erythrocyte is variable. In the later stages of the disease, leukocyte counts increase because of lymphocytosis. During the period of severe anemia, the activity of hepatic enzymes such as alanine and aspartate aminotransferases (ALT and AST) and bilirubin are elevated. Serologic tests are available to assist in the diagnosis of babesiosis; these tests are most useful in carrier animals in which organisms are difficult to find. The indirect fluorescent antibody test for *Babesia* in erythrocytes is highly specific but not very sensitive. Agglutination tests, including hemagglutination, capillary, slide, and card tests, are sensitive methods for the detection of antibodies.

At necropsy, cattle dying of the acute disease have congestion of the spleen, brain, lungs, and skeletal muscle. Jaundice, hemoglobinuria, and subepicardial and subendocardial hemorrhages are also present. The kidneys are swollen, edematous, and dark because of their hemoglobin content. The gallbladder is usually distended with thick bile. A striking feature of *B. bovis* infection is congestion of the gray matter throughout the brain, which is readily visible when compared with the white matter.

Anaplasmosis is a disease of cattle and sheep caused by organisms of the genus *Anaplasma,* order Rickettsiales. In cattle, *A. marginale* causes hemolytic anemia, whereas *A. centrale* is less pathogenic. Bovine anaplasmosis is a significant disease in Australia, the United States, South America, and the former states of the USSR; *A. ovis* (of sheep and goats) causes significant disease in the Mediterranean region. The organisms are transmitted by ticks and, mechanically, by biting flies and hypodermic needles.

Mechanisms of disease induced by *Anaplasma* organisms involve penetration of the erythrocyte; the membrane of the erythrocyte invaginates to engulf the organisms within a vesicle. The parasite then divides by binary or multiple fission to form new infective units. Later, pores form in the erythrocytic membrane, through which organisms escape to infect other cells. It is suspected that the organism can proceed through these stages and exert its effects upon the erythrocyte by release of hydrolytic enzymes. The presence of *Anaplasma* proteins on the erythrocyte results in the formation of antibodies that subsequently affix to the erythrocyte and interact with macrophage receptors. The observation that noninfected erythrocytes are also destroyed would suggest that antibodies are produced that interact with membrane proteins of normal erythrocytes.

Young animals are susceptible to infection but do not develop disease. The immunity that follows infection is tolerant of the carrier state, resulting in a population of domestic and wild ruminants that are a reservoir of infection for other animals. Splenectomy of carrier animals results in marked parasitemia and acute hemolysis of erythrocytes.

The incubation period of anaplasmosis is 1 to 3 months. Affected animals develop a hemolytic anemia and have pale, icteric mucosae, depression, weakness, and reduced exercise tolerance. In contrast to babesiosis, hemoglobinuria is not observed in anaplasmosis because the destruction of erythrocytes occurs within macrophages. Animals may recover completely or remain debilitated with nonregenerative anemia without parasitemia.

Laboratory findings are anemia of varying severity with PCVs as low as 0.10 to 0.15 L per liter (10% to 15%). During this phase of the disease, as many as 50% to 60% of the erythrocytes contain organisms (Fig. 7-7). There

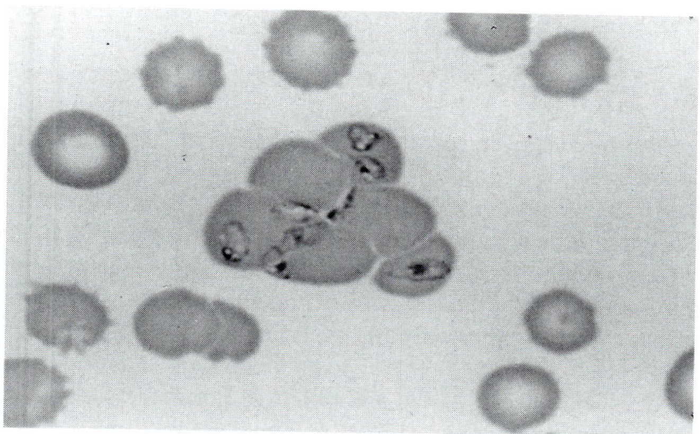

Fig. 7-6 Blood smear; dog. Babesiosis. Wright-Giemsa stain. *Courtesy L.J. Rich.*

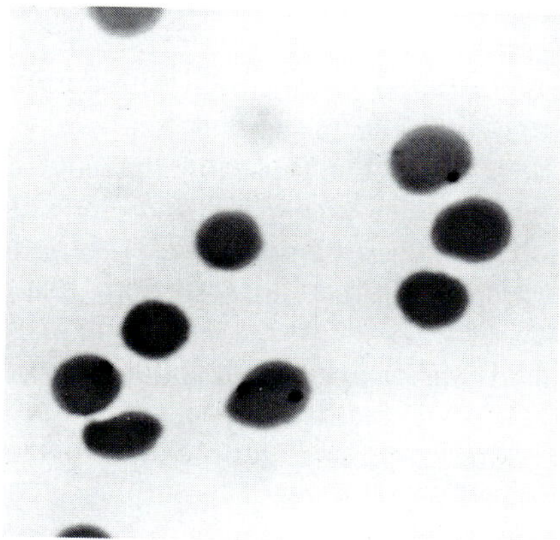

Fig. 7-7 Blood smear; cow. Anaplasmosis. Discrete, round organisms are visible at the periphery of erythrocytes. Wright-Giemsa stain.

may be one or more dark blue to black organisms of uniform size per erythrocyte. They must be differentiated from nuclear remnants, which are usually not as numerous, vary more in size, and occur as single inclusions. The anemia is usually regenerative with abundant polychromasia, basophilic stippling, and reticulocytosis. There may be moderate neutrophilia. During acute hemolysis, a prehepatic hyperbilirubinemia is detectable.

Animals dying of acute anaplasmosis have the nonspecific findings of acute hemolytic anemia with blood of low viscosity, pale to icteric tissues, an enlarged turgid spleen, and an icteric liver with a distended gallbladder.

Eperythrozoonoses are diseases caused by erythrocytic parasites within the order Rickettsiales, family Bartonellaceae. A carrier state exists in sheep, cattle, swine, and llamas and may, on occasion, cause a hemolytic anemia. Transmission of the organisms from animal to animal has not been as extensively studied as that of babesiosis and anaplasmosis, but the greatest incidence of disease in sheep and swine accompanies heavy ectoparasite infestations. The mechanism of disease appears similar to that of other erythrocytic parasites, wherein immune-mediated extravascular hemolysis follows parasite-erythrocyte interaction.

The disease in sheep and swine has a seasonal incidence, corresponding to the peak occurrence of biting insects. However, it can also occur at other times of the year, as a recrudescence in a carrier animal with another disease. In both sheep and swine, sudden death of one or two animals is followed by subsequent detection of other anemic animals within a herd. *Eperythrozoon wenyoni* in cattle is less pathogenic than *E. ovis* and *E. suis;* it appears to be widespread but rarely causes disease.

It is imperative that blood samples and smears be taken from anemic sheep and swine prior to euthanasia, because detection of the organism is difficult after death. In acute disease, the anemia may be severe and significantly regenerative, with many parasitized erythrocytes; in blood smears, organisms are found free among erythrocytes. In less severe infections, the anemia may be mild, and blood smears may have only a few parasitized erythrocytes. Regardless of the degree of parasitemia, infected erythrocytes usually harbor several organisms, frequently within one portion of the cell. The organisms tend to be ring forms with pale centers, except those on the edge of the cell, which appear bacillary (Figs. 7-8 and 7-9). Identification of the organisms requires a good-quality blood film, staining without precipitation, and microscopy using an oil immersion lens.

In animals dying of eperythrozoonosis, the findings are typical of extravascular hemolysis with obvious anemia, icterus, splenomegaly, and gallbladder distention. Bone marrow has varying degrees of hyperplasia, reflecting the duration of erythrocytic destruction.

Trypanosomiasis is caused by flagellated protozoa that occur in the blood and, occasionally, in tissues of animals

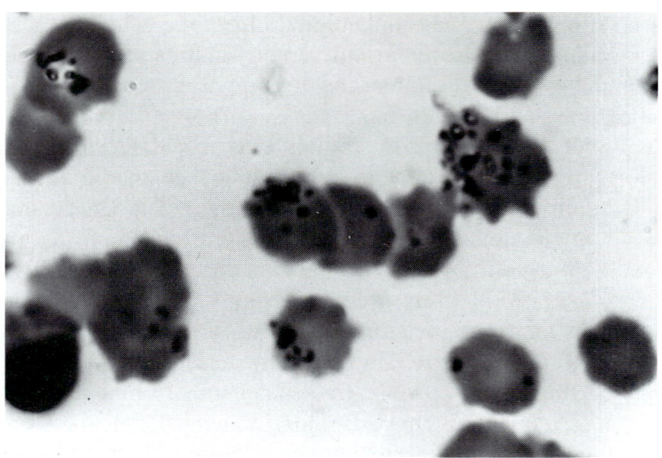

Fig. 7-8 Blood smear; pig. Eperythrozoonosis. Wright-Giemsa stain.

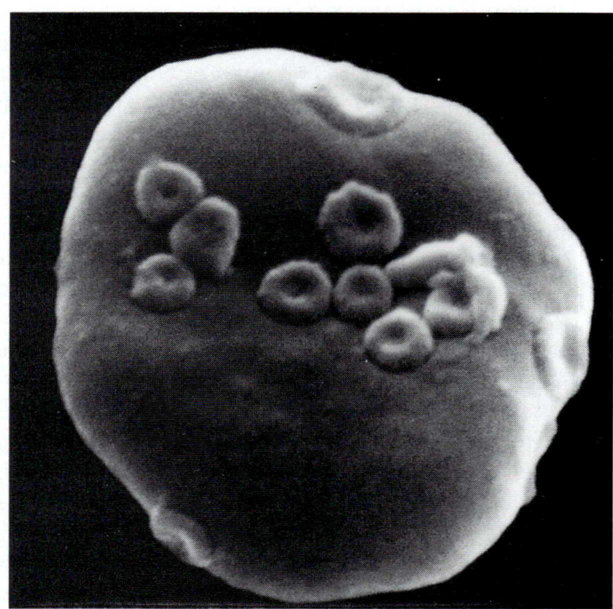

Fig. 7-9 Scanning electron micrograph. Blood; calf. *Eperythrozoon* organisms on an erythrocyte.

and human beings. They have widespread geographic distribution, but cause significant disease in warmer climatic areas, such as Africa and South America. The principal pathogens of animals are *Trypanosoma congolense, T. vivax,* and *T. brucei,* whereas trypanosomes such as *T. melophagium* in sheep and *T. theileri* in cattle are widespread and nonpathogenic. Trypanosomes normally survive and are nonpathogenic in wildlife reservoir hosts. They are transmitted to other animals by arthropod vectors, such as the tsetse fly, in which the organism survives in the salivary glands for the life of the fly. Other biting insects transmit trypanosomes mechanically.

The mechanisms by which trypanosomes cause disease

are complex and incompletely studied. The considerable variation in disease is due to factors such as strain of organism and host immunocompetence. Some trypanosomial species induce rapidly fatal disease, others cause chronic debilitating disease, and some allow complete recovery with significant immunity. Since some African native cattle have considerable resistance to trypanosomes, clearer insight into these parasite-host interactions would be of considerable significance in learning to control infections in more susceptible cattle. Trypanosomes escape from the host's immune response following emergence of new cell membrane proteins, which results in waves of parasitemia and chronic disease.

Cattle with acute trypanosomiasis have significant anemia that initially is regenerative with increased MCV, macrocytosis, reticulocytosis, and marrow erythroid hyperplasia. With time, the anemia becomes less regenerative. Platelets numbers are between 100 to 200 × 10^9/L (100 to 200 × 10^6/mm^3), and the significant leukopenia is caused by neutropenia and lymphopenia. Plasma proteins are low due to hypoalbuminemia. The extent of parasitemia is readily apparent with *T. vivax* infections because the organisms are present in large numbers in the blood. This is in contrast to *T. congolense,* which localizes within the vasculature of the brain and skeletal muscle. Cattle with *T. congolense* infections develop chronic debilitating disease; animals have roughened, scruffy hair coats; appear "potbellied"; and have low-grade fever, intermittent diarrhea, and exercise intolerance. Mortality is greater with *T. vivax* infections, usually owing to intercurrent acute infectious diseases such as salmonellosis.

Necropsy findings in cattle with trypanosome infections include cachexia, generalized edema with increased fluid in body cavities, and generalized lymph node enlargement. Bronchopneumonia, a flabby heart, and serous atrophy of pericardial fat may be present. Liver and kidneys are enlarged. The lymph nodes are enlarged up to four times normal size, and the bone marrow fat is mostly replaced by red hemopoietic tissue. The spleen is enlarged due to lymphoid hyperplasia, but does not ooze blood when incised.

T. cruzi infection (Chagas' disease) occurs in dogs in the southern United States. Reservoir hosts include raccoons, opossums, armadillos, and skunks, and transmission to dogs is by hemipteran insects. Clinical signs include tachycardia, pale mucous membranes, and lymph node enlargement. Laboratory evaluation involves finding trypanosomes in the peripheral blood, buffy coat smears, and lymph node aspirates or biopsies (Fig. 7-10). Postmortem findings include those of cardiac failure, i.e., pulmonary edema, ascites, and chronic passive congestion of the liver. Cardiac lesions, most pronounced in the right heart, include multiple, yellow to white myocardial foci (myocardial necrosis and myocarditis) and, in chronic cases, myocardial flaccidity and dilatation.

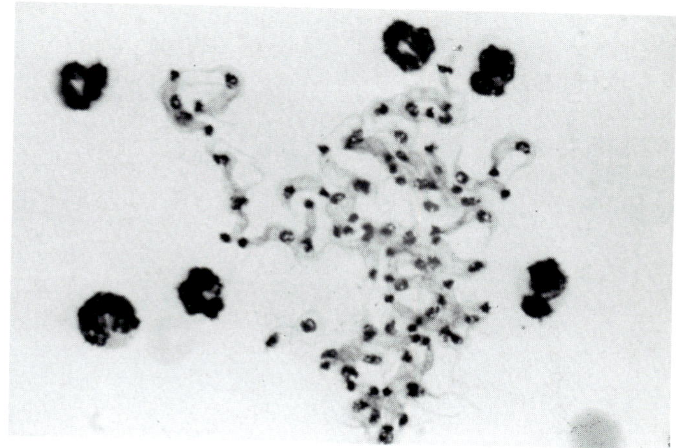

Fig. 7-10 Buffy coat preparation of blood; dog. Trypanosomiasis. A cluster of trypomastigotes of *Trypanosoma cruzi. Courtesy J.C. Fox.*

Haemobartonellosis is caused by organisms (family Bartonellaceae, order Rickettsiales) that resemble *Eperythrozoon* species in most respects. They are widespread geographically and occur in rats, cattle, goats, cats, and dogs but are of most significance in the cat as the cause of feline infectious anemia. Transmission is probably due to bloodsucking arthropods. The protozoa should always be searched for in dogs following splenectomy, but, even if they are present, they may not significantly shorten the life span of erythrocytes.

Haemobartonellosis in the cat may cause an acute hemolytic, regenerative anemia with marked parasitemia. *Haemobartonella felis*–erythrocyte membrane interactions are assumed to provoke immune-mediated erythrophagocytosis in the spleen, liver, and bone marrow. Cats with the acute form of the disease are weak and depressed and have pale, icteric, mucous membranes. Hematologic findings in these cats are a regenerative anemia and PCVs as low as 0.10 L per liter (10%). The degree of polychromasia is assessed to ensure that erythropoiesis is orderly and complete. Determination of the presence of *H. felis* in erythrocytes requires a correctly stained, high-quality blood film and an experienced examiner. The differentiation of the organisms from artifacts may be difficult, especially when the organisms are rod forms on the edge of the erythrocyte. Finding ring forms away from the cell periphery is very helpful in distinguishing organisms from artifacts (Fig. 7-11). When *H. felis* is present on erythrocytes of chronically ill cats with nonregenerative anemia, other underlying diseases, especially feline leukemia and immunodeficiency virus infections, should be investigated.

Cats dying of hemolytic anemia due to *H. felis* have pale mucous membranes with or without icterus. Splenomegaly and bone-marrow hyperplasia are lesions with fatty marrow replaced by red hemopoietic tissue in long bones of limbs.

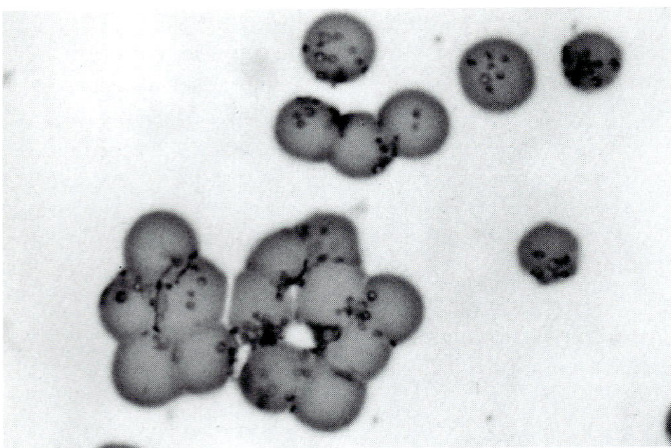

Fig. 7-11 Blood smear; cat. Haemobartonellois. Wright-Giemsa stain.

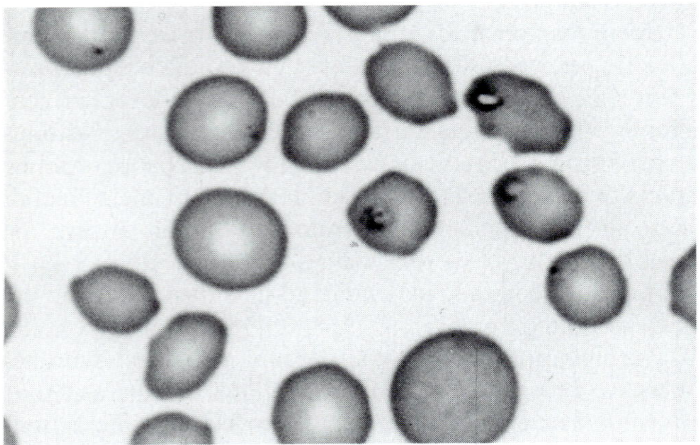

Fig. 7-12 Blood smear; cat. Cytauxzoonosis. The protozoa are bipolar, oval, or "signet ring" forms, 1.0 to 1.5 μm in diameter. Wright-Giemsa stain. *Courtesy D.A. Schmidt.*

Cytauxzoonosis, caused by *Cytauxzoon felis,* a protozoal organism in the order Piroplasmida, family Theileriidae, is an acute, fatal disease of domestic cats in the southern United States. The mechanism of natural transmission is unknown, although arthropods are most likely vectors. Experimental transmission has been achieved by injection of blood or tissue homogenates from infected cats into normal cats. The domestic cat is probably an unusual or "dead end" host for this organism, and the bobcat *(Lynx rufus)* may be the reservoir host.

C. felis undergoes schizogony within monocytes and macrophages. Merozoites are released and enter erythrocytes. Cats become acutely ill with fever, pallor, and icterus and usually die within 2 to 3 days. Laboratory evaluation confirms moderately regenerative anemias. The organisms within erythrocytes are "signet ring" shaped or bipolar oval forms, 1.0 to 1.5 μm in diameter (Fig. 7-12). The protozoal cytoplasm stains light blue, whereas the nucleus stains purple. Impression smears of the spleen are useful for demonstration of protozoa in macrophages.

Hemolytic anemias can be induced by chemicals that inhibit erythrocyte metabolism or that cause denaturation and precipitation of hemoglobin. The erythrocyte, as an anucleate cell, survives by constantly generating ATP from glucose metabolism through the Embden-Meyerhof pathway (see Fig. 7-3). This energy is needed to maintain erythrocyte cation content, iron of hemoglobin in the divalent form, the sulfhydryl groups of hemoglobin and enzymes in the reduced form, and membrane integrity. The erythrocytic membrane consists of a lipid bilayer in which certain proteins are attached to an underlying cytoskeletal network. The latter components provide the membrane with both its strength and its flexibility, allowing it to withstand shearing and deforming stress in the circulation (see Fig. 7-4). Any disruption of this complex protein network may lead to hemolysis.

An important aspect of erythrocyte metabolism, relative to injury by oxidative toxins, is the capacity to maintain a reducing environment by efficient antioxidant mechanisms. These mechanisms involve enzymes such as methemoglobin reductase and glutathione peroxidase, as well as the reduced pyridine nucleotides, nicotinamide-adenine dinucleotide (NADH) and NADH phosphate (NADPH) (see Fig. 7-3). Oxidant injury to erythrocytes in animals usually occurs due to overloading of the reducing environment subsequent to ingestion of the offending substance. Methemoglobin formation appears to be a prerequisite in the evolution and precipitation of denatured hemoglobin to produce Heinz bodies. It is suspected that the precipitated, denatured hemoglobin results in further heme oxidation of membrane proteins and inhibition of several erythrocyte enzymes. The end result is erythrocyte injury, leading to cation leak, loss of deformability, and fixation of immunoglobulin to altered membrane proteins. Both macrophage-mediated erythrocyte destruction and intravascular lysis occur.

Onions contain an agent capable of causing oxidative hemolytic anemia. Indeed, some of the earliest veterinary records of disease and death in North American horses and cattle were associated with the ingestion of wild onions. Poisoning occasionally occurs in cattle when onions are incorporated into the ration and in dogs that ingest onions in cooked feed or chew raw onions. Clinical findings include acute hemolytic anemia with pallor, icterus, and weakness. Hemoglobinuria has occurred in cattle that have ingested large quantities of onions.

Cats are prone to erythrocyte oxidative injury because their globin chains contain more sulfhydryl-containing amino acids than do those of other mammals. For this reason, Heinz bodies are frequently present in feline erythrocytes. **Propylene glycol,** a common additive to commercial pet foods, can induce hemoglobin denaturation and Heinz body formation in feline erythrocytes and a measurable decrease in erythrocyte half-life. Drugs such as aspirin and related products contain strong oxidants that can cause hemolytic anemia in cats.

Hemolytic anemia caused by oxidation of hemoglobin has occurred in horses following the ingestion of leaves and bark of red maple trees. Experimental studies have established significant hemoglobin oxidative injury with Heinz body formation and hemolysis in marine birds following ingestion of crude oil, thus establishing that these phenomena are likely significant in birds involved with oil spills. Heinz body hemolytic anemia may occur in dogs due to zinc toxicity following ingestion of zinc nuts, bolts, and pennies. Hematologic findings in animals with oxidative erythrocyte disorders include varying degrees of anemia and compensatory erythropoiesis. An important diagnostic feature of these anemias is the presence of Heinz bodies in erythrocytes. These are visible in Wright's-Giemsa–stained blood films as discrete protrusions from the cells (Fig. 7-13). These inclusions are more readily visible on new methylene blue–stained preparations. Eccentrocytes, erythrocytes with hemoglobin concentrated in one portion of the cell, also occur subsequent to erythrocytic oxidative injury (Fig. 7-14). Animals dying following hemoglobin denaturation have the nonspecific indications of hemolysis, including generalized pallor and icterus. Pulmonary edema with frothy fluid in the trachea is a usual finding. The spleen is enlarged and turgid. The liver is usually enlarged and icteric, and the gallbladder is distended.

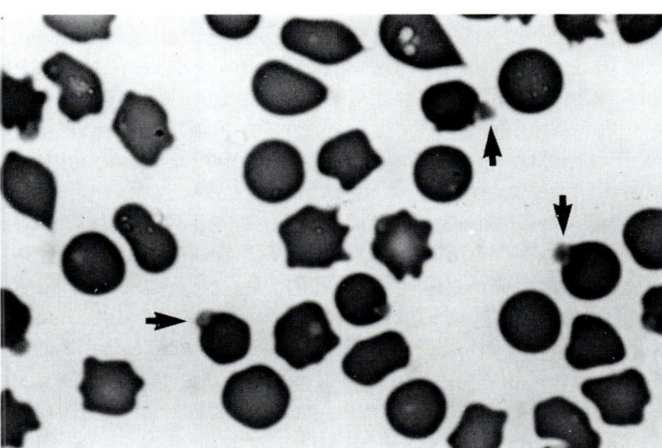

Fig. 7-13 Blood smear; cat. Denatured hemoglobin (Heinz bodies) on feline erythrocytes *(arrows)*. Wright-Giemsa stain.

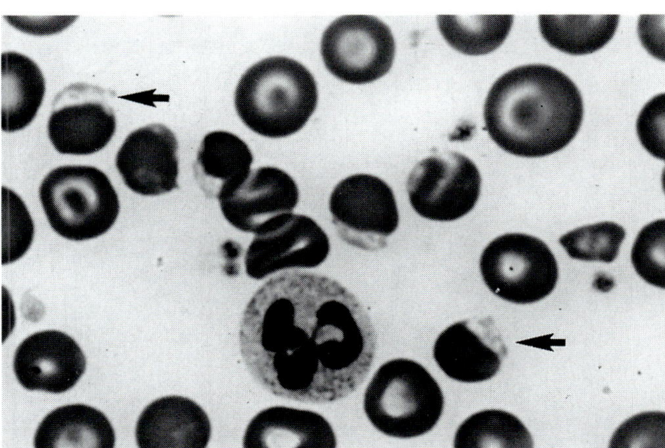

Fig. 7-14 Blood smear; dog. Eccentrocytes *(arrows)* in a dog with hemoytic anemia following ingestion of onions. Wright-Giemsa stain.

Copper poisoning and hemolysis occur when copper is present in the plasma at concentrations exceeding the binding capacity of its transport proteins. This occurs in sheep, cattle, and swine following release of copper from the liver. Sheep are uniquely susceptible to copper toxicity, with rapid sequestration of copper within the liver followed by delayed biliary excretion. Sporadic copper-induced hemolytic anemia occurs in cattle and swine; hemolytic crises have occurred in dogs due to release of copper in the late stages of liver disease. At lower concentrations, copper inhibits erythrocyte enzymes in the Embden-Meyerhof pathway, which causes ATP depletion and lysis. At greater concentrations, it inhibits enzymes within the hexose-monophosphate shunt, leading to impaired glutathione metabolism and Heinz body formation (see Fig. 7-3). Anemia in all species most likely results from a combination of these mechanisms, which lead to hemolysis with hemoglobinemia and hemoglobinuria.

Hemograms from animals with copper toxicity confirm severe anemia. Hemoglobin concentrations may be disproportionately large because plasma hemoglobin is included in the measurement. Blood films confirm severe anemia and Heinz bodies. However, sheep may die from copper toxicity before compensatory erythropoiesis becomes evident.

Hypophosphatemic hemolytic anemias is described as postparturient hemoglobinuria in the dairy cow 3 to 8 weeks after parturition. It also occurs in beef cattle and nonpostpartum cattle on phosphorus-deficient diets. One or two animals with hemolytic anemia may serve as indicators of the underlying nutritional disorder in a herd. Hypophosphatemic hemolytic anemia also occurs in human beings with diabetes mellitus or undergoing withdrawal from alcohol consumption, and following enteric phosphate binding by medicants in patients treated for peptic ulcer disease or renal failure.

Erythrocytes require inorganic phosphorus for incorporation into phosphorylated intermediate molecules within the Embden-Meyerhof pathway and for synthesis of ATP (see Fig. 7-3). Inorganic phosphorus also exerts control over the reaction rate of a key enzyme in the pathway (phosphofructokinase). In phosphate depletion, the erythrocytic glycolytic rate is slowed, and ATP synthesis declines. These erythrocytes are no doubt compromised in many ways relative to structure and function, and when plasma phosphorus concentrations reach a critical level, hemolysis occurs. Intravascular hemolysis indicated by hemoglobinuria is a common finding, but phagocytosis of abnormal erythrocytes by macrophages probably also occurs.

Laboratory findings include hemoglobinemia and hemoglobinuria. The anemia may be very severe, with PCVs as low as 0.10 L per liter (10%). In some animals, the disease is so acute that very few immature erythrocytes are present in blood smears, but in those with hemolysis of several days' duration, moderate to marked reticulocyte responses are seen. Serum phosphorus concentrations in hemoglobinemic animals may be normal, perhaps because phosphates from the hydrolysis of intracellular phosphates of lysed erythrocytes are measured in the assay. In these cases, it is advisable to measure serum phosphorus in other animals in the herd. In the author's experience with a herd of beef cattle with hemolytic anemia and serum phosphorus of 1.40 mmol per liter (4.34 mg/dl) in one cow, serum phosphorus concentrations of 18 animals had a mean of 0.97 mmol per liter (3.00 mg/dl), with a range of 0.38 to 1.65 mmol per liter (1.18 to 5.1 mg/dl) in comparison to normal reference values of 1.08 to 2.76 mmol per liter (3.34 to 8.54 mg/dl).

Animals dying in hemolytic crises have generalized pallor, icterus, watery blood, pulmonary edema, and fluid in serous cavities. The liver is enlarged, turgid, and pale; the gallbladder is distended with bile, and the spleen is enlarged and congested.

Immune-mediated hemolytic anemias are those in which erythrocyte destruction occurs following attachment of antibody to the erythrocytic membrane. It is the most common type of hemolytic anemia in dogs, but the incidence is much lower in other species. The etiology of most cases of canine immune-mediated hemolytic anemia is unknown. It is possible that the offending antibody develops because of alteration of proteins of erythrocytic membranes by infectious agents (such as viruses) or foreign substances (such as drugs). Circulating immune complexes involving these antigens may be adsorbed by erythrocytic membranes. Indirect evidence would suggest that the antibodies lack specificity for a particular erythrocytic antigen; erythrocytes administered to dogs with high titers of antierythrocytic antibody are also destroyed.

The decreased survival of antibody-coated erythrocytes is mostly due to the fact that macrophages, principally in the spleen, but also in the liver and bone marrow, have receptors for the Fc region of IgG. Partial phagocytosis, probably due to removal of portions of the erythrocytic membrane with the greatest concentration of antibody molecules, results in spherocytosis, the hallmark of this disease. This is readily recognized in dogs as small erythrocytes lacking central pallor. It would seem logical that a direct correlation exists between the numbers of spherocytes and the rate of hemolysis. However, when the disease is acute and spherocytes predominate, the phagocytic capacity of the macrophage population, especially those in the spleen, may be temporarily overwhelmed, pending the arrival of monocytes and their maturation to activated macrophages. Spherocytic erythrocytes are at risk for phagocytosis because they are no longer pliable or deformable and are retained in the spleen in close proximity to macrophages. As these cells accumulate, lactic acid from erythrocytic glycolysis produces a drop in environmental pH and adds additional erythrocytic stress.

The IgG class of antibody is the most significant cause of canine immunohemolytic anemia. As demonstrated in human beings, there is most likely a direct correlation between the quantity of IgG bound to erythrocytes and hemolysis. The antibody may also fix complement-enhancing phagocytosis. Occasionally, dogs in hemolytic crisis have hemoglobinemia and hemoglobinuria due to a complement-mediated intravascular hemolysis. IgM antibodies are particularly efficient at binding complement and may also be present on erythrocytes of these animals.

Dogs with immune-mediated hemolytic anemia are frequently acutely ill and recumbent, but the disease may occur in a subclinical form. Affected dogs have pale mucosae, with or without icterus, and some may vomit and have a fever. Should it occur, hemoglobinuria is a grave sign, as it indicates acute and severe hemolysis. These animals should be recognized as emergency cases requiring rapid diagnosis and treatment. When presented with these dogs, the clinician should obtain a drop of blood for the evaluation of agglutination (Fig. 7-15) of erythrocytes.

Determination of the laboratory features of this disease is essential for an accurate diagnosis. The degree of anemia is variable but may be severe, with PCVs of 0.05 to 0.15 L per liter (5% to 10%). Thus, practicing veterinarians must do the studies necessary for diagnosis as there is no time

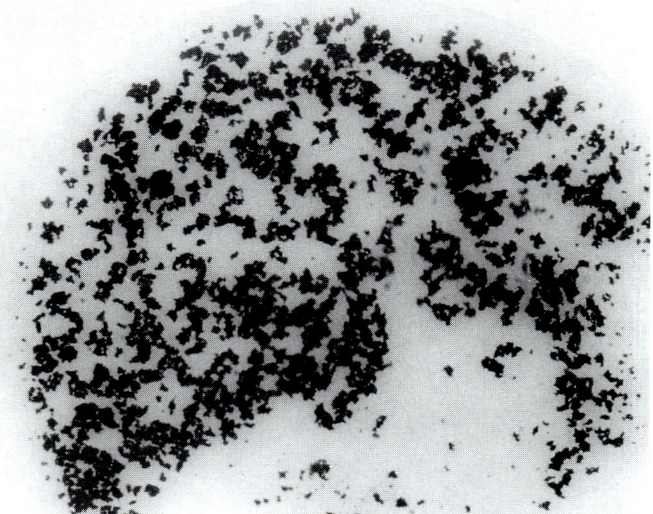

Fig. 7-15 Blood; dog. Immune-mediated hemolytic anemia. Erythrocyte agglutination in a drop of blood.

to send blood to a laboratory. In most dogs, the anemia is regenerative at the time of presentation; however, in a few, very acute cases, the blood film will have spherocytosis without polychromasia. Occasionally, dogs with immune-mediated hemolytic anemia remain reticulocytopenic beyond the time required for compensatory erythropoeisis to be evident in peripheral blood. Bone marrow examination is indicated in these dogs, and samples contain phagocytosed erythrocytes, metarubricytes, and rubricytes, and evidence of marked erythroid hyperplasia (Fig. 7-16). Obviously, the prognosis is guarded in these reticulocytopenic dogs. The blood in the tube and the stained blood film must be critically examined for erythrocytic agglutination. Agglutinated erythrocytes are most easily detected in the thicker areas of the blood smear, occurring in irregular clumps, which must not be confused with the linear formations of erythrocytes in rouleaux. The presence of polychromatophilic erythrocytes in clumps indicates agglutination because they do not participate in rouleaux. One of the most striking features, visible at low magnification, is marked anisocytosis. This extreme variation in erythrocyte diameter is due to the presence of macrocytic, immature erythrocytes plus small spherocytes (Fig. 7-17). Polychromasia is usually pronounced, and metarubricytes and rubricytes may be present (Fig. 7-18). Platelet numbers may be reduced because of concurrent immune-mediated thrombocytopenia. If platelets are not involved, their numbers will be increased, and some may be enlarged. Neutrophilia is also common and appears to accompany the reticulocyte response. A few dogs have leukocyte counts in excess of 50×10^9/L (50,000/mm^3) because of neutrophilia and monocytosis. The monocytosis is a reflection of traffic between the bone marrow and spleen where monocytes become activated macrophages capable of erythrophagocytosis.

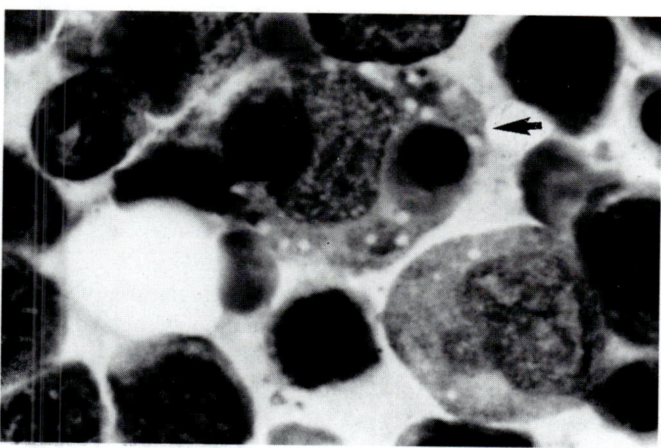

Fig. 7-16 Bone marrow aspirate; dog. A reticulocytopenic dog with immune-mediated hemolytic anemia. Note the macrophage with intracellular, nucleated erythrocytes *(arrow)*. Wright-Giemsa stain.

The direct antiglobulin test (DAT; Coombs' test) is a hemagglutination assay for antibody or complement bound to erythrocytes (Fig. 7-19). Washed saline suspensions of erythrocytes are incubated at 37° C and 4° C with antisera containing goat- or rabbit-derived antibody for canine IgG, IgM, and complement C3. The assay should be conducted in microtiter trays, using serial doubling dilutions of the antisera. This will overcome the prozone effect in which false-negative results occur because excess antibodies prevent the crosslinking necessary for agglutination (Fig. 7-19). The reported titer should be the last dilution causing agglutination of the patient's erythrocytes; this gives a rough estimate of the quantity of antibodies coating the erythrocytes. Although this test is justified as part of the laboratory investigation of this disease, the results must be

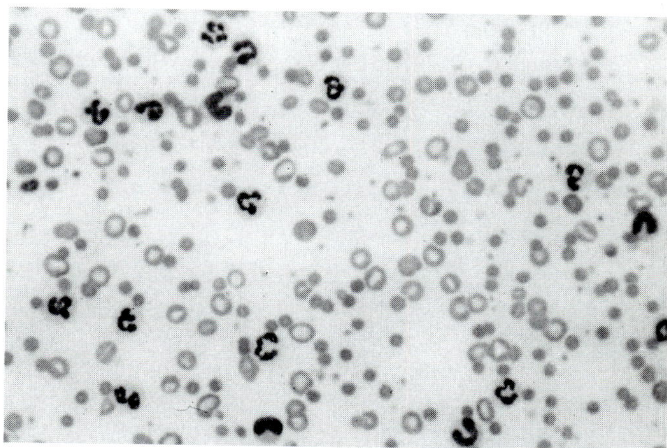

Fig. 7-17 Blood smear; dog. Immune-mediated hemolytic anemia. Neutrophilia and marked anisocytosis due to the presence of both spherocytes and macrocytes. Wright-Giemsa stain.

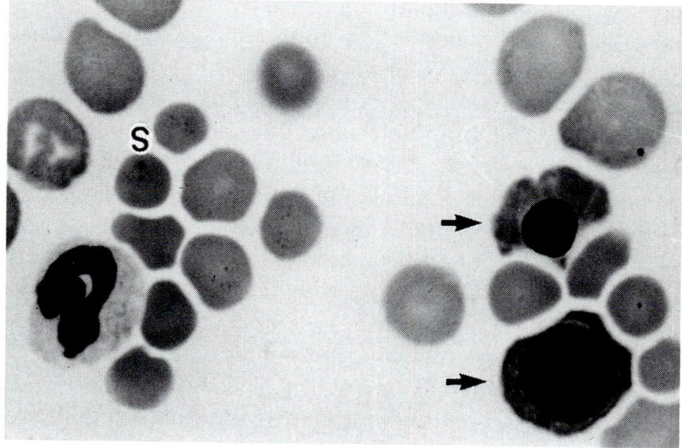

Fig. 7-18 Blood smear; dog. Immune-mediated hemolytic anemia. Nucleated erythrocytes *(arrows)* and spherocytes (*S*). Wright-Giemsa stain.

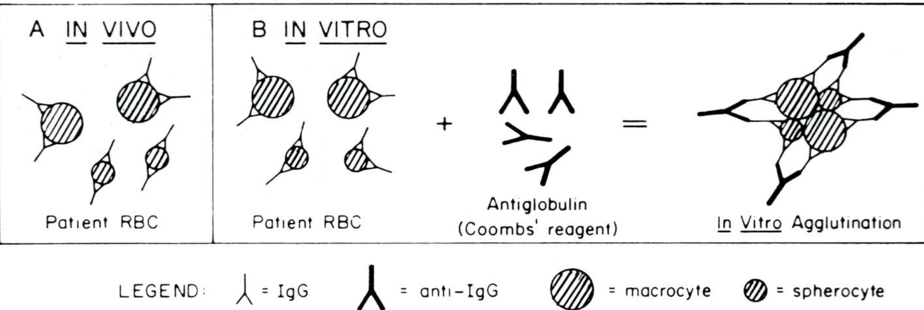

Fig. 7-19 Direct antiglobulin test (DAT). **A**, Red blood cells *(RBC)* of patient are coated with antibody in vivo. **B**, In vitro detection of autoantibody is accomplished by adding heterologous antiglobulin reagent, resulting in cross-linking of RBCs and microscopic or macroscopic agglutination. *From Lewis RM, Picut CA.* Hematologic Disorders. *In: Veterinary Clinical Immunology: From Classroom to Clinics. Philadelphia: Lea & Febiger, 1989:9.*

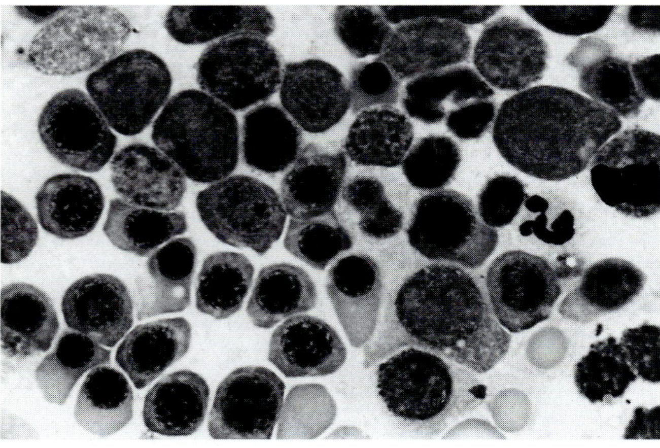

Fig. 7-20 Bone marrow aspirate; dog. Immune-mediated hemolytic anemia. Erythroid hyperplasia. Wright-Giemsa stain.

carefully interpreted in the context of other laboratory and clinical information. Dogs previously treated with glucocorticoid drugs frequently test negative. Negative results may also be obtained when antibody molecules of low avidity are lost during erythrocyte washings or when the numbers of antibody molecules are too low to be detected. A negative DAT in the presence of hematologic and clinical findings consistent with immune-mediated hemolytic anemia should not preclude the diagnosis.

Bone marrow aspirates have erythroid hyperplasia and varying amounts of erythrophagia in the early stages of the disease (Fig. 7-20). Megakaryocyte numbers are usually increased. When the disease is of some duration or following relapses, bone marrow iron content and plasma cells may be increased. In dogs with severe hemolysis, a biochemical profile will include hyperbilirubinemia and elevated activities of enzymes such as ALT, as occurs in hypoxic hepatocyte injury.

Postmortem findings in dogs with immune-mediated hemolytic anemia include pale tissues, mild to moderate icterus, pulmonary edema, and frothy tracheal fluid. The heart may be rounded and dilated if the anemia is of some duration; the liver is usually enlarged and pale and the gallbladder is distended. Lymph nodes are enlarged and hyperplastic in the acute disease but are small in dogs treated with glucocorticoid drugs. Hemorrhages are present on the serosal surfaces and on capsular surfaces of visceral organs in dogs with concurrent thrombocytopenia. The bone marrow has varying amounts of red marrow extending from the ends and endosteal surfaces of long bones, reflecting the long duration of compensatory erythropoiesis.

DATs have been performed on cats with a variety of diseases. The incidence of positive tests has been much greater than the incidence of hemolytic anemia. Most of these cats have nonregenerative anemia due to chronic diseases, such as those resulting from feline leukemia or immunodeficiency virus infections. Blood films from these cats may have erythrocytic agglutination. The combination of erythrocyte agglutination and positive DATs in cats with chronic diseases may be due to adherence of antigen-antibody complexes to erythrocytes.

Occasionally, hemolytic anemias are encountered in horses that have negative tests for equine infectious anemia by the agar-gel immunodiffusion test. An immune-mediated pathogenesis should be suspected and may be associated with occult lymphosarcoma.

Nonregenerative anemias

Anemias due to impaired erythropoiesis are the most common anemias in animals and human beings. For this reason, the hemogram is essential as an integral part of a thorough clinical examination because nonregenerative anemia is an indicator of occult disease. Dogs with hepatic disease, for example, are frequently anemic, and additional laboratory tests will be required to discover the underlying disorder. Bone marrow examination is indicated in animals with significant nonregenerative anemia when an underlying disease is not apparent.

Chronic disease is a common cause of nonregenerative anemias. The causes include inflammatory, renal, hepatic, and neoplastic diseases. Although these entities may share some underlying mechanisms, chronic inflammatory states and nonhemopoietic malignancies have more in common with each other than they do with renal and hepatic disease.

The mechanisms of impaired erythropoiesis in chronic inflammation are obscure and undoubtedly complex. At least three general mechanisms have been implicated in anemias of chronic disorders: iron sequestration in macrophages, shortened erythrocytic survival time, and impaired marrow response to anemia. For many years, a disturbance in iron reutilization for erythropoiesis has been demonstrated in both animals and human beings. This disturbance is characterized by a paradoxic association of hypoferremia and increased iron stores. In normal animals, approximately 80% of the iron salvaged from effete erythrocytes is transported in serum by transferrin to erythroid precursors for incorporation into hemoglobin; the remaining iron is bound to ferritin found in most cells and body fluids. Iron is released from transferrin to be utilized in erythropoiesis, or many ferritin-iron complexes can become coalesced within macrophages to form hemosiderin. Hemosiderin is the least labile form of iron in the body because it is released slowly, in response to demand. In chronic inflammation and neoplasia, movement of iron from tissues to plasma is impaired, and hemosiderin accumulates in macrophages.

The mechanisms responsible for shortened erythrocyte survival time are still unclear, but there is some experimental support for the possibility that binding of immunoglobulin to senescent erythrocytes is accelerated during chronic inflammation. This erythrocyte-associated immunoglobulin will facilitate uptake of erythrocytes by macrophages. Studies of erythrocyte precursors in culture would suggest that a poorly responsive marrow is significant in the pathogenesis of these anemias. Activated macrophage products significantly inhibit erythropoiesis in culture; these would be secreted in most chronic diseases and include tumor necrosis factor (cachectin). Animals in renal failure are frequently anemic owing principally to inadequate production of erythropoietin by damaged kidneys. The mechanisms of anemia in chronic hepatic disease are as yet unknown.

Animals with anemia of chronic disease usually have a mild to moderate anemia with quantitative erythrocyte parameters reduced by 10% to 30% (occasionally lower in dogs with renal failure). Despite the interference with release of iron from macrophages, the erythrocytic indices are usually normal. Alterations in shape of erythrocytes occur in cats and dogs with chronic hepatic disease. Alterations include elongated erythrocytes with short, irregular projections and, occasionally, acanthocytes (Fig. 7-21). In chronic inflammatory disorders, concentrations of plasma proteins are frequently increased, and the albumin/globulin ratio decreased due to increased gamma globulin. Bone marrow aspirates usually have normal granulocyte/erythrocyte ratios. Granulocyte hyperplasia may be present in animals with chronic suppurative inflammation. Hemosiderin deposits visible microscopically as gold, nugget-like clumps in unstained marrow aspirates (Fig. 7-22) may be increased. If these are not visible, iron stores should be assessed using Prussian blue-stained marrow smears, as this reaction stains ferritin as well as hemosiderin.

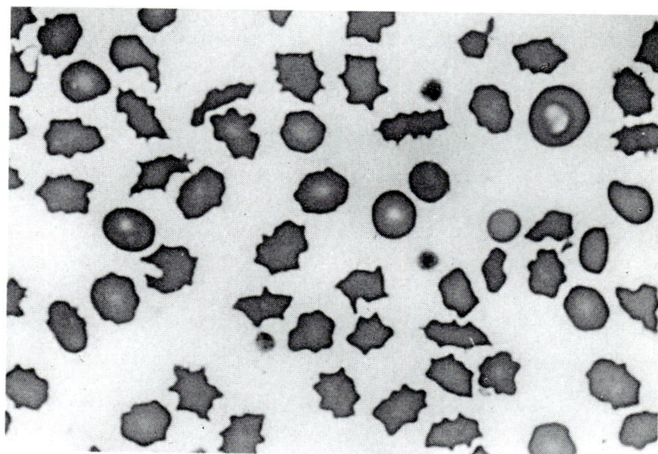

Fig. 7-21 Blood smear; cat. Chronic liver disease. Note the shape alterations of the erythrocytes. Wright-Giemsa stain.

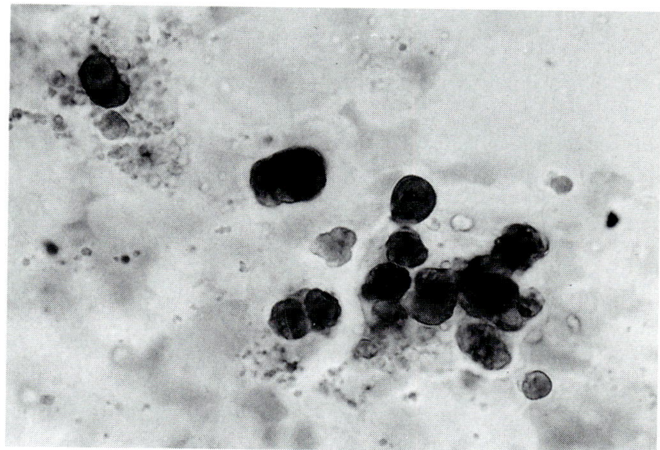

Fig. 7-22 Bone marrow aspirate; dog. Clumps of hemosiderin resemble gold nuggets. Unstained.

Nutritional deficiency anemias are uncommon in domestic animals. Piglets become iron deficient, anemic, and severely debilitated if they do not receive a supplement of iron. Parenteral iron administration is now common in swine, and iron deficiency anemias occur only sporadically when injection of iron to a litter of piglets has been overlooked. Iron-deficient piglets have retarded growth, dyspnea, and lethargy at around 3 weeks of age. The skin and

Table 7-3. Hemogram from a 2-year-old male Corgi dog with mycotic rhinitis, epistaxis, and von Willebrand's disease

Hemogram	Patient values	Reference values
WBC × 10^9/L	9.5	6.0-17.1
RBC × 10^{12}/L	4.41	5.5-8.5
Hemoglobin g/L	97	120-180
PCV L/L	0.28	0.37-0.55
MCV fL	62	60-77
MCH pg	22	19.5-24.5
MCHC g/L	346	320-360
RDW %	15.8	11-12.5
Platelets × 10^9/L	575	200-900
Iron μmol/L	8	16.8-22
RETICS %	10	0-1

WBC, white blood count; *RBC,* red blood count; *PVC,* packed cell volume; *MCV,* mean corpuscular volume; *MCH,* mean corpuscular hemoglobin; *MCHC,* mean corpuscular hemoglobin concentration; *RDW,* red cell distribution width; RETICS, reticulocytes.

mucosae are pale, and edema may be present about the head and forelimbs. Hematologic findings include erythrocyte numbers as low as 3 or 4 × 10^9/L (3.0 or 4.0 × 10^6/mm^3), hemoglobin concentration of 20 to 40 g/L (2.0 to 4.0 g/dl), and PCVs as low as 0.08 L per liter (80%). MCV may be reduced to approximately 40 femtoliters, mean corpuscular hemoglobin (MCH) to 20 picograms, and mean corpuscular hemoglobin concentrations (MCHC) to 280 g/L. Furthermore, the RDWs are increased, and the curves may not be symmetrical, indicating populations of cells of different sizes. Blood films from these animals have microcytic, hypochromic erythrocytes and poikilocytes. Serum iron concentrations are decreased and may be as low as 5 μmol/L (28 μg/dl). Bone marrow aspirates have an accumulation of rubricytes and metarubricytes, caused by decreased hemoglobin synthesis.

Nutritional iron deficiencies are rare in other species, but can occur in some pups of large kennel operations when, because of competition for feed, an occasional pup becomes nutritionally deficient. A more common occurrence is iron deficiency secondary to chronic hemorrhage. This is seen in all species. Hemorrhage may be caused by bloodsucking parasites or chronic bleeding from mucosal surfaces. Thus, when a routine hematologic examination establishes a hypochromic, microcytic anemia, an occult bleeding lesion, such as an intestinal neoplasm, should be suspected. The hemogram in Table 7-3 is an example of iron deficiency, secondary to chronic epistaxis, caused by mycotic rhinitis in a dog with von Willebrand's disease. The MCV is reduced and the erythrocyte distribution width is increased, findings consistent with iron deficiency.

Aplastic pancytopenia

This group of disorders is characterized by hypocellular marrow and pancytopenia. Pure erythrocytic aplasia describes failure of erythropoiesis, with normal granulopoiesis and thrombopoiesis. Dogs with pure erythrocytic aplasia initially may progress to trilineage aplasia. These disorders result from injury to pluripotential stem cells and failure of hemopoiesis, but more precise details of the pathogenetic mechanisms are obscure. A variety of hemopoietic and immunoregulatory defects have been described in human beings; future investigations into the human disease will eventually assist in clarification of bone marrow failure in animals. Traditionally, failures of hemopoiesis have been suspected of being disorders either of stem cell or of stroma (hemopoietic-inductive microenvironment). Recent studies using long-term bone marrow cultures from human patients with aplastic pancytopenia have established that most have atypical, blast-cell colony formation, decreased adhesiveness, and impaired response to recombinant growth factors. Stromal defects are rare. Chemical injury to stem cells by agents such as benzene and related compounds is documented in human beings and experimental animals, and possible exposure to these substances should always be considered. Dogs are particularly prone to estrogen toxicity that may occur as an endogenous hyperestrogenism in dogs with Sertoli cell tumors or that may follow estrogen therapy. Dogs initially have neutrophilia and thrombocytosis followed by thrombocytopenia and anemia. Dogs may recover at any time if serum estrogen concentrations return to normal; the disease, however, becomes irreversible in some dogs, and they become pancytopenic. Viruses have been incriminated as causes of stem cell failure in animals and human beings. Canine and feline parvoviruses and the feline leukemia virus are the most significant viruses in animals.

Pancytopenia from bone marrow failure occurs sporadically in dogs, and the etiology is not known. Immune-mediated stem cell injury has been implicated as a cause in human beings, following the discovery of immunoglobulin stem cell inhibitors and erythropoietin inhibitors and following a favorable response to immunosuppressive therapy. There have been reports of serum immunoglobulin stem cell inhibitors and response to immunosuppressive therapy in dogs.

Dogs with pancytopenia are presented for a variety of reasons, including hemorrhage, infection, lethargy, and depression. Because bone marrow aspirates may have few cells, all fragments of marrow in the needle should be used in making the smear. Marrow tissue frequently consists of stromal cells with low numbers of hemopoietic cells (Fig. 7-23), fibrous tissue, and numerous hemosiderin-laden macrophages. Marrow core biopsies should be obtained for paraffin embedment and hematoxylin-eosin (H & E)–stained sections to more accurately estimate cellularity and fibrous tissue content. As would be expected, these biopsies are hypocellular and have varying amounts of fibrous tissue.

The outcome of these cases varies. In the author's experience, the prognosis has been poor, and some dogs have

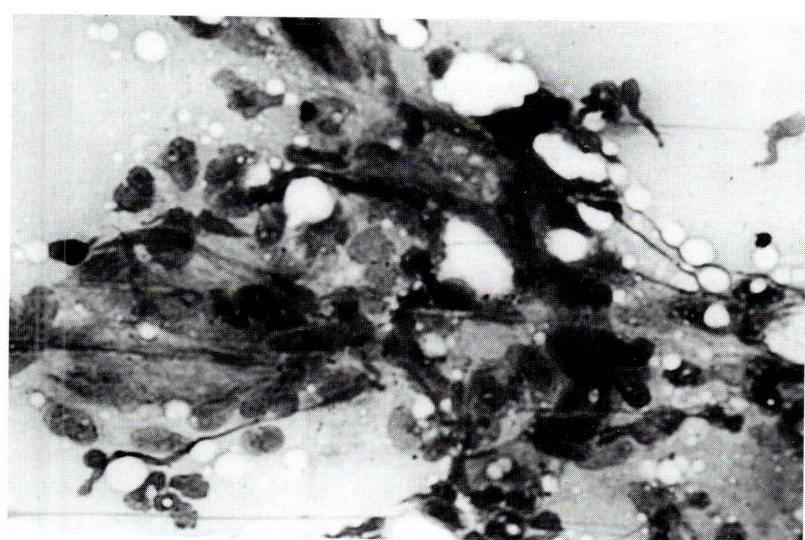

Fig. 7-23 Bone marrow aspirate; dog. Pancytopenia. Note the paucity of hemopoietic cells in the reticular cell stroma. Wright-Giemsa stain.

succumbed to acute bacterial pneumonia. A few dogs either undergo spontaneous recovery or respond to immunosuppressive therapy.

Ehrlichiosis is a tick-transmitted rickettsial disease of dogs and horses. In dogs, the disease is caused by *Ehrlichia canis, E. equi,* and *E. platys,* and, in horses, by *E. equi. E. risticii* causes fever, diarrhea, and leukopenia in horses and is discussed with the gastrointestinal system. *E. platys* causes canine cyclic thrombocytopenia and is discussed with that disorder. These organisms are transmitted by the brown dog tick *Rhipicephalus sanguineus.* Following an incubation period of 8 to 20 days, *E. canis* induces acute disease in which organisms infect monocytes and then spread throughout the mononuclear phagocyte system. This is followed by endothelial invasion and vasculitis. The disease then enters a subclinical phase, from which dogs may either recover or go on to develop pancytopenic marrow failure. In transmission studies using blood from *E. canis*–infected dogs, some dogs developed and, then, spontaneously overcame subclinical infections.

Clinical findings during the acute phase of canine ehrlichiosis are nonspecific and include fever, ocular and nasal discharges, anorexia, and lymph node enlargement. Erhlichial organisms have been found in granulocytes of dogs with acute polyarthritis. The subclinical phase lasts from 40 to 120 days. Ehrlichiosis in German shepherd dogs causes a severe hemorrhagic disorder. This unique susceptibility has been attributed to depressed cell-mediated immunity to *E. canis* in this breed.

Laboratory findings in the acute phase of canine ehrlichiosis include consistent thrombocytopenia, large platelets, and nonregenerative anemia. Concurrent *Babesia canis* infection may be present and can result in regenerative anemia. Morulae of *E. canis* may be visible in neutrophils, lymphocytes, and monocytes in the acute phase of the disease (Fig. 7-24). Examination of buffy coat smears is helpful for finding the organism. Lymphocytosis develops in some dogs as the disease progresses in severity. Pancytopenia develops in the chronic phases of the disease, and bone marrow is depleted of erythrocytic, granulocytic, and megakaryocytic cells but not of plasma cells. Other significant laboratory findings include hypergammaglobulinemia and hypoalbuminemia. Enzymes indicative of hepatic damage are increased in the acute phase of the disease. Serologic confirmation of *E. canis* infection is possible with an indirect fluorescent antibody test. Lesions vary with the stage of the disease and include widespread petechiae and ecchymoses. Lymph nodes and spleen are enlarged in the earlier stages of the disease. Chronically infected dogs are emaciated and have edema of the legs. The bone marrow is pale.

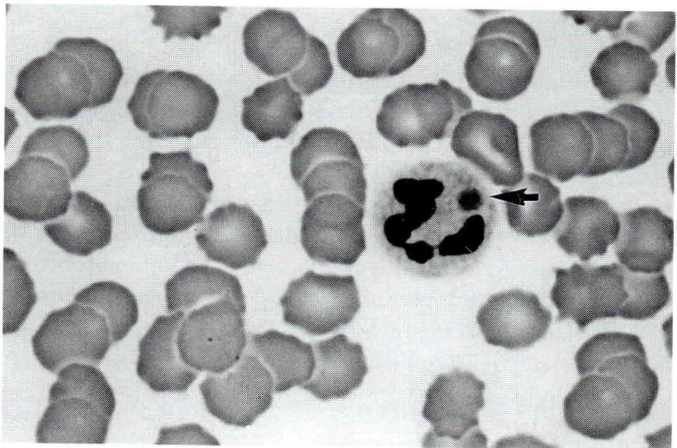

Fig. 7-24 Blood smear; dog. Ehrilichiosis. Morulae of *Ehrlichia canis* within the cytoplasm of a neutrophil. Wright-Giemsa stain. *Courtesy J. Bentinck-Smith.*

E. equi infection in horses produces a disease similar to the canine disease, but mortality is low. Equine ehrlichiosis is characterized by fever, anorexia, depression, edema of the legs, and ataxia. Laboratory findings include a mild anemia, leukopenia, and thrombocytopenia. Morulae of the organisms may be visible in the cytoplasm of neutrophils and eosinophils. Lesions include petechiae, ecchymoses, icterus, and edema. Hemorrhages are confined to subcutaneous tissues and fascia.

Bracken fern poisoning is a pancytopenic disease of cattle and horses that follows several weeks of ingestion of green plants or hay containing the fern. In both species, it causes stem cell injury; in horses, however, the thiamiase in the plant causes nervous system dysfunction prior to significant changes in the hemopoietic system. In cattle, hemorrhage is the main lesion of a disease of low morbidity and high mortality. Laboratory findings include leukopenia and thrombocytopenia. The severity of the anemia reflects the duration of toxic inhibition of stem cells and the amount of hemorrhage resulting from thrombocytopenia. Postmortem findings are dominated by numerous hemorrhages apparent in all tissues. Since animals are leukopenic, hepatic and renal infarcts resulting from bacterial embolism may occur. Bone marrow is obviously nonreactive (appearing pink and watery) and is hypocellular.

Myeloproliferative disorders are bone marrow diseases in which disturbance of one hemopoietic cell type interferes with differentiation of that cell line as well as other hemopoietic cells arising from the same stem cell. An erythrocytic sarcoma, for example, invariably results in anemia and may cause leukopenia and thrombocytopenia. In the same manner, granulocyte and plasma cell sarcomas also interfere with erythropoiesis. The myeloproliferative disorders are discussed in more detail later in this chapter.

PHAGOCYTIC LEUKOCYTE DISORDERS

Total and differential leukocyte counts should be an integral part of clinical evaluations. Correlation of these data with clinical findings can confirm or exclude diseases characterized by significant inflammation and/or necrosis. Knowledge of granulocyte kinetics in health and disease allows assessment of the duration and severity of inflammatory processes. Animals that are ill and under stress or are receiving glucocorticoid drugs have characteristic changes in the leukocyte profile; these include neutrophilia, eosinopenia, and lymphopenia. Monocytosis occurs in the dog under similar circumstances. Reversal of these changes implies recovery from the stressful state and a favorable prognosis. Blood monocyte numbers and morphology provide insight into the activity of the mononuclear phagocyte system; these cells play a vital role in chronic inflammation and hemolytic anemias.

Neutrophils

Because of their significance in defense against infections, evaluation of numbers and age of neutrophils is particularly valuable in disease assessment. To interpret changes in these parameters, one must be cognizant of species variations in neutrophil kinetics in health and disease. Neutrophils or neutrophilic granulocytes are produced in the bone marrow, and it is useful conceptually to consider granulopoiesis as occurring in compartments or pools—the mitotic and postmitotic maturation and storage pools (Fig. 7-25). Progression through these compartments, with release to the blood or circulating pool, requires approximately 110 to 130 hours. The terminology for the morphologic stages of progression through these pools is summarized in Fig. 7-26.

In the circulating compartment, neutrophils may marginate along vascular endothelium or be free in the blood. In the dog, horse, and calf, the two pools are of equal size; in cats, the marginated pool is larger than the circulating pool. The size of the circulating pool, i.e., total neutrophil numbers, is a reflection of the rate at which cells enter the

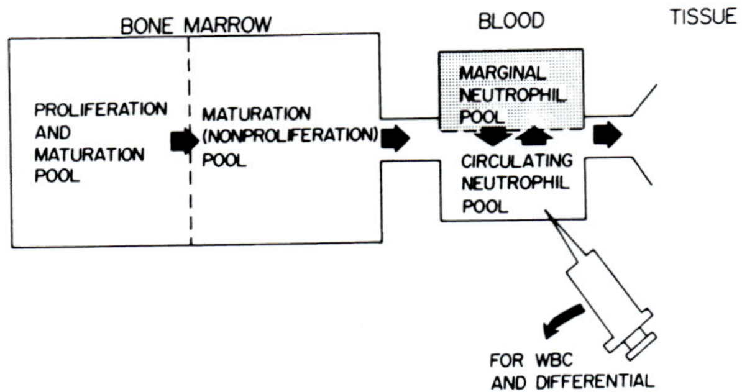

Fig. 7-25 Schema of neutrophil kinetics. Release of neutrophils from the bone marrow to the blood is ordered according to the age of the cells. *From Prasse KW. Disorders of leukocytes. In: Ettinger SJ, ed. Textbook of Veterinary Internal Medicine: Diseases of the Dog and Cat. Philadelphia: Saunders, 1983:2001.*

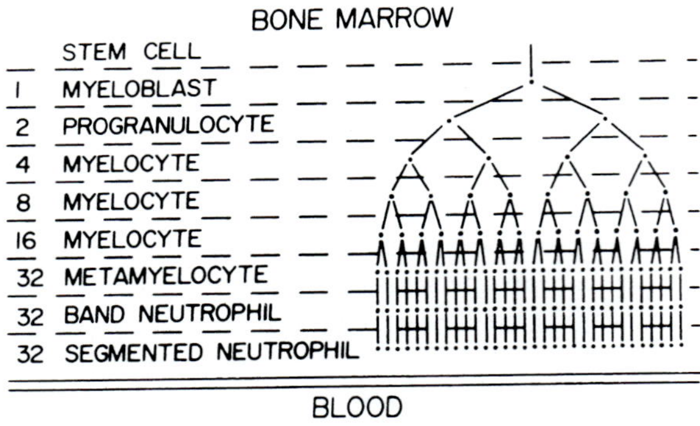

Fig. 7-26 Schema of granulopoiesis, an orderly catenated maturation. Cell division stops at the metamyelocyte stage. Mechanisms for increased neutrophil production, with times for effects to be manifested in the blood, are increased stem cell input (110–130 hours) and increased number of divisions or reduction in cell attrition in the myelocytic compartment (approximately 72–96 hours). Increased rate of release of mature neutrophils into the blood may occur rapidly with appropriate stimuli. *From Prasse KW. Disorders of leukocytes. In: Ettinger SJ, ed. Textbook of Veterinary Internal Medicine: Diseases of the Dog and Cat. Philadelphia: Saunders, 1983:2001.*

blood from the bone marrow and leave the blood to enter the tissues. Blood, therefore, serves as a vehicle to transport neutrophils to tissues, with a transit time of approximately 10 hours. When neutrophils enter tissues, they do not return to the bloodstream. There is continual movement of neutrophils across mucous membranes and into other tissues.

The ability of animals to respond to increased tissue demand for neutrophils varies according to species and can be predicted from the normal numbers of circulating neutrophils or the neutrophil/lymphocyte ratio (Table 7-4). Animals with greater numbers of circulating neutrophils in health are able to release, transport, and sequester the most neutrophils. Animals respond to a greater tissue demand for neutrophils by releasing mature cells from the marrow postmitotic maturation and storage pools, followed, if necessary, by releasing of immature cells that shift prematurely to the circulating pool. At the same time, humoral mediators stimulate differentiation of pluripotent stem cells into the committed neutrophil mitotic pool (see Fig. 7-1). Therefore, the degree of neutrophilia or neutropenia, as well as the total numbers of band and metamyelocyte neutrophils in a given species, provides insight into the duration and severity of an inflammatory process. Reference to Table 7-4 allows one to predict that the severest neutrophilia, without release of band neutrophils in response to inflammation, would occur in the dog; whereas a less severe neutrophilia, with increased need for band neutrophils, would occur in the cow. In very severe inflammations, sequestration of the entire circulating neutrophil pool and most of the marrow postmitotic maturation and storage pool may occur, and circulating band and metamyelocyte neutrophil numbers approximate or exceed mature neutrophils. This is a more common occurrence in the cow and horse than in the dog and cat. From another perspective, these changes occur with less severe inflammatory processes in the cow and horse than in the cat and dog. Table 7-5 presents leukocyte profiles of a cow and a bitch, each with severe mastitis of short duration; depletion of the marrow neutrophil storage pool is obviously greatest in the cow.

The rate of restoration of the marrow neutrophil postmitotic maturation and storage pool and the blood neutrophil pool is determined by the severity of the inflammatory process and the rate and degree to which it is contained. If the infection is rapidly contained, neutrophil numbers return to normal, and band neutrophils disappear. However, if the infection is not contained, stem cell commitment to granulopoiesis continues. Marrow hypertrophy occurs until more neutrophils are released than are required, resulting in neutrophilia. These inflammatory processes can then be considered as moderately severe and of long duration. One could predict that greater neutrophilia would occur in carnivores than in herbivores, with severe to moderately severe inflammatory processes of long duration. A dog with severe inflammation of some duration may have a leukocyte count of 80 to 100 $\times 10^9$/L (80.0 to 100.0 $\times 10^3$/mm^3) with neutrophilia, a mild shift, and monocytosis. Granulopoiesis in such an animal has reached a new steady state, in which neutrophil production per kilogram of body weight per hour is several times greater than normal. In cattle, a total leukocyte count greater than 30 $\times 10^9$/L (30.0 $\times 10^3$/mm^3) because of neutrophilia is unusual. Calves and foals less than 3 to 5 months of age can manifest a greater neutrophilia than their adult counterparts.

A good illustration of granulocyte kinetics in disease is that of a bitch with endometritis, in which the initial leukocyte profile is compared with one 24 to 48 hours following hysterectomy (Table 7-6). Rapid neutrophil sequestra-

Table 7-4. Leukocyte responses in benign diseases

Species	Normal neutrophil/ lymphocyte ratio	Maximum expected leukocytosis $\times 10^9$/L
Dog	2.4	120
Cat	1.5	75
Foal	1.4	70
Horse	1.2	60
Pig	0.7	35
Goat	0.6	30
Sheep	0.5	25
Calf	1.0	50
Cow	0.5	25

From Valli VEO. The hemopoietic system. In: Jubb KVF, Kennedy PC, Palmer N, eds. Pathology of Domestic Animals. Vol. 3, 4th ed. San Diego, Calif.: Academic Press, 1993: 113.

Table 7-5. A species comparison of granulocyte kinetics in mastitis

Hemogram	Cow	Bitch
WBC $\times 10^9$/L	3.18	23.90
Neutrophil $\times 10^9$/L	0.50	18.50
Band neutrophils $\times 10^9$/L	0.78	4.80
Metamyelocytes $\times 10^9$/L	0.35	0.00
Lymphocytes $\times 10^9$/L	1.50	0.60

WBC, white blood cells.

Table 7-6. Comparison of leukocyte profiles from a bitch with endometritis before and 24 hours after hysterectomy

Hemogram	Before hysterectomy	After hysterectomy
WBC $\times 10^9$/L	42.78	72.35
Neutrophils $\times 10^9$/L	28.63	56.73
Band Neutrophils $\times 10^9$/L	9.54	10.32
Lymphocytes $\times 10^9$/L	0.96	1.20
Monocytes $\times 10^9$/L	3.65	4.10

WBC, white blood cells.

tion into the uterus leads to partial depletion of the marrow postmitotic maturation and storage pool; this is evident from the total leukocyte count and mature and band neutrophil numbers. The leukocyte profile following hysterectomy indicates output from the expanded neutrophil mitotic and postmitotic pools. The total leukocyte count is rapidly elevated because the tissue site of sequestration (the uterus) has been removed. The neutrophilia gradually subsides over a 2- to 3-week period.

Neutrophilia with varying degrees of left shift (band neutrophil release) occurs with bacterial and fungal infections, immune-mediated inflammation such as polyarthritis, tissue necrosis, and severe hemolysis.

Neutropenias result from depletion of the circulating and marrow postmitotic maturation and storage pools in animals with overwhelming infections. Although admittedly rare, immune-mediated neutropenias occur and should be considered in chronically neutropenic animals. Bone marrow aspirates may confirm neutrophil phagocytosis. Bone marrow disorders with failure of granulopoiesis result in neutropenia. Parvoviral infections of cats and dogs cause neutropenia due to sequestration of neutrophils into the gut subsequent to epithelial necrosis and impaired granulopoiesis resulting from stem cell injury. Neutropenia also results from all the forms of stem cell injury. Neutropenia is a frequent manifestation of feline leukemia virus infections. In contrast to parvoviral neutropenia, feline leukemia virus neutropenia is of longer duration and can be cyclic. The recently discovered feline immunodeficiency virus is also a significant cause of neutropenia. Bone marrow aspiration and core biopsy are indicated diagnostic tests in persistently neutropenic animals.

Neutrophil dysfunction has been documented in human beings with diabetes mellitus and uremia. As in human beings, impaired neutrophil movement and phagocytic defects probably occur in animals with these diseases. Congenital leukocyte function diseases have been described in human beings, Irish setter dogs, and Holstein cattle. These are characterized by recurrent bacterial and fungal infections and persistent neutrophilia in the young. The neutrophils in these disorders lack all proteins within the surface glycoprotein (CD11/CD18) family; these are responsible for adhesion of neutrophils to surfaces and also serve as receptors for complement C3b. The defect is in the CD18 subunits, which are common to all membranes of the CD11/CD18 family. Recurrent bacterial and fungal infections have also been described in Doberman pinscher dogs, which have neutrophils with normal phagocytic function but impaired bactericidal ability.

Eosinophils

Eosinophilopoiesis in the bone marrow resembles that of neutrophilopoiesis. However, infiltration of tissues by eosinophils occurs somewhat independent of other leukocytes. There is now good evidence that eosinophils are attracted to tissues as part of a T-lymphocyte–mediated immune response to certain antigens, most notably allergens and antigens of helminths. Eosinophils are predominantly tissue cells, especially in those tissues with an epithelial interface with the environment, such as the respiratory and gastrointestinal tracts. Consequently, it is possible to have marked marrow eosinophilopoiesis and tissue eosinophilia without significantly increased numbers of circulating eosinophils, since their blood transit time is short. The principal cytokine responsible for tissue eosinophilia is interleukin-5 (IL-5) (see Fig. 7-1). IL-5 upregulates eosinophil membrane adhesion molecules, resulting in increased adhesion to endothelial cells at the site of inflammation.

Eosinophil granules have constituents similar to those of other granulocytes; however, their specific effector molecules are the most important. Major basic protein, the most abundant cationic eosinophil protein, is toxic to helminths, tumor cells, and host cells. Eosinophil peroxidase is toxic to helminths, protozoa, bacteria, tumor cells, and host cells, and eosinophilic cationic protein has bactericidal and helminthotoxic activities.

It is now apparent that eosinophils defend against large, nonphagocytosable organisms, such as parasites. It would appear that eosinophil numbers, as routinely noted in veterinary hematology, vary depending on geographic locale; this may reflect variations in parasite burdens. Initial binding of eosinophils to helminths can be mediated by antiparasite IgG or IgE antibodies or by C3b deposited on parasite surfaces.

Another function of eosinophils, that is confined to body surfaces, is the modulation of inflammatory reactions involving mast cells, basophils, and IgE antibodies. Products of activated mast cells serve as chemoattractant molecules for eosinophils. At hypersensitivity inflammatory sites, eosinophils neutralize histamine and are capable of inhibiting mast cell degranulation. Eosinopenia is a common occurrence in animals, usually in response to stress or the administration of glucocorticoid drugs. Eosinopenia is most likely due to inhibition of T-lymphocyte subsets that modulate eosinophil movement and functions.

Basophils and Mast Cells

Basophils and mast cells are similar to eosinophils as specialized effector cells of the immune system. They share the membrane glycoprotein CD45 with other leukocytes, an indication that mast cells are derived from hemopoietic stem cells. Mast cells leave the bone marrow as undifferentiated cells to assume their unique structure and function after transport to a tissue site. The mast cell–committed progenitor cell appears to be a nongranulated, mononuclear cell sharing certain properties with monocytes. Basophils and mast cells differ in their expression of cytokine binding sites and, therefore, their response to hemopoietic growth factors.

There is no clear definition of basophil and mast cell functions in some inflammatory states. It is likely, however, that they have critical roles in the expression of host resistance to certain parasites and that this role may vary according to factors such as species of parasite, host, and site of inflammation. Experiments with mast cell–deficient mice have demonstrated that mast cells are essential for certain IgE-dependent cutaneous responses. Basophils and mast cells have IgE binding sites, and, following formation of IgE-antigen complexes, activation of the cells results in secretion of granule contents such as histamine and heparin. Basophilia is rare in animals, but is occasionally seen in conjunction with eosinophilia. Basophils and eosinophils share many immunophenotypic properties. Occasionally, basophils and mast cells are seen with eosinophils in transtracheal washes from dogs and horses with intermittent or chronic bronchitis, presumably due to hypersensitivity disorders. The same combination of cells is seen in transtracheal washes from dogs infected with *Oslerus osleri* larvae.

Monocytes and Macrophages

Monocytes are produced in the bone marrow and then migrate to tissues and body cavities, where they rapidly differentiate into macrophages. Monoblasts, promonocytes, and monocytes can be differentiated in bone marrow, based on recognition of cell surface glycoproteins by monoclonal antibodies (immunophenotyping), and the development of granule enzymes. Newly formed monocytes remain in the bone marrow approximately 24 hours before entering marrow sinusoids. In human beings, blood monocytes are distributed into circulating (approximately 40%) and marginated (approximately 60%) pools. In the normal steady state, the proportion of monocytes migrating to various organs corresponds approximately to the size of the organ. Most macrophages are derived from monocytes, but a small percentage of monocytes/macrophages divide once within 24 hours of arrival in the tissues. After arrival in tissues, monocytes rapidly differentiate into macrophages by undergoing the appropriate biochemical and immunophenotypic changes appropriate to the environment. The morphologic transitions from monocytes to resting and activated macrophages may be evident in fine-needle aspirates of hematomas (Fig. 7-27). Tissue macrophage populations are constantly being renewed; the turnover time for Kuppfer cells is approximately 5 to 6 days. The rate of monocyte migration to inflammatory sites increases (evident as monocytosis) to compensate for increased requirement and turnover of macrophages.

Macrophages play a vital role in the immune response. They display foreign antigens on their surface in a form that can be recognized by antigen-specific T-lymphocytes. T-lymphocytes, in turn, can secrete cytokines that activate macrophages, which are then more efficient at phagocytosis and cytocidal functions. Macrophages and lymphocytes, therefore, are mutually interactive.

Bone marrow macrophages not only secrete growth factors vital to hemopoiesis, but, no doubt, exert local control over stem cells, as components of the hemopoietic inductive microenvironment. Macrophages are the central cells in erythroblastic islands, where they are bound to erythroid precursor cells by means of the cytoadhesive protein fibronectin and they nurture these erythroid precursor cells. The erythroid cells migrate along macrophage membrane extensions until they reach a marrow sinusoid. The island macrophage also ingests nuclei extruded by metarubricytes as they enter sinusoids.

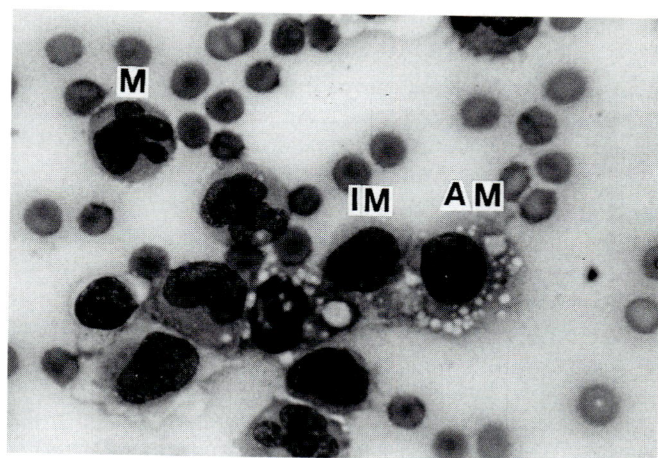

Fig. 7-27 Aspirate from a subcutaneous hematoma on a dog. Note the transition from monocytes *(M)* to immature macrophages *(IM)* and activated macrophages *(AM)*. Wright-Giemsa stain.

Monocytosis in hematologic profiles of animals suggests increased traffic to supply macrophages to the point at which a new steady state of macrophage turnover has occurred. This is especially evident in hemolytic anemias; blood smears from cats with severe *Hemobartonella felis* infection or dogs with immune-mediated hemolytic anemia frequently have numerous monocytes in route to the spleen. Marked monocytosis (2 to 5 $\times$ 10^9/L) (2.0 to 5.0 $\times$ 10^3/mm^3) may accompany established suppurative inflammatory states, such as pyometra in dogs and traumatic pericarditis in cattle. Monocytosis (1 to 3 $\times$ 10^9/L) (1.0 to 3.0 $\times$ 10^3/mm^3) occurs in dogs following administration of glucocorticoid drugs.

MYELOPROLIFERATIVE DISORDERS

This is a useful, but nonspecific diagnosis, meaning proliferation of one or more of the hemopoietic cell lines in the bone marrow. Myeloproliferative disorders may be evident as abnormal cells in peripheral blood, or they may cause pancytopenia due to interference with hemopoiesis. Granulocytic sarcomas, for example, may cause nonregenerative anemia or thrombocytopenia. Lymphosarcomas become myeloproliferative disorders when they involve the bone marrow. The myeloproliferative disorders considered in this section are the erythrocytic, granulocytic, megakaryocytic, and plasma cell sarcomas.

Erythrocytic Sarcomas

Erythrocytic sarcomas (erythremic myeloses) in cats are characterized by lethargy, pallor, and a variety of hematologic abnormalities including a severe, nonregenerative anemia with PCVs as low as 0.06 L per liter (6%). The mean corpuscular volume is frequently high, but reticulocytes are absent or present in inadequate numbers for the degree of anemia. Blood films often contain variable numbers of erythrocyte precursors in various stages of differentiation and atypia. Metarubricytes without polychromasia are present in the blood of some cats, and it is important to recognize this as an arrest at a late stage of erythrogenesis; in other cats, there may be only a few large atypical cells, which are difficult to classify without cytochemical staining (Fig. 7-28). Nuclear-cytoplasmic asynchrony of erythrocyte precursors is often evident in blood and marrow smears of cats with erythrocytic sarcomas. This is a poorly understood manifestation of impaired nuclear division and maturation (simulating cobalamin and folic acid deficiency), which results in asynchronous cell development, evident as an immature nucleus in hemoglobinated cytoplasm (Fig. 7-29). This disturbance in nuclear division results in large erythrocytes that electronic cell counters record as having large MCVs. Bone marrow from cats with erythrocytic sarcomas has many erythrocytic precursor cells, which have displaced other cells (Fig. 7-30). Nuclear-cytoplasmic asynchrony is usually evident in cells with hemoglobin.

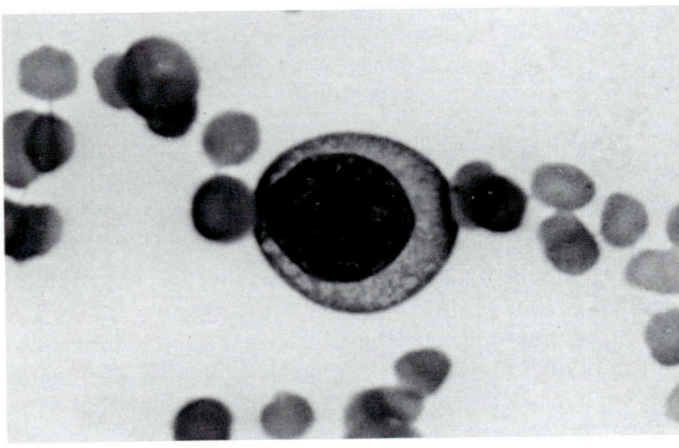

Fig. 7-28 Blood smear; cat. Myeloproliferative disorder. Note the large atypical cell. Wright-Giemsa stain.

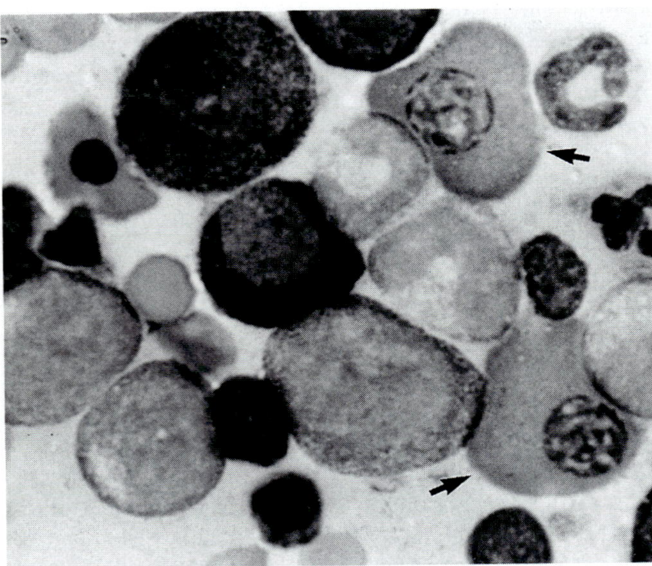

Fig. 7-29 Bone marrow; cat. Erythrocytic sarcoma. Asynchronous nuclear-cytoplasmic maturation in erythrocytic precursors. Note the large, coarse nuclei in cells with fully hemoglobinated cytoplasm *(arrows)*. Wright-Giemsa stain.

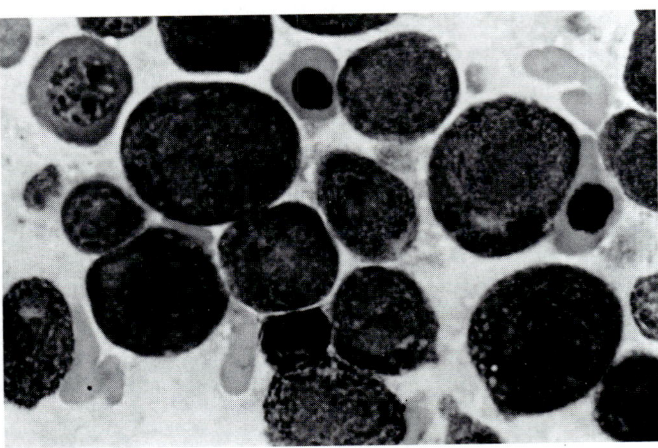

Fig. 7-30 Bone marrow; cat. Erythrocytic sarcoma. Wright-Geisma stain.

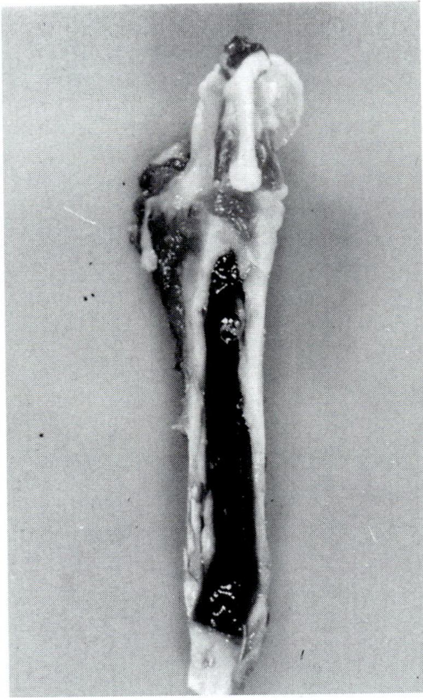

Fig. 7-31 Femur; cat. Erythrocytic sarcoma. Firm tissue completely occupies the bone marrow cavity.

In addition to watery blood at necropsy, striking abnormalities occur in bone marrow cavities. In a split femur, the bone marrow cavity is partially to completely occupied by firm, red tissue. Impression smears should be made and samples placed in fixative for histopathologic evaluation (Fig. 7-31). When examining long bones at necropsy, reference to the hemogram will assist in differentiating hyperplasia from neoplasia. Splenomegaly and hepatomegaly may also be present, most often in cats with large numbers of circulating neoplastic cells.

Granulocytic Sarcomas

Granulocytic sarcomas are rare in animals, but occur in cats infected with feline leukemia virus, usually without leukocytosis, but with bizarre immature cells. The neoplasm seen in dogs is occasionally evident as marked leukocytosis with varying numbers of immature cells. Differentiation from leukemoid reactions—i.e., nonneoplastic neutrophilias—may be difficult. Anemia (of greater severity than expected from chronic inflammation) and thrombocytopenia are expected with this neoplastic disease. Other dogs with granulocytic leukemia will have low, normal, or moderately elevated leukocyte counts and circulating neoplastic cells. These are most easily differentiated from lymphocytes or, in the cat, from neoplastic erythroid precursor cells by the presence of cytoplasmic granules. Differentiation from neoplastic granular lymphocytes may be difficult and requires cytochemical staining. Bone marrow aspirates from dogs with granulocytic leukemia will usually have a dominant population of cells in the granulocytic series (Fig. 7-32). Predominance of less differentiated cells is to be expected in dogs with lower numbers of circulating cells. At necropsy, dogs and cats with granulocytic sarcomas and leukemia have generalized, mild to moderate lymph node enlargement, hepatomegaly, and marked splenomegaly. Large numbers of granulocytes are present in hepatic sinuses and in splenic red pulp. The differentiation of a leukemoid reaction from granulocytic sarcoma can be difficult.

Megakaryocytic Sarcomas

Megakaryocytic sarcomas are rare but do occur in dogs and in cats infected with the feline leukemia virus. Platelet numbers may exceed 2000 × 10^9/L (2000 × 10^3/mm^3) with marked variation in platelet size and shape. The anemia is nonregenerative and neutropenia is mild to moderate (Table 7-7). Bone marrow aspirates have changes of impaired erythropoiesis and nuclear-cytoplasmic asynchrony of erythrocyte precursors. Megakaryocytes are numerous and include all stages of development. At necropsy, these cats have generalized tissue pallor, splenomegaly, hepatomegaly, and bone marrow cavities filled with solid tissue. Microscopically, marked accumulations of megakaryocytes occur in the splenic red pulp, hepatic sinusoids, and lymph nodes (Fig. 7-33).

Table 7-7. Hemogram from a 5-year-old feline leukemia virus-infected cat with megakaryocytic sarcoma

Hemogram	Patient values	Reference values
WBC × 10^9/L	6.9	5.50-9.50
RBC × 10^{12}/L	2.44	5.00-10.00
Hgb g/L	37.0	80-150
PCV L/L	0.16	0.24-0.45
MCV feL	65	39-55
MCH pg	14.7	13-17
MCHC g/L	228	300-360
Platelets × 10^9/L	2040	300-700
Neutrophils × 10^9/L	4.62	2.50-12.50
Lymphocytes × 10^9/L	2.00	1.50-7.00
Metarubricytes × 10^9/L	0.20	—
Protein g/L	84	68-80

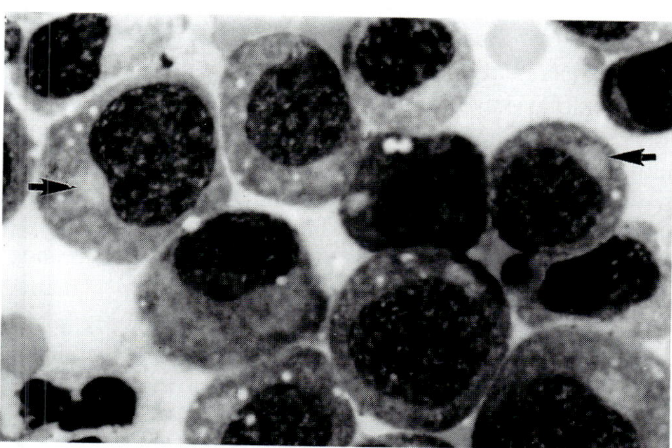

Fig. 7-32 Bone marrow aspirate; dog. Granulocytic sarcoma. A homogeneous population of cells is consistent with that of a sarcoma. The prominent perinuclear Golgi zones *(arrows)* are typical of cells in the granuocytic series. Wright-Giemsa stain.

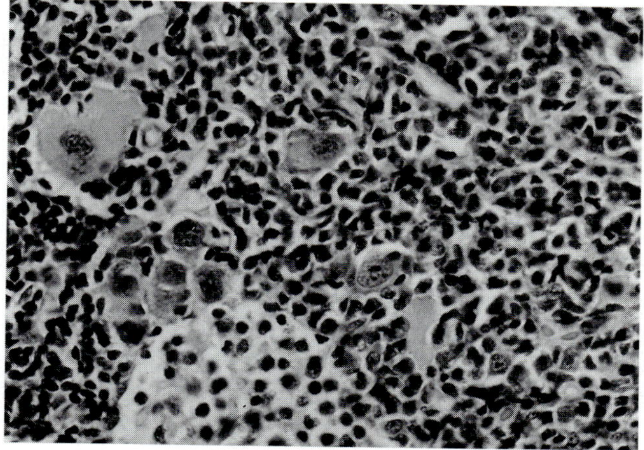

Fig. 7-33 Lymph node; cat. Megakaryocytic sarcoma. Note the accumulation of megakaryocytes. Hematoxylin-eosin (H & E) stain.

Plasma Cell Sarcomas

Plasma cell sarcomas are neoplasms of cells that can produce a variety of paraneoplastic disorders secondary to secretion of partial or complete immunoglobulin molecules. The disease is not common but does occur in dogs. Plasma cell sarcomas in other species are rare.

There is no known etiology for plasma cell neoplasms. However, neoplastic transformation of a clone of plasma cells can follow prolonged antigenic stimulation. Monoclonal gammopathies suggestive of lymphocytic or plasma cell neoplasia have been noted in chronic infections such as Aleutian disease in minks and coccidioidomycosis and erhlichiosis in dogs.

There are two basic disease mechanisms in animals with plasma cell sarcomas: one is caused by neoplastic cell proliferation; the other is the result of protein produced by the neoplastic plasma cells. Although plasma cell neoplasms have been described in other tissues, many arise in the bone marrow and can interfere with hemopoiesis and erode endosteal bone by focal osteolysis. Most plasma cell sarcomas secrete proteins. Since the neoplastic cells arise from transformation of one cell, the protein molecules are similar and represent partial to complete immunoglobulin molecules of one class. Hyperviscosity of the plasma is a reflection of the hypergammaglobulinemia and structural properties of the protein and is, therefore, more severe if cells are producing IgM molecules rather than IgG or IgA molecules. Plasma hyperviscosity causes a variety of clinical signs and lesions; retinal hemorrhages, glomerular disease, and depression have been documented in dogs.

Epistaxis, melena, and bleeding from venipuncture sites have been observed in dogs with plasma cell sarcomas. Bleeding is presumed to be caused by effects of the abnormal protein on platelets and coagulation enzymes. When hyperviscosity is severe, bleeding can result from distention and rupture of small vessels.

In dogs, renal disease is caused by the effects of hyperproteinemia on glomeruli and deposition of protein in tubules. The precise effects on the kidneys depend on the molecular weight of the proteins involved (and, hence, their filterability). Some neoplastic plasma cells fail to assemble normal combinations of light and heavy chain molecules, resulting in release into the circulation of light chains or small-molecular-weight proteins that appear in the urine.

Animals with plasma cell sarcomas have mild to moderate nonregenerative anemias and pancytopenia if marrow involvement is severe. Extensive erythrocytic rouleaux formation and a diffuse, intercellular, proteinaceous precipitate are evident in blood films when protein content exceeds 115 g/L (11.5 g/dl) (Fig. 7-34). Plasma cells are occasionally found in blood smears from dogs with plasma cell sarcomas. Plasma viscosity can be simply assessed by comparing the rate at which the patient's plasma and normal plasma at 37° C drain from warmed pipettes. Marrow aspirates may have increased numbers of well-differentiated plasma cells (Fig. 7-35). In some cases, the differentiation of neoplasm from prolonged antigenic stimulation may be difficult, and all laboratory and clinical findings must be evaluated. If the cells have abnormal morphology (for example, binucleate cells) and if there is interference with hemopoiesis, a diagnosis of neoplasia should be made.

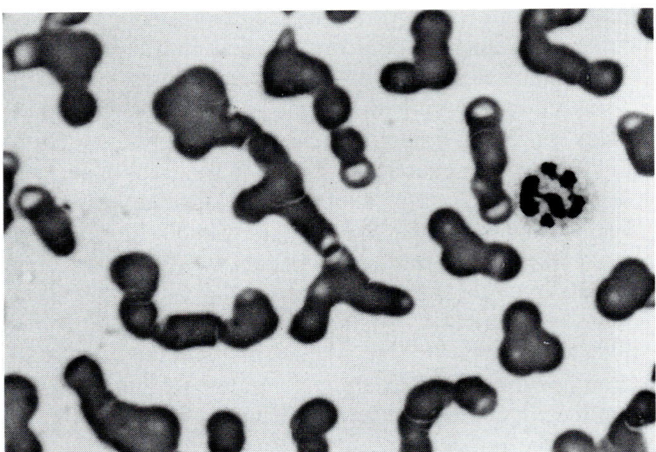

Fig. 7-34 Blood smear; dog. Plasma cell sarcoma. Note the extensive erythrocyte rouleaux accompanying marked hyperproteinemia. Wright-Giemsa stain.

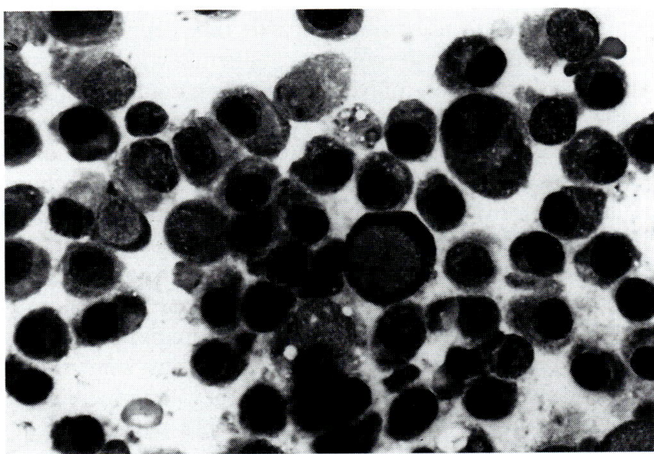

Fig. 7-35 Bone marrow aspirate; dog. Plasma cell sarcoma. Note how normal marrow cells have been displaced by a homogeneous population of plasma cells in various stages of differentiation. Wright-Giemsa stain.

Hyperproteinemia may be a striking abnormality when neoplastic plasma cells are forming proteins. Serum electrophoresis has a sharp, spikelike pattern in the beta or gamma zone in contrast to the large, broad peaks observed in samples from animals with chronic infections (Fig. 7-36). Immunoelectrophoresis should allow characterization of the class of immunoglobulins; IgG, IgM, and IgA hyperproteinemias have all been described in dogs with

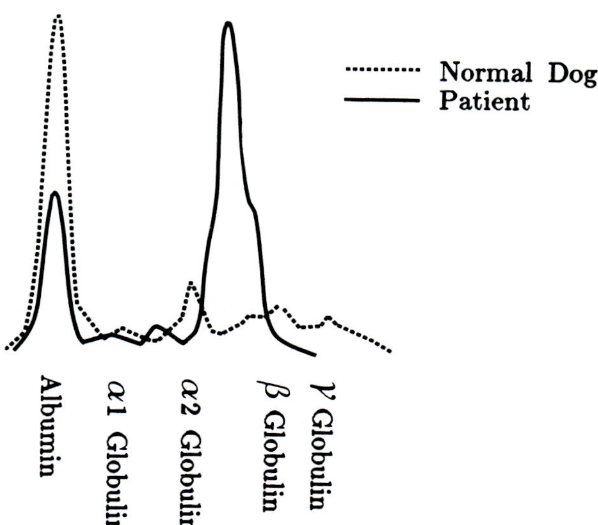

Fig. 7-36 Serum electrophoretogram; dog. Plasma cell sarcoma. Note the spikelike pattern of the protein secreted by the neoplastic cells.

plasma cell sarcomas. Direct immunofluorescence studies can detect the class of antibodies on plasma cell surfaces. In some dogs with plasma cell sarcoma, light immunoglobulin chains appear in the urine and may be quantitated by heat precipitation. More sensitive immunoprecipitation assays would most likely confirm these proteins in a greater number of cases.

At necropsy, plasma cell sarcomas appear as soft, gelatinous, pink to red masses in bone marrow spaces and may be found in vertebrae; some neoplasms cause erosion of bone and extend into the surrounding soft tissue. These masses are composed of sheets of atypic to well-differentiated plasma cells.

PLATELET DISORDERS

Platelets are small, anucleate, granular cells that should be routinely scrutinized when examining blood films. They may vary in size, especially in cats, but are approximately one third to one half the diameter of erythrocytes. Platelets form from megakaryocytes in the bone marrow and circulate for approximately 8 days. Equine platelets stain less prominently and may be difficult to see in blood films.

Although anuclear, platelets are metabolically active and have a cytoskeleton containing actin and myosin. They also have numerous granules, which release their contents during platelet activation into a canalicular system that communicates with the external membrane. Bovine platelets are unique in having a poorly developed canalicular system; they secrete granular constituents directly onto the surface. Following endothelial injury, platelets arrest bleeding by adhering to exposed, subendothelial collagen. Once adhered, the platelets are immediately activated and release granular constituents, causing nearby platelets to aggregate to the adhered platelets to form a platelet plug. The platelet plug is then stabilized by fibrin. When platelet numbers are sufficiently reduced or platelets are functionally impaired, erythrocytes seep through capillary walls. Further consideration of the role of platelets in hemostasis can be found in the discussion on Coagulation Disorders.

Thrombocytosis

Platelet numbers fluctuate in animals and substantially increase in response to most hemopoietic stimuli. This may reflect the intimate apposition of megakaryocytes to sinusoidal walls in the bone morrow and extension of long platelet processes into the lumina. Normal reference values for platelets in animals vary, ranging from 100 to 600 $\times$ 10^9/L (100 to 600 $\times$ 10^3/mm^3) in the horse to 200 to 900 $\times$ 10^9/L (200 to 900 $\times$ 10^3/mm^3) in the dog. Neutrophilia and anemia with reticulocytosis are usually accompanied by thrombocytosis. Thrombocytoses in which platelets exceed 1000 $\times$ 10^9/L (100 $\times$ 10^3/mm^3) are rare but occasionally are observed in cats infected with feline leukemia virus. Thrombosis is a possible consequence of marked thrombocytosis in these animals.

Thrombocytopenia

Thrombocytopenia is an important disorder in animals. When electronic cell counters record low platelet numbers, it is important that this result be confirmed by examination of the blood film because tiny clots commonly occur in animal blood samples and may result in a spurious thrombocytopenia. Microscopic examination of a stained blood film should routinely include the feather edge, where platelet clumps are visible when the sample is partially clotted. The simplest approximation of platelet numbers in a blood film is as follows: each platelet identified in a 1000 magnification oil immersion objective field, containing a monolayer of erythrocytes, represents approximately 20 $\times$ 10^9 platelets per liter (20 $\times$ 10^3/mm^3).

Thrombocytopenia, similar to neutropenia or anemia, may be due to premature cellular destruction or impaired production. Platelet life span may be decreased because of consumption following platelet adhesion to injured vascular endothelium in diseases such as infectious canine hepatitis and hog cholera. Platelet adhesion followed by platelet activation may initiate intravascular coagulation and further platelet consumption. Thrombocytopenia due to phagocytosis may be an isolated, immune-mediated phenomenon, or it may accompany immune-mediated hemolytic anemia and systemic lupus erythematosus. The possible mechanisms resulting in antibody adherence to platelets are similar to those discussed with immune-mediated hemolytic anemias. An isoimmune thrombocytopenia occurs in neonatal piglets at 1 to 3 days following ingestion of colostrum. The syndrome is characterized by severe hemorrhage and high mortality.

An infectious cyclic thrombocytopenia occurs in dogs

due to infection of platelets by *Ehrlichia platys,* an organism presumably transmitted by ticks. Following an incubation period of 8 to 15 days, many platelets contain morulae of *E. platys,* resulting in a marked thrombocytopenia. Platelet numbers return to normal in 3 to 4 days. Parasitemia and thrombocytopenia subsequently recur at 1- to 2-week intervals. *E. platys* antibodies are detected by an indirect serum fluorescent antibody test.

Thrombocytopenia due to failure of platelet production can occur in any bone marrow disorder. More detailed information is presented under Aplastic Pancytopenia and Myeloproliferative Disorders. Estrogen toxicity in dogs is frequently detected clinically by hemorrhages that are typical of thrombocytopenia. The same is true of bracken fern poisoning in cattle.

The cardinal clinical signs of thrombocytopenia are petechiae, best observed on mucosae and ocular sclerae. The skin of affected dogs has tiny to diffuse hemorrhages, which can be detected at grooming. Mucosal bleeding at the free gingival margin and into the intestine is significant in canine thrombocytopenia but may escape detection. Epistaxis is also common in thrombocytopenic animals. Hemorrhage can be severe following either surgery or trauma.

Thrombocytopenic animals with spontaneous bleeding have platelet numbers ranging from undetectable to approximately 50×10^9/L (50×10^3/mm^3). Electronic cell counters will enumerate platelets, determine mean platelet volume, and plot a curve based on range of platelet size. Together, these data and data obtained from blood film examination help to differentiate platelet destruction, accompanied by release of large platelets, from impaired thrombopoiesis with release of small platelets. In animals with myeloproliferative disorders, very large platelets or fragments of megakaryocytic cytoplasm may be found in blood films and probably are the result of bone marrow sinusoidal disturbance.

Animals with thrombocytopenia resulting from platelet destruction have increased numbers of megakaryocytes in various stages of development. Young megakaryocytes are large, mononuclear or binuclear cells with a thin rim of deeply basophilic cytoplasm. In contrast, mature megakaryocytes are larger, with multiple nuclei and abundant granular cytoplasm.

Unlike the erythrocyte direct antiglobulin test, tests for antiplatelet antibody have been difficult to develop. Assays have been developed that have detected increased platelet-associated immunoglobulin in human beings and dogs suspected of having immune-mediated thrombocytopenia. However, platelet alpha granules normally contain immunoglobulin, and the increased amounts most likely are due to increased numbers of large, immature platelets accompanying any form of platelet destruction.

Platelet Function Disorders

Platelet function disorders are characterized by petechiae and mucosal bleeding in animals with normal platelet counts. These disorders may be congenital or acquired and result from impaired platelet adhesion, aggregation, or a combination of both. The adhesion of platelets to subendothelium at high shear rates is mediated by the von Willebrand cytoadhesive protein. This protein may be congenitally absent or decreased, resulting in von Willebrand's disease (discussed below). Platelet adhesion is impaired in uremia, which is responsible for the mucosal hemorrhage that tends to occur in animals with renal failure. The mechanisms responsible may be multifactorial and are currently under investigation. It has recently been reported that, in human beings, expression of platelet glycoprotein Ib, a receptor for von Willebrand protein, and calcium mobilization are reduced in uremia.

Platelet aggregation is the accumulation of additional platelets to adherent platelets to form a platelet plug. Aggregation is mediated by proteins such as fibrinogen, which act as a bridge between adjacent platelets by binding to receptors (GPIIb/IIIa) that are exposed following platelet activation. Like adhesion disorders, impaired aggregation may be congenital or acquired. The in vitro assessment of platelet aggregation using specialized photometers (aggregometers) has facilitated the study of these disorders. Congenital disorders of platelet aggregation occur in basset hounds and Simmental cattle. These animals experience spontaneous mucosal bleeding and severe hemorrhage following minor surgery. In both species, in vitro aggregation fails in response to a variety of agonists. In both species, failure of aggregation occurs despite the binding of normal numbers of fibrinogen molecules in vitro by the activated platelets. However, in flow cytometric studies, delayed binding of fibrinogen to platelets has been found in bleeding Simmental cattle.

Acquired disorders of platelet aggregation occur in uremia and following administration of aspirin and antiinflammatory drugs such as phenylbutazone. Dogs with plasma cell sarcomas may have a tendency to bleed, as proteins secreted by the neoplastic cells may interfere with platelet function.

COAGULATION DISORDERS

Platelet disorders result in seepage bleeding from mucosal surfaces because of inadequate initial plugging at sites of endothelial disruption. Disorders of coagulation result from impaired synthesis of fibrin and inadequate stabilization of the platelet plug. Prolonged bleeding then occurs after temporary occlusion of the injured vessel by the unstable platelet plug.

The familiar cascading sequence of coagulation has undergone significant revision over the past decade. It is now apparent, for example, that platelet and endothelial cell surfaces provide a framework for assembly and appropriate interaction of coagulation proteins. Traditionally, the cascade hypothesis of coagulation has been subdivided into intrinsic and extrinsic pathways; these are now known to be highly interdependent. The general principle, that co-

Table 7-8. Molecular properties of human blood coagulant proteins

	Site of synthesis	Molecular weight	Protein characteristics	Plasma level
Fibrinogen (Factor 1)	Hepatocyte	330,000	Dimeric, with each monomer having three subchains	2.0-4.0 g/L
Prothrombin (Factor II)	Hepatocyte	72,000	Vitamin K-dependent	100 mg/L
Tissue Factor (Factor III)	Many cell types	37,000	Transmembrane protein	0
Factor V	Hepatocyte; megakaryocyte	330,000	Cofactor to factor Xa	10 mg/L
Factor VII	Hepatocyte	55,000	Vitamin K–dependent	0.5 mg/L
Factor VIII	Hepatocyte	330,000	Cofactor to Factor IXa	0.1 mg/L
von Willebrand factor	Endothelial cell; megakaryocyte	220,000 (multimers up to 20 × 10^6)	Carries Factor VIII in plasma	10 mg/L
Factor IX	Hepatocyte	55,000	Vitamin K–dependent	5 mg/L
Factor X	Hepatocyte	55,000	Vitamin K–dependent	10 mg/L
Factor XI	Hepatocyte	160,000	—	5 mg/L
Factor XII	Hepatocyte	80,000	—	30 mg/L
Factor XIII	Hepatocyte	320,000	—	10 mg/L
Protein C	Hepatocyte	62,000	Vitamin K–dependent	5 mg/L
Protein S	Hepatocyte	80,000	Vitamin K–dependent	25 mg/L
Thrombomodulin	Endothelial	75,000 to 105,000	Expressed on endothelial surface	0
Antithrombin III	Hepatocyte	60,000	Forms complex with heparin	150 mg/L
Lipoprotein-associated coagulation inhibitor (LACI)	Endothelial cell	33,000	Circulates in plasma	11.5 mg/L

Modified from Roberts HR, Lozier JN. Hosp Pract 1992; 27:97-112.

agulation events are all directed toward the conversion of fibrinogen to fibrin, remains unchanged. Fibrinogen, an acute-phase reactant, is synthesized in hepatocytes, circulates in plasma, and is located in alpha granules of platelets and megakaryocytes.

Certain coagulation proteins (prothrombin and factors VII, IX and X and proteins C and S [inhibitors of coagulation]) are vitamin K–dependent factors (Table 7-8). In order to become functional, the vitamin K–dependent proteins must undergo carboxylation of selected glutamic acid residues. This reaction is catalyzed within hepatocytes by the vitamin K–dependent enzyme gamma-glutamylcarboxylase. These carboxylated glutamic acid residues avidly bind calcium ions, which in turn maintain the critical shapes of the proteins, necessary for them to bind to phospholipids exposed on activated platelets. Vitamin K–dependent proteins become functional serine proteases following cleavage of a specific activation domain; they then assume a structure that exposes their catalytic domains.

Factors V and VIII are homologous cofactors for the vitamin K–dependent serine proteases (Table 7-8). Both molecules are activated (designated Va and VIIIa) by thrombin. Factor VIIIa participates in assembling Factor IX and calcium in close proximity to Factor X on the platelet surface (Fig. 7-37). This facilitates Factor IXa activation of Factor X. Factor VIIIa is rendered inactive following further cleavage by thrombin or protein C. Factor V activation and inactivation mechanisms are very similar to those of Factor VIII. Factor Va serves to assemble Factor Xa and calcium on platelets so as to facilitate the Factor Xa–catalyzed conversion of prothrombin to thrombin (Fig. 7-37).

It is now evident that cell surfaces play a vital role in coagulation. Platelets have surface receptors for Factors V, VIII, IX, and X, which become exposed following platelet activation by thrombin (Fig. 7-37). Platelet activation also causes exposure of phospholipids normally found on the internal aspect of the platelet membrane. A further event following platelet activation is the release of membrane particles, which most likely also provide sites for assembly of coagulation proteins.

The traditional view of initiation of coagulation by activation of Factor XII in the intrinsic pathway has been modified by recent research into the molecular biology of coagulation. It now appears that essentially all coagulation in vivo is initiated by the extrinsic pathway. A key component of extrinsic pathway activation is tissue factor, a transmembrane polypeptide that acts as a cell surface receptor for Factor VII. It is found on cells surrounding blood vessels; it does not occur on endothelial cells or circulate in plasma. It is, therefore, obvious that binding of Factor VII by tissue factor occurs whenever there is tissue trauma. The extrinsic and intrinsic pathways are now known to be highly interdependent because the tissue factor/Factor VII complex not only activates Factor X but also Factor IX (Fig. 7-37). Tissue factor pathway activity is controlled by a lipoprotein-associated coagulation inhibitor (LACI) also known as extrinsic pathway inhibitor (EPI).

Thrombin is most important in sustaining coagulation

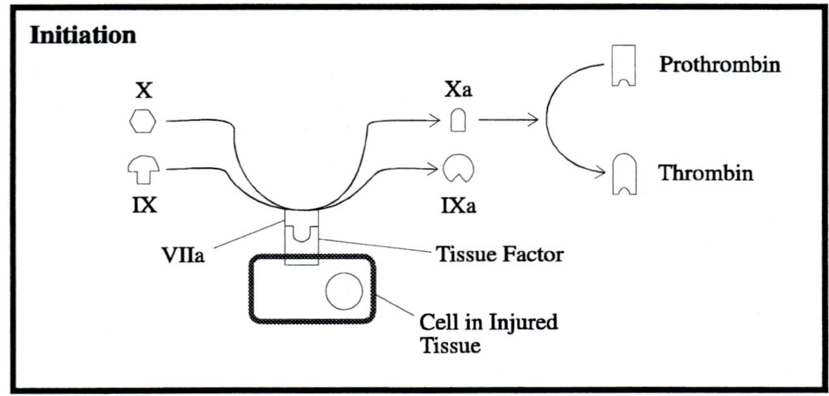

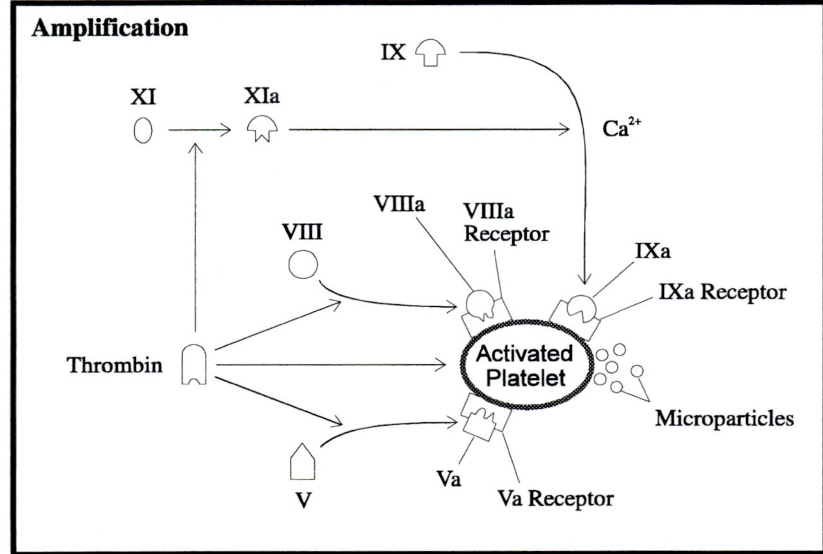

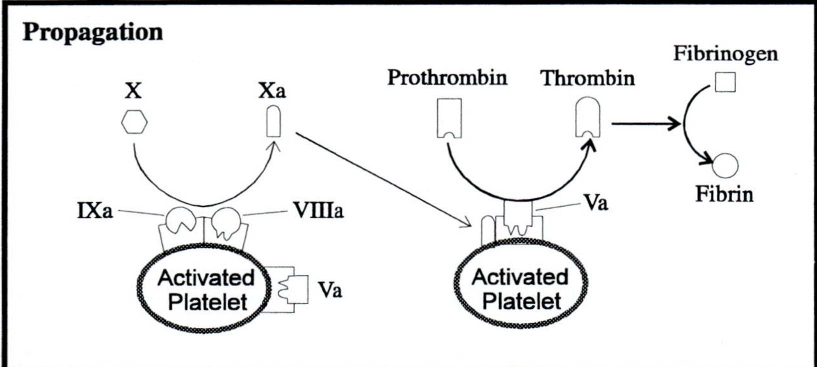

Fig. 7-37 Three-stage model of coagulation is suggested by recent advances in knowledge of the underlying molecular biology. Clotting is initiated *(top)* by tissue factor/Factor VIIa surface complexes, which activate Factor X (and also Factor IX). The result is the generation of a small amount of thrombin. In turn, thrombin activates platelets *(middle)* and promotes the activation and assembly of coagulation factors and cofactors on the platelet surface. In this way, the stage is set for augmented generation of Factor Xa, thrombin, and fibrin *(bottom)*. Not shown are the effects of inhibitors of coagulation: lipoprotein-associated-coagulation inhibitor (LACI), also known as extrinsic pathway inhibitor (EPI), inhibits the TF/VIIa/Xa complex. Antithrombin III controls thrombin in amplification and propagation phases of clotting. *From Roberts HR, Lozier JN. Hosp Pract 1992; 27:97-112.*

and is the chief activator of Factor XI. Thrombin also activates Factors V and VIII as well as Factor XIII (Fig. 7-37). Factor XIII is responsible for the stabilization of fibrin.

Downregulation of coagulation is vital to normal hemostasis and, like the initiation of coagulation, initially occurs on cell surfaces. Endothelial cells are most important because they express the transmembrane protein thrombomodulin, a receptor for thrombin. Thrombin bound to thrombomodulin activates protein C. In turn, activated protein C, with protein S as a cofactor, inactivates Factors Va and VIIIa (Fig. 7-38). Activated protein C also promotes dissolution of clots. Antithrombin III (Table 7-8) is an important inhibitor of coagulation factors by forming complexes with the activated zymogens in the presence of heparin. The fibrinolytic system is a series of reactions similar to those of coagulation, in which zymogens are activated, resulting in proteolysis of fibrin. Fibrinolysis is achieved by a potent plasma proteolytic enzyme, plasmin, which is synthesized in the liver and circulates as an inert zymogen (plasminogen). Plasminogen activators convert plasminogen to plasmin. Plasmin digests fibrinogen and fibrin and also degrades von Willebrand's factor and Factors V and VIII. An intensely proteolytic enzyme such as plasmin must be under constant control; this is achieved primarily by alpha$_2$-antiplasmin, which forms a stable complex with plasmin.

Coagulation disorders, because of inadequate synthesis or altered function of one or more coagulation proteins, may be congenital or acquired. The congenital, inherited disorders usually appear in young animals, but, if the defect is mild, it may not become apparent until severe hemorrhage occurs following injury or surgery. Congenital coagulopathies usually involve a single defect in a single protein; acquired disorders usually affect more than one protein.

Acquired Coagulation Disorders

Toxicities resulting in hemorrhages most commonly follow ingestion of one of a group of related substances—the coumarins. Coumarins are synthesized by molds in sweet clover and are used in rodenticides. Sweet clover poisoning is most common in cattle but can also occur in sheep and horses. Dogs and cats that accidentally ingest rodenticides develop life-threatening bleeding disorders. Development of resistance to the coumarins has initiated development of more potent ''second-generation'' anticoagulant rodenticides. Repeated ingestion of coumarins is necessary to exhaust vitamin K stores, whereas the second-generation an-

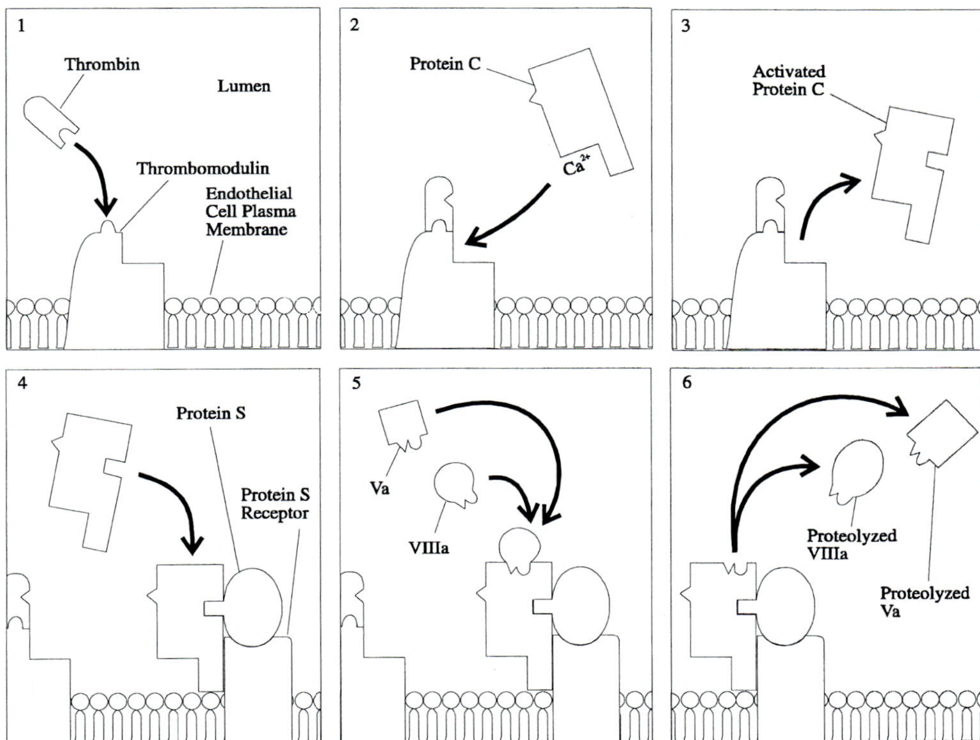

Fig. 7-38 Downregulation of clotting is one of the multiple roles endothelial cells play in hemostasis. Thrombomodulin, an endothelial transmembrane protein, binds thrombin (*1*). The resulting complex captures protein C through electrostatic attraction between calcium ions on protein C and a negative region on thrombomodulin (*2*). The bound protein C is proteolytically activated (*3*); it then binds to nearby protein S on endothelial cells or platelets (*4*). In the C-S complex, activated protein C is capable of inactivating Factors Va and VIIa (*5* and *6*). *From Roberts HR, Lozier JN. Hosp Pract 1992; 27:97-112.*

ticoagulants, such as brodifacoum and bromadiolone, cause significant bleeding following a single exposure.

Coumarins and related compounds interfere with the vitamin K–dependent coagulation Factors II, VII, IX, and X. As described in the review of hemostasis, the calcium and phospholipid binding properties of these proteins follow posttranslational carboxylation of the gamma carbon on glutamic acid. Vitamin K is a cofactor in the carboxylation reaction, becoming oxidized as the reaction proceeds. Coumarin compounds interrupt the vitamin K oxidation-reduction cycle, resulting in exhaustion of the vitamin and incomplete carboxylation of coagulation factors.

Vitamin K–deficient animals have a variety of clinical signs associated with the degree and the location of the hemorrhages. Spontaneous bleeding causes large, superficial hematomas and hemarthroses. Cattle with sweet clover poisoning bleed severely following minor surgery. Calves born to dams ingesting moldy sweet clover may die of internal hemorrhage, although the dam is unaffected. Human infants are also susceptible to vitamin K deficiency and hemorrhage; this is presumably a result of inadequate dietary intake of the vitamin prior to intestinal colonization with vitamin K–producing bacteria and low concentrations of vitamin K in milk.

Rodenticide toxicity in dogs causes a variety of clinical signs resulting from hypovolemia, organ dysfunction, and bleeding into body cavities. Hemorrhage into the brain may produce neurologic dysfunction and, sometimes, sudden death. Hemarthrosis causes acute lameness. Hematomas follow venipunctures and trauma.

Vitamin K–deficient animals have long, one-stage prothrombin times (OSPT). The OSPT may also be used to monitor hemostasis in cattle ingesting sweet clover. The short half-life of Factor VII (relative to prothrombin and Factors IX and X) results in prolongation of the OSPT prior to activated partial thromboplastin time (APTT) prolongation. However, both tests are usually prolonged when animals are presented due to hemorrhages from vitamin K antagonism. Animals that die following coumarin or rodenticide toxicity have massive hemorrhages into body cavities and joints and along fascial planes.

Hepatic disease is a potential cause of severe bleeding due to inadequate synthesis of coagulation factors (Table 7-8). It is apparent that significant depletion of these factors only occurs late in progressive hepatic diseases when most of the organ is destroyed or in instances of acute, overwhelming hepatocyte necrosis. Accurate laboratory assessment of coagulation in animals with hepatic disease is difficult because there may be complications of subnormal platelet function and concurrent disseminated intravascular coagulation with fibrinolysis. Severe acute hepatic disease in dogs may prolong both OSPT and APTT, whereas partially compensated chronic hepatic disease may cause slight prolongation of APTT.

Disseminated intravascular coagulation and fibrinolysis is an important coagulation disorder in animal patients and represents an intriguing array of intermediary mechanisms in neoplastic diseases, overwhelming viral and bacterial infections, severe hemolysis, and other disorders (see Thrombosis and Embolism, Chapter 4).

Congenital Coagulation Disorders

Congenital coagulation disorders result from molecular lesions in coagulation proteins. In the broadest sense, there may be inadequate synthesis of a normal molecule or synthesis of an abnormal molecule in which strategic location of the abnormality may interfere with function. The latter situation may result from a purine or pyrimidine base change in DNA. Most coagulation factors undergo postribosomal modification, such as cleavage of a portion of the molecule before it becomes functional, and this process also may be abnormal.

Factor XII deficiency

Factor XII deficiency occurs in cats as an autosomal recessive trait and has been occasionally reported in dogs. Feline heterozygotes have approximately 50% activity, whereas homozygotes have no measurable Factor XII. Homozygotes have prolonged APTTs but no clinical evidence of bleeding. Recent attempts to characterize the defect have found no apparent deletion of genomic DNA sequences or transcriptional or splicing abnormalities, suggesting that abnormal Factor XII synthesis in cats may be due to premature termination of ribosomal amino acid assembly.

Factor XI deficiency

Factor XI deficiency occurs in Holstein cattle and in Great Pyrenees, English springer spaniel, and Kerry blue terrier dogs. It is transmitted as an autosomal recessive gene in cattle. Spontaneous hemorrhage is insignificant in affected animals but can be severe following surgery. Homozygous Factor XI–deficient animals have prolonged whole-blood clotting times, prolonged APTTs, and lack of Factor XI activity. Heterozygous animals have approximately 50% of normal Factor XI activity.

Factor IX deficiency

Factor IX deficiency occurs in dogs and cats. The inheritance is sex linked, because the gene is present on the X chromosome. Affected males have very low Factor IX activity, and carrier females have 40% to 60% of normal activity. A wide variety of genetic defects account for hemophilia B in different human families. Some patients have normal amounts of Factor IX antigen but low Factor IX activity, i.e., a poorly functioning protein. This can result from a single amino acid substitution that may distort one of the many changes the molecule must undergo prior to becoming functional. For example, in one Factor IX–deficient patient, a strategic amino acid substitution prevents cleavage of a portion of the molecule, which is normally removed as part of the molecular rearrangement necessary for function. The abnormal Factor IX molecule is not only larger but nonfunctional. It should now be apparent that Factor IX and other factor deficiencies in animals may result from a wide range of molecular lesions that have yet to be clarified. Hemorrhage in Factor IX deficiency is mild in cats and small dogs and more severe in large dogs, presumably because of the greater degrees of trauma in large weight-bearing animals.

Laboratory findings in Factor IX–deficient animals are normal OSPTs and prolonged APTTs and activated clotting times (ACTs). In mildly affected animals, it may be necessary to dilute the plasma to establish a prolonged APTT.

Factor VIII deficiency

Factor VIII deficiency is an important disease in dogs and has been described in most breeds and in mongrels. It also occurs in horses and cats. In all species, it is an X chromosome–linked recessive trait. Bleeding may be severe in large dogs and horses. Hemarthroses, subcutaneous hematomas, and bleeding into the CNS and body cavities may occur to varying degrees in Factor VIII deficiency. Laboratory findings include long APTTs and ACTs, low Factor VIII activity, and normal amounts of von Willebrand's factor. Carrier female animals have approximately 50% Factor VIII activity and normal amounts of von Willebrand's factor.

von Willebrand's disease

von Willebrand's disease is an inherited abnormality of the synthesis of von Willebrand glycoprotein. It is generally acknowledged as the most significant hemostatic disorder in human beings and occurs in many breeds of dogs and in cats and horses. It was described in swine in the 1940s, and affected animals have been used extensively in research of von Willebrand's disease.

The von Willebrand protein or factor (vWF) is synthesized as a prepropolypeptide in endothelial cells and megakaryocytes. The human gene encoding the protein is located on chromosome 12. The mature human subunit of 2050 amino acids is glycosylated and joined to other subunits by disulfide bonds to form multimers with molecular weights as great as 10 to 20 $\times 10^6$; very large molecules (Table 7-8). Immunochemical methods used to study this protein in humans have also been used in dogs and cats, and it has similar multimeric patterns. The glycoprotein is found in plasma, megakaryocytes, platelets, subendothelium, and endothelial cells. Plasma von Willebrand glycoprotein forms a complex with Factor VIII. Platelet von Willebrand glycoprotein is primarily located in alpha granules and is secreted onto the surface following platelet activation.

Mature vWF functions to facilitate adhesion of platelets to exposed vascular subendothelium following injury. This is especially important in small vessels with rapid blood flow (high shear rate). The most important platelet vWF receptor is glycoprotein Ib (GPIb). As is frequently true, the occurrence of a bleeding disorder due to quantitative and qualitative disorders of GPIb (Bernard-Soulier syndrome) in humans greatly facilitated our understanding of the function of the von Willebrand glycoprotein. As might be anticipated, the largest vWF molecules have the most GPIb binding sites, and bleeding times are prolonged in human beings and dogs unable to assemble large multimers. Because the vWF binds to Factor VIII in plasma, it appears to protect it from proteolysis. Unlike human beings, however, most dogs with von Willebrand's disease do not have prolonged PTTs due to smaller amounts of Factor VIII.

Laboratory assessment of animals suspected of having von Willebrand's disease is achieved by quantitative and functional assays. The most common quantitative assay is an electroimmunoassay in which plasma samples are added to an agarose gel containing rabbit-derived antibodies to canine vWF or rabbit antihuman vWF antibodies. By convention, the protein measured in this assay is referred to as von Willebrand antigen (vWF:Ag). Assessment of the multimeric structure of the protein is achieved by autoradiographic visualization of electrophoretic gels using radioactive iodine anti-vWF antibodies. Although electroimmunoassay is available at some veterinary colleges and commercial laboratories, autoradiography is confined to research laboratories. von Willebrand glycoprotein functional assays utilize substances such as botrocetin, a viper venom, which induces platelet agglutination in the presence of normal quantities of von Willebrand glycoprotein of normal structure. (This test is referred to as the botrocetin cofactor assay.) von Willebrand glycoprotein is assumed to be the cofactor required for botrocetin to bring about platelet agglutination.

Intensive study of von Willebrand's disease in human beings has established molecular heterogeneity among families, and similar heterogeneity probably occurs among breeds of dogs. This is now becoming apparent, and breed differences are being characterized. Most forms of the disease are one of three types. Type I, the most common in dogs, is characterized by decreased concentrations of a normal multimeric glycoprotein pattern. In type II, dogs lack the large multimers. Type III dogs have very low or no detectable von Willebrand glycoprotein.

It should now be apparent that animals with von Willebrand's disease have a bleeding disorder due to impaired platelet adhesion. Epistaxis, oozing of blood from mucous membranes, petechiae, and serious postoperative hemorrhage are the most common findings. Despite its being a congenital defect, variation in the expression of von Willebrand's disease may result in bleeding in some mature dogs; dogs with mild forms of von Willebrand's disease may only bleed secondary to another disorder such as urinary or intestinal tract carcinomas or inflammation of a mucosal surface (see Table 7-3). Thyroxine and estrogen are examples of hormones that increase concentrations of vWF in plasma. It has long been noted that older hypothyroid dogs may develop signs of von Willebrand's disease.

LYMPHORETICULAR TISSUES

Thymic Disorders

The thymus, a lymphoepithelial organ within the mediastinum of young animals, is essential for the development and function of the immune system. The epithelial portions are derived from branchial pouches, whereas lymphocytes arise in bone marrow. Thymic corpuscles are morphologically distinct clusters of medullary epithelial cells whose function is unknown.

The thymus is essential for the development of T-lymphocytes, which normally constitute 70% to 80% of peripheral blood lymphocytes. Precursor bone marrow–derived lymphocytes or prothymocytes migrate to the thymus, where they undergo differentiation into mature T-lymphocytes. The gland consists of subcapsular, cortical, and medullary zones, and prothymocytes in afferent blood migrate from the subcapsular zone to the medulla before leaving through efferent blood vessels and lymphatics. During this intrathymic migration, some cells proliferate after entering the thymic cortex and many cells die. The cell death ensures that only MHC-restricted and self-tolerant T cells leave the thymus. MHC-restriction ensures that T cells will only interact with those cells that present antigen associated with MHC molecules on their surfaces.

The epithelial cells, bone marrow–derived macrophages, and reticular cells of the thymus provide the unique microenvironment essential for T-lymphocyte development. MHC molecules are expressed by many of the nonlymphoid cells and may be necessary for the selection of the mature T cell repertoire. In addition, thymic hormones are produced by epithelial cells, which are postulated to promote T cell maturation.

During the final stages of T cell development, various subsets of T cells can be delineated. These include CD4 T cells (helper cells) and CD8 T cells (cytotoxic cells). The CD4 and CD8 transmembrane glycoproteins mediate cell-cell adhesion and may be involved in signal transduction. Following release from the thymus, these cells are distributed to splenic periarteriolar lymphatic sheaths and the cortical areas around germinal centers in lymph nodes. The critical balance of production and distribution of T-lymphocytes is extremely important in immune homeostasis, so much so that immunodeficiency or autoimmunity may result from inadequate or overzealous activity of a particular subset.

The thymus is large prior to birth and involutes following sexual maturity; the lymphoid and epithelial components are gradually replaced by loose connective tissue and fat. This organ is therefore no longer required following stocking of peripheral lymphoid organs with a responsive population of T-lymphocytes, which probably live throughout the life of the animal. These cells continually circulate through splenic and lymph node T cell zones. Expansion of the antigenic specific T cells would occur subsequent to antigenic presentation.

Developmental Disorders of the Thymus

Included in this discussion are the congenital disorders that result in inadequate T-lymphocyte function, as well as those resulting in B-lymphocyte and plasma cell dysfunction. Many have been described in human beings and, indeed, have been invaluable in learning more about mechanisms of immunity and immune regulation. The animal counterparts of immunodeficiency serve as valuable models in comparative immunology research. Combined immunodeficiency (CID) disorders are those affecting both B- and T-lymphocytes.

Equine CID is a genetic disorder occurring in Arabian or partly Arabian foals. It is inherited as an autosomal recessive trait, meaning that both the sire and dam are carriers of the defective gene. It has been determined that CID occurs in approximately 2% of Arabian foals and that approximately 25% of Arabian horses carry the gene. There is failure of functional B- and T-lymphocyte production, so foals are remarkably susceptible to a variety of microbial agents and usually die before 5 months of age. Adenoviruses that are typically resisted by normal foals are major causes of death in foals with CID. The viral infection is frequently complicated by various bacterial or protozoal infections that typically result in pneumonia.

The underlying biochemical basis for failure of B- and T-lymphocyte differentiation must occur at an early stage of lymphocyte development. In some children, this is the result of adenosine deaminase deficiency, which may cause impaired DNA synthesis in lymphocytes. This enzyme is not deficient in affected foals; the exact mechanism of lymphocyte stem cell failure is unknown.

Affected foals frequently have profuse nasal discharge, unthrifty hair coat, loss of condition, pneumonia, and, occasionally, diarrhea. Confirmatory diagnosis of CID in such a foal requires evidence of the following: persistent lymphopenia, absence of serum immunoglobulin, or hypoplastic lymphoid tissue. Varying degrees of neutrophilia and left shift and a mild anemia occur and probably result from chronic inflammation. Lymphopenia is marked and persistent and usually less than 0.8 to 1.0×10^9/L (0.8 to $1.0 \times 10^3/mm^3$). Serum IgM, which is normally present in newborn foals, is undetectable. Maternally derived IgG declines to very low concentrations by approximately 3 months of age. Necropsy findings are severe bronchopneumonia in combination with a small spleen and lymph nodes. The thymus may be difficult to identify or may consist of a few isolated lobules within the mediastinal fat. The spleen has marked reduction in the white pulp owing to absence of germinal centers and periarteriolar lymphocyte sheaths. Lymph nodes are similarly depleted of lymphocytes. The thymus usually consists of a few islands of lymphocyte-like cells and thymic corpuscles.

X-linked severe combined immunodeficiency (SCID) has been reported in basset hounds. The affected male pups lack mature, functional T cells. The animals have a normal serum level of IgM but low or undetectable IgG and IgA. The thymus of these dogs is small and often obscured by mediastinal fat. Tonsils, lymph nodes, and Peyer's patches usually cannot be identified at necropsy. Microscopically, the thymic tissue consists of small dysplastic lobules with a variable number of Hassall's corpuscles.

Inflammatory and Degenerative Disorders of the Thymus

Injury to the thymus resulting in variable degrees of immunodeficiency may be caused by infectious agents, toxins, neoplasms, or malnutrition. The feline leukemia and immunodeficiency viruses are examples of agents that infect T-lymphocytes, resulting in chronic respiratory and digestive system infections. Viruses with similar capabilities are those of canine distemper, bovine virus diarrhea, and equine rhinopneumonitis (equine herpesvirus-1). Previous reference has been made to the importance of T-lymphocyte surface glycoproteins; one of these (CD4) is the receptor for attachment of the human acquired immunodeficiency virus. In cats infected with the feline immunodeficiency virus, CD4 lymphocytes are reduced, and there is reversal of the CD4/CD8 T-lymphocyte ratio. As would be anticipated, thymic and lymph node atrophy are apparent at necropsy in animals with these viral infections.

Environmental toxins, such as polychlorinated biphenyls, lead, and mercury, have a suppressive effect on the immune system. Thymic function is impaired in severe protein deficiencies of young animals, leading to reduced immunoglobulin synthesis.

Neoplastic Disorders of the Thymus

Since the thymus has both lymphoid and epithelial components, it is possible for either or both to serve as cells of origin of neoplasms. Thymic lymphosarcoma is a T-lymphocyte neoplasm of young animals, particularly cats and cattle, with a much lower incidence in dogs. Clinical findings reflect the presence of a large mass in the thoracic cavity. Thoracic aspirates contain many medium to large lymphocytes, which frequently have vacuolated cytoplasm, a feature unique to neoplastic lymphocytes in fluid (Fig. 7-39). Cells in mitosis may be present and are a significant indication of neoplasia.

Bovine thymic lymphosarcoma most often occurs in beef cattle 6 to 24 months of age and is characterized by massive thymic enlargement. The etiology is unknown, and the occurrence of a concurrent leukemia is unusual. The thymus is an important site of lymphosarcoma in cats.

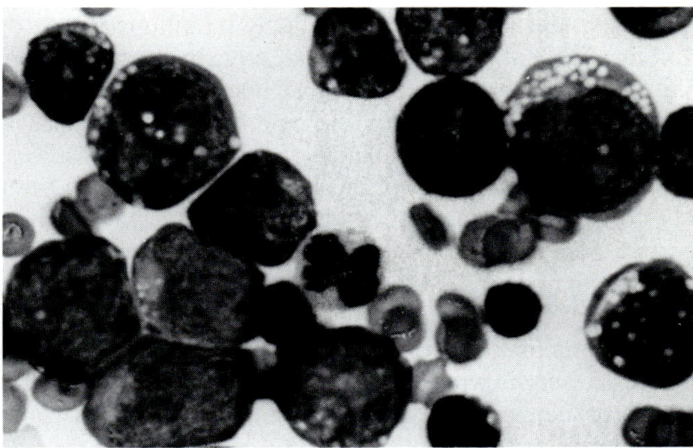

Fig. 7-39 Thoracic aspirate; cat. Thymic lymphosarcoma. Wright-Giemsa stain.

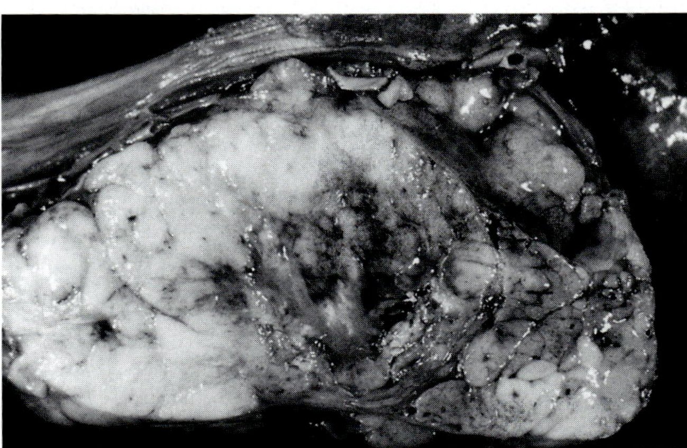

Fig. 7-40 Thymus; cat. Lymphosarcoma. The large tumor has been transected and lies immediately cranial and ventral to the lungs.

The neoplasms are large, white or gray, mediastinal masses that result in displacement of adjacent structures and in fluid accumulation (Fig. 7-40). In cats, the throacic fluid is frequently chylous because of lipid accumulations. Microscopically, these diffuse lymphosarcomas are dominated by lymphocytes that are homogeneous in size, shape, nuclear morphology, and nuclear/cytoplasmic ratio.

Lymphoepithelial thymomas are significantly less common and only distinguishable microscopically by the presence of neoplastic epithelial cells in addition to neoplastic lymphocytes.

LYMPHOCYTE AND LYMPH NODE DISORDERS

Lymph nodes are ideally suited for surveillance and immune function. Lymph transports antigens from a wide area of tissue to lymph nodes, where they are concentrated among phagocytes and lymphocytes. Lymphocytes enter lymph nodes by migrating through walls of specialized venules, and they leave in efferent lymph within a few hours if they do not encounter an antigen they recognize. The successful encounter of lymphocytes with antigen is assisted by antigen-presenting cells that display antigens in highly immunogenic forms. Lymph nodes, therefore, serve to introduce lymph-borne antigens to blood-borne lymphocytes in order to enhance antigen detection and presentation.

Lymph nodes are traditionally divided into three regions: the superficial cortex, the deep cortex or paracortex, and the medulla (Fig. 7-41). From a functional viewpoint, there are three spaces within each region: an intralympatic space, an intravascular space lined by endothelium, and an interstitium.

Afferent lymphatics penetrate the capsule and enter the subcapsular sinus. The subcapsular sinus connects with medullary sinuses that eventually converge on the efferent lymphatics. Unless these sinuses are particularly distended with lymph, they and their thin endothelium are usually microscopically imperceptible. A striking feature of the intravascular space is the concentration of lymphocytes within venules characterized by tall endothelial cells. At these sites, lymphocytes migrate into the interstitium. This controlled migration of blood cells now appears to be mediated by surface glycoproteins, which become expressed on lymphocytes and bind to appropriate glycoproteins expressed on endothelial cells.

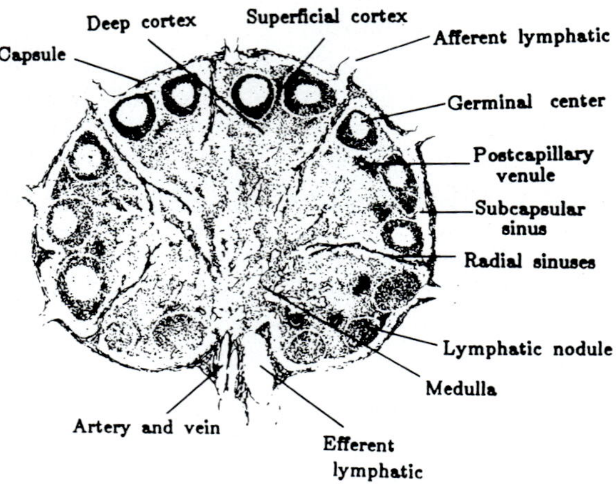

Fig. 7-41 Schema of a lymph node. Afferent lymphatic vessels pierce the capsule, and efferent lymphatics leave the node at the hilus. The superficial cortex consists of spherical lymphatic nodules, some of which contain germinal centers. The deep cortex lies between the nodules and deep to them. Within the center of the node lie the linear medullary cords, converging on the hilus. A subcapsular sinus, into which the afferent lymphatic vessels empty, lies beneath the full expanse of capsule. Radial sinuses run from the subcapsular sinus toward the hilus. They run along the trabeculae, and, in the medulla, between medullary cords. Arteries enter the node at the hilus and branch, richly penetrating the node. Postcapillary venules tend to lie in the cortex. Veins leave the node at the hilus. *From Weiss L. Lymphatic vessels and lymph nodes. In: Weiss L, ed. The Blood Cells and Hematopoietic Tissues. 2nd ed. New York: Elsevier, 1984:256.*

The lymphoid cells within lymph nodes are classified on a morphologic basis as small lymphocytes, large lymphocytes, and plasma cells. Recently developed techniques using monoclonal antibodies for cell surface protein recognition have allowed subclassification of cells within these groups. For example, immunocytochemistry using monoclonal antibodies not only separates helper and cytotoxic T-lymphocyte populations, it also allows determination of their tissue distribution.

Lymphocytes within the superficial cortex form spherical or ovoid lymphoid nodules or follicles. Germinal centers of lymphoid nodules consist of a central, pale zone of large lymphocytes and macrophages within a zone of small lymphocytes (Fig. 7-41).

Most lymphocytes in the follicles of the superficial cortex are B cells, whereas most lymphocytes in the paracortex are T cells. Following migration through tall endothelial venules, B cells proceed to follicular areas, while T cells migrate toward lymphatic spaces. B cells also eventually reach efferent lymph, but much later than T cells. Interaction of B cells with antigens and T cells in germinal centers results in proliferating B cells. These B cells may return to the blood as memory cells, or they may mature into antibody-secreting plasma cells located in the medullary cords (Fig. 7-42).

The accessory or nonlymphoid cells in lymph nodes act in harmony with B- and T-lymphocytes throughout the immune response. There are several groups of accessory cells in lymph nodes that are recognizable mainly by morphology and location. The perception of where they come from relative to their function is of central significance to immunology. The sinus macrophages are differentiated, bone marrow–derived monocytes with morphologic and cytochemical characteristics of macrophages. Interdigitating cells within the paracortex have numerous fingerlike cytoplasmic projections that intertwine with those of their neighbors. They also appear to be of bone marrow origin, but, if they are monocyte-derived, they undergo differentiation to assume characteristics distinct from those of classic macrophages. Follicular dendritic cells are probably non-marrow-derived stromal cells found in follicles following antigenic stimulation. They, too, have numerous branching projections. It seems probable that these accessory cells collaborate in the complex process of digesting and presenting antigenic particles (Fig. 7-43). A particularly interesting concept, which will no doubt become clearer in the future, is the possibility that accessory cells leave the bone marrow as identical precursors and migrate to various tissues where they undergo differentiation and assume characteristics unique to that environment. Ultimately, they may trap antigen and carry it to the nearest lymph node. There is good evidence that the Langerhans'

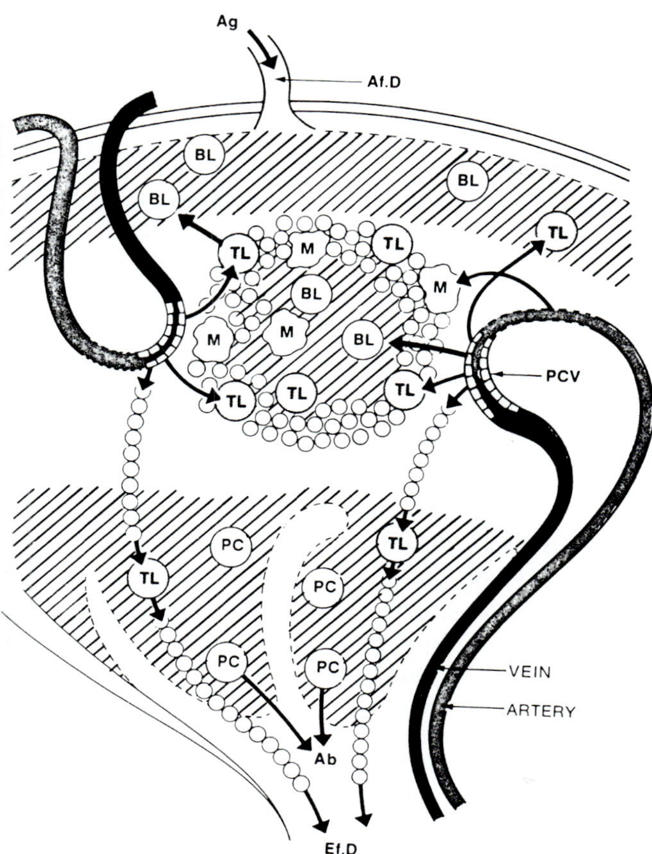

Fig. 7-42 Schematic representation of the approximate location of B- and T-lymphocytes in lymph nodes. Constant recirculation of lymphocytes occurs as they percolate around and through regions containing heavy concentrations of macrophages; this permits interaction among these cells and antigen. The hatched areas represent B-lymphocyte areas, and the areas containing open circles, or unhatched, represent T-lymphocyte areas. Germinal centers form in response to antigens that elicit humoral antibody; they contain B-lymphocytes and their plasmacytic progeny and macrophages. The surrounding mantle zone is composed chiefly of T-lymphocytes. *TL,* T-lymphocytes; *BL,* B-lymphocytes; *PC,* plasma cell; *M,* monocyte-macrophage; *Ag,* antigen; *Ab,* antibody; *Af.D,* afferent lymphatic duct; *Ef.D,* efferent lymphatic duct; *PCV,* postcapillary venule. *Modified from Craddock CG, Longmire R, McMillan R. New Engl J Med 1971; 285:378-384.*

cells of the skin follow such a route and ultimately become interdigitating cells in the nearest lymph node.

Lymph nodes may undergo atrophy or hypertrophy or may become the site of focal or diffuse inflammation (lymphadenitis). They may become enlarged because of lymphoid neoplasia or metastatic tumor cell proliferation. It is essential that enlarged lymph nodes be examined microscopically. For superficial nodes, this is easily accomplished by aspiration using 22- to 25-gauge needles, with expulsion of the cell suspension onto glass slides. The fragility of lymphocytes necessitates gentle spreading techniques to prevent cellular distortion. Aspirates may be stained with Wright-Giemsa or new methylene blue stains. The ease of lymph node aspiration and staining provides veterinary clinicians the opportunity to become proficient in the evaluation of lymph node cytology. Aspirates provide excellent cellular detail, but, for the study of architectural dearrangements, removal of the node for microscopic evaluation is required. The surgeon must handle lymph nodes carefully to minimize artifacts. A portion of one end of the node should be removed and used to prepare impression smears. The remainder of the node should be placed in fixative fluid, with the capsule intact, for 1 hour. This period of fixation hardens the node and prevents artifactual bulging of the tissue through the capsule, which occurs when lymph nodes are cut without prior fixation. The lymph node, if large, should then be sliced into parallel sections to ensure penetration of the fixative fluid.

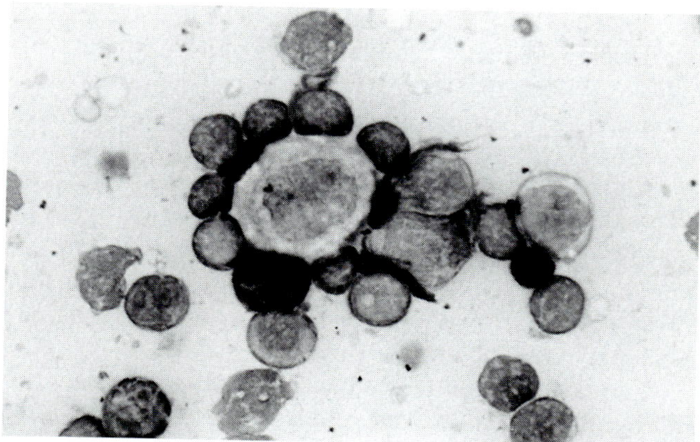

Fig. 7-43 Mesenteric lymph node imprint from a calf. Coccidiosis. The large cell encircled by lymphocytes may be an antigen-presenting cell. Wright-Giemsa stain.

Developmental Disorders of Lymph Nodes

The congenital immunodeficiency syndromes include developmental disorders of lymph nodes, which are discussed in the section on Developmental Disorders of the Thymus.

Degenerative Disorders of Lymph Nodes

Atrophy of lymph nodes and bronchial and gut-associated lymphoid tissues may result from viral infections, toxins, and malnutrition. Examples of these are discussed in the section on Inflammatory and Degenerative Disorders of the Thymus.

Hyperplasis of Lymph Nodes

The arrival of large numbers of antigens into a lymph node results in increased blood supply, increased numbers of macrophages, and recruitment of many lymphocytes. Superficial lymph nodes become palpably enlarged. Lymphocytes transform to lymphoblasts, which undergo cellular division. Depending on the nature of the antigen, lymphoblasts will mature into T-lymphocytes or plasma cells. In comparison to normal lymph nodes, hyperplastic nodes have greater variation in cellular morphology because of increased numbers of large immature cells and increased numbers of macrophages, which may be antigen-presenting cells, and a few neutrophils. Mitotic figures are not common. Plasma cells are usually evident and are valuable indicators of recent stimulation of the lymph node by antigens that stimulate antibody synthesis (Fig. 7-44).

Hyperplastic lymph nodes have changes that reflect the duration of stimulation. The venules with tall endothelium are prominent, reflecting increased lymphocyte adhesion and migration shortly after the arrival of antigen. Germinal centers with numerous debris-laden macrophages become prominent in secondary follicles (Fig. 7-45). The T cell population in the paracortex may be expanded. Within a few days, increased numbers of plasma cells may be detected in the mantle zone and later in medullary cords.

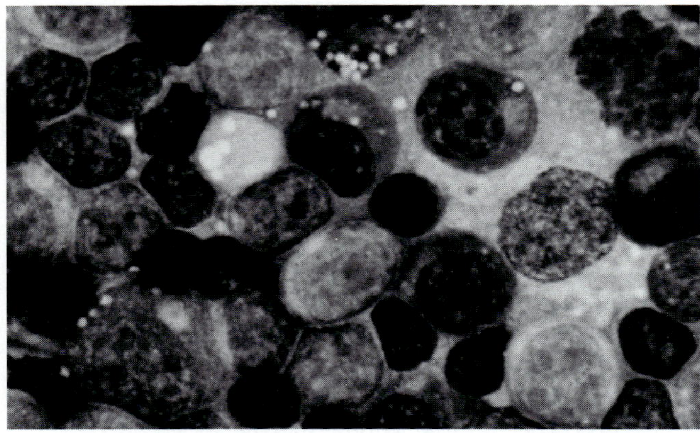

Fig. 7-44 Lymph node aspirate; dog. Hyperplasia. Note the increased numbers of immature lymphocytes and plasma cells. Wright-Giemsa stain.

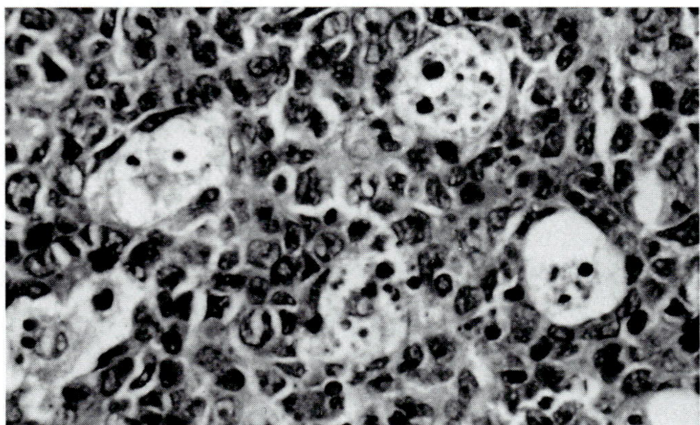

Fig. 7-45 Lymph node. Hyperplasia. Note the debris-laden macrophages in the germinal center of a lymphoid follicle. H & E stain.

Chronically stimulated nodes have increased numbers of follicles with irregular contours. Differentiation of benign hyperplasia from neoplasia may be difficult, but nodal architecture, especially the subcapsular sinus, is retained in hyperplastic nodes.

Inflammatory Disorders of Lymph Nodes

Many of the gross and microscopic findings in lymphadenitis include those of hyperplasia because of the antigenic stimulation. In addition, the numbers of neutrophils, monocytes, and macrophages are increased. Lymph node aspirates and biopsy specimens should be thoroughly examined for the presence of organisms. In some bacterial and mycotic infections, the lymph node is mostly occupied by neutrophils, and incision of the capsule exposes an abscess.

Caseous lymphadenitis

Caseous lymphadenitis is a specific lymphadenitis of sheep and goats caused by *Corynebacterium pseudotuberculosis,* which is also the cause of ulcerative lymphangitis in cattle and horses and pectoral abscesses in horses. It is suspected that the organism lives within the intestine and enters the skin through wounds contaminated with soil containing fecal material or purulent discharges. Abscesses occur in superficial lymph nodes, and these may discharge thick, green pus. Most sheep do not become ill; debilitation occurs only in a small percentage of sheep in which infection involves internal lymph nodes and other organs.

The encapsulated abscesses of ovine cutaneous lymphadenitis are characteristically green and caseous, with concentric rings resembling those of an onion. Similar abscesses may be found in the lungs, especially in older sheep. The abscesses in goats are usually more numerous and frequently involve lymph nodes of the head and neck.

Histoplasmosis

Histoplasmosis is a diffuse disease of the monocyte-macrophage system caused by *Histoplasma capsulatum.* A dimorphic fungus, it grows as a mold in soil and as a yeast in animal tissues. The fungus is distributed throughout the world, in major river valleys in temperate and tropical climates; it grows especially well in soil enriched by bird feces. The greatest incidence of disease is in dogs; the incidence is lower in cats.

In most animals, the organism is inhaled and results in mild, self-limiting infections with hypertrophy of tracheobronchial lymph nodes in asymptomatic dogs and cats. Since the fungus is confined to monocytes and macrophages, spread beyond the respiratory tract is assumed to occur by hematogenous and lymph dissemination of infected cells. Disseminated histoplasmosis in dogs and cats results in gastrointestinal or hepatic disease of long duration. Several reports describe ocular involvement in cats with disseminated histoplasmosis.

Disseminated histoplasmosis is characterized by neutro-

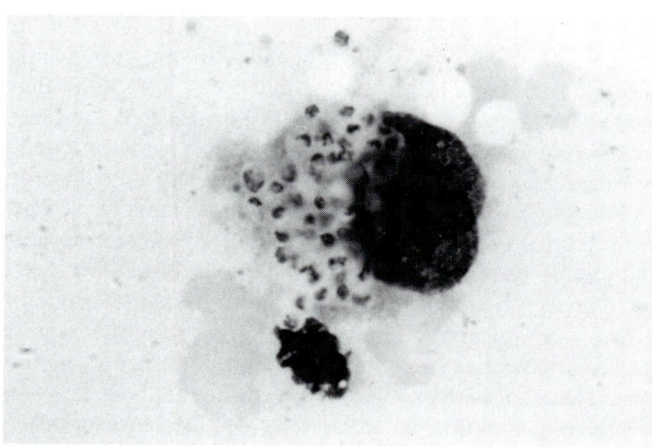

Fig. 7-46 Lymph node imprint; dog. Histoplasmosis. Macrophage-containing *Histoplasma capsulatum* organisms. Wright-Giemsa stain. *Courtesy K.W. Prasse.*

philia and monocytosis in some animals. Nonregenerative anemia is common because of the chronic inflammation. Biochemical changes include elevated activities of alkaline phosphatase and hyperbilirubinemia. The total serum protein may be low, normal, or increased, depending upon factors such as extent and duration of the diarrhea and emaciation. Regardless of the total protein concentration, a shift in the albumin/globulin ratio occurs because of hypergammaglobulinemia and hypoalbuminemia.

Cytology is useful for the diagnosis of histoplasmosis. The least invasive procedures include examination of cells of buffy coat, body fluids, and tracheal wash preparations and aspirates of bone marrow and lymph nodes. The organisms are visible in monocytes and macrophages (Fig. 7-46).

Dogs dying of this disease are emaciated. The large bowel is thickened with mucosal corrugations caused by infiltration of the submucosa and lamina propria by macrophages, lymphocytes, and plasma cells. Lymph nodes are uniformly enlarged and, in contrast to lymphosarcoma, are firm when incised. The spleen and liver are enlarged and firm, and the liver is diffusely gray. Affected organs can be imprinted on glass slides for cytologic examination.

Epizootic lymphangitis

Epizootic lymphangitis or equine histoplasmosis is a chronic suppurative lymphadenitis of solipeds caused by *Histoplasma farciminosus.* It occurs in Mediterranean countries, Asia, and Africa. The fungal organisms exist in the soil and enter the body through contaminated wounds. Fungal spores are also inhaled and cause lesions of the upper and lower respiratory tracts. Keratoconjunctivitis may result from transmission of the organism by flies.

The lesions, in most locations, are nodules that eventually discharge a mucopurulent exudate. The organism is evident in smears of the exudate as globose to oval yeasts 2 to 3 μm in diameter. Spontaneous recovery may occur, but horses are often euthanatized because of debilitation. At necropsy, suppurative and granulomatous lesions are most numerous in the skin, with occasional dissemination to the lungs, liver, and spleen.

Leishmaniasis

Leishmaniasis is a disseminated disease of the monocyte-macrophage system caused by protozoa of the genus *Leishmania.* It occurs in humans, dogs, and other animals and is confined to endemic areas, including parts of Europe, the Mediterranean countries, the Middle East, Africa, and Central and South America. It may be seen in any part of the world in dogs that have resided in endemic areas. The protozoa proliferate by binary fission in the gut of the sand fly and become flagellated organisms that are introduced to mammals by insect bites; they then assume a nonflagellated form in macrophages.

The cutaneous lesions in dogs are ulcers at the site of insect bites. These ulcers are directly attributable to proliferation of the organism within macrophages, the accumulation of neutrophils, lymphocytes, and plasma cells and focal disruption of the dermis and epidermis. In the visceral form of the disease, dogs are emaciated and have generalized enlargement of lymph nodes. Lymph node aspirates contain macrophages with organisms. Dogs have a nonregenerative anemia and a polyclonal hypergammaglobulinemia with total protein concentrations that may exceed 100 g/L (10 g/dl).

At necropsy, dogs with visceral leishmaniasis are emaciated and have enlarged liver, spleen, and lymph nodes. The bone marrow is usually hyperplastic. Imprints made of these enlarged organs have macrophages containing numerous round organisms approximately 2 μm in diameter. They have a vesicular nucleus and a small kinetoplast, which aids in distinguishing them from *H. capsulatum* (Fig. 7-47).

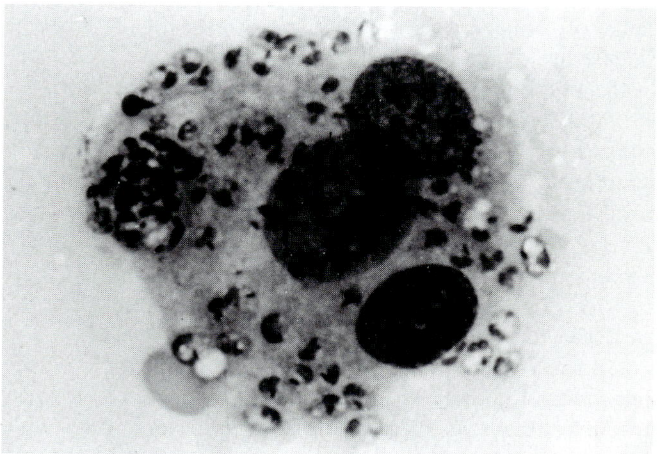

Fig. 7-47 Lymph node aspirate; dog. Leishmaniasis. Macrophage containing numerous *Leishmania* organisms. Wright-Giemsa stain.

Neoplastic Lymphocyte Disorders

Lymphosarcoma is a significant disease in domestic animals, with species-dependent variations in etiology, tumor distribution, and clinical and necropsy findings. Animals with lymphosarcoma may or may not be leukemic, i.e., have neoplastic cells in bone marrow and blood.

The National Cancer Institute Working Formulation classification system for human lymphosarcomas has been applied to animal lymphosarcomas. The precepts of the Working Formulation are that lymphosarcomas of small cells with low mitotic rate have a low rate of progression and, thus, respond poorly to cytoreductive therapy, whereas lymphosarcomas of larger cells with high proliferative rates are potentially curable diseases. The system requires the identification and correlation of tumor cell types and tumor growth patterns. The neoplasms are thus graded as low-grade (indolent clinical course), intermediate-grade, and high-grade (aggressive clinical course) lymphosarcomas.

Canine lymphosarcoma

In dogs, lymphosarcoma occurs predominantly in middle-aged animals. The etiology is unknown, but viruses have been incriminated with the demonstration of reverse transcriptase activity (see discussion of feline leukemia virus) in culture supernatants of dogs with lymphosarcoma. Most canine lymphosarcomas are B-lymphocyte neoplasms with a small percentage of T- and null-lymphocyte tumors. The future application of monoclonal antibodies for recognition of cell surface proteins will enable more specific characterization of the lymphoid neoplasms.

Canine lymphosarcoma occurs in multicentric, alimentary, cutaneous, and mediastinal forms, with the multicentric form being most common. In all forms of the disease, dogs are anorexic and lethargic and gradually become cachectic. The **multicentric** form leads to generalized enlargement of lymph nodes, with or without hepatic and splenic enlargement and infiltration of bone marrow. Because of the size of the neoplasm, dogs with mediastinal disease are dyspneic and have reduced exercise tolerance. In the **alimentary form,** vomition, diarrhea, and blood in the stool are observed. Nodules, plaques, and ulcers are present in the skin of dogs with the **cutaneous form** of lymphosarcoma. Occasionally, dogs are presented to veterinarians because of polyuria and polydypsia. These dogs have hypercalcemia and, frequently, azotemia due to hypercalcemic nephropathy. Hypercalcemia occurs in 10% to 20% of dogs with lymphosarcoma; most of these are T-lymphocyte tumors.

Mild to moderate nonregenerative anemia is observed, and the anemia may be microcytic and hypochromic with mild reticulocytosis, because of iron depletion in dogs with bleeding tumors of the intestines. Dogs with lymphosarcoma may have marrow involvement and be leukemic. In blood films, the cellular populations are variable and range from marked lymphocytosis with counts exceeding 100×10^9/L (100×10^3/mm^3) to leukopenia with the presence of a few large lymphocytes or lymphocytes with abnormal nuclear morphology. These have been classified as either acute lymphoblastic leukemia or chronic lymphocytic leukemia, in an attempt to make comparisons with human leukemias. The lymphoblastic leukemias, characterized by the presence of large lymphocytes, are the most common and tend to occur in younger dogs. The chronic form, with more mature lymphocytes, occurs more frequently in dogs over 8 years of age. The nuclear criteria of malignancy in the large lymphocytes include large nuclei, irregular nuclear shape, homogeneous nucleochromatin, and faint to prominent, multiple irregular nucleoli. Many neoplastic lymphocytes are fragile and may be distorted or completely disrupted during blood film preparation. In chronic lymphosarcoma, the marked lymphocytosis is frequently composed of small lymphocytes.

Bone marrow aspirates should be examined in suspected cases of lymphosarcoma. If the neoplasm is present, marrow particles are often large and fleshy. Low-magnification microscopy of these aspirates provides evaluation of the degree to which the hemopoietic cells have been replaced by lymphocytes (Fig. 7-48). Examination at greater magnification allows identification of the cells. Aspirates of enlarged lymph nodes, liver, and spleen are also valuable. Submandibular lymph node aspirates should be avoided, if other nodes are enlarged, due to the high incidence of hyperplasia in dogs with oral disease. In contrast to those of lymphadenitis and lymph node hyperplasia, the aspirates of neoplastic nodes have homogeneous populations of large lymphocytes similar to those described in blood and bone marrow. Mitotic figures are frequently more numerous in neoplastic nodes in comparison to those enlarged because of hyperplasia.

Necropsy findings in canine lymphosarcoma vary, de-

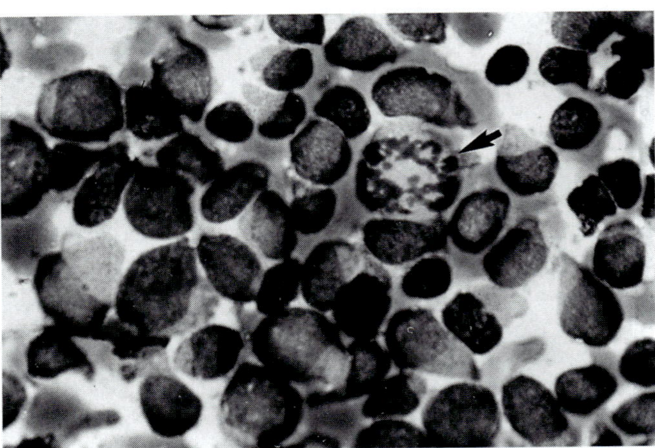

Fig. 7-48 Bone marrow aspirate; dog. Lymphosarcoma. There is complete displacement of hemopoietic cells by neoplastic cells. Note the cell in mitosis *(arrow).* Wright-Giemsa stain.

pending on the form of the disease. Lymph nodes are almost always involved and, when incised, bulge a white-gray, soft tissue. Similar tissue is frequently present in the spleen and liver. Long bones should be examined for replacement of fat and hemopoietic tissue by characteristic tumor tissue.

Feline lymphosarcoma

Lymphosarcoma is one manifestation of several hemopoietic diseases caused by the feline leukemia virus (FLV). The virus is shed in saliva, and cats become infected when virus first colonizes the pharyngeal epithelium and pharngeal lymphoid tissue. This represents the first of six possible stages of FLV infection (Table 7-9). The virus evokes an immune response in most cats, with neutralization of the virus by stage III or IV. Cats that are unable to mount an effective immune response progress through the six stages and shed virus in saliva. Persistent viremia is most likely in kittens, in cats in crowded unsanitary conditions, and in cats that are immunosuppressed.

FLV is a retrovirus that contains a single strand of RNA and the enzyme reverse transcriptase, enclosed in a lipoprotein envelope. Reverse transcriptase enables the virus to make a DNA copy of the viral RNA, which is then incorporated into the host cell's DNA. The viral DNA may be transcribed with host cell DNA or remain dormant and be passed to daughter cells. The virus may replicate at any time, but replication usually follows some form of stress.

Persistently viremic cats are immunosuppressed and may develop other infectious diseases, bone marrow disorders, or lymphosarcomas. The lymphosarcomas have been classified as **multicentric, thymic, alimentary,** and **miscellaneous,** the latter in reference to ocular, renal, and neural forms. Abnormal lymphocytes may be found in blood or bone marrow from cats with any form of lymphosarcoma.

Table 7-9. Pathogenesis of feline leukemia virus (FLV) infection

Stage	Disease progression
1 (2-4 days)	Replication of FLV occurs in lymphoid tissues surrounding the site of exposure (tonsils and pharyngeal lymph nodes by oronasal exposure).
II (1-14 days)	Small numbers of circulating lymphocytes and monocytes are infected.
III (3-12 days)	FLV replication is amplified in the spleen, lymph nodes, and gut-associated lymphoid tissue (GALT).
IV (7-21 days)	Replication progresses to include bone marrow neutrophils, platelets, and intestinal crypt epithelial cells.
V (14-28 days)	Peripheral viremia occurs once FLV has been incorporated into bone marrow–derived neutrophils and platelets.
VI (28-56 days)	Widespread epithelial infection causes excretion of virus in saliva and urine.

From Beck ER, Harris CK, Macy DW. Comp Cont Educ 1986; 8:567-574.

The clinical expression of lymphosarcoma varies with the form of the disease, i.e., the location of the tumor or tumors. Nonspecific signs include pallor of mucous membranes, lethargy, and wasting. Cats with thymic lymphosarcoma have dyspnea and a noncompressible thorax. Cats with internal lymph node enlargement, hepatomegaly, or intestinal lymphosarcoma may have palpable abdominal masses. Cats with renal lymphosarcoma may be presented in renal failure.

Laboratory findings in feline lymphosarcoma include nonregenerative anemia, regardless of the form of the disease. If the marrow is involved, there may be neutropenia, thrombocytopenia, and anemia. Frequently, dyserythropoiesis, due to impaired nuclear maturation, is reflected in a high MCV, despite reticulocytopenia, and the release of a few rubricytes or metarubicytes with asynchronous maturation of nucleus and cytoplasm (discussed with erythrocytic sarcomas). Occasionally, small numbers of *Haemobartonella felis* organisms are evident on erythrocytes, most likely due to the immunosuppressive effects of the virus. Blood films from these animals should be scanned at low magnification to detect abnormal nucleated cells. Agglutination of erythrocytes is also frequently observed, perhaps owing to circulating FLV-antibody complexes. Lymphocytes from cats with lymphosarcoma and leukemia are usually larger than normal large lymphocytes. They have large nuclei with homogeneous nucleochromatin. Nuclear shapes may be irregular; nucleoli are usually not prominent. Aspirates of bone marrow and fine-needle aspirates of palpable masses are indicated in cats suspected of having lymphosarcoma. The marrow aspirates may contain variable numbers of immature lymphocytes, and, in some instances, the hemopoietic cells are completely replaced by tumor cells. Cats with abdominal masses are frequently emaciated, allowing immobilization and fine-needle aspiration of the tumors. If the masses are lymph nodes, the aspirate contains mainly large lymphocytes, some of which are in mitosis. With hepatic and renal lymphosarcomas, aspirates have numerous lymphocytes among hepatocytes and renal tubular epithelial cells. Cats have been described that have large granular lymphocytes in aspirates of tumor masses, consistent with neoplastic transformation of natural killer (NK) cells (Fig. 7-49).

Necropsy findings in cats with lymphosarcoma include enlargement of organs such as the liver or kidneys. They may be diffusely enlarged or have gray-white nodular masses protruding beneath the capsule. Lymph nodes, if enlarged, bulge soft, white tissue from the excised surfaces. With thymic lymphosarcomas, a large, gray, soft mass is present in the thoracic cavity (see Fig. 7-40). Marrow cavities of long bones are occupied by soft pale tissue in an-

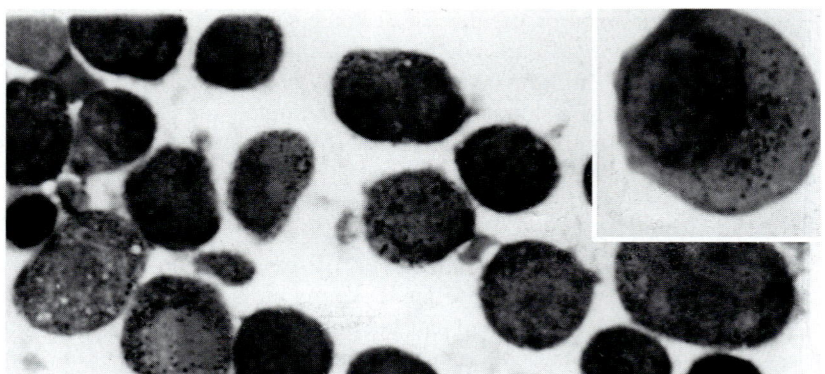

Fig. 7-49 Bone marrow aspirate and blood smear *(inset);* cat. Granular lymphocyte, lymphosarcoma. Wright-Giemsa stain.

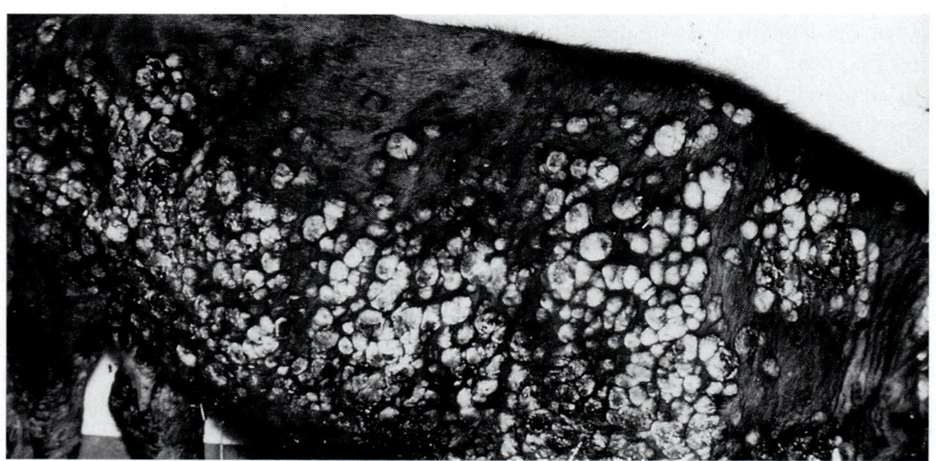

Fig. 7-50 Cutaneous lymphosarcoma.

imals with marrow lymphosarcoma. Imprints should be made of these tissues and included with the microscopic examination of fixed tissues.

Bovine lymphosarcoma

Enzootic bovine lymphosarcoma is a disease of adult cattle caused by the bovine leukemia virus (BLV). **Sporadic bovine lymphosarcoma,** of no known etiology, is a disease of young cattle. BLV is an RNA retrovirus similar to other oncogenic viruses. Its behavior differs from that of the feline virus because of minimal viral expression and persistence within lymphocytes for the life of the animal. Transmission of the virus is mostly horizontal, due to transmission of infected lymphocytes as opposed to free virus in secretions. Blood-sucking arthropods or mechanical means of transferring small numbers of infected lymphocytes are the principal means of spread. The disease has a much greater incidence in dairy cattle in comparison to beef cattle, presumably because dairy cattle husbandry favors viral transmission. Herd surveys have established high incidence of infection but low incidence of disease.

Clinical expression of sporadic bovine lymphosarcoma is different from the enzootic disease. The **thymic form** of sporadic lymphosarcoma is characterized by large cranial thoracic and lower cervical masses, respiratory distress, and weight loss in cattle less than 2 years of age. The **juvenile form** of sporadic lymphosarcoma is disseminated lymphosarcoma in calves 3 to 6 months of age, with generalized lymphadenopathy, depression, and weight loss. The **cutaneous form** is rare, occurs in young cattle, and consists of discrete cutaneous plaques or large scabby lesions (Fig. 7-50).

Clinical expression of enzootic bovine lymphosarcoma reflects the location of tumors. The disease may vary from several days' to several weeks' duration, with loss of condition, weakness, and pallor. Enlargement of superficial lymph nodes is common, and enlarged pelvic and abdominal lymph nodes are found on rectal palpation. Involvement of the digestive tract may cause persistent diarrhea, and congestive heart failure results from lymphosarcoma of the right ventricle. Nervous system lymphosarcoma is most frequently manifested as posterior paresis or paralysis because of pressure by the extradural mass on the cauda equina or on the lumbar cord.

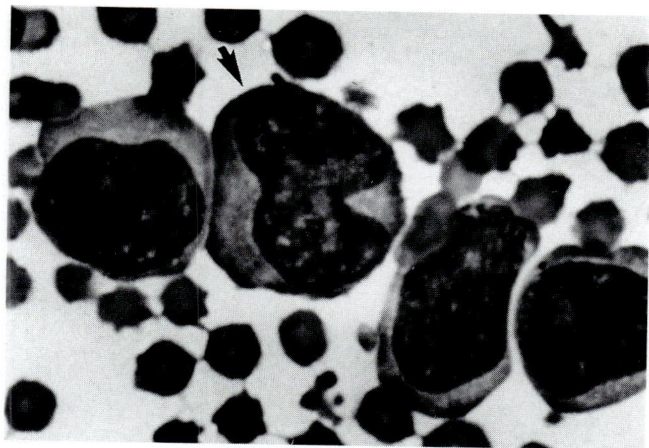

Fig. 7-51 Blood smear; calf. Lymphocytic leukemia. The lymphocytes are very large, and some have irregularly shaped nuclei *(arrow)*. Wright-Giemsa stain.

Cattle with all forms of lymphosarcoma usually have a mild, nonregenerative anemia. In the generalized sporadic form of calves, lymphocytic leukemia with extensive bone marrow involvement may occur (Fig. 7-51). It is important to differentiate leukemia from nonspecific lymphocytosis in calves with chronic inflammatory disease, in which lymphocyte numbers can reach 15 to 20 $\times$ 10^9/L (15 to 20 $\times$ 10^3/mm^3). Neoplastic lymphocytes are large, with large nuclei that may assume irregular shapes resembling monocyte nuclei. Bone marrow aspirates have large numbers of similar appearing cells with variable interference with hemopoiesis. Lymphocytosis occurs in a significant number of BLV-infected cows and may persist for years without tumor development. Most of these lymphocytes have normal morphology, but a few abnormal cells are usually present.

Enlarged lymph nodes, which should always be aspirated or biopsied, have a homogenous population of large lymphocytes. Some cells have irregular nuclei and prominent irregular nucleoli. Microscopic differentiation of diffuse lymphoid hyperplasia from lymphosarcoma can be difficult, but basic nodal architecture is retained in hyperplastic nodes.

Necropsy findings in bovine lymphosarcoma include the presence of characteristic neoplasms with locations depending upon the form of the disease. Enlarged lymph nodes, when incised, bulge soft gray-white tissue that may exude a milky fluid. Large masses, as in thymic lymphosarcoma, may contain areas of necrosis. Calves with juvenile disseminated lymphosarcoma frequently have widespread lymph node enlargement in addition to hepatic, splenic, and renal involvement. In adult cattle, there is usually generalized lymph node enlargement. Cardiac involvement is common, specifically the right atrium, with possible extension to the ventricular myocardium. Abomasal involvement results in a variably thickened wall, with a tendency for mucosal ulceration.

Equine lymphosarcoma

The incidence of lymphosarcoma in horses is lower than that of cattle, dogs, and cats. In the last decade, several reports have described from 1 to as many as 40 cases. The distribution of lymphosarcoma in the horse is variable; reports of concurrent leukemia vary from rare to over 50%. With the exception of the cutaneous disease, most forms result in debility with anemia, hypoproteinemia, and dependent edema.

The **multicentric form** of equine lymphosarcoma is characterized by irregular involvement of peripheral lymph nodes with tumor masses in the mediastinum and abdomen. **Cutaneous lymphosarcoma** in horses, as in other species, is a chronic disease without leukemia or internal organ involvement. The lesions, easily biopsied for cytologic and microscopic evaluation, have a mixture of small and large lymphocytes with few mitotic figures. The **alimentary form** of equine lymphosarcoma is a wasting syndrome, presumably due to involvement of the small intestine, resulting in malabsorption. The neoplastic lymphocytes from the bowel and enlarged adjacent lymph nodes are frequently plasmacytoid; mitotic figures are rare. In some horses, involvement of abdominal organs includes the large intestine and numerous lymph nodes, occasionally including the nodes of the thorax. In contrast to the intestinal form, this form consists of lymphoblasts with numerous mitotic figures. **Splenic lymphosarcoma** in the horse is characterized by massive organ enlargement; some horses are leukemic and have lymphocyte counts in excess of 100 $\times$ 10^9/L (100 $\times$ 10^3/mm^3). Occasionally, in these horses and in those with other forms of lymphosarcoma, hemolytic anemia is suspected because of an elevated MCV, RDW, and marrow erythroid hyperplasia in the absence of hemorrhage. Splenic sequestration of erythrocytes could occur in massively enlarged spleens; however, some horses are positive for the direct antiglobulin (Coombs') test, which is consistent with an immune-mediated mechanism of hemolysis.

SPLENIC DISORDERS

The blood supply to the spleen and its sievelike anatomic structure render it an efficient organ for monitoring viability of cells, particularly erythrocytes. Splenic immune functions include trapping of blood-borne antigens with subsequent macrophage T- and B-lymphocyte interactions and production of antibody and activated B and T cells.

Spleens have been classified as either storage or defense spleens. Although the organ may serve both functions, in many species, one function often predominates. Spleens that are relatively large, rich in smooth muscle, but poor in lymphoid tissue, such as that of the horse, are primarily storage spleens. In contrast, smaller spleens that are poor in trabeculae but rich in lymphoid tissue may be regarded as defense spleens. Spleens of the rabbit and human beings are examples of defense spleens; those of cats, dogs, and cattle have considerable storage capability.

Fundamental to splenic structure and function are the afferent and efferent blood vessels and the white and red pulp. The white pulp consists of lymphocytes and macrophages surrounding central arteries. The red pulp is a meshwork of specialized fibroblast-like cells, called **reticular cells,** with long interdigitating filamentous projections. Interspersed among the reticular cells are numerous macrophages.

The vascular components of the red pulp vary among species, based on the presence or absence of thin-walled venous sinuses. Sinusal spleens of dogs and horses have sinuses one endothelial cell layer thick, through which erythrocytes, leukocytes, and platelets pass on their way to venules. In the feline nonsinusal spleen, cells are deposited from terminal arterioles into the red pulp, where they traverse the reticular cell–macrophage meshwork before entering terminal venules. In both types of spleen, blood may pass through the red pulp rapidly or slowly, depending upon whether the spleen is in a storage state or a contracted state. A particularly dense population of macrophages (the periarteriolar macrophage sheaths) are adjacent to the terminal arterioles in the red pulp. This arrangement favors efficient trapping of antigenic material from the plasma as well as scrutiny of passing erythrocytes. The red pulp–reticular cell and macrophage populations retain immature erythrocytes to allow maturation. Erythrocyte inclusions such as nuclear remnants, Heinz bodies, or rickettsial organisms are removed as they make their way among the macrophages and through sinus walls in sinusal spleens. Indeed, large numbers of nuclear remnants are a good indication of splenic malfunction. Splenic macrophages have IgG receptors, and they remove entire erythrocytes, or portions of erythrocyte membranes, and platelets in immune-mediated hemolytic anemias and thrombocytopenias.

The red pulp–reticular cells in canine and equine spleens have an extraordinarily large complement of filaments, especially intermediate filaments, and these spleens are rich in adrenergic nerve fibers. These contractile reticular cells are ideally suited to shunt blood through the red pulp into the venous circulation or, when appropriate, to store large numbers of erythrocytes and platelets.

Degenerative Disorders of the Spleen

Atrophy and enlargement of the spleen are difficult to distinguish from normal variations in organ size. Atrophy results from mechanisms such as hemosiderosis, old age, wasting diseases, and induration following prolonged congestion. The atrophic spleen is small and firm, with a wrinkled capsule. Accumulation of iron and calcium as siderocalcific nodules is a frequent finding on the surface of the spleen of old dogs (Fig. 7-52). Hemosiderin is frequently visible within splenic macrophages, especially following prolonged congestion. Episodes of hemolysis mediated by splenic erythrophagocytosis and chronic inflammatory states result in increased numbers of hemosiderin-laden macrophages.

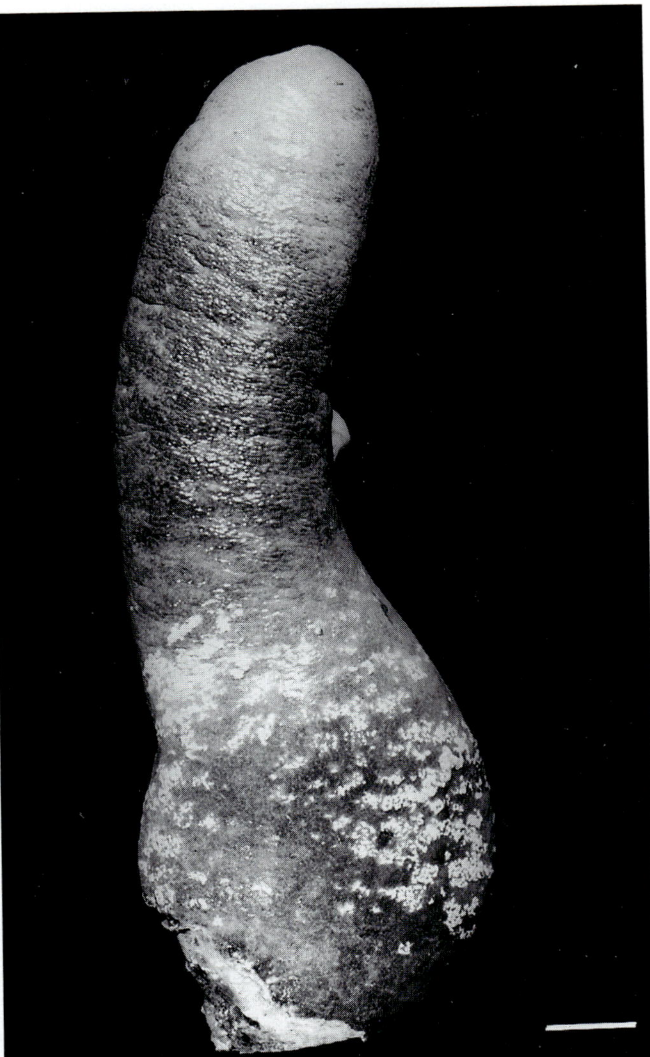

Fig. 7-52 Spleen; dog. Subcapsular siderocalcific nodules formed by deposits of iron and calcium. Bar = 2 cm. *Courtesy Dr. G.L. Mason.*

Rupture of the spleen is a frequent finding in the dog. The spleen may exist in two or more portions with various irregular fibrotic fissures reflecting trauma at some time in the animal's life.

The spleen is one of the organs that is usually involved in systemic AA amyloidosis. The amyloid deposits are initially found in the marginal zone surrounding the lymphoid follicles. In advanced cases, follicles are obliterated by the amyloid deposits. The enlarged follicles may be visible on gross examination of a cross section of the spleen as gray granules.

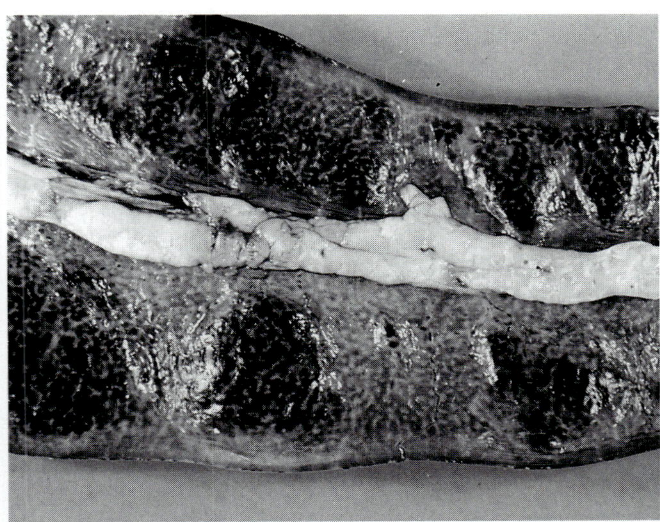

Fig. 7-53 Spleen; pig. Vasculitis. Note the presence of numerous infarcts. *Courtesy E.G. Clark.*

Circulatory Disorders of the Spleen

Congestion of the spleen is common; the enlarged organ has a tendency to bulge and ooze dark blood when incised. The most common cause is enthanasia with barbituates. Congestion also occurs in hemolytic anemias with retention of erythrocytes in the red pulp. Splenic infarction is visible as discrete, deeply congested areas with focal capsular distention (Fig. 7-53). Spleens enlarged for any reason are prone to thrombosis and infarction.

Torsion of the spleen occurs occasionally in the pig and dog, resulting in venous occlusion with marked congestion and enlargement. Torsion of the spleen may or may not accompany gastric torsion. Hemoglobinemia may occur due to intrasplenic erythrocyte lysis and leakage through the devitalized capsule. Erythrocytic charges such as acanthocytes and nuclear remnants are consistent with splenic diseases (see Table 7-1).

Splenic hematomas are common in dogs, but the cause is often not obvious at necropsy. Small hematomas must be differentiated from nodular hyperplasia and large ones from hemangiomas. The latter differentiation requires careful dissection and microscopic examination of tissue specimens.

Inflammatory Disorders of the Spleen

Splenitis as a localized entity is uncommon but may occur by extension of peritonitis, such as occurs in bovine traumatic reticuloperitonitis. The sequence of events following arrival of bacteria and viruses through terminal arterioles varies with the agent. With anthrax, the spleen is classically severely congested, whereas in less acute septicemias, reactive hyperplasia involves the lymphoid tissues of the white pulp and macrophages of the red pulp. The virus of equine infectious anemia, for example, stimulates marked macrophage proliferation, resulting in an enlarged, firm spleen.

Nodular Disorders of the Spleen

The presence of discrete nodules that tend to protrude from the cut surface of the spleen is indicative of benign nodular lymphoid hyperplasia (Fig. 7-54). It is most common in the dog but is seen in all species. The nodules may be up to 2 cm in diameter, and they vary from gray to red pink. The largest nodules may have yellow centers because of necrosis.

Neoplastic Disorders of the Spleen

The spleen is frequently the site of endothelial cell neoplasms, hemangiomas, and hemangiosarcomas. They occur frequently in older dogs of the large breeds and are prone to rupture with development of significant intraperitoneal hemorrhage. The presence of anemia with reticulocytosis in many of these dogs is indicative of bleeding from these tumors over a period of time.

Splenic involvement in bovine lymphosarcoma is variable, but a significant incidence occurs in both the enzootic and juvenile forms of the disease. A high incidence of splenic involvement occurs in canine, feline, and equine lymphosarcoma. In most cases, the organ is uniformly enlarged, and, microscopically, the normal white pulp follicles are displaced and the red pulp is occupied by neoplastic lymphocytes.

Granulocytic leukemia in the dog usually results in marked splenomegaly caused by infiltration and proliferation of neoplastic granulocytes. Plasma cell sarcomas in dogs and mast cell and erythrocytic sarcomas in cats may also involve the spleen. Splenic aspirates are more commonly attempted in dogs, cats, and horses and are a valuable adjunct to bone marrow aspirates for diagnosis of lymphosarcoma. In contrast to aspirates from normal spleens,

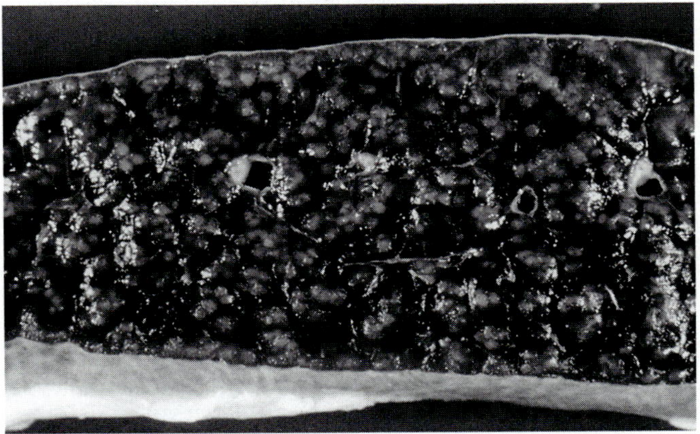

Fig. 7-54 Spleen; pig. Leptospirosis. Nodular hyperplasia. *Courtesy E.G. Clark.*

which have many erythrocytes, lymphocytes of varying age, and a few macrophages, the aspirates from neoplastically infiltrated spleens are dominated by a homogeneous population of sarcoma cells.

Acknowledgments

I wish to thank Ian Shirley and Barbara McCoy for preparation of photographs. The chapter "The Hematopoietic System" written by V.E.O. Valli in the fourth edition of the book, *Pathology of Domestic Animals,* edited by K.V.F. Jubb, Peter C. Kennedy, and Nigel Palmer, was an important source of information and is hereby acknowledged.

Suggested Readings

Abbas AK, Lichtman AH, Pober JS. Cellular and molecular immunology. Philadelphia: Saunders, 1991.

Beutler E. Hemolytic anemia due to chemical and physical agents. In: Williams WJ, Beutler E, Erslev AJ, Lichtman MA, eds. Hematology. 4th ed. New York: McGraw-Hill, 1990:660.

Blue J, Weiss L. Electron microscopy of the red pulp of the dog spleen including vascular arrangement, periarterial macrophage sheaths (ellipsoids), and the contractile, innervated reticular meshwork. Am J Anat 1981; 161:189-218.

Breitschwerdt EB. Babesiosis. In: Greene CE, ed. Infectious diseases of the dog and cat. Philadelphia: Saunders, 1990:796.

Breitschwerdt EB, Brown TT, DeBuysscher EV et al. Rhinitis, pneumonia, and defective neutrophil function in the Doberman pinscher. Am J Vet Res 1987; 48:1054-1062.

Capen CC. The endocrine glands. In: Jubb KVC, Kennedy PC, Palmer N, eds. Pathology of Domestic Animals. Vol 3, 4th ed. San Diego, Calif.: Academic Press 1993:267.

Christopher MM, White JG, Eaton JW. Erythrocyte pathology and mechanisms of Heinz body-mediated hemolysis in cats. Vet Pathol 1990; 27:299-310.

Erslev AJ. Anemia of chronic disorders. In: Williams WJ, Beutler E, Erslev AJ, Lichtman MA, eds. Hematology. 4th ed. New York: McGraw-Hill, 1990:540.

Fossum S, Ford WL. The organization of cell populations within lymph nodes: Their origin, life history, and functional relationships. Histopathology 1985; 9:469-499.

Franks PT, Harvey JW, Calderwood-Mays M et al. Feline large granular lymphoma. Vet Pathol 1986; 23:200-202.

Furie B. Disorders of the vitamin K–dependent coagulation factors. In: Williams WJ, Beutler E, Erslev AJ, Lichtman MA, eds. Hematology. 4th ed. New York: McGraw-Hill, 1990:1510.

George JN. Platelet immunoglobulin G: Its significance for the evaluation of thrombocytopenia and for understanding the origin of alpha-granule proteins. Blood 1990; 76:859-870.

Giger U, Boxer LA, Simpson PJ et al. Deficiency of surface glycoproteins Mo1, LFA-1, and Leu M5 in a dog with recurrent bacterial infections: An animal model. Blood 1987; 69:1622-1630.

Giger U, Harvey JW, Yamaguchi RA et al. Inherited phosphofructokinase deficiency in dogs with hyperventilation-induced hemolysis: Increased in vitro and in vivo alkaline fragility of erythrocytes. J Am Vet Med Assoc 1985; 65:345-351.

Green RA. Hemostatic disorders: Coagulopathies and thrombotic disorders. In: Ettinger SJ, ed. Textbook of Veterinary Internal Medicine: Diseases of the Dog and Cat. 3rd ed. Philadelphia: Saunders, 1989:2246.

Harvey JW. Haemobartonellosis. In: Greene CE, ed. Infectious Disease of the Dog and Cat. Philadelphia: Saunders, 1990:434.

Harvey JW. *Ehrlichia platys* infection. In: Greene CE, ed. Infectious Diseases of the Dog and Cat. Philadelphia: Saunders, 1990:415.

Janik J, Kier A, Ratnoff OD. Molecular analysis of Hageman factor deficiency in cats. Blood 1986; 68:347a (suppl 1).

Kaneko JJ. Porphyrins and the porphyrias. In: Kaneko JJ, ed. Clinical Biochemistry of Domestic Animals. 4th ed. San Diego, Calif.: Academic Press, 1989:235.

Kehrli ME, Schmalstieg FC, Anderson DC et al. Molecular definition of the bovine granulocytopathy syndrome: Identification of deficiency of the Mac-1 (CD11b/CD18) glycoprotein. Am J Vet Res 1990; 51:1826-1836.

Kier AB. Cytauxzoonosis. In: Greene CE, ed. Infectious Diseases of the Dog and Cat. Philadelphia: Saunders, 1990:792.

Johnson GS, Turrentine MA, Kraus KH. Canine von Willebrand's disease. In: Feldman BF, ed. Hemostasis, The Veterinary Clinics of North America. Philadelphia: Saunders, 1988; 18:195-229.

LaCelle PL. Destruction of erythrocytes. In: Williams WJ, Beutler E, Erslev AJ, Lichtman MA, eds. Hematology. 4th ed. New York: McGraw-Hill, 1990:398.

Latimer KS, Meyer DJ. Leukocytes in health and disease. In: Ettinger SJ, ed. Textbook of Veterinary Internal Medicine. 3rd ed. Philadelphia: Saunders, 1989:2181.

Leighton FA, Lee YZ, Rahimtula AD et al. Biochemical and functional disturbances in red blood cells of Herring gulls ingesting Prudhoe Bay crude oil. Toxicol App Pharmacol 1985; 81:25-31.

Losos GJ. Infectious tropical diseases of domestic animals. New York: Churchill Livingstone, 1986:3.

Mullins JI, Hoover EA. Molecular aspects of feline leukemia virus pathogenesis. In: Gallo RC, Wong-Staal F, eds. Retrovirus Biology and Human Disease. New York: Marcel Dekker, 1990:87.

Novotney C, English RV, Housman J et al. Lymphocyte population changes in cats naturally infected with feline immunodeficiency virus. AIDS 1990; 4:1213-1218.

Packam CH, Leddy JP. Acquired hemolytic anemia due to warm-reacting autoantibodies. In: Williams WJ, Beutler E, Erslev AJ, Lichtman MA, eds. Hematology. 4th ed. New York: McGraw-Hill, 1990:666.

Perryman LE. Comparative pathology of immune deficiency disorders. Comp Path Bull 1984; 16:1-3.

Rezanka LJ, Rojko JL, Neil JC. Feline leukemia virus: Pathogenesis of neoplastic disease. Cancer Invest 1992; 10:371-389.

Roberts HR, Lozier JN. New perspectives on the coagulation cascade. Hosp Pract 1992; 27:97-112.

Sandeson GJ. Interleukin-5, eosinophils and disease. Blood 1192; 79:3101-3109.

Schoonderwoerd M, Doige CE, Wobeser GA, Naylor JM. Protein energy malnutrition and fat metabolism in neonatal calves. Can Vet J 1986; 27:365-371.

Slappendel RJ, Greene CE. Leishmaniasis. In: Greene CE, ed. Infectious Diseases of the Dog and Cat. Philadelphia: Saunders, 1990:769.

Stockam SL, Tyler JW, Schmidt DA et al. Experimental transmission of granulocytic erhlichial organisms in dogs. Vet Clin Pathol 1990; 19:99-104.

Tablin F, Weiss L. The equine spleen: An electron microscopic analysis. Am J Anat 1983; 166:393-416.

Tamatani T, Kotani M, Tanaka T et al. Molecular mechanisms underlying lymphocyte recirculation. II. Differential regulation of LFA-1 in the interaction between lymphocytes and high endothelial cells. Eur J Immunol 1991; 21:855-858.

Theilen GH, Madewell BR, Gardner MB. Hematopoietic neoplasms, sarcomas and related conditions. In: Theilen GH, Madewell BR. Veterinary Cancer Medicine. Philadelphia: Lea & Febiger, 1987:345.

Thompson AR. Structure, function, and molecular defects of factor IX. Blood 1986; 67:565-572.

Troy GC, Forrester SD. Canine ehrlichiosis. In: Greene CE, ed. Infectious Diseases of the Dog and Cat. Philadelphia: Saunders, 1990:404.

Valli VEO. The hematopoietic system. In: Jubb KVF, Kennedy PC, Palmer N, eds. Pathology of Domestic Animals. Vol 3, 4th ed. San Diego, Calif.: Academic Press, 1993:101.

van Furth R. Origin and turnover of monocytes and macrophages. In: Iverson OH, ed. Current Topics in Pathology: Cell Kinetics of the Inflammatory Reaction. Berlin: Springer-Verlag, 1989:125-150.

Wang XL, Gallagher CH, McLure TJ et al. Bovine postparturient haemoglobinuria: Effect of inorganic phosphate on red cell metabolism. Res Vet Sci 1985; 39:333-339.

Weiser MG. Erythrocytes and associated disorders. In: Ettinger SJ, ed. Textbook of Veterinary Internal Medicine. 3rd ed. Philadelphia: Saunders, 1989:2145.

Weiss DJ, McClay CB. Studies on the pathogenesis of the erythrocyte destruction associated with the anemia of inflammatory disease. Vet Clin Pathol 1988; 17:90-93.

Weiss DJ, Stockham SL, Willard MD et al. Transient erythroid suppression in the dog: Report of five cases. J Am Anim Hosp Assoc 1982; 18:353-359.

Weiss L. The spleen. In: Weiss L. The Blood Cells and Hematopoietic Tissues. 2nd ed. New York: Elsevier, 1984:544.

Wolf AM. Histoplasmosis. In: Greene CE, ed. Infectious Diseases of the Dog and Cat. Philadelphia: Saunders 1990:679.

CHAPTER

8

Central Nervous System

RALPH W. STORTS

STRUCTURE AND FUNCTION

The central nervous system (CNS) consists of a parenchyma containing neurons, oligodendroglia, astrocytes, microglia, and blood vessels. Neurons are the major component responsible for the transmission of nervous impulses. The first four cellular components have multiple processes that form a very complex tissue network referred to as the neuropil. In hemaloxylin-eosin (H & E)–stained sections, this appears as an eosinophilic meshwork. The different components vary in their susceptibility to injury (e.g., ischemia), with neurons being the most sensitive. Glial cells that survive (particularly astrocytes and microglia) often react to injury by an increase in size and/or number. Because the response of the neuron to injury is frequently death (necrosis) followed by its disappearance, in chronic diseases the response of the glia to injury may be more obvious histologically than changes involving the neurons.

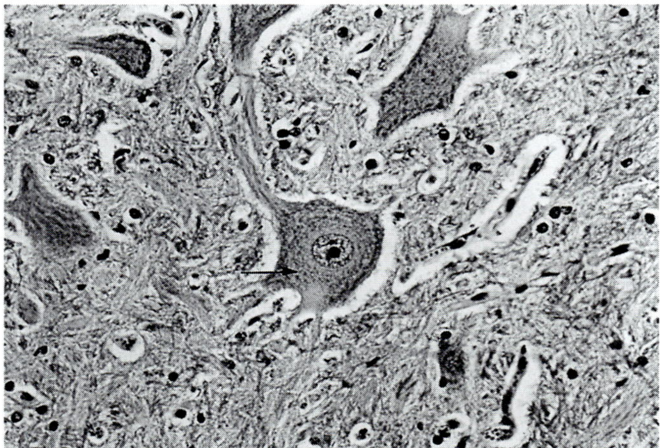

Fig. 8-1 Spinal cord, ventral horn; dog. Normal animal. This normal motor neuron *(center)* has a centrally positioned nucleus and contains cytoplasmic Nissl substance *(arrow).* Hematoxylin-eosin (H & E) stain.

Neurons

Neuronal cell bodies vary considerably in size and shape, from very small, lymphocyte-like granule cells of the cerebellar cortex to the large neurons of the lateral vestibular nucleus and ventral gray matter of the spinal cord. Their nuclei tend to be vesicular to spherical, are centrally located, and, often, particularly in large neurons, contain a prominent central nucleolus. Nissl substance (focal arrays of rough endoplasmic reticulum and polysomes) is also a characteristic feature (Figs. 8-1 and 8-2) and is responsible for the production of proteins involved in many vital processes, including development of cytoskeletal components that are involved in axoplasmic transport (flow of axoplasm along axons) and regeneration of peripheral nerves.

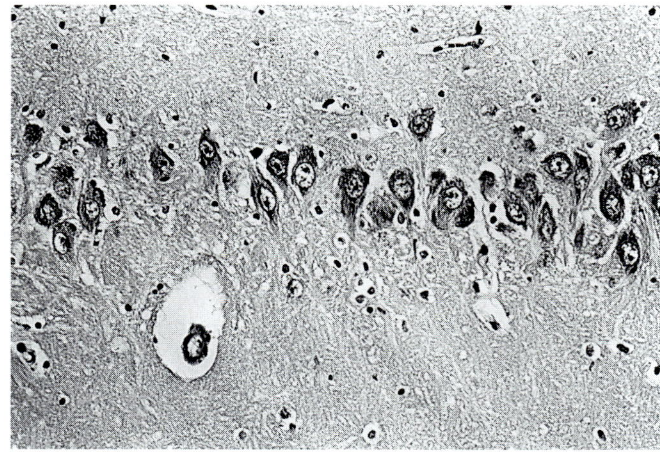

Fig. 8-2 Hippocampus, pyramidal neurons; normal dog. The pyramidal neurons are normal, are smaller, and have less prominent Nissl substance than the motor neurons depicted in Fig. 8-1. H & E stain.

Reaction to injury

The appearance of the neuronal cell body can vary according to the injury. For example, characteristic changes are associated with axonal injury (central chromatolysis), ischemia (ischemic cell change), lysosomal enzyme deficiencies (enlargement of the cell body due to alteration of lysosomes), aging (accumulation of lipofuscin pigment), certain neuronal degenerative diseases (excess accumulation of neurofilaments), certain viral infections (intranuclear and/or intracytoplasmic inclusion body formation, the latter being typical of Negri body formation in rabies), and prominent cytoplasmic vacuolation (caused by the etiologic agents of spongiform encephalopathies such as scrapie).

Response of neurons following injury to their axons that extend to the periphery. This lesion occurs in lower motor neurons of the brain and spinal cord that have cell bodies in the CNS (e.g., neurons of cranial and ventral spinal motor nerves) and axons that extend exteriorly in peripheral nerves, as well as in cell bodies of neurons in the cerebrospinal ganglia that also have peripherally extending processes. Following axonal injury (e.g., crush or transection), the change that occurs in the cell body is referred to as *central chromatolysis* or the *axonal reaction.* The extent to which central chromatolysis develops is related to the degree and location of axonal injury. It is more prominent, and may even be followed by neuronal death, the more severe the axonal injury and the closer to the cell body that it occurs. The time required for recovery of cell bodies can be several months and, in most cases, will vary from 3 to 6 months, depending on the severity of the axonal injury.

Microscopically, central chromatolysis is characterized by swelling of the neuronal cell body, dispersion of central Nissl substance, and peripheral displacement of the nucleus (Fig. 8-3; see Figs. 8-36 and 8-46). It may begin within 24 to 48 hours and reach its maximum in about 18 days following axonal injury. The change in the axon distal to the point of injury, which is referred to as **Wallerian degeneration,** is first evident within 24 hours of injury. Wallerian degeneration is initially characterized by irregular swelling of the axon that is followed (after 48 to 72 hours) by fragmentation along its length. This is followed by degeneration, and, usually, there is no evidence of the axon remaining by the second week postinjury. Changes in the myelin sheath surrounding myelinated axons are evident by 28 to 96 hours after injury, when axonal disintegration is well advanced. Initially, there are irregularities in the sheath, accompanied by folding, lamellar splitting, fracturing, and fragmentation. The fragmented components of the sheath form droplets (termed ellipsoids) that surround and enclose isolated fragments and debris of the former axon. Both axonal and myelin debris are then removed by phagocytosis. Degeneration of myelin is usually completed by the end of the second week, although evidence of myelin debris may be detectable for as long as 3 months following axonal injury.

If the neuronal cell body survives the injury to its axon, regeneration from the proximal stump can occur. The degree of axonal regeneration depends on the status of the endoneurial tube distal to the original point of axonal injury. The normal endoneurial tube and its contents consist (from the outside inward) of (1) a connective tissue investment referred to as the endoneurium, (2) the basement membrane that surrounds the Schwann cell, (3) the myelin sheath of myelinated axons, and (4) the axon. Approximately 24 to 72 hours following axonal injury, the endoneurial tube contains degenerating remnants of the previously existing axon, along with Schwann cells that begin to proliferate and eventually form a longitudinal column of cells referred to as the bands of Büngner. If the endoneurial tube remains intact, as can occur following compression injury to a peripheral nerve, a regenerating sprout from the proximal axonal stump can enter the endoneurial tube and regenerate uninterruptedly along its original pathway to the periphery, where it can reestablish innervation with an end organ (e.g., skeletal muscle). Such axons can also become remyelinated and regain their physiologic function of impulse transmission. Although the rate of axonal regeneration is not uniform along the length of the regenerating axon (the rate being slower the greater the distance the growing tip is from the cell body), it can range from 1-4 mm per day. If the integrity of the endoneurial tube is destroyed, as would occur following complete severance of a peripheral nerve, the proximal axonal stump may not reach the distal endoneurial tube because of fibrous connective tissue proliferation (scar formation) at the site of axonal severance, and regeneration with reestablishment of peripheral innervation may not occur.

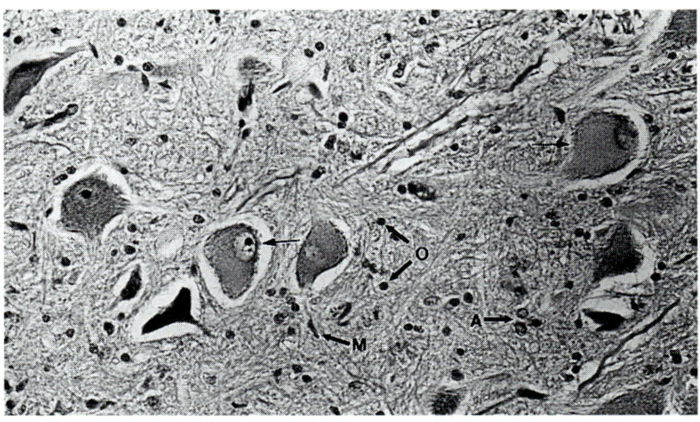

Fig. 8-3 Neurons, facial nucleus; dog. Central chromatolysis. Compare with Fig. 8-1. Three cells have eccentric nuclei *(arrows);* neurons in the center and to the right have pale central cytoplasm. The cell body of the neuron to the right is also swollen. Note the normal astrocytic (*A*), oligodendroglial (*O*), and microglial (*M*) nuclei. H & E stain.

Response of neurons following injury to their axons that remain within the CNS. The response of the cell body following injury of axons that remain within the CNS may vary. Some cell bodies may have central chromatolysis; others

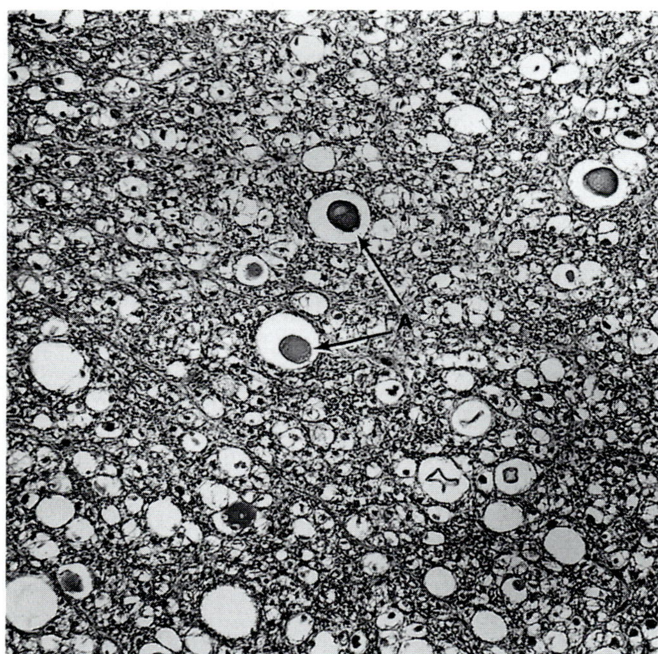

Fig. 8-4 Spinal cord, lumbar; cow with posterior paralysis for 2 days secondary to trauma. Wallerian degeneration of axons in the white matter. Several axons (*A*) are markedly swollen and their myelin sheaths are distended. Empty spaces may indicate absence of axons that have separated at the plane of section. H & E stain.

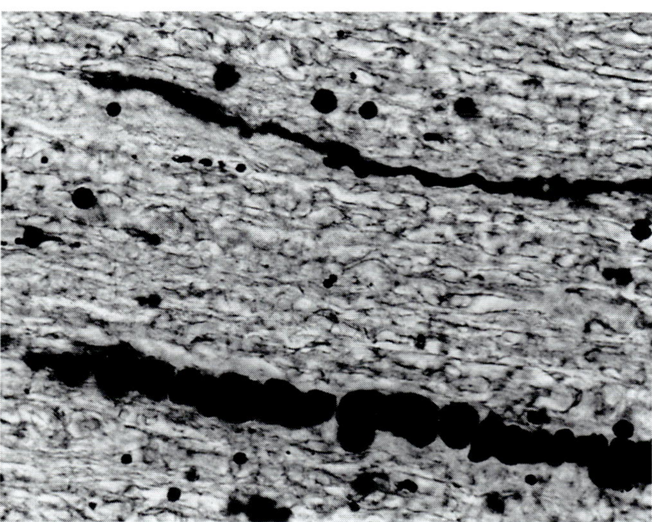

Fig. 8-5 Spinal cord, white matter; cow. Wallerian degeneration. Two myelinated axons are degenerated. The top one is minimally enlarged while the lower axon is markedly swollen and undergoing fragmentation. Marchi method for degenerating myelin. *Courtesy Dr. M.D. McGavin.*

initially have central chromatolysis followed by atrophy and eventual disappearance; and others may just undergo atrophy. Infrequently, central chromatolysis can result from causes other than specific axonal injury (e.g., with avian encephalomyelitis picornaviral infection in the young chicken and dietary niacin deficiency in human beings). Wallerian degeneration within the CNS is similar to that described above for the peripheral nervous system (PNS), except that in the CNS degenerated axons and myelin sheaths may remain for a longer period (e.g., months) before complete removal.

Affected axons and their myelin sheaths undergo a rather characteristic series of changes as they degenerate. Initially, axons form linear and bulbous swellings at, and some distance from, the site of injury (Figs. 8-4 and 8-5). The axonal enlargements can be seen as early as a few hours, especially, at the site of injury, and remain prominent, particularly for the first week or so. The surrounding myelin sheath is usually distended to create a space between the sheath and the axonal swelling (Fig. 8-4). Progressively, such affected axons and myelin sheaths fragment along their length (Fig. 8-5) and form **ellipsoids,** as in the PNS, and eventually are removed through degeneration and phagocytosis, leaving an empty space or one containing myelin debris and/or macrophages. With continued degeneration, most of the lesion will consist of enlarged empty spaces. It should be noted that the absence of swollen axons from such dilated spaces, especially in the early stages following CNS trauma, does not necessarily mean that the entire axon has degenerated and been removed, which may require several months. It may instead represent an area where an enlargement may have separated from the adjacent axon at the level of the section being examined.

Ischemic neuronal injury

Neurons are dependent on a continuous supply of oxygen to remain viable, and, if the supply is interrupted, the most susceptible neurons will degenerate within several minutes. Ischemic neuron injury (also referred to as ischemic cell change) occurs following ischemia, resulting from either obstruction of blood flow or reduction in the available oxygen in the blood and other disturbances (e.g., certain metabolic disorders associated with nutritional deficiency and toxicity that ultimately also interfere with oxygen utilization). In H & E-stained sections, the cell body is shrunken. The cytoplasm stains lightly eosinophilic and has microvacuolation due to swollen mitochondria. The nucleus is reduced in size, often is triangular, and is pyknotic (stains dark blue). The nucleolus may not be detectable. Unstained perineuronal and perivascular spaces are prominent because of swelling of astrocytic processes (Fig. 8-6). For a review of the specific causes and mechanisms involved in ischemic cell change, see the section on Infarction.

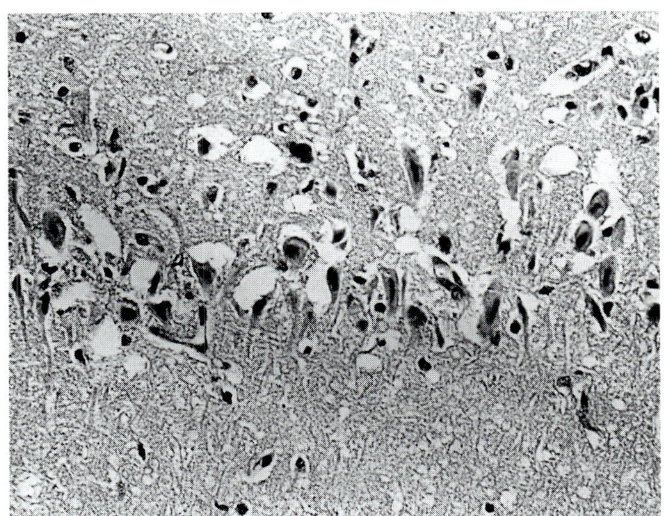

Fig. 8-6 Hippocampus, pyramidal neurons; dog. Cerebral ischemia caused by cardiac arrest. Compare with Fig. 8-2. The hippocampal pyramidal neurons have shrunken cell bodies and dark, shrunken nuclei typical of ischemic cell change. The pericellular space is prominent due, in part, to swelling of astroglial processes. H & E stain.

Astrocytes

Traditionally, astrocytes have been classified, based on morphology, into two main types: fibrous astrocytes located primarily in white matter and protoplasmic astrocytes chiefly present in the gray matter. A more recent classification, based on cell marker and functional studies, has resulted in the designation of type 1 and type 2 astrocytes.

The function of astrocytes in the normal and diseased CNS has only recently received the recognition that it deserves. Astrocytes have several known anatomic features and functions, including (1) forming the innermost subpial covering of the brain and spinal cord **(glia limitans),** (2) being variably prominent in the subependymal area, (3) having processes **(foot processes)** that terminate on vessels within the CNS, (4) participating in the development of the blood-brain barrier, (5) insulating synaptic contacts on the surface of neurons (cell body and dendrites) from each other, (6) providing a structural guide that enables neurons to migrate to their final destination during embryogenesis, and (7) having certain biochemical functions (neurotransmitter regulation, detoxification of ammonia, and regulation of potassium concentration associated with neuronal impulse transmission). Astrocytes are also becoming recognized as important mediators of cell regulation, including immune function and ability to secrete substances (e.g., tumor necrosis factor) that can affect other cells (e.g., cause death of oligodendroglia).

Microscopically, astrocytes have relatively large, pale-staining nuclei, poorly visible nucleoli, and cytoplasm that are usually undetectable with conventional (H & E) staining (see Fig. 8-3). Following special metallic impregnation (with silver or gold) or treatment with monoclonal antibody for glial fibrillary acidic protein (GFAP), the cytoplasm and processes can be seen.

Reaction to injury

Astrocytes react following many and varied types of injury to the CNS. After severe injury, astrocytes swell, lose their processes, and degenerate. When conditions are unfavorable, but less severe, astrocytic nuclei and cell bodies increase in size and number (astrocytosis) without losing processes. Under moderately unfavorable conditions, there is a variable degree of hypertrophy of cell bodies and processes. The cytoplasm is homogeneously pink (H & E staining), the nucleus often is enlarged and eccentric, and the cell outline, in contrast to that of normal astrocytes, is

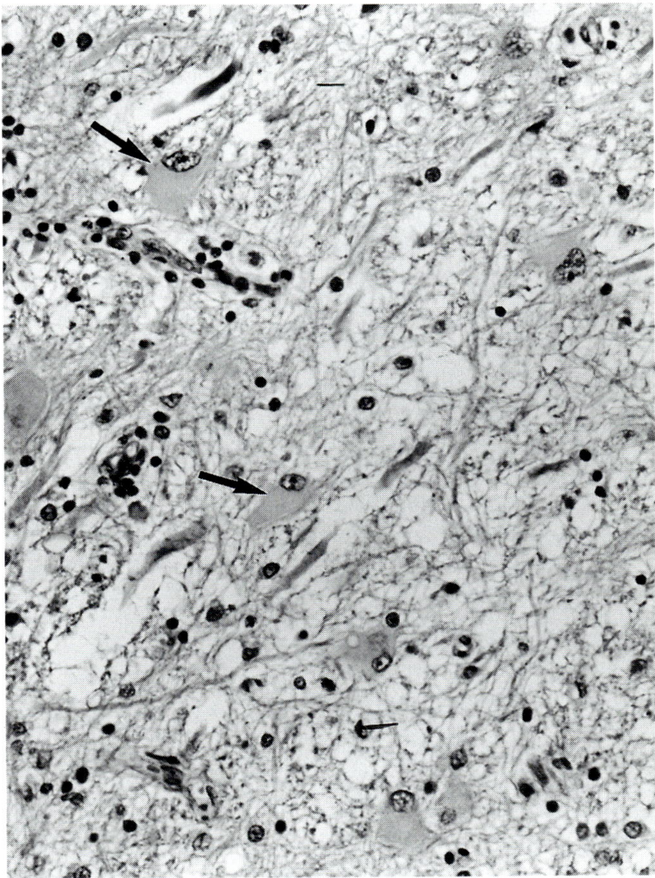

Fig. 8-7 Cerebellum, deep cerebellar white matter; cat. Focal chronic lesion secondary to unilateral inner ear infection. Note the prominent gemistocytic astrocytes *(arrows)* with eccentric nuclei, homogeneous cytoplasm, and extended processes that have developed in the lesion. Holzer's stain.

rather clearly defined in H & E-stained sections. These cells are referred to as **gemistocytes** (Fig. 8-7), which have an increased accumulation of intermediate filaments and an increased synthesis of GFAP, the major glial intermediate filament protein (As-1). With return to favorable conditions, the cell body gradually decreases in size, but the prominent, dense accumulation of astrocytic processes (astrogliosis) remains. When mildly unfavorable conditions exist for some time, the cell body may continue to enlarge to 25 μm or more in diameter and eventually undergoes degeneration.

Oligodendroglia

Normal

Oligodendroglia are located in both the white and gray matter of the CNS. They are prominent in the white matter, where they tend to be aligned in rows parallel to myelinated axons. These oligodendroglia (termed **interfascicular** oligodendroglia) are responsible for the formation and maintenance of the myelin sheaths. Oligodendroglia also occur around neuronal cell bodies (where their accumulation is referred to as *satellitosis*) and around vessels. The mature, small oligodendrocyte has a spherical, hyperchromatic nucleus similar to that of a lymphocyte. As with astrocytes, the cell body and processes of this cell do not stain with conventional (H & E) staining methods (see Fig. 8-3) and can only be demonstrated following special procedures that include metallic (silver) impregnation.

Reaction to injury

Reaction to injury includes degeneration and proliferation. Degeneration of oligodendroglia, which can have several causes (including ischemia, infection by certain viruses, and certain immunologic processes), can result in rather selective degeneration of periaxonal myelin sheaths (**primary demyelination**). Oligodendroglia can also proliferate in response to noncytocidal injury. The significance that oligodendroglia have as perineuronal cells (satellitosis) and the extent to which these cells respond to neuronal injury has not been clarified.

Microglia

Normal

In the mature CNS, microglia are predominantly located at perineuronal, perivascular, and interfascicular sites, with some variation in their size and shape in different regions. They also are present in greater numbers in the gray rather than the white matter. Normally, only the nuclei of this cell can be seen in H & E-stained preparations. Nuclei are hyperchromatic and shaped as small rods, ovoids, or commas, as seen in H & E-stained sections (see Fig. 8-3). With special silver impregnation or specific labeling procedures, a small amount of cytoplasm and several delicate processes can be seen. The cells (nuclei) are smaller than astrocytes, and their nuclear shape distinguishes them from oligodendrocytes.

The precise nature of microglia has been controversial. Recent experimental studies, using specific cell surface markers and sensitive immunochemical methods, have demonstrated that monocytes enter the CNS during the late embryonic and early postnatal periods and differentiate into resident microglia, which have been identified as macrophages. In addition to the resident microglia, macrophages with a different phenotype (and possibly a different function) are also associated with the CNS but exist outside the parenchyma (e.g., in the leptomeninges and choroid plexus). Possible functions of macrophages (including resident microglia) within the CNS include their playing a role in development and remodeling (e.g., direct and opsonin-mediated phagocytosis of cells that normally degenerate during embryogenesis), homeostasis (e.g., neurotransmitter and hormone processing and catabolism), lipid turnover, inflammation and repair (e.g., release of mediators, neutral proteinases, cytotoxic agents, growth factors), and immune functions (e.g., antigen processing, macrophage activation).

Reaction to injury

Following injury to the CNS, there is often a parenchymal accumulation of mononuclear cells (commonly referred to as "microglia," based on their general morphology) that may represent an influx of monocytes from the circulation or an increase in the resident microglial population. Other cells, including neutrophils, lymphocytes, and plasma cells, may also be present, depending on the type of injury. Microglia, conceivably either from hematogenous or of resident CNS tissue origin, may accumulate focally as **glial nodules** or diffusely (diffuse microgliosis) and commonly have typical rod-, oval-, or comma-shaped nuclei. When tissue necrosis occurs, such cells often phagocytose the debris and develop into characteristic lipid-laden macrophages referred to as "gitter cells" (see Fig. 8-20). The extent to which accumulation of mononuclear cells in the CNS involves resident microglia is not clear, although evidence has been advanced to support the fact that they can proliferate. Macrophages that accumulate in response to many injuries that cause inflammation are likely to be monocytes that have migrated into the CNS from the blood.

ANOMALIES AND MALFORMATIONS

General Anomalies

Anencephaly

Anencephaly literally refers to an absence of the brain, but, in many instances, the rostral part of the brain (cerebral hemispheres) is absent or very rudimentary, and, to varying degrees, the brain stem is preserved. Thus, this abnormality is best designated as **prosencephalic hypoplasia** (Fig. 8-8).

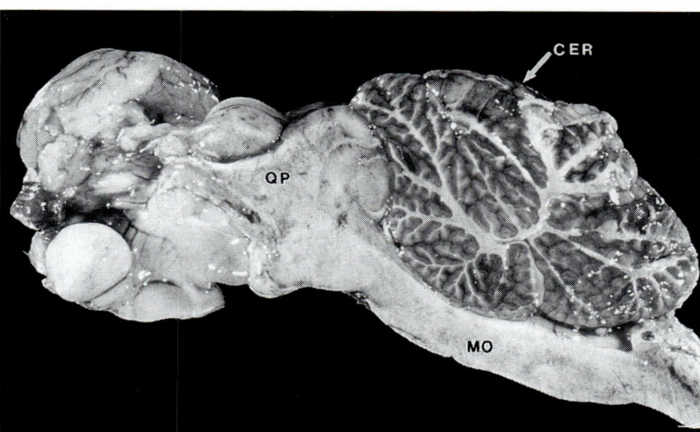

Fig. 8-8 Brain, markedly underdeveloped cerebral hemispheres; quadrigeminal plate (tectum) *(QP),* cerebellum *(CER),* and medulla oblongata *(MO);* calf. Prosencephalic hypoplasia. Only the caudal components of the brain are clearly recognizable.

Such anomalies result from an abnormal development of the rostral aspect of the neural tube.

Hydrocephalus

Hydrocephalus typically refers to an increased accumulation of cerebrospinal fluid (CSF) either solely within the ventricular system (noncommunicating form) or within both the ventricular system and the subarachnoid space (communicating form) due to obstruction. Obstruction within the ventricular system at or rostral to the lateral apertures of the fourth ventricle results in noncommunicating hydrocephalus. An area of particular vulnerability for obstruction is the mesencephalic aqueduct (Fig. 8-9). When congenital, this type of hydrocephalus may be associated with an enlargement (doming) of the cranium caused by separation of the sutures prior to their fusion, and the enlarged head may cause dystocia. Hydrocephalus of this type has a predisposition for certain breeds of dogs, being most common in toy breeds and brachycephalic dogs. Acquired noncommunicating hydrocephalus may be associated with obstruction of any of the following: the lateral apertures of the fourth ventricle, the aqueduct, or the interventricular foramen. Causes of obstruction include inflammation, neoplasia, and, uncommonly, the occurrence of cholesteatomas in the choroid plexus of the horse (Fig. 8-10).

Communicating hydrocephalus is the less common of the two forms. It results from an obstruction preventing outflow of CSF into the venous system and can occur following inflammatory or neoplastic involvement of the subarachnoid space, which interferes with the outflow of CSF through the arachnoid villi.

In a third type of hydrocephalus, referred to as **hydrocephalus ex vacuo,** the increase in size of the lateral ventricles is secondary to absence or loss of cerebral tissue. This type of hydrocephalus can occur any time there is lack of development or destruction and loss of cerebral tissue surrounding the lateral ventricles. Examples include certain anomalies (hydranencephaly) (see Fig. 8-12) and neurodegenerative diseases (e.g., ceroid-lipofuscinosis, a lysosomal storage disease of sheep) and aging of the CNS that are both associated with cerebral atrophy.

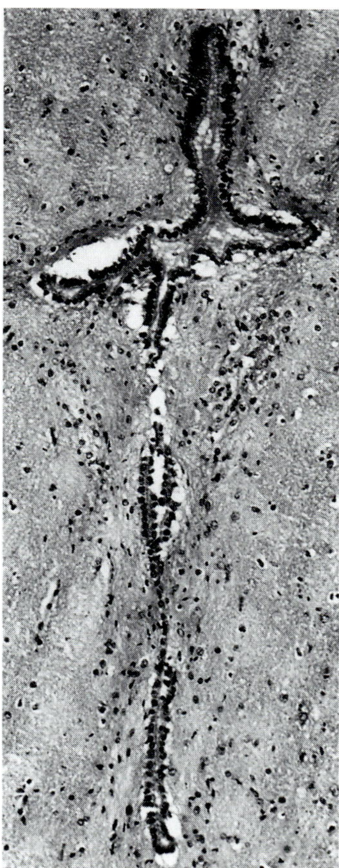

Fig. 8-9 Brain, mesencephalon; young cat. Stenotic mesencephalic aqueduct causing hydrocephalus. Undetermined cause. Note the stenosis and discontinuity of the mesencephalic aqueduct. H & E stain.

Lesions associated with either of the first two forms of hydrocephalus, but particularly the noncommunicating form, include prominent enlargement of the ventricular system proximal to the point of obstruction (Fig. 8-11). White matter adjacent to the dilated lateral ventricles is reduced in thickness, although the gray matter may retain a relatively normal appearance. The ependyma is generally not markedly affected but may be focally discontinuous. Other lesions include atrophy with fenestration of the interventricular septum (septum pellucidum), atrophy of the hippocampus in the floor of the lateral ventricles, flattening

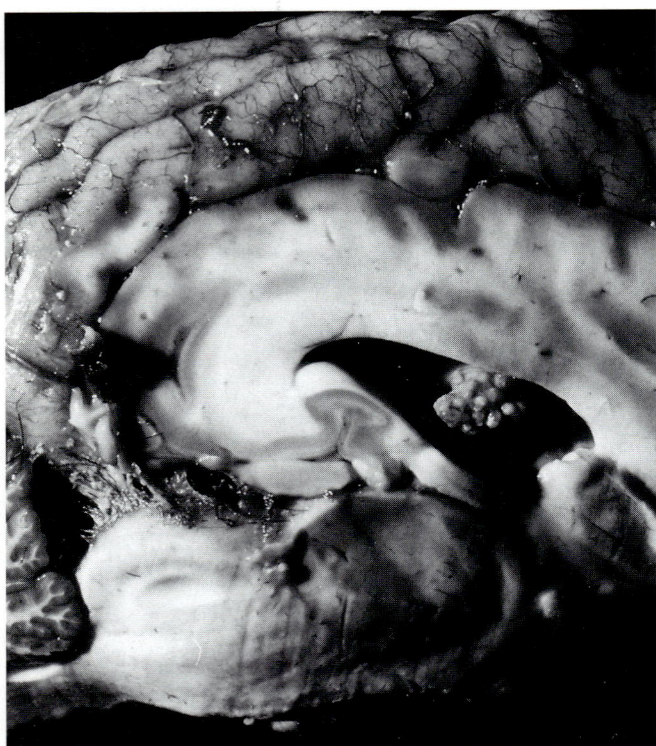

Fig. 8-10 Brain, left lateral ventricle; horse. Cholesteatoma of choroid plexus. A cholesteatoma consists of firm nodules with cholesterol crystals and granulomatous inflammatory tissue. *Courtesy Dr. M.D. McGavin.*

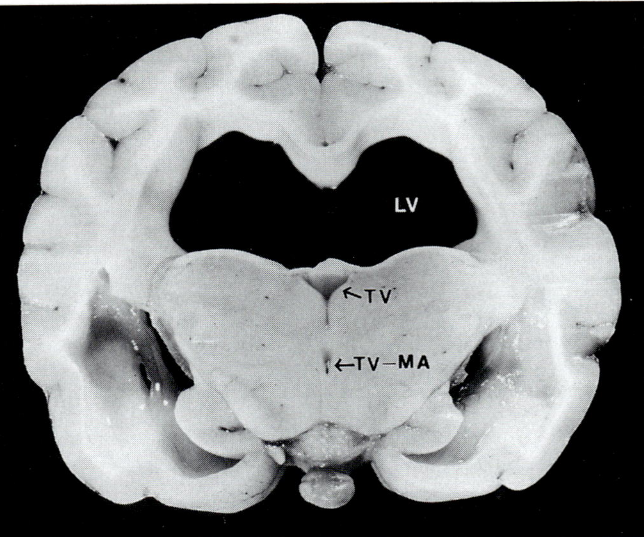

Fig. 8-11 Brain, junction between parietal and occipital lobes, level of thalamus; dog. Hydrocephalus. Bilateral dilatation of lateral ventricles, dorsally *(LV)* and ventrolaterally. The fornix has separated and now lies on the flattened floor of the ventricle. Note that the third ventricle *(TV)* and junctional area between the third ventricle and mesencephalic aqueduct *(TV-MA)* are not markedly enlarged, suggesting that the obstruction may be rostral to this plane of section.

of surface gyri, and posterior positioning of the brain with herniation of the cerebellum through the foramen magnum, resulting in a coning effect that may be accompanied by necrosis caused by circulatory obstruction.

Hydranencephaly

Hydranencephaly, unlike hydrocephalus, is characterized by a cavitation in the area normally occupied by the white matter of the cerebral hemispheres and results from lack of proper development of this part of the cerebrum (Fig. 8-12). Because of the lack of resistance, the ventricles may expand into this space, and the ependymal lining may remain relatively preserved or be variably defective. The cranium and meninges are generally unaltered. The several causes of this lesion include fetal viral infection (e.g., Akabane viral infection in calves and bluetongue and border disease viral infections in lambs) and nutritional copper deficiency (affecting the ovine fetus in utero) that result in destruction of immature progenitor cells whose loss prevents normal development. Another term, **porencephaly,** originally referred to a cyst that extended from the surface of the cerebrum to the ventricle, but, more recently, the term has been used less specifically and can indicate almost any cyst that occurs in the newborn brain.

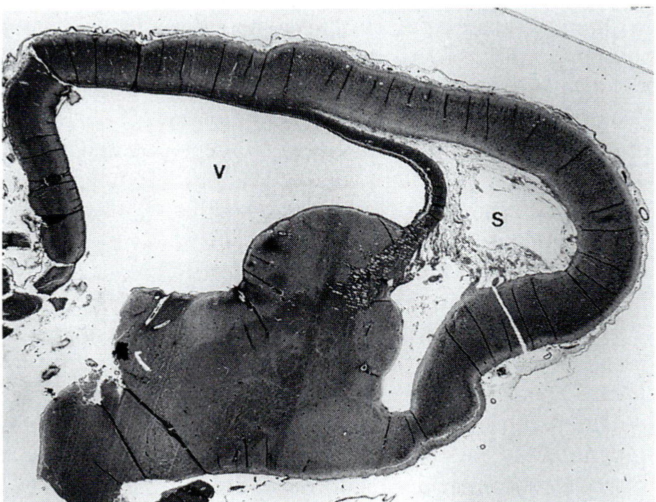

Fig. 8-12 Brain (transverse section), junction between parietal and frontal lobes, level of corpus striatum; lamb infected in utero with Cache valley bunyavirus. Hydranencephaly. A prominent space (*S*) has replaced the central part of the cerebral parenchyma. The lateral ventricle (*V*) is enlarged due to expansion (hydrocephalus ex vacuo). H & E stain. *Courtesy Dr. J.F. Edwards.*

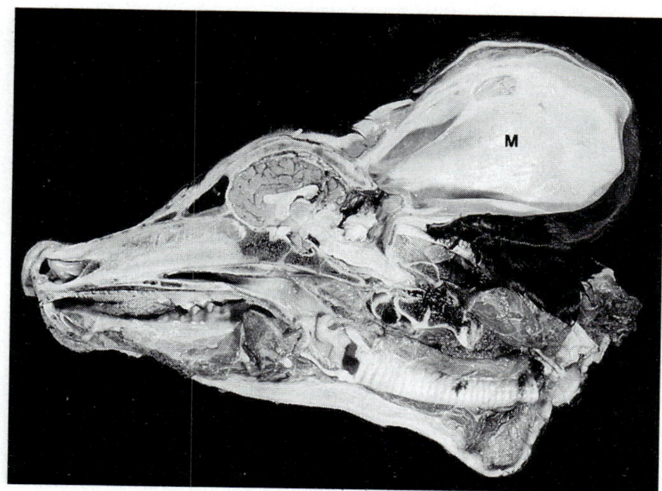

Fig. 8-13 Brain, cranium bifidum; calf. Meningocele (*M*). A defect in the caudal skull has resulted in continuity between the cranial cavity and a large external pouch covered by skin. The pouch is lined by meninges that are continuous with those of the brain.

Cranium bifidum

Cranium bifidum is characterized by a midline cranial defect through which meningeal and brain tissue may protrude. The protruded material, which forms a sac (-cele), is covered by skin and may be lined by meninges (meningocele) (Fig. 8-13) or meninges accompanied by a part of the brain (meningoencephalocele).

Spina bifida

Spina bifida is the spinal counterpart of cranium bifidum. This lesion, which frequently tends to affect the caudal spine, is characterized by a defect in the dorsal spinal column, through which there may be no herniation of the meninges or spinal cord (spina bifida occulta) or herniation of either meninges (meningocele) or meninges and spinal cord (meningomyelocele) into a sac covered with skin. The lesion has been detected in several species, including horses, calves, sheep, dogs (especially the English bulldog), and cats (particularly the Manx breed).

Syringomyelia

Syringomyelia is defined as a tubular cavitation (syrinx) in the spinal cord, separate from the central canal, that is not lined by ependyma and may extend over several segments. The lesion is well known in human beings and has also been described in the dog (weimaraner breed). The syrinx may communicate with the central canal, but should not be confused with hydromyelia, which means dilatation of the central canal. The lesion may extend rostrally and affect the medulla (syringobulbia) and pons (syringopontia) in the human being. The cavity can contain fluid and is unlined, except for varying degrees of mural astrocytosis, which is usually very mild in the weimaraner dog. Proposed causes include presence of an anomalous vascular pattern that results in a low-grade ischemia, as well as trauma, infection, and neoplasia that can lead to parenchymal degeneration and cavitation.

Dysraphic anomalies

Dysraphia literally means an abnormal seam and usually refers to a defective closure of the neural tube during development. This defect, which may occur at any point along the tube, is exemplified by anencephaly and prosencephalic hypoplasia, cranium bifidum, and spina bifida.

Lesions resulting from viral infection of the fetus

Viruses can affect the fetus directly or indirectly (i.e., only the dam or the placenta is infected, and fetal lesions occur secondarily). Direct infection can induce malformation by affecting organogenesis in the developing embryo, immature cells of the fetus, or differentiated cells of the fetus.

Viral effect on organogenesis. Two examples of this type of viral teratology include microencephaly (abnormally small brain) and myeloschisis (proposed to result from failure of the neural tube to close or rupture of a preformed neural tube) caused by influenza viral infection and myeloschisis caused by Newcastle disease viral infection, both in young chicken embryos.

Viral effect on immature cells. Lesions due to **parvoviral infection** have been detected in the rat, hamster, cat, and ferret (rat virus); cat and ferret (feline infectious enteritis virus); and mouse (minute virus). Grossly, there is reduction in size of the cerebellum that varies in severity, depending on the age when the host (e.g., fetus or neonate) is infected. The viruses involved have an affinity for and destroy cells undergoing mitosis (mitocidal virus), and, therefore, the lesions that occur depend on the developmental stage of the brain at the time of infection. The viruses primarily infect cells of the external granular layer of the cerebellum (e.g., in the cat) that are still dividing during the late gestational and early neonatal periods. Necrosis of these cells prevents their normal migration to form the internal granular layer. In addition to the loss of the external granular layer, there is degeneration and loss of Purkinje cells that are postmitotic, but immature (see Fig. 8-43 for a similar lesion). The Purkinje cells may also be malpositioned. Reasons for degeneration of Purkinje cells might include infection by the virus and/or lack of normal development of the cerebellar cortex.

Congenital defects in neonatal calves can result from fetal infection with **bovine virus diarrhea** virus (a pestivirus). The primary lesion is a cerebellar hypoplasia-atrophy (Fig. 8-14), but other lesions of the CNS also can occur, including porencephaly, hydranencephaly (associated with early inflammation), and dysmyelination (see Disorders of Myelin Formation and Maintenance). The type of

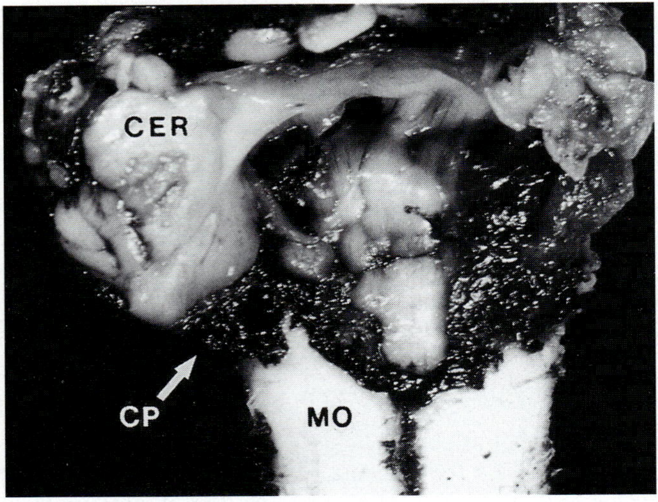

Fig. 8-14 Brain, cerebellum and medulla oblongata; calf. Cerebellar hypoplasia-atrophy resulting from bovine virus diarrhea viral infection. Cerebellar hypoplasia-atrophy. Only a remnant of the cerebellum *(CER)* is present. Note the choroid plexus *(CP)* of the fourth ventricle, and medulla oblongata *(MO)*.

lesion depends on the age of the fetus (and, therefore, the stage of CNS development) at the time of infection. Early retinal inflammation followed by degeneration can also occur when fetuses are infected in utero. The cerebellar lesion, which follows infection at 150 days of gestation (midtrimester), is considered to involve two processes. One is early necrosis of the undifferentiated cells in the external granular layer; the second is marked edema of the folial white matter with focal hemorrhage in the cortex, followed by focal cavitation of the white matter and atrophy, all being due to vascular impairment resulting from vasculitis. Leptomeningitis, characterized by accumulation of lymphocytes and plasma cells and occasional fibroplasia, causes adhesions between adjacent cerebellar folia and focal obliteration of the subarachnoid space.

Hog cholera (swine fever) virus, also a pestivirus, can be teratogenic in the porcine fetus. The best-known neural defects resulting from fetal infection are hypomyelinogenesis (see Disorders of Myelin Formation and Maintenance) and cerebellar hypoplasia, although other lesions of the CNS (e.g., microencephaly) and nonneural tissues have been reported. The mechanism of lesion development has not been definitively determined, but a persistent infection that results in inhibition of cell division and function of selected tissues has been proposed.

Border disease viral infection (also a pestiviral infection) is capable of inducing maldevelopment in the CNS and nonneural tissues (e.g., skeleton) of lambs and goats following natural infection of the dam during pregnancy. One of the characteristic lesions in the CNS is hypomyelinogenesis (see Disorders of Myelin Formation and Maintenance). Other lesions detected in lambs include early inflammation, porencephaly-hydranencephaly, cerebellar malformation including hypoplasia, microencephaly, and reduction in diameter of the spinal cord.

Akabane viral infection (a bunyaviral infection) occurs in cattle, sheep, and goats in Japan, Israel, and Australia. Characteristic lesions of the CNS include porencephaly-hydranencephaly and degeneration (with loss of neurons) of the ventral horns of the spinal cord. Nonsuppurative encephalitis also occurs. Arthrogryposis is a common lesion. The porencephalic-hydranencephalic lesion results from destruction of germinal cells during brain development, and the arthrogryposis is secondary to degeneration of lower motor neurons in the spinal cord, resulting in denervation atrophy of muscles with resultant lack of joint movement.

Bluetongue viral infection (orbiviral infection) of sheep is also known to induce porencephaly-hydranencephaly, plus cerebellar hypoplasia (all or part of the cerebellum), hypoplasia of the spinal cord, and retinopathy (retinal degeneration and dysplasia) following fetal infection during pregnancy. The mechanism involved in the development of the porencephalic-hydranencephalic lesion begins as necrosis of undifferentiated cells (including potential neuroblasts and neuroglia) in the subventricular zone that are required to form the central white matter of the cerebral hemispheres.

Finally, two other fetal viral infections that occur in Africa and are caused by *Rift Valley fever* virus (a bunyavirus) and *Wesselsbron* virus (a flavivirus) have been reported to cause hydranencephaly (e.g., in sheep).

Viral effects on differentiated cells. Infections of neonatal laboratory animals with several viruses that include mumps virus, reovirus type I, and parainfluenza virus types I and II can induce hydrocephalus. *Parainfluenza* virus can cause the lesion in the hamster, mouse, and dog. Although there are some differences among the different viral infections, the basic lesion is an aqueductal stenosis (incomplete closure in the dog) that results in the development of noncommunicating hydrocephalus (see Fig. 8-9). The virus grows in ependymal cells and is initially accompanied by an inflammation that resolves within 2 to 3 weeks. The final lesion (altered stenotic aqueduct) is not associated with a glial response or presence of viral antigen but is replaced by normal-appearing brain tissue and focal accumulations of remaining ependymal cells, all of which suggest agenesis rather than previous viral infection. Infection of adult laboratory animals (e.g., mice with influenza viral infection) also can induce aqueductal stenosis and hydrocephalus, but, in contrast to neonatal infection, there is a persistent glial response in the area of stenosis.

INBORN ERRORS OF METABOLISM

Disturbance of Amino Acid Metabolism

Aminoacidopathy

Two diseases characterized by errors of amino acid metabolism have been described in the neonatal calf. One disease, designated as **maple syrup urine disease,** occurs in young polled Hereford calves (see Disorders of Myelin Formation and Maintenance). The second disease, **bovine citrullinemia,** which was originally described in Australia, occurs in neonatal Friesian calves.

Bovine citrullinemia is a rare, inborn error of metabolism of the urea cycle that results in a pronounced accumulation of citrulline in the body fluids due to a failure of normal synthesis of arginosuccinic acid by the enzyme arginosuccinate synthetase. Grossly, the livers of affected animals have a pale yellow-ochre color. The brains appear normal grossly and have normal weights. Microscopic lesions in the brain are characterized by mild to moderate, diffuse, astroglial swelling in the cerebrocortical gray matter. Liver lesions are characterized by mild to severe hepatocellular hydropic change. The onset of the marked neurologic signs, which occur during the first week of life, is correlated with increasing concentrations of plasma ammonia, and the cerebral lesions have been suspected to be related to the hyperammonemia. However, the pathogenesis of the disease remains undecided.

Lysosomal storage disease *(Table 8-1)*

Lysosomal storage generally refers to a cellular alteration in which an increased amount of material that is normally degraded accumulates within lysosomes of cells, often eventually resulting in cell death. Lysosomal storage diseases were originally thought to result from mutations that result in a reduction in lysosomal enzyme synthesis. More recently, however, it has become clear that several mechanisms may be involved, and they include synthesis of catalytically inactive proteins that resemble active normal enzymes, defects in posttranslational processing of enzyme protein destined for the lysosome, lack of enzyme activator or protector protein, lack of substrate activator protein, and lack of transport protein that is required for elimination of the digested material from lysosomes. Characterization of lysosomal disorders has, therefore, been

Table 8-1. Classification of selected lysosomal storage diseases that involve the CNS of animals

Disease	Storage product	Deficient enzyme	Species	Breed
GM_1 gangliosidosis	GM_1 ganglioside	β-galactosidase	Bovine	Holstein-Friesian
			Canine	Beagle-mix
			Feline	Siamese, Korat, mixed
GM_2 gangliosidosis	GM_2 ganglioside	β-hexosaminidase	Ovine	Suffolk
			Canine	German shorthair pointer
			Feline (Sandhoff-like disease)	Mixed, Korat
			Porcine	Yorkshire
Globoid cell leukodystrophy (Krabbe's-like disease)	Galactosylceramide (galactocerebroside) and galactosylsphingosine (psychosine)	Galactosylceramidase (galactocerebroside β-galactosidase)	Canine	West Highland terrier, Cairn terrier, miniature poodle, blue tick hound, beagle, Pomeranian
			Feline	Domestic shorthair
α-mannosidosis	Mannose-containing oligosaccharide	α-mannosidase	Ovine	Polled Dorset
			Bovine	Angus, Murray gray, Galloway
			Feline	Persian, domestic shorthair
β-mannosidosis	Mannose-containing oligosaccharide	β-mannosidase	Caprine	Nubian
			Bovine	Salers
Ceroid-lipofuscinosis	Ceroid-lipofuscin	Unknown. Mechanisms proposed: (1) increased lipid peroxidation; (2) p-phenylene-diamine-mediated peroxidase deficiency (proposed for humans and English setter dogs); (3) increased levels of dolichol or dolichyl phosphate; (4) accumulation of subunit c of ATP synthase	Canine	English setter, chihuahua, dachshund, cocker spaniel, Saluki, terrier-cross, blue heeler, Yugoslavian shepherd
			Feline	Siamese
			Bovine	Beefmaster
			Ovine	Rambouillet, South Hampshire
			Equine*	
			Primate	Cynomolgus monkey *(Macaca fascicularis)*

*Acquired lipofuscinosis-like disease.

broadened to include any protein that is essential for normal lysosomal function.

The best-known diseases are characterized by accumulation of the substrate and substrate precursors, and/or, sometimes, even the absence of a critical metabolic product for normal lysosomal function. An example of lysosomal storage diseases that affect human beings and animals includes the gangliosidoses (one form of which is referred to as Tay-Sachs disease in human beings). Such diseases are usually transmitted as autosomal recessives. They are also often gene-dose dependent, and, correspondingly, recessive homozygotes manifest the disease, whereas heterozygotes are phenotypically normal but have a reduced amount of the specific enzymatic activity (often approximately 50% of normal).

Accumulation of materials in lysosomes can also be acquired and not initiated by an inherited lysosomal defect. Such lysosomal storage can occur following acquired toxicities (see Plant Toxicities), accumulation of iron (e.g., as hemosiderin after erythrocytic lysis), and accumulation of copper from external sources. One unique lysosomal storage disease, which has several forms, is **ceroid-lipofuscinosis.** Its lysosomal dysfunction has not been completely characterized. The disease resembles other lysosomal storage diseases in that it may have a recessive mode of inheritance but is dissimilar in that it has no gene-dose effect or demonstrated lysosomal enzyme defect.

Many lysosomal storage diseases of human beings and animals affect the CNS and cause neurologic disturbances. The lesions of the different diseases vary, but, within the nervous system, neurons and, occasionally, other cell types are generally affected. Affected neurons often have a foamy (finely vacuolated) or granular-appearing cytoplasm, and the specific features of the stored material can be appreciated by ultrastructural examination. In **globoid cell leukodystrophy,** the primary lysosomal defect appears to be in the oligodendrocytes rather than involving neurons. This results in their destruction, subsequent disturbance of myelin formation and maintenance, and accumulation of globoid cells (see Disorders of Myelin Formation and Maintenance).

Features of some selected lysosomal storage diseases of the CNS of animals are given in Table 8-1 (also see Figs. 8-15 to 8-18).

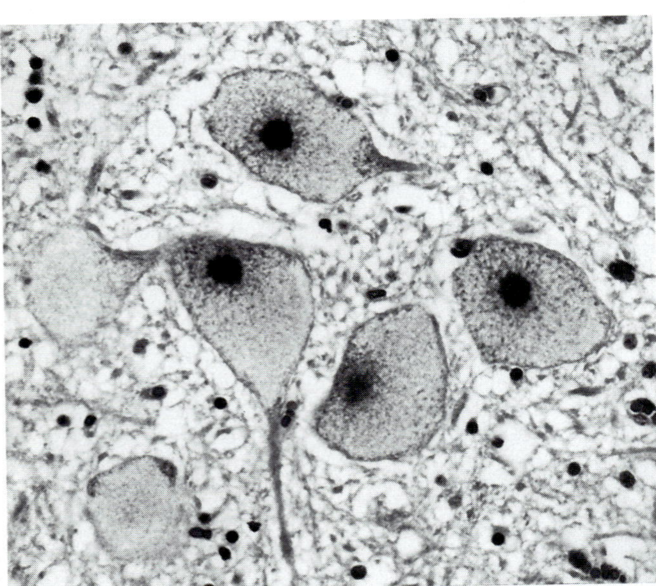

Fig. 8-15 Brain, medulla oblongata, hypoglossal nucleus; pig. GM_2 gangliosidosis. The cytoplasm of swollen neuronal cell bodies (two with displaced nuclei in lower center of photograph) appears finely vacuolated. H & E stain. *Courtesy Dr. C.H. Bridges.*

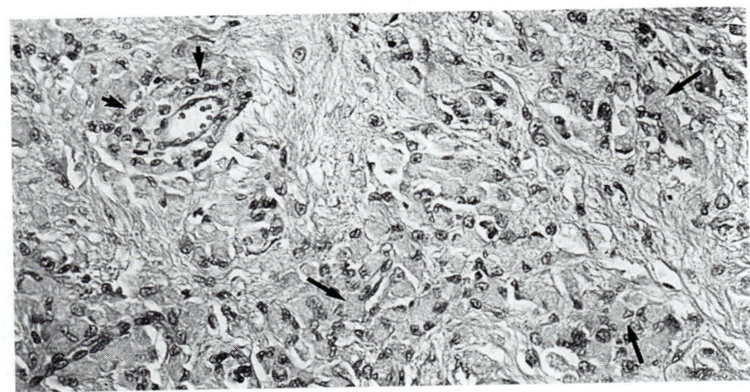

Fig. 8-16 Brain, junction between parietal and frontal lobes, deep cerebral white matter, centrum semiovale; dog. Globoid cell leukodystrophy. Globoid cells have accumulated in the cerebral white matter *(long arrows)* and perivascularly *(short arrows).* H & E stain.

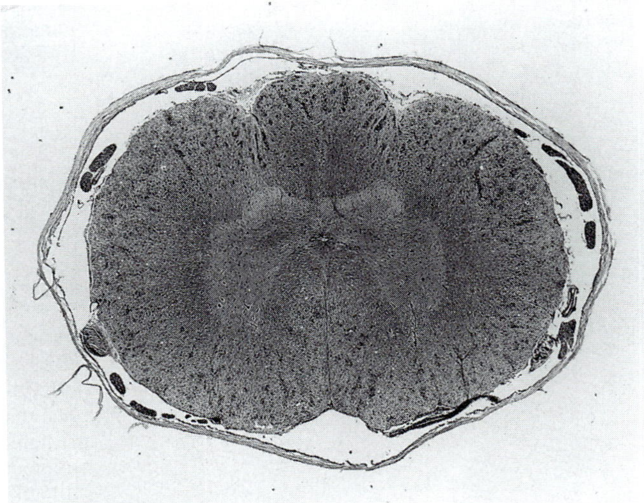

Fig. 8-17 Spinal cord, thoracic level; dog. Globoid cell leukodystrophy. There is peripheral loss of myelin in all funiculi (light staining area). The vessels in affected areas are prominent due to the perivascular accumulation of globoid cells. H & E stain. *Courtesy Dr. M.D. McGavin.*

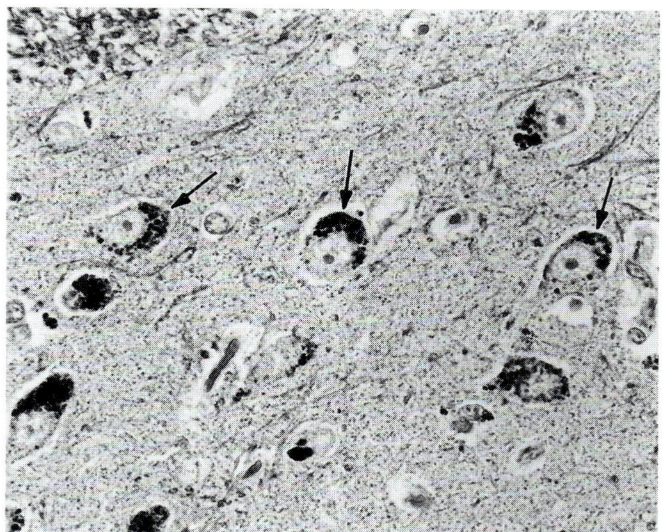

Fig. 8-18 Brain, junction of frontal and parietal lobes, junction of caudate nucleus and internal capsule; Rambouillet sheep. Ceroid-lipofuscinosis. Affected neurons contain variable accumulation of granular pigment *(arrows)* that is sometimes prominent at one pole of the cell body. Sudan black stain for lipid.

PHYSICAL DISTURBANCES

Factors Influencing the Susceptibility of the CNS to Trauma

In general, trauma to the CNS of animals occurs less frequently than it does in human beings. Animals are not exposed as frequently to trauma-causing situations (e.g., automobile travel) as are humans, and there are anatomic differences that help protect the brain of animals.

Among animals, cerebral and spinal cord trauma is probably most frequently encountered in dogs due to automobile-induced injury. Trauma, particularly involving small animals, also can result from falls from significant heights (e.g., high-rise apartment buildings, balconies, roofs), although cats often have remarkably minor injury to the CNS, even after falling from considerable heights. Other examples include fracture of the spinal column or cranium of jumping horses and fractious animals (e.g., horses and ruminants) during restraint.

Predisposition to cerebral trauma is also influenced by anatomic differences. In animals, the percentage of brain mass in relation to skull size is much less than that for primates, and, in some species (e.g., bovine and porcine), the cranial cavity is additionally protected by prominent dorsal frontal sinuses. Also, birth trauma, which can be important in human beings, is essentially insignificant in animals, because in the latter the shoulders and, particularly, the pelvis rather than the head are likely to be compressed in the birth canal. Exceptions to this generalization include brachycephalic breeds of dogs. Several factors also influence the susceptibility of the spinal cord to trauma. The amount of space between the spinal cord and the wall of the vertebral canal is very important in determining the degree of injury following swelling (e.g., edema) or compression (e.g., disk herniation). This space is greater in the cervical area (e.g., in the dog) than at the thoracolumbar level, causing disk herniation at the latter area to often result in more severe spinal cord injury.

Functional factors also play an important role in brain injury. The brain of a freely movable head is much more susceptible to injury than that of a stationary, supported head. This increased susceptibility has been attributed to the ability of the cranium and its contents (the brain) to impact upon each other following trauma. This can occur because the brain does not fill the cranial cavity; there is a small space between the brain tissue and bone. Thus, following an impact upon a stationary freely movable head, the bone will move upon the stationary brain and can result in injury. Also, the mass and velocity of the object striking the head are important. Trauma following impact of a relatively large blunt object can create marked head movement as well as a large-impact injury, whereas a small object (e.g., bullet) moving at a high rate of speed may cause less head movement and a smaller but deeper area of tissue damage.

Factors involved in the protection of the brain include the rigidity of the cranium (dependent upon age), the round shape of the dorsum of the skull, the structure of the cranial bone (two layers of compact bone separated by spongy bone [diplöe]), cranial sutures, sinuses, ridges in the floor of the cranial cavity, meninges, and CSF. The spinal cord is enclosed and protected by the vertebral column, which is surrounded by soft tissues (e.g., adipose tissue and muscle). Other structures that help protect the spinal cord (by absorbing shock) are the intervertebral disks and the cancellous bone of the vertebrae. Vertebral ligaments maintain the alignment of the vertebral column, denticulate ligaments help to maintain the proper position of the spinal cord, and the meninges and the CSF help to cushion against trauma.

Cerebral Trauma

Concussion

Concussion is a clinical designation often characterized by a temporary loss of consciousness with recovery that follows head injury. It should be noted, however, that this type of injury is only part of a spectrum that has been referred to as **diffuse brain injury.** The severity of diffuse brain injury, depending on the degree of trauma, can range from a very mild, reversible concussion, without loss of consciousness, to severe injury that may be accompanied by microscopic lesions, such as hemorrhage and axonal degeneration, and result in a permanent neurologic deficit or even death. Diffuse brain injury involves widespread or global disruption of neurologic function that is usually not associated with gross lesions. Injury of this type results primarily from rotational acceleration forces that cause shear, tensile, and compressive strains throughout the brain.

Concussive injuries of the diffuse type also occur in animals, but there are some differences between animals and human beings. For example, it is difficult to produce severe concussion in animals because the margin between a stunning blow and fatal injury is very small. The smaller the brain, the less vulnerable it is to rotational forces and the larger are the forces necessary to cause concussion. As in the human being, a movable head is much more susceptible to trauma than a fixed, supported one. Application of an appropriate concussive trauma to the mobile head of an animal results in a reversible cerebral dysfunction that lasts for a matter of seconds or, at most, a few minutes; stronger blows cause death. Long periods of coma after a single head injury of the diffuse type (referred to above as diffuse brain injury) have not been readily produced in animals. Microscopic lesions detected in animals have included central chromatolysis, axonal degeneration, and cell loss.

Contusion

In contrast to the diffuse form of cerebral injury, contusion is characterized by **focal brain injury** that is grossly detectable, usually as hemorrhage, and it may, like concussion, result in unconsciousness and even death. In fact, it would be reasonable to assume that the causative factors involved in concussion and contusion may occur together to varying degrees in the same animal. Lesions may be superficial (e.g., cerebral gyri) or more central (e.g., brain stem), and there may be associated skull fracture. Although hemorrhage is the most common lesion, contusion may also include necrosis and tearing of the brain. Two designations are used to identify the location of contusive injury. A **coup contusion** is located at the impact site, and a **contrecoup contusion** at a location on the opposite side of the brain. When the two lesions occur together (e.g., coup-contre-coup or contrecoup-coup), the first term indicates the site of most severe injury.

Many investigations have been made to determine the mechanisms involved in the development of contusive lesions, and the kinetics are complicated and still not completely resolved. Factors considered to be significant include the ability of the head to move freely, the occurrence of a rotational movement of the brain over rough surfaces of the cranial vault, and the development within the cranial cavity of positive and negative pressures as well as gravitational forces. Several neuropathologic principles have been generally accepted regarding craniocerebral contusive trauma in the human being, including the following: (1) a blow to the stationary (but freely movable) head produces a cerebrocortical **coup** contusion beneath the point of cranial impact but, with rare exceptions, causes no cerebrocortical contrecoup contusion opposite the point of cranial impact; (2) an impact of a moving head (moving prior to impact, as in a fall from a standing position) against a firm or unyielding surface causes a cerebrocortical **contrecoup** contusion opposite the point of cranial collision (often at the poles and inferior surfaces of the frontal and temporal lobes), but, with rare exceptions, there is no contusion beneath the point of impact; and (3) falls from great heights, as well as crushing of the head between a strong external force and unyielding surface, are generally not associated with the occurrence of contrecoup lesions. Dawson and coworkers (see Suggested Readings) proposed a mechanism for both contrecoup and coup injury of the human brain that also addressed the specific deficiencies of mechanisms that have been advanced by others. An example explaining the mechanism of contrecoup injury states that when a person falls backward from standing position, due to loss of balance, the gravitational torque acting on the body causes downward acceleration of the head in excess of the acceleration due to gravity. Under these circumstances, the brain lags toward the trailing anterior surface of the cranium prior to impact (dissipating the protective cerebrospinal fluid layer), and at impact of the posterior surface of the cranium, contrecoup compressive stress may occur. Because dissipation of the cerebrospinal fluid at the contrecoup site causes this compressive stress to be nonuniform, a contrecoup shearing stress is generated. In addition, a relative rotational gliding motion between the brain and skull is produced when the impact suddenly stops the skull's motion and rotation, thus creating an additive shearing stress because the fluid lubrication necessary to facilitate gliding of the brain over the cranial surface is reduced. The concentration of this rotational shearing stress is likely to occur beneath the frontal and temporal lobes because of the rough surface of the skull that exists in these locations. In contrast to contrecoup injury, coup contusions occur infrequently in the type of fall being discussed. In such situations, brain lag away from the impact site results in a thickening of the protective cerebrospinal fluid layer over the brain immediately beneath the point of impact, which helps explain the absence of coup injury in typical moving head trauma. Coup injury can occur when a stationary (but freely movable) head is impacted. In this type of trauma, there is neither brain lag nor disproportionate distribution of cerebrospinal fluid prior to impact, which accounts for the typical absence of contrecoup contusions. With regard to falls from great heights, the dynamics involving rotation of the body about a fixed point of ground contact, associated with a fall from a standing position, do not occur. Since gravity places no torque on a freely falling object, no angular acceleration of the body is produced and, therefore, such a fall is a true free-fall state that is associated with an absence of brain lag. For this reason, contrecoup lesions occur infrequently with this type of trauma. One point should be emphasized with regard to the evaluation of coup and contrecoup cortical contusions just described. Displacement of bone associated with skull fracture can contuse the subjacent brain, regardless of the resting or moving status of the head, and such fracture-contusions have nothing to do with the coup-contrecoup mechanisms described. In domestic animals (e.g., dog) coup and contrecoup cerebral injury can also occur following head trauma and even though the basic mechanisms discussed above apply to the human being, they should also be considered when examining cerebral contusions of animals.

Hemorrhage

Following trauma to the head, hemorrhages can develop in the epidural, subdural, and leptomeningeal (subarachnoid space and pia mater) areas and in the brain parenchyma (Fig. 8-19). Such hemorrhages can result from increased forces within the cranial cavity, movement of the brain over bony ridges of the cranium with stretching and tearing of blood vessels and parenchyma, and following the cutting and penetrating action of bone fragments associated with skull fracture. Epidural hemorrhage, which is not commonly described in animals, has been reported in the horse, especially jumpers, resulting from falls while working. Subdural hemorrhage, which is an accumulation of blood between the dura mater and arachnoid membrane, occurs with some frequency in dogs and cats struck by vehicles. Leptomeningeal hemorrhage is probably most common and occurs in dogs and cats following vehicular-induced injury. Parenchymal hemorrhage can result from injury to the brain in a normal or fractured cranium by the mechanisms given above and from penetrating objects (bullets and stab wounds).

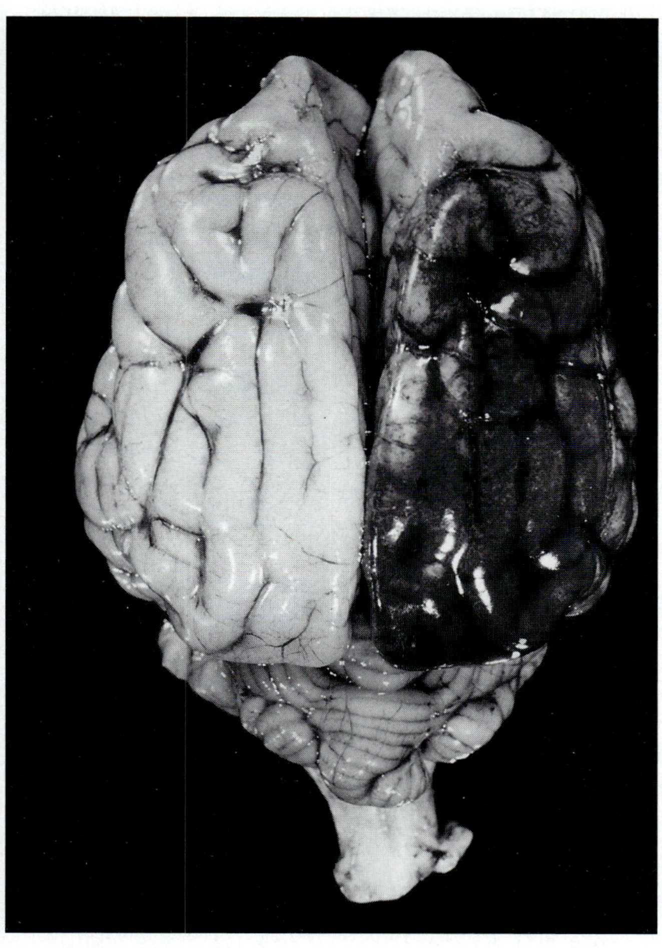

Fig. 8-19 Brain, meninges of right cerebral hemisphere; dog. Leptomeningeal (subarachnoid-pial) hemorrhage over the surface of the right cerebral hemisphere.

Brain swelling resulting from cerebral trauma

Brain swelling, as distinguished from cerebral edema, is thought to represent, at least in part, an unregulated vasodilatation following trauma, and it can cause serious brain damage (even more severe than the primary injury) if not properly controlled. Acute brain swelling can be localized (usually insignificant) when associated with focal lesions or generalized (often serious) when caused by diffuse brain injury. One exception to the importance of focal lesions is extracerebral hemorrhage (e.g., acute subdural hematoma in human beings), which though principally over one hemisphere, may cause more mass effect in the cerebral hemisphere than does the hematoma itself. If a craniotomy is performed to relieve the pressure caused by the subdural hemorrhage, the underlying brain may actually herniate through the craniotomy site following removal of the free blood. The more serious forms of diffuse brain injury are associated with generalized acute brain swelling. It should also be noted that brain swelling, which can initially be detected as soon as 30 minutes after injury in human beings, can be complicated by the development of vasogenic edema after several hours to days.

Spinal Cord Trauma

Evaluation of spinal cord trauma should include examination not only of the spinal cord but also of the vertebral column and spinal nerve roots. Injuries to the spinal cord can involve concussion, contusion, hemorrhage, laceration, transection, and compression.

Concussion

Spinal concussion is the term applied to the immediate and temporary loss of function, which sometimes follows severe direct blows to the spinal column. Loss of function usually affects the long tracts (e.g., ventral motor tracts) and the segmental mechanism, but usually there is no demonstrable external change in the vertebrae or spinal cord.

As with cerebral concussion, there is often only a temporary functional disability of the cord following injury, but permanent neurologic deficits may occur.

Contusion

Contusion is characterized by hemorrhage, necrosis, and tears that are generally focal and grossly visible. It may occur without fracture of the vertebral column, with fracture, and with fracture plus dislocation of the spinal column. The latter combination can result in tearing and transection of the spinal cord.

Hemorrhage

The same types of hemorrhage that affect the brain (epidural, subdural, leptomeningeal, and parenchymal hemorrhage) also occur in the spinal cord and its meninges. Causes in this location would be similar to those affecting the brain, including stretching due to abnormal movement and severance of blood vessels associated with vertebral fracture.

Laceration and transection

Both laceration and transection can occur following vertebral fracture, the former caused by penetration of bony fragments and the transection resulting from severance of the spinal cord by sharp fragments of bone that can be associated with dislocation of the vertebrae.

Compression

Compression of the spinal cord can be caused by pressure that may be either intramedullary (within the spinal cord) or extramedullary (outside the spinal cord). Causes of intramedullary compression include intraparenchymal hemorrhages and neoplasms. Extramedullary pressure may be caused by intervertebral disk herniation in the dog, cervical static myelopathy (wobbler syndrome) in the horse and dog, vertebral fracture and dislocation, and neoplasms of the meninges and/or nerve rootlets.

Intervertebral disk disease occurs in the canine species, particularly dogs of the chondrodystrophic breeds typified by dachshund and Pekingese dogs. Intervertebral disks are present between all vertebral bodies, except for the C1-C2 space and the sacral vertebrae, and they act as absorbers of shock during movement. Intervertebral disks of a significant percentage of dachshund and Pekingese dogs begin to degenerate after approximately 1 year of age, which predisposes them to sudden herniation (Hansen type I herniation) earlier than for nonchondrodystrophic breeds. Disk herniation in nonchondrodystrophic breeds (e.g., large breeds of dogs) occurs more slowly due to dorsal protrusion of a weakened but not ruptured disk (Hansen type II herniation). Herniation of either type occurs most frequently in the thoracolumbar and cervical areas. Intercapital (conjugal) ligaments, which extend across the floor of the vertebral canal over the dorsal aspect of each annulus fibrosus from the T1-T2 through T10-T11 intervertebral spaces, add support and account for the infrequent occurrence of herniation in the thoracic area. Severity of injury to the spinal cord is influenced both by the amount of space existing between the spinal cord and bone of the vertebral canal and by the speed with which herniation occurs. The space surrounding the cervical cord is larger than that in the thoracolumbar area, which generally results in less compression following cervical disk herniation.

Cervical stenotic myelopathy or wobbler syndrome is characterized by stenosis of the cervical vertebral canal that causes compressive trauma to the cervical spinal cord. It has been known for many years to affect horses and, more recently, has been recognized in the dog. The disease in the horse has been referred to by several designations: the wobbler syndrome, wobbles, equine incoordination, and, more recently, cervical stenotic myelopathy. The disease has been described in many breeds. Reports indicate that the disease is not caused by a straightforward mechanism but apparently involves several factors. Cervical stenotic myelopathy in the horse has been divided into two syndromes: cervical static stenosis and cervical vertebral instability.

Cervical static stenosis commonly affects horses 1 to 4 years of age. The spinal cord is compressed at C5-C7 as the result of an acquired dorsal or dorsolateral narrowing of the spinal canal. The stenosis is due to formation of bone that requires time to develop. The compressive effect with this type of stenosis is present regardless of head position. The second form of **cervical stenotic myelopathy** (cervical vertebral instability) occurs in horses ranging in age from 8 to 18 months. It is characterized by a narrowing of the spinal canal during flexion of the neck (e.g., with downward movement of the head) and primarily involves C3-C5 vertebrae.

A disease process with many similarities to that in the horse also affects the dog. It has been known as wobbler syndrome, vertebral instability, vertebral subluxation, and cervical spondylolisthesis. The disease has been most frequently described in the Great Dane and Doberman pinscher breeds but has also been reported to occur in the Saint Bernard, Irish setter, Fox terrier, basset hound, Rhodesian Ridgeback, and Old English sheepdog. Dogs can develop signs between 8 months and 1 year of age, with a range of 1 month to 9 years. Great Danes tend to develop lesions at a young age (e.g., 8 months to 1 year), whereas Doberman pinschers are generally older, often more than 1 year of age. The vertebral and associated spinal cord lesions in the dog have been reported to most often involve the caudal cervical area from C5-C7 vertebrae. An exception is the basset hound in which C3 is affected. The pathogenesis appears to be similar to that in the horse.

Lesions of the CNS associated with intervertebral disk

herniation and cervical stenotic myelopathy are similar. The severity of injury depends upon the speed and degree to which the compression is applied and the specific area of the cord that is involved. Central nervous tissue can tolerate a considerable degree of compression if it is applied slowly (e.g., Hansen type II disk herniation in nonchondrodystrophic breeds of dogs and possibly in equine cervical static stenosis). Rapid compression (e.g., associated with Hansen type I disk herniation in chrondrodystrophic breeds of dogs and possibly following sudden forceful compression in equine cervical instability) can lead to quickly developing hypoxia-ischemia and necrosis. Lesions detected include a spectrum of change characterized by axonal injury (wallerian degeneration), disruption of myelin sheaths, and necrosis of the gray and/or white matter (due to ischemia secondary to interruption of the blood supply), which may be visible grossly from the exterior but particularly on cross section. Microscopically, after a few days, particularly at the site of injury, there is loss of architecture of the neuropil due to necrosis and a beginning accumulation of macrophages (gitter cells) that have phagocytosed the lipid-rich tissue debris (Fig. 8-20). Eventually, the necrotic area is cleared, and a cystic space is formed in its place, which is surrounded by a varying degree of astrocytosis and astrogliosis. Rostral and caudal to this location, the lesion is primarily one of axonal (wallerian) degeneration in the white matter, and the pattern of lesion development seen depends upon the level of the spinal cord that is examined relative to the site of compression. At the site of injury, all parts of the cord (white and gray matter) will be affected (and often are necrotic) if the compressive force is sufficient. Rostral to this site, white matter degeneration is generally limited to the ascending tracts in the dorsal funiculi and the superficial portions of the dorsolateral part of the lateral funiculi, where affected axons are distal to the point of injury. Caudal to the area of injury, white matter degeneration tends to be limited to the descending tracts in the ventral funiculi and the more central portions of the lateral funiculi for the same reason (see Reaction to Injury under Neurons for discussion of Wallerian degeneration).

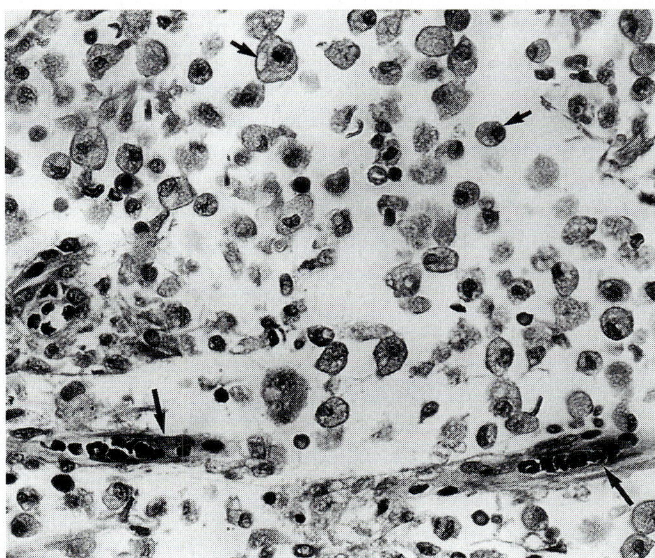

Fig. 8-20 Brain, parietal lobe; dog. Infarction. The lesion has progressed to the stage of liquefaction necrosis, characterized by a predominance of lipid-laden macrophages (gitter cells) *(short arrows)*. Intact blood vessels *(long arrows)*, which are more resistant to ischemia than neurons, oligodendroglia, and astrocytes, are the only tissue components remaining in the lesion. H & E stain. (See Figs. 8-25, 8-33, and 8-34 for the gross appearance of such a lesion.)

CIRCULATORY DISTURBANCES

Rate of Oxygen Deprivation and Development of Lesions

The rate at which ischemia occurs in the CNS determines the degree of injury that follows. The more rapid the onset of ischemia, the more severe the lesion. If the blood flow through an artery is gradually reduced (e.g., due to arteriosclerosis), there is often sufficient time for anastomotic vessels to dilate and compensate. However, if the obstruction is sudden (e.g., caused by an embolus), much of the tissue may die before an adequate anastomotic circulation can be established. This same principle may apply to compressive injury to the CNS that produces a reduction in blood flow. This tissue may compensate rather remarkably if the compression is slow (e.g., slowly developing [Hansen type II] disk herniation in the dog or compression by a slowly growing neoplasm from the exterior, such as meningioma in the dog) when compared with a sudden compressive injury (e.g., rapidly occurring Hansen type I disk herniation in the dog).

Susceptibility of Cells and Specific Anatomic Areas to Ischemia

Cells and tissue structures of the CNS susceptible to ischemia, in decreasing order of susceptibility, are neurons, oligodendroglia, astrocytes, microglia, and blood vessels. Neurons are not all equally susceptible to ischemia, and differences occur in relation to the location of neurons in the CNS. The most susceptible neurons (e.g., cerebrocortical neurons of the third lamina in the human being) will not survive more than 5 to 6 minutes of ischemia, e.g., following cardiac arrest and resuscitation. Purkinje cells of the cerebellar cortex are slightly less vulnerable. Neurons of the basal ganglia can survive up to 10 minutes of ischemia with only minor alterations. The motor neurons of the spinal cord, and apparently also many of the brain stem, can recover following ischemic periods of up to 15 minutes.

Edema of the CNS

The basis of our current understanding of cerebral edema was advanced by Klatzo in 1967 when he proposed two distinct types: the first characterized by an increased extracellular fluid resulting from increased vascular permeability (**vasogenic** type), and the second characterized by an increased intracellular fluid with the vascular permeability remaining intact (**cytotoxic** type). Other types of cerebral edema are **hydrostatic** (or interstitial) edema associated with increased hydrostatic pressure (e.g., resulting from hydrocephalus), and **osmotic edema,** which is dependent on development of abnormal osmotic forces between the blood and nervous tissue.

Vasogenic edema

The underlying mechanism of vasogenic cerebral edema is a breakdown of the blood-brain barrier that results in movement of plasma constituents such as water, sodium, and plasma proteins into the extracellular space, particularly that of the white matter (Figs. 8-21 and 8-22). In addition to extracellular accumulation of fluid, vasogenic edema may also be accompanied by some cellular swelling (e.g., involving astrocytes). Vasogenic edema is the most common type and occurs following vascular injury. It is often associated with hematomas, contusions, infarction, inflammation, certain toxicities, and neoplasia.

Cytotoxic edema

Cytotoxic edema is characterized by the accumulation of fluid intracellularly (e.g., in neurons, astrocytes, oligodendroglia, and endothelial cells) as a result of altered cellular metabolism, often due to ischemia. Affected cells swell within seconds of injury. The mechanism is considered to involve an energy deficit that interferes with normal function of the ATP-dependent Na-K pump, resulting in an abnormal intracellular Na accumulation followed by an increased influx of water. The gray and white matter of the brain are both affected. The fluid taken up by the swollen cells is primarily derived from the extracellular space, which becomes reduced in size and may contain an increased concentration of extracellular solutes. For this lesion to be described accurately as cerebral edema, there must be additional fluid movement into the brain and not merely a change of existing intraparenchymal fluid from extracellular to intracellular compartments. The additional fluid originates from the circulation (by way of the transcapillary fluid exchange) and from the CSF, which has extensive diffusional communication with the extracellular fluid of the brain. The blood-brain barrier remains intact during development of this type of edema, so fluid does not enter the brain by a disturbance in vascular permeability. Specific causes of this lesion include hypoxia-ischemia (particularly in the early stages); intoxication with metabolic inhibitors such as 2,4,dinitrophenol, 6-aminonicatinamide, and ouabain; and severe hypothermia.

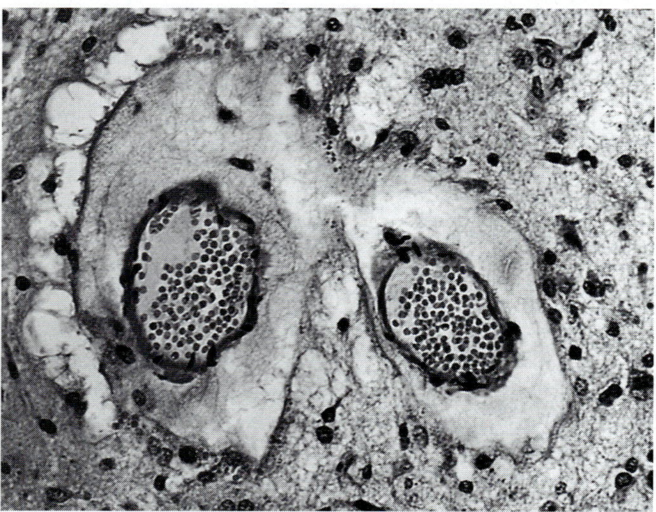

Fig. 8-21 Brain, pyriform lobe; pig. Mercury toxicity. Two vessels with fibrinoid necrosis of their walls are surrounded by fibrin and vasogenic edema fluid. H & E stain. *Courtesy Dr. W.W. Carlton.*

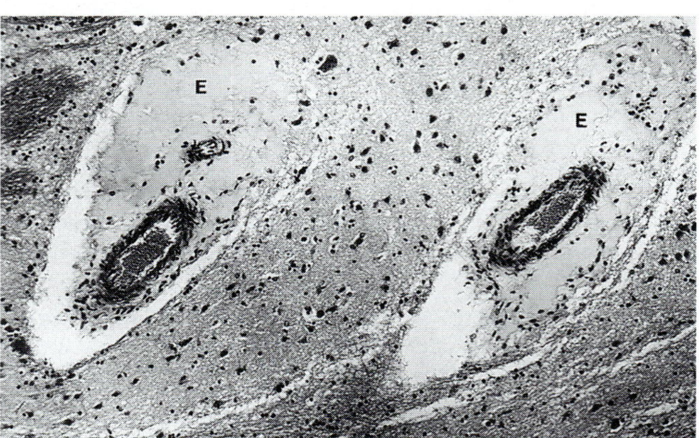

Fig. 8-22 Brain, parietal lobe, level of the thalamus; feeder lamb. *Clostridium perfringens* type D enterotoxemia. Marked perivascular (vasogenic) edema fluid (*E*) surrounds each vessel. H & E stain.

Hydrostatic (interstitial) edema

Hydrostatic edema is characterized by the accumulation of a protein-free fluid in the extracellular space of the brain because of elevated ventricular hydrostatic pressure that can accompany hydrocephalus. Fluid moves across the ependyma of the ventricular wall and accumulates extracellularly in the periventricular tissue (primarily white matter). Unlike the other forms of cerebral edema that cause swelling of affected CNS tissue, hydrostatic edema causes variable degeneration and loss of the periventricular white matter. The blood-brain barrier remains intact.

Osmotic cerebral edema

Cerebral edema has also been associated with "water intoxication," which can result from an increased body hydration caused by (1) excessive, faulty intravenous hydration; (2) compulsive drinking caused by abnormal mental function; or (3) altered antidiuretic hormone secretion. The increased body hydration produces a hypotonic (hypoosmolar) plasma, with subsequent development of an osmotic gradient between the hypotonic plasma and the relatively hypertonic state of the normal cerebral tissue. Fluid moves from the plasma into the brain. In this type of edema, the blood-brain barrier remains intact. If it did not, the change in plasma osmolarity would soon be transmitted to the brain tissue (through vascular leakage) and would abolish the necessary osmotic gradient. Fluid accumulation occurs primarily intracellularly, but may also be present extracellularly. In addition, there typically is a pronounced increase in the rate of formation of CSF originating from the choroid plexus and the extracellular fluid of the brain.

Sequelae of cerebral edema

The gross lesions that accompany cerebral edema are the result of enlargement of an organ in an enclosed, limited space; the degree of swelling obviously determines the type and extent of lesions. In evaluating lesions, it is particularly important initially to examine the brain and spinal cord in the fresh state and in situ.

Because of compression against the cranium, an affected brain has flattened gyri and shallow sulci, and it may have shifted in position. If the edema is confined to one side, there is unilateral displacement, which may be associated with herniation of the cingulate gyrus under the falx cerebri, and the extent of the unilateral intracerebral enlargement can be best appreciated following the examination of coronal (transverse) sections. Diffuse swelling usually causes a caudal shifting that may result in herniation of the brain (parahippocampal gyri of temporal lobes) beneath the tentorium cerebelli or herniation of the cerebellar vermis through the foramen magnum, which can result in a "coning" of the vermis (Fig. 8-23). On cut surface, the white matter is most often affected (frequently with the vasogenic type of edema, which is the most common). It is swollen and soft, has a damp appearance, and is light yellow in the fresh, unfixed state.

Microscopically, in contrast to that of some other tissues such as the lung, the extracellular fluid associated with vasogenic edema is often not detectable, except in instances of marked vascular injury. When the extracellular space-occupying fluid cannot be identified, only its effects (separation of the neuropil, causing reduced staining intensity) can be recognized. Additionally, following prolonged vasogenic edema formation, there may be hypertrophy and hyperplasia of astrocytes, activation of microglia, and demyelination. Cytotoxic edema is characterized by cellular swelling, including swelling of astrocytes.

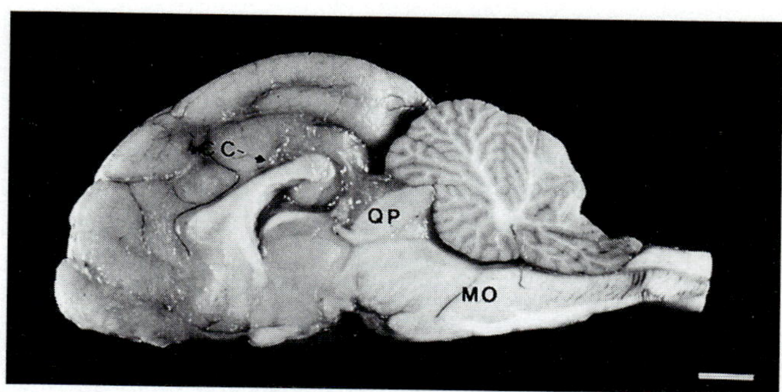

Fig. 8-23 Brain, cerebellum; cat. Coning of the cerebellum (caudal displacement of the caudal cerebellar vermis through the foramen magnum with compression of the medulla oblongata [*MO*]) due to cerebral edema. Note the elevation of the corpus callosum *(CC)* and compression of the rostral cerebellar vermis by the quadrigeminal plate (tectum) *(QP)*. Bar = 5 mm. *Courtesy Dr. D.Y. Cho and International Veterinary Pathology Slide Bank.*

Infarction

Infarction means necrosis of a tissue following obstruction of its arterial supply. There are usually insufficient anastomoses of the arteries that penetrate from the ventral and cortical surfaces of the brain to prevent infarction following sudden occlusion of one or more of these arteries.

Cerebral necrosis, comparable with infarction following vascular occlusion, can also result from other causes, including cessation of cerebral circulation (e.g., caused by cardiac arrest); sudden hypotension (e.g., caused by reduced cardiac output); reduced or absent oxygen in inspired air; altered function of hemoglobin (e.g., due to carbon monoxide poisoning); inhibition of tissue respiration (e.g., cytochrome oxidase system following cyanide poisoning), toxic substances and poisons, and nutritional deficiencies. Although resulting from different mechanisms, the necrosis that occurs has, with some variation, essentially the same gross and microscopic characteristics as that which is associated with classical infarction. Since the above causes of brain injury (excluding arterial obstruction) are not related to the blood supply of one or more specific arteries, the distribution of tissue damage will depend on where the susceptible cells are located. The degree of injury, obviously, will depend upon the severity and duration of the inciting cause.

Areas of cerebral infarction differ somewhat in gross appearance from infarcts in other tissues. The abundance of lipids and enzymes, plus the relative lack of fibrous con-

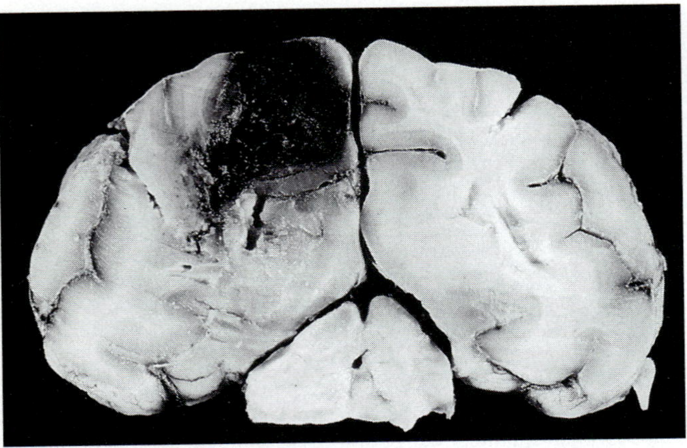

Fig. 8-24 Brain, left dorsal parietal lobe; dog. Cerebral hemorrhagic infarct affecting the cortex and white matter of the endomarginal, marginal, suprasylvian, splenial, and cingulate gyri; and the centrum semiovale.

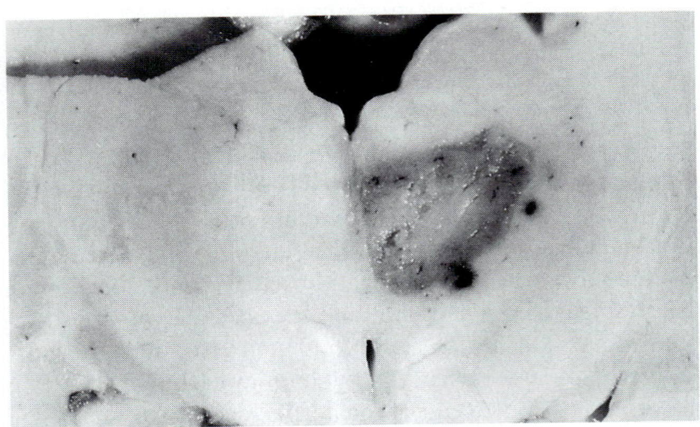

Fig. 8-25 Brain, thalamus; dog. There is a focus of liquefaction necrosis (malacia) in the right midcentral thalamus.

Table 8-2. Chronologic sequence of changes within infarcted tissue (in the living animal) following ischemic event

Time following ischemic event	Tissue change
Immediate (seconds)	Cessation of blood flow (ischemia) and accumulation of waste products
Few minutes	Cellular injury and death; coagulation necrosis, and edema; hemorrhage (especially in gray matter)
20 minutes	First microscopic evidence of neuronal injury (perfusion-fixation)
1-2 hours	First microscopic evidence of neuronal injury (immersion fixation)
2 hours	Pale staining of infarct microscopically (white matter); swelling of capillary endothelium; increase in size of astrocytic nuclei
3-5 hours	Ischemic cell change in most neurons; swelling of oligodendroglia and astroglia; beginning clasmatodendrosis of astrocytes
6-24 hours	Beginning neutrophilic infiltration; alteration of myelin (pale-staining), 8-24 hours; degeneration and decrease of oligodendroglia, 8-24 hours; astrocytic swelling and retraction and fragmentation of processes (clasmatodendrosis), and degeneration;* cytoplasm of astrocytes visible, 8-24 hours;* vascular degeneration and fibrin deposition, 8-24 hours; thrombosis,** 6-24 hours; beginning endothelial proliferation at margin of infarct, 9 hours
8-24 (up to 48) hours	Initial gross detection of infarct unless hemorrhagic; infarct edematous (swollen), soft, pale, or hemorrhagic and demarcated
1-2 days	Swelling of axons and myelin sheaths; prominent neutrophilic infiltration
2 days	Prominent loss of neuroectodermal cells; continued proliferation of endothelial cells; reduced number of neutrophils; beginning increase in mononuclear cells (gitter cells)
3-5 days	Prominent number of mononuclear cells (gitter cells); disappearance of neutrophils; continued endothelial cell proliferation; number of capillaries appear increased; beginning of astrocytic proliferation (often at margin of infarct)
5-7 days	Grossly, swelling of infarct reaches maximum
8-10 days	Reduction in gross swelling of infarct; liquefaction necrosis; prominent number of mononuclear cells (gitter cells); continued endothelial cell proliferation; beginning fibroblastic activity with collagen formation (variable, but most prominent in CNS tissue adjacent to the meninges); beginning increase of astroglial fiber production, 5-13 days
3 weeks-6 months	Mononuclear cells decreased; astroglial fiber density increased (especially at margin); astrocytic proliferation reduced; astrocytes return to original appearance; cystic stage of infarct, 2-4 months; vascular network may be present within cyst; endothelial cell proliferation reduced

*The degree of astrocytic injury will depend on the location (e.g., central or peripheral) of the cells within the infarct.

**Obviously, thrombosis may occur earlier than 6 hours. This is the time when it may initially be prominent.

nective tissue stroma in the brain and spinal cord, results in affected areas eventually becoming soft (often referred to as malacia) because of liquefaction necrosis. The gross appearance of infarction may differ according to location. Lesions affecting the gray matter tend to be hemorrhagic (hemorrhagic infarction) (Fig. 8-24), whereas infarction of the white matter is often pale (pale infarction). This result is probably due in part to the less dense capillary meshwork in the white matter, and in part to the fact that the vessels that supply the white matter have fewer anastomoses than those of the gray matter. Infarcted tissue goes through a characteristic sequence of changes that can permit a relatively accurate determination of the age of the infarct (Figs. 8-24 and 8-25; see also Fig. 8-20). An outline of the chronologic events that occur after an ischemic episode that lasts more than 5 to 6 minutes, and is followed by resuscitation of an animal, is given in Table 8-2. As can be seen, the tissue changes listed below take different periods of time to develop in the living resuscitated animal after ischemia occurs. There may be some variation in the times that specific lesions occur depending on the extent and duration of the initial ischemic event.

Recent advances have improved our understanding of the mechanisms involved in ischemic injury of the CNS. The CNS depends on blood for a continuous, necessary supply of oxygen and glucose, and interruption of this blood flow for only a few minutes will result in the death of certain vulnerable neurons. If the cessation of flow is sustained for a longer period, all types of cells (neurons, oligodendroglia, astrocytes, and microglia) in the affected area will die. It appears that death of neurons involves a process that is more complicated than just a loss of energy and that these cells can also be killed by injurious chemical mechanisms that result from disturbed neurotransmitter function.

When an artery supplying the CNS is suddenly occluded, blood supply to cells at the center of the infarcted area (the core) is rapidly stopped, and, if maintained for a sufficient period, all cells die. Neurons at the border (penumbra) of this area, that lie between the normal tissue and core of the infarct, continue to receive some blood from nonobstructed vessels. It is proposed that the axonal terminals of degenerated ischemic neurons in the core of the infarct release excessive amounts of the neurotransmitter glutamate, that causes injury to still-viable neurons in the penumbra, thus increasing the extent of injury that can occur with infarction. The process involved in neuronal injury begins following the binding of the neurotransmitter glutamate to receptor molecules on viable neurons in the penumbra, which induces an abnormal movement of calcium ions into the recipient cells followed by an increase in intracellular calcium ion concentration. This process results in a buildup of the calcium ion, which contributes to a multifunctional cascade that leads to neuronal death. When infarction is additionally associated with hemorrhage, the mechanical injury from the pressure, plus tissue displacement by the hemorrhage, can cause additional damage.

Vascular Disease

Arteriosclerosis, which means increased arterial firmness, is a general designation for several types of arterial lesions that can be grouped under lipid arteriosclerosis (atherosclerosis) and nonlipid arteriosclerosis (arterial fibrosis, mural mineralization, and amyloidosis). Naturally occurring arteriosclerosis of animals is primarily of the nonlipid type, although lipid forms can occur in nonhuman primates, aged swine, birds, dogs with hypothyroidism, and variably in ruminants. Arteriosclerosis in human beings is primarily of the lipid type (atherosclerosis).

Cerebrovascular lipid arteriosclerosis (atherosclerosis)

Atherosclerosis of cerebral arteries of nonhuman primates can occur in the monkey, chimpanzee, and gorilla. The lesion in swine is usually most severe in older animals (e.g., 8 to 14 years) and can be common. Affected vessels include the aorta and its major branches, extramural coronary arteries, and intracranial (but extracerebral) arteries. Most frequently affected are the internal carotid; middle, rostral, and caudal cerebral; and caudal communicating arteries. Affected arteries are stiff, irregularly thickened, white, or yellow-white. Lumina are narrowed or almost completely obliterated, but there is usually no intimal ulceration, thrombosis, or hemorrhage. Intimal thickenings contain less lipid and have a greater tendency for fibrosclerosis than affected vessels in other areas of the body. The extracerebral atherosclerotic arteries do not continue into the cerebral tissue. Parenchymal arterial lesions are characterized by a nonlipid arteriosclerosis with excess collagen in the adventitia or in all layers of the vessel wall. Infarcts of varying size can occur in the external capsule, putamen, fornix, septum pellucidum, globus pallidus, cau-

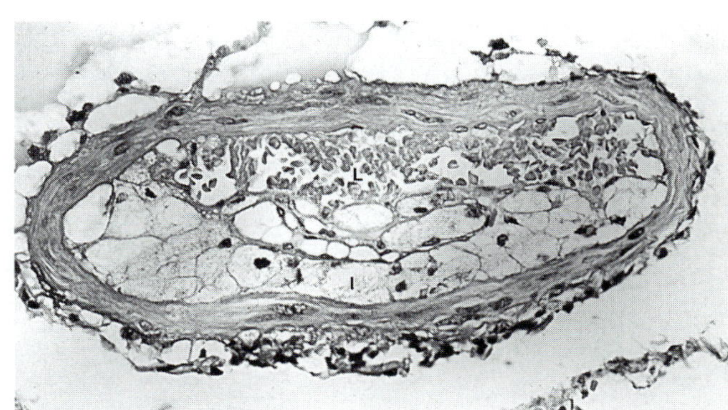

Fig. 8-26 Brain, junction of parietal and frontal lobes, meningeal artery; dog. Atherosclerosis. The lumen (*L*) is narrowed because of accumulation of lipid-laden cells in the intima (*I*) on the lower side of the lumen. H & E stain.

date nucleus (head), internal capsule, perivascular zones of perforating basal ganglial arteries, hippocampus, and thalamus. Atherosclerosis occurs uncommonly in the dog in association with hypothyroidism. Lesions, which occur in extracerebral arteries as well as arteries of other tissues (e.g., coronary and renal arteries), are most pronounced in the media and intima (Fig. 8-26). There may or may not be cerebral infarction, depending on the restriction of blood flow. Atherosclerosis has also been reported in several species of birds, including the pigeon, turkey, chicken, and parrot, but only rarely have changes in cerebral vessels and parenchyma been reported.

Cerebrovascular nonlipid arteriosclerosis

Arterial **fibrosis,** which occurs more frequently in older animals, has been described in cerebral vessels of dogs and horses. In the dog, particularly aged dogs, fibrosis of the intima, media, and adventitia (individually or combined) occurs with some frequency in cerebrospinal vessels of all types and calibers. Changes in small meningeal and intracerebral arteries are characterized by proliferation of the adventitia and, less commonly, by an extension of the connective tissue into the other components of the vessel wall. A preferential site is the choroid plexus. Also, cerebrovascular **amyloidosis** of meningeal and cerebrocortical vessels can occur in aged dogs. Large and small extracerebral and intracerebral vessels, as well as vessels of the spinal cord, of old horses also often have intimal fibrosis, although any or all layers of the vessel wall may be affected. An especially prominent fibrosis of the adventitia and media, particularly of arteries but also of veins, can involve the choroid plexus. **Mineralization** (involving calcium and iron salts) of intracerebral vessels has been detected in the brain of many species, including the horse, cow, dog, and cat. It preferentially affects vessels of the globus pallidus, internal capsule, and dentate nucleus of the cerebellum and, less frequently the hippocampus (horse, cow, and, rarely, the dog), meninges (old cats, old horses, and cattle) and choroid plexus (old cats). Cerebrovascular mineralization (vascular siderocalcinosis) is particularly common in adult horses and can affect arteries, veins, and capillaries (Fig. 8-27). Arterial fibrosis and mineralization, as described above, is infrequently a cause of cerebral infarction in any animal species.

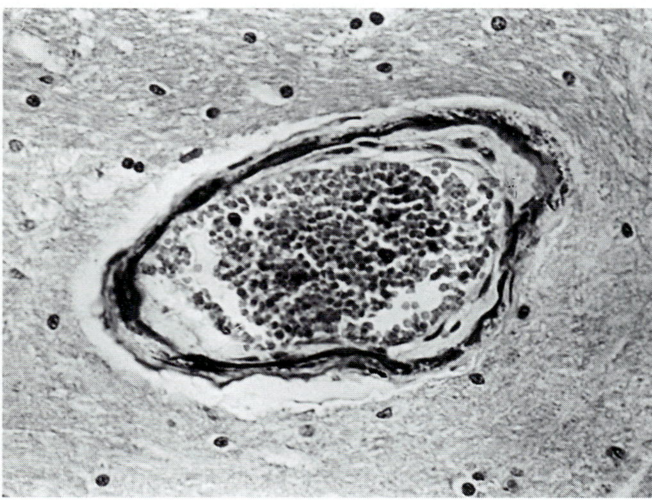

Fig. 8-27 Brain, junction of parietal and frontal lobes, globus pallidus; horse. Vascular siderocalcinosis. The vessel wall contains a prominent amount of dark-staining mineral. H & E stain.

Specific Diseases Associated with Circulatory Dysfunction

Suspected or known vascular-mediated injury of the CNS may be associated with lesions other than arteriosclerosis. Two rather unique diseases, feline ischemic encephalopathy and ischemic (or necrotizing) myelopathy-encephalopathy, are discussed here.

Feline ischemic encephalopathy

Feline ischemic encephalopathy affects cats of any age and is characterized by an acute to peracute onset accompanied by signs that are usually referable to unilateral cerebral involvement.

Lesions consist of variable degrees of usually unilateral but occasionally bilateral necrosis of the cerebral hemisphere. The necrosis may be multifocal in the cortex or may involve up to two thirds of one cerebral hemisphere.

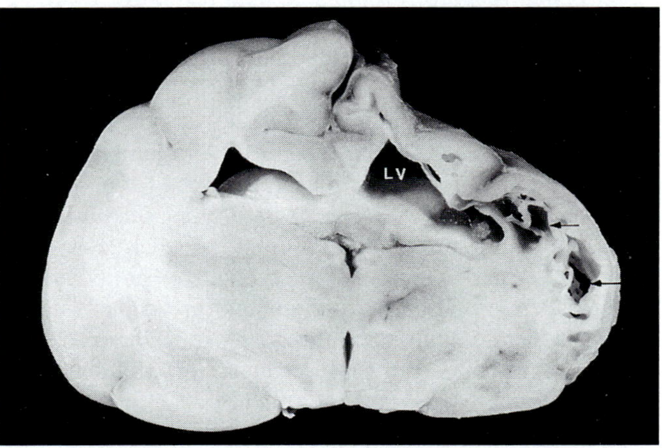

Fig. 8-28 Brain, junction between parietal and occipital lobes, level of thalamus; cat. Chronic feline ischemic encephalopathy with unilateral cerebral degeneration-atrophy. The dorsolateral aspect of the right cerebral hemisphere has undergone necrosis, which was followed by collapse after removal of the necrotic debris. Remaining are spaces *(arrows)* in place of the previously existing parenchyma and an enlarged right lateral ventricle *(LV)* that has expanded into the area of lost tissue (hydrocephalus ex vacuo).

Occasionally, hemorrhages also occur in the parenchyma or in the leptomeninges. Usually the major lesion is in the area supplied by the middle cerebral artery. In chronic cases, cerebral atrophy can occur and is most marked in the vicinity of the middle cerebral artery on the lateral side of the affected hemisphere (Fig. 8-28). Lesions may also occur in the brain stem, especially in the periventricular areas. Microscopically, the lesions are infarction and follow the sequence presented in Table 8-2.

The cause of the disease has not been determined. A vascular-mediated mechanism has been suggested, although specific lesions (thrombosis or vasculitis) have been found in only a few cases. Feline infectious peritonitis virus, which can induce meningeal vasculitis, has been proposed as a possible cause of the disease. Also, affected cats often have a history of a recent upper respiratory infection or other illness with pyrexia, the causes of which are unknown.

Ischemic myelopathy-encephalopathy

A disease process referred to as ischemic (or necrotizing) myelopathy has been described in the dog, cat, horse, pig, and lamb. Clinically, the disease is characterized by sudden onset of a spinal cord deficit and, sometimes, by cerebral involvement in certain species. In the dog, the disease tends to occur in large breeds. Morphologically, there is focal infarction of the spinal cord. All levels of the spinal cord may be affected, although lesions are often present in the cervical and lumbosacral areas. Emboli that are histochemically identical to the fibrocartilage of the nucleus pulposus of intervertebral disks are found within arteries and/or veins of the leptomeninges and parenchyma of the CNS (Fig. 8-29). In the dog, the disease, which has been associated with intervertebral disk degeneration, has been proposed to result from the forcing of fibrocartilaginous material (originating from the nucleus pulposus) into the venous and/or arterial circulation of the spinal cord, where it forms emboli that cause infarction.

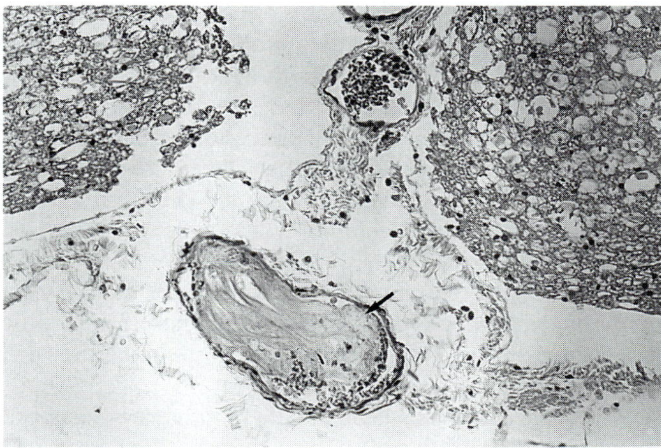

Fig. 8-29 Spinal cord, lumbar level, ventral spinal artery; dog. A fibrocartilaginous embolus *(arrow)* has caused acute infarction in the central gray matter and variable amounts of axonal degeneration in the white matter. H & E stain.

METABOLIC DISTURBANCES

Chemical Toxicities

Sodium chloride toxicity

Sodium chloride (NaCl) toxicity, also referred to as salt poisoning or **water deprivation syndrome,** occurs naturally and has been reproduced experimentally in domestic, wild, and laboratory animals, and poultry. Toxicity occurs primarily in swine (e.g., following freezing of available drinking water) and poultry but also, occasionally, in ruminants. The disease has been studied, particularly in swine. The sodium ion is the toxic principle; various sodium salts (e.g., chloride, carbonate, acetate, sulfonamide, proprionate, sulfate, lactate) can all induce the same disease.

Clinicopathologic findings in swine include an eosinopenia, concluded to be the result of stress, that persists during the course of the disease but disappears during recovery. Affected swine have elevated sodium and chloride concentrations in the blood and CSF.

In swine, gross lesions of the nervous system are not constant but can include cerebral and leptomeningeal congestion and edema. A grossly detectable zone of cerebrocortical necrosis may be evident in sliced sections of the fixed brain. Nonneural gross lesions include gastroenteritis, gastric ulceration, dilatation of the heart, dehydration, cyanosis of skin, degeneration of skeletal muscle, and hydropericardium. Gross lesions in ruminants (e.g., cattle) may be absent or may include gastroenteritis, skeletal muscular edema, and hydropericardium.

Microscopic lesions of the CNS of affected swine in the acute stages of the disease are characterized by variable perivascular accumulations of eosinophils in the cerebral leptomeninges and adjacent cortex. After about 48 hours, these cells can decrease in number or disappear and be replaced by mononuclear cells. Neuronal degeneration (ischemic cell change) occurs within the cerebral cortex, often with a laminar distribution (Fig. 8-30). This may progress to parenchymal necrosis with accumulation of macrophages (gitter cells). Vessels are prominent because of hypertrophy (swelling) and hyperplasia of endothelial cells. The staining density of the subcortical white matter may be reduced because of edema.

Microscopic lesions in ruminants include cortical laminar neuronal degeneration (ischemic cell change) and cortical arteriolar necrosis with mural neutrophilic accumulation. Other lesions are Purkinje cell degeneration (ischemic cell change) and edema of the corpus striatum, thalamus, midbrain, and centrum semiovale. Perivascular accumulation of eosinophils occurs inconsistently. Nonneural lesions include gastroenteritis and cystitis. In sheep, there is gastroenteritis with epithelial necrosis.

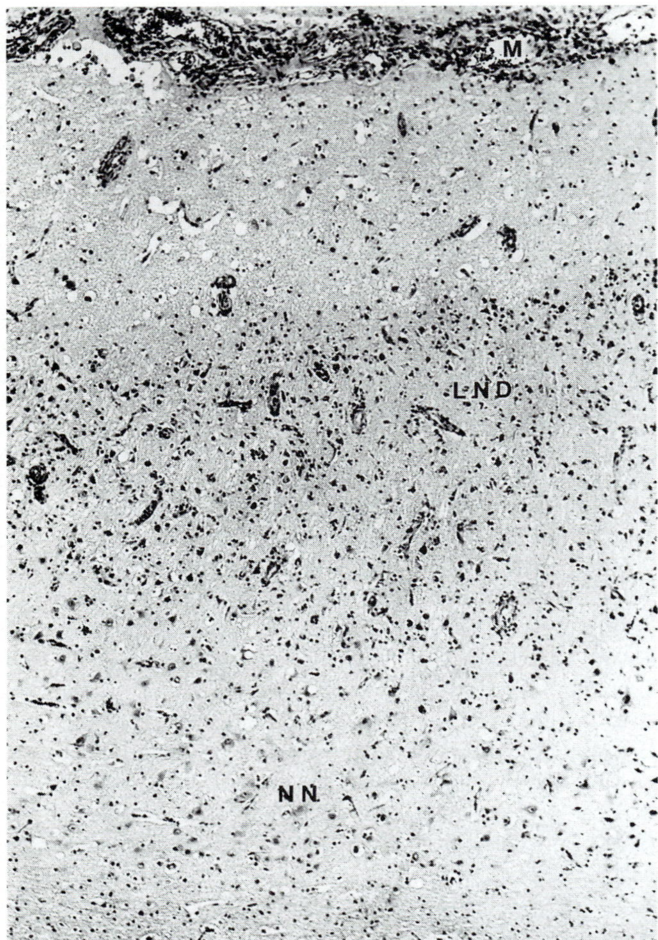

Fig. 8-30 Brain, junction of parietal and frontal lobes, cerebral cortex; pig. Sodium chloride toxicity. Meninges *(M)* are infiltrated with mononuclear cells and eosinophils. The middle of the cerebral cortex has laminar neuronal degeneration *(LND),* increased cellularity, and prominent blood vessels. Normal neurons *(NN)* are present in the lower cortex. H & E stain.

All aspects of the pathogenesis of NaCI toxicity are not known, but, in any species, two significant factors are availability of salt (usually in excess) and deprivation of water. Toxicity in swine may even occur when normal salt levels (usually 0.5% to 1%) of the ration are fed if water intake is severely restricted. However, swine may tolerate high concentrations of salt (2% to 13% of the ration) if they have free access to water.

A proposed mechanism for the disease is as follows. Following the ingestion of an abnormally high-salt diet (with some degree of water deprivation), the animal develops hypernatremia. Because of osmotic forces, interstitial, intracellular, and cerebrospinal fluid of the brain moves into the hypertonic cerebral circulation, resulting in cerebral dehydration. Brain volume can be decreased substantially in 1 hour. The equilibration of NaCl between plasma and the extracellular space of the CNS, unlike that in other tissues, is slow and coincides with the length of time (36 to 48 hours) required for pigs to develop nervous signs. Eventually, when animals are provided free access to drinking water and/or after elimination of Na through the kidneys (osmotic diuresis), the toxicity of the blood becomes reduced and then hypotonic relative to the brain, a mechanism similar to that of osmotic edema. This change can result in movement of fluid into the CNS and development of cerebral edema.

Lead toxicity

Lead poisoning in cattle (calves and adults) can be acute, subacute, or chronic. The acute form occurs more frequently. Calves are very susceptible. The disease in sheep is similar to that in cattle, and acute and chronic forms have been described in the equidae. Young dogs are more frequently affected, primarily because they have a propensity to lick and chew objects.

Lead poisoning affects the CNS, PNS, kidneys, liver, bone marrow, bone, gastrointestinal (GI) tract, blood vessels, and reproductive and endocrine systems. In cattle, acute gross lesions of the CNS include cerebral swelling with flattening of the gyri, intense meningeal congestion, occasional meningeal hemorrhage and occurrence of small malacic foci to prominent cavitation on cut surface of the cerebral cortex. Microscopically, the meninges are congested. In the cortex, there is generalized prominence of capillary endothelial cells, astrocytic swelling, status spongiosus, neuronal degeneration (ischemic cell change) that may be laminar in the cerebral cortex, accumulation of macrophages, and, in severely affected brains, liquefaction necrosis. Additional lesions include edema associated with microcavitation and swelling of glial cells in the cerebral white matter. In the equine species, paralysis of the larynx and facial muscles is compatible with a peripheral neuropathy. Lesions in dogs resemble those of cattle. In the dog, there is obvious and consistent involvement of blood vessels, which are congested and have swollen and sometimes hyperplastic endothelial cells. Other lesions are vascular degeneration with mural hyalinization, necrosis, and thrombosis; neuronal degeneration in the cerebral cortex, hippocampus, and cerebellum (Purkinje cells and various nuclei); demyelination (cerebral white matter); and peripheral neuropathy.

In animals, lead compounds enter the body orally (most common) via the respiratory tract and, when in inorganic form, through the skin. Also, ovine and human fetuses can be exposed transplacentally.

Within the nervous system, lead (1) influences neuronal function and development and (2) causes disturbances in the fluid environment by affecting the blood-brain barrier and astrocytes. Many of the biologic aberrations produced by lead appear related to its ability to alter calcium metabolism, which may involve disturbed mitochondrial function, by modulating the important role of calcium in influencing the release of neurotransmitters from presynaptic nerve endings. This disruption of neuronal activity may adversely affect synaptic function and development, particularly during brain development, and result in various CNS dysfunctions (including cognition in the human).

In acute lead encephalopathy, vasogenic edema resulting from breakdown in the function of cerebral microvasculature produces increased intracranial pressure. When the pressure approaches that of the systemic blood pressure, cerebral perfusion decreases, resulting in cerebral ischemia that may contribute to the neuronal degeneration (ischemic cell change). This disturbance of the blood-brain barrier is thought to result from direct and indirect effects of the toxicity. Lead may directly affect the blood-brain barrier by affecting development (in young animals) and function of endothelial cells, and it may cause injury indirectly by affecting astrocytes that are responsible for the induction and maintenance of the barrier. Lead also can disrupt heme synthesis and thus, possibly, mitochondrial function that could affect energy metabolism, which could result in injury of the blood-brain barrier.

Arsenic poisoning

Arsenic poisoning can result from exposure to harmful concentrations of either inorganic or organic arsenic compounds, which, in general, cause different signs and lesions. Inorganic compounds (e.g., arsenic trioxide, sodium arsenite) are usually associated with signs and lesions referable to the GI tract, liver, kidneys, lungs, and skin, although trembling, stupor, and partial paralysis of the rear limbs have also been reported. Lesions of the CNS and PNS occur with both the acute and chronic toxicities in human beings.

Organic phenylarsonic compounds (the focus of the present discussion) have been used as feed additives to improve weight gain and feed efficiency and to aid in the prevention and control of certain enteric diseases of swine and poultry. Arsanilic acid (or its salt, sodium arsanilate) and 3-nitro-4-hydroxyphenylarsonic acid (3-nitro or roxarsone) have been widely used. Others include 4-nitrophenylarsonic acid (nitarsone) and *p*-ureidobenzenearsonic acid (carbarsone). Toxicity (especially in swine) can be due to accidental overdose from inaccurate preparation of diets, prolonged and excessive administration of these compounds in combination with other drugs, administration to animals with abnormal renal (excretory) function, and restriction of water supply.

Lesions and clinical signs of arsanilic acid and 3-nitro toxicity in swine are not the same, and the two should be considered separately. No gross lesions of the nervous system are detectable following arsanilic acid poisoning. Nonneural lesions include erythema of the skin (e.g., in white pigs). Microscopically, lesions are consistently detected chronologically in the optic nerves, optic tracts, and peripheral nerves (e.g., sciatic nerve and brachial plexus). The basic lesion, which can occur after feeding of arsanilic acid for only a few days (e.g., 4 to 10 days), includes fragmentation of myelin sheaths followed several days later by axonal degeneration. Except for hyperemia of the skin, lesions do not appear to occur in nonneural organs of swine, but, in lambs, renal lesions have been reported.

No significant gross lesions of the nervous system are detectable in swine following 3-nitro poisoning, but similar to signs of arsanilic acid toxicity, integumentary erythema may also occur. Microscopic lesions are largely confined to the spinal cord, although variable changes have also been reported in the peripheral nerves and optic nerve and tracts. Spinal cord lesions, which occur at the cervical and thoracic levels and later in the lumbar area, consist of destruction of myelin sheaths, axonal degeneration, and status spongiosus with little cellular reaction. The distribution of lesions suggests that the distal ends of the long ascending fibers of the fasciculi gracilis and cuneatus are preferentially injured. Peripheral neuropathy, characterized by myelin and axonal degeneration, occurs infrequently in nerves (e.g., radial and sciatic).

The exact mode of action of the organic arsenicals is unclear. However, phenylarsonic compounds may have a different action than inorganic arsenics, which inhibit sulfhydryl enzyme systems essential to cellular metabolism.

Mercury poisoning

Acute inorganic mercury poisoning is characterized by injury to the GI tract, renal tubules, and respiratory tract (following inhalation exposure), whereas chronic inorganic mercury poisoning can be neurotoxic. Organic mercury poisoning, particularly the short-chain alkylmercury compounds that are the most toxic, can cause lesions of the CNS, PNS, digestive system (including the liver, esophagus, and intestine), and urinary tract. This discussion will focus on organomercury toxicity.

Organomercury poisoning of animals is frequently associated with the ingestion of seed grain treated with alkylmercury compounds (particularly methylmercury and ethylmercury compounds) used as fungicides. Swine and cattle are most frequently affected. Cats, because of their fish-eating habits, may become poisoned where high concentrations of mercury (primarily the alkylmercury compound methylmercury) occur in fish.

Lesions induced by alkylmercury compounds vary somewhat among species. In swine, there may be pronounced atrophy of the cerebral hemispheres with a marked reduction in size of gyri and widened sulci. Grossly, the surface of the affected cortex is granular, and it is reduced in thickness. Focal malacia (necrosis) in the caudate nucleus and adjoining internal capsule and hyperemia of leptomeningeal vessels may also occur. Nonneural lesions can involve the GI tract (suppurative to necrotic pharyngitis and esophagitis; ulcerative, hemorrhagic gastritis; hepatic mottling; focal necrosis of cecal and colonic mucosa); presence of serous and serofibrinous fluid in the pleural and pericardial cavities and fibrinous pericarditis; serous atrophy of epicardial fat; and pulmonary congestion. Microscopically, there is a laminar cerebrocortical neuronal degeneration (ischemic cell change) with axonal degeneration in both the gray and white matter. Neuronal degeneration may also occur in the brain stem (extending rostral to the level of the thalamus) and is minimal in the granule cell layer of the cerebellum. Other lesions are astrocytosis or astrocytic degeneration, microgliosis, and, sometimes, prominent lymphocytic cuffing of vessels. Characteristic vascular lesions, particularly in the leptomeninges, are proliferation of the tunica adventitia; thickening of the tunica intima; reduplication, thickening, or fragmentation of the tunica elastica interna; and fibrinoid necrosis that may be accompanied by thrombosis (see Fig. 8-21). The initial neural degeneration is probably the result of a direct effect of mercury, but ischemia secondary to the vascular lesions is a contributing factor. In the spinal cord and peripheral ganglia (e.g., dorsal root and trigeminal) there is also neuronal degeneration, and axonal degeneration occurs in spinal nerves. Nonneural microscopic lesions are compatible with gross lesions in the esophagus, stomach, cecum, and colon. Also, degeneration of proximal convoluted tubules (consisting of random cell necrosis and moderate hydropic degeneration) occurs in the kidney.

Lesions in other species are similar to those described for swine, but there are specific differences. Gross lesions of cerebrocortical atrophy have been reported in the dog but not in the cow or cat. Some differences in microscopic lesions include degeneration and loss of granule and Purkinje cells in the cerebellar cortex in the bovine and feline species. Vascular degeneration appears to occur most prominently in swine, cattle, and dogs. Meningitis occurs in cattle and dogs. Lesions of peripheral nerves are not generally reported in domestic animals other than swine. Nonneural lesions include degeneration of myocardial and Purkinje fibers of the heart and myofibers of skeletal muscle in cattle.

Several specific effects of alkyl organomercury compounds (e.g., methylmercury) have been proposed. Probably the best known is inhibition of protein synthesis (resulting from destruction of ribosomes and rough endoplasmic reticulum), which may be the first alteration to occur. This inhibitory effect may explain a greater susceptibility of smaller neurons (e.g., granule cells of the cerebellar cortex) in certain animals and humans, because of their low ribosomal content. Methylmercury has also been reported to impair the integrity of the blood-brain barrier (probably as a result of injury to cell membranes of endothelial cells), which may be a factor in the development of fibrinoid necrosis of vessels. Vascular lesions, sometimes accompanied by thrombosis, may also lead to ischemia that produces secondary lesions in the CNS. Other disturbances attributed to methylmercury compounds include (1) nuclear injury associated with inhibition of DNA synthesis and chromosomal disturbances, (2) disruption of enzyme systems and destruction of mitochondria, (3) breakdown of biologic membranes, (4) injury to the developing nervous system due to alteration in cell division and migration, and (5) depolymerization of intracellular microtubules (which are essential for cell division).

Organophosphate poisoning

Organophosphorus compounds are commonly used as pesticides (i.e., insecticides) to control parasites on plants and animals. Such compounds are also used as fungicides, herbicides, and rodenticides.

Organophosphates can be divided into two main groups according to their mechanism of action and the type of disease produced. In the first group (typical of most organophosphorus esters), acute clinical disease is produced by inhibition of acetylcholinesterase either directly or indirectly, and clinical signs result from the abnormal accumulation of endogenous acetylcholine at synapses (or nerve-tissue junctions).

These signs vary with the type of animal affected. Domestic food-producing animals may be hyperactive, reflecting excessive stimulation of the CNS, but they rarely convulse. More commonly, severe CNS depression occurs. In small animals, such as dogs and cats, hyperstimulation of the CNS may progress to convulsive seizures, but extreme CNS depression is also common. The immediate cause of death following acute organophosphate poisoning is asphyxia, resulting from respiratory failure associated with bronchoconstriction, increased bronchial secretions, paralysis of respiratory muscles, and depression of the respiratory center. Lesions include bronchoconstriction, pulmonary edema, emphysema, atelectasis, and generalized hyperemia and congestion of tissues.

A second group of compounds, cresyl and related phosphates, cause a different clinical entity known as delayed neurotoxicity, which results from a toxic effect not related to inhibition of acetylcholinesterase. Triorthocresyl phosphate (a cresyl phosphate) is well known to be toxic for humans. Cresyl and related phosphates are components of hydraulic fluids, lubricants, plasticizers, and flame retardants. Toxicity produced by the triaryl phosphate group (used as a high-temperature lubricant and containing triorthocresyl phosphate and other organophosphate compounds) is toxic for several species of animals and humans. Signs of neurotoxicity are characteristically delayed until 1 to 2 weeks following exposure. Young animals tend to be more resistant to the effects of the toxicity because of their ability to compensate more quickly than adults, in which recovery may be slow and incomplete. Species also differ in susceptibility. Susceptible animals include cats, cattle, lambs, adult sheep, goats, water buffalo, chickens, pheasants, and ducks (mallard). Rats, mice, hamsters, gerbils, guinea pigs, rabbits, dogs, and some nonhuman primates are less sensitive.

No specific gross lesions occur with this form of neurotoxicity, but microscopic lesions are characterized initially by a distal axonopathy of both sensory and motor peripheral axons or processes, particularly ones of large diameter. This type of degeneration has been concluded to be of the dying-back type, which is typified by axonal injury extending from the periphery back toward the cell body. This lesion is accompanied by an alteration of calcium homeostasis that results in aggregation and accumulation of tubulin, neurofilaments, and neurotubules, plus proliferation of smooth endoplasmic reticulum. The nerve cell bodies of affected nerves may have central chromatolysis. Axonal degeneration of the distal parts of ascending and descending tracts in the spinal cord also occurs.

It has been demonstrated that organophosphorus compounds causing delayed neurotoxicity have the ability to inhibit the activity of a target enzyme (referred to as **neuropathy target esterase** or **neurotoxic esterase**) in the CNS and PNS whose normal function is not fully understood. It has been proposed that toxic compounds phosphorylate this enzyme and cause its inhibition and that the neural dysfunction results from the effect of the altered target esterase molecule. Recent studies have shown that organophosphorus compounds causing delayed neurotoxicity interact with Ca_2^+/calmodulin kinase II, an enzyme responsible for the endogenous phosphorylation of cytoskeletal proteins (i.e., microtubules, neurofilaments, and microtubule associated protein-2), which eventually results in the disassembly of these proteins that accumulate in the distal portions of the axon. This change is accompanied by axonal swelling and degeneration.

Plant Toxicities

Astragalus, Oxytropis, *and* Swainsona *poisoning*

Astragalus, Oxytropis, and *Swainsona* represent three groups of plants with species that are toxic for livestock. As many as 300 species of *Astragalus* may grow in North America, and the genus is the largest of any legume family in this part of the world. The toxic species of *Astragalus* can be divided into three general categories according to the manner in which they produce their effect. They can be nitro-containing, selenium-accumulating, or of the locoweed type. Only the last group is discussed here. Locoweed poisoning is associated with ingestion of plants belonging to the genera *Astragalus* and *Oxytropis,* considered together here because of their similar actions. Cattle, sheep, and horses are generally affected. The toxicity is generally insidious; signs of poisoning do not occur until an animal has grazed the plant for 14 to 60 days. *Swainsona,* which grows in Australia, like locoweed, produces swainsonine.

There are no significant gross lesions. Microscopically, affected cells are enlarged, often have peripherally displaced nuclei, and have a cytoplasm that appears finely vacuolated (see Fig. 8-15 for comparable lesion). Lesions occur in both central nervous and nonnervous tissues, and neurons throughout the brain and spinal cord are affected. The material that accumulates in the cytoplasm of affected cells does not stain for lipid. In advanced stages, there is death of neurons with subsequent mineralization of cellular remnants. Meganeurite formation (enlargement of proximal axon) and distal axonopathy can be present. Other lesions include mild microgliosis and neuronophagia, vacuolation of neuroglia, and swelling of axons and astrocytic foot processes surrounding blood vessels.

The cytoplasmic change is also detectable in neurons outside the CNS: in the retina and autonomic ganglia of the digestive tract, kidney (proximal convoluted tubules), liver, spleen (reticuloendothelial cells), lymph nodes (reticuloendothelial cells), endocrine glands (adrenal, thyroid, parathyroid), urinary bladder (epithelium), pancreas (acinar cells), placenta, fetus, and circulating lymphocytes and monocytes. Peripheral nerves are not affected.

The mechanism of toxicity has been clarified by the isolation of the indolizidine alkaloids swainsonine and swainsonine N-oxide from *Astragalus lentiginosus.* Both of these compounds inhibit lysosomal α-mannosidase and thus are responsible for the induction of an acquired storage disease (α-mannosidosis) that affects both the nervous and nonnervous tissues and mimics the genetically determined disease (see Lysosomal Storage Disease). In addition, swainsonine interferes with normal synthesis of glycoproteins that contain asparagine-linked complex oligosaccharides. Swainsonine inhibits Golgi mannosidase II, which results in the production of hybrid glycoproteins. The activity of Golgi-apparatus mannosidase II is not known to be affected in inherited α-mannosidosis.

Bacterial Toxins

Encephalopathy associated with Clostridium perfringens *type D enterotoxemia in sheep (pulpy kidney disease, overeating disease)*

C. perfringens type D enterotoxemia, which is associated with epsilon toxin production and, often, with acute death, occurs in sheep throughout the world. Sheep of all ages except newborns are susceptible, and isolated cases have also been reported inoats and calves. Affected sheep are usually on highly nutritious diets and are in very good condition. The highest incidence of the disease is in suckling lambs between 3 and 10 weeks of age and in feeder lambs, soon after being introduced into a feedlot. Neonatal animals are generally considered to be nonsusceptible to the disease; possibly because the proteolytic enzymes necessary for activation of the epsilon toxin are not available in adequate amounts from the pancreas at this age. Also, trypsin inhibitors in the colostrum may provide protection.

Typical gross lesions occur in the internal capsule of the neostriatum, corpus striatum, thalamus, hippocampus, mid-

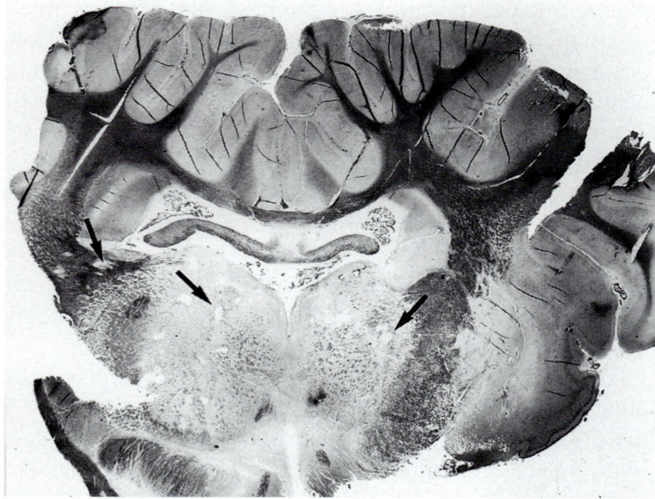

Fig. 8-31 Brain, parietal lobe, level of thalamus; feeder lamb. *Clostridium perfringens* type D enterotoxemia, acute stage of the disease process. Focal edema and necrosis *(arrows)* are present in the thalamus and adjacent white matter (optic radiation and internal capsule). H & E stain.

brain (rostral colliculus and substantia nigra), cerebellar peduncles (especially the middle cerebellar peduncle) or pons, and the white matter of the gyri of the frontal cortex (Fig. 8-31). Lesions are focal, bilaterally symmetrical, vary from yellow-gray to hemorrhagic, and, in advanced stages, have a soft consistency (malacia). Other typical but nonnervous tissue lesions include pulmonary congestion and edema, excess fluid (serofibrinous) in the pericardial sac, petechiation (e.g., of the thymus, epicardium, and endocardium), and pulpy (soft) kidneys.

Microscopically, acute lesions are characterized by perivascular and intercellular edema, which has been proposed to be responsible for the neurologic signs characteristic of the disease (see Fig. 8-22). The edema fluid surrounding blood vessels is frequently rich in protein and stains eosinophilically. Walls of severely affected arterioles are hyalinized. Endothelial cells are occasionally swollen and hypochromatic. Vasogenic (extracellular) edema may cause the neuropil to have a light to pink-stained, spongy appearance. Both the white and gray matter may be affected, but changes are more pronounced in the white matter. There is also pericapillary hemorrhage and degeneration of neurons and neuroglia. As the lesions age, other changes may include mild to moderate accumulation of neutrophils, axonal swelling, accumulation of macrophages (gitter cells), increased prominence of blood vessels (caused by hypertrophy and hyperplasia of endothelium and perithelial cells), occasional lymphoplasmacytic cuffing, and liquefaction necrosis.

Ultrastructural and vascular permeability studies have indicated that lesion development in affected tissues (CNS and non-CNS) involves a binding of epsilon toxin to endothelial surface receptors, resulting in their injury. This is followed by opening of vascular tight junctions (in the CNS), which leads to perivascular and parenchymal edema, swelling of astrocytic processes, and necrosis. Epsilon toxin also has been proposed to increase the permeability of vascular endothelial cells through a mechanism mediated by an adenylcyclase-cAMP system. Necrosis of tissue is due to hypoxia-anoxia.

Enterotoxemic colibacillosis (edema disease) of swine

Typically, edema disease occurs in rapidly growing, healthy pigs receiving nutritious rations producing good growth rates. Affected animals are usually 4 to 8 weeks of age, as the disease usually occurs 1 to 2 weeks after weaning. Most affected pigs die within 24 hours. Animals that develop characteristic CNS lesions (including malacia) generally survive for several days (see the chronologic sequence of infarction, Table 8-2).

The basic lesion in all affected tissues is an angiopathy that is responsible for the other lesions that occur. Grossly, nonneural lesions include accumulation of fluid, particularly in the subcutis, gastric cardial submucosa, gallbladder, mesentery of large intestine, mesenteric lymph nodes, lung, larynx, thorax, and pericardial sac. Hyperemia and, sometimes, hemorrhage may also occur. The characteristic gross lesion of the CNS is necrosis, which is bilaterally symmetrical in the brain stem but may extend rostrally to the level of the caudate nucleus. Lesions are yellow-gray and slightly depressed on the cut surface. Sometimes malacia is almost continuous from the medulla through the caudate nucleus; in other animals, the lesions involve only portions of the brain stem.

The primary microscopic lesion is a degenerative angiopathy, which occurs most frequently and severely in the brain stem (rostrally to the level of the diencephalon) and in cerebral and cerebellar meninges. The lesion is less frequent in the cerebrum, spinal cord, and cerebellum. Initially, there is perivascular edema resulting from early vascular injury. This is followed by necrosis of smooth-muscle cells of the tunica media, which then undergoes fibrinoid necrosis, followed by accumulation of inflammatory cells (macrophages, lymphocytes) in the tunica adventitia (Fig. 8-32). Although endothelial cells and their nuclei become altered and swollen, this layer generally remains essentially intact, and, consequently, thrombosis is not a prominent feature. Therefore, focal necrosis is the result of injury to the vessel itself.

Although *Escherichia coli* is generally accepted as being the cause of edema disease, the exact mechanism by which it participates is still not fully understood. There is good evidence that edema disease is an enterotoxemic colibacillosis in which *E. coli* located in the intestine releases a biologically active substance that is absorbed into the blood and acts elsewhere in the body. It has been proposed that, under certain circumstances, specific serotypes of the organism colonize and proliferate in the small intestine and release a biologically active substance that until recently

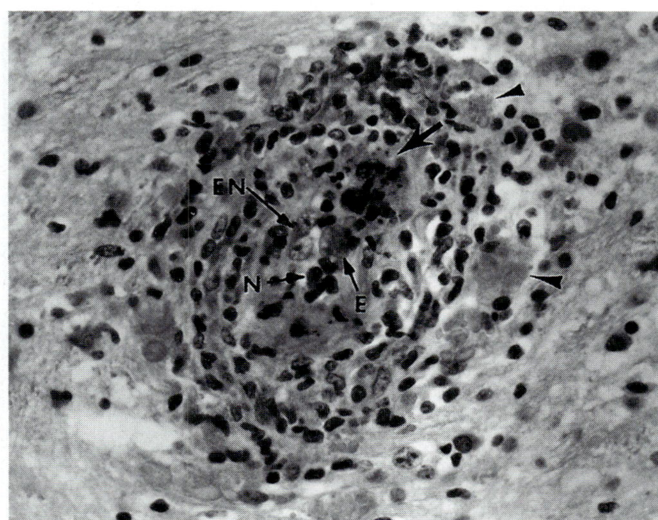

Fig. 8-32 Brain, medulla oblongata; pig. Enterotoxemia (edema disease). There is cerebral vascular necrosis and inflammation with inflammatory cells within, and surrounding, the vessel wall. Also, note the fragmentation of cells within the vessel wall *(thick arrow)* and focal accumulation of edema fluid and fragmented erthrocytes adjacent to the vessel *(arrowheads).* The lumen of the vessel contains a clump of erythrocytes (*E*) and a neutrophil (*N*) and is lined by endothelial cells with enlarged nuclei *(EN).* H & E stain.

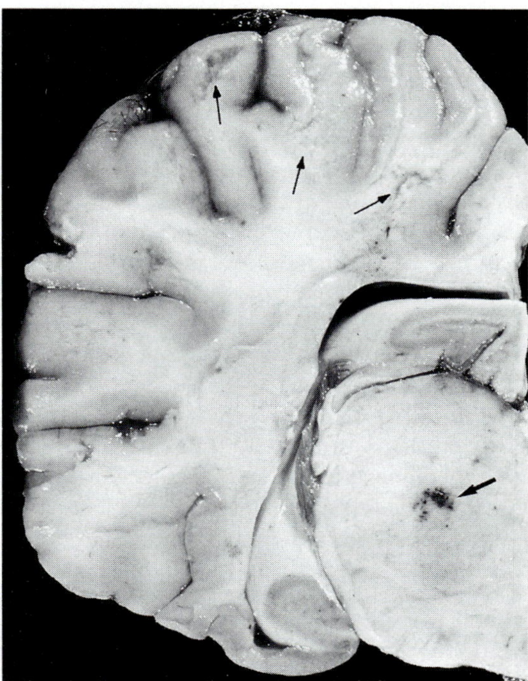

Fig. 8-33 Brain, rostral occipital lobe, level of thalamus; horse. *Fusarium moniliforme*–induced encephalopathy (equine leukoencephalomalacia). There is focal liquefaction necrosis of the cerebral white matter *(thin arrows).* See Fig. 8-20 for illustration of microscopic lesion. There is also focal hemorrhage in the thalamus *(thick arrow).*

was referred to as edema disease principle (EDP), which, following absorption, injures small arteries and arterioles. The substance is now known to be a shiga-like toxin (because of its close similarity to the toxin produced by shigella dysenteriae) and has been specifically designated shiga-like toxin type II variant (SLT-IIv).

Mycotoxins

Fusarium moniliforme–*induced encephalopathy (equine leukoencephalomalacia, moldy corn poisoning)*

F. moniliforme–induced encephalopathy of the horse is an encephalomalacia primarily affecting the cerebral white matter following the ingestion of moldy corn, corn stalks, fodder, or pelleted or nonpelleted feed that is contaminated. Signs of disease develop in less than 2 to several weeks after initial consumption. The clinical course, that often ends in death, ranges in duration from a few hours to several days, with an average of approximately 72 hours.

The characteristic gross lesion is liquefaction necrosis of the cerebral white matter (centrum semiovale) that may be bilateral but not necessarily symmetrical (Fig. 8-33). The cortex over a large lesion may be soft and edematous, and gyri are flattened. The underlying white matter varies in consistency from soft to gelatinous to cystic and ranges in color from gray-yellow to yellow-orange. Varying degrees of hemorrhage and edema are also present in and surrounding the lesion. Lesions may involve white matter of the frontal lobe (possibly most frequently affected) and of the temporal and occipital lobes of one or both hemispheres. Sometimes lesions also occur at the junction of the gray and white matter. Other grossly detectable changes include leptomeningeal edema; cerebrocortical edema, hemorrhage, and necrosis; edema and petechiation of the cerebellar cortex; and focal areas of discoloration or hemorrhage in the hippocampus, medial geniculate body, caudal colliculus, and medulla. The spinal cord may have comparable lesions.

Microscopically, affected cerebral white matter is coagulated or liquefied, depending on the age of the lesion, and has edema, scattered neutrophils, and macrophages (some being gitter cells). The lesion is surrounded by diffuse and/or perivascular edema, perivascular hemorrhage, and variable perivascular cuffing; diffuse cellular accumulation (macrophages, plasma cells, eosinophils); and microgliosis. Vessels in affected areas are degenerated and contain varying numbers of neutrophils, plasma cells, and eosinophils in their walls. Although not often emphasized, thrombosis may also occur. Less characteristic lesions include focal edema and perivascular cuffing in the leptomeninges; focal neuronal degeneration (deeper laminae) to full-thickness necrosis of the cerebral cortex; and hemorrhage, edema, and degeneration in the cerebellar molecular layer, thalamus, hippocampus, and brain stem.

Similar lesions have been reported in the spinal cord, where they occur primarily in the gray matter.

Nonneural lesions are hepatic enlargement and congestion (with mild inflammation and epithelial degeneration), swelling and congestion of the kidney (with early tubular degeneration), hemorrhage and inflammation of the urinary bladder, and hemorrhagic and erosive enteritis.

Recently, it has become clear that this disease in the horse can involve a second process, referred to as the **hepatotoxic syndrome,** which may or may not accompany the neurologic form of the disease. The type of disease that occurs is dose-dependent, with both syndromes being different manifestations of the same toxicity.

F. moniliforme produces a specific toxin, fumonisin B_1, that has been demonstrated experimentally to cause both the cerebral and hepatic lesions. The mechanisms involved in initiating tissue injury are not totally understood, but the initial event appears to be vascular injury that often results in prominent tissue necrosis in the CNS.

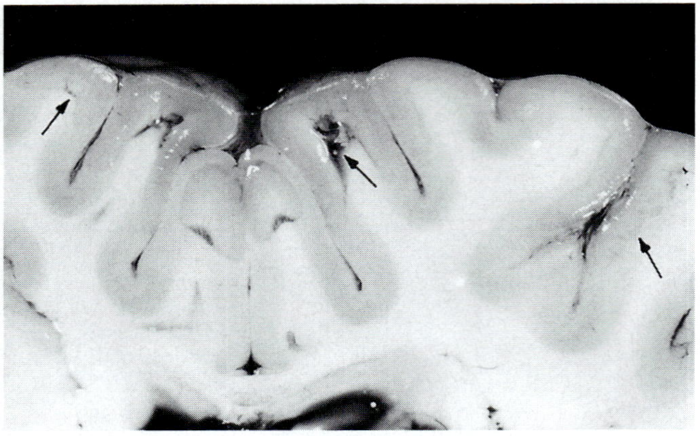

Fig. 8-34 Brain, parietal lobe, level of thalamus; goat. Thiamine deficiency. Cerebrocortical liquefaction necrosis with varying degrees of tissue separation *(arrows).*

Nutritional Deficiencies

Bovine cerebrocortical necrosis (polioencephalomalacia)

Thiamine deficiency in ruminants (cattle, sheep) was first described by Jensen and co-workers in 1956 and designated polioencephalomalacia. The disease has since been recognized in the goat. First noted in Colorado in the United States, the disease occurs in both cattle and sheep at pasture, or, more frequently, when animals are fed primarily concentrate diets. Most ovine cases occur in younger age groups (e.g., 2 to 7 months); for cattle, the most common age range is 6 to 18 months.

Grossly, affected brains are swollen due to edema, which may result in flattening of the cerebral gyri and herniation of the caudal cerebrum beneath the tentorium cerebelli and caudal cerebellum through the foramen magnum. Cerebrocortical lesions range from a slight yellow discoloration (during early stages when distribution of the lesion can be appreciated by its autofluorescence under ultraviolet light) to necrosis (characterized by altered consistency and coloration with liquefaction after 8 to 10 days) (Fig. 8-34). Brains from animals that survived for a longer period of time are reduced in size and have areas that are almost (or totally) devoid of cortex, when only a thin layer of cortex or leptomeninges makes direct contact with the white matter (Fig. 8-35).

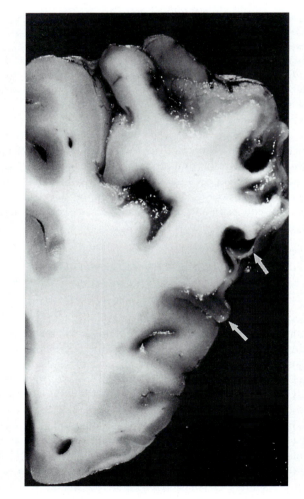

Fig. 8-35 Brain, cerebral cortex of right frontal lobe; steer. Thiamine deficiency. Advanced cerebrocortical necrosis (*upper* and *middle right*) has resulted in only a remnant of outer cortex remaining *(arrows).*

Microscopically, during early lesion development, the cortex has cortical neuronal degeneration (often laminar in distribution) characterized by ischemic cell change. Also, there is variable status spongiosus of both the cortex and the immediately subjacent white matter. Endothelial and perithelial cells of existing capillaries hypertrophy within affected and adjacent tissue, and a few lymphocytes, monocytes, plasma cells, and erythrocytes may be present in the perivascular spaces. In the meninges, particularly over affected parts of the cortex, the vessels are frequently congested, and there is moderate accumulation of lymphocytes, monocytes, plasma cells, and, occasionally, a few neutrophils. With time (after 8 to 10 days), there is liquefaction necrosis of the affected cerebral cortex with eventual removal of necrotic cortical tissue by phagocytes (gitter cells). Additional focal lesions may occur in the cerebellum, midbrain (e.g., colliculi), thalamus, hippocampus, and caudate nucleus.

Polioencephalomalacia has been associated with a disturbance in thiamine metabolism, but the exact basic mechanism involved remains to be clarified. Thiamine has an important function in metabolism of the brain, and is critical for normal glucose metabolism in the nervous system. Possible mechanisms for disturbed thiamine metabolism include inactivation of the vitamin by thiaminase I produced by bacteria in the rumen (e.g., *Clostridium sporogenes* and *Bacillus thiaminolyticus*), production or ingestion of inactive thiamine analogs, ingestion of thiaminases such as bracken fern rhizosomes, impaired absorption or phosphorylation of thiamine, increased fecal excretion of thiamine, and decreased ruminal production of thiamine diphosphate. Diets high in concentrate, which are often associated with this disease, have been suggested to cause a reduction of thiamine in the rumen by reducing the number of microorganisms that synthesize thiamine, as well as by permitting an increase in bacteria that produce thiaminase I. Also, the associated decrease in ruminal pH is near the optimum for activity of bacterial thiaminase I, and histamines accumulate to become a potent cosubstrate for activity of the enzyme. In addition, use of the coccidiostat amprolium and the anthelmintics thiabendazole and levamisole hydrochloride may exacerbate the deficiency.

A proposed, less direct mechanism for development of the cerebrocortical lesion in ruminants is that a thiamine deficiency indirectly causes cerebral swelling by altering function of the Krebs cycle, which is an important pathway for production of ATP that supplies energy for regulation of sodium and water transport mechanisms. It is proposed that intracellular edema results in increased intracranial pressure, which causes reduction in cerebral blood flow, resulting in development of laminar cortical necrosis and polioencephalomalacia.

In recent years, there has been evidence that sulfur-containing diets can also produce a similar cerebrocortical necrosis in the ruminant. High sulfate concentrations in drinking water, consumption of a sulfate-accumulating plant *(Kochia scoparia),* and diets in which sulfate salts or sulfur dioxide was an added ingredient have been incriminated. Hydrogen sulfide production has been proposed as being responsible for producing lesions. Reports that thiamine concentration in the blood, CSF, brain, and liver are not abnormal indicate that a mechanism other than a direct thiamine deficiency (i.e., a sulfide toxicosis) may be involved.

Thiamine deficiency of nonruminants (monogastrics such as the dog, cat, fox, and mink) that depend on exogenous sources of the vitamin can result from the feeding of diets (e.g., fish) that contain thiaminase or ones that are low in the vitamin (e.g., due to heating or incorporation of sulphur dioxide as a preservative). The distribution of gross lesions is somewhat different from that in ruminants and may extend from the medulla to the cerebral hemispheres, including the cortex. Lesions are symmetrical and primarily affect the gray matter, although white matter can be involved. The caudal colliculus is characteristically affected, although there is, in general, some preferential involvement of the periventricular gray matter. Microscopic lesions include status spongiosus (edema), neuronal degeneration, degeneration of myelin, rare axonal degeneration, reduced density of the neuropil, hypertrophy and hyperplasia of endothelial and adventitial cells, and hemorrhage (variable according to species). In advanced lesions, there is fragmentation and edema of the neuropil, with presence of macrophages (gitter cells). Other changes include variable astrocytosis. Margins between affected and normal tissue are distinct. In nonneural tissues, focal myocardial necrosis may also occur in the dog and fox.

Copper deficiency (swayback-enzootic ataxia)

Swayback-enzootic ataxia, which primarily affects sheep (lambs), but also goats (kids), is associated with a nutritional copper deficiency. Ataxia, paresis, and paralysis accompanied by lesions in the spinal cord similar to those that occur in sheep and goats have also been reported in copper-deficient swine.

Swayback-enzootic ataxia has been associated with a simple or conditioned deficiency of copper, the latter involving one or more factors (such as availability of excess molybdenum and sulfate) that participate in inducing the deficiency. The disease manifests in two ways. The congenital (or neonatal) form, which is characterized by lesions in the cerebral hemispheres, affects animals at birth. In comparison, animals with the delayed form have lesions in the brain stem and spinal cord and appear normal at birth. Such animals develop signs from about 1 week to 6 months of age.

The lesions of swayback-enzootic ataxia do not routinely involve the cerebral hemispheres, but are regularly detected in the brain stem and spinal cord. Gross lesions, which are essentially limited to the cerebral hemispheres, occur in lambs with the congenital (or neonatal) form of the disease and can be detected from birth up to 3 weeks of age, but rarely after 8 weeks. The lesions are characterized by cavitation of the centrum semiovale (hydranencephaly), which often contains clear serous fluid resembling normal CSF. There is almost complete absence of white matter, with a thin overlying layer of cortex. In less severe lesions, the subcortical white matter is gelatinous and translucent, revealing (on close inspection) a lacy meshwork of interconnecting trabeculae of residual fibers.

Lesser lesions are confined to the subcortical white matter near the tips of the gyri and consist of either tiny, focal, gelatinous softenings or microcavitations that are occasionally collapsed and slitlike. In some instances, there is only a graying of the white matter with an indistinct demarcation from the gray substance. In addition, there may be dilatation of the lateral ventricles (hydrocephalus ex vacuo) due to the reduced resistance associated with the parenchymal cavitation when it occurs. The lesions are often bilaterally symmetrical and involve white matter from frontal to occipital lobes.

Microscopically, the large cavities of the cerebral white matter are sometimes lined by tissue composed of fibrous glia and nerve fibers, although astrogliosis, as indicated by astroglial scar formation, is infrequently observed. The gelatinous areas consist of a loose glial network with a very fluid matrix in which varying numbers of nerve fibers, many without myelin sheaths, are present. Definitive microscopic lesions in the cerebellum are described by most researchers as either absent or minimal, although they have been reported. With the delayed form, characteristic lesions in the brain stem and spinal cord occur regularly and involve neurons and myelinated axons. Large multipolar neurons of the brain stem and ventral, lateral, and (less frequently) dorsal horns of the spinal cord have mild to prominent central chromatolysis (accompanied by an increased accumulation of cytoplasmic neurofilaments) to acute necrosis (Fig. 8-36). Degeneration of myelinated axons in the brain stem has a rather scattered distribution rostrally, whereas caudally the lesion occurs in recognizable tracts. In the spinal cord, axonal degeneration occurs in the dorsolateral and (less frequently) ventral aspects of the lateral funiculi and in the medial to ventromedial aspects of the ventral funiculi (Fig. 8-37). Such lesions also occur infrequently in the medial (septomarginal) aspect of the dorsal funiculi.

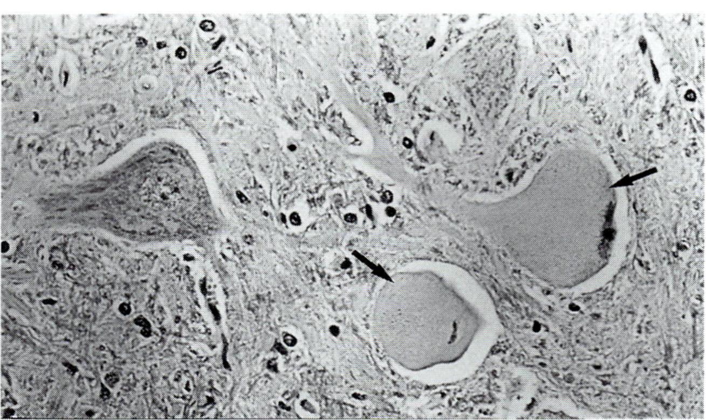

Fig. 8-36 Spinal cord, cervical level; kid. Swayback-enzootic ataxia. Central chromatolysis is present in two motor neurons *(arrows)* of the ventral horn. The other neuron is normal. H & E stain. *Courtesy Dr. R.A. Fiske.*

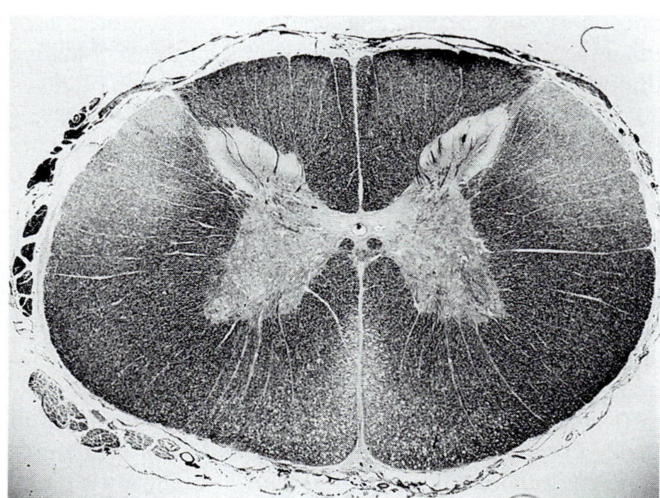

Fig. 8-37 Spinal cord, cervical level; kid. Swayback-enzootic ataxia. Reduction in myelin and axonal degeneration are in the dorsal aspect of lateral funiculi and ventromedial part of the ventral funiculi. Luxol fast blue stain for myelin. *Courtesy Dr. R.A. Fiske.*

Signs and lesions of swayback-enzootic ataxia in kids are similar to those of lambs, except that lesions (gross or microscopic) of the cerebrum are generally not reported, and the cerebellum is more frequently affected, with the primary change being cortical hypoplasia. Variable axonal degeneration of ventral spinal roots and peripheral nerves also may occur.

The mechanism(s) involved in the development of lesions associated with this disease remain(s) incompletely explained. The cerebral lesion has been suggested to result from a loss of immature cells at an appropriate period of gestation, similar to the mechanism involved in the induction of hydranencephaly following viral infection, or to involve a neurodysgenesis resulting from a biochemical disturbance. Axonal degeneration, induced by a deficiency of the copper-containing enzyme cytochrome oxidase could, therefore, possibly occur early in development and affect normal cerebral formation. Likewise, axonal degeneration in the brain stem and spinal cord may occur during a later stage of development from the same cause. Axonal degeneration has been proposed to initially occur distally and be followed by central chromatolysis and degeneration of neuronal cell bodies. Other suggested mechanisms that might be involved in the brain stem and/or spinal cord lesions are that low copper concentrations may result in altered chemical stability of myelin followed by degeneration (brain stem–spinal cord), and that a function of copper may be to protect lipids of myelin from peroxidation by circulating molecular oxygen (spinal cord).

DISORDERS OF MYELIN FORMATION AND MAINTENANCE

Terminology

Disorders of myelin formation include hypomyelinogenesis and dysmyelination. Hypomyelinogenesis (hypomyelination) is a process in which there is underdevelopment of myelin. Dysmyelination refers to the abnormal formation of myelin which may be chemically defective. Demyelination, which means degeneration and loss of myelin already formed, can be divided into primary and secondary types. Primary demyelination, which will be the type discussed in this section unless otherwise indicated, refers to a disease process in which the myelin sheath is relatively selectively affected, with the axon remaining essentially intact. Secondary demyelination, a designation criticized by some, refers to a process in which degeneration of myelin occurs along with injury to the axon, as in Wallerian degeneration, and is not a selective injury of the myelin sheath.

Hereditary Diseases

Hypomyelinogenesis and dysmyelination

Most diseases characterized by hypomyelinogenesis and dysmyelination occur in the early postnatal period and have similar clinical and pathologic features, although there are some differences in their lesions and the mechanisms by which they develop. Some diseases that occur in domestic animals are outlined in Table 8-3.

Globoid cell leukodystrophy

Globoid cell leukodystrophy is unique in that it is a lysosomal storage disease with one of its primary lesions being demyelination. Brain, spinal cord, and peripheral nerves can be affected. The disease, which is inherited as an autosomal recessive, is generally seen in younger animals, often under 1 year of age. Oligodendroglia are deficient in the lysosomal enzyme galactosylceramidase that normally is responsible for the degradation of galactosylceramide (galactocerebroside) and galactosylsphingosine (psychosine), which accumulate within these cells. Galactosylsphingosine is toxic and causes death of oligodendroglia. Consequently, there is a cessation of additional myelin formation and a degeneration of the myelin already formed before the death of the myelin-forming cells. The other product (galactosylceramide), which is nontoxic and is released into the extracellular space during degeneration of oligodendroglia, appears to stimulate the accumulation of macrophages that phagocytose the material. Such cells are referred to as globoid cells (see Fig. 8-16). Gross lesions of the CNS are characterized by a grayish discoloration of the affected white matter (e.g., centrum semiovale of cerebral hemispheres and spinal cord), the latter espe-

Table 8-3. Hypomyelinogenesis and dysmyelination in animals

Species	Breed	Disease designation	Genetic cause	Infectious cause	Metabolic cause
Canine	Dalmatian	Hypomyelinogenesis			
	Chow Chow	Dysmyelination	Suspected		
	Springer spaniel	Shaking pups (hypomyelination)	Sex-linked recessive		
	Samoyed	Tremor (hypomyelination)	Suspected		
	Lurcher	Tremor syndrome (hypomyelination)			
	Weimaraner	Hypomyelination	Suspected		
Bovine	All breeds	Bovine virus diarrhea (dysmyelination)		Bovine virus diarrhea (pestivirus)	
Porcine	Landrace	Congenital tremor (myelin agenesia)	Sex-linked recessive		
	Saddleback	Congenital tremor	Autosomal-recessive		
	Chester-white	Myoclonia congenita	Autosomal-recessive suspected		
	All breeds	Congenital tremor (dysmyelinogenesis and cerebellar hypoplasia)		Hog cholera virus (pestivirus)	
	All breeds	Congenital tremor (dysmyelinogenesis)		Unknown virus suspected	
	All breeds	Congenital ataxia and tremor (hypomyelinogenesis and cerebellar hypoplasia)			Trichlorfon (acaricide)
Ovine	All breeds	Border disease (hypomyelinogenesis-dysmyelination)		Border disease virus (pestivirus)	

cially in the dog (see Fig. 8-17). Microscopically, such areas have pronounced loss of myelin. Peripheral nerves are also affected, and lesions are typified by demyelination and axonal degeneration.

Spongy degeneration

Under the heading of spongy degeneration is a group of disease processes of young animals characterized by a spongy lesion (referred to here as **status spongiosus**) that primarily occurs in the white matter of the CNS. Ultrastructurally, the lesion, when described, is characterized by a splitting or separation of the myelin sheath at the intraperiod line (e.g., in the dog), with the formation of large intramyelinic spaces. In some instances, there may also be a deficiency of myelin formation.

Some species and breeds affected include the canine (Labrador retriever, Saluki, silky terrier, Samoyed), feline (Egyptian Mau), and bovine (Jersey, Shorthorn, Angus-Shorthorn, Hereford), and an autosomal recessive mode of transmission has been proposed for some forms of the disease. A form of the disease described in polled Hereford and Hereford calves, designated **maple syrup urine disease,** results from a branched chain ketoacid decarboxylase deficiency, which results in an elevated concentration of the branched chain amino acids valine, isoleucine, and leucine in the serum, plasma, CSF, and urine. The unique odor associated with urine of affected animals is caused by isoleucine. Calves are affected within 2 days of birth with a severe, generalized CNS disorder characterized by dullness and weakness that progresses to recumbency and opisthotonus. A mechanism proposed for causing the characteristic status spongiosus (splitting of the myelin sheath) involves the formation of a toxic metabolite from the oxidative decarboxylation of α-keto acids.

A general overview of the lesion referred to here as **status spongiosus** is warranted at this point. This lesion can be associated with several different disease processes, including splitting of the myelin sheath (as described above, or as an early stage of demyelination); accumulation of extracellular fluid; swelling of cellular (e.g., astrocytic, neuronal) processes; and axonal injury (e.g., Wallerian degeneration) when swollen axons are no longer detectable within distended spaces (see Fig. 8-4).

Metabolic Diseases

Several toxic compounds, including triethyltin, hexachlorophene, isoniazid (isonicotinic acid hydrazide), and cuprizone, are also characterized by production of prominent status spongiosus within the CNS that results from splitting of the myelin sheath at the intraperiod line. A reduction in total myelin content has also been demonstrated following administration of certain compounds (e.g., cuprizone). In addition, myelin of the peripheral nervous system may be affected by some of the toxicities.

Circulatory and Physical Disturbances

Circulatory disturbances

It is well known that extracellular edema (i.e., vasogenic and hydrostatic) that occurs secondary to inflammation, tumors, trauma, and hydrocephalus can cause degeneration of myelin sheaths. The underlying mechanisms for this injury are multiple and include creation of a hypoxic-anoxic environment, degeneration of oligodendroglia, and alteration in stability of the myelin sheath, permitting entry of injurious proteolytic enzymes from the surrounding environment.

Physical disturbances

Physical compression of CNS tissue, which can result from various causes, can also induce demyelination. Some possible mechanisms include compression on myelin sheaths and oligodendroglia, as well as interference with circulation.

Infectious Diseases (Confirmed as or Suspected of Being Caused by Viruses)

Progressive Multifocal Leukoencephalopathy and Mouse Hepatitis Virus-4 Infection

Some viruses have the ability to induce demyelination within the CNS by directly infecting and destroying oligodendroglia. One of these diseases (progressive multifocal leukoencephalopathy), which occurs rarely in humans and the nonhuman primate, is caused by the JC (human) or SV40 (nonhuman primate) strain of papovavirus. The disease has been associated with immunosuppression, but, in some instances, there is no obvious predisposing cause.

A murine infection, caused by mouse hepatitis virus-4 (JHM virus), a coronavirus, is considered to exert a similar effect, although recent evidence also indicates tropism for other neuroglia (astrocytes) and macrophages. The white matter of the brain (particularly the brain stem) and spinal cord may be variably affected. This same murine virus may also cause a persistent infection accompanied by demyelination in the mouse and rat. An immune mechanism may be involved in the infected rat.

Canine distemper

Canine distemper, which has a worldwide distribution and has been one of the most important diseases of the canine species, is caused by a morbillivirus (family Paramyxoviridae). Lesions of the disease do not appear to always result from straightforward viral infection with injury of susceptible cells and may also involve other (possibly immunologic and cytotoxic) factors. The virus is pantropic and has a particular affinity for lymphoid and epithelial tissues (e.g., lung, GI tract, urinary tract, skin) and the CNS (including the optic nerve and eye). Lymphoid involvement (characterized by lymphoid depletion and necrosis) is particularly important, because it can result in immunosuppression (affecting both the humoral and cell-mediated response), which makes the animal less able to combat the primary viral, as well as secondary bacterial, infections.

Following aerogenous infection, the virus infects macrophages and monocytes located in or on the respiratory epithelium and tonsils. After a brief replication, virus spreads through lymphatics and blood to other lymphoid tissues, where additional replication takes place. This is followed by cell- or noncell-associated virus spreading hematogenously to epithelial tissues and to the CNS approximately 8 to 9 days after infection. It is at this stage of the infection that the host's immune response determines the outcome of the disease. Any one of three results can occur. First, the animal may die from an acute fulminating infection in which there is unrestricted spread of the virus throughout the body. Death generally results from secondary bacterial infection or prominent involvement of the CNS. A second type of infection is characterized by a more delayed progression of the disease accompanied by a modest immune response, possible subtle early signs, and variable development of later neurologic signs. Finally, dogs may recover from the infection and remain clinically normal.

Initial infection of the CNS has been proposed to occur via the hematogenous route, which is followed by a noninflammatory or inflammatory process. The noninflammatory lesion has been primarily characterized by neuronal infection, whereas the inflammatory lesion of the CNS has been typified by the presence of virus in perivascular lymphocytes, neurons, ependyma, and meninges. Lesion development that begins with inflammation, as just described, will be the focus of this discussion. The early inflammation subsides and is undetectable by about 20 days after infection. The next stage of lesion development is characterized by the virtual absence of inflammatory cells, status spongiosus, astrocytic hypertrophy and hyperplasia with focal and variable syncytial formation, reduced numbers of oligodendroglia, variable neuronal degeneration, and demyelination (Fig. 8-38). Inclusion bodies (cytoplasmic, nuclear, or both) are detectable, particularly in astrocytes, which are important target cells for the distemper virus, but also in ependymal cells and, occasionally, neurons (Fig. 8-39). The earliest evidence of myelin injury is a ballooning change resulting from a split in the myelin sheath or more degenerative changes, including axonal swelling. This lesion is also variably associated with astroglial and microglial proliferation. This initial injury of the myelin sheath, which has been suggested to be a result of perturbed astrocytic function following viral infection, is followed by a progressive removal of compact myelin sheaths by phagocytic microglial cells (that infiltrate the myelin lamellae), and variable axonal necrosis. A late stage of lesion development is similar to the above, but demyelination is more pronounced and there is nonsuppurative inflammation (perivascular cuffing, leptomeningitis, and choroiditis), which can be accompanied by tissue degeneration and the accumulation of gitter cells (macrophages) (Fig. 8-40). During this stage, immunoglobulin-bearing cells and IgG bound to degenerated tissue are present in lesions of the white matter.

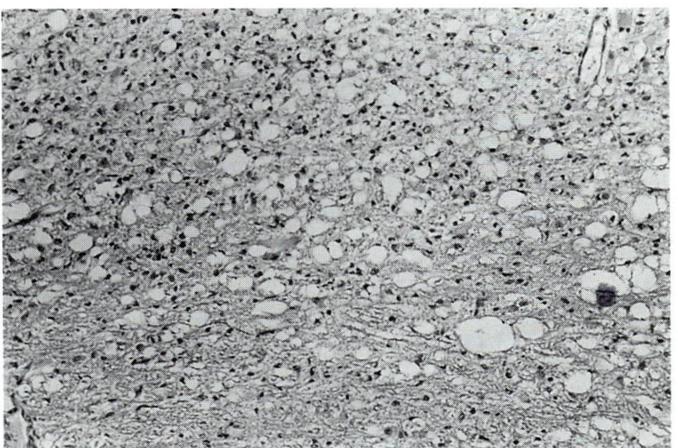

Fig. 8-38 Brain, deep cerebellar white matter; dog. Noninflammatory stage of demyelination associated with canine distemper infection. A demyelinated area *(top),* typified by reduced staining intensity and status spongiosus, borders a myelinated area *(below).* Status spongiosus is present in both the demyelinated as well as the myelinated areas. H & E stain.

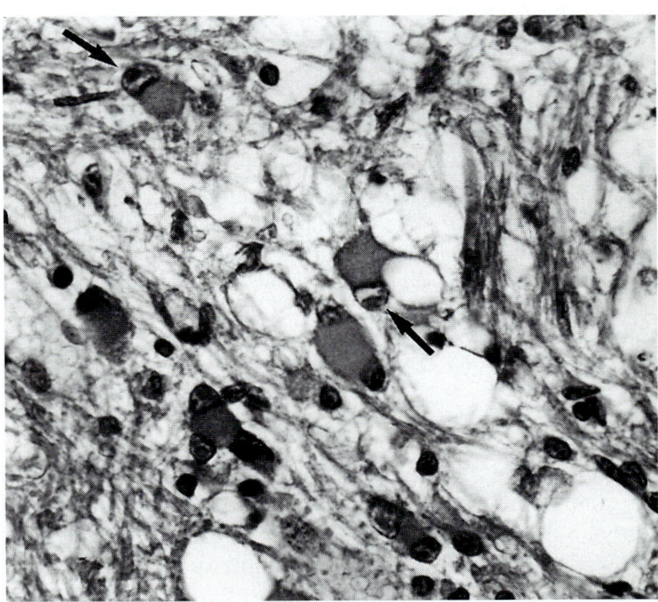

Fig. 8-39 Brain, deep cerebellar white matter; dog. Noninflammatory stage of demyelination associated with canine distemper infection. Note the prominent status spongiosus and presence of gemistocytic astrocytes containing intranuclear inlusion bodies *(arrows).* H & E stain.

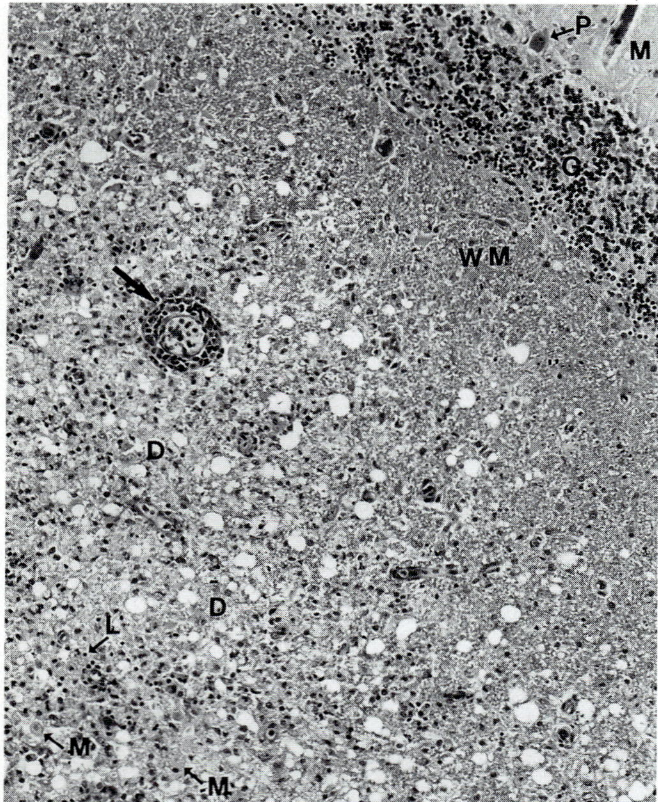

Fig. 8-40 Brain, cerebellar follum; dog. Late stage of canine distemper infection. Cerebellar cortex-molecular layer (*M*); Purkinje cell layer (*P*); and granular cell layer (*G*) are at top right. Folial white matter (*WM*) is normal, except for focal status spongiosus. There is also perivascular cuffing (*large arrow*) and demyelination (*D*). In the areas of demyelination, there are scattered lymphocytes (*L*) and gitter cells (↑ *M*).

Of the above-mentioned lesions affecting the white matter, status spongiosus (empty spaces in the neuropil) and demyelination (uniformly pale-stained areas of the neuropil) warrant special clarification. Status spongiosus can be associated with several different disease processes that are reviewed above under Spongy Degeneration. Demyelination (primary demyelination) refers to a loss of the myelin sheath and is characterized microscopically by a uniform reduction in, or an absence of, myelin staining, with the majority of the axons remaining intact. Such affected areas specifically appear pale pink following H & E staining, or unstained when stained with the luxol fast blue procedure for myelin. Status spongiosus may occur within areas that are demyelinated or myelinated.

Lesions characteristically occur in the cerebellum (medullary area and folial white matter), medulla oblongata (particularly in the subependymal area of the fourth ventricle), subpial white matter of the cerebellum, cerebellar peduncles (with white and sometimes gray matter involvement of the pons), rostral medullary vellum, cerebrum (both white and gray matter), optic nerves, optic tracts, spinal cord, and meninges.

The pathogenesis of the demyelination associated with canine distemper infection is not completely understood. However, several possible mechanisms have been proposed based on investigations conducted both in vitro (e.g., in tissue culture of CNS cells) and in vivo.

There is accumulating evidence that demyelination in canine distemper results from injury to the oligodendroglia, the myelin-forming cells of the CNS. Although oligodendroglia can become infected, the extent of infection appears to be much less than that for other cells of the CNS, such as astrocytes, macrophages, and ependymal cells, and to not be sufficiently significant to explain the demyelinating lesion. For this reason, other less direct mechanisms that might explain oligodendroglial injury have been examined, including (1) the ability of macrophages to produce injurious reactive oxygen species in response to the interaction of anti–canine distemper viral antibody with viral antigen (e.g., incorporated on the surface of infected astrocytes) and the ability of astrocytes and macrophages to produce tumor necrosis factor, which can cause degeneration of oligodendroglia; (2) **bystander demyelination,** which is defined as a process in which T cells, macrophages, or both secrete factors (e.g., neutral proteases, including plasminogen activator, from macrophages) during their reaction to viral antigens that cause demyelination; and (3) **antibody-dependent cell-mediated cytotoxicity** during the later stages of distemper infection when inflammation becomes a prominent part of the response. This process involves lysis of infected cells that have antibody attached to viral antigen expressed on their cell surface following exposure to certain types of cells (e.g., NK cells, macrophages).

Old-dog encephalitis

Old-dog encephalitis occurs rarely in mature adult dogs with clinical signs of dementia and is considered to be caused by distemper virus. Lesions occur primarily in the cerebral hemispheres and brain stem. Microscopic lesions are characterized primarily by a disseminated, nonsuppurative encephalitis with variable (sometimes prominent) lymphoplasmacytic perivascular cuffing, microgliosis, astrogliosis, and variable leptomeningitis and neuronal degeneration. Nuclear and cytoplasmic inclusions, positive for distemper viral antigen, have been detected in neurons and astrocytes in the cerebral cortex, thalamus, and brain stem but, in contrast to distemper, not in the cerebellum. Demyelination also occurs but is not prominent. Although the virus has the same general polypeptide composition as the one causing conventional distemper, some differences among peptides have been reported.

The mechanisms involved in development of lesions are

not known, but it has been proposed that the disease results from a persistent viral infection.

Visna

Visna (which means wasting) is a slowly progressive, transmissible disease of sheep. The disease, which is caused by a lentivirus (family Retroviridae), was originally described in Iceland, but sheep with similar lesions of the CNS have been detected in Europe (Netherlands), Kenya, the United States, and Canada. Related lentiviral infections (maedi and ovine progressive pneumonia) also may be accompanied by lesions of visna. CNS signs include an abnormal hind-limb gait that progresses to incoordination and rear-limb paresis over a period of weeks or months.

Early lesions primarily affect the gray and white matter subjacent to the ependyma of the ventricular system of the brain and central canal of the spinal cord. These lesions are characterized by a nonsuppurative encephalomyelitis accompanied by pleocytosis, variable edema, parenchymal necrosis, astrocytosis, choroiditis, and nonsuppurative leptomeningitis. Degeneration of myelin sheaths also occurs at this time but is often accompanied by axonal degeneration, suggesting that it may be a secondary lesion such as the one that accompanies Wallerian degeneration. Neuronal cell bodies and oligodendroglia are normal during this stage of the disease. The latter cells can become infected, however, which leads to later development of demyelination. Primary demyelination (particularly in the spinal cord) has been described in animals infected for prolonged periods (months to years). Such animals also have periventricular inflammation. Infected sheep may also develop inflammation in the mammary gland and arthritis (of the carpus or hind limb joints), although the latter is apparently a rare complication. Irrespective of the target organ, the lesions are characterized by infiltration and proliferation of mononuclear cells.

In recent years, understanding of the factors associated with infection, including the mechanism of lesion development, has improved. Visna is a persistent viral disease that probably results from the ability of the virus to form provirus (integration of viral and host genome). The virus can also change its antigenic characteristics (antigenic drift), which enables it to escape the effects of the host's immune response. However, antigenic drift does not appear essential for persistence of virus or occurrence of demyelination. The visna virus replicates in circulating monocytes and in tissue macrophages, but can also be present in oligodendrocytes and astrocytes located in foci of demyelination. It has been suggested that virus gains access to these cells via close contact with monocytes. The primary demyelination that occurs during the late stages of the disease process (½ to 8 years after infection) has been proposed to result from such oligodendroglial infection. The main sources of excreted virus are the udder and lung (as mainly cell-associated virus), and transmission occurs most readily between the dam and lamb via the milk and between confined individuals, probably via respiratory secretions. It is also of importance to note that no profound immune deficiency occurs with visna, as in HIV (AIDS) infection, also caused by a lentivirus, since the visna virus does not affect and deplete T cell populations.

Caprine leukoencephalomyelitis-arthritis (caprine arthritis encephalitis or CAE)

This disease was first described in the United States and has since been recognized in other parts of the world. The infection can be readily transmitted by colostrum and milk following birth. The disease is caused by a lentivirus similar to the visna virus described above. A close relationship exists between the visna virus of sheep and the CAE virus, but genomic differences between them can be demonstrated.

The pattern of disease in CAE is age-dependent. Neurologic manifestations are usually seen in young kids 2 to 4 months of age, but, unlike visna in sheep, there is a more rapid progression, and signs progressing to quadriplegia may develop within weeks to months. As with visna, affected goats have pleocytosis.

Gross lesions in the nervous system include tan to salmon-colored foci of necrosis and inflammation that can occasionally be detected in the brain and spinal cord, most prominently in the spinal cord. Microscopic lesions of the nervous system are similar to those of visna. Nonneural lesions include interstitial pneumonia of moderate severity in some affected kids. Such lungs fail to collapse completely and are mottled red or blue. In adult goats, the primary target tissue is the synovium of the joints, and animals that survive the initial infection develop lymphoproliferative synovitis and arthritis. Also, some affected animals (adults) develop aseptic lymphocytic mastitis.

Immune-Mediated Disorders

This category of demyelinating disease involves the development of a type IV hypersensitivity. The best-known representative of this group is an experimental model referred to as **experimental allergic encephalomyelitis (EAE)** that is produced by inducing a hypersensitivity to myelin or, more specifically, to myelin basic protein. If appropriate laboratory animals are inoculated with white matter or myelin basic protein (suspended in complete Freund's adjuvant), they become paralyzed after 2 to 3 weeks and have lesions characterized by perivascular (perivenular) demyelination accompanied by accumulation of lymphocytes and macrophages. A similar process, referred to as **post-vaccinal encephalomyelitis,** occurred occasionally when human rabies vaccine contained central nervous tissue. The opportunity for this process to occur decreased after 1957 when duck embryo rabies vaccine came into use. A third situation in which this type of demyelination occurs is after infection with certain viruses (e.g., rubeola) in humans. This disease, which is rare and designated **postinfectious encephalomyelitis,** is also characterized by development of lesions in the CNS comparable to those of EAE. Although such a naturally occurring process is not commonly recognized in animals, there is little reason to doubt that it can occur.

NEURODEGENERATIVE DISEASES

Neurodegenerative diseases, often referred to as **primary neuronal degenerations,** represent a group of disorders in which neurons of a particular type or in a particular region undergo degeneration. The specific causes and mechanisms of the majority of these diseases still remain to be clarified, although examples in humans and animals are known to be genetically transmitted. A word that has been used in association with this group of diseases is **''abiotrophy,''** introduced by Gowers in 1902 to mean a lack of (''a'') a vital (''bios'') nutrition (''trophy'') required to sustain life of a tissue, and is particularly applied to diseases of the nervous system. The method by which neurodegenerative diseases are classified varies somewhat according to the specific emphasis intended. The classification used here, which is not intended to be all-inclusive, attempts to place emphasis on the location of the most significant lesion(s) that occur.

Neurodegeneration of the Brain (with General Involvement)

Striatonigral and cerebello-olivary degeneration of the Kerry blue terrier

This hereditary disease is clinically characterized by signs of caudal ataxia, hypermetria of rear and front limbs, stumbling and falling, and atrophy of appendicular and epaxial muscles (apparently resulting from reduced use). Initial onset of signs ranges from 5 weeks to 5.5 months of age. Gross lesions include a slight reduction in the size of the cerebellum, with a shortening and thinning of the folia, and granularity of the cut surface of the cortex in advanced cases (likely associated with astroglial scarring) (Fig. 8-41). Other lesions that occur in the more advanced stages of the disease include focal softenings of the caudal olivary nucleus, caudate nucleus, putamen (infrequently), and substantia nigra (Fig. 8-42). Microscopic lesions in chronologic sequence involve degeneration with loss of neurons in the cerebellum (Purkinje cells and granule cells) (Fig. 8-43), caudal olivary nucleus, caudate nucleus and putamen, and substantia nigra. This change is accompanied by varying degrees of astrocytosis and astrogliosis, which, in advanced lesions, are particularly prominent in the Purkinje cell and molecular layers of the cerebellar cortex. The pathogenesis of the disease is proposed to involve neuronal degeneration caused by possible abnormal (increased) action of the excitatory neurotransmitter glutamic acid released from the glutaminergic axons of granule cells and cerebrocortical neurons, which synapse with Purkinje cells and caudate neurons, respectively. Neuronal degeneration in the caudal olivary nucleus and substantia nigra has been proposed to result from secondary transsynaptic degeneration.

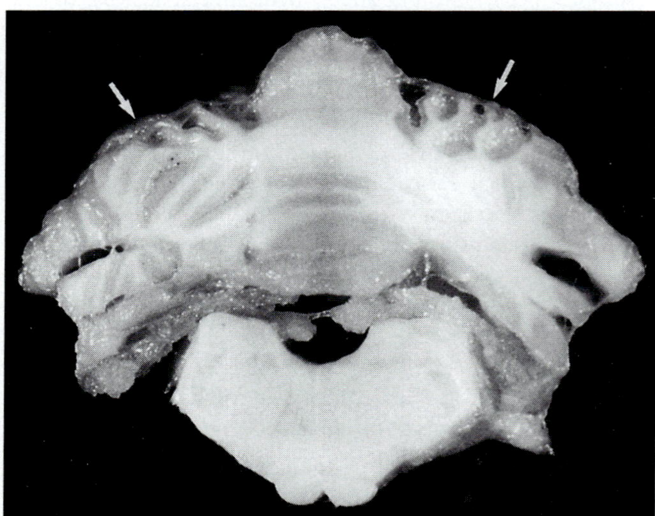

Fig. 8-41 Brain, cerebellum; Kerry blue terrier. Striatonigral and cerebello-olivary degeneration. Marked atrophy of folia of dorsal cerebellum *(arrows)* has resulted in increased width of sulci. *Courtesy Dr. D.L. Montgomery.*

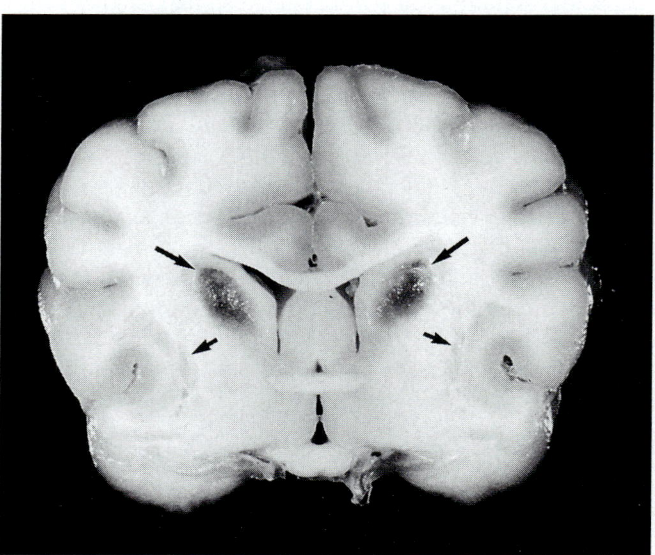

Fig. 8-42 Brain, rostral parietal lobe, at level of corpus striatum; Kerry blue terrier. Striatonigral and cerebelloolivary degeneration. Note liquefaction necrosis of caudate nuclei *(long arrows)* and putamen *(short arrows). From Montgomery DL, Storts RW. Vet Pathol 1983; 20:143-159.*

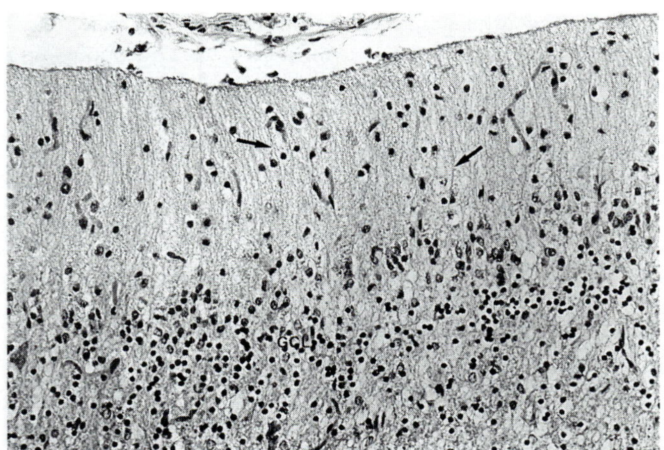

Fig. 8-43 Brain, cerebellar cortex; Kerry blue terrier. Striatonigral and cerebello-olivary degeneration. Cerebellar cortex has absence of Purkinje cells, depletion of the granular cell layer *(GCL),* and mild to moderate hypertrophy of vertical processes of Bergmann astroglia *(arrows).* H & E stain. *Courtesy Dr. D.L. Montgomery.*

Multisystem neuronal degeneration of the red-haired cocker spaniel

This disease, which is suspected of being inherited, is characterized clinically by progressive ataxia and mental deterioration, which can occur during the first year of life. Bilaterally symmetrical lesions that are present in the gray and white matter of the brain include diffuse nerve cell loss, astrogliosis, and development of small numbers of dystrophic (enlarged) axons in several nuclei (e.g., septal nuclei, globus pallidus, subthalamic nuclei, substantia nigra, tectum, medial geniculate bodies, and cerebellar and vestibular nuclei). Lesions in the white matter, which consist of intense astrogliosis, moderate numbers of axonal spheroids, perivascular accumulations of macrophages, and a discrete loss of myelin, were most prominent in the central cerebellar white matter, corpus callosum, thalamic striae, and some areas of the subcortical white matter (particularly subcallosal gyri).

Neurodegeneration of the Brain (with Significant Cerebellar Involvement)

Neonatal syndromes

Neonatal degeneration that primarily affects the cerebellum has been reported in the canine (beagle, Samoyed, Irish setter), ovine (Welsh mountain and Corriedale), and bovine (Hereford, Hereford cross, and Ayrshire) species. Signs are present at birth (ovine and bovine species) or at time of ambulation (canine species), and an inherited mode of transmission is known or suspected in some instances. Lesions vary regarding cellular involvement and degree of injury among affected species and breeds, but overall include degeneration or absence of Purkinje cells and/or their axons, proximal swelling of Purkinje cell axons, variable depletion of granule cells, cortical astrocytosis and astrogliosis (see Fig. 8-43 for comparable lesion), and degeneration of deep cerebellar medullary nuclei.

Postnatal syndromes

Animals affected with postnatal syndromes are generally normal at birth or at the time they first begin to ambulate. Onset and progression of signs vary from slow (weeks to months) to rapid (few days), with a static course or a slow progression. Species affected include the dog (breeds given below), cow (Holstein-Friesian, Hereford cross), pig (Yorkshire), horse (Arabian and Arabian crosses), pony (Gotland), and sheep (Merino). Grossly, the cerebellum may be normal to reduced in size. Microscopic lesions are degenerative and usually affect Purkinje cells, with variable degeneration of granule cells (see Fig. 8-43 for comparable lesion) and occasionally neurons of the cerebellar medullary nuclei (rough-coated collie dog, Merino sheep) and brain stem (rough-coated collie dog, Merino sheep). Other lesions include cortical astrogliosis (Holstein calf, severely affected Gordon setter dog, and Merino sheep); swelling of proximal Purkinje cell axons (rough-coated collie dog and Yorkshire pig); axonal degeneration in the cerebellum, brain stem, and spinal cord (rough-coated collie dog and Merino sheep); and loss of ventral horn neurons in the spinal cord (rough-coated collie dog). In several instances, these disorders are suspected, or are known, to have an autosomal recessive mode of transmission.

Canine breeds that have been reported to be affected include the Airedale, German shepherd, Gordon setter, rough-coated collie, Border collie, Finnish terrier, Bernese mountain dog, Bern running dog, Labrador retriever, golden retriever, cocker spaniel, Cairn terrier, and Great Dane.

Neurodegeneration of the Brain and Spinal Cord

Neuraxonal dystrophy

Neuraxonal dystrophy, which is characterized by prominent axonal swelling in different areas of the brain and spinal cord, has been reported among domesticated animals such as the dog (Border collie, Chihuahua, Rottweiler), cat, sheep (Suffolk breed), and horse (Morgan breed). Onset of clinical signs varies with the different species and ranges from 4 weeks to 3 years but, generally, is before 1 year of age. Lesions also differ somewhat in degree and distribution but are basically characterized by prominent axonal swelling in various nuclei (often sensory) in the brain stem, cerebellum (including cortex), and spinal cord of some species (e.g., Rottweiler and Border collie dog and Suffolk sheep). Variable lesions of the cerebellum (loss of Purkinje and granule cells in the Rottweiler dog and the cat) and loss of brain stem neurons (cat) have also been reported. The basic process has been suggested to be a distal axonopathy.

Lesions of this disease entity should be compared with the similar occurrence of dystrophic axons in brain nuclei discussed in the section on Multisystem Neuronal Degeneration of the Red-haired Cocker Spaniel.

Multisystemic neuronal degeneration of the Cairn terrier

This disease, which has features of an inherited disorder, is characterized clinically by onset of progressive signs (including cerebellar ataxia, spastic paresis and ataxia, and collapse) between 2.5 and 5 months of age. Lesions include widespread central chromatolysis of multiple neuronal systems involving the CNS and PNS. Affected neurons are located in the brain stem motor and sensory nuclei, roof nuclei of the cerebellum, ventral and dorsal gray columns of the spinal cord, and spinal and autonomic ganglia. Other lesions include degeneration in the lateral and ventral funiculi of the spinal cord, with necrosis of the substantia gelatinosa and adjacent white matter (caudal thoracic and cranial lumbar segments) and degeneration in the dorsal and ventral nerve roots and peripheral nerves.

Neurodegeneration of the Spinal Cord (with Significant Gray Matter Involvement)

In most degenerative diseases of animals in which lesions of the spinal cord are prominent, there is primary involvement of either the gray or white matter, and, in some, there is also involvement of the brain. In diseases that primarily affect the gray matter, signs often occur in young animals, and the disease may have a suspected or confirmed genetic cause. Older animals may be affected and the cause may be a known or suspected extraneous influence. Many of the diseases can be classified as motor neuron diseases. Lesions are usually characterized by degeneration and loss of motor neurons in the ventral horn, although lesions involving neurons of the brain stem (Brittany spaniel, Swedish Lapland, and Rottweiler dogs), cerebellum (Swedish Lapland and Rottweiler dogs), tracts of the spinal cord (Swedish Lapland dog), and PNS (Swedish Lapland and Rottweiler dogs) have been described. In growing animals, the lack of motor ability, together with muscle atrophy, can lead to severe deformations, such as arthrogryposis. In addition to the degenerative diseases of the Brittany spaniel, Rottweiler, and Swedish Lapland dogs, similar diseases have been reported in other breeds of dogs (sheepdogs of the collie type, collie, pug, dachshund, fox terrier, Saint Bernard or bloodhound crosses with the Great Dane, German shepherd), the cat (Siamese and other breeds), pig, calf, zebra, and horse.

The disease in the calf, referred to as the **shaker calf syndrome,** can occur in newborn, horned Hereford calves and causes a tremulous shaking of the head, body, and tail. Lesions include a marked accumulation of neurofilaments within neurons of the central, peripheral, and autonomic nervous systems. The spinal cord (all segments) in shaker calves is most severely affected. Neurons in the ventral horns, substantia gelatinosa, Clarke's column, and intermediolateral nucleus have swelling of the cell bodies and distention of neuronal processes. Axonal degeneration occurs in the ventral roots and intramedullary rootlets, as well as in the white matter of the spinal cord, as a result of degeneration of neuronal cell bodies supplying the affected axons. Similar lesions occur less prominently in the brain stem. Purkinje cells of the cerebellum are swollen, and degenerate neurons are present in the lateral geniculate body and frontal cortex. Pedigree analysis suggests that the disease is an inherited disorder.

A recently described motor neuron disease of the horse (referred to as **equine motor neuron disease**) is characterized clinically by signs of generalized weakness, muscle fasciculations, muscle atrophy, and weight loss that progresses over 1 to several months in young and old horses of different breeds. Lesions include degeneration and loss of motor neurons in the spinal cord and brain stem with axonal degeneration in the ventral roots and peripheral (including cranial) nerves, and atrophy or denervation of skeletal muscle. Affected spinal neurons are swollen, have central chromatolysis, and contain neurofilamentous accumulations. The cause of the disease is unknown, but because of the varying ages, breeds, and origins of affected animals, the disorder is considered to likely be acquired in most, if not all, instances.

A common feature of several of the above described diseases is the increased accumulation of neurofilaments in the cytoplasm of affected neuronal cell bodies (more prominently in the proximal axon in the Brittany spaniel dog). This change, which has been attributed to impairment of neurofilament protein transport, has been suggested to be one response of neurons to a variety of disease processes, with causes that range from genetic to acquired (e.g., copper deficiency [swayback-enzootic ataxia] of sheep and goats).

Neurodegeneration of the Spinal Cord (with Significant White Matter Involvement)

Generally, degenerative diseases of the white matter of the spinal cord are characterized by various degrees of paresis and ataxia, which often begin in the hind limbs.

Degenerative myelopathy in the German shepherd

The German shepherd is the breed best known to be affected by degenerative myelopathy, but a similar syndrome has also been reported in other breeds of large dogs. The disease generally first manifests itself in animals over 5 years of age and is more prevalent in dogs older than 8 years. Lesions, which are diffuse or multifocal, are most extensive in the thoracic spinal cord and can involve degeneration of all funiculi of the white matter, although lesions have been described as being more pronounced in the dorsal part of the lateral funiculi and ventromedial aspect

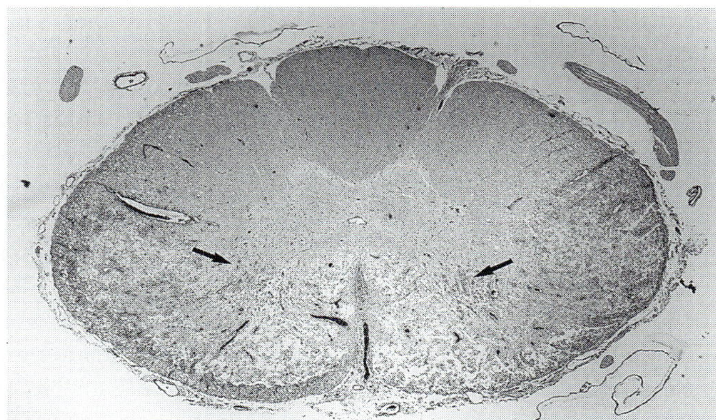

Fig. 8-44 Spinal cord, caudal thoracic level (T12); dog. Afghan myelopathy. There is severe degeneration of white matter in the lateral and ventral funiculi. Intact neuronal cell bodies are present in the ventral horns *(arrows).* H & E stain.

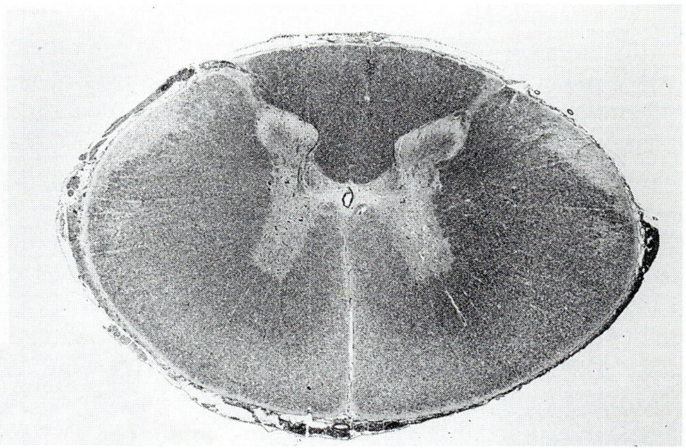

Fig. 8-45 Spinal cord; thoracic level; horse. Degenerative myeloencephalopathy. There is marked loss of myelin in the dorsolateral aspect of the lateral funiculi and less pronounced changes in the remainder of the lateral funiculi and ventromedial aspect of the ventral funiculi. Luxol fast blue stain. H & E stain. *Courtesy Drs. J.F. Edwards and A. DeLahunta.*

of the ventral funiculi. Dorsal roots and peripheral nerves may also be affected, and neuronal loss in the gray matter of the spinal cord may occur.

Although the exact mechanism involved in this disease is unknown, it has been proposed that an autoimmune process involving abnormal suppressor cell activity may play a role.

Inherited necrotizing myelopathy of the Afghan hound

Onset of clinical signs occurs between 3 and 13 months. There is prominent destruction of the white matter that involves the dorsal (variable) and ventral funiculi of the cervical cord, all funiculi of a large part of the thoracic cord, and ventral funiculi of the lumbar cord. There may also be necrosis, perivascular accumulation of macrophages, and astrocytosis of the neuropil in the cranial olivary nucleus of the brain stem. Neuronal cell bodies of the spinal gray matter and ventral roots remain morphologically unaffected (Fig. 8-44). The disease is suggested to be transmitted by an autosomal recessive mode of inheritance. The mechanism of lesion development is unknown.

Degenerative myeloencephalopathy in the horse

Several breeds of horses and even zebras can be affected. The onset of clinical signs varies with the following age incidence: 50% before 7 months of age, 25% between 7 and 14 months of age, and the remainder in older animals. The spinal cord appears normal grossly. Microscopically, there is a diffuse degeneration in all funiculi of the spinal cord, but it is more pronounced in the dorsolateral (dorsal spinocerebellar tract) and ventromedial funiculi of the thoracic spinal cord (Fig. 8-45). Lesions are least evident in the dorsal funiculi. Myelin loss can be the most visibly detectable lesion and is accompanied by variable astrocytosis and axonal degeneration. Swollen axons and, less frequently, central chromatolysis of neurons are present in the gray matter, especially in the nucleus of the dorsal spinocerebellar tract (Clarke's nucleus) in thoracic segments, and in the nucleus gracilis and cuneatus of the medulla. Axonal and/or neuronal cell body degeneration also occurs variably in the lateral cervical, olivary, vestibular, oculomotor, pretectal, and thalamic nuclei. The disease has been classified as a multisystemic degeneration of the CNS. Proposed causes include a nutritional deficiency (e.g., vitamin E deficiency), toxicity, or familial mechanism (suggested for the Appaloosa breed).

Progressive degenerative myelopathy in Brown Swiss cattle

Initial clinical signs of progressive degenerative myelopathy occur at 5 to 8 months of age and are characterized by hind leg weakness, ataxia, and dysmetria. Microscopic lesions are confined to the CNS. The white matter of the spinal cord is most consistently affected, with no significant changes occurring in the gray matter or spinal ganglia. The extent and degree of involvement vary with location. The peripheral parts of the lateral and ventral funiculi are more severely affected than areas closer to the gray matter. Dorsal funiculi, in general, are more uniformly affected throughout. In the thoracic segments, the most severe lesions occur ventromedially. Lesions in the white matter are characterized by axonal degeneration at all levels of the spinal cord, although they are most severe in the thoracic region. Lesions also occur in the medulla oblongata (axonal degeneration) and cerebellum (primarily degeneration of Purkinje cells). The disease is considered to be a familial degenerative disease of the CNS.

INFLAMMATION OF THE CNS

Infectious agents can spread to the CNS (1) hematogenously (most commonly); (2) within the axoplasm of peripheral axons; (3) from the olfactory mucosa (containing receptor cells whose processes synapse within the CNS), as well as direct spread from the nasal submucosa into the CSF via focally exposed subarachnoid space; and (4) by direct spread resulting from trauma (skull or vertebral fracture), various paracranial and paravertebral infections associated with inner ear infection, sinusitis, inflammation of the ethmoid and nasopharyngeal areas (including the guttural pouches in equidae), vertebral osteomyelitis, and following docking of lambs. Within the CNS, infectious agents may spread in the interstitium, within neurons and neuroglia, by mobile infected leukocytes that enter from the circulation, and in the CSF.

Four commonly occurring changes, associated with inflammation of the CNS from many different causes, are leptomeningitis, perivascular cuffing, microgliosis, and neuronal degeneration. Less common, but important additional lesions include ganglioneuritis involving the PNS (e.g., in rabies); vasculitis, which may be accompanied by edema and thrombosis (e.g., *Haemophilus somnus* infection of cattle); parenchymal necrosis (e.g., in pseudorabies of swine); and demyelination (e.g., in canine distemper).

The type of inflammatory response can vary with the cause. A rather simplistic guideline (to which there are always exceptions) that compares the type of inflammation with different etiologic agents is as follows: suppurative (or purulent) response—several species of bacteria; nonsuppurative (lymphocytic, monocytic [macrophage], plasmacytic) response—viruses and certain other infectious agents (e.g., protozoa such as *Toxoplasma gondii*) and parasitic infestations; and granulomatous response—fungi and some bacteria (e.g., *Mycobacterium* species).

Viral Infections

Rabies

Rabies virus is one of the most neurotropic of all viruses infecting mammals. Gross lesions of infected central nervous tissue are often absent. Microscopic lesions of the CNS are typically nonsuppurative and include a variable leptomeningitis and perivascular cuffing with lymphocytes, macrophages, and plasma cells; microgliosis (which sometimes is prominent); variable (often not severe) neuronal degeneration; and ganglioneuritis (Fig. 8-46). Emphasis should be given to the fact that infected neurons often are minimally altered morphologically, even though they may be infected. Also, some species (e.g., canine) are reported to have a tendency to develop a more severe inflammatory reaction than others (e.g., bovine), in which little if any inflammation may occur. Nonneural lesions include variable nonsuppurative sialitis accompanied by necrosis and presence of Negri bodies (e.g., dog) in salivary epithelial cells.

Negri body formation within neurons of the CNS and even in the peripheral ganglia has long been the hallmark of rabies infection, although it is not detected in all instances. The inclusions are intracytoplasmic and initially develop as an aggregation of strands of viral nucleocapsid, which rather quickly transforms into an ill-defined granular matrix. Mature rabies virions, which bud from the nearby endoplasmic reticulum, may also be located around the periphery of the matrix. With time, the body becomes larger and detectable by light microscopy. Classically, in H & E-stained sections, the Negri body has one or more very small, light clear areas called inner bodies that form due to invagination of cytoplasmic components (that includes virions) into the matrix of the inclusion (Fig. 8-47). Inclusions that do not possess inner bodies have been referred to as Lyssa bodies, but they are actually Negri bodies

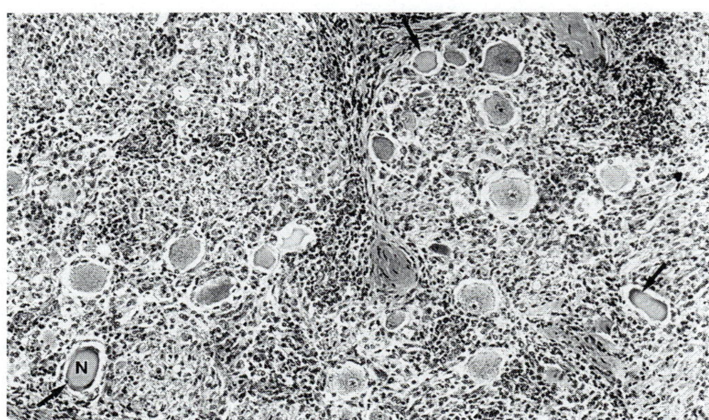

Fig. 8-46 Trigeminal (gasserian) ganglion; steer. Rabies. There is ganglioneuritis with focal accumulation of mononuclear cells and varying degrees of degeneration of neuronal cell bodies *(arrows)*. A neuron with central chromatolysis and an eccentric nucleus (*N*) is at the lower left. H & E stain.

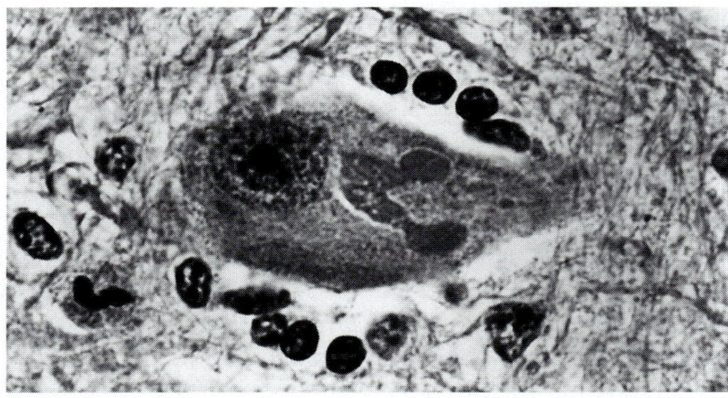

Fig. 8-47 Brain, medulla oblongata; steer. Rabies. A neuron of the medulla oblongata contains a large C-shaped Negri body. The small light areas in the inclusion represent "inner bodies." H & E stain.

without cytoplasmic indentation. It should also be noted that both fixed viruses (adapted to the CNS by passage) and street viruses (that produce the naturally occurring disease) produce the same ultrastructural features, except fixed viral strains generally cause severe neuronal degeneration that precludes the development, and thus the detection, of Negri bodies. Negri bodies also tend to occur more frequently in large neurons (e.g., pyramidal neurons of the hippocampus and large neurons of the medulla oblongata) than in small ones. Also, inclusions are reported as often being present in neurons that are not located in areas of inflammation.

A spongiform lesion, indistinguishable qualitatively from the lesion characteristic for several of the spongiform encephalopathies (see Scrapie), was described for the first time in 1984 by Charlton. The lesion has been detected in animals with the experimental and naturally occurring disease. The lesion, which occurs in the neuropil of the gray matter (especially the thalamus and cerebral cortex), develops initially as intracytoplasmic membrane-bound vacuoles in neuronal dendrites (less commonly in axons and astrocytes), enlarges with compression of surrounding tissue, and ultimately may rupture with formation of a tissue space. Although the mechanism responsible for the development of this lesion has not been determined, it is thought to result from an indirect effect of the rabies virus on neural tissue (possibly involving an alteration of neurotransmitter metabolism).

Rabies is generally transmitted by a bite from an infected animal, although respiratory infection has been uncommonly reported (e.g., following exposure to virus in bat caves and resulting from accidental human laboratory exposure to the virus). Following inoculation of rabies virus (e.g., rear leg of an animal), the virus may enter local myocytes where it can replicate and remain for a variable period. Also, it appears that the virus may directly enter peripheral nerve terminals without first infecting nonnervous tissue, such as skeletal muscle. After the virus enters the axoplasm of peripheral nerves, it moves by axoplasmic transport (apparently via sensory or motor nerves) to the CNS. With sensory axons, the first cell bodies encountered are in the dorsal root or cranial sensory ganglia; for motor axons, the cell bodies of the ventral motor neurons are the ones initially infected. It is not known whether viral infection and replication in dorsal root ganglial neurons is essential for infection of the CNS. Virus then moves into the spinal cord and spreads to the brain. Neuron-to-neuron spread (by budding of virions from the plasma membrane) has been demonstrated to occur in a direction opposite to that of impulse transmission (from the infected cell body or dendrite into an axonal terminal that synapses on the cell surface). Virus spreads in this manner because axons do not possess the rough endoplasmic reticulum necessary for viral replication. Viral spread within the CNS may be quite rapid, and, although neurons are the primary cell affected, there is evidence that the infection can also involve the leptomeninges, ependyma, oligodendroglia, and astrocytes. During the spread of virus in the CNS, there is simultaneous centrifugal movement of virus peripherally via axons, which results in infection of various tissues, including those of the oral cavity and salivary gland, permitting transmission of the disease in the saliva. During centrifugal spread, there is also infection of neurons of dorsal root ganglia, with widespread involvement of ganglia occurring terminally. Affected ganglia have a moderate to severe nonsuppurative inflammatory response that may be accompanied by a neuronal degeneration (more frequently occurring than in the CNS). An additionally important feature of rabies is that infection of specific areas of nervous and nonnervous tissues (i.e., limbic system and salivary glands, respectively), during the same time period, results in affected animals having the required behavior, with the required viral inoculum (in the right location), to transmit the disease.

When conducting a necropsy on an animal suspected of having rabies, it is important to remember (1) to provide adequate protection for the prosector and (2) to collect the proper CNS tissues (cerebral hemisphere that includes hippocampus, cerebellum, and medulla and, optionally, the spinal cord) for viral examination (by immunofluorescence and, sometimes, mouse inoculation).

Pseudorabies

Several species of domestic and wild animals are susceptible to infection with pseudorabies virus. The disease in susceptible species other than swine is generally fatal. Although swine (particularly young, suckling animals) can die from infection, most mature pigs remain persistently infected and act as carriers.

Gross lesions in swine occur in several nonneural tissues, including the respiratory tract, lymphoid system, digestive tract, and reproductive tract. Focal tissue necrosis also occurs (e.g., liver, spleen, adrenal), particularly in young, suckling pigs, and mortality in such animals can be high. The CNS may be free of gross lesions except for leptomeningeal congestion. Microscopic lesions in swine are characterized by a nonsuppurative meningoencephalomyelitis with ganglioneuritis. Injury to CNS tissue can be marked, with neuronal degeneration and parenchymal necrosis. Intranuclear inclusion bodies are not commonly detected in swine but can be present in neurons, astrocytes, oligodendroglia, and endothelial cells.

The route of natural infection in swine is intranasal (by direct contact or aerosolization), followed by reproduction of virus in the upper respiratory tract. The virus then travels to the tonsil and local lymph nodes by way of the lymphatics. Following replication in the nasopharynx, the virus invades bipolar olfactory cells (and other nerve terminals) and is then transported in their axoplasm to the brain or spinal cord. In latently infected pigs, the oronasal epithe-

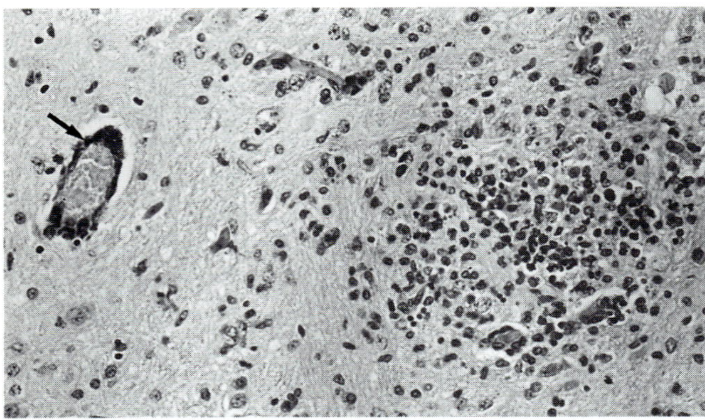

Fig. 8-48 Brain, deep cerebellar white matter; sheep. Pseudorabies. Nonsuppurative inflammation with perivascular cuffing *(arrow)* and focal and diffuse microgliosis *(right)*. H & E stain. *Courtesy Dr. E.B. Janovitz.*

lium can be recurrently infected by virus spreading from the nervous system, and infectious virus may then be excreted in oronasal fluid. The virus can also spread hematogenously, although in low titer, to other tissues of the body.

Infection of secondary hosts (e.g., cattle, sheep, dogs, cats) with virus involves direct or indirect contact with swine. Infection can occur by ingestion, inhalation, and wound infection. Dogs and cats usually become infected by ingesting virus-infected pig carcasses. The pathogenesis involving axonal spread to the CNS is comparable to that of swine, with lesions that include nonsuppurative encephalomyelitis accompanied by ganglioneuritis (Fig. 8-48; see Fig. 8-46). Intranuclear inclusion bodies of neurons, either eosinophilic or basophilic in their staining characteristics, have been described in neurons of the brain.

Enterovirus-induced porcine polioencephalomyelitis

Several diseases of swine (e.g., Teschen disease, Talfan disease, and others) caused by porcine enteroviruses (family Picornaviridae) are characterized by polioencephalomyelitis. Clinical manifestations of the different diseases vary in severity from being marked and associated with death of affected animals (Teschen disease occurring sporadically in Europe and Africa) to being less severe with signs that include fever, diarrhea, and paralysis (sometimes most severe in the hind legs) in pigs in North America and some other regions of the world.

No gross lesions are detectable. All forms of the disease are characterized microscopically by a nonsuppurative polioencephalomyelitis. The sequence of changes in degenerating neurons includes acute swelling, central chromatolysis, necrosis, neuronophagia, and variable resultant axonal degeneration. Astrocytosis and, particularly, astrogliosis also occur, especially in the later stages of the infection. Cerebral and cerebellar involvement is variable with the different forms of the disease. Ganglioneuritis, particularly of dorsal root ganglia of the spinal cord, and variable leptomeningitis of varying severity also occur.

Natural infection occurs by the oral route and is followed by viral localization and replication in the tonsil and intestinal tract (primarily ileum, large intestine, and mesenteric lymph nodes). Following replication in the intestine, virus travels hematogenously to the brain and spreads into the parenchyma.

Hemagglutinating encephalomyelitis viral infection of swine

In 1958, a disease of nursing pigs, characterized by high morbidity, vomiting, anorexia, constipation, and severe progressive emaciation, was reported in Ontario, Canada. The etiologic agent has been determined to be a coronavirus.

Gross lesions are limited and include cachexia and enlargement of the abdomen caused by gaseous distention of the stomach and intestine. Microscopic lesions occur in the respiratory tract, stomach, CNS, and PNS. Lesions in the CNS, which are most pronounced in the gray matter, are characterized by a nonsuppurative meningoencephalomyelitis and neuronal degeneration. The caudal brain stem (particularly the medulla and pons) and spinal cord are affected. In the peripheral ganglia, there is a nonsuppurative inflammation and neuronal degeneration.

Infection by the oronasal route, which has been demonstrated experimentally, is followed by viral replication in epithelial cells of the nasal mucosa, tonsils, lungs, and small intestine. After local replication, the virus spreads to the CNS by way of the peripheral nerves, including the trigeminal and olfactory nerves, vagus, and extensions from intestinal plexuses to the spinal cord. Neurons of peripheral ganglia may also be infected. Viral antigen is restricted to the cytoplasm of neurons. The vomiting associated with the disease is presumed to result from altered function of neurons (in the vagal nucleus and its ganglion and gastric intramural plexuses) secondary to viral infection.

Borna disease

Borna disease (named after Borna, a town in Saxony) is an encephalomyelitis caused by an uncharacterized RNA virus (with properties of an enveloped virus) that has been recognized in Central Europe for more than 250 years. The naturally occurring infection, which has no seasonal incidence, occurs in horses, sheep, cattle, goats, and deer and has an incubation period that can be relatively long, weeks to several months. The infection is also considered to be a persistent infection of the CNS in certain species, and behavioral abnormalities can accompany infection.

There are no significant gross lesions. Microscopic lesions, which are limited to the nervous system, are characterized by a nonsuppurative encephalomyelitis that may be pronounced and accompanied by neuronal degeneration. Lesions are confined largely to the gray matter, although white matter may also be affected, and are most severe in the midbrain, midbrain-diencephalon junction, and hypothalamus. Marked inflammation also occurs in the hippocampus. In addition, lesions occur in the cerebral cortex (especially laterobasal areas, olfactory bulb, caudate nucleus, and periventricular gray matter). Inflammation of the meninges and spinal cord is generally mild. A vascular necrosis accompanied by focal hemorrhage has also been described. Small, round to oval, eosinophilic intranuclear inclusions occur in neurons of the brain stem, hippocampus, and cerebrospinal ganglia. In the PNS, there is inflammation of cranial, spinal, and autonomic ganglia and peripheral nerves.

Experimental evidence indicates that infection of the CNS via olfactory nerves can follow intranasal viral exposure. The agent is highly neurotropic, similar to the rabies virus, and is transported to the CNS from the periphery intraaxonally, although nonneuronal infection (of astrocytes, ependyma, and Schwann cells) may occur and possibly contribute to viral replication (e.g., in astrocytes and Schwann cells) during the chronic stage of the disease. Similar to rabies, infection of the CNS can be prevented by severance of peripheral nerves proximal to a distal site of inoculation (e.g., footpad). Viral antigen can be demonstrated in neuronal nuclei, perikarya, dendrites, and axons, with the majority of viral assembly occurring within the cytoplasm and presence of little infectious virus in nuclei.

The specific lesions that develop in the CNS appear to depend upon a viral-induced cell-mediated immune mechanism. Infected laboratory rodents that are immunosuppressed do not develop the disease or lesions despite high titers of virus in the CNS, but transfer of cells (spleen or lymph node origin) from diseased animals into immunosuppressed recipients can induce encephalitis and clinical disease. Antibody to Borna disease virus does not appear to play any significant role in the disease process.

Equine encephalomyelitis

Infection of horses with Eastern, Western, or Venezuelan equine encephalomyelitis (EEE, WEE, VEE) viruses produces a range of clinical manifestations. The viruses are members of the family Togaviridae, genus alphavirus. In addition to in horses, Eastern encephalomyelitis has also been reported in the bovine and porcine species.

Lesions of the CNS induced by all three viruses are similar, but there are some differences. Overall, gross lesions include cerebral hyperemia, edema, petechiation, focal necrosis, and leptomeningeal edema. Microscopic lesions are most prominent in the gray matter of the brain and spinal cord and are characterized by perivascular cuffing (with lymphocytes, macrophages, and neutrophils), variable neutrophilic infiltration of the gray matter parenchyma, microgliosis, neuronal degeneration, focal parenchymal (cortical) necrosis, perivascular edema and hemorrhage, necrotizing vasculitis, thrombosis, choroiditis, and leptomeningitis.

Neutrophils are detectable during the early stages (2 days) of clinical EEE and VEE. Vasculitis, thrombosis, and cerebrocortical necrosis have been associated particularly with VEE but also with EEE. Peripheral ganglia (e.g., Gasserian or trigeminal ganglion) appear to be unaffected.

Following inoculation (by mosquito), the virus initially infects several tissues hematogenously, including bone marrow, lymphoreticular tissue, muscle, and connective tissue. In some tissues (e.g., lymphoid and myeloid [bone marrow]), there may be cellular depletion, necrosis, or both. A second viremia results in hematogenous infection of the CNS. Experimental evidence suggests that the virus may replicate in endothelial cells before entering the nervous system and infecting neurons, for which it has an affinity. There is also evidence that viruses of this group (e.g., VEE virus) may be associated with alteration in the metabolism of neurotransmitters of the CNS, which has been cited as possibly explaining clinical signs that occur.

Japanese encephalitis

Japanese encephalitis is a particularly important disease in humans, but infection also occurs in animals (e.g., horses, swine, cattle, and sheep). Its geographic distribution is restricted to eastern and southeastern Asia. The causative virus is classified as a member of the family Flaviviridae and is transmitted by mosquitoes, mainly *Culex tritaeniorhynchus*. In nature, infection is maintained in a cycle involving vector mosquitoes, birds, and mammals.

Although young susceptible pigs may have signs, detectable illness is not a feature of viral infection in adult or pregnant swine. However, fetal infection during pregnancy may result in mummification and still-birth of fetuses or in birth of weak live pigs with nervous signs accompanied by nonsuppurative encephalitis and neuronal degeneration.

Well-documented outbreaks of meningoencephalomyelitis in horses have been reported. Young or immature horses are reported to be more susceptible to infection than older animals. Lesions are limited to the nervous system. Grossly, they include mild leptomeningeal congestion, hyperemia, and occasional areas of hemorrhage within the brain and spinal cord. Microscopic lesions are characterized by an early leptomeningitis and encephalitis in which neutrophils predominate, followed by nonsuppurative inflammation, neuronal degeneration, focal hemorrhage, and focal malacia. The lesions are distributed diffusely throughout the nervous system but affect the gray matter more than the white.

Factors that may be involved in the pathogenesis of this viral infection include the recent finding that the susceptibility of laboratory animals (e.g., rat) to the virus is closely associated with neuronal immaturity. Such an age-dependent susceptibility of brain to viral infection has also been noted with other flaviviruses, including St. Louis encephalitis virus and yellow fever virus. The fact that fetal and neonatal swine and young horses appear to be more susceptible than adult animals suggests that such a correlation may also possibly exist in naturally occurring infections of animals.

Louping ill

Louping ill is primarily a disease of sheep, but it may also occur in cattle, horses, pigs, goats, red deer, and dogs. It is caused by a flavivirus and is mainly limited to the British Isles, although reports of infections resembling louping ill have also been reported in southern and western Europe. The disease occurs in the spring and summer.

No significant gross lesions are present. Microscopic lesions are characterized by a meningoencephalomyelitis that is primarily nonsuppurative, although neutrophils may be present. Specific changes also include neuronal degeneration. The most consistent and pronounced lesions, which include inflammation and degeneration of Purkinje cells, occur in the cerebellar cortex and have been proposed to be at least partially responsible for the unique clinical signs (peculiar leaping gait) displayed by affected ataxic animals. Prominent lesions, although more variable, also occur in the medulla oblongata and spinal cord. Other areas of the CNS may also be affected but less prominently. No inflammation of spinal ganglia occurs, but inflammation has been detected in peripheral (e.g., sciatic) nerves.

Following infection by the tick *Ixodes ricinus,* the virus replicates in lymphoreticular tissue (e.g., lymph nodes and spleen), resulting in development of a high titered viremia. A subsequent infection of the CNS (primarily of neurons) probably occurs hematogenously. Excretion of the virus in milk of infected ewes and goats has also been reported, with the suggestion that transmission by ingestion is of possible significance in suckling kids.

Scrapie

Scrapie is the prototype of a group of diseases referred to as **subacute spongiform encephalopathies.** Until relatively recently, the group included scrapie, transmissible mink encephalopathy (scrapie infection in mink), and chronic wasting disease (mule deer and elk) of animals, and the human diseases kuru, Creutzfeldt-Jakob disease, and Gerstmann-Strüssler-Scheinker syndrome. A more recent addition to this group includes **bovine spongiform encephalopathy** (BSE), which was originally identified in Great Britain in 1986, but was likely first evident there as early as April 1985. This disease was subsequently confirmed to exist in cattle in Northern Ireland and the Republic of Ireland and was identified in cattle exported from England to Oman. Additional cases (in native cattle) have been diagnosed in the Channel Isles and Isle of Man, France, and Switzerland. The bovine agent has also experimentally produced disease in swine, but only following the use of highly infectious inoculum given simultaneously by multiple routes. Finally, a BSE-like encephalopathy has been identified in the domestic cat and several zoo ruminants (kudu, Arabian oryx, nyala, gemsbok, and eland) in Great Britain.

Scrapie is best known as a disease of sheep but also occurs naturally in the domestic goat. The name is derived from the characteristic clinical signs of pruritus, which often results in loss of wool in sheep. The disease progresses inexorably, with signs that include incoordination, recumbency, and eventual death. Signs that accompany BSE include behavioral, gait, and postural abnormalities that usually begin with evidence of apprehension, anxiety, and fear. Following the onset of clinical signs, affected cattle deteriorate until they either die or require euthanasia. This period usually ranges from 2 weeks to 6 months. All cases of the disease in cattle have occurred in adult animals, with an age range of 3 to 11 years, but most animals develop clinical signs between 3 and 5 years of age.

Scrapie is quite different from other conventional viral infections. First, it is caused by a very unique agent that is still being characterized and is discussed in more detail below. Second, the disease has a variable incubation period that depends on the species affected (e.g., from 2 months in laboratory hamsters to 2 years or more in sheep). Further, the disease lacks a typical immune response and is not accompanied by any significant inflammation within the infected CNS.

Grossly, in sheep and goats, there is variable loss of body condition, and skin lesions as a result of pruritus. Other than a reported increase in the CSF, no gross lesions of the nervous system are detectable.

Significant microscopic lesions in sheep and goats are limited to the CNS and are most commonly present in the diencephalon, brain stem, and cerebellum (cortex and deep nuclei), with variable lesions in the corpus striatum and spinal cord. Except for some minor changes, the cerebral cortex is essentially unaffected. The characteristic lesions include neuronal degeneration, astrocytosis, and variable spongiosus (generally affecting the gray matter) (Figs. 8-49 and 8-50). The type of neuronal degeneration can vary and commonly is characterized by shrinkage with increased basophilia and cytoplasmic vacuolation (Fig. 8-49), although other changes (e.g., central chromatolysis and ischemic cell change) variably occur. Astrocytosis in affected areas of the brain, including the cerebellar cortex, may be pronounced. There has been speculation whether the astrocytic reaction is a primary or a secondary response, and recent results have helped clarify this problem. An abnormal protein (prion amyloid protein) first accumulates in astroglial cells in the brain during scrapie infection, which could mean that this cell is the primary site of replication. The spongiform change tends to affect the gray matter, and greater severity of this lesion has been associated with long

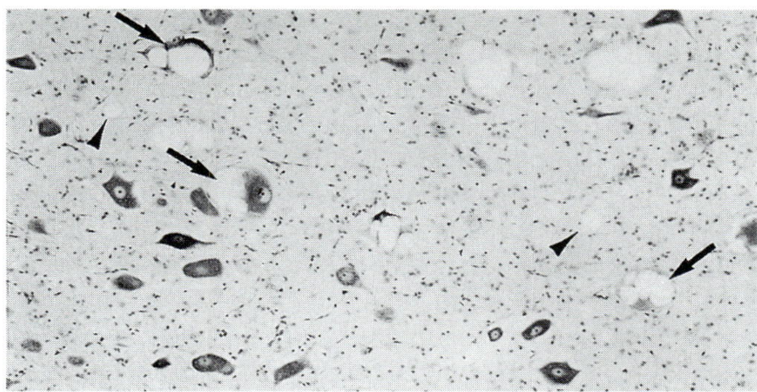

Fig. 8-49 Brain, red nucleus of mesencephalon; goat. Scrapie. There is prominent neuronal vacuolation *(arrows)* and focal status spongiosus *(arrowheads)*. H & E stain. *Courtesy of Dr. W.J. Hadlow.*

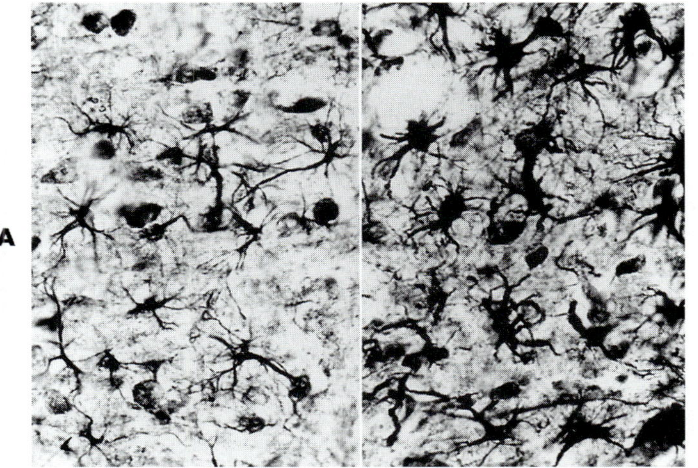

Fig. 8-50 Brain, medulla oblongata; mouse. **A**, Normal brain. Compare the size, shape, and density of normal astrocytes with, **B**, scrapie. The pronounced hypertrophy and hyperplasia of astrocytes are characteristic of scrapie. Cajal's gold sublimate impregnation. *Courtesy Dr. W.J. Hadlow.*

incubation periods. The lesion, when occurring in the gray matter, has been identified as resulting from dilatation of neuronal processes, although other causes, including vacuolation of neuronal and astroglial perikarya, swelling of astrocytic processes, dilatation of the periaxonal space, and splitting of myelin sheaths, have also been reported. Another lesion that occurs variably in experimentally infected animals and with the other spongiform encephalopathies is amyloid plaque formation. Cerebrovascular amyloidosis also has been detected in the naturally occurring disease in sheep.

A proposed pathogenesis of the natural infection in Suffolk sheep has been advanced by Hadlow and coworkers. Following oral infection at an early age, there is an extremely long eclipse phase (about 1 year) before the virus can be detected in infected animals. At this time virus occurs in low titers in the tonsil, suprapharyngeal (medial retropharyngeal) lymph node, and lymphoid tissue of the intestine. Virus then spreads to regional lymph nodes and eventually to other lymph nodes and the spleen. Other extraneural tissues are not significantly infected. The virus continues to replicate in the extraintestinal and intestinal lymphoid tissues for many months or even a year or more before it reaches the CNS, which is the target organ. It has been proposed that the CNS in sheep is infected by hematogenous spread, although axonal spread has also been advanced as a mechanism following study of the disease in experimental laboratory animals. Virus first appears in the CNS, initially in the medulla oblongata and diencephalon, when infected sheep are clinically normal. It then spreads to other parts of the CNS and replicates to titers higher than those in nonneural tissues. Infection in nonneural tissues remains, where moderate titers persist until death of the animal. Clinical disease usually occurs when sheep are 3 to 4 years of age, when high concentrations of virus are present in the CNS, especially in the diencephalon, brain stem, cerebellar cortex, spinal cord, and, sometimes, the cerebral cortex. Interestingly, the last two areas are not ones in which microscopic lesions are frequently detected. The pathogenesis of the natural disease in goats appears to be comparable with that in sheep. With regard to bovine spongiform encephalopathy, there is epidemiologic evidence that strongly suggests that this disease was caused initially (during the early 1980s) by the feeding of rations containing meat and bone meal supplements contaminated with the scrapie agent.

One of the most intriguing features of scrapie concerns the uniqueness of its etiologic agent. Unlike conventional viruses, the agent has unusual resistance to inactivation by heating and ultraviolet irradiation, and no structures resembling virions can be detected ultrastructurally. Three main concepts have been advanced regarding the nature of the infectious agent. First, some researchers have suggested that the agent is a virus whose protein(s) is coded by its nucleic acid, but morphologic and biochemical studies of purified preparations of the agent have failed to demonstrate viral particles or nucleic acids. A second hypothesis proposes that the scrapie nucleic acid is too small to code for protein and that the agent's protein required for infectivity is coded for and produced by the infected cell. The name *virino* has been proposed for such an agent. A third proposal is that the agent is a proteinaceous infectious particle (prion) without evidence of an associated nucleic acid and that it appears to accumulate selectively in neurons. A specific protein referred to as PrP (prion protein), a 27 to 30 kilodalton polypeptide, seems to be required for and inseparable from prion infectivity. It should be noted that normal cells of the body produce a normal prion protein, whose normal function is unknown. It is expressed throughout the body and is the product of a highly conserved gene found in organisms as diverse as the fruit fly and the human. An abnormal form of PrP is present in animals and humans who develop the characteristic spongiform encephalopathy. Although the mechanism by which the abnormal form (PrPsc) develops is not known, it has been proposed that in some way there is posttranslational modification of the normal noninfectious PrP (by the infectious form) to produce PrPsc.

Although scrapie can be caused by an infectious agent, host genetic factors also have a considerable influence on the development of the disease. Investigations suggest that all sheep carry a gene, referred to as *Sip,* which controls the scrapie incubation period. There is good evidence that the *Sip* gene may also be the homologue of the *Sinc* gene in mice, and, if this is true, it could control neuroinvasion and subsequent events in the nervous system upon which development of the clinical disease depends.

Equine herpesvirus 1 infection

Alpha-herpesviruses, designated equine herpesvirus 1 (EHV-1) with subtypes 1 and 2 (the latter formerly known as equine herpesvirus 4) and equine herpesvirus 3, have been identified as causes of disease in horses. More recently, a new subtype of the abortigenic EHV-1, subtype 1, has been identified as subtype 1b.

Equine herpesvirus 1, subtype 1, is the important cause of equine abortion, perinatal foal infection and death, and encephalomyelitis but can also cause rhinopneumonitis. Equine herpesvirus 1, subtype 2, causes respiratory disease almost exclusively, but the virus has also been isolated from cases of sporadic abortion. Equine coital exanthema is caused by equine herpesvirus 3. An additional virus, a beta-herpesvirus designated equine cytomegalovirus (or equine herpesvirus 2), also has been isolated from horses with respiratory disease.

The neurologic form of EHV-1 has a worldwide distribution and may affect other equidae, including the zebra, but the disease appears to be relatively uncommon when compared with the incidence rate of abortion and upper respiratory disease caused by EHV-1.

The characteristic lesion in the CNS caused by herpesvirus 1 infection is a vasculitis (affecting arterioles, capillaries, and venules) accompanied by thrombosis and focal parenchymal necrosis (infarction). Lesions occur in both the gray and white matter of the spinal cord, medulla oblongata, mesencephalon, diencephalon, and cerebral cortex. The endothelium appears to be the site of involvement, with the subsequent occurrence of intimal and medial degeneration, hemorrhage, thrombosis, extravasation of plasma proteins into the perivascular space, neuronal degeneration (e.g., axonal swelling with ballooning of the myelin sheath and degeneration of the cell body), and variable mononuclear cellular cuffing. Other lesions include cerebrospinal ganglioneuritis and vasculitis in nonneural tissues including the endometrium, nasal cavity, lung, uvea of the eye, hypophysis, and skeletal muscle.

The disease begins with infection of the respiratory mucosa. The neurologic disease has been experimentally reproduced by intranasal inoculation of the virus (EHV-1, subtype 1), which can replicate in the epithelium of the respiratory or intestinal tracts following infection (with intranuclear inclusions in the nasal mucosa). This is followed by infection of mononuclear leukocytes (predominantly but not exclusively T-lymphocytes) and, then, a cell-associated viremia. The virus has been shown to be endotheliotropic and can localize in small arteries and capillaries of the CNS and some other tissues following direct spread from the circulating mononuclear cells to vascular endothelium. Inflammation of the vascular wall then results in vasculitis, thrombosis, and infarction of the neural tissue supplied by the thrombosed vessel. Equine herpesvirus 1, subtype 1, does not appear to be neurotropic, which is in contrast to some herpesvirus encephalitides of other species in which the virus replicates in neurons (e.g., herpes simplex viral infection in the human, infectious bovine rhinotracheitis viral infection in calves, and pseudorabies viral infection in swine). In addition to having vasculitis as the principal lesion, the infection in the horse also differs somewhat from most other herpetic infections of the CNS in being primarily a disease of the adult (although young animals can be affected).

Bovine malignant catarrhal fever

Malignant catarrhal fever is a highly fatal disease of cattle and other ruminants, including deer, buffalo, and antelope. The primary target tissues affected are the lymphoid organs, epithelial tissues (particularly the respiratory and GI tracts), and the vasculature. Involvement of the kidney, liver, eye, joints, and CNS may also occur. Three distinct patterns of the disease are recognized, and from only one has a virus (*alcephaline herpesvirus 1,* a member of the subfamily Gammaherpesviridae) been definitively identified. This form of the disease occurs in Africa and in zoos; it affects cattle (sometimes involving many animals) and susceptible wild ruminants following transmission of the virus from the wildebeest. A second form of the disease occurs worldwide, including Africa, and has been referred to as the sheep-associated form. This disease affects cattle and especially deer, which are also susceptible to the first form described. Only irregular transmission of the sheep-associated form of the disease between cattle has been achieved, and identification of the agent capable of reproducing the disease has remained elusive, although more recent evidence (e.g., that sheep have antibody to *alcephaline herpesvirus 1*) is supportive of it being a herpesvirus. A third form of the disease, also described as malignant catarrhal fever, has been reported in feedlot cattle in North America in the absence of contact with sheep. The identity and source of a virus remain to be clarified.

Gross lesions of the CNS include congestion and cloudiness of the meninges. Microscopically, the lesion is a nonsuppurative meningoencephalomyelitis that can be associated with a vasculitis. Lymphocytic perivascular cuffing and varying degrees of necrotizing vasculitis occur in all parts of the brain and occasionally in the spinal cord, with the white matter being most consistently involved. Other lesions in the affected CNS include variable neuronal degeneration, microgliosis, leptomeningitis, hemorrhage, choroiditis, necrosis of ependymal cells, and ganglioneuritis.

It is generally accepted that cattle and other susceptible ruminants contract the disease naturally (following respiratory or oral infection) during association with infected wildebeest (and other wild ruminants) or sheep (particularly at the time of parturition of carrier animals). An immune-mediated (e.g., cell-mediated) process has been proposed to be involved in lesion development.

Hog cholera (swine fever)

This disease of swine is caused by a pestivirus and has a worldwide distribution, except for several countries (including the United States) from which it has been successfully eradicated.

Lesions of the acute disease, which primarily result from a tropism of the virus for vascular endothelium with subsequent hemorrhage, are present in many organs, including the kidney, intestinal serosa, lymph nodes, spleen, liver, bone marrow, lungs, skin, heart, stomach, gallbladder, and CNS. Lesions of the CNS are characterized by swelling, proliferation, and necrosis of endothelium; perivascular lymphocytic cuffing; infrequent hemorrhage and thrombosis; microgliosis; neuronal degeneration; choroiditis; and leptomeningitis. Lesions occur in both gray and white matter and tend to be most prominent in the brain stem (medulla oblongata, pons, colliculi) and thalamus, but also occur in the cerebrum, cerebellum, and spinal cord.

Infection under natural conditions occurs by the oronasal route. The virus initially infects epithelial cells of the tonsilar crypts and surrounding lymphoreticular tissue, then spreads to draining lymph nodes, where it replicates. Extension continues via the circulation to the spleen, bone marrow, visceral lymph nodes, and lymphoid tissue of the intestinal tract, where high titers are attained. Hematogenous spread of the virus throughout the infected pig (including the CNS) is usually completed in 5 to 6 days.

Feline infectious peritonitis

Feline infectious peritonitis (FIP), which is caused by a coronavirus and has a worldwide distribution, is mainly a disease of domestic cats, although wild felidae can be affected. It generally occurs sporadically in cats of all ages (with a peak incidence between 6 months and 5 years) and can be clinically significant, as it can result in death. The disease manifests itself in **effusive** or **noneffusive** forms.

The basic lesion of both forms of the disease is a pyogranulomatous inflammation (with a tendency to be surface-oriented) accompanied by vasculitis and variable necrosis. The **effusive form** is typified by serositis, accumulation of fluid in the abdominal and thoracic cavities, with varying degrees of inflammation of visceral tissue. Lesions of the **noneffusive form** more frequently include leptomeningitis, chorioependymitis, focal encephalomyelitis, and ophthalmitis, although involvement of other tissues (kidney, hepatic and mesenteric lymph nodes, and, less frequently, serosa and other abdominal viscera) may occur.

There has been speculation concerning the origin of the FIP virus: whether it is a separate entity in nature, or whether it can arise periodically as a mutation of feline enteric coronavirus. Probably both situations occur to some extent.

The FIP virus may be shed and transmitted to other susceptible cats. The virus may be spread by the oronasal route or by direct inoculation (via cat bite, licking open wounds, etc.) following contact with carrier cats, although in utero transmission has also been proposed. The route of virus shedding is probably via excretions from the bowel. Following infection, the virus replicates in the intestinal epithelium, which is followed by hematogenous spread of virus-infected phagocytic cells. There is preferential infection of phagocytes of the body (in the liver; visceral peritoneum and pleura, uvea, meninges, and ependyma of the brain; and spinal cord). The possible relationship between the surface orientation of the lesions in this disease and phagocytic spread of the organism is discussed below (see Other Bacterial Infections of the CNS).

Following dissemination of the virus in the body, the development of disease appears to depend on the type and degree of immunity that develops. Virus containment, with resistance to disease, is thought to be due to development of a strong, cell-mediated immunity. Humoral immunity by itself is not protective and, in some instances, actually enhances the severity of the disease. The effusive form occurs only in cats that mount a humoral response. Noneffusive FIP, in comparison, is thought to occur when partial cell-mediated immunity develops, and it represents an intermediate stage between nonprotective humoral immunity alone and protective cellular immunity. This is supported by the fact that cats that develop the noneffusive form of FIP following experimental infection usually have a preceding and transient bout of effusive-type disease. In addition, there is evidence to support the theory that cats recovered from FIP are immune by a process of "infection immunity" or "premunition." Once these cats no longer retain such infections, they seem to also lose protective (cell-mediated) immunity and are, in fact, more sensitive to a subsequent challenge exposure, due to the presence of humoral antibody.

It should also be noted that an Arthus-type reaction involving antigen-antibody complex formation (with fixation of complement) has been proposed as being involved in lesion development with FIP, although more recent evidence, indicating that decomplementation of inoculated cats may have no appreciable effect on the resulting disease, suggests that the mechanism involved may not be completely resolved.

Chlamydial Infections

Sporadic bovine encephalomyelitis

Sporadic bovine encephalomyelitis, an uncommon disease that is now recognized as being caused by a *Chlamydial* organism, was originally described in the United States but also occurs in several other countries.

Young animals (under 6 to 12 months of age) are uniformly more susceptible to the disease than older animals. The hallmark lesions of sporadic bovine encephalomyelitis are serofibrinous serositis and nonsuppurative meningoencephalomyelitis, although fibrinous arthritis may also occur. Grossly, lesions of the CNS are not present or include congestion and edema of the leptomeninges. Microscopically, there is a diffuse nonsuppurative inflammation of the CNS that can extend from the cerebral cortex to the lumbar spinal cord and includes the leptomeninges. Additional lesions include neuronal degeneration, focal necrosis, and vasculitis.

Lesions of the CNS, particularly neuronal degeneration and focal necrosis, presumably result from a primary insult to the vasculature that causes ischemia. Immune-mediated mechanisms have also been proposed as being involved in development of lesions in the CNS.

Protozoal Infections

Sarcocystosis

Equine protozoal encephalomyelitis (*Sarcocystis neurona* infection) generally occurs in young adults. The pathogenesis is unknown. Although lesions occur throughout the CNS, there is a definite predilection for the spinal cord. Gross lesions, when present, are often clearly visible and consist of necrosis frequently accompanied by hemorrhage (Fig. 8-51). Microscopic lesions include prominent necrosis; hemorrhage; perivascular cuffing with lymphocytes and macrophages; presence in the neuropil of gitter cells, eosinophils, multinucleated giant cells, and varying numbers of neutrophils; gemistocytic astrocytosis; neuronal degeneration with axonal swelling; and, sometimes, leptomeningitis. The etiologic agent is small and crescent-shaped to round, has a well-defined nucleus, and is often arranged in aggregates or rosettes. Organisms can be difficult to detect but can occur in the cytoplasm of capillary pericytes, neuronal cell bodies and axons, macrophages, and neutrophils, as well as extracellularly.

The causative agent, the coccidian *S. neurona,* has recently been isolated in tissue culture and characterized. The organism, which develops in the host cell cytoplasm and divides by endopolygeny, is characterized by development of schizonts that contain merozoites arranged in a rosette around a prominent residual body. The organism differs from those of the genera *Toxoplasma, Isospora, Eimeria, Besnoitia, Hammondia,* and *Neospora,* but resembles organisms of the genera *Sarcocystis* and *Frenkelia.* At present, only asexual stages of the parasite are known, and no information is available on its life cycle or transmission. One unique feature is that the schizonts of *S. neurona* are generally not seen in the endothelium of affected horses, whereas schizonts of all other infections by this genus (in nonequine species) infect this cell of blood vessels throughout the body.

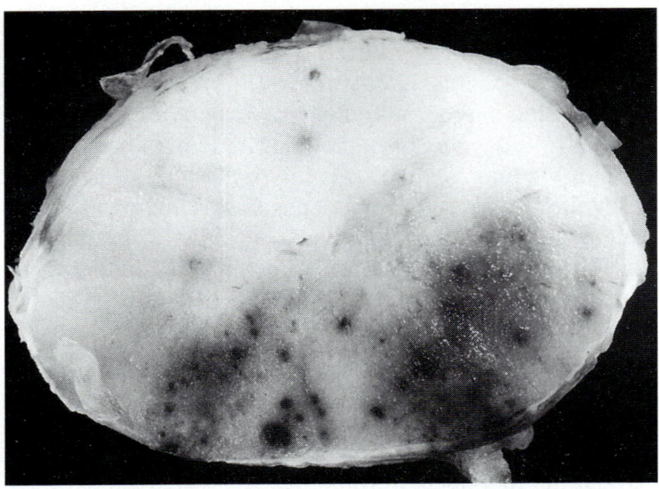

Fig. 8-51 Spinal cord, lumbar level; horse. Myelitis due to *Sarcocystis neurona* infection. Prominent focal hemorrhage and necrosis are present in the right lateral funiculus and in the right and left ventral funiculi.

Sarcocystosis in nonequine species involves organisms similar to *S. neurona.* Such organisms have also been associated with encephalomyelitis in the bovine, ovine, and canine species, plus the raccoon, but such infections apparently are often sporadic. Lesions have additionally been detected in the CNS of infected fetuses (e.g., bovine species).

Toxoplasmosis

Toxoplasma gondii, which is ubiquitous, can infect many animals as intermediate hosts, including fish, amphibians, reptiles, birds, humans, and other mammals (dogs, cats, sheep, cattle, swine, plus several other domestic, laboratory, and wild animals). Cats are unique in that they are "complete" hosts for the organism, being able to serve as both definitive and intermediate hosts. New World monkeys and Australian marsupials are the most susceptible to toxoplasmosis, while Old World monkeys, rats, cattle, and horses are highly resistant.

T. gondii is indiscriminate in the type of cell it parasitizes in the intermediate host and can cause lesions in such tissues as the lung, lymphoid system, liver, heart, skeletal muscle, pancreas, intestine, eye, and nervous system.

Gross lesions involving the nervous system are limited and include occasional submeningeal hyperemia and hemorrhage, hemorrhagic infarction, cerebral edema that can be sufficiently severe to cause displacement and herniation, and ventricular dilatation. Early microscopic lesions are characterized by degeneration of vessel walls and edema. Subsequent parenchymal invasion of organisms is accompanied by tissue necrosis (with variable hemorrhage) that can be striking. Other lesions include nonsuppurative inflammation (microgliosis, perivascular cuffing); degeneration of astrocytes, oligodendroglia, and neurons; focal astrocytic hypertrophy; and leptomeningitis (Fig. 8-52). Lesions are distributed throughout both the gray and white matter of the CNS (brain and spinal cord). Radiculitis may also occur.

Following ingestion, bradyzooites from tissue cysts or sporozoites from oocysts penetrate the intestinal epithelial cells and multiply in the intestine. There is evidence that *T. gondii* invades host cells by active penetration (e.g., following disruption of the plasma membrane by organism-secreted lytic products) and not by phagocytosis. Organisms may then spread locally to mesenteric lymph nodes, Peyer's patches, and other cells, where they multiply as tachyzoites (within a parasitophorous vacuole) by repeated intracellular endodyogeny during the acute phase of the infection. There is continued spread to distant organs via the lymphatics and the circulation following vascular invasion. Infection of the CNS occurs hematogenously (with neurons and astrocytes being target cells). In utero infection in animals (with cats being more resistant), as well as humans, can also occur, and lesions may occur in the fetal CNS (e.g., ovine fetus in which the incidence may be 90%). With chronicity and increased antibody titer, tachyzoites of *T. gondii* transform into slowly growing bradyzoites that replicate within tissue cysts.

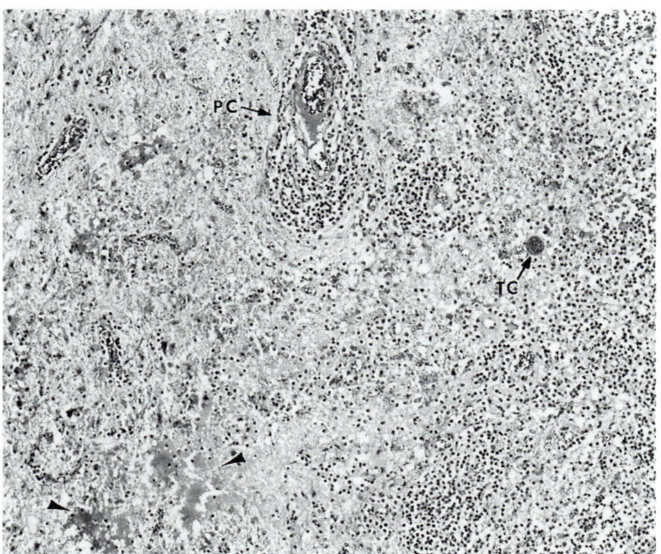

Fig. 8-52 Brain; parietal lobe, dorsomedial thalamus; cat. Toxoplasmosis. Nonsuppurative encephalitis with perivascular cuffing *(PC),* diffuse accumulation of macrophages and plasma cells *(right side),* focal edema *(arrowheads),* and a *Toxoplasma* cyst *(TC)* are present. H & E stain.

Immune-mediated mechanisms have been proposed as explanations for vascular injury (type III hypersensitivity) and cellular necrosis (type IV hypersensitivity). Immune cytotoxic T-lymphocytes (CD8+ T cells), which play a defensive role because of their ability to lyse infected cells, could also potentially be involved in causing tissue damage. Intracellular growth of tachyzoites has also been advanced as a cause of necrosis. The organism does not produce a toxin.

Neosporosis

A newly described protozoal disease, caused by a recently identified parasite, *Neospora caninum,* was first recognized in 1988 as affecting the nervous and other systems of the dog. In addition to the dog, natural infections can also occur in neonatal sheep and the equine fetus. Similarly, a naturally occurring *N. caninum*–like infection has been demonstrated to cause fetal and neonatal infection (with CNS involvement) in the bovine species. Experimental infection has also been produced in the dog, cat, sheep, and laboratory animals (e.g., mouse) resulting in lesions of the CNS in all these species. The organism *N. caninum* has some features that are similar to those of *T. gondii,* including its microscopic morphology, division of tachyzoites by endodyogeny, and having both proliferative (tachyzoite) and tissue cyst stages of development, but there are also some characteristics that distinguish the two organisms (e.g., *N. caninum* does not develop within a cytoplasmic parasitophorous vacuole in vivo as does *T. gondii,* the walls of tissue cysts of *N. caninum* are much thicker than those of *T. gondii,* and there is a lack of immunologic cross-reactivity). Organisms can infect different cell types, including neurons; ependymal cells; mononuclear cells of the spinal fluid; endothelial cells, intima, and media (plus connective tissue) of blood vessels (including those of the CNS); skeletal and myocardial myofibers; macrophages; neutrophils; and fibroblasts. Organisms have also been detected in spinal nerves. Other than for transplacental transmission, which has been either demonstrated or proposed for the canine, feline, ovine, and equine species (and associated with lesions of CNS in the first three species listed), the mechanism of infection is unknown. Likewise, the life cycle also remains to be determined.

Both young and adult dogs can be affected. The predominant signs in young dogs (often most severely affected) are ascending paralysis, with the hind limbs being more severely affected due to polyradiculoneuritis and polymyositis. In adult dogs, signs are consistent with involvement of the CNS as well as with polymyositis, myocarditis, and dermatitis. Also, the administration of corticosteroids has been demonstrated to exacerbate acute and chronic neosporosis in experimentally infected dogs.

Neurologic lesions include meningoencephalomyelitis accompanied by sometimes prominent vasculitis and focal necrosis. The causative organism (both proliferative and cystic forms) is variably present in lesions of the CNS. The inflammation is characterized by microgliosis, and perivascular cuffing (with accumulations of macrophages, lymphocytes, plasma cells, and variable neutrophils). In addition, radiculoneuritis can also occur. Nonneural lesions variably include myositis, hepatitis, pancreatitis, dermatitis, myocarditis, pneumonia, lymphadenitis, nephritis, and necrosis of the gastric mucosa. All the lesions except nephritis include necrosis. Tachyzooites replicate intracellularly in many cell types of dogs and other species and appear to destroy cells by active multiplication. The cyst form of the organism appears to occur only in the CNS in the dog and other species.

Bacterial Infections

Haemophilus somnus *infection in cattle (thromboembolic meningoencephalitis [TEME], infectious thromboembolic meningoencephalitis, infectious emboli encephalitis)*

Haemophilus somnus infection of cattle was first described in 1956 as infectious embolic meningoencephalitis and has since been detected in many areas of the United States, Canada, and other countries. The disease occurs most frequently in feedlot cattle in the United States but also can affect animals on pasture, and dairy cattle. The majority of affected animals range in age from 5 to 18 months, and CNS involvement, even in its mildest form, occurs in only a small percentage of infected animals.

Although *H. somnus* infection is characterized by involvement of several systems (e.g., causing pneumonia, infertility, abortion, septicemia, and arthritis), only lesions of the CNS are discussed here.

Gross lesions include irregularly sized areas of hemorrhagic necrosis disseminated throughout the brain (seen both externally and on cross section) and occur more frequently in the cerebrum (often at the cortical–white matter junction) but also irregularly in the spinal cord (Fig. 8-53). Other lesions detected are flattening of the gyri secondary to cerebral edema, and cloudiness of the CSF caused by fibrinopurulent leptomeningitis.

The microscopic lesions are similar in all organs affected and consist of a marked vasculitis and thrombosis that often result in infarction. In the brain, as in other tissues, vasculitis is an early event, followed by accumulation of edema fluid and inflammatory cells (primarily neutrophils but also some macrophages) in the surrounding neurophil (Fig. 8-54). Although little is known about the chemotactic signals involved, infections with *H. somnus* and related organisms provoke a vigorous accumulation of inflammatory cells. Bacterial colonies are frequently present within thrombi (associated with the vasculitis), in and around affected vessels, and in areas of necrosis. Fibrinopurulent leptomeningitis also usually accompanies the encephalitis and occasionally constitutes the major lesion.

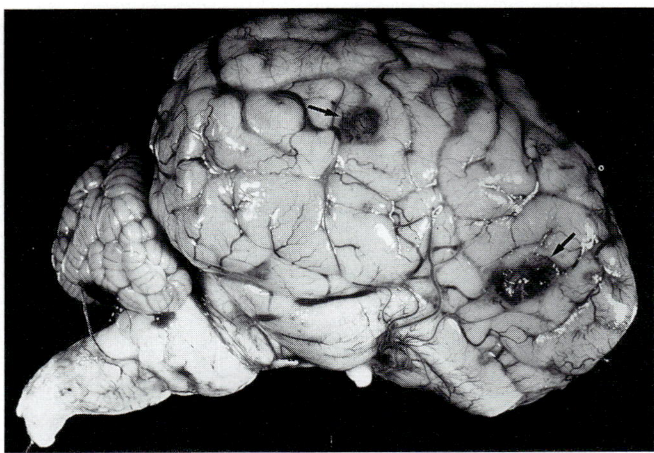

Fig. 8-53 Brain; steer. *Haemophilus somnus* infection. Foci of parenchymal hemorrhage, edema, and necrosis extend to the surface of the brain (*arrows*). *Courtesy Dr. H.W. Leipold.*

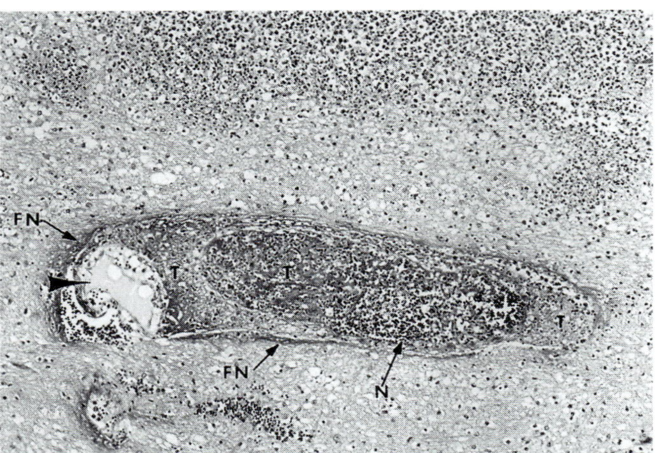

Fig. 8-54 Brain, parietal lobe, thalamus; steer. *Haemophilus somnus* infection. There is pronounced vasculitis of a large cerebral vessel whose lumen is occupied by a thrombus (*T*) and neutrophils (*N*) in various stages of degeneration. Note the fibrinoid necrosis *(FN)* of the cell wall. Varying degrees of neutrophilic accumulation are in the peripheral areas *(top)*. A side branch of the vessel can also be seen *(arrowhead)*. H & E stain.

The pathogenesis of *H. somnus* infection remains incompletely understood. Many cattle carry the organism without signs; yet, under some circumstances, it invades to cause severe disease. The mechanism(s) by which the organism enters the bloodstream is not definitively known, but invasion from the respiratory tract has been proposed. Stress and bacterial colonization on the surface of the mucous membrane, which can be influenced by release of growth factors by normal flora, should be considered as factors that may influence the invasive process. Once the organism enters the circulation, it appears to have a special ability to adhere to endothelial cells, which results in their contraction and desquamation. Large areas of subendothelial collagen are thus exposed, leading to thrombosis, vasculitis, infarction, and tissue invasion, including that of the CNS. The effect of *H. somnus* on host cells also importantly influences the degree of lesion development that occurs. It has been shown that bovine neutrophils, blood monocytes, and alveolar macrophages are incapable of killing *H. somnus* and that the organism can injure macrophages, including those of the lung. Also, a toxic factor (a lipooligosaccharide or LOS) may be involved in resistance of the organism to host factors during infection.

Listeriosis

Listeriosis, an infectious disease caused by *Listeria monocytogenes,* is a significant disease of sheep, goats, and cattle. Listeriosis can occur in three forms: infection with CNS involvement; infection of a pregnant animal associated with abortion or stillbirth; and septicemia, which primarily develops in young animals, probably as a result of in utero infection. The encephalitic and genital forms rarely occur together in the same animal or even in the same flock of sheep.

Gross lesions are usually not detected in the CNS, but, when present, they include leptomeningeal opacity, necrosis in the caudal brain stem, cerebral congestion, and an increase in CSF, which may be cloudy. Microscopic lesions are typified by a meningoencephalomyelitis that characteristically affects the gray and white matter of the brain stem (pons and medulla), but may extend from the diencephalon to the caudal medulla or rostral cervical spinal cord. The smallest and probably the earliest parenchymal lesion consists of loose clusters of microglia, which become larger and which contain variable numbers of neutrophils. There is early necrosis, and bacteria can be detected in the cellular foci. The next stage is characterized by the predominance of neutrophils, tissue necrosis, and accumulation of gitter cells (Fig. 8-55). Numerous bacteria (gram-positive bacilli) are present within and around these lesions. Although neutrophils are a characteristic feature of the listerial lesion, they are not present in all areas of inflammation, and, in some instances, macrophages may predominate. Other changes include neuronal degeneration (particularly in the pons and medulla) and leptomeningitis, which is regularly present (often marked) and characterized by the accumulation of macrophages, plasma cells, lymphocytes, and neutrophils. Additionally, a peripheral neuritis occurs that particularly involves the trigeminal nerve and ganglion (ganglioneuritis).

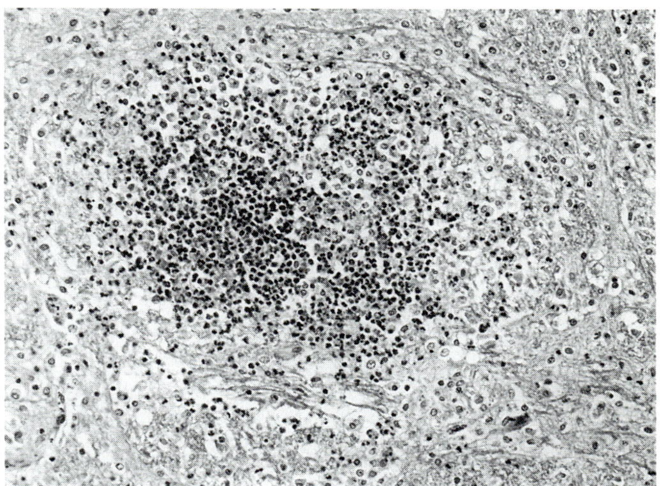

Fig. 8-55 Brain, medulla oblongata; goat. Listeriosis. There is focal accumulation of neutrophils and a loss of parenchyma. H & E stain.

Pathogenetically, there is good evidence to support invasion of the organism through the oral epithelium and into branches of the trigeminal nerve. This is followed by intraaxonal migration to the trigeminal ganglion and brain (pons) from which the disease may spread rostrally and caudally. The exact mechanism involved in tissue injury associated with *L. monocytogenes* infection is not fully understood, but evidence has been presented indicating a correlation between the degree of cell-mediated immunity and lesion development in the CNS. Other factors cited as contributing to development of disease include the presence of listeriolysin (an extracellular hemolysin produced by all pathogenic strains of *L. monocytogenes*) as an essential virulence factor required for the intracellular multiplication of the organism in host tissues. Although cell-mediated immunity has been proposed as the principal type of immunity mounted against *L. monocytogenes,* humoral immunity has also recently been implicated as playing a role.

Other bacterial infections of the CNS

The primary bacteria to be discussed under this heading include: *Escherichia coli, Streptococcus, Salmonella, Pasteurella,* and *Haemophilus.* Although there are individual differences among organisms and the diseases that develop in infected animals, some common features of these infections are that they occur in young farm animals (calves, foals, lambs, and pigs) and that they tend to produce fibrinopurulent inflammation in membranous tissues of the body (e.g., leptomeninges, ependyma, choroid plexus of the CNS; synovia [of joints]; uvea [of the eye]; and serosa [peritoneum, pleura, and pericardium]). Some of these lesions tend to be caused by specific organisms. For example, serositis is primarily associated with *Haemophilus parasuis* and *Streptococcus suis,* type 2, infection in swine, although *E. coli* may also be a cause. It has been proposed that the surface-relatedness of these infections results from the transport of bacteria in monocytes (with low bactericidal activity) that migrate by normal pathways to maintain significant surface populations of macrophages.

In the calf, infections with *E. coli, Streptococcus,* and *Pasteurella* generally occur in young animals, ranging in age from 2 days to 1 month. Infections can occur during the first 1 to 2 weeks of life, although *Pasteurella* may also affect older animals (1 to 2 years). Of the above group of organisms, *E. coli* appears to be the most frequent cause. In addition to fibrinopurulent leptomeningitis (Fig. 8-56), other lesions include purulent ventriculitis, ependymitis, choroiditis *(E. coli, Pasteurella),* encephalitis and/or meningitis with vasculitis and thrombosis *(E. coli),* synovitis-arthritis *(E. coli, Streptococcus),* perioptic neuritis *(E. coli),* and ophthalmitis *(E. coli, Streptococcus).*

In the foal, important bacteria include *E. coli,* streptococci, and *Salmonella.* Foals infected with *E. coli,* which appears to have become more significant as a cause of neonatal infection, have signs at or shortly after birth, and foals with meningitis may live to 3 to 14 days of age. Besides leptomeningitis, lesions include ventriculitis with extension into the adjacent parenchyma, polyarthritis, and effusions containing exudate in the serous sacs. Chronic synovitis may also occur in some animals. Streptococcal infections of foals, accompanied by meningitis, may occur in the neonatal period, with signs present at birth or during the first 12 hours. Such animals may die within 24 to 48 hours. Other animals are older (possibly more common) and develop fibrinopurulent infection of serous sacs and arthritis. *Salmonella* infection, accompanied by septicemia and leptomeningitis, generally affects animals 1 to 6 months of age, and *Salmonella typhimurium* is most frequently isolated. In addition to leptomeningitis (accompanied by vasculitis), lesions include abscess formation, ventriculitis-ependymitis, and choroiditis. Extraneural lesions include synovitis-arthritis.

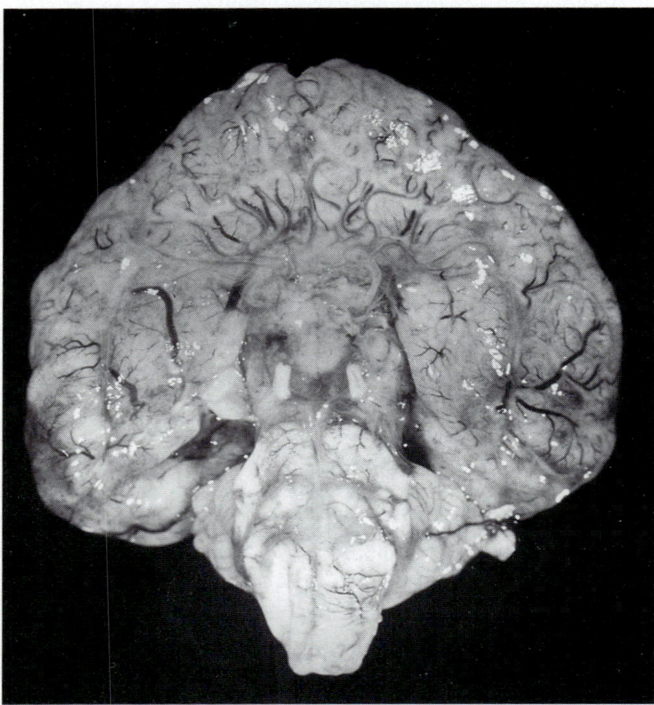

Fig. 8-56 Brain, leptomeninges; calf. Purulent leptomeningitis. The meningeal opacity is due to the presence of purulent exudate in the leptomeninges (that include the subarachnoid space).

In the lamb, significant organisms include *E. coli* and *P. multocida.* The age of lambs infected with *E. coli* ranges from 1 day to 8 weeks, and they have a clinical course that ranges from 2 to several days. Lesions include purulent leptomeningitis with vasculitis, purulent ventriculitis with focal loss of lining ependyma, occasional cerebral and cerebellar necrosis accompanied by inflammation, fibrinopurulent peritonitis, and arthritis. *P. multocida* has been reported to cause purulent meningitis in ewes and lambs.

Bacterial infection in swine is frequently caused by streptococci, often *Streptococcus suis.* It has become clear during the past several years that there are more strains of *S. suis* capable of causing disease than was originally appreciated. Reports over the years have indicated that *S. suis* type 1 generally affects suckling pigs ranging in age from less than 1 week to 6 weeks, whereas *Streptococcus suis* type 2 generally infects weaned pigs from 6 to 14 weeks. *Streptococcus suis* type 2 has become recognized as one of the more important serotypes causing meningitis (as well as other lesions) in young pigs and also in human beings, particularly individuals working with pigs or handling porcine tissues. Recent reports have additionally incriminated other serotypes of *S. suis* (e.g., serotypes ½, 3), as well as untypeable isolates, as the cause of serious disease (including meningitis) in pigs. *S. suis* type 1 can produce a septicemia resulting in lesions that include fibrinopurulent meningochoroiditis with extension of the inflammatory process to the subpial and subependymal tissues. Also, the meningitis can extend to the cranial and rostral spinal nerve roots, and the central canal of the spinal cord may contain exudate. Some affected animals also have liquefaction necrosis of the parenchyma (cerebellum, brain stem, and cervical cord). *S. suis* type 1 can additionally cause fibrinopurulent arthritis. *S. suis* type 2 infection is also capable of producing a septicemia, lesions comparable to those of serotype 1 (including cerebellar necrosis), and polyserositis. *H. parasuis,* which can be frequently isolated from the nasal cavity of healthy pigs, causes fibrinopurulent leptomeningitis, serositis (peritonitis, pleuritis, pericarditis), and synovitis-arthritis in 2- to 4-month-old pigs (Fig. 8-57). The outcome of infection is believed to depend upon the immune status of the pig and stress factors

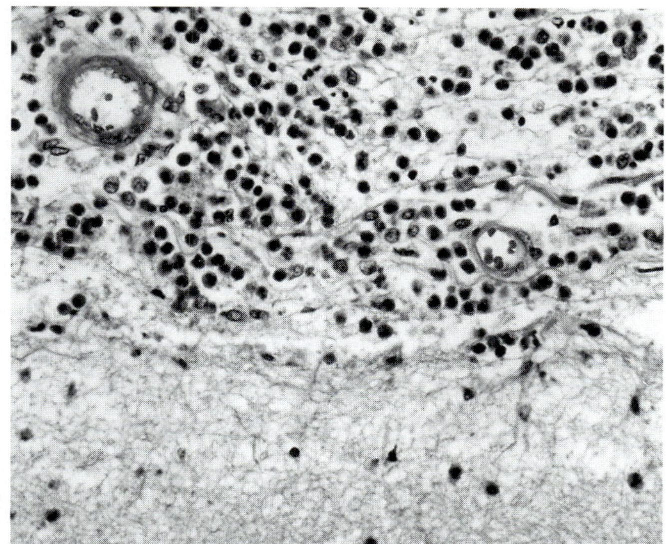

Fig. 8-57 Brain, parietal lobe, leptomeninges; pig. Purulent leptomeningitis caused by *Haemophilus parasuis* infection. There is a marked accumulation of neutrophils in the leptomeninges *(top)* that includes the subarachnoid space.

(e.g., related to transport). In addition, specific features of pathogenic strains of the organism have been identified. In addition to streptococcus other organisms include *E. coli,* which can cause a septicemia accompanied by a diffuse purulent leptomeningitis and fibrinous serositis in early-weaned pigs, and *Erysipelothrix rhusiopathiae,* which can induce a leptomeningitis and vasculitis that are generally not frankly purulent, even though a few neutrophils may be present. Neurologic lesions associated with *Salmonella choleraesuis* infection occur in the brain and spinal cord. They differ from those discussed above and are characterized by nonsuppurative meningoencephalomyelitis accompanied by vasculitis and choroiditis. Encephalitic lesions may be marked, with severe vasculitis surrounded by microgranulomas accompanied by necrosis. Ophthalmitis can also accompany *E. coli, Salmonella,* and *Erysipelothrix* infections in the pig.

Pathogenetic mechanisms for the above involve entrance of bacteria into the body by several possible routes. This is followed by bacteremia and the development of lesions in the CNS and elsewhere. Depending upon the circumstances, infection can occur following oral, umbilical, intrauterine, or aerogenous exposure.

Mycotic Infections

Cryptococcosis

Cryptococcus neoformans has a particular affinity for the leptomeninges and parenchyma of the CNS but may also affect other tissues of the body. Of the domestic animals, the cat, dog, horse, and cow can have neural involvement.

Grossly, the leptomeninges vary from normal to cloudy gray in appearance. The tissue may be thickened and sometimes contains nodules. The exudate in affected meninges often has a viscous consistency caused by the mucopolysaccharide capsule of the organisms. Multiple small cysts can occur in the parenchyma, and there may be thickening of the choroid plexus. Microscopically, meningeal spaces are widely dilated and contain encapsulated organisms in a weblike network within which are hyperplastic histiocytes, variable numbers of giant cells, lymphocytes, plasma cells, neutrophils, eosinophils, and collagen. The meningeal reaction can also extend for some distance along cranial, spinal, and optic nerves and may result in wallerian degeneration of axons. Within the parenchyma, similar cellular accumulations may be accompanied by neuronal degeneration, choroiditis, and ependymitis-ventriculitis. Also, cysts that develop within the nervous tissue contain organisms. Depending on the immune status of the host, the microscopic features of the infection may vary from one having no significant cellular reaction, even though many organisms are present (e.g., when the animal is immunocompromised), to one that is characteristically granulomatous with macrophages, giant cells, lymphocytes, and a fibrous stroma (e.g., in the presence of a stronger immunocompetent state).

It has been proposed that the organism enters through the respiratory tract, where it initiates a respiratory (possibly pulmonary) infection and then spreads hematogenously to various tissues, including the CNS.

Parasitic Infestations

Lesions resulting from parasitic infestation of the CNS vary in degree and distribution. There may be gross lesions of hemorrhage or necrosis, if sufficient injury occurs. Microscopically, the lesions often have a tract formation (resulting from migration) and are characterized by variable necrosis, hemorrhage, and nonsuppurative inflammation accompanied by variable numbers of eosinophils. The degree of host response will, to a large extent, depend on the degree of trauma induced by the parasite, following its entrance in the CNS, and the degree of sensitivity that the host has for parasitic antigens.

Insect larval infestations

Among the common larvae of this group are those of *Oestrus ovis* and *Hypoderma bovis.* The larvae of *O. ovis* normally develop in the nasal cavity of sheep but may occasionally penetrate into the cranial cavity through the ethmoid bone. The larvae of *H. bovis* can enter the spinal canal during their migration in cattle and penetrate the spinal cord. Such larvae can also migrate into the CNS (brain) in the horse. The larvae of *Cuterebra* species, usually an infestation of rabbits and rodents, may invade the CNS of dogs and cats.

Cestode infestations

Coenurus cerebralis, which is the larval form of the dog tapeworm *Multiceps multiceps,* most commonly infests sheep, which are the intermediate host. Other ruminants may also be affected. It is assumed that the intermediate larval form reaches the CNS hematogenously, where it frequently locates in the brain and forms cysts. Another tapeworm, *Taenia solium,* has the human as its definitive host, with the chief intermediate host being the pig. The larval stage, *Cysticercus cellulosae,* generally forms in porcine muscle but can also occur in the meninges and brain.

Nematode infestations

Several nematodes have been reported to produce lesions in the CNS. One disease, setariasis, has been known for many years to affect goats, sheep, and horses in the Far East, where it is referred to as **"kumri."** The causal parasite is *Setaria digitata,* which has cattle and water buffalo as natural hosts and in whose abdominal cavities it resides without causing injury. Mosquitoes transmit the larvae. In unnatural hosts, such as the goat, sheep, and horse, the parasite passes through the nervous system, where it produces lesions. A cerebrospinal nematodiasis considered to be caused by *Setaria* species in the horse has also been reported in the United States.

Halicephalobus deletrix (Micronema deletrix) is a rhabditiform parasite that can cause lesions in the nasal cavity, kidney, and CNS of the horse. Microscopically, lesions and parasites are prominently associated with blood vessels along which the organisms apparently migrate through the CNS.

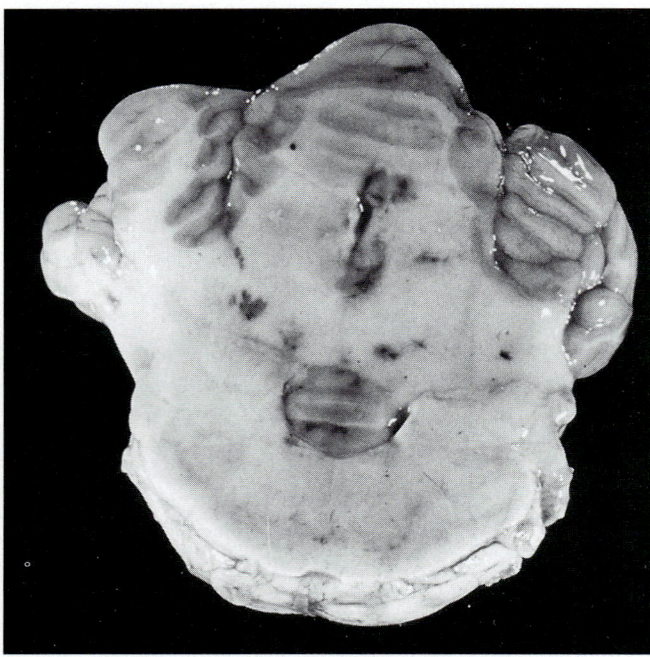

Fig. 8-58 Brain, cerebellum, and medulla oblongata; horse. *Strongylus vulgaris* migration. Several small foci of hemorrhage and necrosis in the cerebellar white matter are sites of larval migration.

Parelaphostrongylus tenuis infestation of sheep and goats can involve migration of the parasite into the CNS. Lesions in sheep and goats are particularly found in the spinal cord. The natural host of this infestation is the white-tailed deer, and, although the parasite normally migrates to the meninges in this species, there is generally no clinical evidence of disease.

The larvae of *Strongylus* species (e.g., *Strongylus vulgaris*) can also aberrantly invade the CNS of the horse and have been incriminated as one of the most common causes of equine cerebrospinal nematodiasis in North America (Fig. 8-58).

MISCELLANEOUS PROCESSES

Reticulosis

Reticulosis has been reported to occur in several species but is most common in the dog. The term reticulosis, which is at best a somewhat imprecise designation and used here in order to give a historical perspective of the spectrum of the lesions involved, includes three disease processes: **inflammatory (granulomatous) reticulosis, neoplastic reticulosis,** and **microgliomatosis.** Inflammatory and neoplastic forms have been considered by some to represent two opposing ends of a spectrum, with intermediate or transitional forms falling in between. Microgliomatosis is described as distinct from the other two types. Recently, an additional designation, **granulomatous meningoencephalomyelitis,** has been used to describe a process that is considered to be analogous, at least in some instances, to the inflammatory form of reticulosis. Ophthalmic lesions may also accompany this form and involve the optic nerve, optic disk, and retina.

Microscopically, the **inflammatory** form of **reticulosis** is characterized by perivascular accumulation of well-differentiated lymphocytes, monocytes, plasma cells, and epithelioid cells, with occasional occurrence of neutrophils and giant cells, plus reticulin fibers and collagen (Fig. 8-59). Not infrequently, cells will be predominantly epithelioid in type. With the **neoplastic** form of **reticulosis,** cells are arranged around vessels and are also usually present in the neuropil. The cells are less differentiated than with the inflammatory form of the disease, and mitotic figures are common. Also, prominent, concentrically arranged reticulin fibers are present around vessels and around cells in the parenchyma. **Microgliomatosis,** which has been classified as a proliferative neoplastic disease, has some features that are quite distinct from the above cited inflammatory and neoplastic forms of reticulosis. The cells, which infiltrate the parenchyma without topographic perivascular arrangement, resemble microglia in that their nuclei, which vary in size and shape and have prominent chromatin, are the only visible cellular component follow-

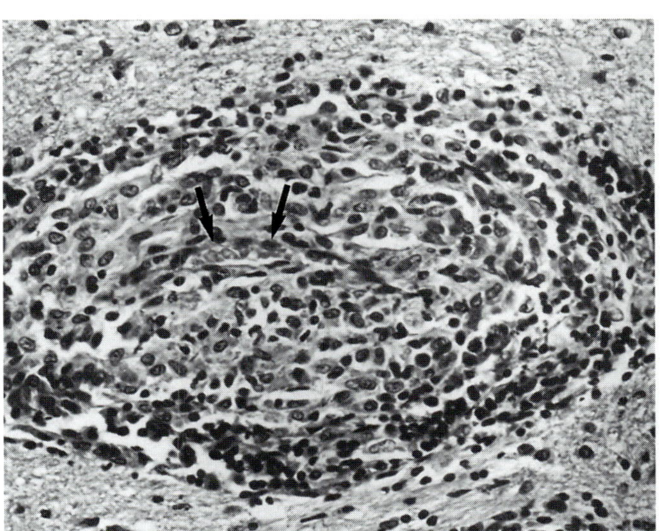

Fig. 8-59 Brain, junction between parietal and occipital lobes, thalamus; dog. Inflammatory reticulosis (granulomatous meningoencephalomyelitis). Perivascular epithelioid cells are located centrally and other mononuclear cells (plasma cells, lymphocytes, and monocytes) have accumulated peripherally. Arrows indicate vascular lumen. H & E stain.

ing conventional staining. Also, mitoses may be common, and there is no accompanying reticulin fiber formation, as occurs with the other two forms described.

When present, gross lesions of the three forms are rarely discrete. They frequently are gray-white to red, expansive areas within the brain parenchyma with loss of structural detail. However, they can have a gelatinous or rubbery consistency with irregular, well-defined margins, or they may appear granular.

When considering all forms of reticulosis as a group, there appears to be no strong breed predilection, although the poodle and terrier-type breeds, including the Airedale, are mentioned as possibly being more frequently affected. Age of affected dogs is variable and ranges from 9 months to 10 years. In three separate studies, involving a total of 85 dogs with reticulosis (including all three forms), the sex distribution was 56 females and 29 males.

NEOPLASMS

Neoplasia of the CNS of animals is not as rare as was once believed. In fact, such neoplasms occur with a frequency and variety, at least in the dog, that is similar to those in humans. The majority of the neoplasms described have been in the dog and cat, and a large portion of these have been in the older population, which is examined more frequently in these species.

The intention of this discussion is to present the reader with a brief overview of the more common or better-known neoplasms that occur in the CNS of animals and not to attempt to be all-inclusive.

Primary Neoplasms of Neuronal Cells

Medulloblastoma

This neoplasm has characteristics similar to the less frequently occurring neuroblastoma, and both are considered to arise from cells of the neuronal lineage. The cell of origin for the medulloblastoma has not been definitely determined, but it has been proposed that the tumor may arise from primitive cells originating in the neuroepithelial roof of the fourth ventricle that give rise to the external granular cell layer.

In animals, the medulloblastoma has been reported in the canine and bovine species, in which young animals of both groups tend to be affected, and in the cat and pig. The neoplasm chiefly occurs in the cerebellum of puppies and calves and sometimes also in adult dogs. The tumor is well circumscribed, soft, and gray to pink and usually does not contain hemorrhage, cysts, or necrosis. The growth may compress the fourth ventricle and cause hydrocephalus and may also infiltrate adjacent structures, including the leptomeninges. It may spread (metastasize) through the CSF in the ventricular or meningeal areas. Microscopically, the tumor is highly cellular and consists of round to elongated nuclei that contain prominent chromatin and ill-defined cytoplasm. The cells may be arranged in sheets or broad bands and also can form pseudorosettes. Mitoses may be common.

Primary Neoplasms of Neuroglial Cells

Astrocytoma

This neoplasm, which can occur in the canine, feline, and bovine species, is best known in the dog. It is possibly the most common neuroglial tumor in the dog and is described here in the canine species. The tumor occurs most frequently in brachycephalic breeds (Boston terrier, boxer) and in the range of 5 to 11 years of age. Common sites of involvement include the pyriform lobe, convexity of the cerebral hemisphere, thalamus-hypothalamus, midbrain, and, less frequently, the cerebellum and spinal cord. The tumors do not grow into the leptomeninges or ventricular system, nor do they metastasize.

Grossly, the area of the CNS involved will be enlarged, and there may be displacement of normal tissue. A characteristic feature of the less malignant forms is that there is no clear demarcation between the neoplasm and normal parenchyma (Fig. 8-60). Such tumors are rather solid or firm and gray-white in color. More rapidly growing forms are softer in consistency and may contain necrosis, hemorrhage, edema, and cystic degeneration. They may also be more readily distinguished from the surrounding parenchyma. Microscopically, astrocytomas have been classified in humans according to degree of cytologic malignancy from grades 1 to 4 or as differentiated and undifferentiated. The more undifferentiated malignant forms (e.g., grades 3 and 4) have also been classified by some as **glioblastoma multiforme.**

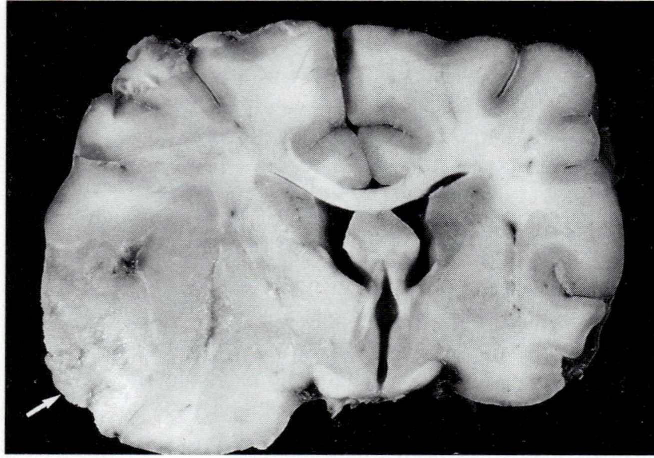

Fig. 8-60 Brain, rostral parietal lobe, level of corpus striatum; dog. Astrocytoma. The neoplasm *(to right of arrow)* is characterized by a diffuse enlargement of the left pyriform lobe with lack of peripheral demarcation.

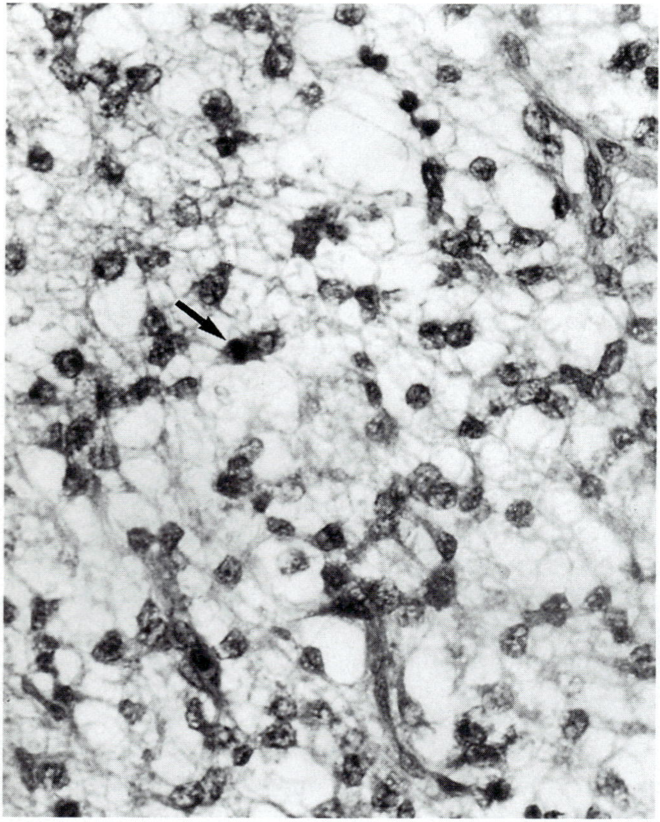

Fig. 8-61 Brain, pyriform lobe; dog. Astrocytoma. The many processes of the loosely arranged cells form a fine intercellular network. Note the characteristic nuclei and the occasional mitotic figure *(arrow)* in this moderately well differentiated astrocytoma. H & E stain.

Microscopically, the more differentiated neoplasms consist of a rather uniform cell type that has a loose arrangement. The cell size varies somewhat, and often distinct, ramifying processes can be seen (Fig. 8-61). Nuclei vary in size and shape and often contain more chromatin than is normal. Cells tend to be arranged around and along blood vessels of the tumor, and growth along boundaries with normal parenchyma is not sharp. Different cell types (e.g., fibrillary, protoplasmic, gemistocytic, and pilocytic) have been described, with the fibrillary form being the most common. In the more undifferentiated neoplasms, cells are more pleomorphic, and there may be mononuclear or multinuclear giant cell formation. Mitoses are also frequent, and degenerative changes (e.g., hemorrhage, necrosis, edema, and cyst formation) are often present.

Oligodendroglioma

Oligodendroglioma occurs most commonly in the dog but has also been reported in cattle and the cat of the domestic animals. The reported incidence of the tumor in the dog is variable; some reports say it is the most common of the neuroectodermal tumors, while others state that it occurs less frequently. As with astrocytomas, there is predilection for occurrence in brachycephalic dogs (e.g., Boston terrier, boxer, bulldog). Affected dogs generally range in age from 5 to 11 years. Tumors occur in the frontal, pyriform, olfactory, and temporal lobes and the brain stem. Other locations include the parietal and occipital lobes and the interventricular septum. Tumors have a tendency to break through to the ventricular or meningeal surfaces, but they spread only exceptionally through the CSF.

Grossly, the tumors are generally demarcated from the surrounding parenchyma. They can vary in size, are soft and gray to pink-red, and often have a gelatinous consis-

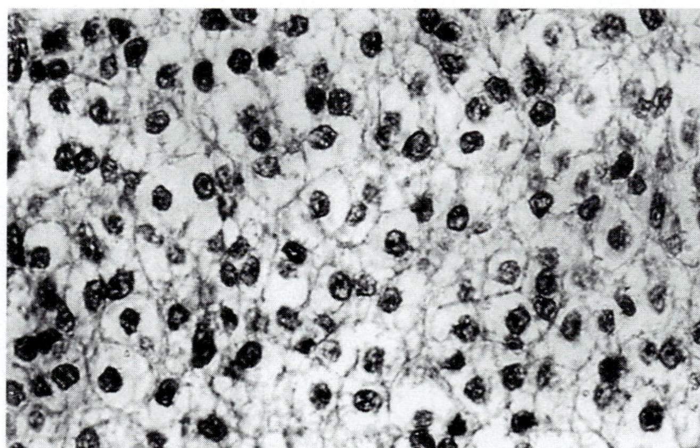

Fig. 8-62 Brain, cerebral hemisphere; dog. Oligodendroglioma. The cells are densely packed and have a characteristic light zone (halo) between the hyperchromatic nucleus and plasma membrane. H & E stain.

tency accompanied by hemorrhage. Microscopically, tumors are highly cellular with cells packed densely against one another. The cytoplasm stains faintly or not at all, and the nuclei are generally hyperchromatic and situated in the center of the cell, creating a perinuclear halo effect (Fig. 8-62). Other patterns that can occur include the arrangement of cells in rows (especially in the areas of peripheral infiltration) or in semicircles. Mitoses are generally infrequent. Regressive changes include mucoid degeneration, edema, cyst formation, and occasional mineralization. Extensive necrosis occurs uncommonly.

Ependymoma

Ependymoma, which is one of the less frequently occurring tumors in animals, has been reported in dogs, cats, cattle, and horses of the domestic species. In the dog, some reports indicate a predilection for brachycephalic breeds (e.g., boxer). Ependymomas, as would be expected, are related to ependymal surfaces and occur primarily in the lateral ventricle and less frequently in the third and fourth ventricles. They also occur in the central canal of the spinal cord. The neoplasm may spread via the CSF within the ventricular system of the CNS and within the subarachnoid space. In the dog, the average age of involvement ranges from 6 to 12 years, but occurrence in younger animals (e.g., 1.5 years in the cat and 5 months in the calf) has also been reported.

Grossly, the neoplasm is an expansive growth that can invade adjacent tissue and be destructive. The tumor tissue is soft and ranges from gray-white to red, depending upon the blood content. Regressive changes include gelatinous degeneration and cyst formation. Microscopically, the tissue is highly cellular and well vascularized. The cells have hyperchromatic nuclei with scant to undetectable cytoplasm. The nuclei are round to oval to slightly elongated; they may form rosettes and be arranged around vessels so that a zone containing processes of tumor cells separates their nuclei from the vessel wall (Fig. 8-63). Another pattern includes the formation of sheets and bands of cells. The numbers of mitoses vary. Hemorrhage of varying degree, mucinous and cystic degeneration, and capillary proliferation may also occur. More malignant changes include evidence of invasion, frequent mitoses, and anaplasia.

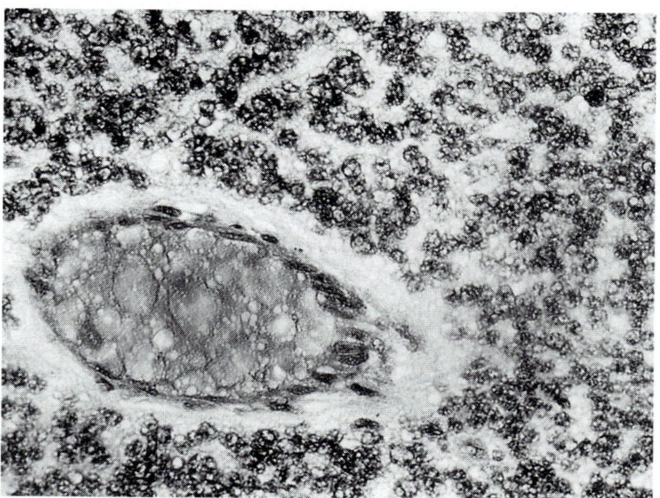

Fig. 8-63 Brain, left lateral ventricle; dog. Ependymoma. Cells with moderately hyperchromatic nuclei and poorly defined cytoplasm are arranged in irregular rows and form a nuclear-free zone around a blood vessel. H & E stain.

Primary Neoplasms of the Choroid Plexus

Choroid plexus papilloma and carcinoma

Choroid plexus papilloma occurs most commonly in the dog but has been reported in the horse and in cattle. In contrast to the neuroglial neoplasms of the dog, there is no predilection for brachycephalic breeds. In the dog, the neoplasm occurs most frequently in the fourth ventricle, but it also can be located in the third and lateral ventricles. The age range of affected dogs in one study was 5 to 13 years, except for one that was 2 years of age.

Grossly, the neoplasm is a well-defined, expansive, granular to papillary growth that is gray-white to red and may compress the adjacent nervous tissue. Some tumors cause hydrocephalus. Microscopically, these neoplasms generally resemble the choroid plexus and are characterized by an arborizing vascular connective tissue stroma that is covered with a cuboidal to columnar epithelial layer. Mitoses are not present in the benign form. A more malignant variety, choroid plexus carcinoma, is characterized by invasiveness, presence of mitosis, additional occurrence of solid tumor growth, and a tendency to spread to involve the brain and/or spinal cord. Metastasis can occur within the ventricular system, or exteriorly into the subarachnoid space (through the lateral apertures), where implantation on the ependyma or meninges, respectively, may occur.

Primary Neoplasms of Mesodermal Tissue

Meningioma

Meningioma is the most common mesodermal tumor of the CNS of animals. It occurs most frequently in the dog and cat but has been reported in other species of domestic animals, including horses, cattle, and sheep. In the dog, this tumor occurs in several breeds, with dolicocephalic animals being frequently represented. The majority of meningiomas in dogs occur between 7 and 14 years of age and in cats 10 years or older. Sites of occurrence in the dog include the basal area of the brain, the area over the convexity of the cerebral hemispheres, the cerebellum-tentorium area, the lateral surface of the brain, the falx cerebri, and the surface of the spinal cord. Retrobulbar involvement (originating from the optic nerve sheath) can also occur. In the cat, the tumor uniquely occurs in the tela choroidea of the third ventricle but also occurs over the cerebral hemispheres, along the falx cerebri, over the cerebellum and tentorium, and, rarely, at the base of the brain. Spinal location is not common. The neoplasm has been reported to arise from arachnoid "cap cells," which are on the external surface of the arachnoid membrane.

Grossly, tumors in the dog are solitary and vary in size. The neoplasms are well defined, variable in shape (e.g., spherical, lobulated, lenticular, or plaquelike), firm, encapsulated, and gray-white. Sometimes on cut surface there are soft, red, brown, or gray areas of hemorrhage and necrosis. The tumors usually grow by expansion, causing pressure atrophy of the adjacent nervous tissue. They can be invasive, and, sometimes, there is hyperostosis of the overlying bone. In the cat, meningiomas vary in size from barely detectable to 2 cm in diameter. Cats, and occasionally cattle, may have more than one tumor. Other characteristics are comparable with those described in the dog (Fig. 8-64).

Microscopically, several patterns of tumor formation can occur, and more than one may be present in a given specimen. The more common pattern is characterized by the formation of nests, islands, or laminated whorls of cells (Fig. 8-65). The cells have large cell bodies with abundant cytoplasm, ill-defined cell boundaries, and elongated, oval, open nuclei with peripherally located chromatin. The number of cells making up a whorl can vary from a few to many, and, in the center of such structures, there may be mineralized material (referred to as psammoma bodies). A second pattern is characterized by strands or streams of elongated cells with a rather irregular or parallel orientation. Regressive changes include hemorrhage and cavernous vascular formations. Invasive growth may occur but is less common than growth by expansion.

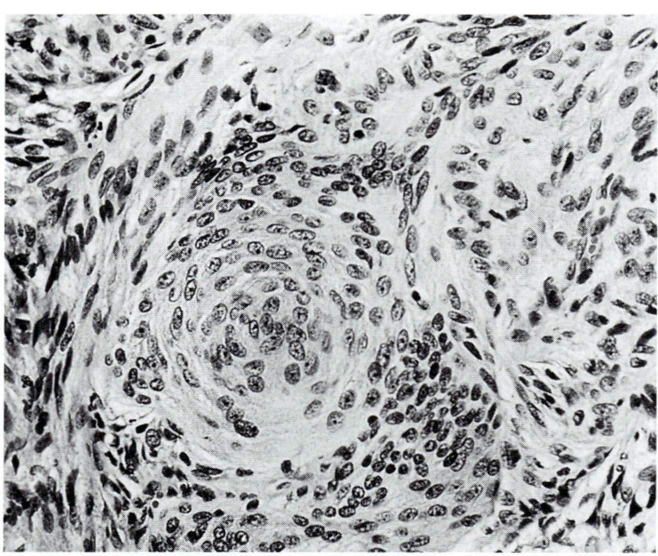

Fig. 8-65 Brain, left dorsal occipital lobe; cat. Meningioma. The cells are arranged in a characteristic whorl pattern. H & E stain.

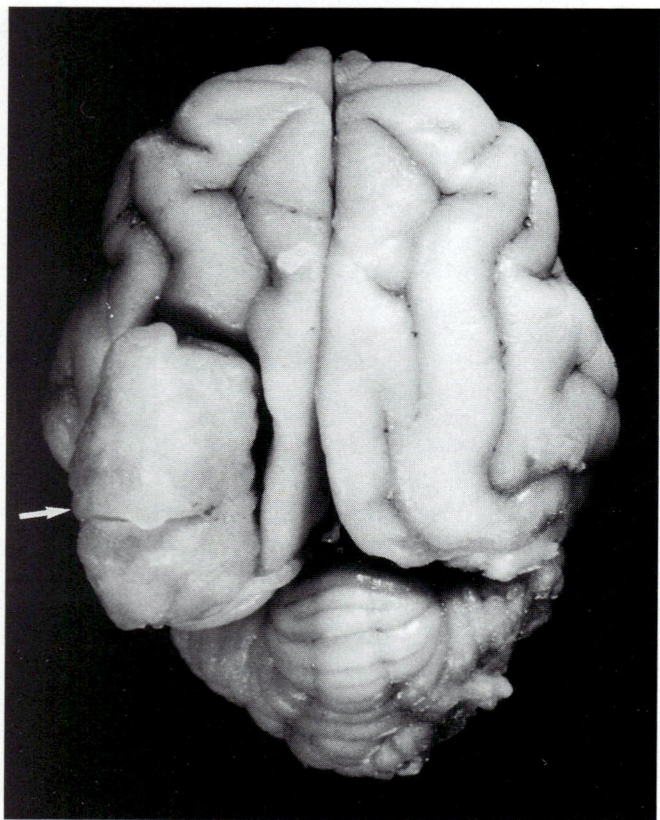

Fig. 8-64 Brain, occipital and parietal lobes of left cerebral hemisphere; cat. Meningioma. The meningioma *(arrow)* has markedly compressed the left dorsal occipital and parietal lobes.

Reticulosis

The neoplastic forms of the reticulosis group are discussed above.

Secondary Neoplasms

Secondary neoplasms of the CNS can occur following growth from adjacent bone, from direct extension of adjacent tumors through the bone or foramina, or by hematogenous metastasis.

Benign growths include osteomas, chondromas, and osteochondromas, which may cause compressive injury to the brain or spinal cord. One neoplasm (chondroma rodens) has been described as originating from the periosteum of the canine skull. Also, malignant neoplasms adjacent to the cranium or spinal column may cause injury by direct invasion. Some examples include extracranial osteosarcoma and fibrosarcoma in the dog. Also, malignant melanoma, of the oral cavity (soft palate) in the dog and involving the

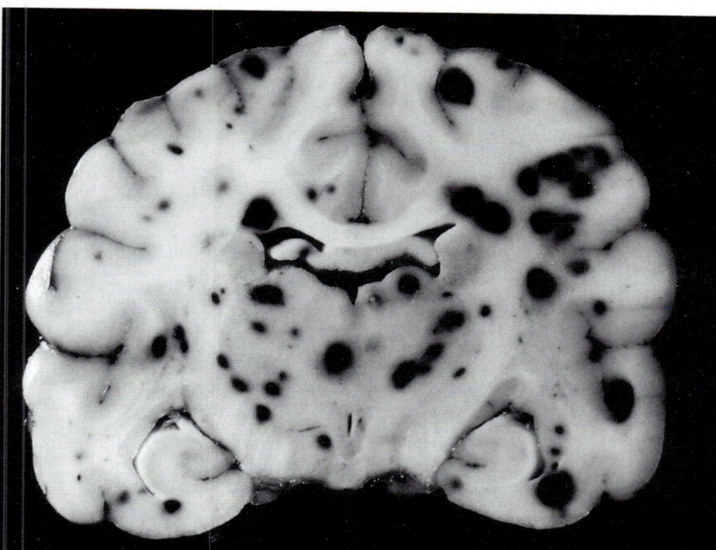

Fig. 8-66 Brain, junction between parietal and occipital lobes, level of the thalamus; dog. Hemangiosarcoma. Note the prominent hematogenous metastases. *Courtesy Dr. M.D. McGavin.*

paravertebral lymph nodes in the horse, may invade adjacent CNS tissue. Other examples of direct extension include lymphosarcoma affecting the spinal cord in the bovine species (and, less frequently, involving the spinal cord or brain in the dog and cat) and carcinomas of the ethmoidal area and nasal cavity.

Hematogenously metastasizing neoplasms also occur and affect the brain more often than the spinal cord. The species in which metastasis has been most commonly reported is the dog; the next most frequent is the cat. Of the carcinomas, the mammary carcinoma in the dog has been reported to occur most frequently, although others have been described. Hemangiosarcoma is one of the most commonly occurring sarcomas in the dog (Fig. 8-66); others are the mesenchymal component of the mixed mammary tumor, lymphosarcoma, fibrosarcoma, and malignant melanoma. In the cat, the neoplasms that metastasize to the CNS include mammary carcinoma and lymphosarcoma.

Suggested Readings

General

DeFelipe J, Jones EG, eds. Cajal's Degeneration and Regeneration of the Nervous System. New York: Oxford University Press, 1991.

Fankhauser R, Luginbühl H. Zentrales Nervensystem. In: Dobberstein J, Pallaske G, Stünzi H, eds. Joest's Handbuch der speziellen pathologischen Anatomie der Haustiere. Vol 3. Berlin: Verlag Paul Parey, 1962:191-436.

Fenner F, Bachmann PA, Gibbs EPJ, et al. Veterinary Virology. New York: Academic Press, 1987.

Haymaker W, Adams RD, eds. Histology and Histopathology of the Nervous System. Springfield, Ill.: Charles C Thomas, 1982.

Sunderland S. Nerve and Nerve Injuries. London: E & S Livingstone, 1968.

Neurons and neuroglia

David S. Reactive gliosis: Characterization of injury-induced changes in astrocytes. In: Norenberg MD, Hertz L, Schousboe A, eds. The Biochemical Pathology of Astrocytes. Alan R. Liss, 1988:123-134.

Frei K, Siepl C, Groscurth P, et al. Immunobiology of microglial cells. Ann N Y Acad Sci 1988; 540:218-227.

Lieberman AR. The axon reaction: A review of the principal features of perikaryal responses to axon injury. Int Rev Neurobiol 1971; 14:49-124.

Hatten ME, Liem RKH, Shelanski ML, et al. Astroglia in CNS injury. Glia, 1991; 4:233-243.

Jenkins LW, Povlishock JT, Lewelt W, et al. The role of postischemic recirculation in the development of ischemic neuronal injury following complete cerebral ischemia. Acta Neuropathol 1981; 55:205-220.

Perry VH, Gordon S. Macrophages and microglia in the nervous system. TINS, 1988; 11:273-277.

Raff MC. Glial cell diversification in the rat optic nerve. Science 1989; 243:1450-1455.

Anomalies and malformations

Brown TT, de Lahunta A, Bistner SI, et al. Pathogenic studies of infection of the bovine fetus with bovine viral diarrhea virus. I. Cerebellar atrophy. Vet Pathol 1974; 11:486-505.

Johnson RT. Viral Infections of the Nervous System. New York: Raven Press, 1982:203-236.

Inborn errors of metabolism

Jolly RD, Martinus RD, Shimada A, Fearnley IM, Palmer DN. Ovine ceroid-lipofuscinosis is a proteolipid proteinosis. Can J Vet Res 1990; 54:15-21.

Physical disturbances

Dawson SL, Hirsch CS, Lucas FV, et al. The contrecoup phenomenon. Reappraisal of a classic problem. Human Pathol 1980; 11:155-166.

Gennarelli TA. Cerebral concussion and diffuse brain injuries. In: Cooper PR, ed. Head Injury. Baltimore: Williams & Wilkins, 1982:83-97.

Minckler J, Bailey OT, Feigin I, Jervis G, Lindenberg R, Neubuerger KT, eds. Pathology of the Nervous System. New York McGraw-Hill, 1971:1705-1831.

Circulatory disturbances

Go KG. The classification of brain edema. New York: Wiley 1981:3.

Zivin JA, Choi DW. Stroke therapy. Sci Am 1991; 265:56-63.

Kornegay JN, Oliver JE, Gorgacz EJ. Clinicopathologic features of brain herniation in animals. J Am Vet Med Assoc 1983; 182:1111-1116.

Metabolic disturbances

Abou-Donia MB. Biochemical toxicology of organophosphorous compounds. In: Blum K, Manzo L, eds., Neurotoxicology. New York: Marcel Dekker, 1985:423-444.

Abou-Donia MB, Lapadula DM. Mechanisms of organophosphorus ester-induced delayed neurotoxicity: Type I and type II. Ann Rev Pharmacol Toxicol 1990; 30:405-440.

Bressler JP, Goldstein GW. Commentary: Mechanisms of lead neurotoxicity. Biochem Pharmacol 1991; 41:479-484.

Christian RG, Tryphonas L. Lead poisoning in cattle: Brain lesions and hematologic changes. Am J Vet Res 1971; 32:203-216.

Gould DH, McAllister MM, Savage JC, Hamar DW. High sulfide concentrations in rumen fluid associated with nutritionally induced polioencephalomalacia in calves. Am J Vet Res 1991; 52:1164-1169.

Smith DLT. Poisoning by sodium salt—a cause of eosinophilic meningoencephalitis in swine. Am J Vet Res 1957; 18:825-850.

Wilson TM, Ross PF, Rice LG, et al. Fumonisin B_1 levels associated with an epizootic of equine leukoencephalomalacia. J Vet Diagn Invest 1990; 2:213-216.

Disorders of myelin formation and maintenance

Appel MJG, Gillespie JH. Canine distemper virus. In: Gard S, Hallauer C, Meyer KF, eds. Virology Monographs. Vol 11. New York: Springer-Verlag, 1972:1.

Cork LC. Differential diagnosis of viral leukoencephalomyelitis of goats. J Am Vet Med Assoc 1976; 169:1303-1306.

Griot C, Burge T, Vandevelde M, Peterhans E. Antibody-induced generation of reactive oxygen radicals by brain macrophages in canine distemper encephalitis: A mechanism for bystander demyelination. Acta Neuropathol 1989; 78:396-403.

Harper PAW, Healy PJ, Dennis JA. Maple syrup urine disease as a cause of spongiform encephalopathy in calves. Vet Rec 1986; 119:62-65.

Krakowka S, Axthelm MK, Johnson GC. Canine distemper virus. In: Olsen RG, Krakowka S, Blakeslee JR, eds. Comparative Pathology of Viral Diseases. Vol. 2. Boca Raton, Fla.: CRC Press, 1985:137-164.

Narayan O, Jolly P. Ovine-caprine lentiviruses: infection and pathogenesis. Dev Biol Stand 1990; 72:203-205.

Raine CS. The neuropathology of myelin disease. In: Morell P, ed. Myelin. 2nd ed. New York: Plenum, 1984:259.

Selmaj KW, Raine CS. Tumor necrosis factor mediates myelin and oligodendrocyte damage in vitro. Ann Neurol 1988; 23:339-346.

Summers, BA, Appel MJG. Demyelination in canine distemper encephalomyelitis: An ultrastructural analysis. J Neurocytol 1987; 16:871-881.

Tabira T. Cellular and molecular aspects of the pathomechanism and therapy of murine experimental allergic encephalomyelitis. Crit Rev Neurobiol 1989; 5:113-142.

Zink MC, Narayan O, Kennedy PGE, et al. Pathogenesis of visna/maedi and caprine arthritis-encephalitis: new leads on the mechanism of restricted virus replication and persistent inflammation. Vet Immunol Immunopathol. 1987; 15:167-180.

Neurodegenerative diseases

de Lahunta A. Abiotrophy in domestic animals: a review. Can J Vet Res 1990; 54:65-76.

de Lahunta A. Comparative cerebellar disease in domestic animals. Comp Cont Educ Pract 1980; 2:8-19.

Montgomery DL, Storts RW. Hereditary striatonigral and cerebello-olivary degeneration of the Kerry blue terrier. I. Gross and light microscopic central nervous system lesions. Vet Pathol 1983; 20:143-159.

Vandevelde M. Degenerate diseases of the spinal cord. Vet Clin North Am Small Anim Pract 1980; 10:147-154.

Inflammation of the central nervous system

Charlton KM, Garcia MM. Spontaneous listeric encephalitis and neuritis in sheep. Vet Pathol 1977; 14:297-313.

Charlton KM. The pathogenesis of rabies. In: Campbell JB, Charlton KM, eds. Rabies: Developments in Veterinary Virology. Norwell, Mass: Kluner Academic, 1988:100-150.

Dubey JP, Davis SW, Speer CA, et al. *Sarcocystis neurona* n. sp. (Protozoa: apicomplexa), the etiologic agent of equine protozoal myeloencephalitis. J Parasitol 1991; 77:212-218.

Gronstol H. In: Gyles CL, Thoen CO, eds. Pathogenesis of Bacterial Infections in Animals. Ames: Iowa State University Press, 1986:48-55.

Hadlow WJ, Kennedy RC, Race RE. Natural infection of Suffolk sheep with scrapie virus. J Infect Dis 1982; 146:657-664.

Johnson RT. Viral Infections of the Nervous System. New York: Raven Press, 1982:203-236.

Kimberlin RH. Transmissible encephalopathies in animals. Can J Vet Res 1990; 54:30-37.

Allen GP, Bryans JT. Molecular epizooitology, pathogenesis, and prophylaxis of equine herpesvirus-1 infections. Prog Vet Microbiol Immunol 1986; 2:78-144.

Storz J. Overview of animal diseases induced by chlamydial infections. In: Barron AL, ed. Microbiology of Chlamydia. Boca Raton, Fla.: CRC Press, 1988:167-192.

Dubey JP, Beattie CP. Toxoplasmosis of Animals and Man. Boca Raton, Fla: CRC Press, 1988:1-220.

Parasitic infestations

Fankhauser R, Luginbühl H. Zentrales Nervensystem. In: Dobberstein J, Pallaske G, Stünzi H, eds. Joest's Handbuch der speziellen pathologischen Anatomie der Haustiere. Vol 3. Berlin: Verlag Paul Parey, 1962: 191.

Miscellaneous processes

Fankhauser R, Fatzer R, Luginbühl H. Reticulosis of the central nervous system (CNS) in dogs. Adv Vet Sci Comp Med 1972; 16:35-71.

Neoplasms

Cordy DR. Tumors of the nervous system and eye. In: Moulton JE ed., Tumors in Domestic Animals. 2nd ed. Berkeley: University of California Press, 1978:430-455.

CHAPTER

9

Muscle

M. DONALD McGAVIN

Structural and physiologic features of skeletal muscle determine much of its response to injury. Although muscle cells are frequently called ''muscle fibers'' or ''myofibers,'' they are, in fact, multinucleated cells of considerable length, which in some animals may approach 1 meter (m). This multinucleation has a significant effect on the processes of necrosis and, later, regeneration, as under favorable conditions, myofibers are able to restore themselves after a segment has become necrotic. Also, the physiologic attributes of a myofiber—its rate of contraction, type of metabolism (oxidative, glycolytic, or mixed)—are determined not by the myofiber itself but by the neuron responsible for its innervation, the ventral horn cell of the spinal cord (Fig. 9-1), or the brain stem motor neuron. This fact is significant in evaluating histologic changes in myofibers. It is possible to divide changes in myofibers into two major classes, **neuropathic** and **myopathic.** Neuropathic changes are those that are determined by the effect or the absence of the nerve supply, e.g., atrophy after denervation. However, the term **myopathic** should be reserved for those muscle diseases where the primary change takes place in the myofiber, not in the interstitial tissue and not secondary to effects from the nerve supply. Myopathies include some types of myofiber degeneration (for example, metabolic myopathies and muscular dystrophies), myofiber necrosis, and some inflammatory conditions that are initiated in the myofiber itself.

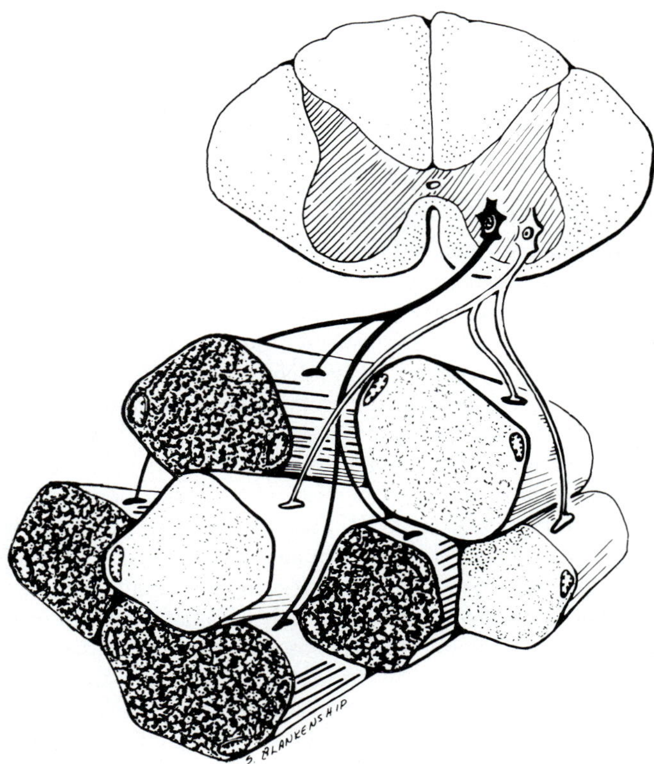

Fig. 9-1 Schematic diagram of motor unit and muscle fiber types. All myofibers innervated by the one motor neuron are of the same fiber type. Thus, the motor neuron determines whether the myofibers are type I (light) or type II (dark).

Muscle pathology has developed into a subspecialty with its own extensive literature. Inevitably, over decades, this has resulted in the development of its own terminology. Pathologists based some names on the then-current anatomic and histologic terms, but, when anatomic nomenclature changed, pathologists frequently retained the older term. A good example is the term ''sarcolemma.'' In muscle pathology, this term has been used for decades for the tube visible by light microscopy following removal of the contents of the muscle fiber by, for example, segmental necrosis (see Fig. 9-5, *A*). Electron microscopy reveals that the myofiber's plasmalemma is applied closely to a basal lamina, and outside of this is an interlacing network of fine collagen fibrils that form the endomysium. Exactly what constitutes the sarcolemma of light microscopy is a little unclear. It is certainly not just the basal lamina, which would not be visible by light microscopy, and, most likely, it includes the basal lamina and reticular fibers. These are collagen fibers that do not stain with eosin or with conventional collagen stains, such as trichrome stains, but only with silver reticulum stains. Over a decade ago, histologists applied the term "sarcolemma" to the myofiber's plasmalemma, thus setting the stage for confusion in the literature. The result has been that in one multiauthored text book on muscle pathology, the word "sarcolemma" was used in three different ways: for the plasmalemma alone, for plasmalemma plus basal lamina, and for the endomysium plus basal lamina. Also the convention in muscle pathology is to call those myofiber nuclei that lie at the periphery of the myofiber **sarcolemmal nuclei,** as opposed to nuclei in the center of the myofiber (a primitive state), which are called **central nuclei.**

The key structure in the "sarcolemma" of muscle pathology is the basal lamina. In myofiber necrosis, the myofiber's plasmalemma disappears, but the basal lamina remains; this is the basis of the so-called sarcolemmal tube. The basal lamina is resistant to insults that destroy the myofiber but is able to be penetrated by macrophages that enter to remove necrotic debris and is responsible for orderly regeneration (see Regeneration). In this chapter, the term "sarcolemmal tube" will be used for this tube formed by the basal lamina.

PHYSIOLOGIC FEATURES

Mammalian muscles are composed of muscle fibers of different contractile properties. The classification of these fibers is based on three major physiologic features: (1) rates of contraction (fast or slow), (2) rates of fatigue (fast or slow), and (3) types of metabolism (oxidative, glycolytic, or mixed). The last feature is the basis for histochemical methods that demonstrate either the concentration of myosin ATPase or mitochondrial enzymes such as succinic dehydrogenase and nicotinamide adenine dinucleotide-tetrazolium reductase (NADH-TR), although the latter is not confined to mitochondria. Fortunately, the physiologic and histochemical classifications are compatible, although this has not been proven for all species. In 1970, the World Federation of Neurology recommended a basic division into type I and type II fibers (Table 9-1). Type I fibers are low in myosin ATPase, rich in mitochondria, oxidative in metabolism, slow contracting, and slow fatiguing. Type II fibers are rich in myosin ATPase, have fewer mitochondria, and are glycolytic, fast-contracting fibers. Type II fibers were later subdivided into type IIA and type IIB. Type IIB are the fast-contracting, fast-fatiguing, glycolytic fibers (FF) that depend upon glycogen for their energy supply. Type IIA are mixed oxidative-glycolytic and, therefore, although fast contracting are also slow fatiguing (FR). Thus, type IIA fibers are "intermediate" in the concentration of mitochondria and myosin ATPase activity between type I and type IIB and, in some classifications, are known as "intermediate" fibers.

Most muscle fibers contain type I and type II fibers, and these are conveniently demonstrated in frozen sections by the myosin ATPase reaction (see Fig. 9-9, *B*). The percentage of each fiber type varies from muscle to muscle and within the same muscle (Fig. 9-2). There is some correlation with function. Type I fibers (slow contracting, slow fatiguing, oxidative) are plentiful in those muscles whose main function is to maintain posture, support the weight of

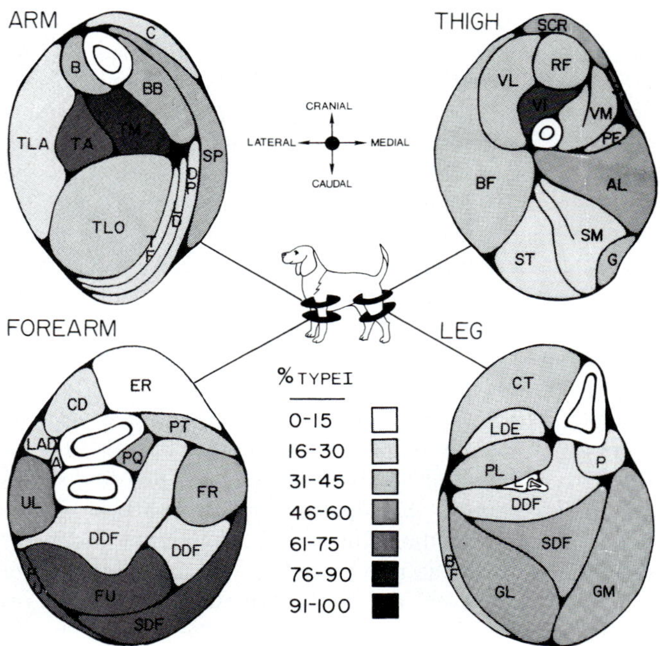

Fig. 9-2 Muscles; dog. Schematic representation of the percentage of type I and type II myofibers in limb muscles in the dog. Note the wide variation from muscle to muscle. The extensor carpi radialis has the lowest percentage of type I fibers (< 15%), and the vastus intermedius the highest (91% to 100%). *Courtesy Dr. R.B. Armstrong et al. Am J Anat 1987; 163:87-98.*

Table 9-1. Relationship between histochemical and physiologic classifications of myofiber types

Dubowitz and Brooke	Peter and co-workers	Burke and co-workers
Type I: low myosin ATPase activity, heavy mitochondrial staining	SO = slow twitch oxidative	S = slow contracting
Type IIA: intermediate ATPase activity, heavy mitochondrial staining	FOG = fast twitch oxidative-glycolytic	FR = fast contracting, fatigue resistant
Type IIB: high ATPase activity, light mitochondrial staining	FG = fast twitch glycolytic-glycolytic	FF = fast contracting, fast fatiguing

the animal, and slow locomotion. Muscles that contract quickly for sprinting contain more type II fibers. Muscles that contract slowly and continuously, e.g., some of the ruminants' masticatory muscles, contain a high percentage of type I fibers. Only rarely are muscles composed of only one fiber type (e.g., ovine vastus intermedius). Athletic training causes some type IIB fibers to be converted to type IIA. There are also variations within breeds and differences in the same muscle in different species, e.g., the dog has no type IIB fibers.

METHODS OF EXAMINATION OF MUSCLES

Frequently, lesions in muscles can be detected and evaluated only by microscopic examination. Muscle is prone to form artifacts, and, thus, successful histologic and electron microscopic examination of muscle tissue depends upon their prevention. Unfortunately, the most common change in muscle samples submitted for routine histopathologic examination is artifact. This problem is so severe that Harriman stated that

> . . . for many years the histopathology of skeletal muscle attracted little interest or effort. Its reactions in disease were limited, and too easily obscured by artifact. A lump of muscle hastily excised and dropped immediately into acid formalin provided a disorderly mass of hypercontracted muscle fibers, impossible to orientate.

Gross Examination of Muscle

Gross examination includes evaluation of changes in shape, color, texture, and volume (atrophy or hypertrophy). Subjective evaluation of size can be highly unreliable unless control muscles, e.g., from normal animals or from the opposite sides, are available for weighing and measuring. Colors of muscles also can be misleading. The variation in the percentage of type I and type II fibers affects the muscle's color. Type II fibers are light (so-called white fibers), and type I fibers are dark (so-called red fibers). Muscles that are formed of predominantly type II fibers (see Fig. 9-2), such as the semimembranosus and semitendinosus, are naturally pale. Conversely, muscles in which type I fibers predominate, such as the diaphragm and the masticatory muscles, are naturally dark. Therefore, a pale muscle is not necessarily undergoing degeneration. However, muscles undergoing necrosis are pale, and these may appear as distinct streaks or foci. If necrotic areas calcify, they contain glistening, chalky-white foci that may coalesce. Muscles infiltrated by fat (e.g., in steatosis) are also pale. Other discolorations detectable grossly are hemorrhages, as in myorrhexis; serosanguineous exudate, as in clostridial infections; focal lesions from parasites, e.g., *Sarcocystis;* and green discolorations in eosinophilic myositis. Thus, a complete necropsy will include palpation of and careful multiple incisions into muscles. Multiple slices should be made in the direction of the fibers, although this is difficult or impossible to do in those muscles where the fibers do not all run in the same direction (e.g., temporalis). Incisions should be less than 1 cm apart in order not to overlook small foci, such as the very early lesions of blackleg. At necropsy, a desirable procedure is to sample a mixture of muscles, including active ones (tongue, diaphragm, intercostal), inactive (psoas), proximal (biceps femoris, vastus lateralis, triceps brachii [lateral head]), and distal (extensor digitorum longus, tibialis cranialis). For purposes of biopsy, certain muscles are easy to sample because of their myofiber orientation. Recommended muscles include triceps brachii, superficial digital flexor, vastus lateralis, biceps femoris, extensor digitorum longus, and tibialis cranialis. Clinical findings should be used to determine which muscles are most likely to have lesions.

Microscopic Examination

Muscle is designed to contract when stimulated, and, if it is still irritable when placed in fixative, it will contract, often violently, forming contraction artifacts. As well as shortening fibers, these can obscure lesions. Myofibers in the very early stages of degeneration are even more susceptible. Hypercontracted fibers are rounded and deeply eosinophilic and, in cross section, have been confused with hyalinized fibers. To avoid these problems, contractions should be prevented during fixation. This will not be a problem in the fixation of muscles from emaciated animals (see Rigor) or in muscles from which rigor has passed. Fresh muscle needs to be clamped or, in an emergency, ligated to a strip of wood, then excised and fixed. Even with these restraints, highly irritable muscles can still contract, in some cases shredding the fibers. Placing the clamped muscle in physiologic saline for 15 to 30 minutes before fixation reduces contraction artifacts. For optimal histologic results, muscle samples must not be overstretched, twisted, or allowed to overcontract during fixation. Muscles taken during rigor will have moderately to strongly contracted sarcomeres, and uncontracted fibers adjacent to these will be thrown into zigzag folds. Adams recommends that the ideal time for sampling is when rigor vanishes.

Both transverse and longitudinal sections should be cut from each muscle sampled. The longitudinal section should be cut carefully so that muscle fibers are parallel and straight. Muscle fiber diameters and the percentage of affected fibers are most reliably evaluated in transverse sections. However, longitudinal sections reveal the extent of segmental necrosis and changes, such as the length of nuclear rows.

Enzyme Histochemistry

Histologic examination of fixed muscle is suitable for recognition of inflammatory and some degenerative diseases but does not allow staining for enzyme histochemistry, which is required for fiber typing. Therefore, changes in specific fiber types cannot be detected in routine formalin-fixed, paraffin-embedded, hematoxylin-eosin (H & E) sections. For fiber-type staining, tissues need to be frozen soon after biopsy or necropsy. Fortunately, muscles stored at 0° C retain adequate levels of active enzymes for about one day and so samples can be shipped, on ice, to a laboratory. Fiber-type staining is absolutely essential for the complete evaluation of muscle. It is most useful in demonstrating preferential involvement of a fiber type, as in some muscular dystrophies or neuropathic changes such as those due to denervation and reinnervation, which result in fiber-type grouping. For the routine histochemical examination of myofibers, sections are stained for myosin APTase (Fig. 9-9, *B*) at three different pHs and for NADH-TR and succinic dehydrogenase (SDH) for mitochondrial activity. Full evaluation requires morphometric examination with calculation of the percentage of each fiber type and the mean diameter and standard deviation of each fiber type. By these means, changes in the percentage of each fiber type and atrophy or hypertrophy can be documented.

RIGOR MORTIS

Immediately after the death of an animal (somatic death), the muscles are still alive biochemically. However, as energy stores are used, a sequence of changes takes place which, after a short period of relaxation, results in contraction and in stiffening of muscles that fix the positions of joints. Muscles are usually affected in a specific sequence: jaws, trunk, and then extremities. Rigor passes off in the same order as onset and does not return. Classically, onset begins 2 to 6 hours after death, reaches a maximum at 24 to 48 hours, and passes off in another 48 hours—a total of approximately 4 days. However, rigor mortis is so variable in routine autopsy material that there is little value in its interpretation. Variation in the rapidity and severity of rigor can be understood once the basic mechanism is defined.

According to the "sliding-filament" theory, which postulates that, in muscle contraction, actin and myosin filaments slide past each other powered by myosin heads attaching to actin-binding sites, ATP (adenosine triphosphate) is necessary for muscle relaxation after normal contraction. Rigor occurs when the majority of the myosin heads remain attached to actin-binding sites at the end of the "power stroke," owing to a deficiency of the ATP necessary for their release. ATP can be reconstituted from adenosine diphosphate (ADP), the energy being supplied either by glycolysis or by phosphocreatine. Factors that control the rate of onset of rigor mortis include the amount of glycogen stores, pH of muscle, and body temperature. Thus, if glycogen stores have been reduced by starvation or vigorous muscle contractions, as occurs in animals dying from tetanus, from strychnine poisoning, or during hunting, onset of rigor mortis is rapid. However, in cachectic animals with little or no energy stores, rigor may be slight or, in extremely emaciated cases, may not even occur at all. Rigor disappears by autolysis or putrefaction (bacterial decomposition). Thus, the basic factor in the delay in onset and the strength of rigor is the energy stores of the muscle in the form of ATP, phosphocreatine or glycogen, at the time of death. One major practical effect of rigor is to interfere with the histologic examination of muscle.

RESPONSE OF MUSCLE TO INJURY

The response of any organ to injury is the summation of the responses of each of the tissues or cells that compose it. Muscle is composed of myofibers surrounded by blood vessels and fibroblasts (endomysium) and penetrated by nerves. The primary cell to respond to injury is the myofiber. Unfortunately, its range of response to insults is extremely limited, and, apart from those involving the nerve supply, the major response of the muscle fiber is degeneration, necrosis, and regeneration. These are the end result of a wide variety of insults; trauma, ischemia, infarction (e.g., bluetongue in sheep due to vasculitis), metabolic diseases caused by nutritional deficiencies (e.g., vitamin E, selenium), toxic myopathies (e.g., *Cassia occidentalis* poisoning), and infections such as gas gangrene. Because of this stereotyped response, it is frequently not possible to determine the etiology based on gross or histopathologic lesions alone. Supplementary tests and clinical histories are essential. Thus, classification of muscle diseases based on lesions alone is not very satisfactory, and many classifications are based on etiology (e.g., toxic myopathy, nutritional myopathy).

Degeneration

The term "degeneration" in pathology implies a potentially reversible injury. In muscle pathology, it is loosely and ambiguously applied and includes reversible changes such as the vacuolar degenerations caused by hypokalemia and hyperkalemia, autophagic vacuoles, and, sometimes, necrosis. No less an authority than Adams states that "degeneration means the destruction of cells or tissue or a change in appearance of such a degree that recognition is no longer possible." In this chapter, the term will be used for changes that may or may not lead to myofiber death and also for some miscellaneous categories, such as calcification and ossification, which are included by convention.

The categories of degeneration include the following:

1. Pigmentations: lipofuscin, melanin, myoglobin
2. Calcification
3. Ossification
4. "True degenerations": cloudy swelling, hydropic, vacuolar, granular, and fatty
5. Other degenerations

Pigmentation

The most important pigment is **lipofuscin**—the so-called wear-and-tear pigment that accumulates in secondary lysosomes, which are later converted to small, compact aggregates known in electron microscopy as residual bodies. The propensity to store lipofuscin is not the same in all domestic animals. It is highest in the skeletal muscles of cattle, particularly old, high-producing dairy cattle. The masseter and diaphragm (two hard-working muscles) are the most frequently affected, although, in badly affected animals, all muscles may be discolored tan to brown. The lesion is of no clinical significance. It is most frequently seen in packing plants where it is known incorrectly as "xanthomatosis" or "xanthosis." Its significance at necropsy in muscle, as well as in other organs such as myocardium, neurons, liver, kidney, and adrenal cortex, is as an indicator either of old age or of past or present episodes of cachexia or starvation. The characteristic microscopic appearance in skeletal muscle is rounded granules of yellow-brown to dark brown pigment at the two poles of the nucleus of the myofiber.

Occasionally, **melanin** will discolor the fascial sheaths and epimysium of muscles as part of the syndrome of congenital melanosis in calves, in which melanocytes are present within the fascial sheaths and epimysium. The pigment appears grossly as black foci or streaks. Muscle fibers themselves are unaffected.

Myoglobin may discolor muscles after extensive muscle necrosis, a process known as rhabdomyolysis (see below). Damage to the myofiber's cell membrane allows myoglobin to leak into the adjacent tissues. This is seen only if the muscle necrosis is extensive and sudden, as in crush injuries. Another cause of localized colored areas in muscle is from injections of medicaments, e.g., tetracycline (yellow) or iron dextran (dark brown).

Calcification

The causes of calcification are the following:

1. Calcification of necrotic muscle fibers
2. Calcification of fibers in extreme old age
3. Rare cases of macroscopic calcification of unknown cause of parts or most of a muscle

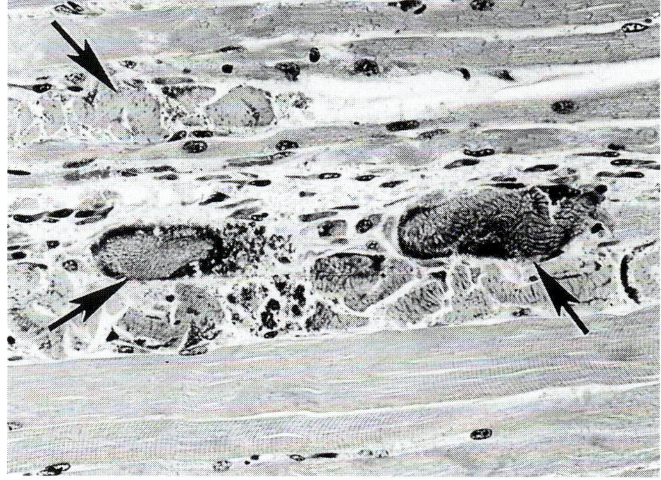

Fig. 9-3 Muscle; horse. Segmental necrosis undergoing calcification *(arrows)*. Hematoxylin-eosin (H & E) stain. ×250.

Calcification is the next step in the sequence of necrosis of individual myofibers (Fig. 9-3) and is prominent in some domestic animals, e.g., sheep. These deposits may be so dense as to be visible grossly as glistening, chalky-white foci. Calcification of myofibers has been a common finding in burros over 40 years of age. Macroscopic calcification of a large portion of a muscle is a rarity. It has been reported in a steer and can cause clinical stiffness. The cause is unknown. Ingestion of toxic plants that contain an active vitamin D metabolite *(Cestrum diurum, Solanum malacoxlyn)* causes widespread calcification that sometimes includes tendons and ligaments *(C. diurum* in horses) but apparently does not involve skeletal muscles.

Ossification

In the past, ossification was termed **myositis ossificans,** which in its broadest sense means the formation of nonneoplastic bone and/or cartilage in extraosseous sites, which may or may not be in muscle. It is essentially a metaplasia to bone. The disease has been reported in horses, pigs, dogs, and cats and is subdivided into progressive and localized forms. The generalized form is better termed **fibrodysplasia ossificans progressiva,** rather than myositis ossificans progressiva, because it is a disorder of connective tissue associated with skeletal muscle, and the muscle itself is only secondarily involved. It has been described in pigs and cats. The porcine disease is inherited, but this has not been proven in cats. Lesions may replace large portions of the muscle. The histologic appearance is of interlacing bundles of dense, fibrous connective tissue, sometimes containing dense accumulations of calcium, cartilage, and bone. The hyperplastic connective tissue compresses the adjacent skeletal muscles, which undergo atrophy. The localized form is confined to a single muscle or a single group of adjacent muscles and may or may not be associated with a history of trauma, after either single or multiple insults. This type has been seen in horses and dogs. The lesion may have zones. The central zone contains proliferating undifferentiated cells and fibroblasts; the middle one, osteoblast-depositing osteoid and immature bone; and the outer one, trabecular bone that may be being remodeled by osteoclasts.

True degenerations

When muscle is insulted metabolically from a wide variety of causes, the final result is frequently segmental necrosis. The muscle fiber may go through a series of degenerations before becoming frankly necrotic, or, in some less severely affected fibers, the degenerations may be reversed and the fiber returned to normal. The earliest detectable change starts in the individual myofiber as extremely fine vacuoles that are barely visible by light microscopy. After hours to a day, these vacuoles become larger and are then relatively easy to detect microscopically (Fig. 9-4). If the

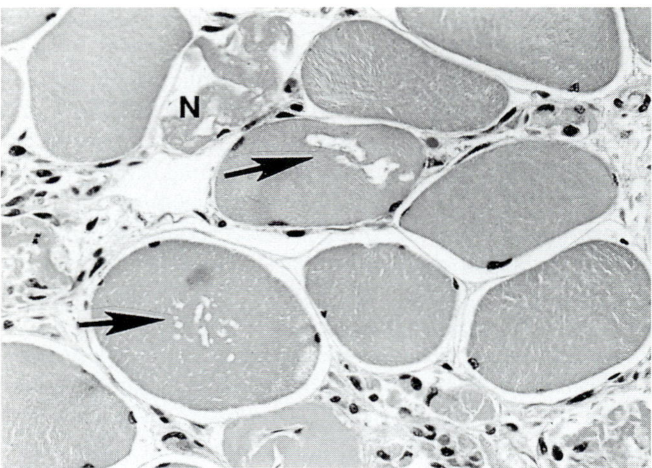

Fig. 9-4 Muscle; ox. Early vacuolar degeneration *(arrows)* has already progressed to segmental necrosis (*N*) in an adjacent myofiber. H & E stain. ×250

degeneration is not reversed, the fiber or a segment of it will progress to later stages of what have been termed floccular, granular, hyaline, and Zenker's "degenerations," but all of which represent different stages of necrosis.

Vacuolar degenerations are caused by swelling of organelles or accumulation of glycogen or fat within the myofiber. Exactly which organelle is involved varies. If there is a mild damage to the myofiber, the vacuoles may be autophagic. These are membrane-bound vacuoles in which damaged organelles undergo autodigestion by fusion with a lysosome. Glycogen vacuoles occur in Pompe's disease, a glycogen-storage disease in cattle. Neutral lipid droplets are present in myofibers in lipid-storage diseases, e.g., that caused by carnitine deficiency. Both hypokalemia and hyperkalemia cause vacuolar degeneration of myofibers.

Other degenerations

Muscle pathologists recognize a variety of degenerations peculiar to myofibers. These include target fibers, central cores, moth-eaten fibers (myofibrillar whorls), tubular aggregates, and rods. Some of these are visible only in histochemical preparations (e.g., target fibers in sections treated with oxidative enzyme stains), and, in other cases, the lesions are visible only by electron micrography.

Necrosis

As myofibers are long, local physical insults cause necrosis of only a segment. Toxic, metabolic, and nutritional myopathies also cause segmental necrosis. Total necrosis of myofibers is rare, occurring in extensive infarcts, massive trauma, and large burns. Thus, segmental myofiber necrosis is present after many different types of insults—a type of "final common pathway." This stage of necrosis quickly merges into the stages of regeneration, described below. Necrotic portions of myofibers have several different histologic appearances. The earliest is the hyaline fiber, which is hypercontracted, rounded in cross section (normal fibers are polygonal), with an increased fiber diameter and increased staining with eosin. Some hyalinized fibers are artifactual and are caused by excessive contraction of normal fibers at the time of fixation. Necrotic portions of the fiber may become floccular or granular as that portion of the myofiber starts to fragment. The normal portion of the fiber can separate from the necrotic segment, forming so-called retraction caps. Early in infarction, the necrotic myofiber may fracture at "Z" lines, causing discoid degeneration. Occasionally, necrotic segments of myofibers will be mineralized (see Fig. 9-3).

Once the plasma membrane of the myofiber is damaged or a segment of the myofiber becomes necrotic, some of the contents of the muscle cell will "leak out" and be taken up into the blood. The concentrations of some of these components are used as an index of the extent of myofiber damage. The most commonly used is creatine kinase (CK). Serum glutamic-oxaloacetic transaminase (SGOT) is also released, but it is not as specific an indicator of muscle damage because it is also present in hepatocytes. Myoglobin is also released. As it has a low renal threshold, it is quickly excreted in the urine. If muscle damage is extensive, myoglobinuria will result. The term rhabdomyolysis has been applied to this process, but it is really no more than muscle necrosis of sufficient extent to produce myoglobinuria. Clinically, rhabdomyolysis and myoglobinuria are used as synonyms.

Necrosis secondary to systemic disease

It is well over 100 years since Zenker described segmental hyaline degeneration (Zenker's necrosis) in the muscles of human patients dying of typhoid. Similar changes may occur in other acute infections in human beings and animals. The pathogenesis is not understood. Some may be secondary to toxemia. Experimentally, *Escherichia coli* endotoxin has been shown to cause myofiber necrosis. Lesions are usually not visible grossly and may be difficult to find histologically because they consist of scattered small segments of necrosis and regeneration. Because the necrosis leaves sarcolemmal tubes intact and the necrotic segments are small, regeneration is fast and effective. Segmental necrosis is also present in toxic and endocrine myopathies, and, in human beings, has been reported secondary to liver disease and cancer. Necrosis can be due to infarction caused by a vasculitis (sheep with blue tongue) or bacterial emboli (*Haemophilus agni* in lambs) (see Bacterial Myositides).

Regeneration

Skeletal muscle has considerable ability to regenerate, and, under optimum conditions, a necrotic segment of a muscle fiber can be repaired so that it is indistinguishable from a normal one. However, the success of regeneration depends on the extent and nature of the injury and whether or not the integrity of the supporting stroma around the muscle fiber (sarcolemmal tube) is intact. It is convenient to first consider the sequence of events that take place under optimal conditions.

If a portion of the muscle fiber is damaged by, say, a toxin, and the sarcolemmal tube is intact, the sequence of events is as follows, although it has been recognized that some "stages" will overlap with others. These are depicted schematically in Fig. 9-5.

1. In the necrotic segment, the muscle nuclei disappear, and, in H & E-stained sections, the sarcoplasm and myofibrils become hyalinized (eosinophilic, amorphous, and homogeneous), indicating the loss of normal myofibrillar structure (Fig. 9-5, *B*). The necrotic portion may separate from the adjacent viable myofiber during contraction (Figs. 9-5, *C* and 9-6, *A*). In some species, the necrotic fiber may be mineralized (see Fig. 9-3).
2. Within 24 to 48 hours and usually between 1 to 4 days, monocytes emigrate from capillaries, become macrophages, and enter the necrotic portion of the myofiber (Fig. 9-5, *D* and 9-6, *B*). Neutrophils may also be present initially, but they rapidly disappear as they die off. Concurrently, the satellite cells, normally located between the basal lamina and the myofiber's plasmalemma, begin to swell (Fig. 9-5, *C*), become vesicular with prominent nucleoli, and then undergo mitosis.
3. The proliferated satellite cells move from the peripheral location to the center of muscle fiber, among the macrophages (Figs. 9-5, *D*, 9-6, *B*, and 9-6, *C*).
4. Macrophages lyse and phagocytose necrotic debris and form a clear space in the sarcolemmal tube. At the same time, the plasmalemma disappears, and the shape of the sarcolemmal tube is maintained by the basal lamina.

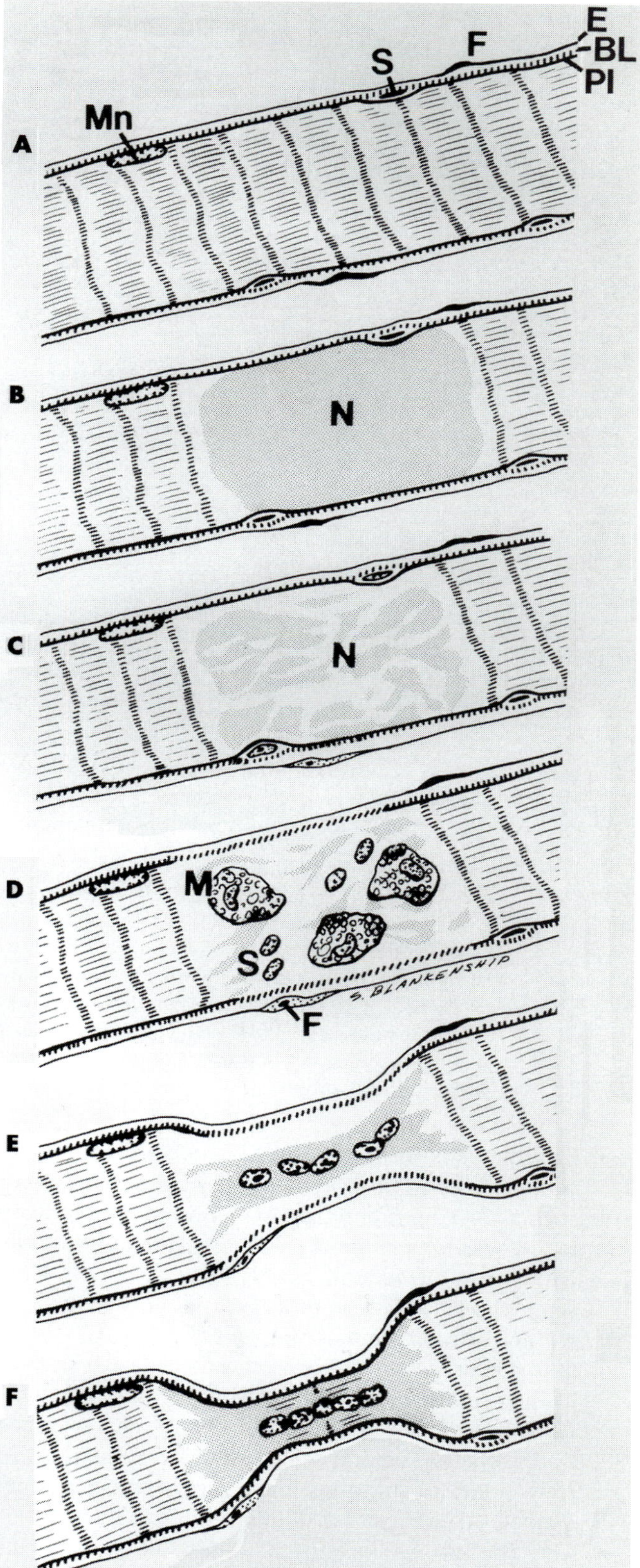

Fig. 9-5 Schematic representation of segmental myofiber necrosis and regeneration. **A**, Longitudinal section of normal muscle fiber. *BL*, basal lamina; *E*, endomysium; *F*, fibroblast; *Pl*, plasmalemma; *Mn*, muscle nucleus; *S*, satellite cell, which lies between the basal lamina and plasmalemma. **B**, Segmental necrosis. Coagulation necrosis (*N*). **C**, The necrotic segment of myofiber (*N*) has become floccular and detached from the adjacent viable portion of the myofiber. The satellite cells are enlarging. **D**, The necrotic segment of the myofiber has been invaded by macrophages (*M*) and satellite cells (*S*). The latter will develop into myoblasts. The plasmalemma of the necrotic segment has disappeared. **E**, Myoblasts have formed a myotube, which has produced sarcoplasm. This extends out to meet the viable ends of the myofiber. The integrity of the myofiber is maintained by the sarcolemmal tube formed by the basal lamina and endomysium. **F**, Regenerating myofiber. Note the reduction in myofiber diameter and central rowing of nuclei. There is early formation of sarcomeres (cross-striations), and the plasmalemma has reformed. Such fibers stain basophilically with H & E.

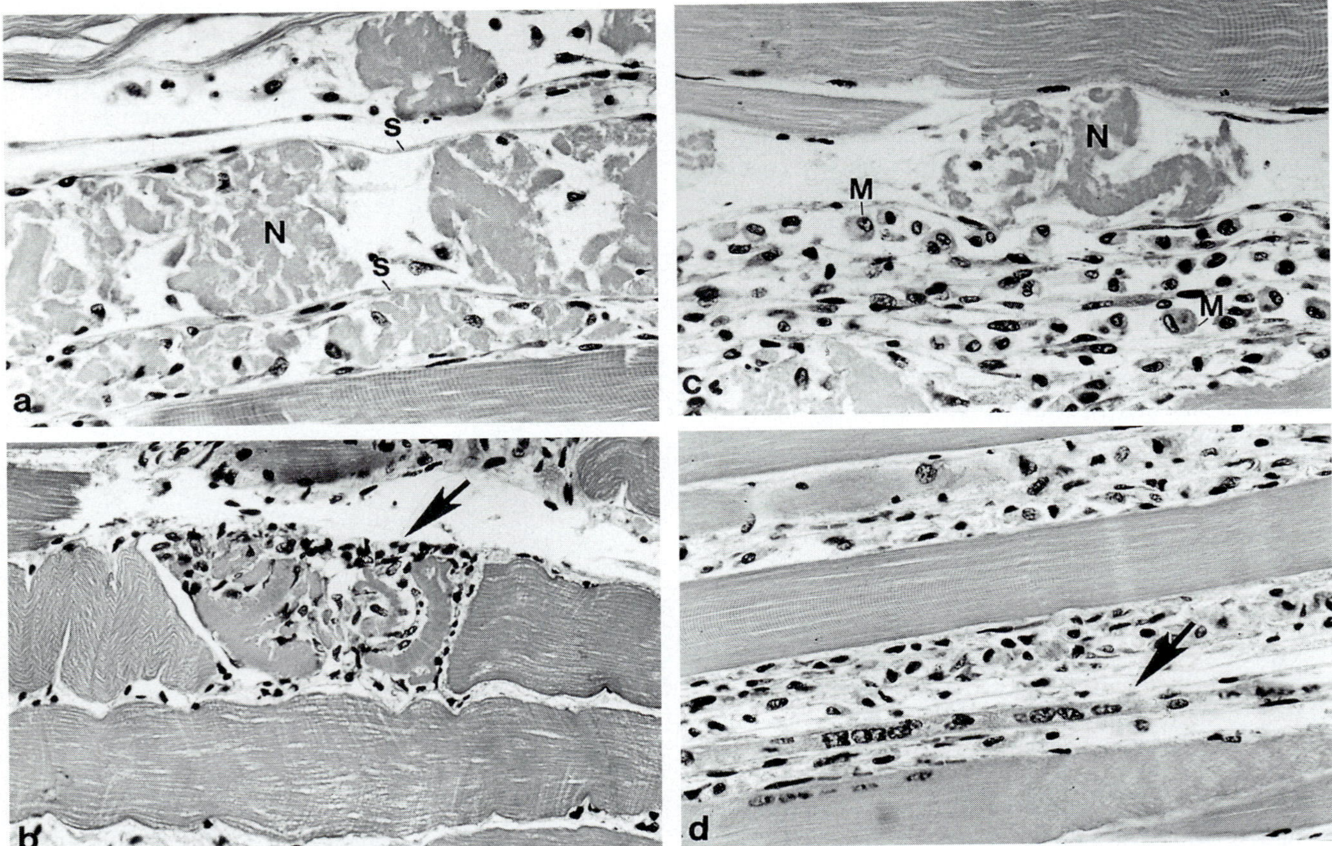

Fig. 9-6 **A**, Segmental necrosis. *N*, necrotic segment undergoing "floccular" degeneration. *s*, sarcolemma. H & E stain. ×250. **B**, Segmental necrosis. At this stage, the necrotic segment is heavily infiltrated by macrophages and myoblasts, the latter formed from satellite cells. H & E stain. ×250. **C**, *N*, necrotic segment of myofiber. In the two fibers below this, necrotic debris has been removed by macrophages (*M*). The other mononuclear cells in the sarcolemmal tubes are satellite cells. H & E stain. ×250. **D**, Regenerating fiber *(arrow)*. Note the rows of central nuclei, the narrow diameter, and the dark cytoplasm (which is due to basophilia). Above the regenerating fiber are two necrotic myofibers heavily infiltrated by macrophages and satellite cells. Between them is a normal myofiber. H & E stain. ×250.

5. Satellite cells form myoblasts, which are embryonic cells, defined as those containing myofibrillar protein such as myosin. These fuse with one another to form myotubes, which are thin, elongated muscle cells with a row of central, closely spaced nuclei. They send out cytoplasmic processes in both directions within the sarcolemmal tube (see Fig. 9-5, *C*). When the processes contact each other or a viable portion of the original muscle fiber, in most cases they fuse. At this stage, the regenerating fiber is characterized by basophilia, central nuclei that are sometimes in rows, a lack of striations, and a narrower than normal diameter (see Figs. 9-5, *F* and 9-6, *D*).
6. The fiber grows and differentiates. Its diameter increases, and longitudinal and cross-striations appear, indicating the formation of sarcomeres.
7. Between 2 to 3 weeks after the initial injury, the muscle nuclei move to the "sarcolemmal" or peripheral position—the normal position for muscle nuclei in mature mammalian muscle.

The success of regeneration depends upon the following:

1. The presence of an intact sarcolemmal tube to act as a scaffold and guide the proliferating myotube cells. The integrity of the basal lamina of the sarcolemmal tube is also responsible for keeping fibroblasts out.
2. The availability of viable satellite cells as a source of nuclei to undergo mitosis to form myonuclei necessary to initiate the production of sarcoplasm. Normal mature myonuclei have lost this ability. Thus, segmental necrosis in which sarcolemmal tubes are preserved, as in metabolic (nutritional and toxic) myopathies, regenerate very successfully. However, the situation when large areas of satellite cells are killed, say, by heat or infarction, is very different. In this case, a return to normal will not be possible, and healing will be chiefly by fibrosis.

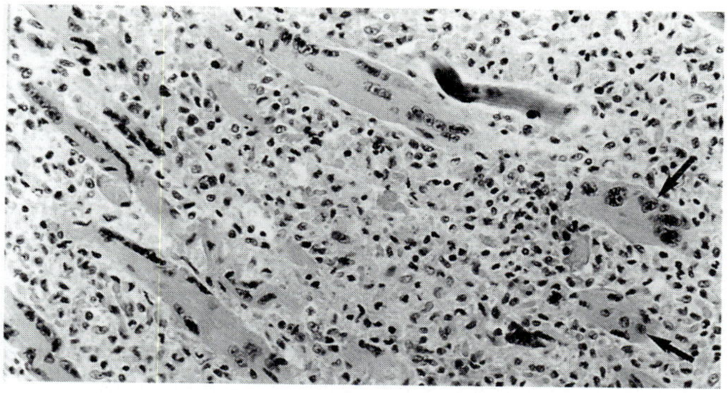

Fig. 9-7 Muscle, gracilis; greyhound dog. The muscle ruptured during racing, 4 weeks prior to euthanasia. Note that healing is by muscle giant cells *(arrows)* and fibrosis. H & E stain.

Regeneration by budding

If the insult to the muscle is sufficient to disrupt the myofiber's sarcolemmal tube, as occurs in destructive lesions such as those caused by trauma, infarction, or injection of irritants, regeneration in those myofibers is by budding. As the myoblasts proliferate and extend to the end of the ruptured tube, sarcoplasm bulges from its cut end and becomes club-shaped, with numerous central nuclei—so called muscle giant cells (Fig. 9-7). Similar cells can also arise from satellite cells remaining in scattered fragments of ruptured muscle fibers. Thus, the presence of muscle giant cells indicates that conditions for regeneration are not optimal. Myotubes are said to be able to bridge gaps of 2 to 4 mm, but any larger ones will be healed by fibrosis, which reduces the elasticity and the efficiency of contraction of the muscle.

Histopathologic interpretation

Because segmental necrosis and regeneration are such a common result of a wide variety of insults, e.g., overexertion, vitamin E deficiency, and the effects of toxins such as monensin, a histologic diagnosis of ''segmental necrosis'' is often not very helpful in determining the cause of the disease. However, the limited usefulness of this histologic diagnosis has been overcome by Kakulas, who realized the significance of (1) the difference between lesions confined to one or multiple sites; and (2) whether lesions were all at one stage (e.g., segmental necrosis without macrophages) or at different stages (e.g., segmental necrosis and regeneration). As a result, he introduced the concept of **monofocal** versus **multifocal** and **monophasic** versus **multiphasic lesions** Monofocal lesions are those confined to one site and could be due to a single incident of trauma, such as an intramuscular injection. Most systemic diseases cause necrosis at multiple sites. However, the concept of monophasic versus multiphasic is more useful. If there were only one insult, e.g., a single episode of overly strenuous exercise (exertional myopathy) or a toxin being fed on one occasion (e.g., brief access to a poisonous plant such as *Cassia occidentalis*), then at autopsy, all lesions would be at the same stage of necrosis or regeneration. However, if the insult were ongoing, such as occurs in vitamin E–selenium deficiency or in continuous feeding of a toxin, then new lesions (segmental necrosis) would form at the same time that regeneration was taking place; in other words, it would be a multiphasic disease. Using this approach, it is sometimes possible to rule out a diagnosis; e.g., vitamin E–selenium deficiency could be ruled out if the lesions were monophasic.

Changes in Myofiber Size

Atrophy

The major types of atrophy are the following:

1. Denervation
2. Disuse
3. Malnutrition, cachexia, and senility

The term ''atrophy'' is used to imply a reduction either in the diameter of the muscle as a whole or in the diameter of a myofiber. In the early stages of atrophy, it may be difficult or impossible to detect loss of muscle mass by gross observation, and morphometric evaluation of fiber diameters may be required. During growth, additional sarcomeres are added to increase length, and additional myofilaments are added to increase diameter. During atrophy, myofibrils are removed by disintegration, and this results in the sarcolemma being too large; consequently, it is thrown into redundant folds. The rate of atrophy depends not only on the lack of use but also on whether or not the muscle is still receiving tropic impulses from nerves.

Denervation atrophy. This atrophy, also known by the misnomer ''neurogenic atrophy,'' is not uncommon in veterinary medicine. Examples are so-called equine roarers, due to laryngeal hemiplegia secondary to damage to the left recurrent laryngeal nerve (Fig. 9-8, *D*), and radial paralysis in dogs. However, any interference with the nerve supply to any muscle will result in atrophy. Under some circumstances, a motor nerve supply can be reestablished, thus reversing the atrophy. Denervation atrophy is particularly rapid, and over half the muscle mass of a completely denervated muscle can be lost in a few weeks. The histologic picture is best considered from two points of view: the sequence in the degenerated myofibers and, secondarily, the changes in the muscle as a whole. The loss of a nerve fiber to a muscle results in atrophy of all myofibers innervated by that nerve. The change is even more dramatic when a whole motor unit is denervated. A motor unit consists of either a ventral horn or a brain stem motor neuron and all the myofibers innervated by it. Because the motor neuron determines the histochemical type, all the atrophic myofibers are of the same histochemical type (type I or type II) (see Fig. 9-1).

Following denervation, fibers become progressively smaller in diameter as peripheral myofibrils disintegrate. If an atrophic fiber is surrounded by normal fibers, it may be pressed into an angular shape, the so-called small, angular

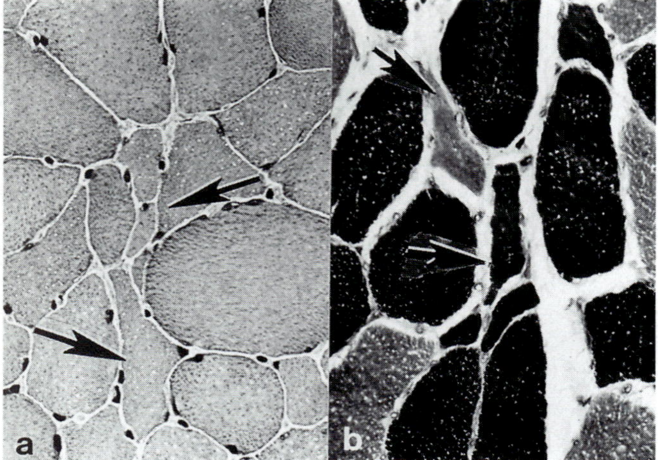

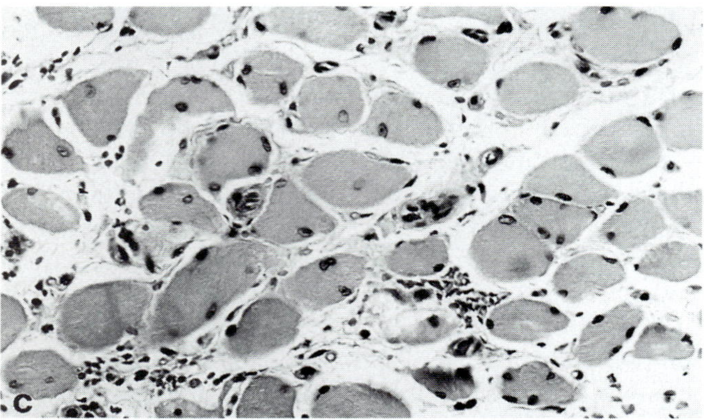

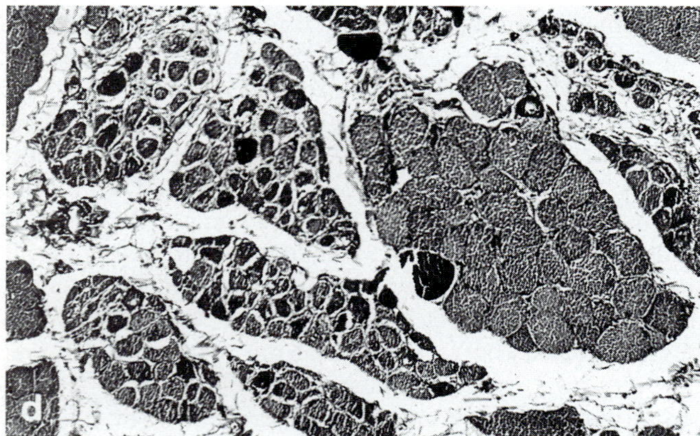

Fig. 9-8 Muscle denervation atrophy. **A**, Early denervation atrophy of several small, angular fibers *(arrows)*. H & E stain. ×250. **B**, Serial section of the same muscle stained with myosin ATPase (pH = 9.8). The atrophic angular fibers *(arrows)*, type I (light) and type II (dark) are a feature of denervation atrophy. ×250. **C**, Vocalis muscle; dog. Several months after denervation. All myofibers are atrophic, rounded, and separated from each other and have numerous muscle nuclei. H & E stain. ×250. **D**, Left cricoarytenoideus dorsalis muscle; horse. Fasciculi are partially or wholely affected and contain atrophic myofibers. H & E stain ×80. ***D**, Courtesy Dr. W.J. Hadlow.*

dark fibers (Fig 9-8, *A*, *B*). However, if atrophic fibers are not compressed, they become round in cross section (Fig. 9-8, *C*). These are very obvious once denervation has advanced to the stage that atrophic fibers are not in contact with other fibers. The most striking change is the increase in the concentration of myofiber nuclei (see Fig. 9-8, *C*). Although myofibrils disappear, muscle nuclei do not do so at the same rate and generally not for a year or so. Thus, the end-stage of a denervated myofiber is a cell devoid of myofibrils but consisting of a row of nuclei. As the muscle fibers atrophy, the fibrous stroma of the endomysium and, particularly, the epimysium becomes more prominent, due to condensation rather than proliferation. Finally, the contractile elements completely disappear, initially leaving aggregates of myofiber nuclei and, later, empty spaces surrounded by endomysium. Eventually, the endomysium compacts, and the end result is a muscle that consists completely or almost completely of fibrous tissue. Occasionally, atrophic myofibers will be replaced by fat, which can cause the muscle to become larger than normal, a condition termed **pseudohypertrophy.**

The extent of changes in the muscle fasciculi will depend on how many motor units have been denervated. If all are affected, then all the muscle fibers will atrophy. Such a change could be secondary to the severance of a major nerve, such as a radial nerve. However, if some of the motor units are still intact, then the muscle fasciculi will have a mixture of atrophic and normal myofibers (Fig. 9-8, *D*). If the nerve damage does not incapacitate the animal and the muscle can still be used, say, for locomotion, the innervated myofibers will not only retain their normal diameter but may even undergo hypertrophy as a result of the increased work load. However, if the animal is incapacitated and cannot use the muscle, then the innervated motor units will undergo disuse atrophy, and, thus, the muscle itself will have a mixture of myofibers undergoing both disuse and denervation atrophy.

If the damage is to a single motor unit, e.g., from destruction of its motor neuron or by transection of its nerve fiber, then atrophic fibers will be scattered through one or more fasciculi, depending on the number of myofibers innervated by a single neuron, i.e., the size of the motor unit (see Figs. 9-1 and 9-8, *D*). Motor units of muscles that have fine motor control, such as the extrinsic muscle of the eye, are small, with as few as 10 myofibers. In large muscles of locomotion where only coarse control is necessary, a motor unit may contain hundreds or even up to 2000 myofibers. Obviously, then, the death of a single ventral horn cell innervating a gluteal muscle would cause extensive denervation atrophy. Loss of a single motor neuron will result in a change in the normal checkerboard appearance of a myosin ATPase–stained cross section. Initially, all the atrophic fibers will be of the same fiber type. However, denervated muscle fibers can be reinnervated by subterminal sprouting of fibers from adjacent normal nerves. Frequently, these nerves will be from a neuron that innervates a different type of myofiber, and, as muscle fiber type is a function of the motor neuron, the newly reinnervated muscle fiber will take on the fiber type determined by that neuron. This results in a loss of the normal mixture of type I and II myofibers, with the formation of groups of the same fiber type adjacent to each other—so-called **fiber-type grouping** (see Fig. 9-29). If the effect is widespread in a fasciculus, it can result in fiber-type predominance.

Disuse atrophy. This results in a less rapid atrophy of muscle than that due to denervation. The cause can be anything that stops the use of the muscle: fractured limbs, failure to use a painful leg, upper motor neuron damage, or recumbency. The loss of the myofibrils has similarities to that of denervation atrophy, but there are differences. Histochemical examination reveals that type II fibers atrophy faster (Fig. 9-9, *A* and *B*). In fact, this occurs so rapidly and frequently that a diffuse type II atrophy is not regarded as having any diagnostic specificity. Disuse atrophy is reversible except when atrophy has been so severe and prolonged that myofibers have been lost.

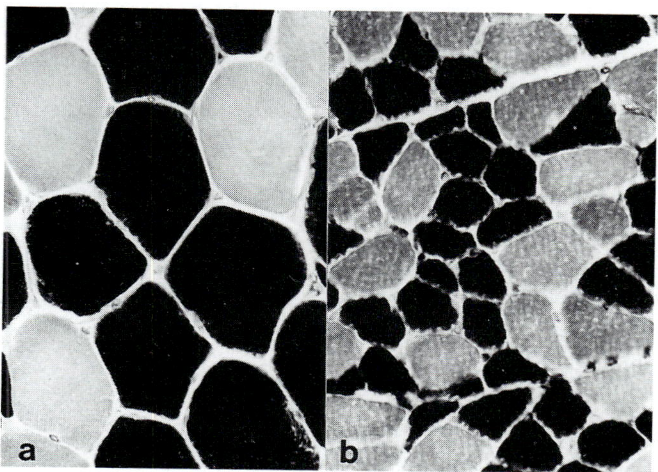

Fig. 9-9 Disuse atrophy; dog. **A**, Normal biceps femoris muscle. **B**, Same muscle. 60 days after forced disuse. Both type I (light) and type II (dark) fibers are atrophic, but the type II fibers are more severely affected. Myosin ATPase (pH = 9.8). ×250.

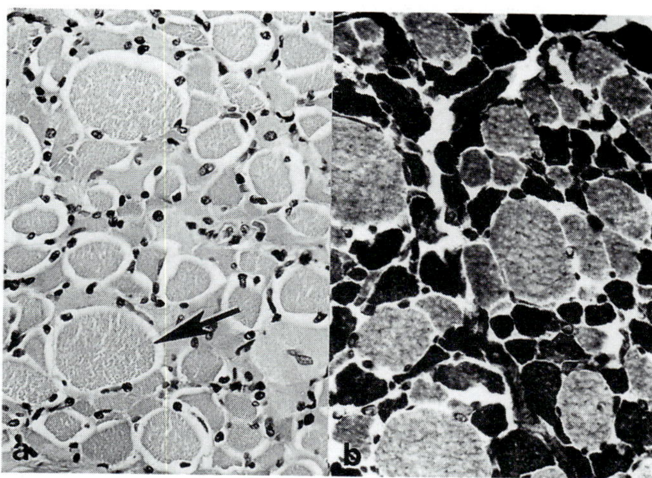

Fig. 9-10 Biceps femoris muscle; dog. Emaciation. **A**, All fibers are atrophic, but some are less severely affected. Note the increased concentration of muscle nuclei. H & E stain. ×250. **B**, Both types I and II fibers are atrophic, but type II (dark) are more severely affected. Some type I (light) fibers *(arrows)* are only mildly atrophic. Myosin ATPase (pH = 9.8) stain. ×250.

Atrophy due to malnutrition, cachexia, and senility. In starvation, muscle protein is metabolized to supply the need for nutrients. This type of muscle atrophy occurs gradually, except in the cachexia associated with some febrile diseases. All muscles of the body are not affected to the same degree (Fig. 9-10, *A*). Postural muscles are spared, and, in these, type I fibers are not only spared (Fig. 9-10, *B*) but sometimes a small percentage actually hypertrophy, no doubt a compensatory hypertrophy due to increased work load. Unlike in muscles undergoing denervation atrophy, some muscle nuclei disappear as the volume of the myofiber is reduced. On gross examination, muscles are smaller, thinner, darker, and flabbier than normal, and no fat remains. In muscles with lipofuscinosis, the brown pigment is concentrated, intensifying the brownish discoloration (see Lipofuscinosis).

Hypertrophy

This term is used in two ways: for an increase in the diameter of the muscle as a whole and for an increase in myofiber diameter even if the muscle diameter itself is not enlarged. Increase in muscle fiber diameter is basically caused by an increased work load on those fibers. Hypertrophy is subdivided into two types: **work hypertrophy** and **compensatory hypertrophy.** Work hypertrophy implies an increase in normal physiologic work, as occurs in muscles

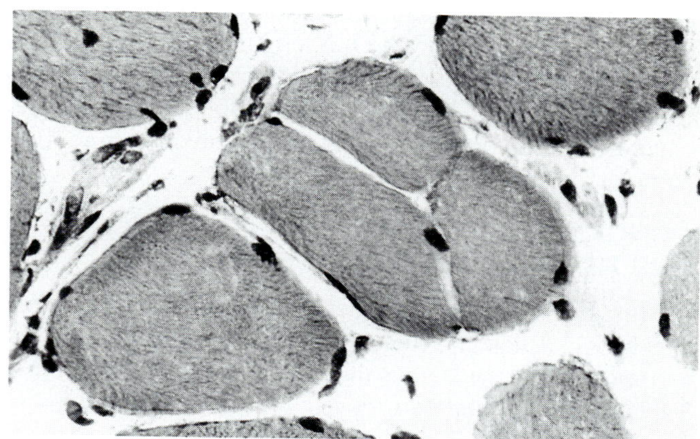

Fig. 9-11 Muscle; cat. Muscular dystrophy. Longitudinal myofiber splitting. The hypertrophic myofiber has been divided into three segments, and other myofibers have marked variation in their diameters. H & E stain.

Table 9-2. Hereditary, congenital, or neonatal defects of muscle of domestic animals

Defect	Etiology, lesion
Muscular hyperplasia in cattle and rarely in sheep	Autosomal recessive with variable penetrance; myofiber hyperplasia; increased percentage of type IIB fibers which are hypertrophied.
Limber leg of Jersey cattle	Autosomal recessive, sublethal, no histologic lesions found.
Myotonia in sheep, goats, dogs	Defined clinically by persistence of voluntary contractions; in goat, defect believed to be located in the sarcolemma.
Daft lambs of Border Leicester	Autosomal recessive hypertrophy of some type-I fibers; others smaller than normal; defect in intramuscular nerves.
Mitochondrial myopathy of dogs	Possible recessive X-linked, ultrastructurally abnormal mitochondria.

Based on Bradley R, Fell BF. Myopathies in animals. In: Walton J, ed. Disorders of Voluntary Muscle. 4th ed. Edinburgh: Churchill Livingstone, 1981: 824-872.

during athletic training and in less obvious sites, such as the internal abdominal oblique muscle of pregnant ewes. Compensatory hypertrophy, which is really a type of work hypertrophy by individual fibers, is in response to an increased work load caused by the loss or absence of fibers in a muscle. This type of hypertrophy can be induced by denervation atrophy of adjacent myofibers in a muscle fasciculus. Thus, compensatory hypertrophy can be secondary to denervation atrophy, muscular dystrophies, cachectic atrophy, and extensive necrosis in nutritional or toxic myopathies in which muscles have lost many myofibers.

The exact mechanism modulating hypertrophy is unknown. Myofibers are increased in diameter by the addition of myofilaments. Fibers undergoing compensatory hypertrophy may enlarge to over 100 μm in diameter. One of the effects of increased work load is to cause longitudinal fiber splitting. In histological cross sections of muscle, these fibers have a characteristic appearance. The myofiber is divided into 2 to 4 segments (Fig. 9-11) that resemble the pieces of a pie. These pieces are usually of different sizes, but all still lie within one endomysial tube. However, the split may not extend the full length of the fiber. Not all longitudinal fiber splitting is believed to be due to increased work load. Some is caused by faulty myofiber regeneration with failure of individual myoblasts to fuse completely.

CONGENITAL, NEONATAL, AND HEREDITARY DISEASES

Muscle is subject to numerous hereditary, congenital, and neonatal defects. Space will not allow a detailed description of all these, and they have been summarized in Tables 9-2, 9-3 and 9-4, based on the classifications of Bradley and Fell, whose review should be consulted. Several of the diseases warrant additional description.

Muscular dystrophy

The term muscular dystrophy is highly ambiguous in veterinary literature. It was introduced in human pathology

Table 9-3. Congenital or neonatal defects of muscle of unknown or complex etiology*

Defect	Etiology
Congenital articular rigidity (CAR)	
Cattle	Teratogens: akabane virus, *Lupinus* species
Horses	Muscle cell hypotrophy, ? myogenic
Sheep	Teratogens: *Astragalus* (locoweed)
	Viruses: akabane, wesselsbrom, Rift Valley Fever
	Chemicals
	Diets deficient in vitamin E or selenium
Pigs	Heritable: simple autosomal recessive
	Vitamin A and manganese deficiencies
	Plants
	Nicotiana tabacum (tobacco)
	Datura stramonium (thorn apple)
	Conium maculatum (hemlock)
	Prunus serotina (black cherry)
Rigid lamb syndrome (Rhodesia)	Lesions: neuron degeneration, arrest of myelination, and underdeveloped muscles
Congenital myopathy of lambs (Scotland)	Possible vitamin E deficiency
	Myodegeneration and calcification
Myofibrillar hypoplasia (spayleg), piglets	Etiology unknown, possibly multifactorial
	Deficiency of myofibrils
Myofibrillar hypoplasia, calf (1 case)	Etiology unknown, lesion as for piglets

Based on Bradley R, Fell BF. Myopathies in animals. In: Walton J, ed. Disorders of Voluntary Muscle. 4th ed. Edinburgh: Churchill Livingstone, 1981: 824-872.

Table 9-4. Familial or hereditary muscle defects manifested after the neonatal period in domestic animals

Muscular dystrophies
Diaphragm myopathy of Meuse-Rhine-Yssel cattle
Ovine progressive muscular dystrophy
Canine muscular dystrophy
Feline muscular dystrophy
Mink muscular dystrophy
Mouse muscular dystrophy
Syrian hamster muscular dystrophy
Myotonic syndromes in sheep, goats, and dogs
Type II myofiber deficiency in the dog
Weaver syndrome of Brown Swiss cattle
Porcine asymmetric hindquarter syndrome

Based on Bradley R, Fell BF. Myopathies in animals. In: Walton J, ed. Disorders of Voluntary Muscles. 4th ed. Edinburgh: Churchill Livingstone, 1981: 824-872.

to define a group of inherited progressive muscle diseases. Unfortunately, in the 1930s, the term *nutritional muscular dystrophy* was applied to nutritional myopathy due to vitamin E deficiency, which should have been termed *nutritional myopathy* or *nutritional myodegeneration.* Muscular dystrophy has been defined by Adams as a progressive, hereditary, degenerative disease of skeletal muscles. The innervation of the affected muscles is sound. The relative inadequacy of regenerative activity is a fundamental characteristic. Thus, it is presumed that the primary defect in muscular dystrophy is in the myofiber itself. The progressive nature of the disease separates it from the benign, relatively nonprogressive congenital muscle disorders, such as central core, nemaline, mitochondrial, and myotubular myopathies. Muscular dystrophies are a subgroup within the inherited diseases of muscle.

Muscular dystrophy in animals has been recognized in cattle, sheep, mice, chickens, hamsters, dogs and cats. In human beings, the disease is divided into major subtypes based on age of onset, group of muscles affected, histologic appearance, and type of inheritance. Of these, Duchenne type and myotonic dystrophy have approximate animal models. As in human beings, muscular dystrophy in animals also preferentially involves groups of muscles (vastus intermedius in sheep, diaphragm in Meuse-Rhine-Yssel cattle) and, sometimes, a specific fiber type (type I in sheep).

A disease resembling Duchenne type dystrophy has been described in golden retrievers and Irish terriers. The X-linked disease of the golden retriever has been studied extensively by Cooper and co-workers. Clinically, at 2 months of age, pups are weak, have a stiff gait, and tire easily. These difficulties increase in severity over the next several months, but dogs can live longer than 6 years. Some have cardiomyopathy. Affected muscles include extensor carpi radialis, sartorius, and diaphragm. Both type I and type II fibers are affected. Histologic lesions consist of myofibers undergoing degeneration, necrosis, and attempts at regeneration (Fig. 9-12). Ultimately, because of the unrelenting necrosis, there is loss of muscle mass, and the increased load on the remaining myofibers causes compensatory hypertrophy of some of the fibers. Individual myofiber splitting is common. Affected dogs are deficient in dystrophin, a plasmalemma-associated protein that can be demonstrated in sections by immunoperoxidase staining (Fig. 9-13). Its absence is diagnostic of the disease.

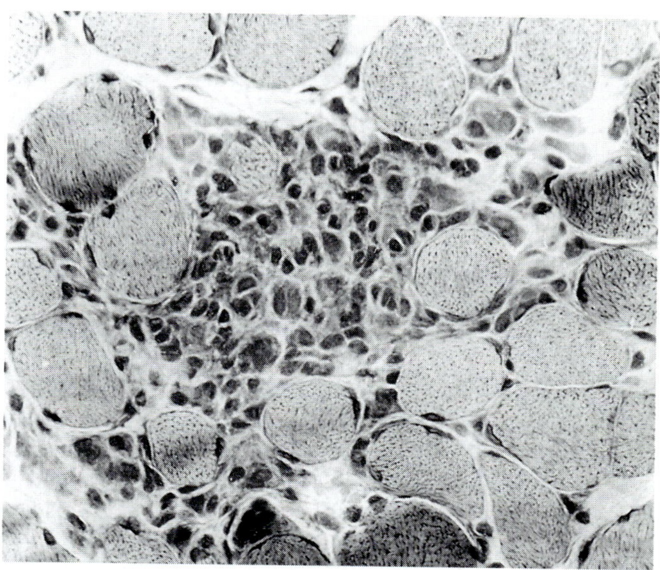

Fig. 9-12 Muscle; dog. X-linked muscular dystrophy. Note that some myofibers are necrotic and are infiltrated by macrophages and others are regenerating. H & E stain. *Courtesy Dr. B.J. Cooper.*

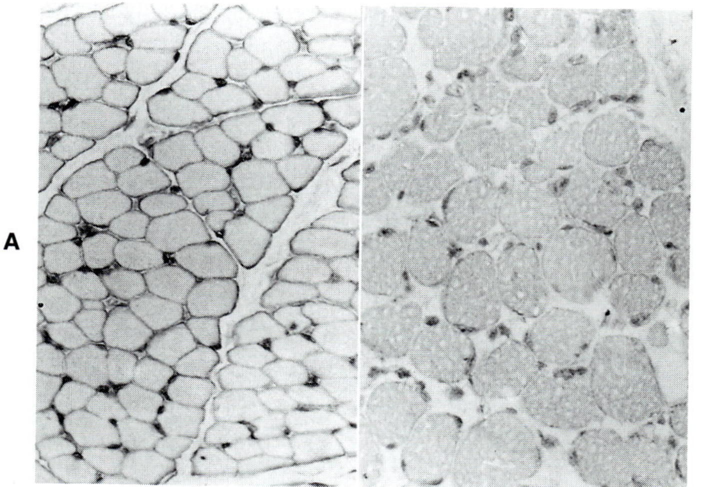

Fig. 9-13 Muscle; dog. X-linked muscular dystrophy. Note the dark staining of the dystrophin at the periphery of the myofibers in the normal control (**A**) and the lack or partial lack of dystrophin in the myofibers of the muscular dystrophy dog (**B**). Immunoperoxidase staining for dystrophin. *Courtesy Dr. B.J. Cooper.*

Storage Diseases

The term ''storage disease'' is somewhat of a misnomer, as the word ''storage'' frequently implies a desirable, useful trait. However, storage diseases are really caused by accumulation of excess metabolite, an undesirable situation, because of some defect in metabolism. These are usually inherited, the result of a missing or defective enzyme. Muscle storage diseases involve the metabolism of glycogen and fat.

Glycogenoses

There are several types of glycogen storage diseases, based on the deficient enzyme (Table 9-5). Of these, six cause glycogen accumulation in muscle, but only types II, III, and VII have been recognized in animals.

Type II glycogenosis, caused by a deficiency of acid maltase, is of economic importance in breeding stock of Shorthorn cattle. Affected animals have muscular weakness and incoordination. Glycogen is stored in the central nervous system (CNS), heart (Purkinje fibers), and skeletal muscle. Neurons of the thalamus and cerebellar nuclei are swollen and vacuolated by glycogen. In muscle, both type I and type II myofibers have vacuoles containing glycogen.

Type III glycogenosis, caused by a deficiency of the debranching enzyme, occurs in dogs. Gross lesions are hypertrophic cardiomyopathy and hepatomegaly. Glycogen is present in neurons, hepatocytes, and cardiac and skeletal muscle.

Phosphofructokinase (PFK) deficiency has been reported as an inherited disease in English springer spaniel dogs. Because there is nearly a complete lack of muscle PFK activity, exercise results in a life-threatening crisis because of a glycolytic block. Muscles become completely depleted of phosphocreatine and ATP. Affected dogs usually do not have muscle lesions, but, in one dog, there were some granular deposits of an amylopectin-like polysaccharide.

Myasthenia Gravis

This neuromuscular disease has been reported in human beings, dogs, and cats. Diagnosis is usually based on clinical findings of muscle weakness and fatigue exacerbated by exercise and response to injection of anticholinesterase drugs. This last potentiates the effect of acetylcholine, the neurotransmitter at the neuromuscular junction, thus indicating that this is the site of the defect. Both acquired and congenital (inherited) forms have been described in dogs, and, because of the similarities, it is convenient to discuss both here. **Acquired canine myasthenia gravis,** usually found in adult dogs, is generally associated with megaesophagus and dysphagia, which can result in a secondary aspiration pneumonia. It is an autoimmune disease in which antibodies are directed against the acetylcholine receptors (AChRs) of the neuromuscular junction. The result is a reduction in the numbers of AChRs to mediate the transmission at the neuromuscular junction. The initial cause is still unclear, but bacteria have been implicated in human myasthenia gravis. Subunits of the AChR and *E. coli, Proteus vulgaris,* and *Klebsiella pneumonia* have been found to share antigenic determinants.

Congenital myasthenia gravis, inherited as an autosomal recessive, has been reported in Jack Russell terriers, springer spaniels, and smooth fox terriers. Although there is a deficiency of AChRs, there is no evidence of an autoimmune-mediated disease. The histologic changes in muscle are nonspecific, being disuse atrophy and fibrosis, or no changes at all.

Steatosis

This disease, also sometimes called lipomatosis or hypoplasia lipomatosa, is a curiosity, occasionally seen in cattle, pigs, and sheep, usually at a packing plant or necropsy. This lesion is believed to be congenital. Because of defective muscle fiber development, lost myofibers are replaced with fat (Fig. 9-14, *B*). The most severely affected muscles are usually in the loin and back (Fig. 9-14, *A*). Gross lesions are bilaterally symmetrical, and muscles retain their normal shape or may be larger than normal. If the body has been chilled, extremely affected muscles appear almost like soap. Less severely affected muscles are speckled, streaked, or partially replaced by fat. The fat can be stained and confirmed in macroscopic specimens by fat

Table 9-5. Types of glycogenoses in domestic animals

Type of glycogenosis	Enzyme deficiency	Disease	Domestic animals affected
II	Acid maltase (α-1,4-glucosidase)	Pompe's disease	Corriedale sheep Shorthorn cattle Brahman cattle (Australia) Lapland dog
III	Debranching enzyme (amylo-1,6-glucosidase)	Cori-Forbes' disease	Dogs (German shepherd) Japanese quail Cats
VII	Muscle phosphofructokinase	Tarui's disease	Dog

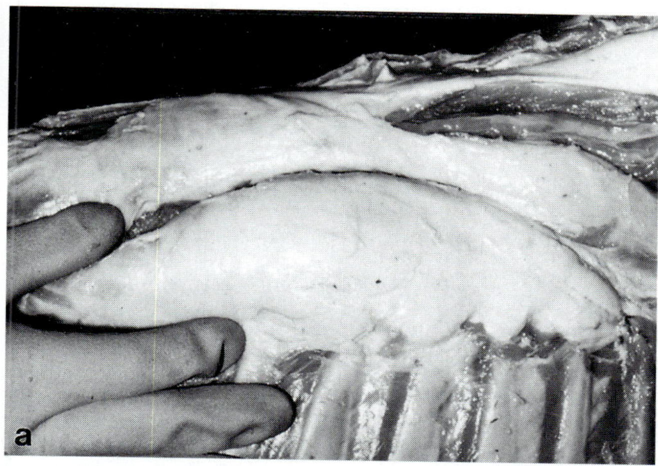

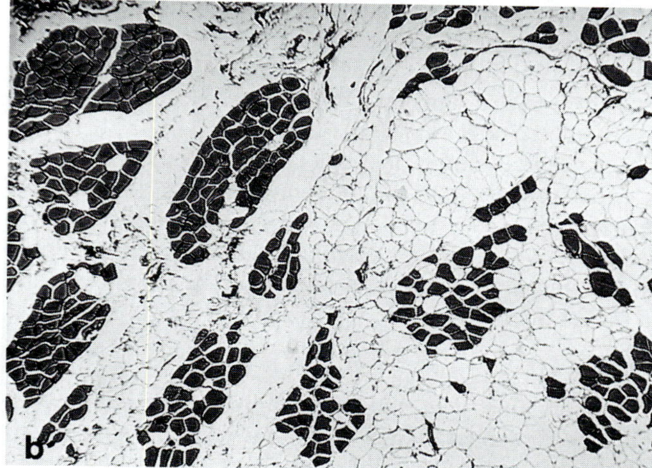

Fig. 9-14 Muscle; ox. Steatosis. **A**, Longissimus muscles are enlarged and almost completely replaced by fat. **B**, Longissimus muscle. Cross section. Many myofibers in fasciculi have been replaced by fat cells. H & E stain. ×30 ***B**, Courtesy Dr. W.J. Hadlow.*

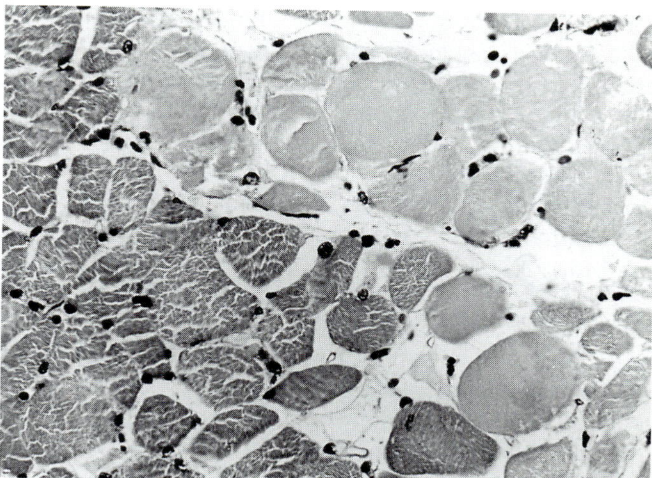

Fig. 9-15 Muscle. Infarct. Note that in the infarcted area *(upper right),* all myofibers are necrotic (rounded, hyalinized), and all stromal nuclei are pyknotic, indicating necrosis. H & E stain. ×250.

''stains'' used in histology, e.g., oil-red-O. The disease appears to be of no clinical significance, but the appearance of a badly affected muscle at a packing plant is likely to be of great interest.

DISTURBANCES OF CIRCULATION

Congestion

Passive congestion of muscles due to localized or generalized stasis results in dark red to very dark red muscles, as in the congestion of muscles cranial to the thoracic inlet as the result of bovine ruminal tympany—''bloat''. The congestion may be so severe as to resemble hemorrhage on gross examination.

Ischemia

If animals are exsanguinated at necropsy or slaughter, their muscles are pale, actually revealing the true color of muscle. Similarly, anemic animals have pale muscles. Because muscle's relatively small energy stores of glycogen and lipid are rapidly exhausted during exercise, myofibers are well supplied with capillaries. The density of capillaries is greater for type I fibers, which depend upon aerobic metabolism, than for type II fibers, which are either glycolytic or mixed-oxidative glycolytic. Athletic training also increases the density of capillaries. The basic factor in determining the effect of ischemia on muscle is the differential susceptibility of the various cells forming the muscle as a whole. Myofibers are the most sensitive, satellite cells less sensitive, and fibroblasts the least sensitive to anoxia. Thus, infarction of an area of muscle leads first to segmental necrosis, then to death of satellite cells, and, finally, to the death of all cells, including the stromal cells (Fig. 9-15). The loss of satellite cells precludes rapid regeneration, because they are not available to form myoblasts. Satellite cells have to be recruited from the edges of viable myofibers. Because all cells in the infarcted muscle die, the result is that most healing takes place by fibrosis and scar formation. Disrupted myofibers at the periphery of the lesion may attempt regeneration by budding.

The basic causes of ischemia are the following:

1. Occlusion of the vascular system
2. External pressure on a muscle
3. Swelling of a muscle in a nonexpandible compartment

Vascular occlusion

Because of the numerous capillary anastomoses within the muscle and the well-developed collateral circulation, infarction from embolism is rare. Blockage of the iliac arteries by aortic-iliac thrombosis in the horse and of the aortic bifurcation by a ''saddle'' thromboembolus in the cat can cause ischemia. In the cat, the feet may be cool and cyanotic, and muscles undergo segmental necrosis before the collateral circulation can be established.

Occasionally, in dogs, *Dirofilaria immitis* (heartworm) may cause a proliferative arteritis and thrombosis of the external and internal iliac arteries and their branches. These lesions produce thromboemboli, some of which cause scattered foci of necrosis (infarcts) in the muscles of the hind limbs.

One cause of muscle infarction in sheep is vasculitis caused by the bluetongue virus. Grossly, these infarcts appear as fine gray streaks, and foci or hemorrhages may be so small as not to be visible.

Equine purpura hemorrhagica is a sporadic, noncontagious disease of horses, characterized by subcutaneous edema and widely scattered hemorrhagic foci in skin and muscles. The muscle lesions are infarcts due to a vasculitis, believed to be immune-mediated. The disease occurs sporadically in horses recovering from streptococcal infections such as strangles. Muscle infarction may be so extensive as to cause myoglobinuria.

The size of infarcts depends on the size of the vessel obstructed and the duration. Blockage of capillaries causes segmental necrosis, usually multifocal and, possibly, multiphasic. However, when larger arteries are blocked, whole areas of muscle, including the satellite cells needed for regeneration, are killed. Healing is by fibrosis. Intermittent obstruction to a major vessel causes two changes in muscle: (1) myofiber necrosis, and, if these fibers are not regenerated, then the result will be compensatory hypertrophy, chiefly of type I myofibers, which are responsible for bearing much of the weight of the animal; and (2) ischemia of the legs, which may cause a peripheral neuropathy. If nerves are irreversibly damaged, denervation atrophy of the muscles will result.

External pressure on muscle

Prolonged periods of recumbency, such as during anesthesia or in animals unable to rise, or too-tightly fitting plaster casts or bandages can put external pressure on muscles. Postanesthesia myopathy is seen, particularly in horses anesthetized for long periods. The location of the lesions depends on the position of the horse during anesthesia. If dorsal recumbency, the gluteals and the longissimus muscles are ischemic; in lateral recumbency, lesions are in the lower legs: triceps brachii, pectoralis, deltoideus, and brachiocephalicus. The basic mechanism is that the pressure in the muscle exceeds the perfusion pressure in the capillaries. Muscle infarction is frequently seen in ''downer'' cows, where the weight of the body of the animal in ventral recumbency causes ischemia of the pectoral muscles and any muscles of the fore or hind limbs tucked under the body. Ewes in advanced pregnancy with twins or triplets develop an ischemic necrosis of the internal abdominal oblique muscle, and this can lead to rupture.

The duration of ischemia determines the severity of necrosis and the success of regeneration (see Necrosis). In the case of the postanesthesia myopathy, the lesion is a monophasic, multifocal necrosis. In the downer cow, the lesions are also multifocal but may be polyphasic if the animal has been recumbent for days to weeks.

Swelling of muscle in a nonexpandable compartment

In human beings, an **anterior tibial syndrome** or anterior tibial compartment syndrome sometimes follows exercise. The pathogenesis is believed to be due to swelling of the pretibial muscles, which are surrounded (cranially) by the inelastic anterior fascial sheath and (caudally) by the tibia. Swelling impedes the blood supply, and, in very severe cases, unless the pressure is relieved by fasciotomy, the muscle will become infarcted. A similar mechanism causes infarction of the supracoracoid muscle of some breeds of turkeys and chickens after they flap their wings. Thus, vigorously exercised muscles enclosed in thick fascial sheaths may be susceptible to this type of infarction. It should be realized, however, that even normal myofibers may be damaged by contraction during extremely strenuous exercise. Evidence of this is the rise in serum creatine kinase in the 24 hours following vigorous exercise.

MYOSITIS

Inflammation of muscle, termed **myositis** (plural: myositides), can be caused by a wide array of agents—bacteria, viruses, protozoa, helminths, immune-mediated mechanisms—or can be idiopathic.

Bacterial Myositides

Bacterial infections of muscle are not numerous, but bacteria may cause suppurative (pyogenic bacteria), serohemorrhagic (clostridia), or granulomatous lesions. Infection may be introduced by direct penetration (wounds or injections), hematogenously, or by spread from an adjacent cellulitis, fasciitis, tendinitis, arthritis, or osteomyelitis.

Pyogenic bacteria introduced into a muscle usually cause a localized suppuration and myofiber necrosis (Fig 9-16; Table 9-6). This may resolve completely or become localized to form an abscess, or, in some cases, the infection may spread down the facial planes. For example, a nonsterile intramuscular injection into the gluteal muscles may cause a myositis that extends down the facial planes of the muscles of the femur and tibia and erupt to the surface through a sinus, proximal to the tarsus. Although the majority of inflammation is serous or seropurulent and involves facial planes, some bacteria extend into and cause necrosis of adjacent muscle fasciculi. *Streptococcus equi* (horses), *Actinomyces pyogenes* (cattle and sheep), and *Corynebacterium pseudotuberculosis* (sheep and goats) are

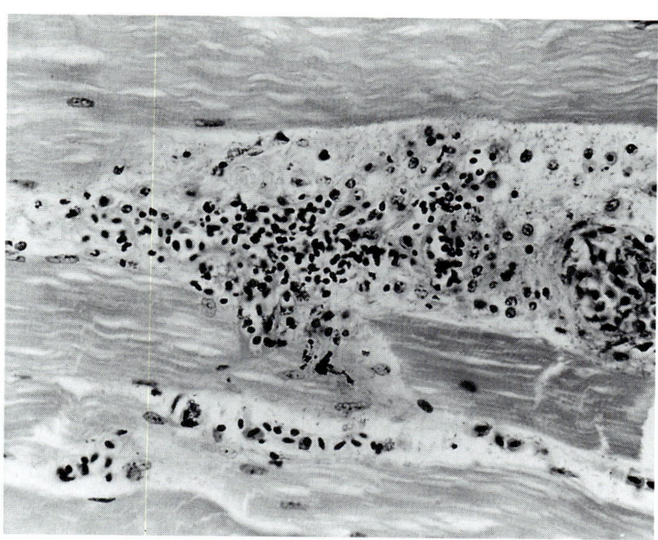

Fig. 9-16 Cranial pectoral muscle; ostrich. Purulent myositis caused by *Pseudomonas aeruginosa* from a penetrating wound. H & E stain. *Courtesy Dr. C. Lenghaus.*

Table 9-6. Pyogenic bacterial infections of muscle

Bacterium	Species of animal	Route of infection
Streptococcus equi	Horses	Hematogenous
Actinobacillus equuli	Foals	Hematogenous
Actinobacillus lignieresi	Cattle	Direct penetration
Actinomyces bovis	Cattle	Extension from bone
Haemophilus somnus	Cattle	Hematogenous
Corynebacterium pseudotuberculosis	Sheep and goats	Hematogenous
Haemophilus agni	Lambs	Hematogenous
Pasteurella multocida	Cats	Hematogenous

common causes of muscle abscesses. Cats are more likely to develop a cellulitis *(Pasteurella multocida)* that extends into the adjacent muscle. Clostridia may produce a serous or serohemorrhagic cellulitis or cellulitis and myositis.

Clostridial myositis may be caused by two completely different mechanisms: by penetrating wounds, in which case the disease is designated **gas gangrene,** or, in the case of cattle and sheep, by the activation of spores of *Clostridium chauvoei* disseminated from the GI tract to muscles, a disease termed **blackleg.**

Gas gangrene and malignant edema are caused by clostridia such as *C. septicum, C. perfringens, C. novyi,* and *C. chauvoei.* These bacteria exist as spores in the soil, and, for their germination and growth to the vegetative form, they require an alkaline environment and low oxygen tension. These conditions are produced in deep, penetrating wounds. The clostridia produce a serohemorrhagic myositis. If the lesions are confined to the subcutis and fascia, i.e., without an involvement of muscle, the lesion is termed **malignant edema.** Death is due to toxemia and septicemia and is rapid. Gas gangrene was responsible for enormous numbers of battle casualties before the introduction of vaccines in the earlier part of the twentieth century.

Blackleg

Blackleg, an economically important disease of cattle and sheep, is caused by the activation of spores of *Clostridium chauvoei* lying latent in muscles. Spores in the intestinal tract of herbivores are apparently able to cross the intestinal mucosa and be disseminated via the blood throughout the body, to a wide variety of tissues, including muscles. If the local environment becomes suitable, e.g., if muscle is devitalized and becomes anaerobic, spores can germinate and the bacilli proliferate.

Blackleg classically affects the fattest cattle, 9 to 24 months old, on pasture. There may be a seasonal incidence, usually in the summer. Because of the rapid induction of toxemia, clinical signs may not be observed and animals may be found dead. If sick animals are seen, then the clinical signs are referable to either toxemia or the muscle lesions. Toxemia is caused pyrexia, depression, circulatory collapse, and pulmonary edema. Muscle lesions result in lameness, crepitus, and hot, swollen muscles, which later may become cool, as the muscle becomes necrotic.

Pathogenesis and gross lesions. Once the vegetative form of *C. chauvoei* proliferates, it produces powerful toxins that can damage capillaries, produce a serohemorrhagic exudation, and cause necrosis of muscle in which proliferating clostridia produce gas, causing emphysema and crepitus. The edema fluid and gas increase the pressure within the muscle and dissect along fascial and epimysial planes to spread lengthwise. The gross appearance of the muscle varies with the age of the lesion. In early stages, which are at the periphery of the lesion, the muscle is dark red and markedly distended by serous or serohemorrhagic exudate, which separates the fibers. The cut surface is wet, and exudate may drip out. The oldest stage, at the center of the lesion, is dry, reddish-black, and porous, because of gas bubbles (Fig. 9-17, *A*). The odor is characteristically reminiscent of that of rancid butter (butyric).

Gross changes elsewhere in the body are directly referable to either toxemia or proliferation of bacilli. Because of the pyrexia, cadavers bloat rapidly and undergo rapid postmortem decomposition. Yellow subcutaneous fluid, with or without gas bubbles, may be associated with affected muscles. Pelvic, pectoral girdle, gluteal, femoral, and humeroscapular muscles are frequently involved; but, lesions can be present in any striated muscle, including heart, crura of the diaphragm, tongue, and masticatory muscles. Lesions may be very small and may be detected only if muscles are incised at not more than 1-cm intervals.

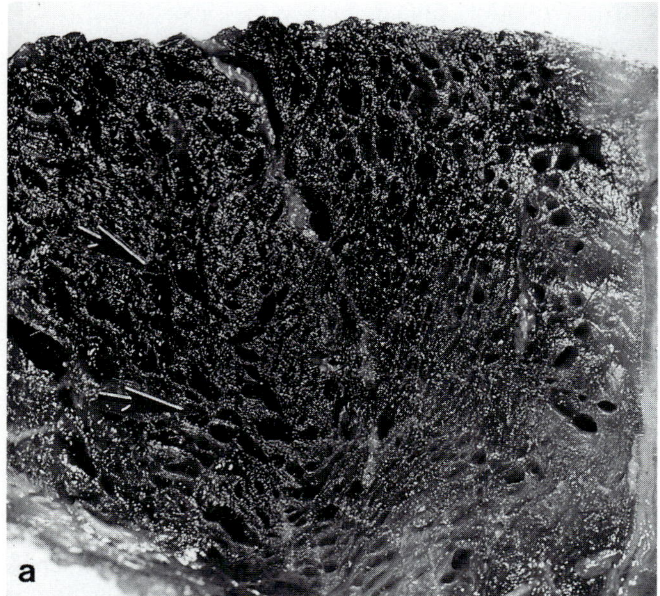

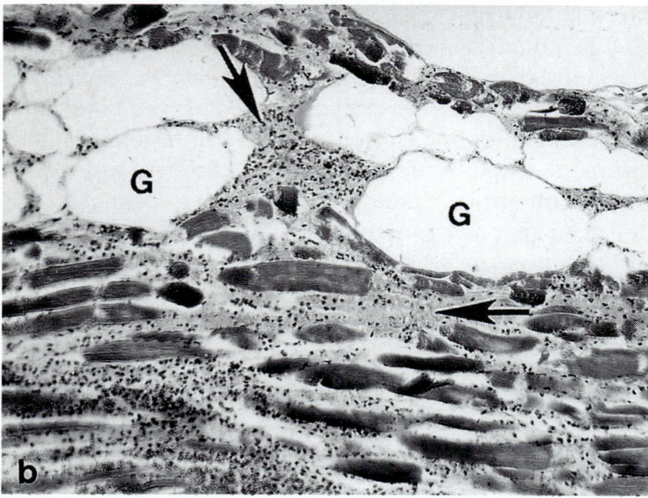

Fig. 9-17 Muscle; cow. Blackleg. **A**, Cut surface of a late stage. Note the dark, dry surface with numerous gas bubbles *(arrows).* **B**, Early stage. Serohemorrhagic exudate (arrow) and gas bubbles (*G*) separate myofibers. H & E stain. ×85. ***B**, Courtesy Dr. W.J. Hadlow.*

Histopathologic Lesions. Obviously, these depend on the stage. In the early "wet stage," the myofibers are separated by serous or serohemorrhagic exudate (Fig. 9-17, *B*) and undergo coagulation necrosis. Thus, nuclei are absent, but the shape of the fibers is retained. In the latest stage (dry stage), the muscle fibers fragment and are separated by gas bubbles. Gram-positive bacilli (*Clostridium chauvoei*) are seen relatively infrequently, although clumps of them may be found.

Diagnosis. Necropsy confirmation of a diagnosis of blackleg depends upon both the isolation of *C. chauvoei* and on the presence of the characteristic lesions. Because latent spores can be harbored in muscles, recovery of the organism alone does not confirm the diagnosis. However, attempts should be made to culture *C. chauvoei* from the lesion and subcutaneous fluid and to check for septicemia by culturing heart blood and parenchymatous organs. Unfortunately, *C. septicum* tends to proliferate rapidly after death and obscure *C. chauvoei.* For this reason, necropsy should be done immediately after euthanasia or death.

Granulomatous Myositides

This usually takes the form of single or multiple granulomas (focal granulomatous myositis) and is relatively rare. It may be caused by *Mycobacterium bovis* (tuberculosis), usually in cattle and swine, *Actinobacillus lignieresi* (cattle), *Actinomyces bovis* (cattle), and *Staphylococcus aureus* (botriomycosis in horses).

Tuberculosis is rare in North America. Lesions are yellowish, variably sized spherical nodules with yellowish, caseous contents usually enclosed in a thick fibrous capsule. Microscopically, the lesion is a granuloma with central necrosis surrounded by epithelioid and giant cells.

Actinobacillosis *(Actinobacillis lignieresii)* (wooden tongue in cattle) is usually due to the direct penetration of the tongue by the bacterium, which produces small, pale granulomas which contain "sulfa granules" composed of masses of gram-negative rods. This disease has also been reported in the tongue and the muscles of the rear limbs of a dog.

Actinomycosis bovis produces a granulomatous osteomyelitis in the mandible or maxilla of cattle. The lesion may extend into adjacent muscles, including the masseter. Lesions have caseous to suppurative centers, surrounded by epithelioid cells and giant cells. The central exudate contains "sulfa granules" containing gram-positive rods and branching filaments.

Botryomycosis

In horses and pigs, *Staphylococcus aureus* can cause a low-grade, persistent infection that becomes granulomatous. The disease is called botryomycosis and is usually the result of wounds in the horse. Lesions are fibrous nodules present in the muscles of the head, sternocephalicus, pectoral region, and, less often, the back and thighs. In pigs, the lesions may be in castration wounds or mammary glands. The nodules are hard and have a fibrous capsule that encloses a cavity containing yellow-brown pus and granules. Histologically, the lesions are encapsulated granulomas containing central "club" colonies in which there are demonstrable staphylococci. The granulomas can extend peripherally to involve adjacent muscles.

Fungal granulomatous myositis

This rare disease is mentioned here for convenience. Occasionally, *Blastomyces dermatitidis* causes lesions in the laryngeal mucosa. This may extend into the adjacent

Table 9-7. Viruses causing lesions in muscles of domestic animals

Disease	RNA viruses	
	Family	Causal agent
Porcine encephalomyelitis	Picornaviridae	Enterovirus
Foot-and-mouth disease	Picornaviridae	Rhinovirus
Bluetongue	Reoviridae	Orbivirus
Akabane disease	Bunyaviridae	Akabane virus

intrinsic muscles of the larynx, causing a granulomatous myositis. It has not been determined whether the infection is spread hematogenously or by direct penetration of fungi coughed up from the lung.

Viral Myositides

Relatively few of these are recognized in veterinary medicine. Spontaneous ones are listed in Table 9-7. Gross lesions may or may not be visible, and, if present, are small, poorly defined, pale foci or streaks. Muscle lesions induced by viruses are either infarcts secondary to a vasculitis, as seen in bluetongue in sheep, or multifocal necrosis, presumably because of a direct effect of the virus on the myofibers. The latter type of lesion is seen in infections by different enteroviruses (porcine encephalomyelitis, coxsackievirus, and poliovirus) and foot-and-mouth disease virus, a picornavirus.

Porcine encephalomyelitis

Porcine encephalomyelitis is due to a coronavirus of the *Enterovirus* genus. Besides the destruction of the neurons, which results in paralysis, the virus may also cause multifocal necrosis of myofibers, accompanied by a focal interstitial and perivascular infiltrate of lymphocytes, macrophages, and a few neutrophils.

Foot-and-mouth disease

The major lesions are vesicles in the skin and mucous membranes. Besides these, the heart and skeletal muscles may have yellow streaks and gray foci, which microscopically are areas of segmental myofiber necrosis accompanied by an intense lymphocytic and neutrophilic infiltration.

Akabane virus of the family Bunyaviridae can produce a nonpurulent myositis in the bovine fetus.

Bluetongue

Bluetongue, caused by a virus of the family Reoviridae, is a noncontagious, insect-borne viral disease that causes vasculitis in a wide array of tissues, particularly the oral mucosa. Gross lesions in muscles are foci of necrosis (infarctions) and hemorrhage. Depending on the age of the lesions, necrosis, calcification, or regeneration may be present. Because of the size of the infarcts, regeneration is usually by muscle giant cells and fibrosis.

Polymyositis (Idiopathic Myositis)

While the word ''polymyositis'' etymologically simply means inflammation involving more than one muscle, the term is often reserved for those inflammatory myopathies (myositides) for which the pathogenesis is unknown or has not yet been fully elucidated. It is likely that an immune-mediated mechanism is involved.

Canine polymyositis

This does not include masticatory muscle myositis, which is described below. Canine polymyositis is a recognized but uncommon clinical entity in the dog. Dogs have fever, muscle pain, and weakness, which is more severe in the hind limbs. As the inflammatory response frequently consists of microscopic foci of lymphocytes, plasma cells, and, sometimes, eosinophils with few or no neutrophils, an immunologic cause is suspected. The inflammatory foci involve only a portion of the fasciculus (Fig. 9-18) in which, depending on the age of the lesions, myofibers are necrotic or regenerating. A muscle biopsy is useful in diagnosis, but a single biopsy may be inadequate to detect the lesions, which are focal and scattered. The lesions are also similar to those caused by *Toxoplasma gondii,* and the presence of this protozoan must be ruled out before canine polymyositis is diagnosed.

Canine bilateral extraocular polymyositis

Carpenter and co-workers described a distinctive disease in two golden retrievers as canine bilateral extraocular polymyositis, characterized clinically by acute bilateral ex-

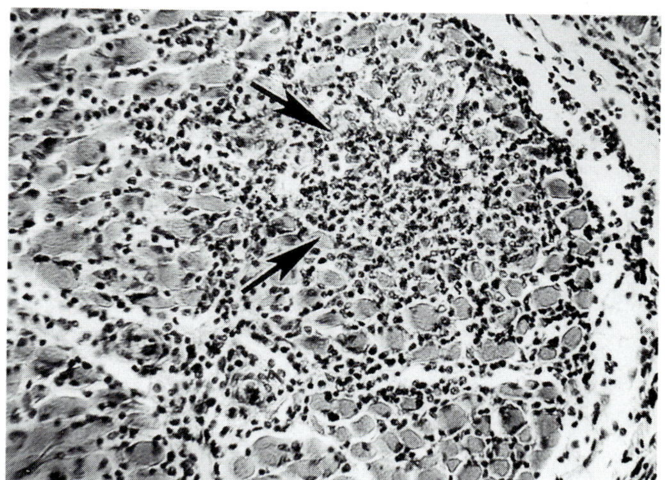

Fig. 9-18 Muscle; dog. Polymyositis. Note that this affects only a portion of the fasciculus and is characterized by a lymphocytic infiltrate *(arrows)* and loss of myofibers by necrosis. H & E stain. ×200. *Courtesy Dr. W.J. Hadlow.*

ophthalmos. All extraocular muscles—except the retractor bulbi, which was unaffected—were swollen and pale. Microscopically, there was a nonpurulent myositis with multifocal myofiber necrosis. The cellular infiltrate consisted of lymphocytes, histiocytes, plasma cells, and a few neutrophils. Localization in these specific muscles and the types of inflammatory infiltrate strongly suggest an immune-mediated myositis.

Bovine and ovine eosinophilic myositis

On the basis of the definition of "polymyositis," the eosinophilic myositis of cattle, sheep, and, sometimes, pigs should be included under this term. The major inflammatory cell is the eosinophil, and this type of inflammatory response suggests an immune-mediated inflammation. The etiology is unknown. Lesions are relatively rare, occur in animals of all ages, and are usually detected at slaughter. The disease is important in meat inspection, as the green discoloration of the muscles renders them esthetically unacceptable. There is mounting evidence that degeneration of *Sarcocystis* spp. is the cause, but this has not been proved. The gross lesions consist of well-demarcated, green discolored areas and streaks that can be small, a few millimeters wide, or in patches up to 7 cm wide. Lesions may be in muscles anywhere, but those of the back and thighs are often affected. Microscopically, lesions are infiltrations of masses of eosinophils. These are responsible for the green color. In the early stages, most of the eosinophils lie between the fasciculi, with small numbers around the myofibers. Muscle fibers may degenerate and disappear, and the space in the fasciculus is filled with eosinophils (Fig. 9-19). In older lesions, there is endomysial fibrosis, myofiber atrophy, little regeneration, and a cellular infiltrate consisting of lymphocytes, plasma cells, macrophages, and few eosinophils. Occasionally, a portion of a muscle containing sarcocysts will become necrotic and evoke a granulomatous response, and the necrotic muscle is enclosed in a palisade of macrophages surrounded by eosinophils. Later, a collagenous capsule will form.

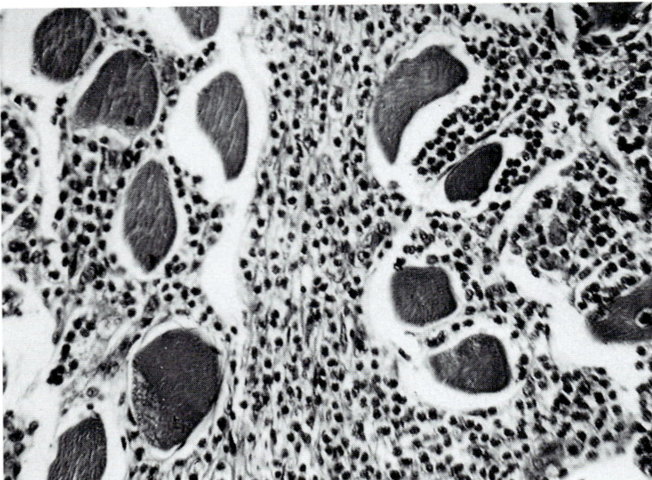

Fig. 9-19 Muscle; cow. Eosinophilic myositis. Atrophic muscle fibers are separated by an exudate consisting chiefly of eosinophils. H & E stain. ×200. *Courtesy Dr. W.J. Hadlow.*

Immune-mediated Myositides

Two types of myositis have been shown to be immunologically mediated—masticatory muscle myositis and dermatomyositis, both in dogs.

Masticatory muscle myositis (MMM)

Two forms of this disease are recognized clinically: an acute stage known as **eosinophilic myositis** and a chronic stage, **atrophic myositis.** It is unclear whether they are two separate diseases or merely different stages of the same entity. Clinically, the acute disease is characterized by extremely swollen, hard, painful masticatory muscles, while, in the chronic disease, there is marked atrophy of the same

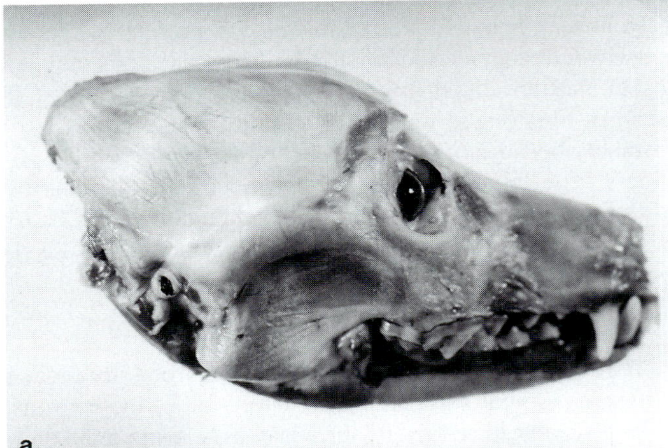

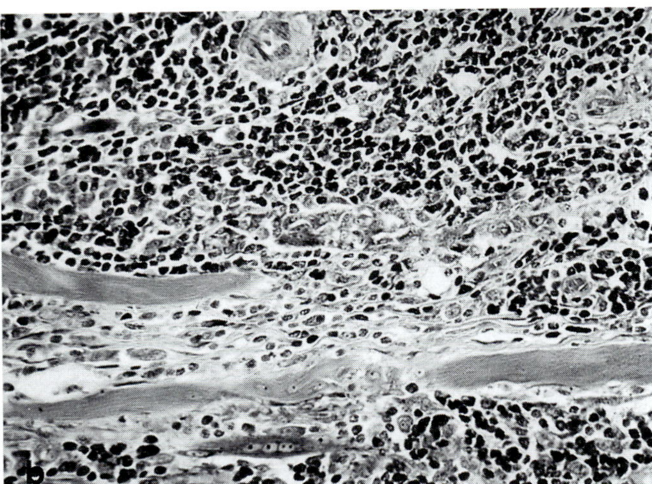

Fig. 9-20 Muscle; dog. Masticatory muscle myositis. **A**, Muscle, temporalis, chronic stage, with marked atrophy. **B**, Acute stage. An extensive infiltrate of chiefly lymphocytes lies between myofibers. H & E stain. ×200. *Courtesy Dr. W.J. Hadlow.*

muscles (Fig. 9-20, *A*). However, atrophy can occur without a prior acute attack.

Lesions. Acute cases are rarely autopsied. The lesions are bilateral but not necessarily symmetric. Initially, affected muscles are enlarged and edematous, and, later, they become dark red and doughy to firm and may contain reddish-brown streaks and yellowish areas.

The microscopic lesions vary with the stage of the disease. In early acute lesions, the infiltrate is chiefly eosinophils with some lymphocytes, plasma cells, and monocytes (Fig. 9-20, *B*). After several attacks of the disease, plasma cells predominate. Myofibers become necrotic, atrophy, and attempt to regenerate. In the chronic stage, the major changes are atrophy of the myofibers with shrunken fasciculi and an apparent increase in endomysium, probably due to condensation of the existing stroma rather than a proliferation. Cellular infiltrates, chiefly plasma cells and lymphocytes, are focal rather than diffuse.

Pathogenesis. The canine temporalis, masseter, and pterygoideus (lateralis and medialis) are composed of type I fibers and a variant of type IIC fibers, now designated type IIM. Thus, the myofibers that form these muscles are different from those of other muscles of the body. In MMM autoantibodies are developed against type IIM fibers, which contain different myosin light and heavy chains to those in the limb muscles (Fig. 9-21). This difference is postulated to be the basis for the immune-mediated inflammation that selectively attacks the masticatory muscles. Sensitization of the immune system to the myosin of the type IIM fibers may be due to previous bacterial infections. Myosin shares antigenic determinants with some bacteria, and, thus, antibodies produced against these bacteria could also be directed against the type IIM fibers of the masticatory muscles (see Fig. 9-21).

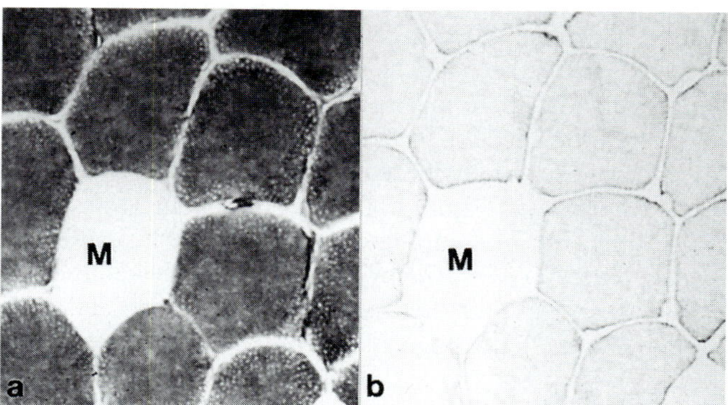

Fig. 9-21 Muscle, temporalis, normal; dog. **A**, Type I myofibers are light, and the type II are dark. Myofibrillar ATPase (pH = 9.8) stain. **B**, The section was incubated with staphylococcal protein A–peroxidase conjugates (SPA-HRPO) following incubation with serum, diluted 1:50, from a dog with masticatory muscle myositis (MMM). The type I fibers are unstained, whereas the type II fibers are positively stained, indicating their involvement in MMM. *Courtesy Dr. G.D. Shelton.*

Canine Dermatomyositis

This familial disease has been reported in collies and Shetland sheepdogs. The muscle lesions are similar to those of polymyositis, described above. In addition, there may be degeneration of blood vessels and, as a result, microinfarcts in muscles. Usually, muscle involvement is generalized, but the temporalis can be affected the most severely.

Parasitic Myositides

Parasitic infections of the skeletal muscles of domestic animals are not common (Box 9-1). The incidence is high in fish. Most diseases are of little economic importance, with the exception of *Trichinella spiralis* in swine.

Helminthic myositides

Trichinosis. This disease is of considerable public health importance in many parts of the world where meat inspection is poor. There are several *Trichinella* species but *T. spiralis,* which parasitizes dogs, cats, pigs, and human be-

Box 9-1 PARASITIC MUSCLE DISEASES

- **I. Helminthic agents**
  - A. Nematodes
    - 1. *Trichinella* spp. larvae: carnivores, omnivores
      - a. *T. spiralis:* north temperate
      - b. *T. pseudospiralis:* temperate, noncoiling
      - c. *T. nativa:* arctic
      - d. *T. nelsoni:* tropical
    - 2. *Ancylostoma* spp. larvae: paratenic hosts
    - 3. *Dirofilaria immitis:* dogs
      - a. Ischemic myopathy
    - 4. *Ascarid larvae:* intermediate and paratenic hosts
  - B. Trematode larvae
    - 1. *Alaria alata:* swine
  - C. Cestode larvae
    - 1. Cysticercosis, coenurosis, hydatid disease
      - a. *Taeniarhynchus saginatus:* cattle (cysticercosis)
      - b. *Taenia solium:* swine, human beings (cysticercosis)
      - c. *T. ovis:* sheep (cysticercosis)
      - d. *Multiceps serialis:* rabbits, primates, etc. (coenurosis)
      - e. *Echinococcus granulosus:* herbivores, human beings (hydatid)
  - D. Acanthocephalan larvae
  - E. Pentastomid larvae
- **II. Protozoal agents**
  - A. *Toxoplasma gondii*
  - B. *Neosporum caninum*
  - C. *Coccocystis* sp.
  - D. *Trypanosoma cruzi*
- **III. Athropod agents**
  - A. Dipterous larvae causing myiasis
    - 1. *Hypoderma* spp.: cattle

ings in the warmer and hotter portions of the world, is the most common. Bears, mice, and raccoons may also be infected. The adult worm inhabits the mucosa of the small intestine and produces larvae that enter the bloodstream and are carried to muscles, where they enter the myofibers. Here, protected from the host's immune system, the larvae grow and form coils that distend the myofibers. They are not normally seen grossly, but dead calcified parasites may be visible as 1 × 0.5-mm oval nodules in rows parallel with the myofibers of a muscle, such as in the diaphragm. There is a predilection for active muscles, such as the tongue, masseter, diaphragm, intercostal and laryngeal, and those of the eye, although the mechanism for this is unknown. Larvae migrating in the muscles and penetrating the myofibers cause a focal myositis characterized by the presence of neutrophils, lymphocytes, and eosinophils. Once the larva is protected in the myofiber, inflammation subsides, although small accumulations of eosinophils and mononuclear cells may linger around some parasites (Fig. 9-22). Larvae may persist for many years or may die and be calcified. Once the infected meat, e.g., pork, is eaten, the larva is released from the cyst by the digestive juices and develops into an adult worm, which continues the cycle. Thus, an infected animal is host both to the adult in the intestine and the larvae in the muscle.

***Ancyclostoma caninum* larva migrans.** The larval forms of *A. caninum* migrate somatically, and, on entering the muscles of paratenic hosts, development is arrested. The larvae cause inflammation and myonecrosis. As they continue to migrate, they leave a trail of segmentally necrotic myofibers and inflammation.

Visceral larva migrans. This has been defined as "the invasion of, and migration through, any of the tissues of the animal body by nematode larvae." *Toxocara canis* larvae migrate through numerous tissues of the dog. Some larvae

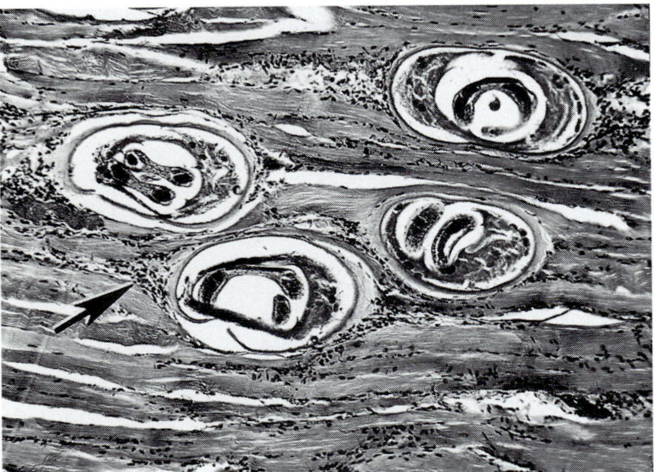

Fig. 9-22 Diaphragm; rat. Trichinosis. Larvae are present within the myofibers. Note the localized mononuclear cell infiltrate *(arrow)*. H & E stain. ×100. *Courtesy Dr. W.J. Hadlow.*

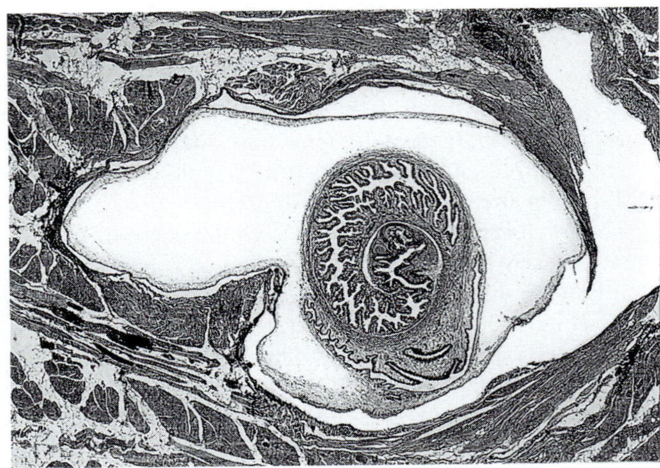

Fig. 9-23 Tongue; pig. Cysticercus—presumably, *C. cellulosae* in the tongue muscles. H & E stain. ×50. *Courtesy Dr. W.J. Hadlow.*

are arrested, and granulomas form around them. These have been found in a wide array of tissues, including kidney, liver, lung, myocardium, and skeletal muscle. The lesions in muscle is a focal granulomatous myositis, with the larvae and granulomas lying between myofibers.

Dirofilaria immitis. In dogs, larvae of this nematode may be present in the external and internal iliac arteries and their branches. Thromboemboli from debris and parasites may cause multiple infarcts in the muscles of the hind limbs (see Ischemia).

Cysticercosis. A cysticercus is a larva with a solid caudal portion and a bladderlike proximal portion. It is the intermediate stage in the life cycle of several tapeworms. *Taenia solium* and *T. saginata,* both tapeworms of human beings, have a cysticercus stage in the pig *(Cysticercus cellulosae)* and cattle *(C. bovis)*, respectively. These cysticerci preferentially lodge in the heart, masseter, and tongue, where they appear as small white or gray cysts. Histologically, there is displacement of myofibers by the cyst but little myositis; there may be a few lymphocytes, macrophages, and eosinophils around the cyst, which lies in the interstitial tissue, not in the myofiber (Fig. 9-23). With time, the immunologic system of the host kills the cysticercus. *C. cellulosae* in pigs may become calcified. *C. ovis* in the heart and shoulder muscles of sheep and goats is the intermediate stage of *Taenia ovis,* a tapeworm of dogs.

Protozoal myositides

The protozoa recognized as causing muscle lesions include *Toxoplasma gondii, Neosporum canium,* over a dozen species of *Sarcocystis,* and several species of *Trypanosoma, Babesia bovis,* and *Hepatazoon.*

Toxoplasmosis. This disease is caused by *T. gondii,* which uses the cat as the definitive host. Oocysts are produced in

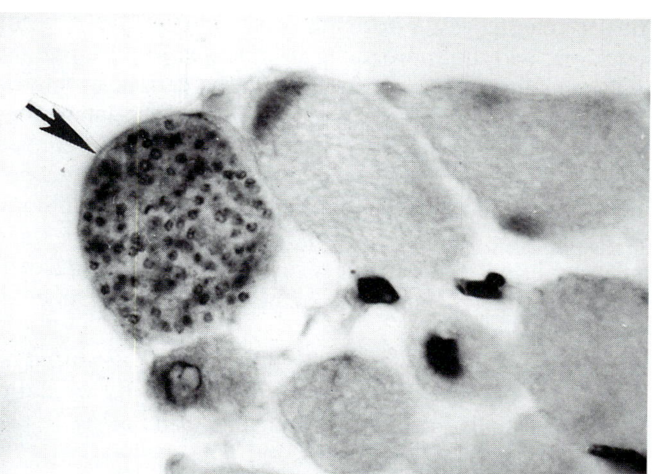

Fig. 9-24 Extraocular muscles; chinchilla. Toxoplasmosis. Cyst *(arrow)* containing bradyzoites. Note the absence of an inflammatory response. H & E stain. ×1125. *Courtesy Dr. W.J. Hadlow.*

the cat's intestinal mucosa by schizogany. These pass out with the feces and infect the intermediate host, which can be most birds and mammals. Tachyzoites are disseminated throughout the intermediate host's body, with the brain, myocardium, lungs, lymph nodes, intestine, and liver being commonly affected. Muscle is frequently not involved. Lesions from tachyzoites are classically necrotizing, and, thus, muscle lesions consist of a multifocal necrotizing myositis. These foci of necrosis, up to 10 μm in diameter, result in segmental necrosis of adjacent myofibers. Infiltration of lymphocytes and plasma cells and, depending on the stage, neutrophils takes place. Because tachyzoites are extremely small, they may not be seen in histologic sections stained with H & E, although they can be identified by immunoperoxidase techniques. However, cysts containing bradyzoites may develop later and, because of their relatively large size, are relatively easily detected histologically, although they do not evoke an inflammatory response (Fig. 9-24). Myofibers with segmental necrosis may regenerate.

Neosporosis. This disease, caused by the coccidian-type protozoan *Neosporum caninum* was confused for many years with *Toxoplasma.* There are some morphologic differences: the *N. caninum* cysts are thinner walled than those of *T. gondii* and are confined to the CNS. The two protozoa can be separated by immunoperoxidase staining techniques. *N. caninum* is pathogenic to dogs, cats, sheep, horses, and cattle, but the life cycle and source of infection are not known. The protozoa cause a necrotizing inflammation in organs, tissues, and muscles over the entire body. The myositis is more severe than that of toxoplasmosis. When meronts escape from the myofiber, they cause myofiber necrosis and an infiltrate containing numerous macrophages and plasma cells.

Sarcocystosis. The mature cysts (sarcocysts, previously called sarcosporidia) have been recognized in the muscles of herbivores and swine for approximately 100 years but are now known to be the intermediate stage of an intestinal coccidium. Because they do not elicit any inflammatory response, they were thought to be of no importance. Work in the last two decades has revealed that *Sarcocystis* produces a significant clinical disease in cattle, sheep, and swine, although muscle lesions may be minor. *Sarcocystis* is a two-host protozoan parasite that uses a carnivore (dog, cat, or human being) as the definitive host and birds, reptiles, small rodents, herbivores, or swine as intermediate hosts. When a herbivore ingests oocysts, sporozoites are released from the sporocysts in the gut. They invade tissues, and schizonts are formed in the endothelial cells of blood vessels of most organs.

In the pathogenesis of the disease, three phases can be recognized. In stage 1, 3 to 5 weeks after infection, schizonts are either free or in the endothelial cells of capillaries and small blood vessels. Perivascular and interstitial mononuclear cell infiltrates, chiefly composed of lymphocytes with a few macrophages, eosinophils, and plasma cells, form in skeletal muscle, lung, liver, and kidneys. During stage 2, muscle lesions develop. Their extent depends on the numbers and the pathogenicity of the organism. In many cases, muscle lesions are minimal or absent. Myositis may develop 1 to 2 months after infection and is secondary to merozoites, which develop from the schizonts, entering the myofibers where they cause a striking focal and segmental muscle necrosis with or without mineralization. The muscles of the tongue, esophagus, and diaphragm, and the intercostal, masseter, semitendinosus, and suprascapsular muscles are affected. However, lesions are most severe in the masseter and the diaphragm. Myofiber segmental necrosis is accompanied by a nonpurulent myositis with infiltrates of lymphocytes, plasma cells, and macrophages between and within the individual myofibers. The presence of inflammatory cells helps to differentiate these lesions from the segmental necrosis of metabolic and toxic myopathies.

In the third stage, which starts approximately 5 weeks after infection, the metrocytes in the cyst mature and develop into bradyzoites, which are infective for the definitive host. Clinically, the third stage is one of convalescence. Inflammatory foci, consisting chiefly of macrophages and plasma cells, are present. Later, these subside to a thin layer of lymphocytes and monocytes around sarcocysts. Finally, the histologic appearance of skeletal muscle is one in which there are numerous sarcocysts to which there is no inflammatory response (Fig. 9-25). Thus, muscle lesions are chiefly a myositis in stage 2 and early stage 3, due to the merozoites in the myofibers.

Trypanosomiasis. *Trypanosoma cruzi,* the etiologic agent of Chagas' disease in America, most frequently parasitize cells of the monocyte-macrophage system, but can cause

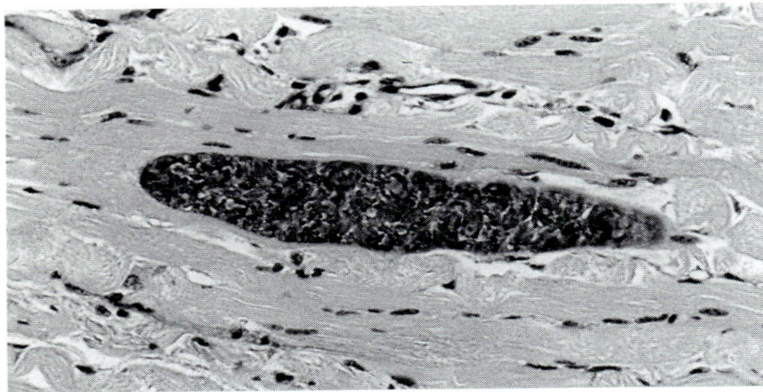

Fig. 9-25 Muscle, avian; gamecock. Sarcosporidiosis. Note the elongated cyst within the myofiber and the lack of inflammation. H & E stain.

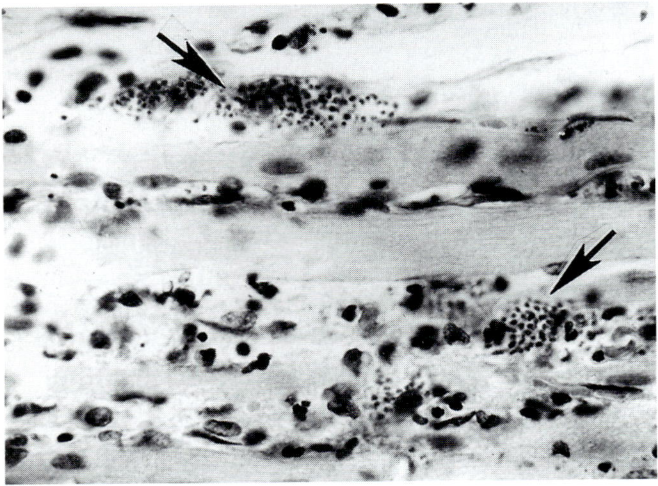

Fig. 9-26 Muscle; dog. Chagas' disease. Amastigotes of *Trypanosoma cruzi (arrows)* are present in myofibers. There is a slight mononuclear infiltrate. H & E stain. ×470. *Courtesy Dr. W.J. Hadlow.*

muscle lesions. Mononuclear infiltrates may occur in almost every body tissue, including skeletal muscle. Cats, dogs, and pigs may be infected or act as reservoirs. In dogs, *T. cruzi* causes a disseminated myocarditis and focal myositis (Fig. 9-26). The parasite penetrates the striated muscle and lies directly between the myofilaments. As amastigotes redifferentiate into trypomastigotes, myofibers may degenerate. Some amastigotes are surrounded by an infiltrate of lymphocytes and macrophages.

Babesiosis. *Babesia bovis* infection in cattle, which causes an acute hemolytic anemia, may cause muscle necrosis. A similar lesion occurs in malaria in human beings. Vascular occlusion of capillaries in the muscle is unlikely, and tumor necrosis factor A, a known myotoxin, is considered to be involved.

Hepatozoonosis. *Hepatozoon canis,* a protozoan, infects dogs, cats, jackals, and hyenas. Sporozoites are carried by the brown dog tick *(Rhipicephalus sanguineus).* When the tick is ingested by a dog, the sporocysts are freed in the intestine; and the sporozoites are released to penetrate the intestine, enter the bloodstream, and be carried to numerous organs, including skeletal muscles. In the latter, they develop into characteristic cysts, and a few of these contain schizonts and merozoites. In some cases, a well-developed pyogranulomatous myositis develops. The pyogranulomas consist of approximately equal parts of macrophages and neutrophils with occasional eosinophils, a few plasma cells and lymphocytes, and rows of neutrophils lying interstitially between myofibers.

Arthropods. The most significant lesions are produced by the larvae of *Hypoderma bovis,* the warble fly of cattle. Larvae normally burrow subcutaneously and along fascial planes but occasionally burrow into muscles.

TOXIC, ENDOCRINE, NUTRITIONAL, AND EXERTIONAL MYOPATHIES

Toxic Myopathies

These may be caused by ingestion of toxic plants, drugs (including feed additives), chemicals, and mycotoxins.

Toxic plants

Plants incriminated include *Cassia occidentalis* (coffee senna) in horses, cattle, sheep, and goats; *Karwinskia humboldtiana* (coyotillo) in sheep and goats; and, possibly, *Eupatorium rugosum* (white snakeroot) in cattle. Both coffee senna and coyotillo produce lesions in skeletal and cardiac muscles. Gross lesions are ill-defined, pale areas in muscle, but necrosis can be so extensive in coffee senna poisoning as to cause myoglobinuria. Histologically, there is segmental myofiber necrosis without mineralization (Fig. 9-27). Regeneration occurs if the animal lives long enough.

Gossypol is a toxic component in cotton seeds, and most,

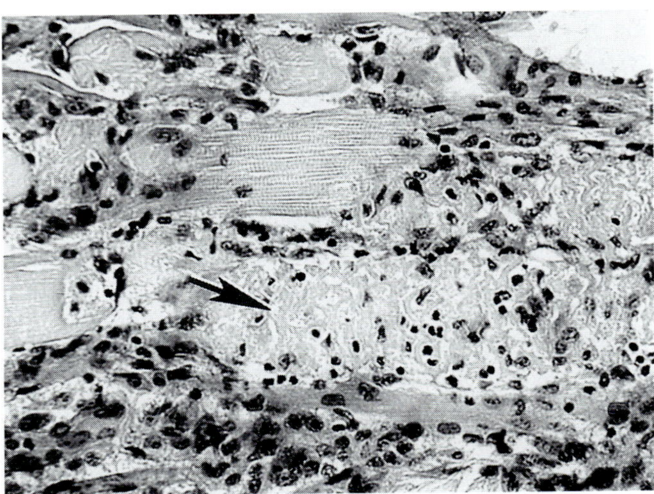

Fig. 9-27 Muscle; sheep. *Cassia occidentalis*–induced segmental necrosis *(arrow).* The necrotic segments are infiltrated by macrophages. H & E stain. ×200. *Courtesy Dr. W.J. Hadlow.*

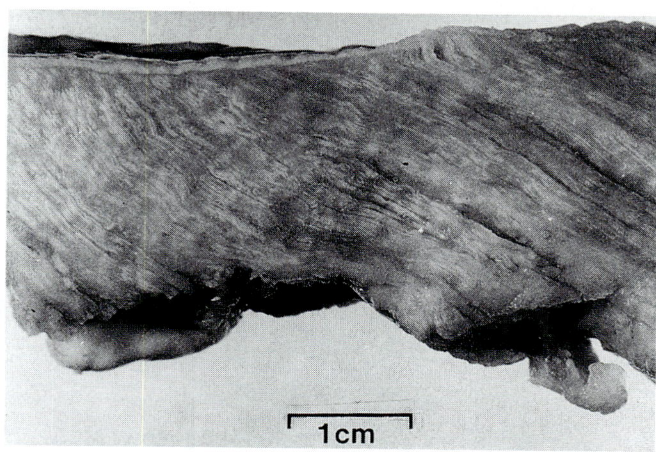

Fig. 9-28 Loin muscle; pig. 4 days after a dose of monensin. The pale streaks are necrotic myofibers. *Van Vleet JF, Amstutz HE, Weirich WE, et al. Am J Vet Res 1983; 44:1460-1468.*

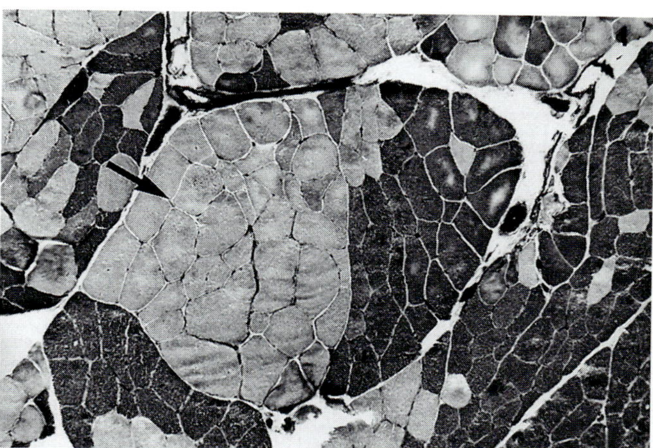

Fig. 9-29 Muscle, triceps brachii; dog. Myofiber type grouping, the result of denervation and subsequent reinnervation secondary to several years of treatment with steroids. Note the loss of the "checkerboard" appearance and the groupings of type I (light) and type II fibers (dark). Myofibrillar ATPase (pH = 9.8) stain.

but not all, of it is removed during manufacture of cotton seed meal. Both cardiac and skeletal muscle are affected. Swine are most susceptible, but dogs have been poisoned. Histologically, there is segmental necrosis.

Drugs and feed additives

A partial list of these includes adriamycin, cholinesterase inhibitors, corticosteroids, monensin, vincristine, and dimethyl sulfoxide (DMSO).

The feed additive *monensin,* an antibiotic and growth promoter in ruminants, has caused myofiber necrosis in equidae (horses, mules, donkeys, and zebras) and in cattle, sheep, dogs, and birds. Gross lesions are ill-defined, pale streaks in the myocardium and skeletal muscle (Fig. 9-28), with a preference for the muscles of the hind limbs. Lesions are segmental myofiber necrosis and, if the animal lives sufficiently long, regeneration.

Toxic substances can also reach the muscle in the form of an intramuscular injection. Local anesthetics such as lidocaine, and antibiotics such as chloramphenicol and oxytetracycline—may produce local muscle necrosis; oxytetracycline causes severe myonecrosis and hemorrhage. Because sarcolemmal tubes are disrupted and satellite cells killed, regeneration is chiefly by fibrosis (scarring), with some budding.

Chemicals

Intramuscular injections of iron dextran and copper acetate cause localized necrosis of muscle fibers.

Mycotoxins

Certain types of staggers in animals are caused by the ingestion of tremorgens, which are mycotoxins produced by species of the genera *Penicillium* and *Aspergillus.* Metabolites cause sustained tremors in domestic animals. Syndromes include paspalum staggers, rye grass staggers, and Bermuda grass staggers. Gross and microscopic lesions are restricted to skeletal muscles. These are minute foci of segmental necrosis. It is thought that these lesions are secondary to extreme, sustained muscular contractions, a form of exertional myopathy.

Endocrine Myopathy

Corticosteroid myopathy

Muscle weakness is a recognized clinical sign of natural and iatrogenic hyperadrenocorticism in human beings and animals. Weakness is followed by muscle wasting and atrophy of type II myofibers. Type II atrophy is not a specific change and is seen in response to inactivity and disuse of muscles. However type IIB (fast twitch, glycolytic) fibers are preferentially affected in hyperadrenocorticism. Prolonged administration of corticosteroids (months to years) has another effect on muscles. A peripheral neuropathy may develop and result in denervation atrophy of many myofibers. However, reinnervation occurs, resulting in fiber-type grouping (Fig. 9-29) (see Denervation Atrophy).

Hypothyroidism

This causes a marked type II atrophy in dogs and, in one case, a reduction in the percentage of type II fibers. Type II fiber atrophy is present in inactivity and has little diagnostic value.

Nutritional Myopathy

This disease—also known as **nutritional myodegeneration, white muscle disease** (because of the grossly visible, calcified necrotic areas), and, incorrectly, **nutritional muscular dystrophy**—is one of the most economically important muscle diseases in animals. It affects chiefly sheep, cattle, and pigs; occasionally, foals, zoo ungulates, and ranch mink; and, rarely, carnivores and possibly adult horses. The disease is due to a deficiency of selenium, vitamin E, or both. However, frequently there is a precipitating factor, such as rapid growth, unaccustomed exercise, or a dietary factor (such as the presence of an unsaturated fatty acid, e.g., from rancid or oxidized fish liver oil). The precipitating factor is presumed to be the "straw that broke the camel's back," being sufficient to cause disease in what had been a borderline case of deficiency. The disease, found worldwide, occurs on selenium-deficient soils but is not confined to them.

Vitamin E and selenium are both involved with the protection of cellular membranes from free radicals, which cause peroxidation of membrane lipids. The mechanisms by which vitamin E and selenium do this are different. Selenium is an essential component of the enzyme glutathione peroxidase, an intracellular enzyme involved in neutralizing free radicals. As an antioxidant, vitamin E can act either extracellularly or intracellularly. It also scavenges free radicals. If these mechanisms are defective or inadequate, then the cell membranes become physiologically defective and allow the influx of calcium into the cytosol; this results in the accumulation of calcium in the mitochondria. Damaged mitochondria are then unable to supply the energy for the cell to maintain homeostasis; and, the result is cell death or, in the case of a multinucleated muscle cell, segmental necrosis. Myoglobin and muscle enzymes such creatinine kinase leak into the plasma. The concentration of the latter in the serum is used to monitor the extent of myofiber necrosis.

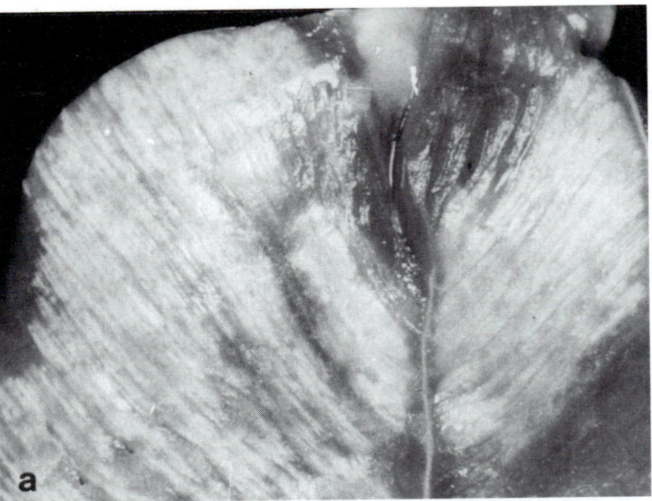

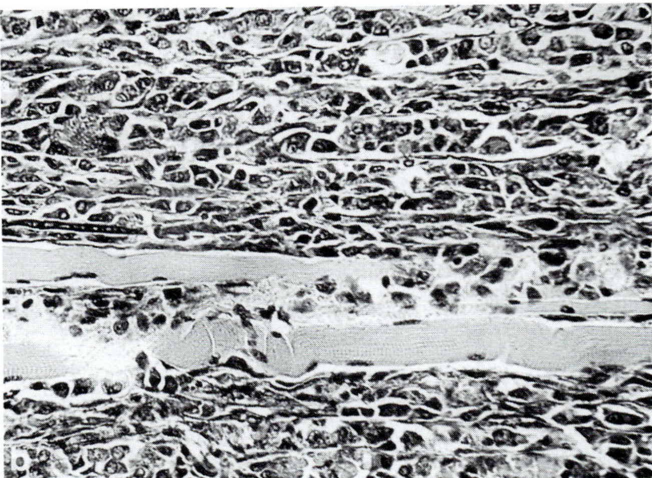

Fig. 9-30 Leg muscles; lamb. **A**, Nutritional myopathy. The numerous gray and white streaks are areas of segmental necrosis and calcification. **B**, Muscle, nutritional myopathy; calf. Sarcolemmal tubes are intact and filled with myoblasts and macrophages—early regeneration. The calf, which died, had extensive lesions in heart and muscles. H & E stain. ×200. *Courtesy Dr. W.J. Hadlow.*

Gross lesions

Lesions are usually bilaterally symmetric and located in the harder-working muscles. Exactly which muscles are involved varies with the age of the animal. Thus, the tongue and neck muscles are affected in neonatal suckling lambs, but the thighs, back, neck, and respiratory muscles are affected in older lambs. In calves, the shoulder and thigh muscles (particularly the biceps femoris), intercostal, and diaphragm are affected. In pigs with vitamin E–selenium deficiency, the striking lesions in the liver (hepatosis dietetica) and heart (mulberry heart disease) are far more obvious grossly than the muscle lesions. Gross lesions in any animal may vary in severity. Early lesions appear as pale areas and streaks (Fig. 9-30, *A*). Early ones may be easily overlooked, particularly in normally pale muscles. However, once calcification takes place, lesions become opaque, white, and far more obvious.

Histologic lesions

The characteristic lesions are segmental necrosis (see Figs. 9-5 and 9-6) and, possibly, calcification and regeneration. Because regeneration is able to proceed in spite of the dietary deficiency, animals that live for days to weeks have all stages of both segmental necrosis and regeneration (multifocal, multiphasic). The success of regeneration depends on the integrity of the sarcolemmal tubes. In nutritional myopathy, these tubes are frequently intact in the early stages, so the muscles of animals treated with vitamin E–selenium regenerate quickly and effectively and may return to normal (Fig. 9-30, *B*). However, once necrosis continues and segmental necrosis becomes widespread, myofibers break under the stress of contraction, fracture the sarcolemmal tubes and this results in regeneration by budding and fibrosis. Thus, the characteristic histologic appearance of a late stage of an untreated case is a muscle with lesions at all stages: segmental necrosis, calcification, regeneration with intact sarcolemmal tubes, regeneration by budding, and diffuse fibrosis.

Diagnosis

The lesions of segmental myonecrosis are characteristic but not diagnostic of this disease. However, the clinical findings, e.g., of young, rapidly growing animals and some associated stress, all support the diagnosis. Confirmation requires the analysis of tissues for selenium and tocopherol levels (renal cortex and liver for selenium and liver for tocopherol). Because erythrocyte glutathione peroxidase activity is highly correlated with the blood selenium levels, activity of this enzyme in blood can be used to evaluate the selenium status of the animal. Analyses of both selenium and tocopherol concentrations are useful, because they identify those cases of segmental myonecrosis caused by something other than vitamin E–selenium deficiency.

Exertional Myopathies

These have been recognized in horses after unaccustomed exercise or inadequate training, in cattle running wild, sheep chased by dogs, in racing greyhounds and during the capture of wildlife (capture myopathy). A separate clinical entity, porcine stress syndrome (malignant hyperthermia), has been recognized in pigs.

Equine Rhabdomyolysis

Two clinical syndromes have been recognized in horses: an acute form—*azoturia* (paralytic myoglobinuria, Monday morning disease)—and a less severe form—*tying-up* (acute rhabdomyolysis, transient exertional rhabdomyolysis). The term ''equine rhabdomyolysis'' is used to cover all these conditions, now generally recognized as a single syndrome, although they may vary in clinical severity. The etiology is still unclear, although exercise is the precipitating factor. In horses, carbohydrate overloading has been blamed for over 50 years, but this is now questioned. In azoturia, the lumbar, gluteal, and femoral muscles become hard and swollen, and this is soon followed by myoglobinuria. At necropsy, the appearance of muscles depends on survival time. Initially, muscles are salmon pink (from rhabdomyolysis), but, after a few days, these muscles are dark, moist, swollen, and sometimes have pale streaks. In tying-up, the milder form, muscles are grossly normal. Histologically, both forms have segmental myofiber necrosis, which affects both type IIA and type IIB fibers, but the type IIB fibers are preferentially affected in the acute disease. In azoturia, either isolated type I fibers or foci of fibers (Fig. 9-31, *A*), which includes both type I and type II fibers, are affected. Inflammatory reaction and calcification are slight. The necrosis is usually multifocal and monophasic. However, susceptible horses may have mul-

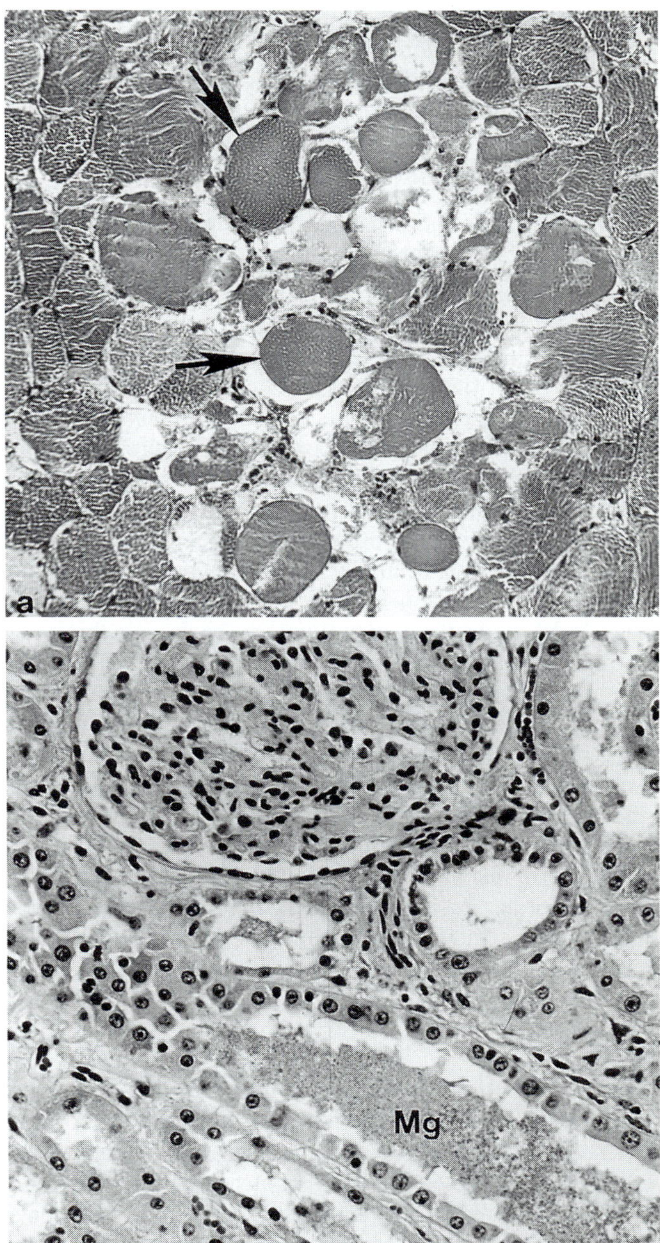

Fig. 9-31 Muscle cross section; horse. Equine rhabdomyolysis. **A**, A focus of hyalinized necrotic myofibers *(arrows)* are surrounded by viable myofibers. H & E stain. ×175. **B**, Kidney. Myoglobinuria. A myoglobin cast *(Mg)* is present in the lumen of a distal tubule. H & E stain. ×250. *A, Courtesy Dr. W.J. Hadlow.*

tiple attacks, days to weeks apart. In those cases, the lesions would be multiphasic. The myoglobinuria may be so severe in azoturia as to induce a myoglobin nephrosis (Fig. 9-31, *B*) and possibly renal failure. In both forms, regeneration takes place depending on the conditions described above in the section on Regeneration.

Porcine stress syndrome (malignant hyperthermia)

This disease has been seen in pigs, human beings, and dogs. It is believed to be a cellular defect, a deficiency of inositol 1,4,5-triphosphate phosphatase, which results in a high intracellular concentration of calcium ions. This activates myofibrillar ATPase, produces rapid intracellular glycolysis, and a consequent increase in body heat. The excess calcium in the myofiber causes hypercontraction, and the increased body heat denatures the proteins of the myofibers. Thus, the cell is metabolically dead, and fluid escapes into the intermyofiber spaces to cause edema. At necropsy, after stress, the muscles are pale, moist, and swollen; this condition is known as pale, soft, exudative pork (PSE). Muscles of the shoulder, back, and thigh are preferentially affected. Histologically, the changes are segmental hypercontraction and, if the pig lives long enough, monophasic, multifocal segmental necrosis. Both type I and type II fibers are affected, although the muscles preferentially affected, such as the longissimus and semitendinosus, are ''white'' muscles that consist mainly of type II fibers. The disease is inherited, and affected pigs are identified by response to halothane anesthesia as there are no gross or microscopic changes in the muscles of unstressed pigs. Under field conditions, the hyperthermia is initiated by stress such as handling, transportation, or slaughter.

TRAUMA

External trauma to muscle includes bruising (crushing with hemorrhage), laceration (tearing), surgical incisions, burns, gunshot and arrow wounds, and certain injections. Some of these may result in complete or partial rupture. The latter is common as the result of automobile accidents where the diaphragm is frequently ruptured secondary to a sudden increase in intraabdominal pressure. A partial rupture of a muscle results in a rent in the fascial sheath, through which the muscle can herniate during contraction. In racing greyhounds, spontaneous rupture of muscles such as the longissimus, quadriceps, biceps femoris, gracilis, triceps brachii, and gastrocnemius can occur during strenuous exercise. Tearing (**myorrhexis**) of muscle fibers occurs in the adductor muscles of cattle doing the ''splits'' on a slippery floor.

Healing of these traumatic wounds follows the principles laid down above in the section on Regeneration. As there is often extensive interruption of sarcolemmal sheaths, most of the healing will take place by budding and fibrosis (see Fig. 9-7), with resultant compromise in the physiologic efficiency of the muscle. Collagen is inelastic, and, thus, large scars will inevitably reduce the contractability of adjacent myofibers. Cleanly transected fibers will heal by scarring, and this will result in essentially two separate contractile units joined by a scar whose work efficiency will be less than that of the original single myofiber. If muscle trauma is accompanied by fractures of bones, and the animal moves the limb, this may result in further trauma by the sharp bone fragments. Similarly, a fractured wing of the ilium can traumatize gluteal muscles.

Thus, in muscle trauma, damage is due to direct transection of myofibers, compression of myofibers with destruction of the sarcoplasm, and secondarily from hemorrhage. The latter may increase intramuscular pressure, resulting in ischemia and further necrosis (infarction).

NEOPLASIA

Theoretically, neoplasms arising in muscle can form from any of the components of muscle: myofibers; mesenchymal tissue such as fibrous, myxomatous, or adipose tissue; blood vessels; or nerve sheaths. Actually, neoplasms of skeletal muscle—benign, malignant, or metastatic—are rare in domestic animals. The majority of benign muscle tumors, **rhabdomyomas** in the pig ox and sheep, have been cardiac; but laryngeal rhabdomyomas are recognized in the dog. Because of the granular eosinophilic cytoplasm and the large numbers of mitochondria seen by electron microscopy, these tumors were originally diagnosed as oncocytomas. Grossly, the tumors are unencapsulated and lobulated. Microscopically, they are composed of large granular cells that stain positively for myoglobin and desmin by immunoperoxidase techniques. Z-band material can be seen by electron microscopy.

Rhabdomyosarcomas are rare. Most cases have been in dogs. These tumors are usually highly malignant and metastasize either via the lymphatic or venous routes. Thus, metastases appear in lymph nodes, lungs, and spleen and also in heart and skeletal muscles. Grossly, they are pink masses with no encapsulation. The histologic appearance of rhabdomyosarcomas varies enormously. Some have cells in which the characteristic cross-striations are found easily, while others are composed of undifferentiated cells with no visible striations (Fig. 9-32). Many pathologists feel uncomfortable in diagnosing a rhabdomyosarcoma without seeing striations. These can be revealed most clearly in histologic sections with iron hematoxylin (Weigert's or Heidenhain's) or with Mallory's phosphotungstic acid–hematoxylin (PTAH) stains. However, searching for cross-striations in undifferentiated tumors is time consuming and not always fruitful. A rapid, reliable method of diagnosing muscle tissue is to demonstrate the presence of myoglobin using the immunoperoxidase method, as only cardiac and skeletal muscle contain myoglobin.

Muscles can also be locally invaded by carcinomas and sarcomas as they proliferate and increase in size. In dogs,

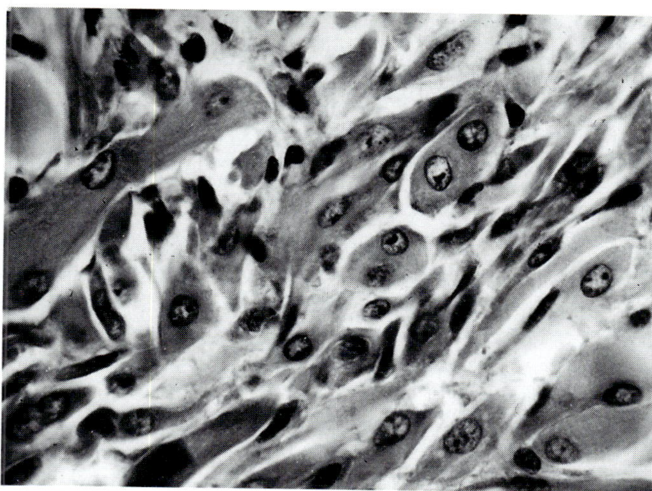

Fig. 9-32 Thigh muscles; mouse. Rhabdomyosarcoma. Multinucleated pleomorphic cells. Cross-striations are not evident. H & E stain. ×475. *Courtesy Dr. W.J. Hadlow.*

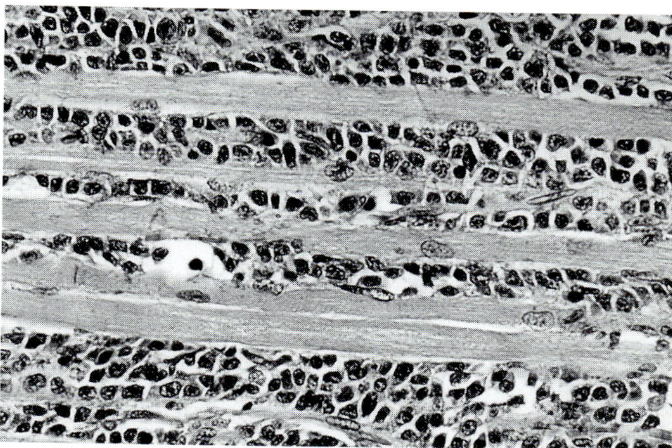

Fig. 9-33 Muscle, periorbital; monkey. Malignant lymphoma. Numerous lymphoid cells lie between the myofibers, which subsequently atrophy and disappear.

squamous cell carcinomas of the vulva may extend into the pelvic musculature. Bovine extraocular squamous cell carcinoma may infiltrate into the adjacent orbicularis oculi muscle. Canine mammary adenocarcinomas and mast cell tumors have occasionally involved the cutaneous muscle.

Infiltrative lipomas are tumors of mature adipocytes in dogs. They are usually deep in the subcutis or muscles. The tumor cells tend to infiltrate along fascial planes but also extend into muscles. Grossly, muscles are soft, and muscle fasciculi are separated by yellow fat. Histologically, the mass consists of well-differentiated adipose cells. The tumor is benign, but, because the margins are difficult to determine, it is difficult to excise and can recur.

Rarely, skeletal muscle is invaded by local mesenchymal tumors such as hemangiosarcomas, fibrosarcomas, and myxosarcomas that have arisen either in adjacent tissue or in the muscle's stroma. Tumors metastatic to muscle are rare, but malignant lymphoma (Fig. 9-33), hemangiosarcoma, pulmonary adenocarcinoma (Fig. 9-34), and pulmonary squamous cell carcinoma have occurred in the dog.

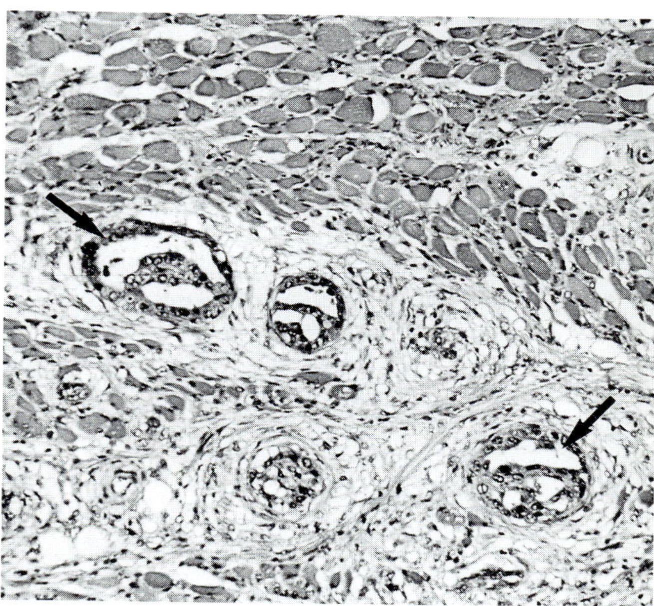

Fig. 9-34 Muscle, diaphragm; dog. Bronchiogenic carcinoma. The neoplasm had extended into the parietal pleura and diaphragm.

Suggested Readings

Adams RD. Diseases of muscle. 3rd ed. Hagerstown, Md: Harper & Row; 1975.

Armstrong RB, Saubert CW IV, Seeherman HJ, Taylor CR. Distribution of fiber types in locomotory muscles of dogs. Am J Anat 1982; 163:87-98.

Bradley R, Fell BF. Myopathies in animals. In: Walton J, ed. Disorders of Voluntary Muscle. 4th ed. Edinburgh: Churchill Livingstone, 1981; 824-872.

Burke RE, Levine DN, Zajac FE III, Tsairis P, Engle WK. Mammalian motor units: Physiological-histochemical correlations in three types in cat gastrocnemius. Science 1971; 174:709-712.

Carpenter JL, Schmidt GM, Moore FM, Albert DM, Abrams KL, Elner VM. Canine bilateral extraocular polymyositis, Vet Pathol 1989; 26:510-512.

Dubowitz V, Brooke MH. Muscle biopsy: A modern approach. London: Saunders, 1973.

Hadlow WJ. Myopathies in animals. In: Pearson CM, Mostofi FK, eds. The Striated Muscle. Baltimore: Williams & Wilkins, 1973; 3640.

Harriman DGF. Muscle. In: Adams JH, Corsellis JAN, Duchan LW, eds. Greenfield's Neuropathology. 4th ed. New York: Wiley, 1985; 1026.

Hulland JJ. Muscles and tendons. In: Jubb JVF, Kennedy PC, Palmer N, eds. Pathology of Domestic Animals. 4th ed. Orlando, Fla.: Academic Press, 1993; 183-265.

Kakulas BA. Experimental myopathies. In: Walton J, ed. Disorders of Voluntary Muscle. 4th ed. Edinburgh: Churchill Livingstone, 1981; 389-416.

Orvis JS, Cardinet GH III. Canine muscle fiber types and susceptibility of masticatory muscles to myositis. Muscle Nerve 1981; 4:354-359.

Peter JB, Barnard RJ, Edgerton VR, et al. Metabolic profiles of three fiber types of skeletal muscle in guinea pigs and rabbits. Biochemistry 1972; 11:2627-2634.

Shelton GD, Cardinet GH III. Pathophysiologic basis of canine muscle disorders. J Vet Intern Med 1987; 1(1):36-44.

Valentine BA, Winand NJ, Pradhan D, Moise NS, de Lahunta A, Kornegay JN, Cooper BJ: Canine X-linked muscular dystrophy as an animal model of Duchenne muscular dystrophy: A review. Am J Med Genet 1992; 42:352-356.

Van Vleet JF, Amstutz HE, Weirich WE, et al. Acute monensin toxicosis in swine: Effect of graded doses of monensin and protection of swine by pretreatment with selenium–vitamin E. Am J Vet Res 1983; 44:1460-1468.

Van Vleet JF, Ferrans VJ, Herman E. Cardiovascular and skeletal muscle system. In: Haschek-Hock WM, Rousseaux CG, eds. Handbook of Toxicologic Pathology. Orlando, Fla.: Academic Press, 1991; 539-624.

CHAPTER

10

Diseases of Bone and Joints

CECIL E. DOIGE
STEVEN E. WEISBRODE

DISEASES OF BONE

Normal Structure and Function

Bone at the cellular level

Various cell types, including endothelial cells, adipocytes, hemopoietic cells, chondrocytes, osteoblasts, osteocytes, and osteoclasts, can be seen in a section of bone viewed with the light microscope. The last three cell types are considered here.

Osteoblasts are mesenchymal cells that arise from bone marrow stromal stem cells under the influence of appropriate paracrine and endocrine stimuli. Osteoblasts line bone-forming surfaces and are responsible for production of bone matrix (osteoid) and initiation of matrix mineralization. When active, osteoblasts are plump, cuboidal cells (Fig. 10-1) with abundant basophilic cytoplasm (rich in rough endoplasmic reticulum). Inactive osteoblasts are flattened with little cytoplasm due to the reduction in cytoplasmic organelles. Osteoblasts send cytoplasmic processes out into the matrix, and some of these make contact with the cytoplasmic extensions of osteocytes. This interconnecting network of osteoblasts and osteocytes forms a functional membrane that separates the extracellular fluid bathing bone surfaces from the general extracellular fluid and regulates the flow of calcium and phosphate ions to and from the bone fluid compartment (Fig. 10-2). It is postulated that calcium diffuses into the bone fluid compartment by moving between osteoblasts. An intracellular pump (within osteoblasts) moves calcium outward across the cell membrane to the general extracellular fluid compartment. Osteoblast membranes are rich in alkaline phosphatase, and an indirect estimate of osteoblast synthetic activity can be determined by measuring the activities in blood of the bone isoenzyme of alkaline phosphatase. The function of this enzyme in the osteoblast is uncertain, but it may play a role in mineralization and in pumping calcium across cellular membranes. Osteoblasts have recep-

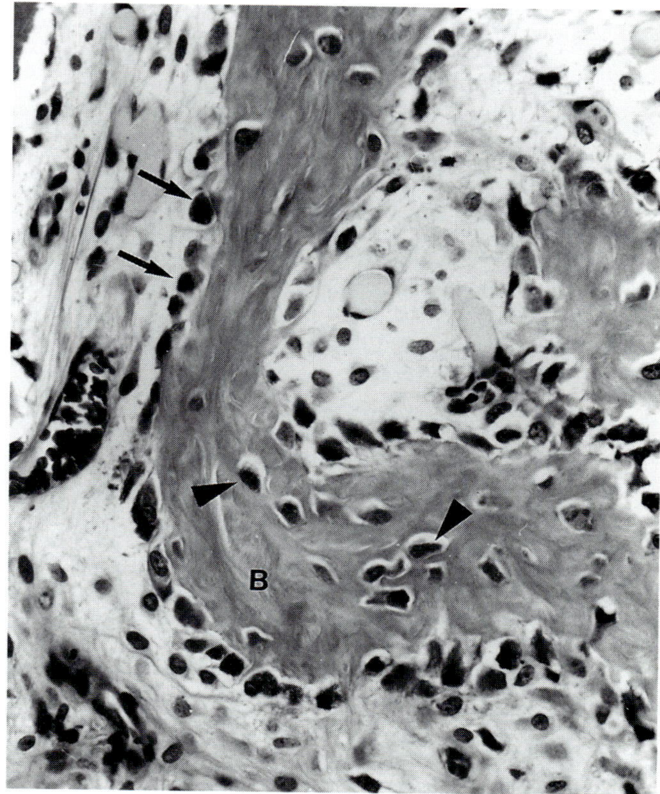

Fig. 10-1 Bone, reactive (repair) woven bone (*B*) at a fracture site. Bone surfaces are lined by plump osteoblasts *(arrows)*; large, irregularly arranged osteocytes *(arrowheads)* are located in lacunae and are surrounded by osteoid with coarsely bundled collagen. Hematoxylin-eosin (H & E) stain.

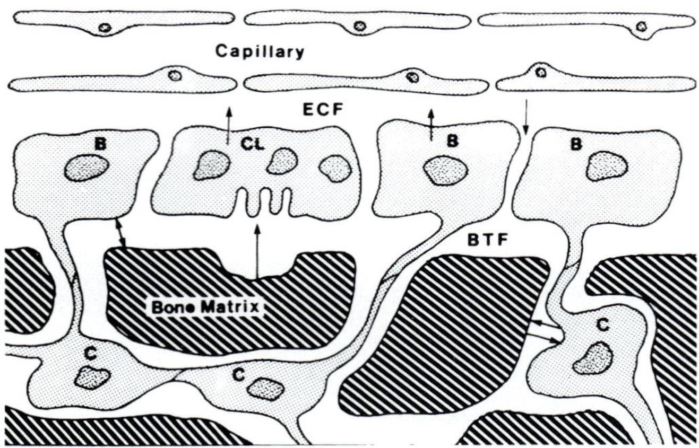

Fig. 10-2 Diagram showing hypothesized calcium movement *(arrows)* and relationships of osteoblasts (*B*), osteocytes (*C*), and osteoclasts *(CL)* to blood vessels, extracellular fluid *(ECF)*, and bone tissue fluid *(BTF)* compartment. *Redrawn from Matthews JL, Vander Wiel C, Talmage RV. Bone lining cells and the bone fluid compartment: An ultrastructural study. Adv Exp Med Biol 1978; 103:456.*

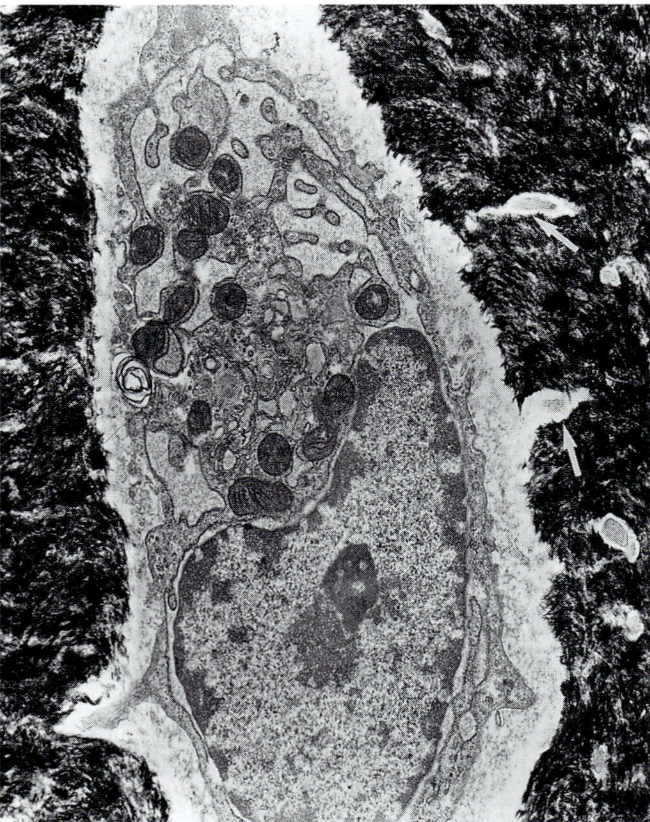

Fig. 10-3 Bone, tibia; rodent. Transmission electron micrograph. A recently embedded osteocyte has residual synthetic organelles used during its osteoblastic period. Cell processes are extending into the mineralized matrix (black) through tunnels called ''canaliculi'' *(arrows)*. Uranyl acetate and lead citrate stain.

tors for parathyroid hormone (PTH), and activation of these receptors increases the activity of the osteoblast calcium pump and initiates bone resorption by the osteoclast (see below).

Osteocytes are osteoblasts that have been surrounded by mineralized bone matrix. They occupy small spaces in the bone called lacunae (singular: lacuna) and make contact with osteoblasts and other osteocytes by means of long cytoplasmic processes that pass through thin tunnels (canaliculi; singular: canaliculus) in mineralized bone matrix (Fig. 10-3). Osteocytes likely play a role in regulating the composition of the fluid in the bone fluid compartment and might be capable of removing bone mineral ions from perilacunar bone. Because of the large surface area of perilacunar and canalicular bone available for rapid ion exchange, it is possible that significant amounts of calcium could be made available to the bone fluid compartment and, eventually, the extracellular fluid compartment without causing structural changes within the bone. Under conditions of extreme stress to calcium homeostasis, osteocytes might have the ability to resorb perilacunar mineral and matrix, causing enlargement of the lacuna (osteocytic osteolysis). This apparently is rare and likely does not contribute significantly to development of bone lesions. Osteocytes also retain a limited capacity for bone formation. The role of osteocytes in maintenance of mature bone is uncertain because dead cortical bone can persist for long periods without losing structural integrity.

Osteoclasts are multinucleated cells responsible for bone resorption (Fig. 10-4). They are derived from hematopoi-

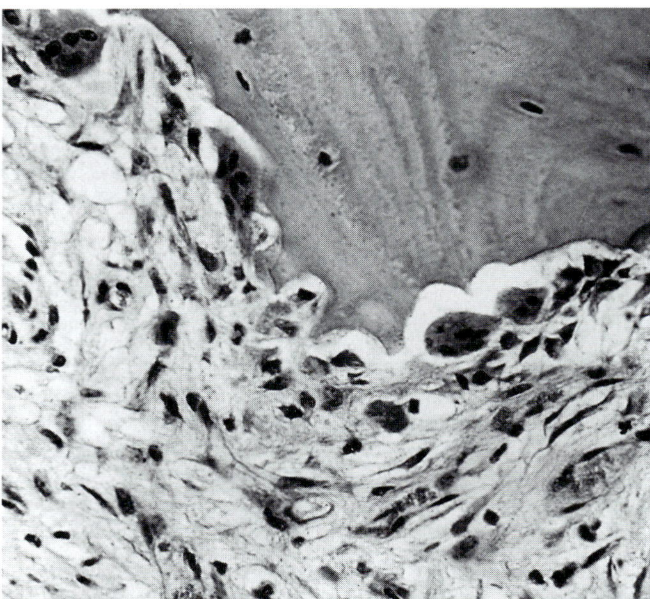

Fig. 10-4 Bone. Necrotic bone with pyknotic osteocytes is undergoing osteoclastic resorption. Numerous Howship's lacunae are present, an indication that bone has been removed.

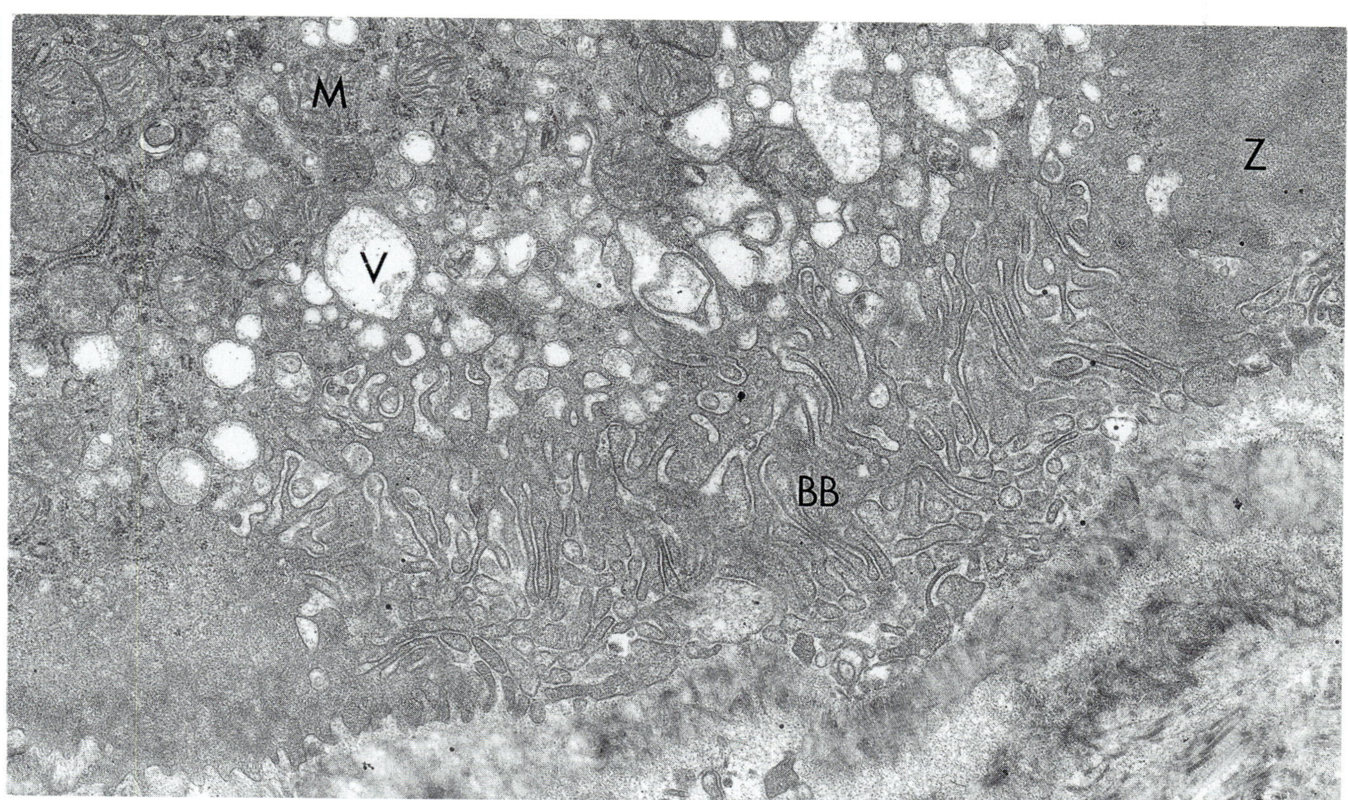

Fig. 10-5 Bone, tibia; rodent. Transmission electron micrograph. Brush border *(BB)* of an osteoclast. A dense zone (*Z*) adjacent to the brush border binds the cell to the bone's surface and prevents diffusion of the digestive process to other surfaces. Mitochondria (*M*) and numerous vesicles (*V*) containing lysosomal enzymes are present. Uranyl acetate and lead citrate stain.

etic stem cells, likely of the granulocyte-monocyte series. They have abundant eosinophilic cytoplasm with a specialized brush border adjacent to the bone surface undergoing resorption (Fig. 10-5). Osteoclasts resorb bone in two stages. Initially, the mineral is dissolved by secretion of hydrogen ions through a proton pump on the brush border. These hydrogen ions are derived from carbonic acid produced within the osteoclast from water and carbon dioxide by the enzyme carbonic anhydrase. Next, the collagen is cleaved into polypeptide fragments by proteinases released from the numerous lysosomes in the osteoclast and secreted through the brush border. The concavity in the bone created by the resorption is called a Howship's lacuna.

PTH is a potent systemic stimulator of osteoclastic bone resorption. In response to PTH, osteoclasts increase in number, and their brush borders become more abundant. Most investigations, however, have found that osteoclasts do not have receptors for PTH and that osteoblasts, which do have receptors for PTH, control the initiation of resorption. In response to PTH, osteoblasts contract and leave exposed bone surfaces on which the osteoclasts can attach. The activated osteoblasts secrete or activate collagenases that remove a thin layer of normal unmineralized fibers so the osteoclast can attach to a fully mineralized surface. Osteoclasts are unable to resorb unmineralized matrix. In addition, osteoblasts release cytokines that attract and stimulate inactive osteoclasts in the local environment. Calcitonin is a systemic inhibitor of osteoclasts. Osteoclasts have receptors for calcitonin and respond by involuting their brush border and detaching from the bone surface. The stimuli for osteoclastic bone resorption in local disease processes are under the influence of cytokines and prostaglandins released not only from inflammatory cells such as the macrophage but, likely also, from a great variety of hyperplastic, neoplastic, and degenerated tissues.

Bone at the matrix and mineral level

Bone matrix consists of type I collagen and "ground substance." Type I collagen polymers are secreted by osteoblasts and assembled into fibrils that are embedded in the ground substance prior to mineralization. Type I collagen molecule is composed of three intertwined amino acid chains. Unique to these chains is the hydroxylated form of the amino acid proline (hydroxyproline). Type I collagen molecules have extensive cross-linkages among the amino acid chains within the molecule and between adjacent molecules. Within the collagen fibers, collagen molecules are deposited in rows with a gap between each molecule and with the rows staggered so that the molecules overlap by one fourth of their length. This specific packing of the collagen molecules and the cross-linkages contribute to the strength and insolubility of the fibrous component of the bone matrix. Other than in rapidly deposited reactive bone (woven bone, discussed below), primary trabeculae, and bone of early fetal development, collagen fibers are arranged in lamellae (singular: lamella). The orientation of the collagen fibers in each lamella is slightly different, giving a herringbone-like pattern. In Haversian (osteonal) bone, lamellae are arranged in concentric layers. In trabecular bone, the lamellae usually are arranged parallel with the surface. The collagen content of bone and its lamellar arrangement give bone its strength. The mineral content gives bone its hardness. The ground substance of bone consists of noncollagenous proteins, proteoglycans, and lipids. Many of the noncollagenous proteins are cytokines capable of influencing bone cell activity. These cytokines, such as **transforming growth factor beta,** may play pivotal roles in controlling the extent of bone formation and resorption in normal remodeling and in disease. Also, among the noncollagenous proteins are enzymes that may function in degradation of collagen (e.g., collagenases) in bone resorption and may destroy inhibitors of mineralization (e.g., pyrophosphatases). Other noncollagenous proteins in the matrix can function as glues and help bind cells to cells, cells to matrix, and mineral to matrix. Examples are osteonectin and osteocalcin. The role of proteoglycans in bone matrix is uncertain. They might play a role in inhibiting mineralization and promoting cell matrix interactions. Lipids can assist in binding calcium to cell membranes and in promoting calcification.

Bone mineral in fully mineralized bone is approximately 65% of the bone and consists, in part, of calcium, phosphorus, carbonate, magnesium, sodium, manganese, zinc, copper, and fluoride. The production of osteoid (organic matrix) by osteoblasts is followed by a period of maturation, after which mineral is deposited at the expense of water. The process of mineralization is gradual and might not be complete for several months, at least, in reactive bone. Mineralization is initiated within cytoplasmic blebs of osteoblasts in the osteoid (Fig. 10-6), and these vesicles have phospholipids and enzymes such as alkaline phosphatase and adenosine triphosphatase (ATPase) on their membranes. These enzymes can act to destroy inhibitors of mineralization, such as inorganic pyrophosphates, that are present in the osteoid and, along with the membrane phospholipids, concentrate calcium and phosphorus within the matrix vesicle. The mineral within the matrix vesicle initially is amorphous and, after reaching critical mass, becomes crystalline. The crystalline hydroxyapatite pierces the matrix vesicle and has access to the gaps between collagen molecules, described above. It is within these holes that the mineral crystals are first deposited within collagen. The process overflows the holes, and mineral crystals eventually are bound by noncollageneous proteins (e.g., osteonectin) to all surfaces of the collagenous fibers and even in the spaces between collagen fibers. Initiation of mineralization in lamellar bone might not require matrix vesicles. Glycoproteins such as sialoprotein and osteonectin can act as the nidus for the mineralization process.

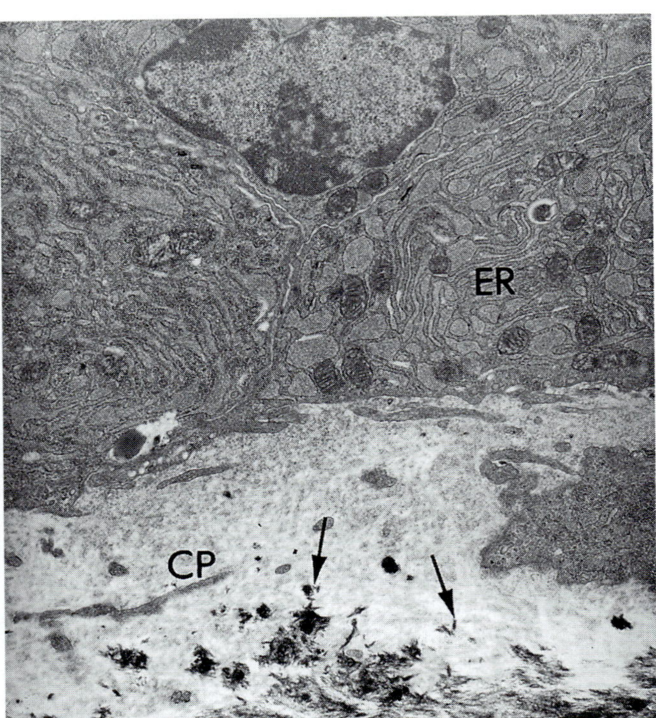

Fig. 10-6 Bone, tibia; rodent. Transmission electron micrograph. Osteoblasts with abundant endoplasmic reticulum *(ER)* are on an actively mineralizing surface. Cell processes *(CP)* of the osteoblasts extend into the osteoid. Mineralization (black spicules) is initiated within matrix vesicles *(arrows)* then grows onto the adjacent collagen. Uranyl acetate and lead citrate stain.

Bone as a tissue

The cellular, organic matrix, and mineral components of bone are organized at the tissue level into osteons or Haversian systems in the remodeled compact bone of the cortex and in subchondral bone of larger animals. In cortical bone, osteons are longitudinally orientated cylinders of concentric layers of lamellae that contain centrally located blood vessels. Haversian or compact bone is made up of numerous osteons that are cemented by interstitial lamallae and surrounded by circumferential lamellae (Fig. 10-7). The osteonal system provides channels for the vascular supply to thick bone of the cortex and also acts as tightly bound cables, giving the cortical bone strength yet limited flexibility. In contrast to the dense compact bone of the

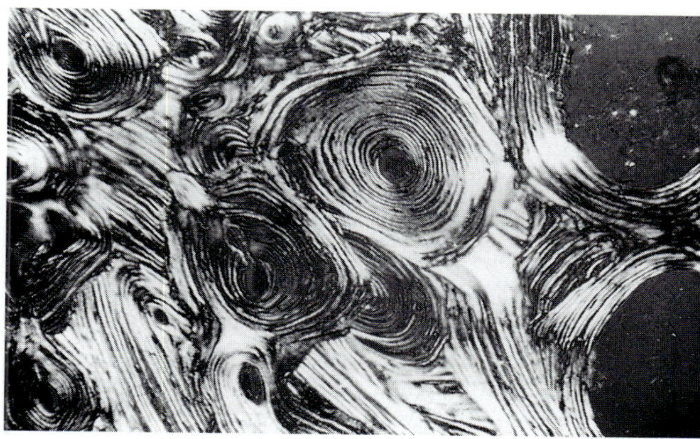

Fig. 10-7 Bone. Polarized light micrograph. Mature lamellar bone has osteons composed of collagen fibers that are aligned in a parallel fashion. Unstained and fully mineralized.

cortex and the subchondral bone plates, the bone in the medullary cavity is in the form of anastomosing plates or rods and is called cancellous, trabecular, or spongy bone. The orientation of the trabecula usually reflects adaptation to stresses applied to the bone. The lamellae within a trabecula usually are arranged parallel with the surface of the trabecula. They are not arranged into tubes or osteons, as in cortical bone.

Other than bone in early fetal life and the bone matrix deposited on the primary trabeculae in endochondral ossification of prenatal and postnatal growth, bone is deposited in lamellae, as described above, and called lamellar bone. Bone rapidly produced in response to injury, inflammation, or neoplasia and the bone of the primary trabeculae and early fetus are woven bone. In woven bone, the collagen fibers are haphazardly arranged, and this bone is of inferior strength when compared with lamellar bone (Fig. 10-8).

The process of activation of bone resorption coupled with subsequent bone formation and replacement of units of bone is referred to as skeletal remodeling. This turnover of old bone to new bone allows for the repair of accumulated microscopic damages in the bone (microfractures). Not all species undergo bone remodeling; small, short-lived animals such as the mouse and rat do not remodel their cortical bone. It is common to find unremodeled cortical bone in aged small dogs and cats. The name of the remodeling unit of cortical bone is the osteon, and, for trabecular bone, it is called the basic structural unit. The shape of the osteon is described above. The basic structural unit is shaped like a shallow bowl. The term "modeling" is used to describe change of the shape or contour of a bone in response to normal growth or disease. In modeling, there is no combining of bone resorption and formation, which allows the shape of bone to change or drift. This process allows the medullary cavity to enlarge and the overall shape of the bone to be maintained while the bone is growing. Both modeling and remodeling are under programmed genetic control but can be markedly altered by disease and changes in use of the bone. Changes in modeling and remodeling secondary to changes in mechanical use might be mediated by stretch receptors on bone cells and piezoelectrical activity. Piezoelectrical activity refers to bioelectrical potentials induced when collagen fibers and mineral crystals are deformed by mechanical forces. This piezoelectric activity affects cell function (bone formation and resorption) and structure (bone mass and orientation of osteons and trabeculae) and is important in the development and maintenance of the skeleton. It results in bone structures that oppose mechanical forces in the most effective manner. It follows that inactivity associated with disuse or weightlessness leads to bone loss. All bone surfaces can be classified as to activity as formative, resorptive, or resting. It is the balance among these activities, over time, that determines bone mass. Normally, there is an increase in bone mass during growth. In the adult bone, removal and replacement continue, but bone mass tends to decline

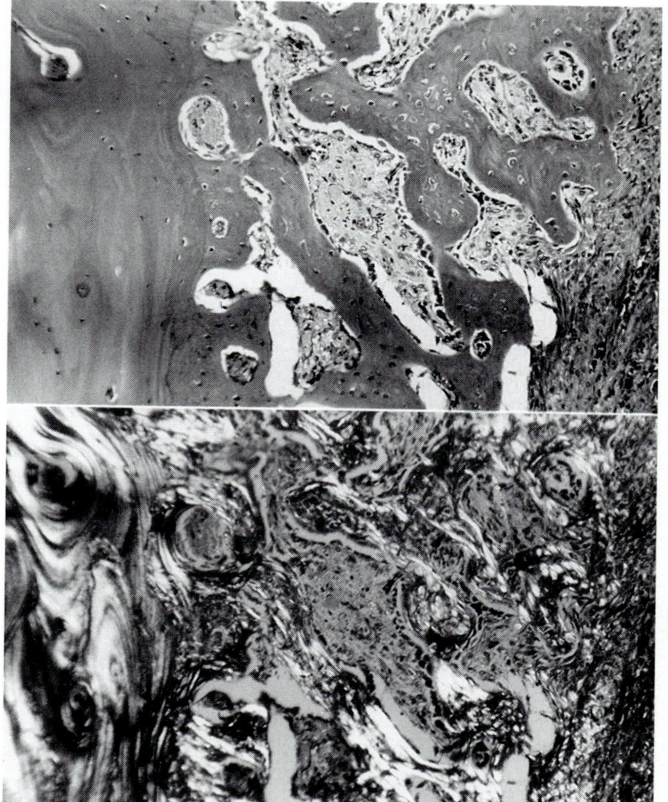

Fig. 10-8 Bone; dog. Reactive periosteal bone formation (woven bone) viewed with brightfield (**A**) and polarized light (**B**). The preexisting lamellar bone is to the left in both **A** and **B**. Both woven bone and lamellar bone polarize, but the pattern is patchy in the woven bone due to the irregular arrangement of the collagen fibers. H & E stain.

in old age due to incomplete formation after resorption in the remodeling process.

Bone as an organ

Individual bones of the skeleton vary in their manner of formation, growth, structure, and function. Flat bones of the skull develop by the process of intramembranous ossification, in which mesenchymal cells differentiate into osteoblasts and produce bone directly. Cartilage is not involved. Most bones develop from cartilaginous models by the process of endochondral ossification. Cartilaginous models are invaded by vessels, and primary (diaphyseal) and secondary (epiphyseal) centers of ossification develop and provide for further growth and increasing strength.

The long appendicular bones and the vertebral bodies are divided anatomically into epiphyses, metaphyseal growth plates (physes), metaphyses, and diaphyses (Fig. 10-9). Some long bones have only one metaphyseal growth plate. The epiphysis is cartilaginous in the fetus, with ossification beginning centrally and progressing to where it is entirely bony and bounded by articular cartilage and the metaphyseal growth plate. Growth of the epiphysis contributes to the overall length of the bone and is accomplished by endochondral ossification involving the articular-epiphyseal cartilage complex and, in some cases, the epiphyseal aspect of the metaphyseal growth plate.

The metaphyseal growth plate, or physis, consists of hyaline cartilage. It is often supported on its epiphyseal aspect by a thin transverse plate of bone, whereas the chondroosseous junction on the metaphyseal aspect is a fragile lattice of bone-covered spicules of calcified cartilage. Cartilage of the metaphyseal growth plate is divided into a reserve or resting zone, a proliferative zone, and a hypertrophic zone (Fig. 10-10). The hypertrophic zone is sometimes further subdivided into zones of maturation, degeneration, and calcification. The resting or reserve zone serves as a source of cells for the proliferating zone where cells multiply, accumulate glycogen, produce matrix, and become arranged in longitudinal columns. This replication of cells results in the overall lengthening of the bone. In the hypertrophic zone, chondrocytes increase their size and begin to lose glycogen. The cytoplasm becomes vacuolated, the nuclear and outer cell membranes fragment, and mitochondria lose stored calcium. The current view is that hypertrophic chondrocytes are not passive cells; rather, they are highly differentiated, active cells that secrete macromolecules that modify capillary invasion, matrix mineralization, and endochondral bone formation. Initial calcification occurs in the longitudinal septae of cartilaginous matrix between col-

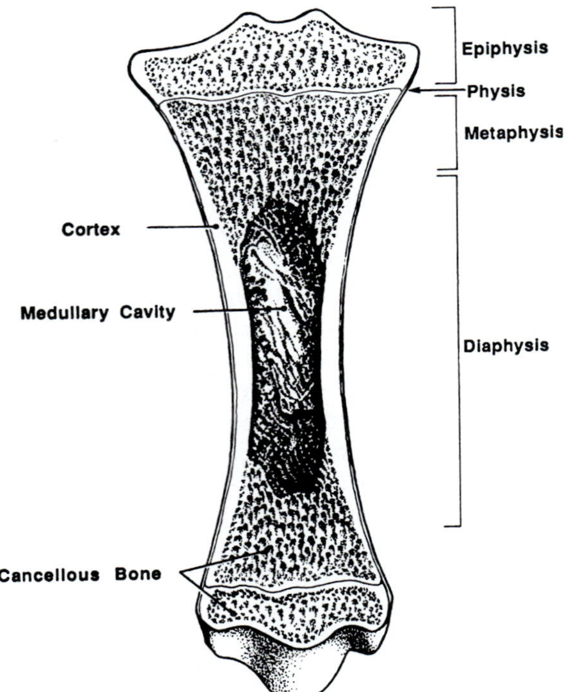

Fig. 10-9 Diagram showing the anatomic components of a long bone.

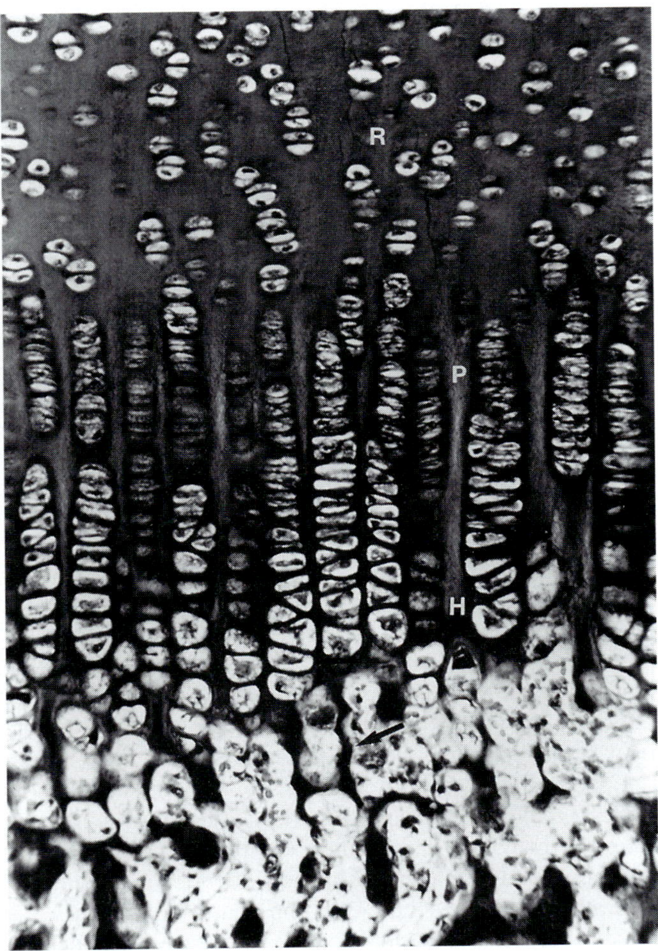

Fig. 10-10 Bone, growth plate; dog. Resting (*R*), proliferating (*P*), and hypertrophic (*H*) zones of the growth plate are present. Invading vessels and chondroclasts release degenerating chondrocytes from their lacunae and leave the remaining septae *(arrow)* as a basis of the primary trabeculae. H & E stain.

umns of cells. Matrix vesicles form in the hypertrophic zone and are important in the process of mineralization.

Growth plates are widest when growth is most rapid; as growth slows, the plate becomes narrow and closes (it is entirely replaced by bone) at skeletal maturity. Androgens and estrogens play a major role in determining the time of growth plate closure.

The metaphysis is bounded on one end by calcified cartilage of the physis and by the shaft (diaphysis) on the other. The sides of the physeal-metaphyseal junction are supported by a fibroosseus structure called the perichondral ring. The metaphysis is composed centrally of primary and secondary trabeculae. The former consists of mineralized spicules of cartilage covered by osteoid. The secondary spongiosa is the next zone toward the diaphysis and consists of enlarged trabeculae, some of which may still contain cartilaginous cores. The metaphyseal cortex beneath the perichondral ring is normally very thin, as its surfaces are the sites of very active osteoclastic bone resorption in the growing bone. Structurally, this is the weakest part of the bone. The diaphysis or shaft of the bone has a thick cortex, and, often, there is only a little trabecular bone along the endosteal surfaces. The medullary cavity of the diaphysis houses adipose and hemopoietic tissues.

Aside from areas covered by structures such as articular cartilage and intervertebral disks, the surfaces of bones are covered by periosteum. This is a thin membrane that is loosely attached to underlying bone except at heavy fascial attachments on bony prominences and at tendon insertions, where its attachments are strong and are associated with large vessels penetrating the underlying bone. Microscopically, it is composed of an outer fibrous layer that provides structural support and an inner osteogenic or cambium layer capable of normal lamellar appositional bone formation on the cortex of the growing animal and abnormal woven bone formation in response to injury. The periosteum is well supplied with lymph vessels and with fine myelinated and nonmyelinated nerve fibers that are responsible for the intense pain when the periosteum is injured.

Blood supply to bone

Arterial blood from the systemic circulation enters bones through nutrient, metaphyseal, and periosteal arteries (Fig. 10-11). A vascular circle supplies periarticular structures and the epiphysis. Nutrient arteries penetrate the cortex under strong, protective fascial attachments; once within the medulla, these arteries divide into proximal and distal intramedullary branches. Multiple smaller proximal and distal metaphyseal arteries also penetrate the cortex and anastomose with the terminal branches of the nutrient arteries. These anastomoses protect against infarction if the nutrient artery is obstructed.

Small periosteal arteries also pass through the diaphyseal cortex at sites of fascial attachment, and, although there is much variation from bone to bone, they supply one quarter

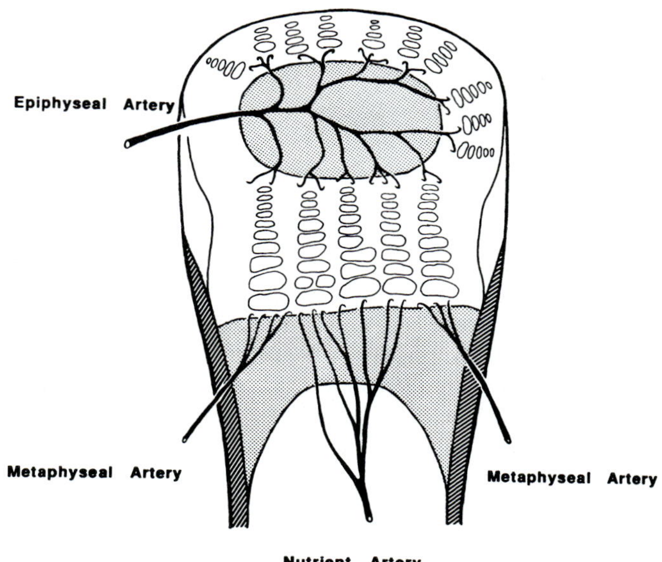

Fig. 10-11 Diagram of the major blood supply to the articular-epiphyseal cartilage complex and the metaphyseal growth plate. *Redrawn from Brighton CT. Structure and function of the growth plate. Clin Orthop 1978; 136:23.*

to one third of the outer cortex and anastomose with the terminal branches of the medullary arteries. These periosteal arteries are not capable of replacing the function of intramedullary or metaphyseal vessels.

Normally, afferent blood flow through diaphyseal cortical bone (from nutrient arteries) is centrifugal (from medulla to periosteum), owing to higher pressures in the intramedullary system. Efferent metaphyseal vessels (veins) pass from the medulla to the periosteal surface. Blood flow is greater in the immature animal than in the mature animal, as the periosteal blood supply is reduced. The epiphyseal surfaces of metaphyseal growth plates are supplied by epiphyseal arteries; the metaphyseal aspect is supplied by branches of metaphyseal and nutrient arteries. As capillaries approach the metaphyseal side of the growth plates, they make abrupt turns (loops); the diameter of the vessels on the venous side of the capillary bed is much larger than that of the vessels on the arterial side. Transphyseal vessels are common.

Postmortem Examination and Evaluation of Bones

The entire skeleton is rarely examined at necropsy. Rather, the extent of the examination is dictated by the clinical history. Antemortem clinical and radiographic findings are invaluable and should be in hand before the postmortem examination is begun. It should remembered that a lesion responsible for lameness may involve the skeleton, or it may involve other systems, such as muscle or the nervous system. Arthritis, osteomyelitis, and fractures are common causes of lameness, but injury to a tendon insertion, compression of a spinal nerve as it exits from the vertebral canal, and a small abscess in the sacroiliac joint are examples of important but easily overlooked lesions. Pathologists should routinely examine certain areas of the skeleton. This provides completeness to the necropsy and leads to familiarity with normal osseous structures. At least one long bone (preferably the femur) should be cut longitudinally and examined at necropsy. This examination should include an assessment of fat cell stores, hemopoietic activity, thickness of cortical bone, cancellous bone density, thickness and uniformity of metaphyseal growth plates, articular surfaces, and tendon insertions. Osseous structures are more readily seen if bone marrow contents are flushed out with a jet of water.

Postmortem changes do not usually pose major problems in the evaluation of the skeleton at necropsy. Postmortem bacterial invasion is less rapid than in most other tissues, and bone marrow cultures may be useful in detecting bacteremia. Bones may be fractured at euthanasia and by postmortem transport and handling.

Reactions of Bone to Injury

Bone, like other tissues when exposed to injury, has predictable reactions and mechanisms of repair. Bone tissue consists mostly of mineral and collagen, which are extracellular and, other than having the ability to fracture, cannot respond to injury without being altered by changes in the activity of bone cells. As with those of any organs, the cells in bone can undergo atrophy, hypertrophy, hyperplasia, metaplasia, neoplasia, degeneration, and necrosis. The amount of inorganic bone material present then is a direct effect of the net activity of these cells. Bone resorption and bone formation can be increased at the periosteum, but, if the hyperplasia, hypertrophy, and functional activity of osteoclasts exceed that of osteoblasts, the net effect will be a loss of cortical bone. Changes in bone cell number, size, and activity can alter the modeling and remodeling of bone as well as cause focal lytic or productive lesions.

Response to physical injury and changes in mechanical use

Direct physical injury to the periosteum is accompanied by pain and by new bone formation due to activation and proliferation of osteoblastic cells, the osteogenic (cambium) layer of the periosteum. Such exostoses can remodel and regress, or they can persist. Removal of the periosteum at surgery is not harmful, if areas of heavy fascial attachment or muscles that carry intramedullary vessels are left opposed to the bone. Mechanical lifting of the periosteum, either by surgery or due to displacement by underlying hemorrhage, edema, inflammation, or neoplasia, is followed by new bone formation. Because there is a balance of pressure and tension between the periosteum and the physis, circumferential incision of the periosteum (as in the fracture of a long bone) can cause a spurt of longitudinal bone growth. Further, if the periosteum is incised on one side of the limb, there is an ipsilateral increase in longitudinal bone growth, a feature utilized by surgeons in treating angular limb deformities. Mechanical disruption of the perichondral ring can lead to peripheral extension of physeal cartilage and the formation of osteocartilaginous nodules on the surface of the bone. These resemble naturally occurring, multiple cartilaginous exostoses in dogs, and they become more distant from the physis as longitudinal growth occurs.

Tension and compression (weightbearing) are important mechanical factors that affect bone mass. Normal mechanical use is required for maintenance of the structure of the skeleton. For example, in the adult skeleton, normal mechanical use causes a suppression of bone resorption. Decrease in mechanical use results in a release of this inhibition and a slight inhibition of bone formation. The net effect of decreased mechanical use is less bone due to increased resorption with inadequate formation (Fig. 10-12).

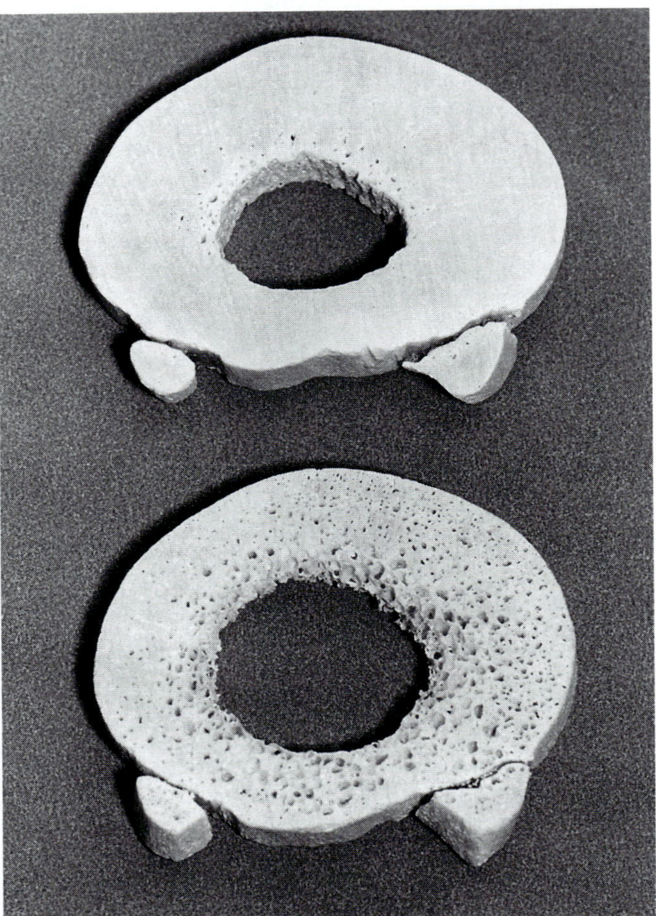

Fig. 10-12 Bone, metacarpus, cross sections; horse. Radial nerve injury and paralysis of the right foreleg, 7 months' duration. There is disuse osteopenia (atrophy of bone) of the right metacarpus *(lower specimen).* Note the enlargement of the medullary cavity and increased intracortical porosity of the bone from the affected limb.

These cellular affects are likely mediated through stretch receptors of bone cells that are attached to the matrix as well as through changes in piezoelectric forces (bioelectric potentials) and blood flow.

Irradiation causes direct injury to bone cells, with osteocytes being most resistant. Necrosis can occur if the dose is large, and sarcomas might develop.

Fracture repair

Broken bones are a common occurrence. It is important to understand how and why fractures heal, and, more important, why they do not. Fractures can be classified as traumatic (normal bone broken by excessive force) or pathologic (an abnormal bone broken by minimal trauma or by normal weightbearing). Osteomalacia, osteomyelitis, and bone neoplasms are examples of lesions that can weaken a bone and predispose it to fracture. Fractures can be classified in many other ways: closed or simple, if the skin is unbroken; open or compound, if the skin is broken and the bone is exposed to the external environment; comminuted, if the bone has been shattered into several small fragments; avulsed, if the fracture was caused by avulsion or pull of a ligament; greenstick, if one side of the bone is broken and the other side is only bent so that there is no separation or displacement; and transverse or spiral, depending on the orientation of the fracture line.

The events that normally occur in the healing of a closed fracture of a long bone are summarized below. The reader should appreciate that this represents a summary of a complex process that is subject to a great deal of variation. At the time of fracture, the periosteum is torn, the fragments are displaced, soft tissue is traumatized, and bleeding occurs at the fracture site (Fig. 10-13). A hematoma forms in and around the fracture site, and necrosis involves any isolated fragments of bone at the broken bone ends and of medullary elements. Mesenchymal cells with osteogenic potential from the periosteum, endosteum, medullary cavity, and, possibly, from metaplasia of endothelial cells proliferate in the hematoma and form a loose collagenous tissue. These cells mature into osteoblasts and later produce woven bone. The term ''callus'' refers to an unorganized meshwork of woven bone that forms following a fracture (Fig. 10-14). It can be external (that formed by the periosteum) or internal (that formed between the ends of the fragments and in the medullary cavity). Necrotic bone is

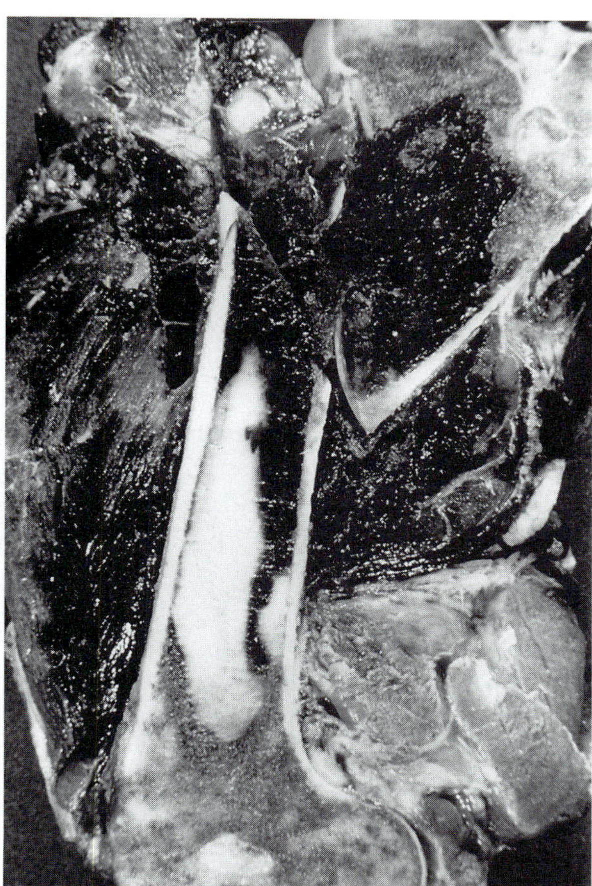

Fig. 10-13 Bone, femur; pig (sow). Recent oblique fracture of the proximal diaphysis. Note the extensive hemorrhage and soft tissue injury. A calcium deficiency has resulted in a pathologic fracture associated with osteoporosis.

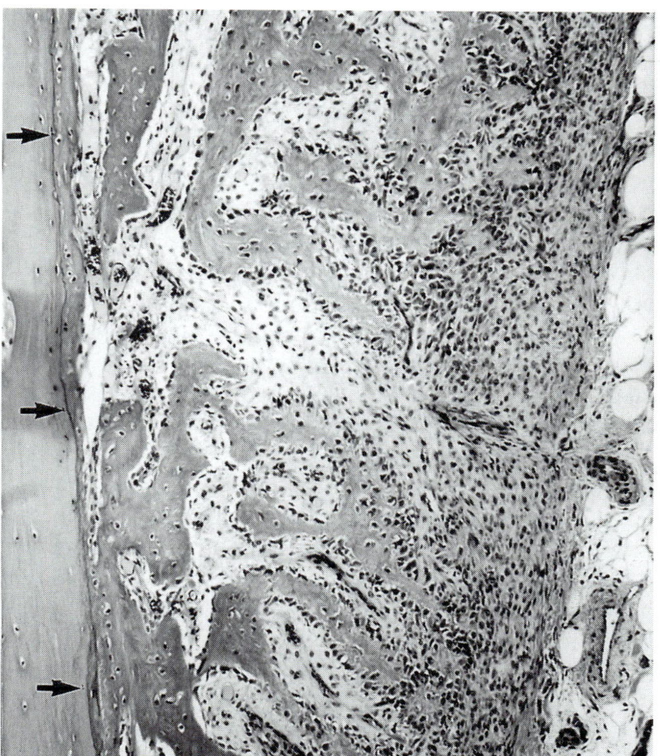

Fig. 10-14 Bone. External callus on the periosteal surface *(arrowheads)* of cortical bone in fracture repair. The callus is composed of coarse trabeculae of woven bone covered with a hypercellular cambium layer of the periosteum. H & E stain.

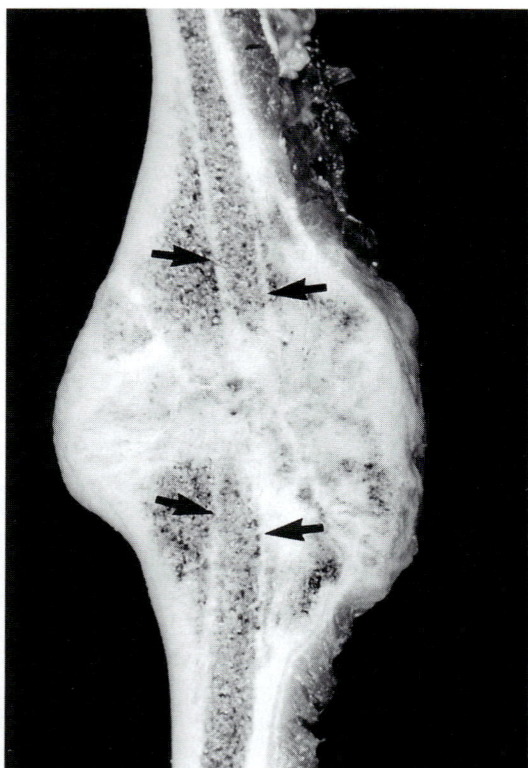

Fig. 10-15 Bone, rib; horse. Fracture of unknown duration. Note the abundant external callus and the original cortex *(arrows).*

removed by osteoclasts, a process that extends over a long period. This ''primary'' callus should bridge the gap, encircle the fracture site, and stabilize the area (Fig. 10-15). Callus can contain hyaline cartilage. Cartilage formation in the callus is likely to increase if the oxygen supply is not optimal. This cartilage does not provide as strong a callus as woven bone, but it will eventually undergo endochondral ossification and, therefore, ultimately contribute to the bony callus. An adequate blood supply and stability of the bone fragments are of prime importance in fracture repair. Local environmental factors, such as oxygen tension, mechanical tension, and compression at the fracture site, influence the reparative process. Minimal movement of the bone edges in contact with one other (slight compression) and a good blood supply favor direct bone formation with minimal periosteal callus. Excessive movement and tension favor the development of fibrous tissue. Mature fibrous tissue is not wanted in the callus because it does not stabilize the fracture and, unlike cartilage, will not act as a template for bone formation. Excessive fibrous tissue between bone ends in a fracture might result in a nonunion. In time, woven bone at the fracture site is replaced by stronger, mature lamellar bone (secondary callus), and, depending on the mechanical forces acting on the site, the callus can eventually be reduced in size by osteoclasts until the shape of the bone is restored to normal. This process, however, might take years.

A number of factors can interfere with the normal repair process. Malnutrition, loss of adequate blood supply to the fracture site, excessive movement of the fragments, too large a gap between fragments, the presence of bacterial infection and associated osteomyelitis, and the interposition of large fragments of necrotic bone, muscle, or other soft tissue all interfere with the healing process and might lead to delayed union or nonunion (Fig. 10-16). Some areas of the skeleton that have a poor blood supply and little surrounding soft tissue might fail to develop an adequate blood supply at the fracture site. In these cases, fibrous tissue rather than callus might develop and persist as a fibrous union. Inadequate immobilization, with repeated movement and shearing of small vessels as they develop, favors the formation of cartilage and fibrous tissue. In time, bony ends can become smooth and move in a pocket of fibrous tissue and cartilage to form a false joint or pseudoarthrosis (Fig. 10-17). The use of fixation devices that cause rigid immobilization of the fractured segments can alter the repair process, and external callus might be minimal with direct bone formation between bone ends.

Metallic implants used in fracture stabilization can have a number of different effects on the skeleton. Metallic devices that are too large deprive the bone (stress shielding) from normal mechanical forces and result in bone loss. Intramedullary fixation devices have the potential to damage the blood supply. Implanted material (metal, plastics, and bone cement) often is separated from the surrounding bone by a thin layer of fibrous tissue, sometimes with metaplastic cartilage that forms in response to operative trauma, implant mobility, or corrosion of the implant. Particulate

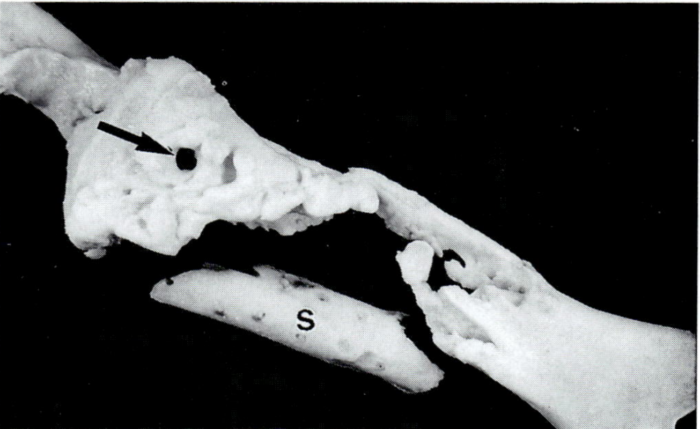

Fig. 10-16 Bone, proximal radius and ulna; horse. A nonunion fracture and osteomyelitis, with irregular new bone formation at the fracture site and around a screw hole *(arrow).* A large necrotic fragment, isolated from its blood supply had formed a sequestrum (*S*).

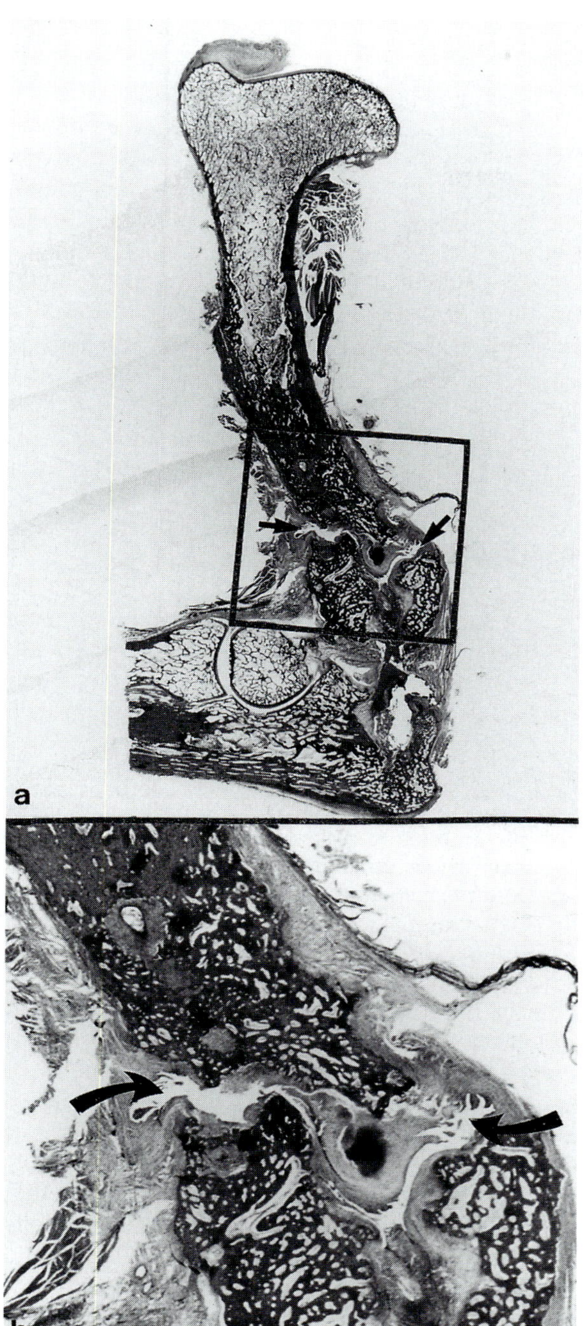

Fig. 10-17 Bone, humerus and elbow joint; dog. **A**, A nonunion fracture of the distal humerus has formed a pseudoarthrosis (false joint) that is lined at its periphery by synovial membrane *(arrows)*. **B**, Detail of the affected area. H & E stain. *Courtesy Dr. W. Riser.*

debris (''wear debris'') elicit a macrophage or giant cell response that can lead to bone resorption and deterioration at the bone-implant surface. A few cases of neoplasia associated with the use of metallic fracture fixation devices have been reported in the veterinary literature.

The factors and mechanisms that initiate the repair of bone are incompletely understood, but growth factors present in the blood clot and from damaged soft tissue likely play a major role in stimulating and recruiting osteoblasts and osteoclasts into the region. In addition, macrophages are attracted to the site by chemoattractants from the clot and damaged tissue. Macrophages contain cytokines that can modulate bone cell activity.

Abnormalities of Growth and Development

Given the complexity of the process, it is not surprising that a vast array of errors occur during the development of the skeleton. A list of definitions is given in Table 10-1 for terms commonly used in describing abnormal skeletal development. Examples of both localized and generalized lesions are cited in the following text. The subjects of hormone-mediated disturbances of growth and angular limb deformities are also included here.

The physis (growth plate) is a fragile structure whose activity and shape are affected by the blood supply it receives and by the mechanical forces applied. In the face of multiple nutrient deficiencies, such as occur in debilitating disease or general malnutrition, the growth plate becomes narrow (growth is impaired) and the metaphyseal face of the plate can be sealed by a layer of bone. If growth resumes, this layer of bone is carried into the metaphysis as a layer of dense, interconnecting spicules (transverse tra-

Table 10-1. Some terms used to describe skeletal abnormalities

Term	Definition
Dystrophy	A disorder arising from faulty or defective nutrition
Dysplasia	Abnormality of development
''Spondylo''	Denotes a relationship to a vertebra or to the vertebral column
Amelia	Absence of a limb or limbs
Hemimelia	Absence of a longitudinal segment of a limb
Phocomelia	Hypoplasia of limbs, hands, and feet attached directly to the body
Synostosis	Osseous union of bones that are normally distinct
Syndactyly	Fusion of adjacent digits
Kyphosis	Abnormal dorsal curvature of the spine
Scoliosis	Lateral deviation or curvature of the spine
Kyphoscoliosis	Abnormal dorsal and lateral curvature of the spine
Lordosis	Abnormal ventral curvature of the spine

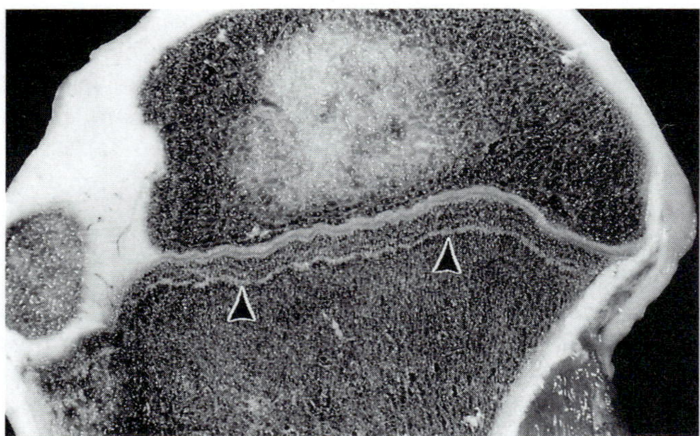

Fig. 10-18 Bone, proximal humerus; cow (newborn). Arrest lines *(arrowheads)* parallel to the physis indicate previous temporary cessation of longitudinal growth.

beculations) of bone. These are visible to the naked eye and are called arrest lines or Harris lines (Fig. 10-18). They are nonspecific in terms of etiology; they simply reflect a period of arrested or retarded longitudinal growth.

Impairment of osteoclastic activity within the primary trabeculae can result in the retention of elongated primary trabeculae that fail to model into secondary and tertiary trabeculae. These will continue to elongate as long as production by the growth plate continues. The retention of the primary trabeculae results in a dense band beneath the growth plate, called a growth retardation lattice. The band is apparent because normally many of the primary trabeculae are removed in the process of modeling. Their persistence results in a dense collection of thin, mineralized spicules that are apparent grossly and on radiographs. Examples of diseases that cause growth retardation lattices are canine distemper and bovine viral diarrhea. In addition, toxic damage to osteoclasts, such as with lead poisoning, can cause a growth retardation lattice (lead line). The name, growth retardation lattice, is inappropriate because the main lesion is in modeling of the trabeculae rather than in longitudinal growth.

Weakening or destruction of the matrix of the physeal cartilage can lead to premature closure of growth plates in animals with hypervitaminosis A or with a manganese deficiency. If the entire plate is affected, no further longitudinal growth is possible. If closure is focal, epiphyseal-metaphyseal bony bridges act as anchors to retard longitudinal growth and can give rise to deformity of the adjacent articular surfaces (Fig. 10-19).

The response of the physis to specific nutritional deficiencies is highly variable. Vitamin C deficiency (scurvy) leads to arrested osteoblastic activity; naked spicules of calcified cartilage remain (scorbutic lattice) as a very fragile support for the metaphyseal area, which often becomes

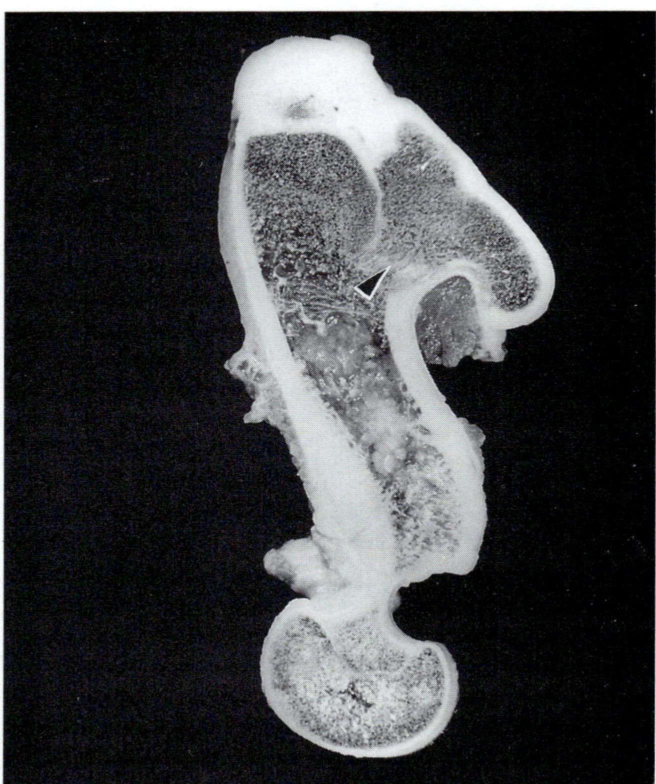

Fig. 10-19 Bone, humerus; cow. There is focal closure *(arrowheads)* of the proximal metaphyseal growth plate. An epiphyseal-metaphyseal bony bridge has deformed the humeral head.

the site of fracture and hemorrhage. Thickening (due to failure of removal) of physeal cartilage or cartilage of the articular-epiphyseal complex occurs in rickets, in osteochondrosis, and in association with metaphyseal osteomyelitis or any other situation in which there is obstruction of vessels that supply the metaphyseal face of the physis. Such thickenings can become necrotic and cause a cystlike lesion or can create instability of the physeal-metaphyseal junction and result in a pathologic fracture. Obstruction of the blood supply to the epiphyseal side of the physis leads to narrowing and premature closure of the physis. Once it is closed, for whatever reason, no further longitudinal growth is possible.

Malformations are primary structural defects due to localized errors in the embryonic period; **deformities** are alterations in shape or structure of a previously normally formed part, and they usually arise late in fetal life. Although the cause is often not apparent, teratogenic substances, such as thalidomide, chromosomal abnormalities, and local in utero factors (such as amputation by amniotic bands in humans) may be responsible. Some lesions, such as syndactyly in cattle, are inherited.

A number of generalized abnormalities in development are characterized by defective cartilage development and are classified as **chondrodysplasias.** Affected animals are short-legged, and the disproportionate dwarfism is variable in severity. Growth is disproportionate because the growth of bones formed in cartilage is retarded, whereas growth of other bones and soft tissues may be normal.

Osteopetrosis

This is an osteosclerotic (increased bone mass) disease that occurs in dogs, sheep, horses, cattle, and some laboratory animals and is described by some as a metaphyseal dysplasia. The basis for the disease is failure of osteoclasts to resorb (remodel) the primary spongiosa. As a result, spicules of bone with central cores of calcified cartilage fill the medullary cavity. This effects all bones that develop in a cartilaginous model. Affected bones are very dense (have no medullary cavity) but are susceptible to fracture (Fig. 10-20). In Angus cattle, it is inherited as an autosomal recessive trait. Affected calves are typically stillborn a few weeks premature and have brachygnathia inferior and impacted molar teeth.

Congenital cortical hyperostosis

This disease of newborn pigs (an example of diaphyseal dysplasia) is characterized by new periosteal bone formation on major long bones of the limbs. Lesions may be a consequence of disorganization of the perichondral ossification groove. Affected limbs (one or more) are visibly thickened by edema and by radiating spicules of bone that form on the periosteal surface. Piglets are stillborn or die shortly after birth because of other defects.

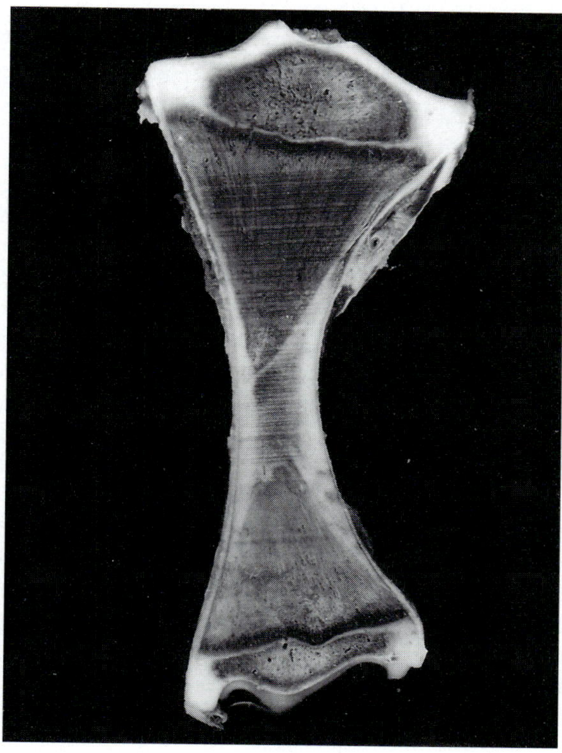

Fig. 10-20 Bone, tibia; cow (Aberdeen Angus calf). Osteopetrosis with failure of modeling. Trabeculae fill the entire medullary cavity.

Osteogenesis imperfecta

An osteopenic disease described in Holstein and Charolais cattle, it involves bone, dentin, and tendons. Clinically, affected calves might have multiple fractures, joint laxity, and defective dentin. Tissues have reduced concentrations of type 1 collagen and osteonectin.

Abnormalities in growth might have an endocrine basis. Defective development of the pituitary gland, resulting in a deficiency of growth hormone, and inadequate amounts of somatomedin occur in German shepherd dogs, in which there is delayed growth of all skeletal and soft tissue; hence, proportionate dwarfism occurs. As in hypothyroidism, both delayed bone maturation (delayed ossification) and growth plate closure are observed. Foals with hypothyroidism have mandibular prognathism and delayed ossification of carpal and tarsal bones, which can predispose to angular limb deformity. Hyperthyroidism is accompanied by accelerated skeletal maturation and osteoporosis.

Angular limb deformity

This term refers to lateral deviation of the distal portion of a limb. These deformities can occur in any species, but are most common in foals. The deviation might originate at various locations, such as the distal radial physis, the carpus, or the distal metatarsal physis. It can be present at birth or can be acquired later in life. It is common in active, well-muscled foals, especially the quarter horse. Causative factors that have been implicated include malpositioning of the fetus in utero, excessive joint laxity, hypothyroidism, trauma, poor conformation, overnutrition, and defective endochondral ossification of epiphyses of carpal, tarsal, and long bones. Joint instability due to laxity of periarticular soft tissues (ligaments) is common at birth and often is self-correcting in a short time. Animals with goiter and in utero hypothyroidism have delayed ossification of carpal and tarsal bones. These bones might be predisposed to injury at birth because they are largely cartilaginous rather than osseous. Deformity, hypoplasia, and osteochondritis dissecans of carpal bones can be associated with angular limb deformity originating at the carpus; the third carpal bone is most commonly affected. Angular limb deformities can also develop because of unequal growth across an epiphysis, such as the distal radius. This can be due to trauma and focal disruption of the blood supply to either the epiphyseal side of the physis or the articular-epiphyseal complex. For example, disruption of the lateral portion of the blood supply causes unilateral retardation of longitudinal growth and lateral deviation of the limb distal to the affected physis. In a similar manner, disruption (retardation) of growth on one aspect of the articular-epiphyseal cartilage complex can lead to malformation of the epiphysis and the associated articular surface and, eventually, to angular limb deformity.

Metabolic Bone Diseases

These are systemic skeletal diseases, generally of nutritional, endocrine, or toxic origin. Structural abnormalities occur in both growing and adult skeletons during normal modeling and remodeling processes. The classical metabolic osteodystrophies are osteoporosis, fibrous osteodystrophy, rickets, and osteomalacia. These terms imply specific pathologic changes but do not necessarily imply a specific cause. For example, osteoporosis can be due to a calcium deficiency, glucocorticoid therapy, or physical inactivity. Osteodystrophies can coexist in the same skeleton, e.g., it is possible for the same skeleton to have evidence of both osteoporosis and osteomalacia. Further, it is important to realize that some osteodystrophies are not definitive entities. A calcium deficiency can lead to osteoporosis, but, if severe and if accompanied by excess dietary phosphorus, it might evolve into fibrous osteodystrophy. In practice, most nutritional deficiencies in domestic animals do not involve a single element; more often, deficiencies are multiple and often not severe, and lesions are often not those produced under experimental conditions. The term ''osteodystrophy'' is a general one and implies defective bone formation.

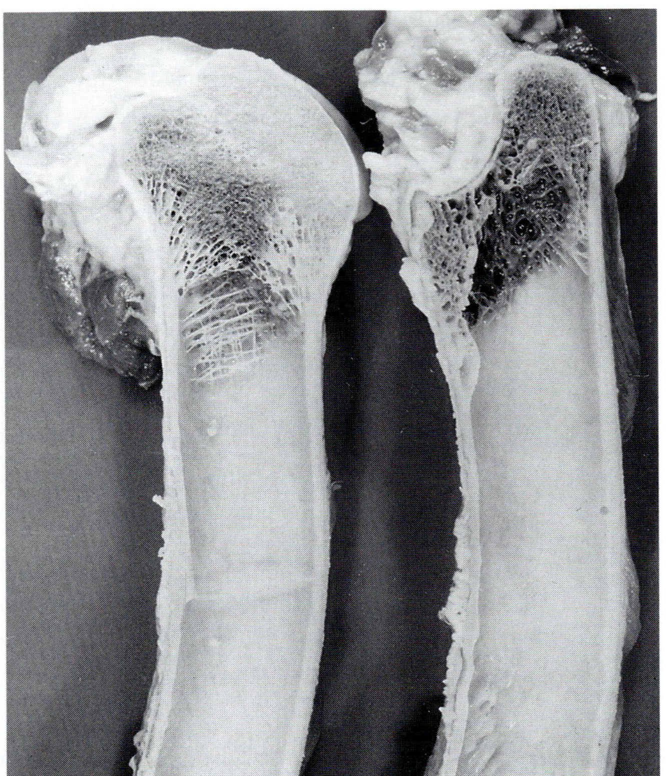

Fig. 10-21 Bone, femur; sheep (ewe). Osteoporosis associated with cachexia of chronic disease. Note the reduced amounts of cortical and trabecular bone. The marrow has been flushed from the specimen.

Osteoporosis

This term refers to the clinical disease of bone pain and fracture characterized microscopically by a reduction of bone mass (osteopenia) but with the remaining bone normally mineralized. The cortical bone is reduced in thickness and increased in porosity (see Fig. 10-12; Fig. 10-21). Trabecular bone becomes thinner, and perforations develop within the plates. Eventually, trabeculae are lost due to imbalance between formation and resorption. The medullary cavity becomes enlarged due to endosteal resorption and removal of metaphyseal cancellous bone. The end result is a bone that lacks normal density and that is easily fractured. In growing animals, osteoporosis is potentially reversible. In adults, however, once trabecular bone is lost, it cannot be regenerated. Some of the causes include calcium deficiency, starvation, physical inactivity, and the administration of glucocorticoids. A calcium deficiency can lead to hypocalcemia, which is corrected by increased PTH output and increased bone resorption. It is not clear why this does not result in fibrous osteodystrophy, as described below. Starvation and malnutrition lead to arrested growth and osteoporosis, largely owing to reduced bone formation because of deficiencies of protein and mineral. Reduced physical activity (disuse or immobilization osteoporosis) leads to an increase in bone resorption and a decrease in bone formation that might be mediated through changes in piezoelectrical activity and stretch receptors. Loss of bone mass associated with long-term paralysis or immobilization is not necessarily progressive; rather, the skeleton stabilizes at a new (reduced) level. Postmenopausal osteoporosis is a common and important disease in women; it often leads to vertebral deformity or collapse and pathologic fractures of the femoral neck. Declining concentrations of estrogens, physical inactivity, reduced muscle tone, and inadequate calcium intake are factors that can modify this disease. Interestingly, ovariohysterectomy in the bitch is not associated with clinical osteoporosis. Experimental studies have found transient osteopenia in ovariectomized dogs, but they confirm years of veterinary clinical observations that spayed dogs are not at risk for developing osteoporosis.

Rickets and osteomalacia

These diseases of the immature and mature skeleton, respectively, are characterized by failure of mineralization,

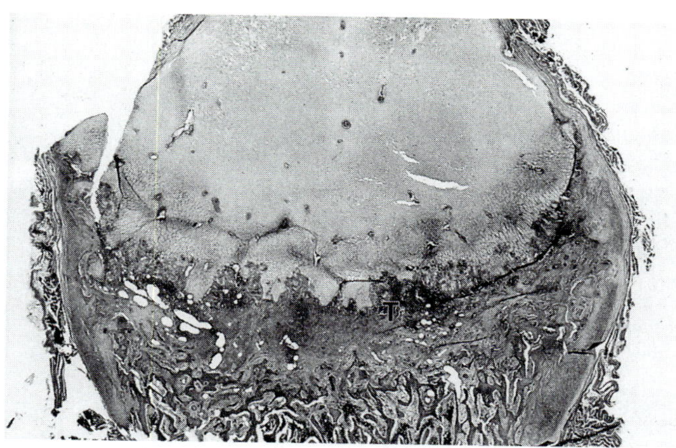

Fig. 10-22 Bone, costochondral junction; pig. Rickets. There is irregular retention (thickening) of the growth plate, with infractions and fibrosis in the region of the primary trabeculae. H & E stain.

with subsequent bone deformities and fractures. In the growing animal, rickets is a disease of bone and cartilage undergoing endochondral ossification. In the adult, osteomalacia is a disease only of bone, most commonly caused by deficiency of vitamin D or phosphorus. However, failure of mineralization and osteomalacia may occur in chronic renal disease and in chronic fluorosis. The microscopic lesions of rickets reflect the generalized failure of endochondral ossification; these are malalignment, disarray, and irregular thickening of physeal chondrocytes (Fig. 10-22). The thickening of the physeal plate is secondary to its failure to mineralize. In mammals, without mineralization of the chondroid matrix, blood vessels with accompanying chondroclasts will not invade the physis. Since the ability of the chondrocytes to proliferate and hypertrophy is at least partially retained in rickets, the plate thickens because there is normal production but a failure of removal. It is uncertain if the cartilage malalignment in vitamin D–deficiency rickets is due to a primary affect of vitamin D metabolites (specifically, 24,25-dihydroxyvitamin D) or a mechanical consequence of the failure of endochondral ossification. Metaphyses contain excess unmineralized osteoid, islands of surviving chondrocytes, and fibrous tissue. Unmineralized bone matrix is resistant to osteoclastic resorption and can accumulate. Abnormally wide seams of osteoid occur on bone-forming surfaces of the trabeculae. Hypocalcemia can develop in a vitamin D deficiency, and lesions of secondary fibrous osteodystrophy and hyperparathyroidism can be present. Soft bones, pathologic fractures, enlargement or flaring of the metaphyses of the long bones and ribs, bowing of the long bones, and reduced bone ash characterize the rachitic skeleton. The flared metaphyses reflect the thickening of the physis and failure of the normal modeling of the metaphysis (cut-back zone) because the poorly mineralized matrix is resistant to resorption.

Osteomalacia develops over time in the new bone formed in the process of skeletal remodeling. The disease is similar to rickets, except that physeal cartilage and associated lesions are not present in the adult skeleton. Microscopically, there are wide seams of unmineralized osteoid; clinically, affected animals have bone pain, pathologic fractures, and deformities such as kyphosis, scoliosis, or both. Phosphorus-deficient animals often have reduced feed intake, are unthrifty, and have impaired reproductive performance.

Fibrous osteodystrophy

This term describes the skeletal lesions of widespread increased osteoclastic resorption of bone and replacement by fibrous tissue that occur in primary and secondary hyperparathyroidism. Weakening of bones leads to lameness, pathologic fractures, and deformities. In domestic animals, primary hyperparathyroidism, as in cases of parathyroid adenoma, parathyroid carcinoma, or idiopathic bilateral parathyroid hyperplasia, is rare. Secondary hyperparathyroidism is more common and can be either nutritional or renal in origin. Nutritional hyperparathyroidism is caused by factors that tend to decrease the concentration of serum ionized calcium and to increase the output of PTH. It is most common in young, growing animals that are fed rations deficient in calcium and with a relative overabundance of phosphorus. Unsupplemented cereal grain rations fed to swine, all-meat diets fed to dogs and cats, and bran fed to horses are examples of low calcium–high phosphorus diets that can cause secondary hyperparathyroidism and, eventually, fibrous osteodystrophy. Increased concentrations of dietary phosphorus are important in the evolution of fibrous osteodystrophy, perhaps by interfering with the intestinal absorption of calcium. The lesions of fibrous osteodystrophy are increased osteoclastic resorption of cancellous and cortical bone, together with the proliferation of fibrous tissue. These changes are due to increased amounts of PTH rather than the direct effect of altered serum electrolytes. Sometimes, the proliferation of fibrous tissue is exuberant and associated with increased external dimension of the bone. This is more common in the maxilla and mandible and might reflect the response to the intense mechanical stress of mastication. Bones affected with fibrous osteodystrophy might fracture, their articular surfaces may collapse, and the vertebrae and ribs might be deformed (Figs. 10-23 and 10-24). Clinical signs vary from a mild lameness to multiple fractures resulting in an inability to stand. Growth plates are normal in fibrous osteodystrophy unless there is an accompanying vitamin D deficiency, in which case in young animals the lesions of rickets can be superimposed.

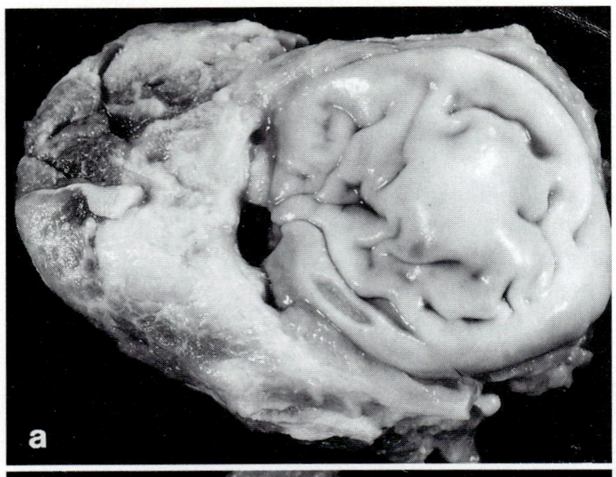

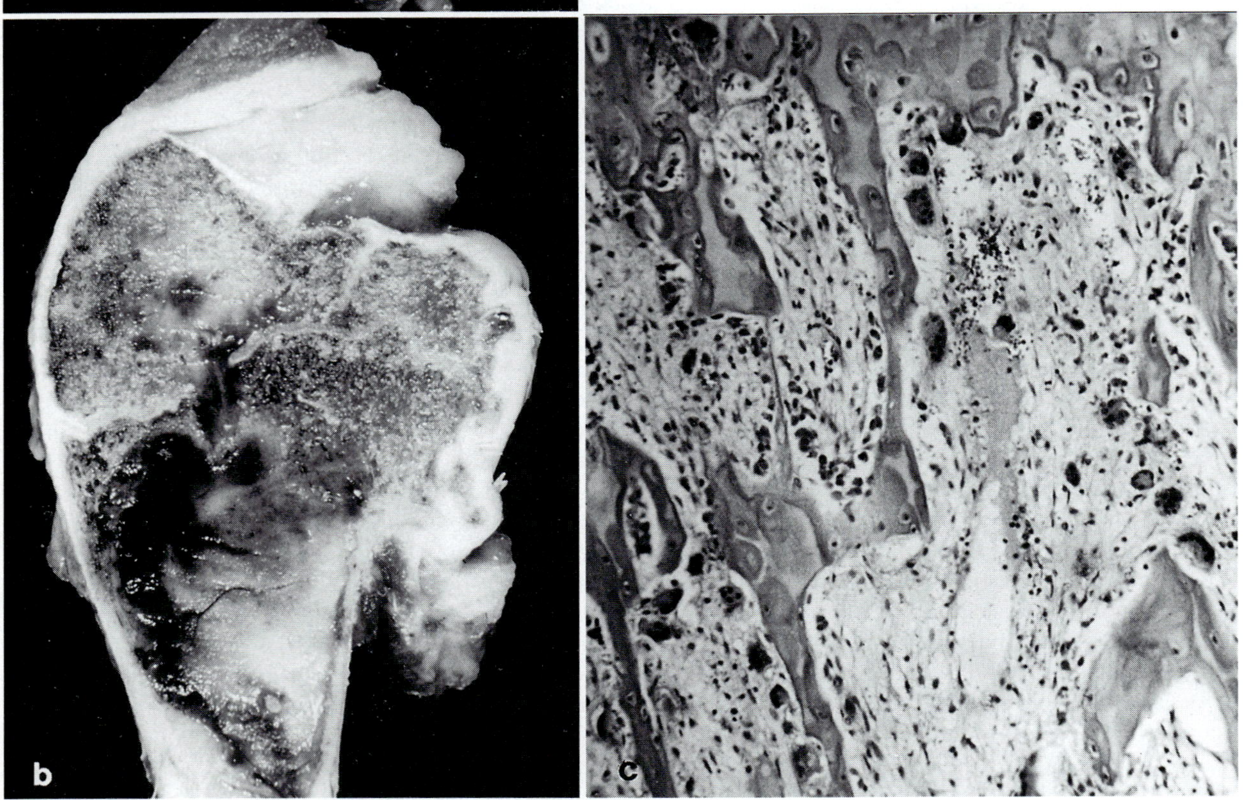

Fig. 10-23 Bone, humerus; pig. **A**, Fibrous osteodystrophy. Creases in the humeral head. **B**, Areas of cartilage have collapsed due to loss of supporting subchondral bone. **C**, The metaphysis has numerous osteoclasts and bone spicules with proliferation of fibrous tissue characteristic of response of bone to increased secretion of PTH. H & E stain.

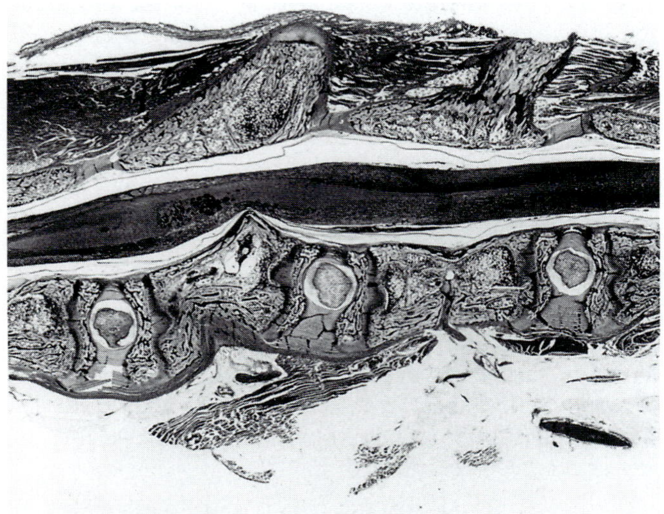

Fig. 10-24 Bone, vertebral column, longitudinal midsagittal section; cat. A pathologic folding fracture, secondary to nutritional fibrous osteodystrophy, of one vertebra has resulted in spinal cord compression. *Courtesy Dr. W. Riser*

Renal osteodystrophy

This is a general term that refers to the skeletal lesions (Fig. 10-25) that develop secondarily to chronic, severe renal disease. Osteomalacia and fibrous osteodystrophy occur singly or together in association with chronic renal disease in human beings, whereas fibrous osteodystrophy, which is sometimes complicated by osteomalacia, is reported in the dog, the animal most commonly affected with renal osteodystrophy. Dogs can have bone pain (lameness) and loss of teeth and deformity of the maxilla or mandible due to the loss of bone and replacement by fibrous tissue. The pathogenesis of the renal osteodystrophies is complex and, likely, varies depending on the extent and nature of the renal disease present and the availability of dietary vitamin D. Loss of glomerular function, inability to excrete phosphate, inadequate production of 1,25-dihydroxyvitamin D by the kidneys, and acidosis are central to the development of renal osteodystrophy. Phosphate retention because of decreased secretion leads to hyperphosphatemia, hypocalcemia, increased PTH output, increased bone resorption, and fibrous osteodystrophy. The reduced production of 1,25-dihydroxyvitamin D by the kidneys, together with impaired mineralization in the uremic, acidotic animal, explains the development of osteomalacia.

Toxic osteodystrophies

A number of different substances are toxic to bone and/or cartilage. Lesions that develop are described as toxic osteodystrophies. A portion of ingested **lead** can be bound to the mineral phase of bone and cartilage, and, in young animals after exposure to a bolus dose, this can manifest itself as a radiodense transverse band of increased density in the metaphysis parallel to the physis. This ''lead line'' (a growth retardation lattice, as described above) is not due to lead itself, which is present in very small amounts, but to lead-induced malfunction of osteoclasts. Osteoclasts in the area can contain acid-fast inclusion bodies.

Hypervitaminosis D can produce bone lesions of osteosclerosis when the intake is prolonged. In acute, massive exposures, death is due to widespread soft tissue mineralization and hypercalcemia; bone lesions are not apparent. In long-term exposures to smaller doses, such as is seen in ruminants ingesting plants containing water-soluble glycosides of 1,25-dihydroxyvitamin D (e.g., *Cestrum diurnum* in the southern United States), the persistent hypercalcemia causes chronic lowering of PTH and elevation

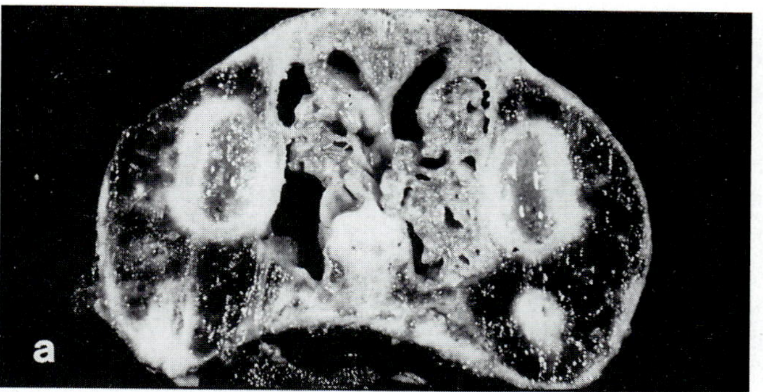

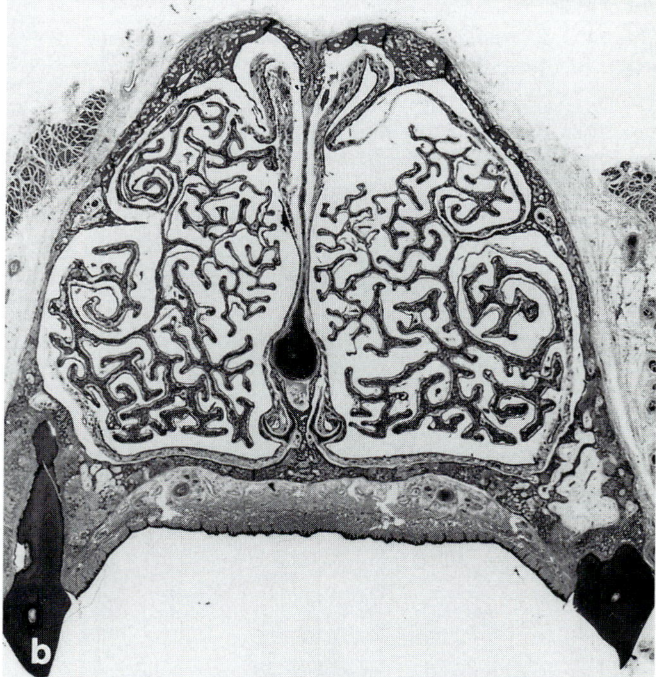

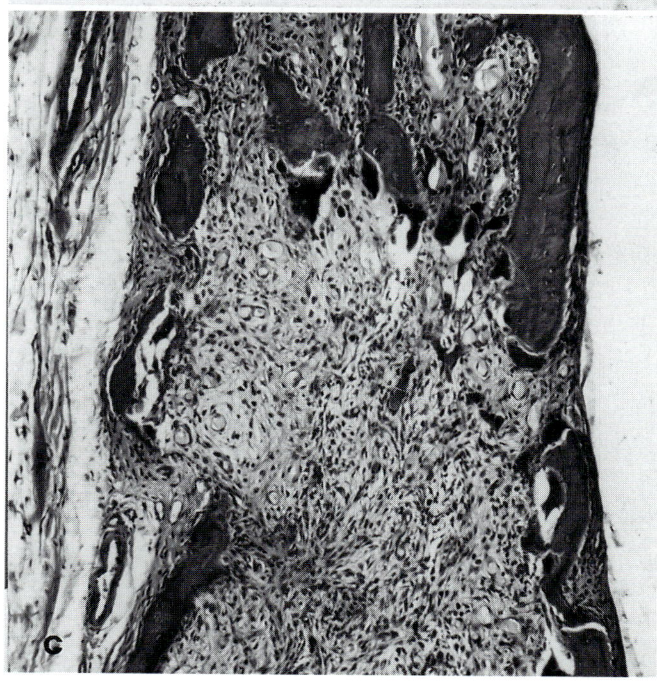

Fig. 10-25 Bone, maxilla; dog. Renal osteodystrophy in two dogs. **A**, Maxillary enlargement due to proliferation of vascular and fibrous tissue that has replaced resorbed bone. **B**, Extensive bone resorption and fibrous tissue replacement, without enlargement of the skull. **C**, The histologic detail of the maxilla in **B** shows much of the preexisting bone replaced by fibrous tissue. Numerous osteoclasts are present. H & E stain. *Courtesy Dr. W. Riser.*

of calcitonin. This combination effectively stops bone resorption. In addition, vitamin D apparently has a direct stimulatory effect on osteoblasts. The inhibition of bone resorption and stimulation of bone formation result in a denser skeleton. The matrix produced in some cases of hypervitaminosis D is abnormal with the process dose-dependent. The matrix is woven and stains variably basophilic after decalcification. Paradoxically, mineralization of the bone may be incomplete, possibly a consequence of abnormal ground substance.

Aseptic Necrosis of Bone

Aseptic necrosis of bone in human beings occurs in a variety of clinical situations, including occlusive vascular disease, hypercorticism, fat embolism, nitrogenous embolism, sickle cell anemia, and intramedullary neoplasms. In domestic animals, aseptic necrosis of bone has been associated with intramedullary neoplasms and various nonneoplastic lesions. Increased bone marrow pressure and decreased venous flow are important factors in the pathogenesis of ischemic or aseptic necrosis of bone. It occurs as a disease entity in the femoral head of dogs. On gross examination, necrotic cortical bone has a dry, chalky appearance, and the periosteum can be easily removed. In longitudinal section, necrotic bone can be yellow-white and involve scattered areas of the endosteal and cancellous bone, or necrosis might be obvious as large, pale areas of infarction surrounded by a zone of hemorrhage. Microscopically, the hallmark of bone necrosis is cell death and loss of osteocytes from their lacunae. Following an episode of ischemia, the cellular elements of the marrow lose their differential staining, and circular spaces (pooled lipid) develop within a few days. Vascular, newly formed fibrous tissue and macrophages advance from the margin of the lesion (Fig. 10-26). The marrow might eventually regenerate entirely, or a scar might form and remain. Dead osteocytes elicit very little reaction; their nuclei become pyknotic, but their disappearance from lacunae is slow and might not be complete for 2 to 4 weeks. The necrotic matrix remains fully mineralized and might even ''hypermineralize'' due to calcification of the dead osteocytes and

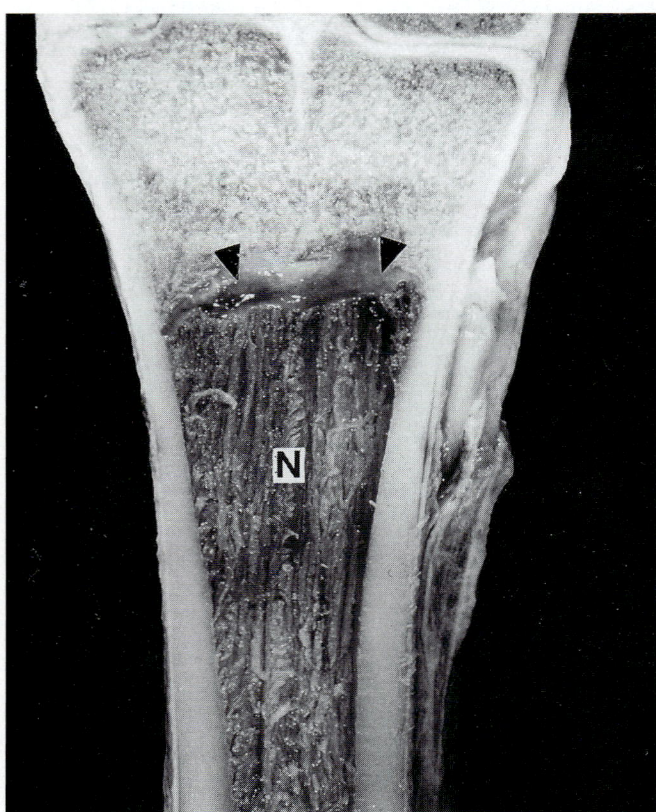

Fig. 10-26 Bone, proximal metacarpus; cow (calf). Ischemic necrosis (*N*) of the distal portion of the bone caused by external pressure of a tightly fitted cast. A reactive zone of fibrous tissue and inflammatory cells is at the margin *(arrowheads)* of viable tissue.

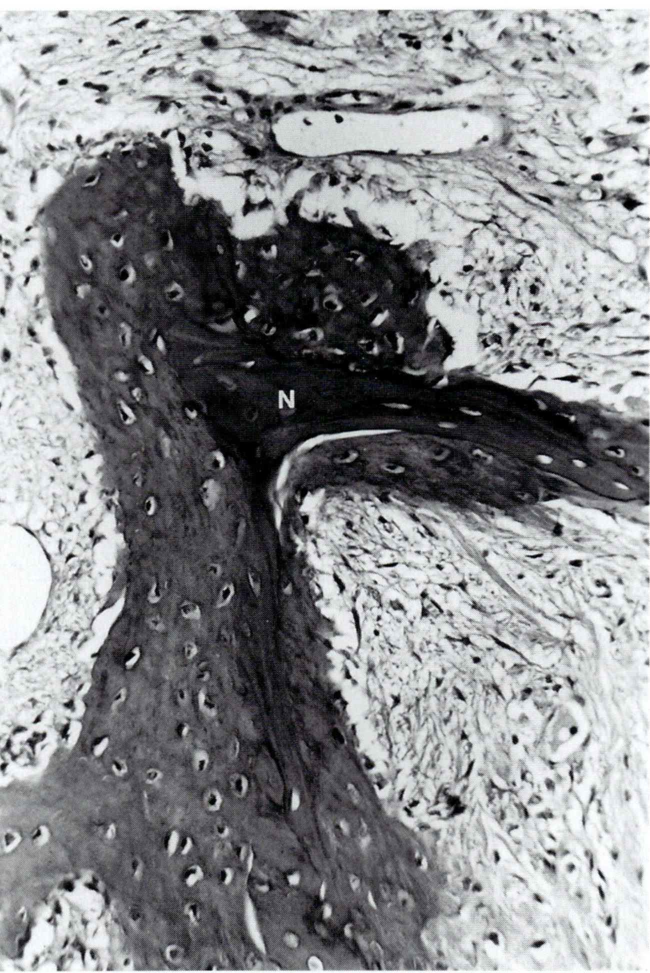

Fig. 10-27 Bone, femoral head; pig. Necrosis experimentally induced by ligature around the femoral head of a piglet. Woven bone with peripheral fibrosis of the marrow surrounds a spicule of necrotic bone (*N*), with many empty osteocyte lacunae.

their lacunae. Some of the necrotic bone can be removed by osteoclasts if the blood supply is reestablished. Large areas of necrotic cortical bone may remain for years. In necrotic trabecular bone, that portion which is not removed by osteoclasis is surrounded by new woven bone. This sandwich of central dead bone covered by woven bone can persist for months and give the necrotic region a radiodense appearance (Fig. 10-27). The slow resorption of necrotic bone with simultaneous replacement by new bone is termed "creeping substitution." The process is slow and often incomplete. Bone necrosis might not be detected clinically or radiographically. In the femoral heads of young, small, and miniature breed dogs, aseptic necrosis is associated with clinical signs because of the collapse of the articular cartilage due to resorption of the necrotic subchondral bone (Legg-Calvé-Perthe's disease). The cause of this infarction is usually not determined but might be due to venous compression. Although the chronic use of steroids in human beings has been associated with necrosis of the femoral head, steroid-induced osteonecrosis does not appear to be a problem in animals.

Inflammation of Bone

Osteitis

Inflammation of bone is designated osteitis: **periostitis** if the periosteum is involved and **osteomyelitis** if the medullary cavity of the bone is involved. These are common, sometimes life-threatening lesions that require early diagnosis and vigorous treatment. Osteomyelitis is often a chronic, disfiguring process characterized by necrosis and removal of bone and by the compensatory production of new bone, the two processes often proceeding simultaneously over a prolonged period. As such, osteitis is often a painful process leading to debilitation of the affected animal. Osteitis and its extensions in animals are usually caused by bacteria, although viral, fungal, and protozoal agents may be involved. *Actinomyces pyogenes* and other pyogenic bacteria are common causes of suppurative osteomyelitis in farm animals.

Bacteria can be introduced directly into bone at the time of a compound fracture, or infection can extend directly from surrounding tissues, as in sinusitis, periodontitis, or otitis media. More commonly, osteomyelitis develops as an extension from suppurative arthritis. Suppurative arthritis can be accompanied by destruction of articular cartilage, with direct extension of the process into subchondral bone. Alternatively, the process can penetrate the thin metaphyseal-epiphyseal cortex in the area of insertion of the joint capsule. In theory, hematogenous osteomyelitis can arise in any capillary bed in bone where bacteria lodge and survive. In practice, it occurs most commonly in young animals, with localization typically occurring in the metaphyseal area of long bones and vertebrae where capillaries make sharp bends to join medullary veins. Bacterial localization at these sites is apparently facilitated by slow flow and turbulence of blood in the larger, descending limbs of the capillary loops, the lack of phagocytic capacity in the venous side of the capillary bed, and the poor collateral circulation in the area. Obstruction of vessels and local tissue necrosis are important in the evolution of bacterial osteomyelitis. The composition of the exudate in metaphyseal osteomyelitis is determined by the infectious agent, but, in domestic animals, it is typically purulent (Fig.

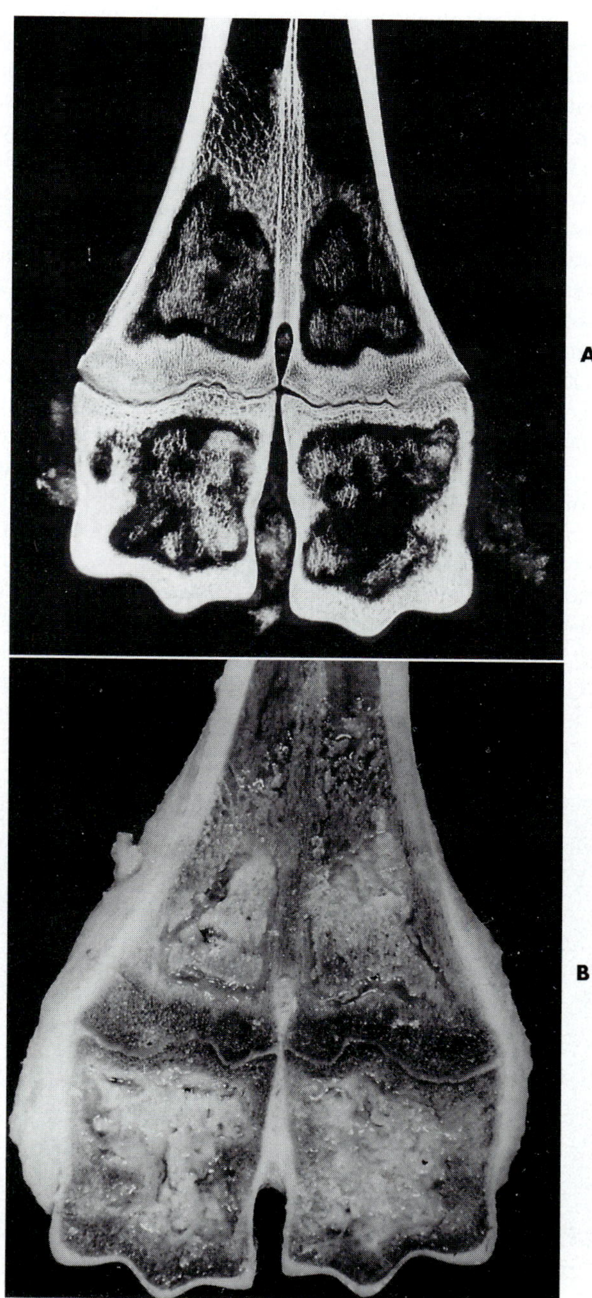

Fig. 10-28 Bone, metacarpus; cow (calf). **A**, Extensive purulent hematogenous osteomyelitis in the epiphyses and metaphyses. **B**, Radiograph. The location of the marked resorption of bone corresponds with the location of the exudate.

10-28). Exudate accumulates in the intertrabecular spaces and spreads; the increased intramedullary pressure causes vascular compression, thrombosis, and necrosis of intramedullary fat, bone marrow, and bone. Local hyperemia, prostaglandin production, and cytokine release by local tissue and inflammatory cells stimulate osteoclastic bone resorption. Obstruction of metaphyseal vessels interferes with the removal of cartilage, and the physeal cartilage can thicken. Lack of drainage and persistence of the offending agent in areas of necrotic bone account for the chronicity of the process. Bacteria can persist for years in cavities and areas of necrosis. Inflammation can spread in the medullary cavity, penetrate cortical bone, and undermine the loosely attached periosteum, further disrupting the blood supply to the bone. Chronic periostitis is characterized by multiple spreading pockets of exudate and areas of irregular new bone formation. Additional sequelae to osteomyelitis include extension to adjacent bone, hematogenous spread to other bones and soft tissue, pathologic fractures, and development of sinus tracts that penetrate cortical bone and drain to the exterior (Fig. 10-29).

Occasionally, fragments of bone become isolated from their blood supply and surrounded by a pool of exudate (bone sequestrum). Sequestration of necrotic fragments can occur when bone fragments are contaminated at the site of a compound fracture, when the fragments at a fracture site become infected hematogenously, or when fragments of necrotic bone become isolated in osteomyelitis. These isolated fragments of bone (sequestra) and associated exudate can become surrounded by a dense collar of reactive bone (the involucrum). Sequestra can persist for long periods (they are isolated from osteoclastic removal) and interfere with repair. They often take on a pale, chalky appearance and lack the glistening appearance of normal bone (Fig. 10-30).

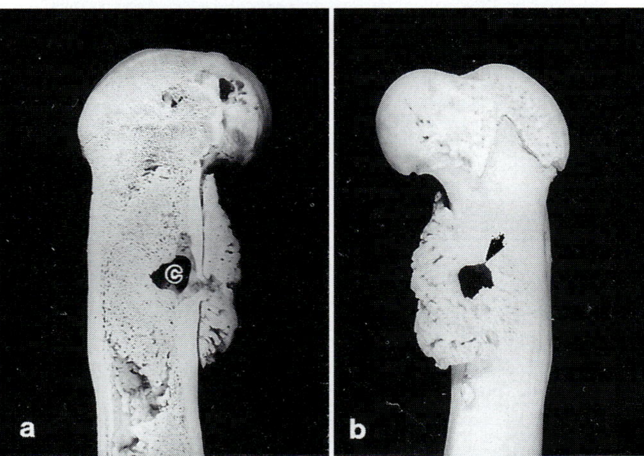

Fig. 10-29 Bone, femur. **A**, Chronic osteomyelitis characterized by central cavitation (*C*) surrounded by dense (osteosclerotic) reactive bone in the medullary cavity. **B**, A tract penetrates the cortex *(arrow),* giving rise to periostitis and new bone formation when viewed from the outer surface.

Hematogenous bacterial osteomyelitis is uncommon in dogs and cats, but it is common in farm animals. As an example, hematogenous vertebral osteomyelitis caused by *Actinomyces pyogenes* is a common cause of posterior weakness or paralysis in swine, and the bacteremia is secondary to bacterial infections of sites of trauma of the skin, tail, and feet. These primary lesions can have healed by the

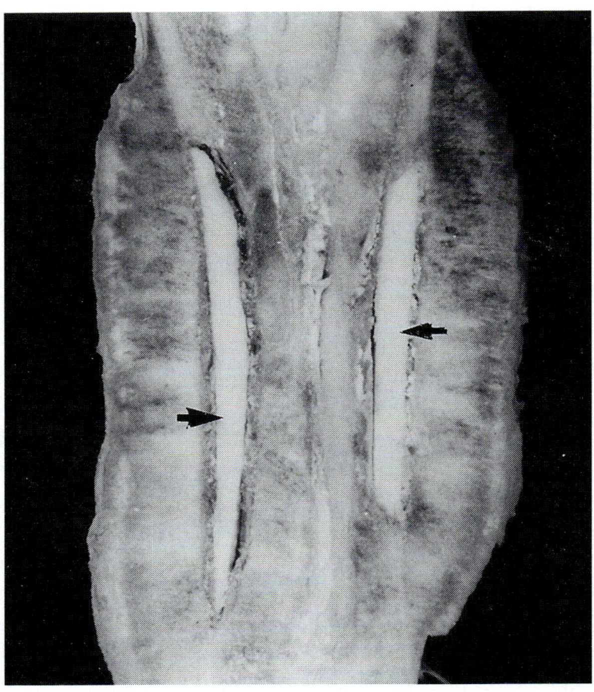

Fig. 10-30 Bone, dog. Exuberant callus formation of fracture repair associated with sequestration of cortical bone fragments *(arrows).*

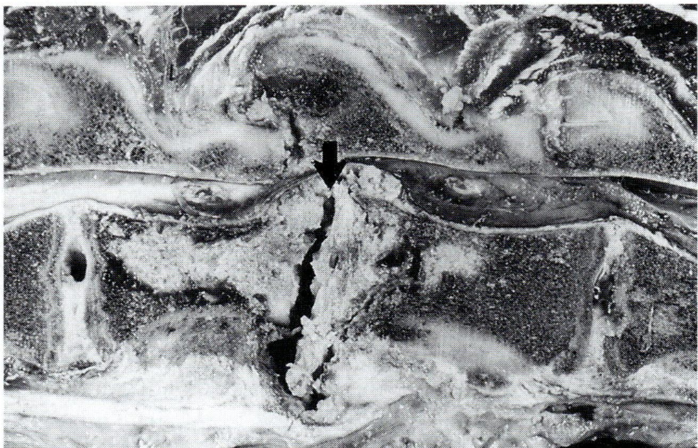

Fig. 10-31 Bone, vertebral column; pig. There is extensive destruction of bone, pathologic fracture, and compression of the spinal cord *(arrow)* due to bacterial osteomyelitis.

time vertebral osteomyelitis becomes clinically apparent. As in the long bones, localization of bacteria (in vertebrae) is often in the metaphyses, with subsequent bone necrosis and cavitation leading to pathologic fractures, displacement of the vertebral body, and compression or laceration of the spinal cord (Fig. 10-31). Occasionally, the periosteum of the vertebral canal is elevated by the exudate, causing compression of the spinal cord; in other areas, the inflammatory process extends outward to cause large paravertebral abscesses.

Mandibular osteomyelitis and periostitis

This disease, caused by *Actinomyces bovis,* occurs in cattle (Fig. 10-32). *A. bovis* is a soil-borne, gram-positive filamentous bacterium. Oral mucosal ulceration and eruption of teeth allow the organism entrance to the osseous tissues of the mandible, where chronic pyogranulomatous inflammation develops. Necrosis and loss of bone, new bone formation, scar tissue, formation of small abscesses, and multiple draining fistulae characterize the disease. The affected mandible is irregularly enlarged; teeth can loosen and fall out.

Mycotic agents such as *Coccidioides immitis* and *Blastomyces dermatitidis* frequently localize in bone to produce granulomatous lesions that cause bone lysis and irregular new bone formation. Various viral agents also localize in bone, and their effects are not all the same. The viruses of hog cholera and infectious canine hepatitis may cause endothelial damage, resulting in metaphyseal hemorrhage and necrosis, and acute inflammation. Osseous localization of the distemper virus injures osteoclasts, causing metaphyseal bone to accumulate (growth retardation lattice). The feline leukemia virus has been associated with myelosclerosis (increased density of medullary bone) in cats.

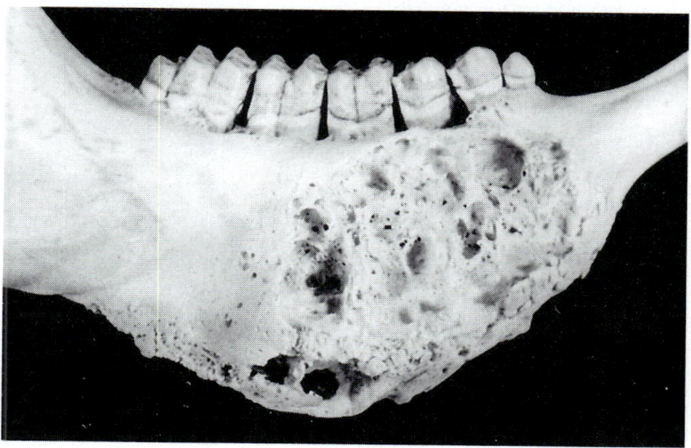

Fig. 10-32 Bone, mandible; cow. Osteomyelitis due to *Actinomyces bovis.* The cavities within the reactive bone indicate the location of pockets of pyogranulomatous exudate surrounding colonies of bacteria. Macerated and bleached.

Hypertrophic osteodystrophy

Also termed metaphyseal osteopathy, this is a disease of young, growing dogs of the large and giant breeds. The cause and pathogenesis are unknown; both nutritional factors and infectious agents have been incriminated. Clinically, it is characterized by lameness, fever, and swollen, painful metaphyses in long bone. Radiographically, metaphyseal zones of increased lucency and increased density are adjacent to the physes; other lesions are metaphyseal enlargement, "lipping," and bone formation in the periosteal areas of the metaphyses. Lesions are usually bilaterally symmetric. Microscopic findings include widespread suppurative inflammation and necrosis of the metaphyseal marrow and bone cells. The death of osteoclasts and osteoblasts results in persistence of long, thin primary trabeculae that are not reinforced by apposition of bone matrix. These then collapse and fracture without external distortion of the bone (infractions). Inflammation may also be present in the periosteum. Most animals recover spontaneously.

Proliferative and Neoplastic Lesions

Surprisingly, bone, as a tissue, offers little resistance to an expanding or invading neoplasm, and many skeletal

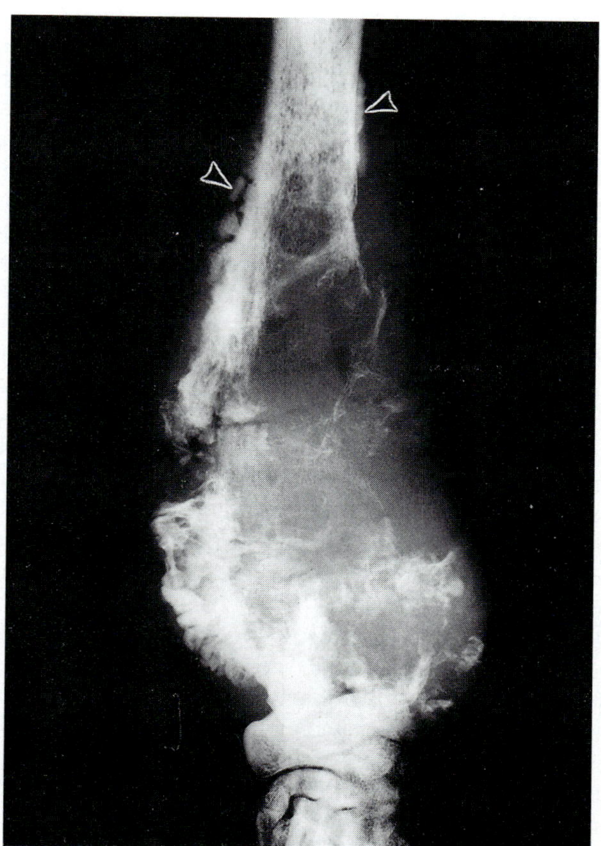

Fig. 10-33 Bone, distal radius; dog. Radiograph. Osteosarcoma with extensive destruction of preexisting bone and some new bone formation on the periosteal surface *(arrowheads).*

neoplasms are accompanied by both bone resorption and new bone formation (Fig. 10-33). Pain, hypercalcemia, and pathologic fracture are other possible manifestations of a skeletal neoplasm. New bone formation occurs, at least in part, in response to stress on a weakened cortex and is prominent in neoplasms that have a marked fibrous stroma, whereas it is minimal in neoplasms with little stroma, such as plasma cell myeloma and lymphosarcoma. Tumor-associated bone destruction is largely accomplished by osteoclasts. Prostaglandins, cytokines, acid metabolic byproducts, and lytic enzymes released by inflammatory or neoplastic cells might be responsible for local bone resorption and formation in response to a neoplasm. Hypercalcemia, due in part to bone resorption induced by release of bone-resorbing factors from extraskeletal neoplasms, is well documented (humoral hypercalcemia of malignancy). The most common example in animals is carcinoma of the apocrine glands of the anal sac in the dog, and this neoplasm produces PTH-related protein. This neoplasm metastasizes widely, but rarely to bone.

Nonneoplastic proliferative and cystic lesions

Lesions considered here vary widely in their cause, structure, and ultimate effect on the host. Remember that new bone formation (often excessive) also occurs in fracture repair, in chronic osteomyelitis, and in degenerative joint disease in the form of periarticular osteophytes. The term **exostosis** or **osteophyte** refers to a usually nodular, benign, bony growth projecting outward from the surface of a bone. In addition to the content of bone, there can be variable amounts of cartilage. Hyperostosis is used to indicate that the dimension of the bone has increased and, usually, implies more uniform growth on the periosteal surface rather than the nodular appearance of an osteophyte. An **enostosis** is a bony growth within the medullary cavity, usually originating from the cortical-endosteal surface, and can result in obliteration of the marrow cavity. All the above are nonneoplastic proliferative lesions in which growth is seldom continuous. Some exostoses can remodel and regress. In general, primary neoplasms of bone can cause damage by acting as space-occupying lesions, by invading and destroying surrounding tissues, or by metastasizing and injuring tissues distant to the primary neoplasm.

Biopsies of reactive lesions or regions of early fracture repair can be mistaken for an osteosarcoma. This statement serves to underline the problem of making a morphologic diagnosis from a biopsy specimen without benefit of a clinical history, radiographic findings, and other laboratory data. Because a neoplasm invades and weakens the cortex, considerable new periosteal bone can form in this area. This new bone is not part of the neoplasm but can constitute a part or all of the biopsy material submitted. Hence, biopsy instruments must penetrate reactive bone and enter the neoplasm itself. One must also remember that more than one process might be active at any one site; e.g., osteosarcoma might be complicated by fracture repair or by osteomyelitis.

Hypertrophic pulmonary osteopathy and **craniomandibular osteopathy** are poorly understood diseases in which there is proliferation of new bone on periosteal surfaces. Hypertrophic pulmonary osteopathy occurs in human beings and in domestic animals, with the dog most commonly affected. The disease is characterized by progressive, bilateral, periosteal, new bone formation in the diaphyseal regions of the distal limbs (Fig. 10-34). The word "pulmonary" is included because most cases have intrathoracic neoplasms or inflammation. Other, less commonly associated lesions or agents are endocarditis, heartworms, and rhabdomyosarcoma of the urinary bladder in

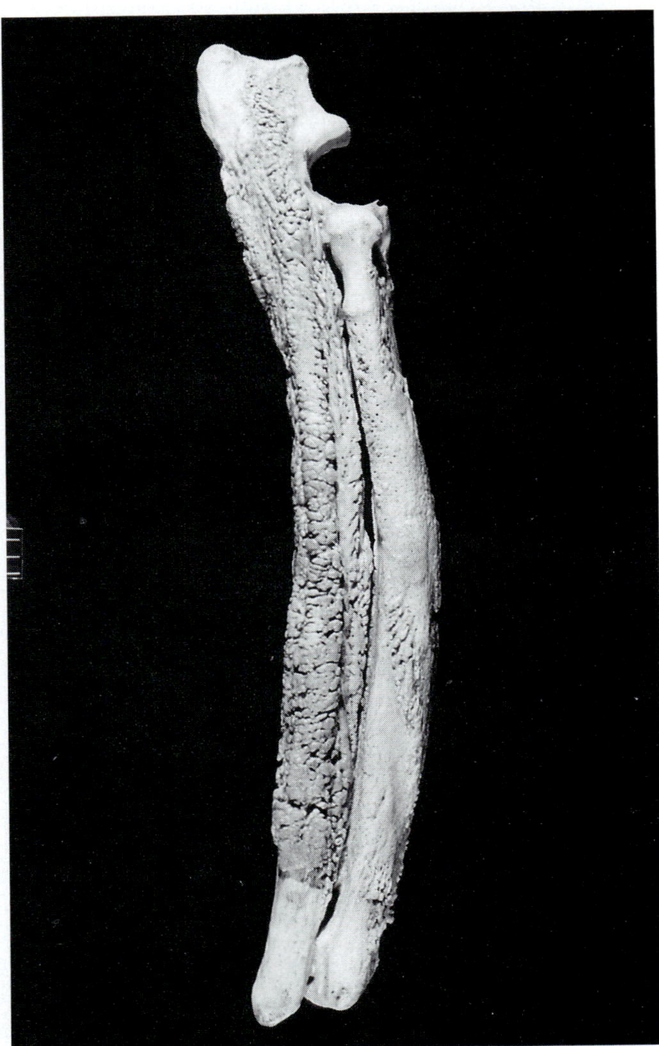

Fig. 10-34 Bone, radius and ulna; dog. Hypertrophic pulmonary osteopathy. The soft tissue has been removed, revealing the highly irregular surface that has resulted from periosteal proliferation of woven bone. Macerated and bleached.

young giant breed dogs and ovarian neoplasms in the horse. Although the association between the pulmonary lesions and the proliferation of new periosteal bone on the extremities is not clear, it has been postulated that pulmonary lesions lead to reflex vasomotor changes (mediated by the vagus nerve) and to increased blood flow to the extremities. New bone formation with thickening of the limbs can occur very rapidly but can regress if the primary lesion is removed. Regression occurs after vagotomy. Increased arterial pressure, hyperemia, and edema of the periosteum lead to thickening of the periosteum both by fibrous tissue and, later, by new bone formation. Lesions can be reproduced in dogs by creating shunts that allow blood to bypass the pulmonary circulation, thereby increasing the stroke volume of the left heart and increasing the blood flow to peripheral tissues.

Craniomandibular osteopathy (also known as "lion jaw") typically occurs in West Highland white or Scottish terrier dogs. Lesions are bilaterally symmetric and consist of new periosteal bone formation, irregular resorption, and overall irregular thickening of the rami of the mandibles, the occipital and temporal bones, and, occasionally, other bones of the skull (Fig. 10-35). The tympanic bullae are often severely affected. Less commonly, new periosteal bone formation may occur on the bones of the limbs. Numerous, thin, basophilic cement lines associated with bone resorption and formation give affected bone a characteristic mosaic appearance at microscopic examination. The disease often becomes apparent at 4 to 7 months of age and can regress after some time. In affected animals, mastication is painful and difficult, and the muscles of the skull become atrophic. The etiopathogenesis of this disease is unknown.

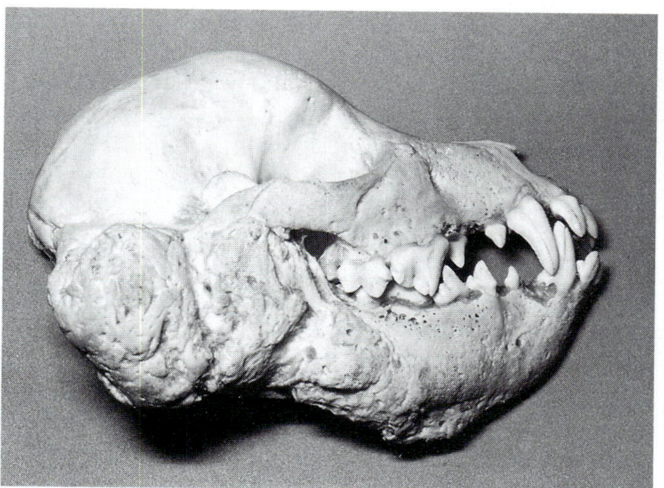

Fig. 10-35 Bone, head; dog. Craniomandibular osteopathy in a West Highland white terrier. Note extensive periosteal bone reaction, with bony bridging of the craniomandibular joint. Macerated and bleached. *Courtesy Dr. W. Riser.*

Osteochondromas (multiple cartilaginous exostoses) occur in dogs, cats, and horses and reflect a defect in skeletal development rather than a true neoplasm. This lesion is inherited in dogs and horses, and lesions are present at an early age (shortly after birth). Osteochondromas project from bony surfaces as eccentric masses that are located adjacent to metaphyseal growth plates (Fig. 10-36). They arise from long bones, ribs, vertebrae, scapulas, and bone of the pelvis and may be numerous. Microscopically, they

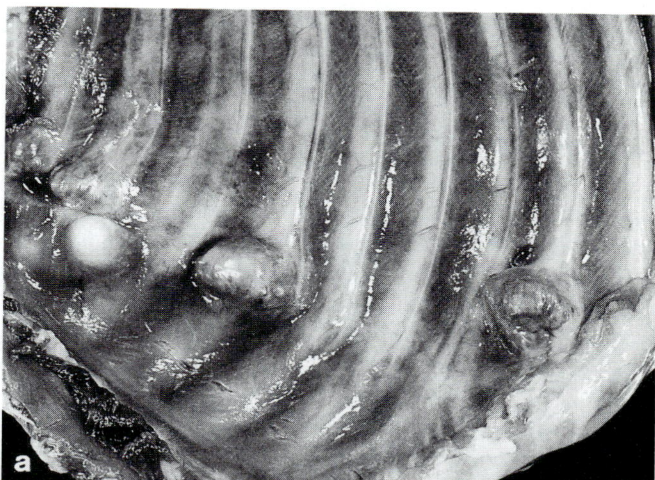

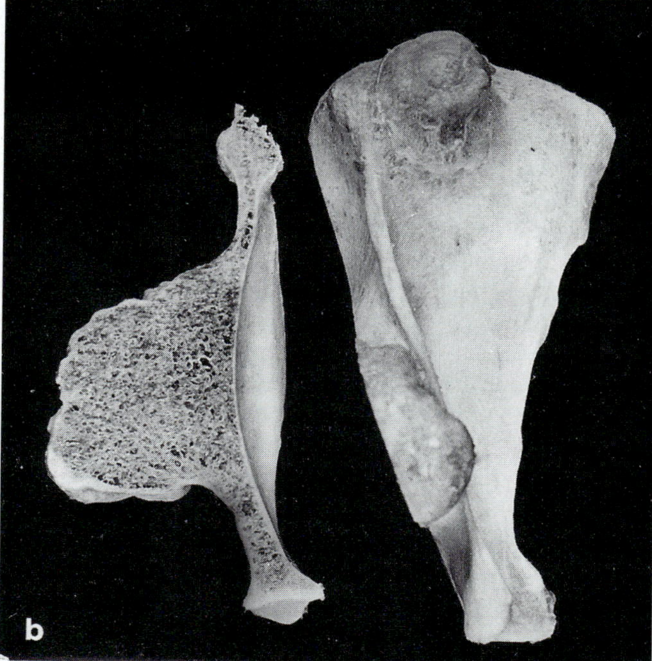

Fig. 10-36 Bone, ribs and scapula; dog. Nodules of multiple cartilaginous exostoses are present on the inner surface of the ribs, **A**. **B**, In the cross section of the scapula (left) the trabecular bone of the nodule is continuous with the medullary trabeculae of the scapula.

have an outer cap of hyaline cartilage that undergoes endochondral ossification to give rise to trabecular bone that forms the base of the lesion. Trabecular bone and bone marrow are continuous with those of the parent bone. Normally, growth ceases at skeletal maturity when the cartilage cap is replaced by bone. Although the origin of osteochondromas is not clear, some arise secondary to a defect in the perichondral ring as peripheral pieces of physeal cartilage are pinched off and carried away from the growth plate by longitudinal growth. Clinically, their importance is threefold. They might interfere mechanically with the action of tendons or ligaments; they can act as space-occupying masses that protrude into the vertebral canal and cause spinal cord compression; and they can undergo malignant transformation and give rise to chondrosarcomas. Osteochondromas in cats are different in that they develop in mature animals, tend to involve the flat bones, do not have orderly endochondral ossification and might be viral in origin. Osteochondromas in cats, like those in horses and dogs, can undergo malignant neoplastic transformation.

Fibrous dysplasia is an uncommon lesion that has been reported at various sites (skull, mandible, long bones of limbs) in several species. The lesion occurs in young dogs, may be a developmental defect, and may be single or multiple. Typically, preexisting bone is replaced by an expanding mass of fibroosseous tissue that may weaken the cortex and enlarge the normal contours of the bone. The lesion is firm, often has evidence of mineralization when sectioned, and can have multiple cysts that contain sanguinous fluid. Microscopically, well-differentiated fibrous tissue contains trabeculae of woven bone. Osteoblasts are not recognizable on trabecular surfaces, a feature that helps to distinguish this lesion from ossifying fibroma.

Bone cysts are classified as subchondral, simple, or aneurysmal. All represent expansile, lytic areas in the bone without radiographic or gross evidence of aggressive growth. Subchondral cysts are sequelae to osteochondrosis and degenerative joint disease. The category of simple bone cysts may overlap substantially with that of fibrous dysplasias, and a clear distinction between them may be artificial. Simple bone cysts may contain clear, colorless, serum-like fluid, or the contents can be markedly serosanguinous. The wall is composed of variably dense fibrous tissue and woven to lamellar bone. Bone peripheral to this has undergone modeling to accommodate the expansile growth of the cyst. Aneurysmal bone cysts consist of spaces filled with blood or serosanguinous fluid. Tissue adjacent to the spaces can vary from well-differentiated fibrous or fibroosseous tissue to marked proliferation of undifferentiated mesenchymal cells admixed with osteoclast-like multinucleated cells. Hemorrhage and hemosiderosis are frequent. An endothelial cell lining is usually not present. The cause of simple and aneurysmal bone cysts is unknown. They may be consequences of ischemic necrosis, hemorrhage, or congenital or acquired vascular malformations. Caution should be exercised in the interpretation of microscopic lesions in biopsy specimens, and these data should be correlated with radiographic findings to rule out cystic cavitation in a neoplasm before the diagnosis of bone cyst is made.

Primary neoplasms of bone

Benign neoplasms arising in the fibrous tissue of bone are not common in animals.

Ossifying fibromas are uncommon and occur as large, nodular, often heavily mineralized neoplasms on the maxillae and mandibles of horses and cattle. Although they are considered benign, they destroy adjacent cortical and trabecular bone by expansile growth. Microscopically, they are composed of well-differentiated fibrous tissue that contains scattered spicules of woven bone covered by osteoblasts (Fig. 10-37). Bone density increases with time, and, ultimately, the histologic appearance approaches that of an osteoma.

Fibrosarcomas are malignancies of fibroblasts that produce collagenous connective tissue but not bone or cartilage. Cells may be arranged in a whirling or interlacing pattern. Central fibrosarcomas arise from fibrous tissue within the medullary cavity, whereas periosteal fibrosarcomas arise from periosteal connective tissue. In general, central fibrosarcomas grow more slowly, are accompanied by less formation of reactive new bone, are slower to metastasize, and produce a smaller tissue mass than osteosarcomas. Grossly, fibrosarcomas are gray-white, fill part of the medullary cavity, and replace cancellous and cortical bone.

Chondromas are benign neoplasms of hyaline cartilage. They often arise from flat bones, are multilobulated, and have blue-white cut surface. Chondromas are uncommon neoplasms of dogs, cats, and sheep; they tend to slowly but progressively enlarge and may cause thinning of underlying bone. Microscopically, they are composed of multiple lobules of well-differentiated hyaline cartilage. Endochondral ossification of the neoplastic cartilage is possible. They are difficult to distinguish from low-grade, well-differentiated chondrosarcomas. Chondromas that arise in the medullary cavity are called enchondromas.

Chondrosarcomas are malignant neoplasms in which the neoplastic cells produce cartilaginous matrix but never osteoid or bone. They are most common in mature dogs of the large breeds and in sheep but probably occur in all species. In sheep, they arise from the ribs and sternum; in dogs, the major sites of origin are the nasal bones, ribs, and pelvis. In general, chondrosarcomas most frequently arise in the flat bones of the skeleton. Chondrosarcomas can evolve from multiple cartilaginous exostoses in dogs and in human beings. Most arise in a medullary cavity and destroy preexisting bone. Given time, they become very large, lobulated neoplasms with gray or blue-white cut surface. Some neoplasms are gelatinous on sectioning, and

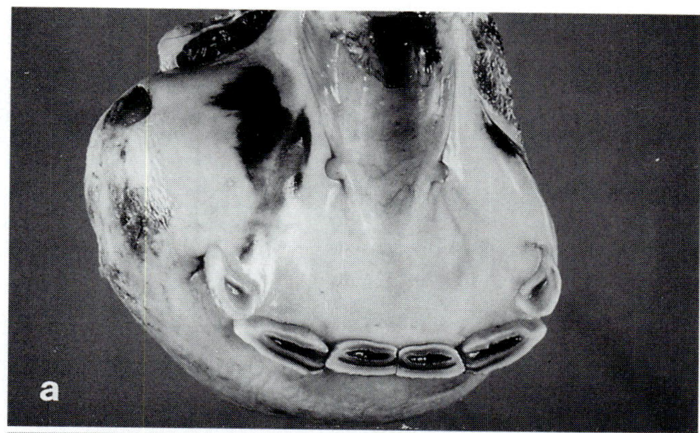

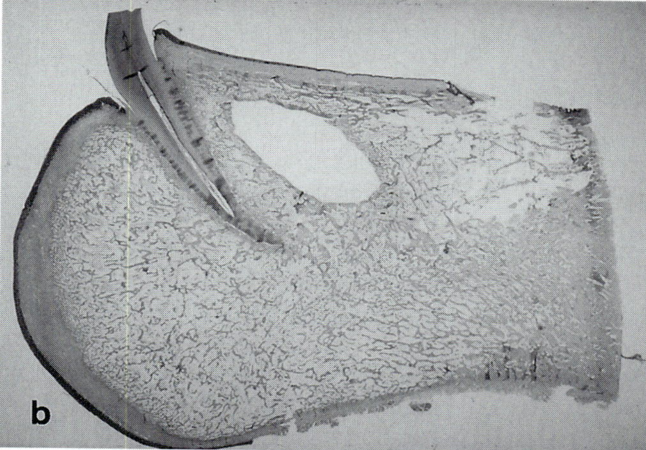

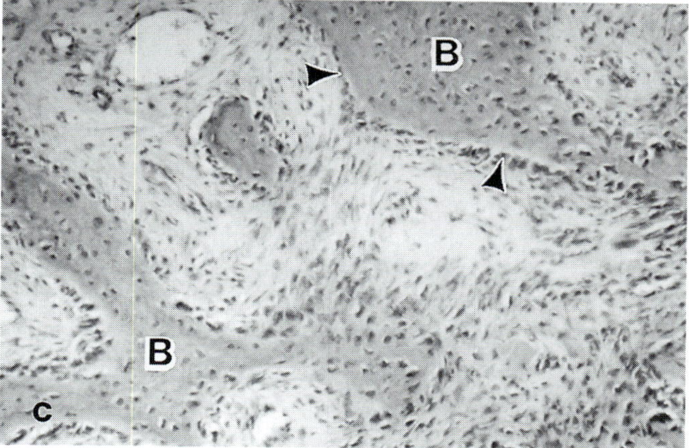

Fig. 10-37 Bone, mandible; horse. **A**, Ossifying fibroma distorts the mandible when viewed from the dorsal aspect. **B**, Low magnification. Sagittal section. The mass consists mostly of fine, bony trabeculae. **C**, High magnification. Active osteoblasts *(arrowheads)* line the trabeculae (*B*). H & E stain. *Courtesy Dr. J.C. Woodard.*

some have large areas of hemorrhage and necrosis. Microscopically, the range of differentiation of neoplastic cells is wide: some neoplasms are well differentiated and are difficult to distinguish from chondroma; other neoplasms are composed of highly anaplastic cells and have only a few areas in which differentiation into chondrocytes and chondroid matrix is apparent. Chondrosarcomas have a longer clinical course, grow more slowly, and develop metastases later than osteosarcomas.

Osteomas are uncommon benign neoplasms that usually arise from bones of the head. They occur as single, very dense masses that project from the surface of the bone. They do not invade or destroy adjacent bone; their growth is slow and progressive but not necessarily continuous. Microscopically, osteomas are covered by a thin layer of bone and are composed of cancellous bone that becomes more dense with time. Trabeculae are covered by well-differentiated osteoblasts and osteoclasts, and intertrabecular spaces contain delicate fibrous tissue, adipocytes, and hemopoietic tissue.

Osteosarcomas are malignant neoplasms in which neoplastic cells form bone and/or osteoid. They are classified as simple (bone formed in a collagenous matrix), compound (both bone and cartilage are present), or pleomorphic (anaplastic, with only small islands of osteoid present). Classification may also be based on cell type and activity (osteoblastic, chondroblastic, or fibroblastic), radiographic appearance (lytic, sclerotic, or mixed), or origin (central, juxtacortical, or periosteal). An uncommon form of osteosarcoma is the telangiectatic type that grossly resembles hemangiosarcoma. Microscopically, these neoplasms are composed of osteoblasts, osteoid, and large cystic, blood-filled cavities lined by malignant cells. Osteosarcomas are common neoplasms, comprising approximately 80% of all the primary bone neoplasms in the dog. They arise most commonly at metaphyses (distal radius, distal tibia, and proximal humerus are the most usual sites). However, they can occur in ribs, vertebrae, bones of the head, and various other parts of the skeleton. Rarely, they arise in soft tissues. Typically, they occur in mature dogs of the large and giant breeds. Growth of the neoplasm is often rapid and painful. Grossly, central or intraosseous osteosarcomas have a gray-white appearance and contain variable amounts of mineralized bone. Neoplastic tissue tends to fill the medullary cavity locally and can extend proximally and distally but, typically, does not penetrate metaphyseal growth plates. Osteosarcomas do not invade joint cavities, although they can surround a joint. Cortical bone is usually destroyed, and neoplastic cells penetrate and undermine the periosteum and can extend outwardly as an irregular lobulated mass (Fig. 10-38). Destruction of cortical bone is accompanied by varying amounts of new reactive periosteal bone. Large pale areas surrounded by zones of hemorrhage (areas of infarction) and irregular areas of hemorrhage are common in rapidly growing intramedullary neoplasms. Microscopically, variable amounts of woven bone or osteoid are visible. Bone formation can be obvious and widespread, or it can be minimal, as in anaplastic neoplasms that are composed of sheets of poorly differentiated mesenchymal cells. Neoplastic bone must be

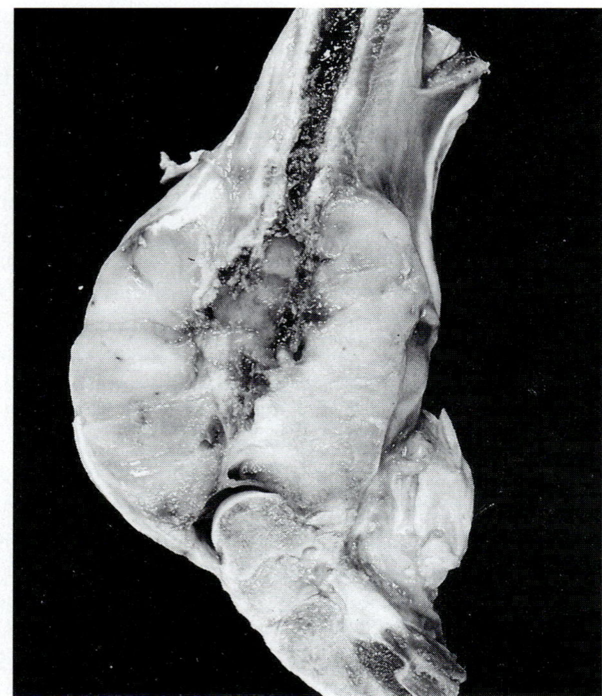

Fig. 10-38 Bone, radius; dog. An osteosarcoma has destroyed the cortices but has not bridged the joint space.

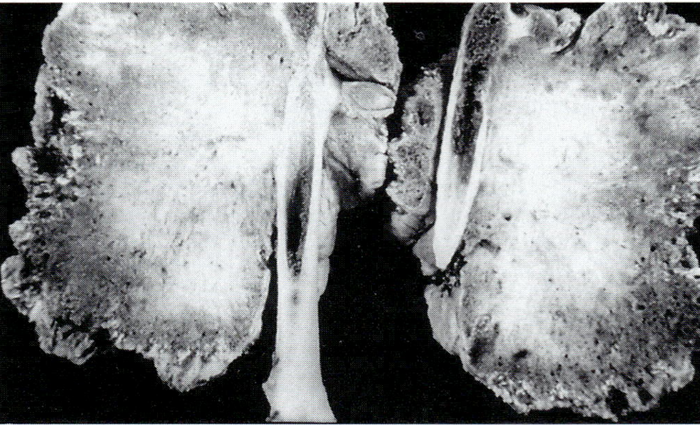

Fig. 10-39 Bone, femur; cat. A juxtacortical osteosarcoma is mostly exophytic, with little destruction of the subjacent cortex. *Courtesy Dr. S. Friend.*

distinguished from reactive bone. The cells, not the matrix, of the neoplasm must be evaluated to determine the malignancy of the neoplasm.

In terms of biologic behavior, osteosarcomas are characterized by aggressive local invasion and, except for those arising in bones of the head, early hematogenous pulmonary metastasis, which are frequently present at the time of diagnosis. Although pulmonary metastasis is common and occurs early, metastasis can be widespread and can involve both soft tissues and other bones.

The above description relates to central or intraosseous neoplasms. Osteosarcomas also may be juxtacortical (parosteal) in origin (Fig. 10-39). These neoplasms arise on the external surface of a bone and form an expansive mass that adheres to and surrounds the underlying cortex. Invasion of the shaft or metastasis is a late event, so early en-bloc excision might effect a cure. Although uncommon, these neoplasms occur in dogs and cats. It is important to distinguish these neoplasms from central osteosarcomas because parosteal osteosarcomas have a more favorable prognosis.

Multiple skeletal osteosarcomas that occur in human beings and dogs may represent a primary neoplasm that has metastasized to bone. The lesions have a random distribution, and pulmonary metastases are likely to be present. Alternatively, multiple skeletal osteosarcomas may represent a multicentric origin. In some cases, there might be no initial pulmonary metastasis, lesions have a symmetric distribution, and neoplasms appear to have arisen in metaphyses of several long bones.

Although the cause of naturally occurring osteosarcomas in human beings and animals is largely unknown, osteosarcomas can develop in association with other disease processes. Osteosarcomas have been associated with bone infarctions, previous fractures, and the use of metallic fixation devices in human beings and domestic animals. Osteosarcomas of viral origin are reported in mice.

Multilobular osteosarcomas (chondroma rodens) occur in dogs and, less commonly, in the horse. These are single, nodular, smooth-contoured, immovable masses on the flat bones of the skull. Neoplastic tissue is firm, the cut surface being composed of multiple, gray, partially mineralized foci set in a background of fibrous tissue. These neoplasms are slow growing and locally invasive; they metastasize to the lungs late in the clinical course, and the metastases are frequently small and clinically silent. The microscopic appearance consists of multiple lobules, each having centrally located cartilage or bone surrounded by plump mesenchymal cells that blend into well-differentiated interlobular fibrous tissue.

Various other neoplasms such as liposarcomas, giant cell tumors, and hemangiosarcomas may arise in bone, and neoplasms such as lymphosarcomas and plasma cell myeloma may involve the bone marrow and surrounding bone.

Secondary Neoplasms of Bone

At autopsy, 60% of (human) cancer patients have skeletal metastases. These are predominantly in red bone marrow, where the vascular sinusoidal system is vulnerable to cancer cells. The true incidence of skeletal metastasis in animals is unknown and might be very low because early euthanasia shortens the course of the disease. However, bone scanning techniques and detailed necropsies might es-

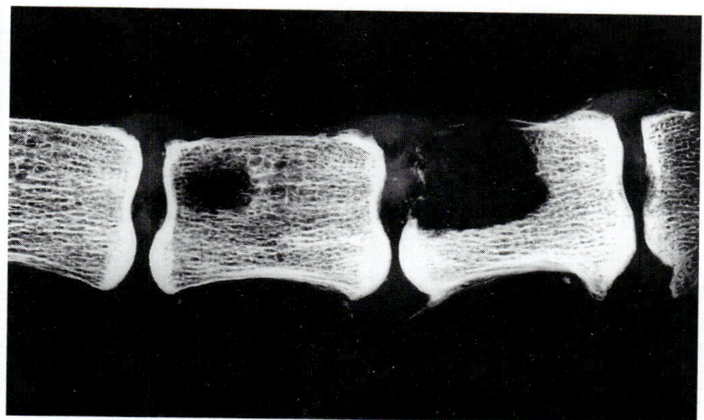

Fig. 10-40 Bone, lumbar vertebrae; dog. High-detail radiographs. Multiple foci of osteolysis due to metastatic osteosarcoma.

tablish that skeletal metastases are more common than presently estimated. Metastatic neoplasms can be associated with pain, hypercalcemia, lysis of bone, pathologic fracture, and reactive new bone formation. Rib shafts, vertebral bodies (Fig. 10-40), and humeral and femoral metaphyses are common sites of metastatic neoplasms in dogs.

DISEASES OF JOINTS

Normal Structure and Function

Joints (articulations) join skeletal structures, provide for movement, and, in some cases, have shock-absorbing functions. Most of the material in this section is confined to the synovial joints.

Synovial joints occur in both the axial and appendicular skeleton. Such joints allow for a variable degree of movement and, anatomically, are composed of two bone ends bound together by a fibrous capsule and ligaments. The inner surface of the joint capsule is lined by a synovial membrane, and the bone ends are covered by articular cartilage. The joint space contains synovial fluid and fibrocartilaginous menisci are present at some sites. Synovial joints operate with very low coefficients of friction and are self-lubricating, self-sustaining units. Articular cartilage serves as the bearing substance, subchondral bone as the supporting material. Articular cartilage functions to minimize friction created by movement, to transmit forces to underlying bone, and to maximize the contact area of the joint under load. Joints receive and absorb energy of impact. Both articular cartilage and subchondral bone deform under pressure, but it is bone and periarticular structures that have the most significant force-attenuating properties.

Articular (hyaline) cartilage is normally a white to blue-white material with a smooth, moist surface. Cartilage thickness is greatest in the young and at sites of maximum weightbearing. Thinning and yellow discoloration occur in old age. At its margins, articular cartilage merges with the periosteum and the insertion of the joint capsule. Nonarticulating depressions known as synovial fossae are often present on the articular surface (Fig. 10-41). These are normal, bilaterally symmetric structures present in the larger joints of the horse, pig, and ruminants and are easily mistaken for lesions. Articular cartilage contains no nerves or blood or lymph vessels, and its nutrition is obtained by diffusion from synovial fluid and, to a lesser extent, from subchondral vessels. In the immature skeleton, articular cartilage overlies the still growing cartilage of the epiphysis (epiphyseal cartilage). The epiphyseal cartilage will undergo endochondral ossification and, thereby, contribute to the growth of the epiphysis. Defects at the junction of the articular cartilage and epiphyseal cartilage (the articular epiphyseal complex) occur in osteochondrosis. At skeletal maturity, the epiphyseal cartilage has been replaced by a bony subchondral plate. The deeper regions of the articular cartilage mineralize and remain, as they are not removed by endochondral ossification. The junction between the unmineralized articular cartilage and the deeper mineralized cartilage is called the tidemark. The mineralized cartilage serves to anchor articular cartilage to subchondral bone and limits the diffusion of substances between bone and cartilage. Articular cartilage is 70% to 80% water by weight. It is a viscoelastic, hydrated fiber-reinforced gel that contains chondrocytes, type II collagen fibers, and proteoglycan ag-

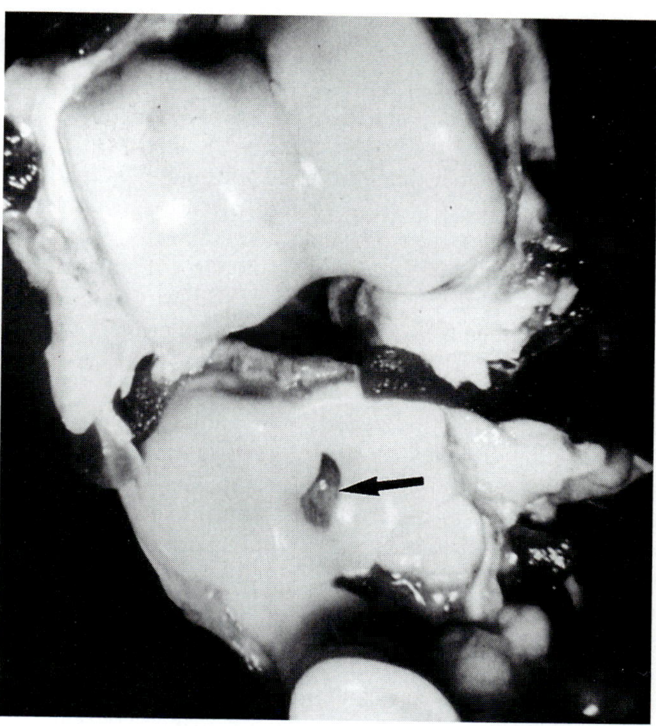

Fig. 10-41 Bone, elbow joint; pig. Disarticulated specimen. Note the normal articular surfaces. The depression in the proximal radius is a normal structure called a ''synovial fossa'' *(arrow)*.

gregates. Chondrocytes are responsible for the production, maintenance, and turnover of intercellular substances. Normal turnover is enzymatic and is balanced by enzyme inhibitors. Disease occurs if there is increased destruction or decreased synthesis of components of the matrix. It is important to remember that compared with bone, which normally renews itself by remodeling, in cartilage only the proteoglycans turn over. The cells and collagen of cartilage are infrequently, if ever, replaced. Chondrocyte mitotic activity is minimal in adult animals and cellularity of articular cartilage declines with age. Collagen fibers provide tensile strength and are arranged in arcades so that the tops of the arcades are parallel to the articular surface and the sides are perpendicular to the surface and parallel with the radial layer of chondrocytes. Proteoglycan aggregates are macromolecules composed of hyaluronic acid and protein cores and attach to glycosaminoglycan molecules of keratin and chondroitin sulfate. By binding water, proteoglycans provide stiffness to resist compression and impede the outflow of water when cartilage is under load. Functionally, the superficial zone of articular cartilage resists shearing forces, the middle zone functions in shock absorption, and the base serves to attach articular cartilage to the bone. In scanning electron micrographs, the surface of articular cartilage is not smooth but rather has numerous depressions that may serve as reservoirs for synovial fluid.

Joint lubrication depends on the microscopic roughness, elasticity, and hydration of articular cartilage and on the presence of mucin (hyaluronate and glycoprotein) in synovial fluid. Lubrication of the synovial membrane itself is hyaluronate-mediated boundary lubrication. Lubrication of articular cartilage is accomplished by the complementary action of weeping (squeeze-film) and boundary lubrication. In weeping lubrication, the loaded articular surface is supplied with pressurized fluid that carries most of the load. Only a small part is carried by cartilage-to-cartilage surface contact, which is lubricated by a glycoprotein-facilitated boundary system. Boundary lubrication implies that a substance sticks to the surface and minimizes contact. Joint stiffness is often due to inability of periarticular soft tissues to lengthen, rather than to intraarticular friction.

The joint capsule consists of outer fibrous and inner synovial tissue layers. The outer layer is a heavy sheath that contributes to joint stability and attaches to bone at its insertion at the margins of the joint and, thereby, encloses a segment of bone of variable length within the joint cavity. It is well supplied by blood vessels and nerve endings. The synovial membrane covers all the inner surfaces of the joints except for that of the surface of the articular cartilage. The synovial membrane is normally a very thin membrane, barely visible to the naked eye. Tiny surface projections (villi) are normally present and are more prominent in some areas than in others. Synovial intimal or lining cells, one to four cells thick, form a discontinuous surface layer. They are designated as "A" cells (phagocytic cells that produce hyaluronate); "B" cells (fibroblast-like cells, rich in rough endoplasmic reticulum), which may produce glycoprotein; and "intermediate" cells, which have some of the characteristics of both. A cells are of bone marrow origin and may be part of the monocyte-macrophage cell system. The synovial subintima may be classified according to the type of predominant tissue (areolar, adipose, or fibrous). It contains blood and lymph vessels that supply and drain the intraarticular structures. Adipose tissue sometimes accumulates within the synovium, forming fat pads that serve as soft cushions in joint cavities.

Synovial fluid is a protein-free dialysate of plasma that nurtures and lubricates intraarticular structures. Normally, it is a clear, colorless to pale yellow, viscous fluid.

Postmortem Examination and Evaluation

Several large synovial joints should be opened and examined routinely at necropsy. If the clinical history suggests disease in any one joint, all the articular and periarticular structures of that joint should be examined in detail. Joints should be disarticulated so that articular surfaces, synovial fluid, and all associated structures are clearly visible. Articular cartilage must be examined as soon as the joint is opened, because dehydration of cartilage occurs rapidly on exposure to air. Villous hypertrophy is best evaluated if the specimen is submerged in water. Microscopic examination of synovium might be required to confirm the presence of synovitis. The joint fluid can be collected and centrifuged, and the resulting pellet cultured for bacteria. Joint fluid is readily contaminated with blood when joints are opened, and this should not be confused with hemarthrosis. Thin, longitudinal, sagittal slabs of tissue that contain articular cartilage, subchondral bone, the joint capsule, and its insertion should be collected for microscopic examination.

Reactions to Injury

Although articular cartilage contains metabolically active cells, it has a limited response to injury and minimal capacity for repair. Superficial cartilage defects that do not penetrate into subchondral bone persist for long periods. Clusters or clones of chondrocytes (evidence of local chondrocyte replication) are present but are ineffective in filling the defect. Some flow or spreading of cartilaginous matrix into the defect might also occur. This phenomenon of matrix flow is likely facilitated by loadbearing and joint movement. In short, superficial injuries to articular cartilage neither heal nor necessarily progress, although progression can occur when there is stiffened subchondral bone. However, if a cartilaginous defect extends into subchondral bone, the defect is quickly filled with vascular fibrous tissue that often undergoes metaplasia to fibrocartilage. Repair by the formation of true hyaline cartilage is infrequent. Formation of fibrocartilage can be hastened in full-thickness cartilaginous defects by exercise or continuous pas-

Table 10-2. Summary of some of the cells and substances involved in joint injury

Substance	Source	Action
Prostaglandin E_2	Macrophage Synovial fibroblast	Inhibits proteoglycan synthesis Promotes fever, pain and inflammation
Interleukin-1	Type A synovial cells Macrophage in synovium or pannus	Attract B- and T-lymphocytes Stimulate synovial fibroblasts to produce PGE_2 and collagenase Stimulate synovial cells and chondrocytes to produce proteases
Neutral proteases	Chondrocytes Inflammatory cells in synovial membrane Synovial lining cells	Attack protein core of proteoglycan aggregates Damage tendon and ligaments
Superoxide radical and H_2O_2	Monocytes Granulocytes	Degrade of hyaluronic acid, collagen, and cartilage

sive motion. Injury to articular cartilage is not painful unless the synovium or subchondral bone is involved. Having no blood supply, articular cartilage does not participate in the inflammatory response, although it can be injured by inflammation in nearby synovial tissue. Given that the alternate compression and release of normal weightbearing facilitates the diffusion of fluid and nutrients into and out of articular cartilage, it follows that constant compression or lack of weightbearing leads to thinning of articular cartilage.

Examples of mediators of injury to articular cartilage and their origin are presented in Table 10-2. Sterile injury to cartilage can be a consequence of trauma, joint instability, or lubrication failure because of changes in synovial fluid and synovial membrane. Lysosomal enzymes (collagenase, cathepsins, elastase, arylsulfatase) and neutral proteases, which are capable of degrading proteoglycan or collagen, can be derived from inflammatory cells, synovial lining cells, and chondrocytes. Intraarticular PGE_2 concentrations are increased in degenerative and inflammatory joint disease. These substances inhibit proteoglycan synthesis and mediate loss of articular cartilage. Interleukin-1 is a cytokine secreted by stimulated macrophages (synovial type A cells or subintimal macrophages); it stimulates secretion of prostaglandins and neutral proteases from synovial fibroblasts and chondrocytes, thereby increasing the degradation of proteoglycans of the cartilage. The loss of proteoglycans from cartilage alters the hydraulic permeability of the cartilage, thereby interfering with joint lubrication and leading to further mechanically-induced injury to cartilage. Enzymatic injury to cartilage also occurs in bacterial arthritis, in immune-mediated arthritis such as rheumatoid arthritis, in hemarthrosis, and in some types of degenerative joint disease.

The loss of proteoglycans, with subsequent inadequate lubrication of the articular surface, leads to disruption of collagen fibers on the surface of articular cartilage. Affected areas of cartilage are yellow-brown and have a dull, slightly roughened appearance. As more proteoglycans are lost, the collagen fibers condense, and fraying of surface

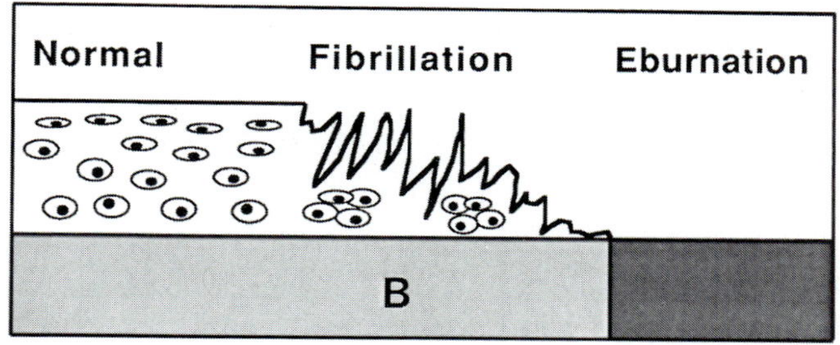

Fig. 10-42 Diagram showing the structural changes that characterize fibrillation of articular cartilage and eburnation of subchondral bone. Subchondral bone (*B*) is dense (eburnated) in the area where the overlying cartilage is completely ulcerated.

collagen fibers extends along the sides of the arcades as multiple vertical clefts (fibrillation). Fibrillation is accompanied by surface loss, overall thinning of articular cartilage, necrosis of some chondrocytes, and attempted, but ineffective, regenerative hyperplasia of chondrocytes (chondrone formation). Loss of articular cartilage can become complete with exposure of subchondral bone (ulceration). Continued rubbing on subchondral bone causes it to become dense, polished, and ivory-like (eburnation) (Fig. 10-42).

Degenerative changes in articular cartilage are often accompanied by the formation of periarticular osteophytes and by some degree of synovial inflammation and hyperplasia. The synovitis is characterized by the presence of variable numbers of plasma cells, lymphocytes, and macrophages in the synovial subintima and the accumulation of hemosiderin-laden macrophages, and by hyperplasia and hypertrophy of synovial lining cells. Osteophytes form as multiple outgrowths of dense trabecular or compact bone, and originate at or near the junctional zone—the zone where articular cartilage, periosteum, and the insertion of the joint capsule merge. Osteophytes do not grow continuously, but once formed, they persist as multiple periarticular spurs of bone that cause joint enlargement (see Figs. 10-48 and 10-51). Osteophytes can also arise sec-

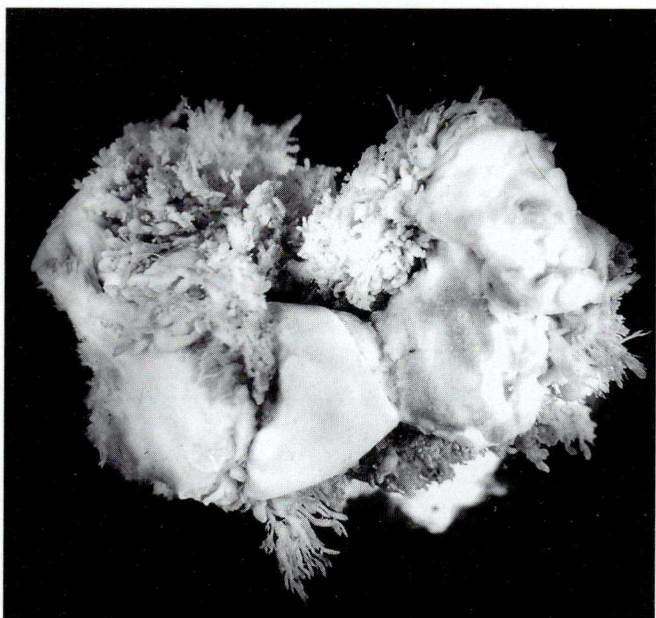

Fig. 10-43 Bone, distal humerus; dog. Hyperplasia and hypertrophy of the synovium. The synovial membrane has formed numerous thickened villi. These are dramatic when seen floating in a fluid medium, as in this example photographed submerged in water.

ondarily to the stretching or tearing of the insertions of the joint capsule or ligaments.

The synovial membrane commonly responds to injury by villous hypertrophy and hyperplasia, hypertrophy of lining cells, and pannus formation. Villous hypertrophy (Fig. 10-43) occurs with and without synovitis. The proportions of A and B cells in the synovium also may change in various disease processes. Fragments of articular cartilage may adhere to the synovium, where they are surrounded by macrophages and giant cells. Larger pieces of detached cartilage (as in osteochondrosis) can float free and survive as ''joint mice'' that continue to be nurtured by synovial fluid. Inflammatory cell infiltration in the synovial membrane may impair fluid drainage from the joint, and joint fluid may lose some of its lubricating properties because hyaluronic acid may be degraded by the superoxide-generating systems of neutrophils.

Pannus may develop in association with chronic infectious nonsuppurative synovitis and with some immune-mediated diseases, such as rheumatoid arthritis. Pannus is a fibrovascular and histiocytic tissue that arises from the insertion of the synovial membrane and spreads over adjacent cartilage as a velvety membrane. The histiocytes transform into macrophages, and, they, along with the collagenases from the fibroblasts cause lysis of cartilage. As the pannus spreads, the underlying cartilage is destroyed. In time, if both opposing cartilaginous surfaces are involved, the fibrous tissue can unite the surfaces, causing fibrous ankylosis (immobilization) of the joint. Pannus can also arise from subchondral marrow and dissect the cartilage from the subchondral bone.

Glucocorticoids are sometimes injected into joints for their antiinflammatory effect. Injection is sometimes followed by the rapid progression of degenerative changes within the joint and is designated ''steroid arthropathy.'' These degenerative changes relate to the antianabolic effects of glucocorticoids on chondrocytes. They reduce the synthesis of cartilaginous matrix, lead to proteoglycan depletion, retard repair, and reduce the mechanical strength of cartilage.

Marked modeling of the osseous and cartilaginous components of the joint can occur over time in chronic diseases. This is secondary to changes in weightbearing and altered mechanical use. Cartilage is capable of dramatic alterations in structure, but yet it is inadequate at repair.

Abnormalities of Growth and Development

A number of congenital neuromuscular disorders that are characterized by restricted articular movement occur in animals. In many cases, this restriction can be relieved by sectioning tendons or the joint capsule. Congenital malformation of articular surfaces or fusion of joints is uncommon; the former can be secondary to restricted articular movement. Restricted or reduced articular movement can be mild and self-correcting or can be severe and crippling. The term ''arthrogryposis'' implies persistent congenital flexure or contraction of a joint. It has been associated with inactivity or paralysis of the fetus in utero, spinal dysraphism, maternal ingestion of poisonous plants (lupine poisoning in cattle, poison hemlock *[Conium maculatum]* in swine), and intrauterine viral infections (Akabane virus and bluetongue virus) in cattle and sheep. Alkaloids in poison hemlock (coniine) and lupine plants (anagyrine) are believed to cause sustained contraction of uterine muscle, and fetal deformity might be due to external compression and reduced fetal movement. Arthrogryposis in cattle can be associated with other lesions such as scoliosis, torticollis, and cleft palate. A syndrome of arthrogryposis and palatoschisis occurs in Charolais cattle as a congenital, inherited, neuromuscular disorder characterized by congenital articular rigidity, muscular hypotonia, and limbs being fixed in either flexion or extension.

Hip dysplasia occurs in dogs and in cattle. In the dog, it is a major inherited (polygenic) orthopedic problem and is most common in large and giant breeds. Many different theories regarding the etiopathogenesis have been advanced, but most agree that it is a biomechanical disease in which inadequate muscle mass leads to joint laxity (instability) and, eventually, to degenerative joint disease. The lesions are not present at birth, but can be well advanced by 1 year of age. The severity of the lesions varies but can be reduced by restricting the rate of skeletal growth. Joint laxity, subluxation, and flattening of the dorsal rim of the

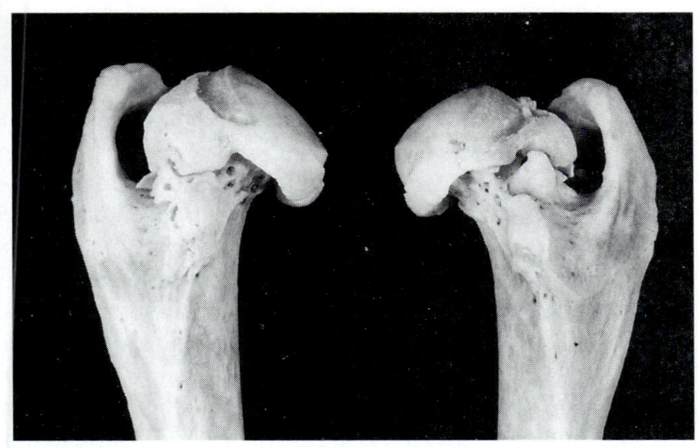

Fig. 10-44 Bone, femur; dog. Hip dysplasia. The femoral heads are markedly flattened, with prominent osteophyte formation at the periphery, resulting in bony "lipping." Macerated and bleached.

acetabulum lead to a shallow but wide acetabulum. In time, the lesions consist of erosion of articular cartilage, eburnation of underlying bone, malformation of articular surfaces, and formation of periarticular osteophytes (Fig. 10-44). The joint capsule is stretched and thickened, and areas of osseous and cartilaginous metaplasia can develop within it. The round ligament of the femoral head can rupture, and luxation can occur. Hip dysplasia, which might be inherited, also occurs in bulls of some beef breeds. Affected animals have a shallow acetabulum, joint laxity, and instability, which lead to degenerative joint disease early in life.

Inflammatory Lesions

The term **arthritis** implies inflammation of intraarticular structures, while the term **synovitis** is restricted to inflammation of the synovium. Arthritis is characterized by the presence of inflammatory cells in the synovial membrane, but the nature of the inflammatory process is often reflected in the volume and character of the joint fluid. Joint diseases are classified as inflammatory or noninflammatory, in recognition of the fact that sometimes striking secondary lymphohistiocytic synovitis occurs in "noninflammatory" diseases such as degenerative joint disease. Arthritis can be classified as to cause, duration, and the nature of the exudate produced (serous, fibrinous, purulent, lymphoplasmacytic). The term "arthropathy" is all-encompassing and refers to any joint disease. Like osteomyelitis, arthritis can be a serious threat to the well-being of an animal. It is painful and can lead to permanent deformity and crippling. Synovitis can be due to the intraarticular localization of an infectious agent, to the presence of foreign material such as urates in gout, or to trauma to intraarticular structures; or it can be partially or entirely immune mediated. Chronicity can be due to an inability of the animal to remove the causative agent or substance, repeated trauma, persistence of bacterial cell wall material, or ongoing immune-mediated processes. Injury to intraarticular structure can be directly due to the offending agent or substance, to the inflammatory process, or to proteolytic enzymes released from cells of cartilage or synovial tissues. Varying degrees of defective joint lubrication, degeneration of cartilage, synovial cell injury, and impaired synovial fluid drainage can be observed. Various substances associated with inflammation (prostaglandins, interleukins, neutrophilic lysosomal enzymes, and products of the activated coagulation, kinin, complement, and fibrinolytic systems in synovial fluid) have the potential to injure intraarticular structures.

Bacterial arthritis is uncommon in dogs and cats but is common in food animals, where it is often hematogenous and polyarticular. Neonatal bacteremia secondary to omphalitis or oral-intestinal entry commonly leads to polyarthritis in lambs, calves, piglets, and foals. Bacteria can also reach the joint by direct inoculation, as in a puncture wound, by direct extension from periarticular soft tissues, or by extension from bone. Bacterial-induced osteomyelitis can extend through the metaphyseal cortex into the joint, or epiphyseal osteomyelitis can lyse directly through articular cartilage. The duration of bacterial arthritis is variable. Some organisms are rapidly removed, and synovitis is short-lived. In other instances, bacteria can persist, and the inflammatory process can become chronic. In some cases, it is postulated that the initial bacterial synovitis can lead to chronic immune-mediated arthritis because of cross-reactivity between antigens in the breakdown products of bacterial cell walls and normal antigens within the joint. In addition, there appears to be cross-reactivity between bacterial heat-shock proteins and articular glycosaminoglycans. These concepts are significant for they explain how an arthritis that began as an infectious process might persist as a sterile immune-mediated one. The extent and mechanism of cartilaginous destruction differ in fibrinous and purulent arthritis. Acute fibrinous arthritis is characterized by synovitis and deposition of fibrin within the synovial membrane and on the surface of intraarticular structures. The process can resolve early with complete fibrinolysis and repair without residual defects. However, if deposits of fibrin are extensive, they can be invaded and replaced by fibrous tissue, leading to restricted articular movement (Fig. 10-45). Fibrinous arthritis of long duration is often accompanied by marked villous hypertrophy, pannus formation, and progressive destruction of cartilage. In summary, articular cartilage can remain intact in fibrinous arthritis unless destroyed by pannus. In contrast, purulent arthritis is accompanied by progressive and often extensive lysis (necrosis) of articular cartilage, with the process commonly extending into adjacent subchondral bone. Proteolytic enzymes derived from large numbers of neutrophils present in the joint are likely responsible. *Actinobacillus pyogenes* is a common cause of purulent arthritis in cattle and swine.

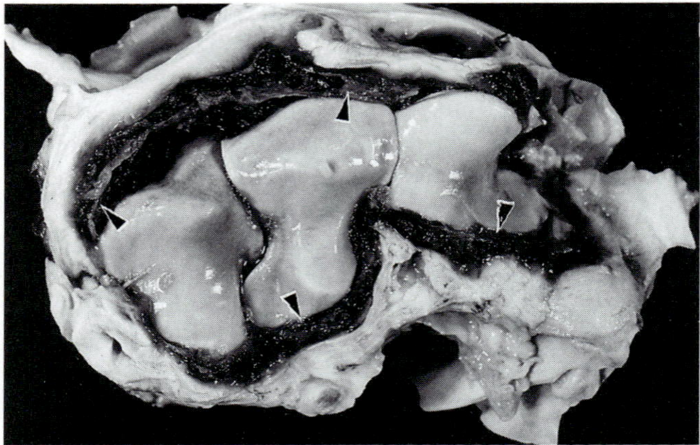

Fig. 10-45 Bone, carpus; cow. Fibrinous synovitis with fibrin *(arrowheads)* limited to the synovium at the periphery of the joint.

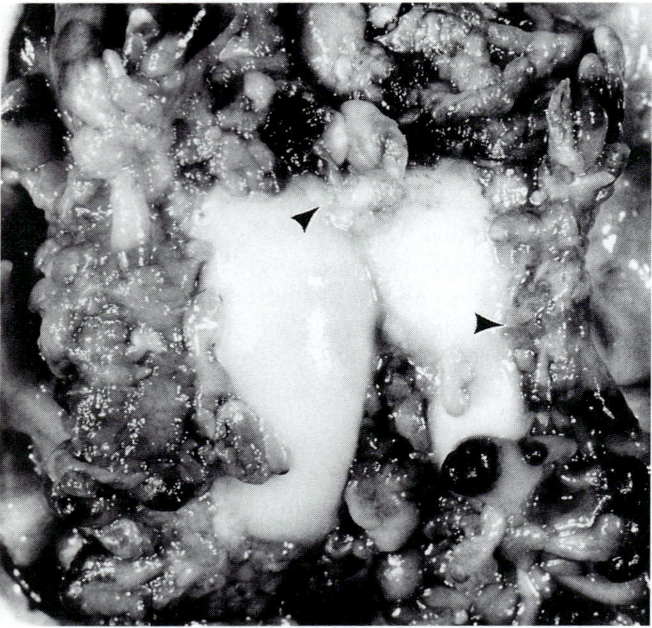

Fig. 10-46 Bone, distal femur; pig. Chronic fibrinous synovitis due to *Erysipelothrix rhusiopathiae* has villous hypertrophy of the synovial membrane and pannus formation *(arrowheads)*. Hemorrhage and necrosis characterize the tips of some villi. *Courtesy Dr. K. Johnston.*

Erysipelothrix rhusiopathiae causes septicemia in swine. Survivors can have lesions associated with localization of the organism in the skin, synovial joints, valvular endocardium, or intervertebral disks. Chronic painful polyarthritis is a common sequela. Initially, the arthritis is fibrinous, and, later, it is lymphoplasmacytic with marked villous hypertrophy of the synovial membrane (Fig. 10-46). Pannus formation, accompanied by destruction of articular cartilage, and fibrous ankylosis of joints can occur. Localization of the organism in the terminal vessels of the annulus fibrosus of the intervertebral disks is common and leads to inflammation and destruction of the vertebral disks, followed by fibrous replacement of the vertebral disks and surrounding structures (discospondylitis).

Many different infectious agents cause arthritis in animals. For example, *Escherichia coli* and streptococci cause septicemia in neonatal calves and piglets and localize in joints, meninges, and, sometimes, serosal surfaces. Synovitis is acutely serofibrinous and often becomes more purulent with time. *Haemophilus parasuis* causes Glasser's disease in swine 8 to 16 weeks of age. Lesions consist of fibrinous polyserositis, polyarthritis, and meningitis. Acute serofibrinous polyarthritis is seen frequently in cattle dying of thromboembolic meningoencephalitis caused by *H. somnus. Mycoplasma bovis* causes fibrinous polyarthritis in feedlot cattle, and the disease is characterized by lameness and swelling of the large synovial joints of the limbs that can contain large volumes of serofibrinous exudate. *M. hyorhinis* causes fibrinous polyarthritis and polyserositis in weanling swine. Chronic cases can develop pannus formation and synovial villous hypertrophy. *M. hyosynoviae* causes polyarthritis in older (more than 3 months old) swine.

The caprine arthritis-encephalitis virus (a retrovirus) causes chronic arthritis in older goats. The disease is characterized by debilitating lameness, carpal hygromas, and distention of major synovial joints. Advanced cases have marked synovial villous hypertrophy with necrosis and mineralization and mononuclear cell infiltration, pannus formation, and destruction of articular cartilage.

Arthritis in the dog is often classified as erosive or nonerosive. Rheumatoid arthritis in the dog is an uncommon, chronic, erosive polyarthritis that resembles the disease in human beings. In human beings and dogs, the cause is unknown, although it is clear that the process is immune mediated (involves humoral and cell-mediated immunity). Antibodies (rheumatoid factor) of the IgG or IgM classes are produced in response to an unknown stimulus. Alterations in the stearic configuration of IgG, persistent bacterial cell wall components that cross-react with normal proteoglycans, anticollagen antibodies, and defective suppressor T cell activity are factors that might be involved. Immune complexes are ingested by neutrophils. These release lysosomal enzymes, which sustain the inflammatory reaction and injure intraarticular structures. Additionally, interleukin-1 is released from synovial type A cells and from macrophages in a pannus and in subsurface areas of the synovial membrane. This cytokine stimulates chondrocytes and the synovial cells and macrophages themselves to release substances that degrade cartilaginous matrix and also stimulate synovial fibroblasts to produce PGE_2. The prostoglandin reduces chondrocyte proteoglycan synthesis and contributes to the production of pain, fever, and intraarticular inflammation. Cytotoxic T cells are also found in the joint fluids in rheumatoid arthritis. Antibodies against normal and altered collagen from articular cartilage are present in human cases of rheumatoid arthritis and might be important mediators of the ongoing joint inflammation and injury that occur in this disease. In dogs, rheumatoid arthritis is characterized by progressive lameness involving the peripheral joints of the limbs. Grossly, the lesions consist of marked villous hypertrophy of the synovial membrane, erosion of cartilage, pannus formation, formation of periarticular osteophytes, and, when severe, fibrous ankylosis of affected joints. Microscopically, the alterations are hyperplasia of synovial lining cells as well as infiltration of large numbers of plasma cells and lymphocytes into the subsurface synovium. Foci of necrosis, exudation of fibrin, and infiltration of neutrophils indicate that the process is chronic but active. Large numbers of neutrophils are present in the joint fluid.

Chronic nonerosive arthritis occurs in dogs with systemic lupus erythematosus, and such dogs may have anemia, thrombocytopenia, polymyositis, or glomerulonephritis. Nonerosive polyarthritis also occurs in dogs in association with chronic disease processes such as pyometra or otitis externa. Immune complexes may localize in joints and lead to local intraarticular inflammation. In these diseases, villous hypertrophy is minimal, pannus formation does not occur, and destruction of articular cartilage is not to be expected. The exudate in these diseases is neutrophilic, with only a small lymphocytic component.

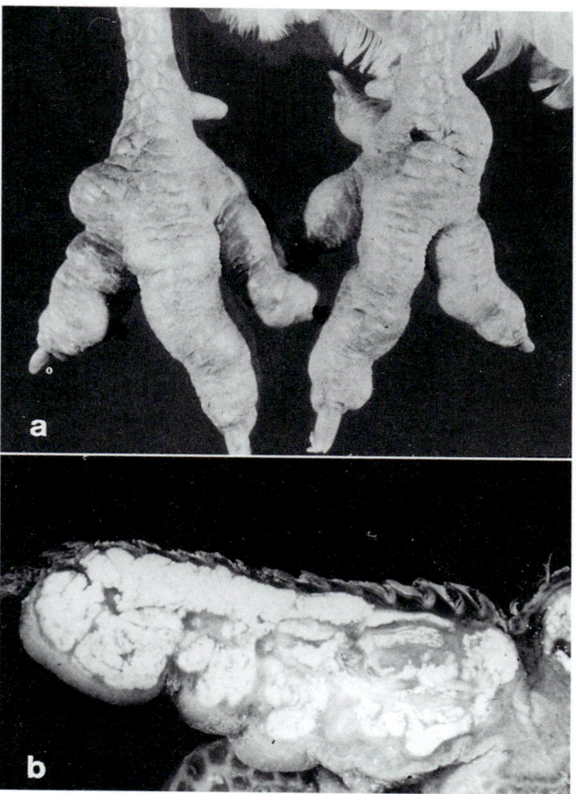

Fig. 10-47 Bone, digits; bird. A, The joints are swollen with uric acid deposits, which on cross section (B) can be seen as white, pasty material.

Crystal-induced synovitis and degeneration of articular cartilage occur in gout when urate crystals are deposited in and around joints in which they incite an acute or chronic inflammatory reaction. Gout occurs in species that do not have the enzyme uricase (human beings, birds, reptiles). Deposits of urate, called tophi, are white, caseous, and periarticular foci and can be grossly visible (Fig. 10-47). Periarticular and intraarticular deposits of calcium pyrophosphate (pseudogout or calcium pyrophosphate deposition disease) and calcium phosphate (calcium phosphate deposition disease) have been reported as a cause of synovitis and lameness in dogs and nonhuman primates. Single or multiple joints can be involved.

Degenerative Joint Disease

Degenerative joint disease (osteoarthritis, osteoarthrosis) is an ancient disease of synovial joints that occurs in all animals with a bony skeleton. It is a destructive disease of articular cartilage characterized by focal erosion and fibrillation of articular cartilage, formation of osteophytes, and osteochondral modeling. It can be monoarticular or polyarticular, can occur in immature or mature animals, and can be symptomatic or represent an incidental finding. Affected animals have variable degrees of joint enlargement and deformity, pain, and articular malfunction. The etiopathogenesis of degenerative joint disease is incompletely understood, and it is likely that the term encompasses a variety of diseases that have a common end stage. Initial changes might occur as injury to articular cartilage, inflammation of the synovium, or increased stiffness of the subchondral bone. The progression of degenerative joint disease is often associated with sclerosis of subchondral bone; but some investigators consider stiffness in subchondral bone as the initial lesion, and this stiffness predisposes the cartilage to mechanical damage. The initial change in articular cartilage is loss of proteoglycan aggregates, which leads to improper binding of water and a net increase in the water content of the cartilage. The increased water and its improper binding lead to softening (chondromalacia). Core proteins of proteoglycan aggregates are susceptible to the action of neutral proteoglycanases, which are increased in early degenerative joint disease. In electron micrographs, the findings include focal loss of the amorphous layer covering the surface and fraying of the superficial collagen fibers. Proteoglycan loss interferes with joint lubrication and allows further mechanical disruption of fibers and vertical cleft formation (fibrillation). Loss (erosion) of cartilage may be progressive, and, eventually, ulceration of the cartilage exposes the underlying subchondral bone (Fig. 10-42). With use of the joint, the subchondral bone becomes smooth and hard (eburnation and sclerosis). Subchondral bone cysts can develop in degenerative joint dis-

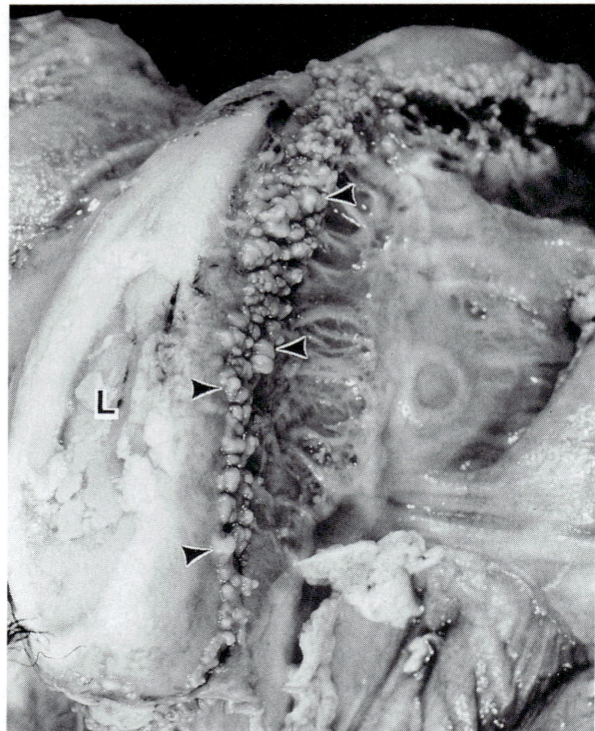

Fig. 10-48 Bone, femur; cow. Degenerative joint disease of the lateral trochlear ridge. Note extensive loss (*L*) of articular cartilage and numerous small, periarticular osteophytes *(arrowheads).*

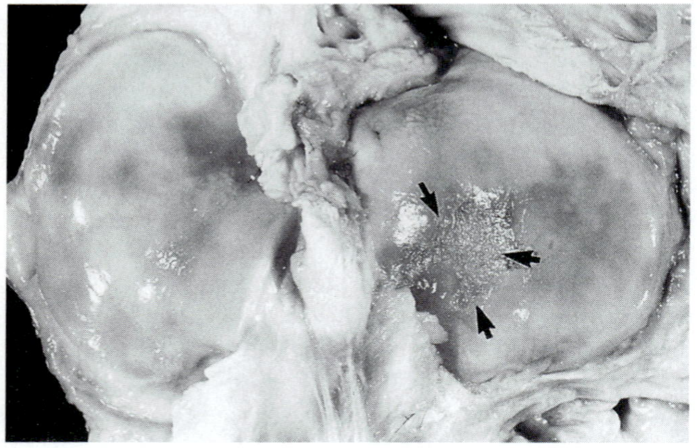

Fig. 10-49 Bone, tibia; horse. The proximal condyles have areas *(outlined by arrows)* of degeneration of cartilage that are roughened and discolored and have softened the cartilage (chondromalacia and fibrillation).

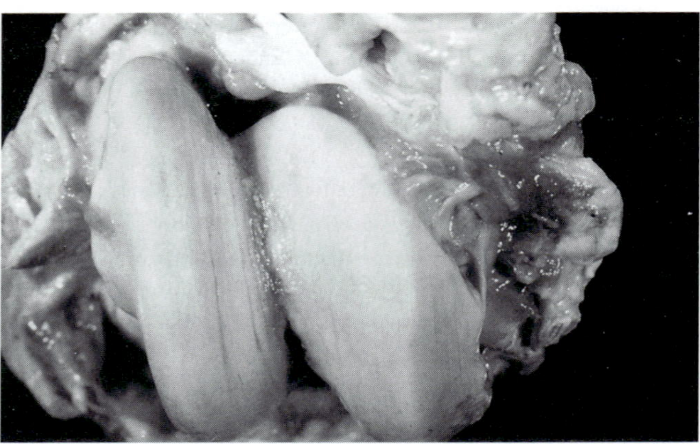

Fig. 10-50 Bone, tibial tarsal; horse. Degenerative joint disease. Linear erosions are present on the articular surface.

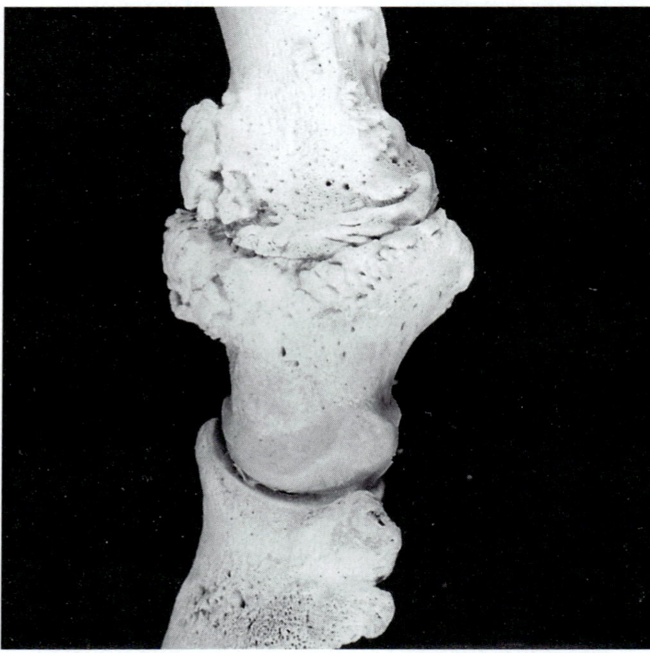

Fig. 10-51 Bone, phalanges; horse. Extensive osteophytic formation due to degenerative joint disease of the interphalangeal joint, called ''ring-bone'' in the horse. Macerated and bleached.

ease, but these are less common in animals than in human beings. The pathogenesis of cyst formation on weight-bearing surfaces is not understood. Marginal (periarticular) osteophytes (Figs. 10-48 and 10-51) are a prominent feature, and synovitis is characterized by villous hypertrophy, hyperplasia of lining cells, and infiltration of plasma cells, lymphocytes, and macrophages. Synovitis occurs secondarily to the release of cartilaginous breakdown products and their phagocytosis by synovial lining cells. Proteases released by cells of the inflamed synovium cause additional joint injury. Grossly, degenerate cartilage initially has a matte finish associated with focal softening and fibrillation and often is yellow or yellow-brown (Fig. 10-49). Lesions can be diffuse but often are focal; in hinge-type joints, they can occur as linear grooves (Fig. 10-50). Advanced lesions can have marked modeling of the subchondral and metaphyseal bone (Fig. 10-51).

Age-related degeneration of articular cartilage is common in all species and can be of minimal clinical significance. Lesions are of greatest importance when they occur at an early age and progress rapidly. Some of the causative factors that have been implicated in the evolution of degenerative joint disease include repeated trauma to articular cartilage, abnormalities in conformation, joint instability, and joint incongruence. In addition, degeneration of cartilage occurs secondary to inflammatory arthritis and diseases such as osteochondrosis that disrupt the articular surface.

Osteochondrosis

The osteochondroses consist of a heterogeneous group of lesions in cartilage of growing animals and are characterized by focal or multifocal failure (or delay) of endochondral ossification. As such, osteochondrosis involves the metaphyseal growth plate and the articular-epiphyseal cartilage complex. The diseases are common and represent an important orthopedic entity that has a number of different clinical manifestations in poultry, pigs, dogs, horses, cattle, and rats. The broad term "dyschondroplasia" implies defective cartilaginous growth and includes the lesions of osteochondrosis. Many authors have pointed out that the word "osteochondrosis," which implies degeneration of cartilage and bone, is inappropriate because the lesions are primarily in the cartilage. Lesions of osteochondrosis are often multiple and bilaterally symmetric; in swine, suspected precursor lesions can be identified shortly after birth of the pigs. Some lesions undergo rapid and complete repair. Others can progress to clinically detectable disease.

In the simplest form of osteochondrosis, lesions appear grossly as white, often wedge-shaped areas of retained cartilage in the metaphyseal growth plate and in the articular-epiphyseal cartilage complex (Fig. 10-52). Microscopically, these areas are composed of hypertrophic, sometimes poorly aligned chondrocytes without evidence of mineralization or vascular invasion. Necrosis of cartilage associated with degenerative and necrotic changes in vessels in the cartilage canals has been proposed as the early lesions of osteochondrosis. However, similar changes have been observed in pigs that do not develop osteochondrosis. Focal disruption of endochondral ossification and longitudinal bone growth has the potential to alter the shape of articular surface and, subsequently, may be responsible for angular limb deformities. In a similar manner, alteration of articular surfaces might lead to joint incongruence and predispose to the development of degenerative joint disease. It has also been proposed that osteochondrosis might play a role in the maldevelopment of articular surfaces that occurs in hip dysplasia and in the equine "wobbler syndrome."

Clefts can develop in these region of retained cartilage. These clefts might form along lines of necrosis, possibly

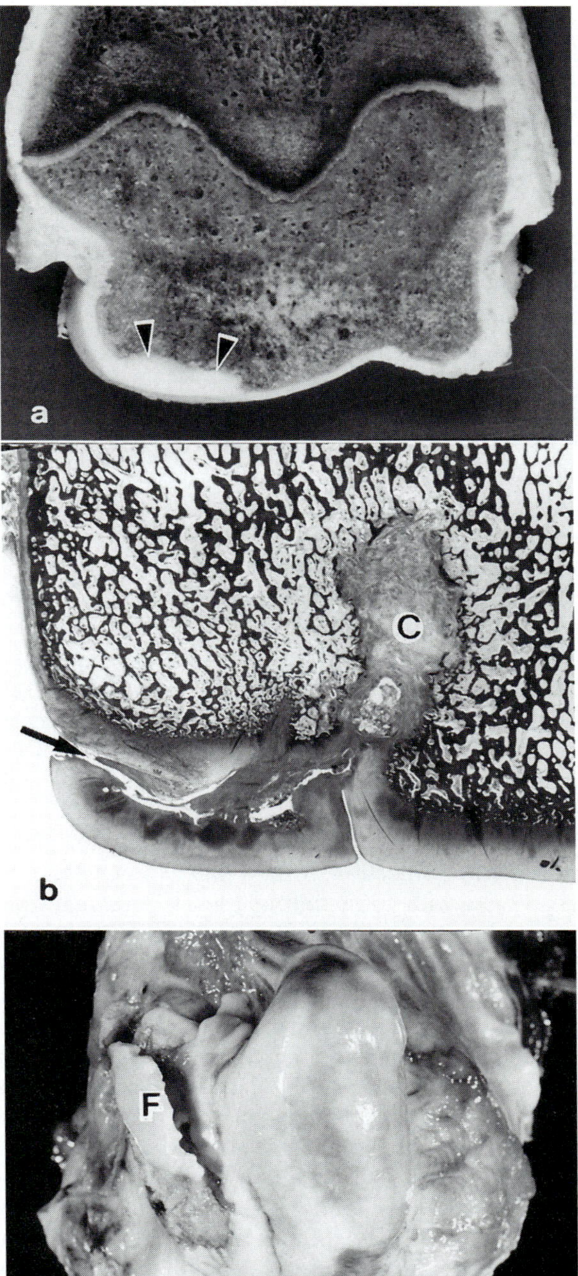

Fig. 10-52 Bone. Distal radius. **A**, Osteochondrosis is present as focal retention of hypertrophic cartilage *(arrowheads)* of the articular-epiphyseal complex. **B**, Femoral condyle. A cleft *(arrow)* in the deeper regions of retained cartilage has formed a flap, characteristic of osteochondritis dissecans. A "cyst" (*C*) is present in the subchondral bone due to focal failure of normal bone formation due to osteochondrosis and degeneration of the retained cartilage. **C**, Femur. Osteochondritis dissecans with a cartilaginous flap (*F*) is present in the lateral trochlear ridge of the femur. *Courtesy Dr. W. Riser.*

induced by pressure or failure of nutrient diffusion, or they might follow acellular streaks within the cartilage. These streaks appear microscopically as eosinophilic lines of variable contour and direction. They apparently are composed of condensed collagen with minimal proteoglycans. They might represent residual cartilage vascular canals or zones of "physiologic" necrosis of chondrocytes. These streaks are found in normal cartilage, but they can appear exaggerated in some lesions of osteochondrosis. Cleft formation can cause mechanical instability and lead to separation within cartilage or of cartilage from the underlying bone. Separation of the articular-epiphyseal cartilage complex from epiphyseal bone gives rise to flaps or free intraarticular fragments of cartilage (joint mice); this process is termed **osteochondritis dissecans** (OCD) (see Fig. 10-52). The lesions of OCD develop in various synovial joints, including those of the facets of the vertebral column. They can be accompanied by pain, joint effusion, and nonsuppurative synovitis. Free-floating "joint mice" occasionally interfere with mechanical movement of the joint. Common sites of OCD are the humeral head in the dog, the anterior intermediate ridge of the distal tibia in horses, and the medial condyles of the distal femur and distal humerus in swine. The disease is a significant cause of lameness in young breeding swine. It is clear that the lesions of OCD can be slow to heal, are accompanied by synovitis, and, in time, lead to degenerative joint disease.

The retained cartilage of osteochondrosis can undergo endochondral ossification, form a flap as in OCD, or may undergo lysis with formation of a cyst. This may be the pathogenesis of some subchondral bone cysts.

Epiphysiolysis is often listed as a lesion of osteochondrosis, but it is not associated with retention of cartilage. Epiphysiolysis represents separation of the epiphysis from the metaphyseal bone and, likely, involves some degree of trauma acting on a degenerate metaphyseal growth plate. The femoral head may be involved in market-weight swine and in young gilts. In young sows, separation of the ischial tuberosity at its growth plate is a common cause of posterior weakness and inability to stand. In dogs, the process of epiphysiolysis may be the basis for an ununited anconeal process and an ununited or fragmented coronoid process.

The cause of osteochondrosis is unknown. The fact that there is a very high incidence in such species as modern commercial swine that are bred and fed to achieve maximal body weight at a minimal age suggests that it might be a mechanical complication superimposed on "normal" multifocal defects of endochondral ossification. Presumably, uneven patterns of endochondral ossification are common occurrences, and most go undetected. Only in animals selected for rapid weight gain might these develop into clinically significant lesions. There is little evidence that the lesions of osteochondrosis represent a specific nutritional deficiency. However, copper deficiency, perhaps conditioned by excess dietary zinc, has been documented in Thoroughbred suckling foals with lysis of the articular-epiphyseal complex and formation of thin flaps of cartilage. Also, lesions of cartilage retention are less frequent in foals when their mares are fed increased dietary copper. Osteochondrosis-like lesions have been reported in growing dogs fed high-calcium diets.

Degeneration of Intervertebral Disks

Degeneration of the intervertebral disks is often an age-related phenomenon in many species. In general, loss of water and proteoglycans, reduced cellularity, and an increase in collagen content of the nucleus pulposus occur, so that the distinction between the nucleus pulposus and the annulus fibrosus becomes difficult. The central part of the disk is yellow-brown and is composed of friable fibrocartilaginous material (Fig. 10-53). These degenerative changes are likely caused by various metabolic and mechanical insults that lead to depolymerization of proteoglycan in the nucleus pulposus and to degenerative changes in the annulus fibrosus. Both rotational and compressive types of movement injure the annulus fibrosus. Changes in structure and function of the nucleus pulposus, together with a weakened annulus, often lead to concentric and radial tears or fissures in the annulus that allow bulging or herniation of the nucleus pulposus material (Fig. 10-54). Herniation is usually dorsal in domestic animals. In human beings (rarely in domestic animals), disk material can be extruded through the end-plate into the vertebral body, producing a lesion known as Schmorl's node.

In chondrodystrophic breeds of dogs such as the dachshund, chondroid metaplasia of the nucleus pulposus is followed by calcification during the first year of life. This can lead to disk prolapse, with total rupture of the annulus fibrosus and extrusion of disk material into the vertebral ca-

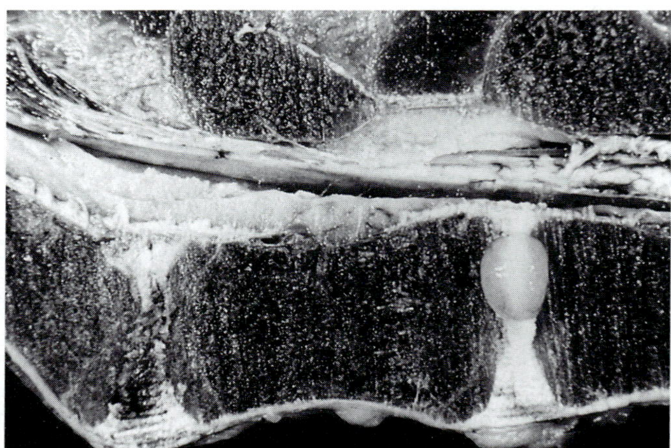

Fig. 10-53 Bone, lumbar vertebrae; pig. The disk on the left is degenerate (narrow, friable, and darkly discolored) compared with the normal disk on the right, which is white and bulging from cut surface.

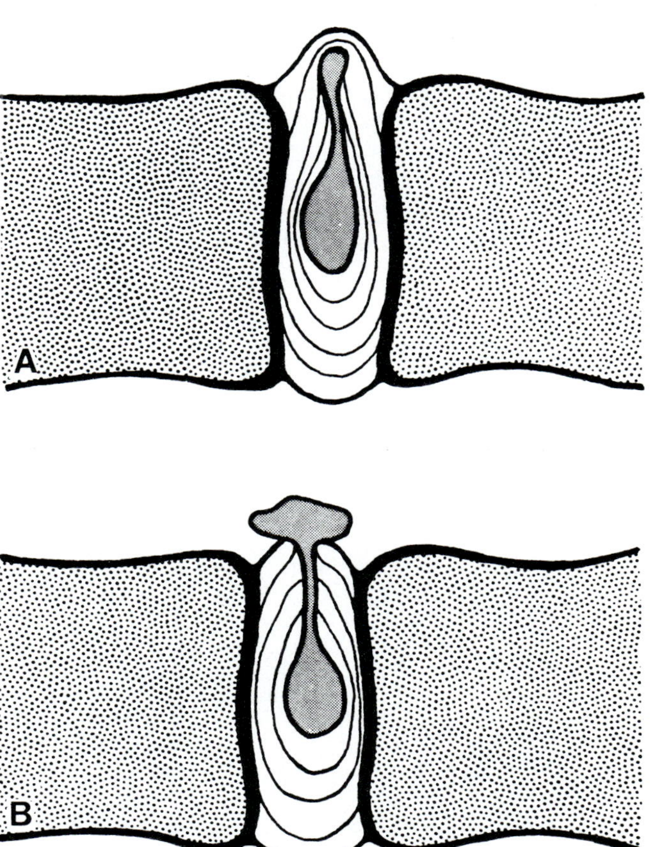

Fig. 10-54 Prolapse of intervertebral disk material may be incomplete with partial rupture of the annulus fibrosus (**A**) or total rupture of the annulus fibrosus may allow extrusion of disk material into the vertebral canal (**B**).

nal at sites of mechanical stress, such as the cervical and thoracolumbar vertebrae.

Senile degenerative disk disease is independent of breed in the dog and also occurs in human beings, pigs, and horses. These lesions are characterized by progressive dehydration and collagenization of the nucleus pulposus and degeneration of the annulus fibrosus. The lesion develops slowly, and calcification is rare. Prolapse of the disk is secondary to partial rupture of the annulus fibrosus and is characterized by bulging of the dorsal surface of the disk into the vertebral canal. There are a number of important consequences of degeneration of intervertebral disks. Prolapse or herniation can be dorsal (spinal cord compression) or lateral (spinal nerve compression and entrapment). Fibrocartilaginous disk material can enter vessels and cause infarction in the spinal cord, although fibrocartilaginous embolism can occur with minimal evidence of disk disease. Given that each intervertebral joint is a three-joint complex, it follows that the reduced disk thickness that occurs with degeneration and dehydration allows overriding of the articular facets and development of joint instability. This contributes to the evolution of degenerative disease with enlargement of articular processes, which can also cause spinal cord compression or spinal nerve entrapment. Degeneration of intervertebral disks and the ensuing intervertebral joint instability can lead to the development of osteophytes on vertebrae at intervertebral spaces (spondylosis) in many species, such as dogs, cattle, pigs, and horses. Vertebral osteophytes are usually ventral and lateral; if dorsal, they can cause stenosis of the vertebral canal.

Suggested Readings

Bonucci E, Motta PM. Ultrastructure of skeletal tissues. Boston: Kluwer Academic, 1991.

Brighton CT. Structure and function of the growth plate. Clin Orthop 1978; 136:22-32.

Brighton CT, Hunt RM. Early histological and ultrastructural changes in medullary fracture callus. J Bone Joint Surg 1991; 73A(6):832-847.

Bullough PG. Atlas of orthopedic pathology with clinical and radiographic correlations. Philadelphia: JB Lippincott, 1992.

Cornell CN, Lane JM. Newest factors in fracture healing. Clin Orthop 1992; 277:297-311.

Fitzgerald RH, Jr. Pathogenesis of musculoskeletal sepsis. In: Sean PF, Hugh RH, Fitzgerald JP, eds. Musculoskeletal Infections. Chicago: Year Book Medical, 1986: 14.

Galasko C. Skeletal metastasis. Clin Orthop 1986; 210:18-30.

Hamerman D. The biology of osteoarthritis. New Engl J Med 1989; 320:1322-1330.

Hughes S, McCarthy ID, Hooper G. The vascular system in bone. Its importance and relevance to clinical practice. Clin Orthop 1986; 210:31-36.

Jones JP, Jr. Etiology and pathogenesis of osteonecrosis. Semin Arthroplasty 1991; 2(3):160-168.

Jones TC, Mohr U, Hunt RD. Monographs on pathology of laboratory animals. Cardiovascular and musculoskeletal systems. Boston: Kluwer Academic, 1990.

Marks SC, Popoff SN. Bone cell biology: The regulation of development, structure and function in the skeleton. Am J Anat 1988; 183:1-44.

Misdorp W, van der Heul RO. Tumours of bones and joints. Bull World Health Organ 1976; 53:265-282.

Mohan S, Baylink DJ. Bone growth factors. Clin Orthop 1991; 263:30-48.

Narayan O, Zink MC, Gorrell M, McEntee M, Sharma D, Adams R. Lentivirus induced arthritis in animals. J Rheumatol 1992; 19:25-32.

Olsson S-E, ed. Osteochondritis in domestic animals. Acta Radiol Suppl (Stockh) 1978; 358:1-306.

Palmer N. Bones and joints. In: Jubb KVF, Kennedy PC, Palmer N, eds. Pathology of Domestic Animals. 4th ed. San Diego: Academic Press, 1992.

Pool RR. Tumors and tumor-like lesions of joints and adjacent soft tissues. In: Moulton JE, ed. Tumors in Domestic Animals. Berkeley: University of California Press, 1990.

Revell PA. Pathology of bone. New York: Springer-Verlag, 1986.

Rosol TJ, Capen CC. Biology of disease: Mechanisms of cancer-induced hypercalcemia. Lab Invest 1992; 67:680-702.

Sumner-Smith G. Bone in clinical orthopedics: A study in comparative osteology. Philadelphia: Saunders, 1982.

Teitelbaum SL, Bullough PG. The pathophysiology of bone and joint disease. Am J Pathol 1979; 96:283-354.

Vaes G. Cellular biology and biochemical mechanism of bone resorption: A review of recent developments on the formation, activation and mode of action of osteoclasts. Clin Orthop 1988; 231:239-271.

Woodward JC, Montgomery CA. Musculoskeletal system. In: Benirschke K, Garner FM, Jones TC, eds. Pathology of Laboratory Animals. New York: Springer-Verlag, 1978: 663.

Ziff M. Role of the endothelium in chronic inflammatory synovitis. Arthritis Rheum 1991; 34(11):1345-1352.

CHAPTER

11

Integumentary System

ANN M. HARGIS

GENERAL CONSIDERATIONS

Overview

The study of the skin bridges the disciplines of clinical medicine and pathology. The gross evaluation of the skin is synonymous with a clinical or dermatologic evaluation of the skin. The majority of cases presented to many veterinary hospitals are for cutaneous problems. This is due, in part, to the fact that the skin is one of the largest organs in the body, it is potentially altered by a variety of exogenous and endogenous factors, and cutaneous lesions are easily seen by owners. The skin, therefore, has significant economic importance in small animal veterinary practice due to the number of cases presented for evaluation. The skin also has significant economic importance in large animal practice as well. Some cutaneous parasites in food animals, e.g., cause anemia; blemish hides; decrease production of meat, wool, and milk; predispose to secondary bacterial infections; annoy animals; and cause paralysis, unthriftiness, downgrading at market, and death.

Functions

The skin participates in temperature and blood pressure regulation, protects against fluid and electrolyte loss, serves as a barrier to physical, chemical, and microbiologic agents, produces vitamin D, is a sensory organ, and stores fat, water, vitamins, carbohydrates, protein, and other nutrients. Although absorption is not a primary function, many substances can be absorbed by the skin. In addition, the epidermal keratinocyte is a major source of cytokines and is now considered to be an integral part of the immune system. Cytokines produced by keratinocytes include some interleukins (IL), colony stimulating factors (CSF), tumor necrosis factor (TNF), and growth factors. These cytokines comprise an interactive network and play a significant role in mediating inflammation and immune responses of the skin. The production of cytokines by keratinocytes is regulated to maintain homeostasis, and malfunction of cytokine production or release may result in cutaneous disease.

ANATOMY AND HISTOLOGY OF THE SKIN

General

The skin, a large and complex organ that has haired and hairless portions (Figs. 11-1 and 11-2), consists of epidermis, dermis, hair follicles, digital appendages, and sebaceous, sweat, and other glands. Histologic structure varies greatly among different sites and among different species of animals. The haired skin is thickest over the dorsal aspect of the body and on the lateral aspect of the limbs and is thinnest on the ventral aspect of the body and the medial aspect of the thighs. The skin of large animals is generally thicker than that of small animals. The subcutis connects epidermis and dermis with the underlying fascia and musculature.

Epidermis

Haired skin has a thinner epidermis, whereas nonhaired skin of the nose and foot pads has a thicker epidermis (see Figs. 11-1 and 11-2). The epidermis of haired skin consists of four basic layers, whereas that of hairless skin consists of five layers. The cells that form keratin are referred to as keratinocytes. The outermost epidermal layer, the stratum corneum, consists of many sheets of flat keratinized cells. The stratum lucidum of hairless skin is absent in haired areas and is a thin layer of compacted fully keratinized cells covering the granular layer, the stratum granulosum, which consists of effete cells with basophilic keratohyalin granules. Under these layers is the stratum spinosum, the spinous layer, which consists of a zone of polyhedral cells attached by desmosomes. During processing for microscopic examination, the cells contract, except where they are attached at desmosomal junctions, thus creating the appearance of ''spines'' or intercellular bridges and providing the name for this epidermal layer. The stratum spinosum in haired areas is thinner in dogs and cats and thicker in cattle, horses, and pigs. The innermost layer of the skin is the germinal layer or stratum basale, consisting of a single layer of cuboidal to columnar cells.

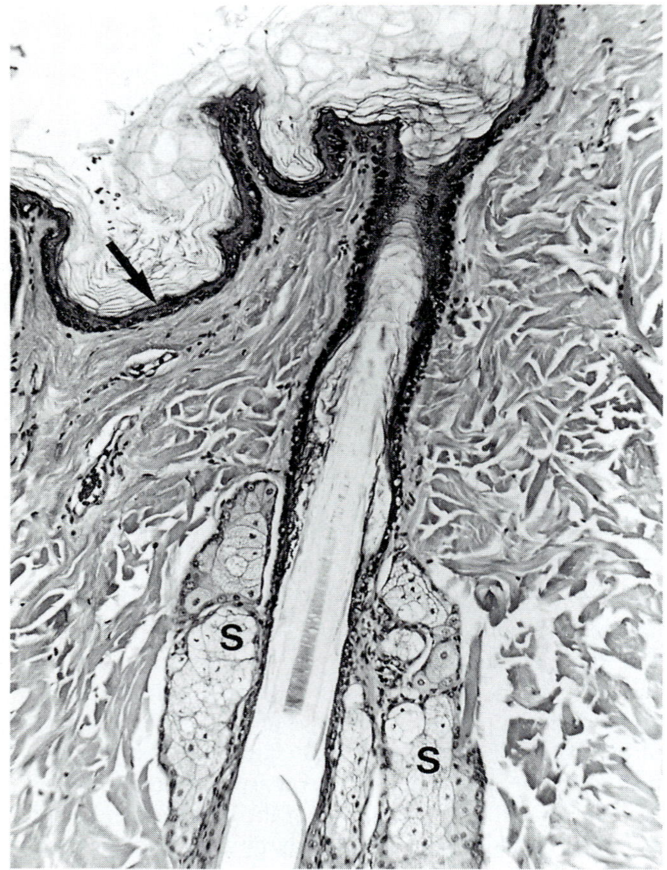

Fig. 11-1 Skin, haired; dog. Normal. The epidermis is thinner in haired than hairless skin *(arrow),* and hair follicles and sebaceous glands *(S)* are present. Hemaloxylin-eosin (H & E) stain.

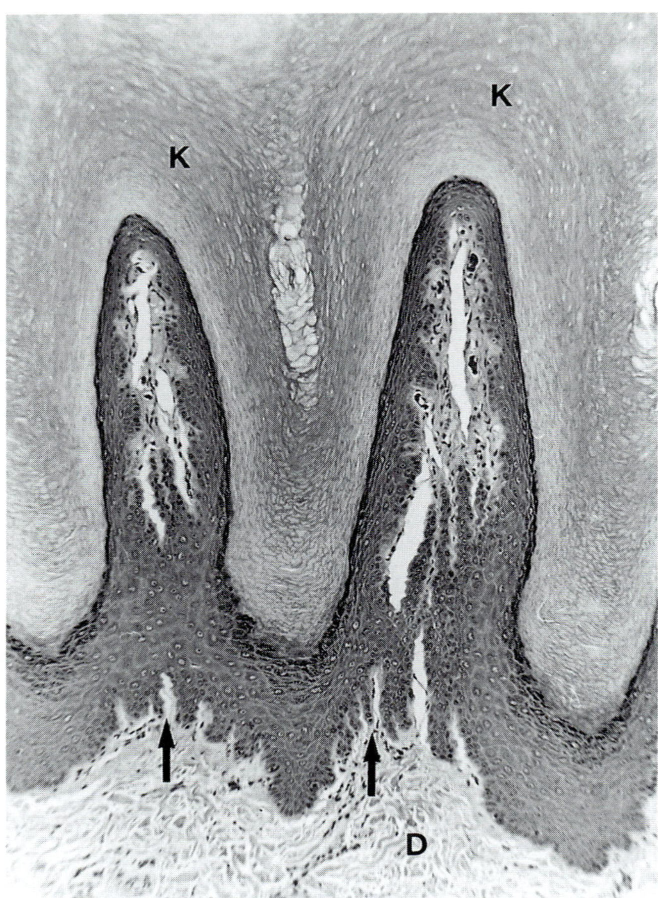

Fig. 11-2 Skin, hairless; dog. Normal. The epidermis is thick and interdigitates *(arrows)* with the dermis *(D).* Note dense zone of keratin (*K*). H & E stain.

Intermixed in the basal cell layer are melanocytes, Langerhans' cells, and Merkel's cells. Melanocytes, derived from the neural crest, are also present in lower layers of the stratum spinosum and produce melanin pigment, giving color to skin and hair. Melanocytic granules, transferred to keratinocytes and distributed as caplike clusters above the nuclei, help protect the nuclei from ultraviolet light. Langerhans' cells derived from bone marrow are important in modulating and mediating immunologic responses. They are related to cells of the monocyte-macrophage system and process and present antigen to sensitized T cells. Merkel's cells, neuroendocrine cells of the basal layer, function as slowly adapting mechanoreceptors and, by a paracrine role, regulate the function of adjacent epidermal and adnexal structures. Intraepidermal lymphocytes, known to be T cells in the human and mouse, probably monitor the skin surface, as do similar lymphocytes in the respiratory and gastrointestinal tissues.

The epidermis and dermis are separated by a basement membrane. In hairless areas such as the foot pads and nasal planum, this junction is irregular due to epidermal projections that interdigitate with dermal papillae, thus strengthening the attachment of the epidermis to the dermis. In densely haired areas, the junction is smooth, and the anchoring function is provided by hair follicles. The more sparsely haired skin of human beings and pigs have more epidermal-dermal interdigitations (rete ridges) and fewer hair follicles.

Dermis

The dermis (corium), consisting of collagen and elastic fibers in a glycosaminoglycan ground substance, supports hair follicles, glands, vessels, and nerves. The superficial layer of the dermis is comprised of fine collagen fibers and is wider in the skin of cattle and horses than in the skin of dogs and cats. The deep layer of the dermis is comprised of larger collagen bundles than is the superficial dermis. Skeletal muscle fibers, partly responsible for voluntary skin movement, extend from the cutaneous muscle to the dermis. Fibroblasts, mast cells, lymphocytes, plasma cells, macrophages, and, rarely, eosinophils and neutrophils can be found in normal dermis.

Vessels and Nerves

Cutaneous arteries give rise to three vascular plexuses, which supply the subcutaneous, cutaneous, and subpapillary regions of the skin. Lymph capillaries arise in the superficial dermis and connect with a subcutaneous plexus. The lymph vessels then converge to form larger channels that eventually reach peripheral lymph nodes.

Nerve supply to the skin consists of motor and sensory fibers. Visceral efferent sympathetic nerves supply the smooth muscle of blood vessels, the arrector pili muscles, and myoepithelial cells of glands. The rich supply of nerves to the epidermis and dermis is mostly general somatic, afferent, myelinated, and nonmyelinated fibers. A dermatome is the area of skin supplied by the branches of one spinal nerve.

Hypodermis (Subcutis, Panniculus)

The hypodermis attaches the dermis to subjacent muscle or bone and consists of adipose tissue and collagenous and elastic fibers, which provide flexibility. Adipose tissue can insulate against temperature variation and, in the case of foot pads, serve in shock absorption.

Adnexa

The adnexa consists of hair follicles and glands (sebaceous, sweat, and specialized).

Hair follicles

Growth of hair is seasonal in animals, with the time of growth and mitotic activity termed the anagen phase. A transitional phase, during which cellular proliferation ceases, is the catagen phase. The follicle then enters a resting state, the telogen phase, after which mitotic activity and new hair production resume and old hair is shed. Anagen follicles have their hair bulbs more deeply positioned and fully formed with invaginated follicular papilla, fully developed inner root sheath, and trichilemmal keratinization (eosinophilic, compact, few if any keratohyalin granules) limited to the follicular isthmus. Catagen follicles are smaller and shorter, have loss of the inner root sheath, and have regression and keratinization of the outer root sheath. The early telogen stage has loss of the inferior portion of the hair follicle and a jagged zone of trichilemmal keratinization around the base of the hair shaft. The late telogen stage has no hair shaft or trichilemmal keratinization and consists of a narrow base of outer root sheath cells and a thin strand of germinal cells in contact with the follicular papilla. The hair cycle is controlled by number of daylight hours, environmental temperature, and genetic factors.

The arrector pili muscles extend from the connective tissue sheath of the hair follicles to attach to the superficial dermis. Arrector pili smooth muscles are well developed on the back of animals, especially dogs. Muscle contraction causes erection of hairs and expression of sebaceous glands.

Forms of hair follicles vary in different animals. Cattle and horses have evenly distributed simple follicles with one large follicle usually with sebaceous and sweat glands and arrector pili muscles. Pigs have simple follicles grouped in clusters. Goats, dogs, and cats have compound follicles that consist of primary follicles associated with smaller secondary follicles. Sheep have simple follicles in hair-growing areas and compound follicles in wool-growing areas. Tactile hairs include sinus and tylotrich hairs. Sinus hairs—simple follicles with a sinus containing blood, located between the inner and outer layers of the dermal sheath (whiskers or vibrissae)—generally occur on the muzzle, above the eyes, on the lips, on the throat, and on the palmar aspect of the carpus of cats. Sinus hairs function as slow-adapting mechanoreceptors. Tylotrich hairs function as rapid-adapting mechanoreceptors and are scattered among the regular body hairs.

Sweat glands

Apocrine glands (epitrichial glands), located throughout haired areas of skin, are tubular or saccular coiled glands lined by cuboidal to low columnar epithelium with a luminal cytoplasmic protrusion and surrounded by myoepithelial cells. Apocrine gland activity is grossly visible in horses as they sweat after exercise or during a high temperature. Other apocrine glands include the interdigital glands of small ruminants, glands of the external ear canal and eyelids of domestic animals, anal sac glands of dog and cats, and the mental organ of pigs. Eccrine glands (atrichial glands) are merocrine in secretion and, in contrast to ducts of apocrine glands, the ducts open directly onto the surface of the epidermis. They are tubular glands lined by cuboidal epithelium surrounded by myoepithelium and are confined mainly to foot pads of dogs and cats, frog region of ungulates, carpus of pigs, and nasolabial region of ruminants and pigs.

Sebaceous glands

Sebaceous glands are simple, branched, or compound alveolar glands that are holocrine in secretion, with ducts opening into hair follicles except at some mucocutaneous junctions where the glands open on the surface of the skin. Well-developed sebaceous glands are found in the supracaudal gland of dogs and cats; the infraorbital, inguinal, and interdigital regions of sheep; the base of the horn of goats; the anal sac glands of cats; the preputial glands of horses; and the submental organ of cats.

Specialized structures

Some specialized cutaneous structures, such as the anal sacs, are especially prone to lesions. These bilateral diverticula, located between internal and external sphincter muscles of the anus, have ducts that open onto the anus at the level of the anocutaneous junction. Ducts and sacs are lined by stratified squamous epithelium; in cats, the sac wall has sebaceous and apocrine glands, but, in dogs, the wall has only apocrine glands.

Circumanal (hepatoid, perianal) glands occur most commonly near the anus but are also present in skin near the prepuce, tail, flank, and groin. They have nonpatent ducts and are comprised of peripheral reserve cells surrounding lobules of large polyhedral cells with abundant acidophilic cytoplasm. These cells resemble hepatic cells.

Claws and hooves are digital organs. The claws shield the third phalanx and consist of a wall (dorsal and lateral sides) and sole (ventral side), both of which are stratified squamous keratinizing epithelium. The wall consists of hard keratin and the sole of softer keratin. The dermis of the claw consists of dense collagen, elastic tissue, and blood vessels that can bleed profusely if the claw is trimmed too short. The dermis is continuous with the ungual crest of the third phalanx and extends distally as the periosteum of the phalanx. The claw fold is a fold of skin that covers the wall laterally and dorsally for a short distance. Hooves consist of the wall, sole, and frog in solipeds; and a wall, sole, and prominent bulb in ruminants and pigs. These structures are composed of keratin. The wall consists of three layers, and the inner layer interdigitates with the dermis, anchoring the hoof to the dermis. In general, the deeper portion of the dermis blends with the periosteum of the third phalanx.

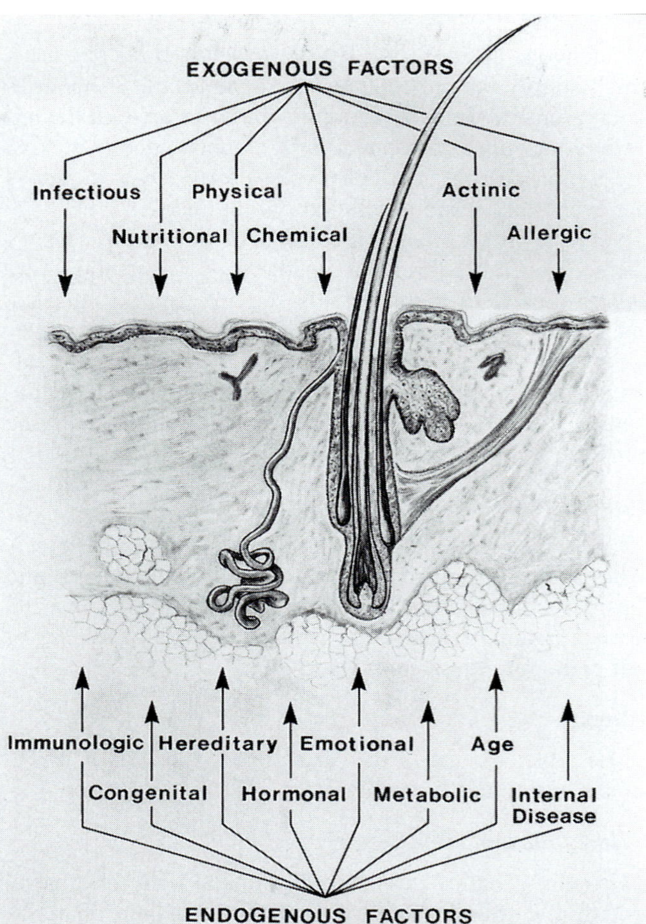

Fig. 11-3 Skin diagram. A myriad of exogenous and endogenous factors influence the gross and microscopic appearance of the skin. Because the skin can respond to these factors in a limited number of ways, different skin disorders may have a similar appearance.

RESPONSE TO INJURY

Numerous endogenous and exogenous factors cause significant alterations in the skin (Fig. 11-3), an organ with a limited spectrum of responses to injury. Because of this limitation of responses, it is often necessary to obtain a thorough history; perform thorough cutaneous and systemic physical examinations; consider anatomic distribution patterns, age, and breed predilections; and perform diagnostic tests relating to cutaneous and systemic disease to determine the cause of a lesion. Cutaneous biopsies may be useful to arrive at a definitive diagnosis, especially if an etiologic agent is present in specimens.

Microscopic changes can be an aid to diagnosis, as patterns of inflammation may suggest specific etiologic agents or classes of cutaneous disease. Systems have been developed for the recognition of histopathologic patterns to facilitate diagnosis in veterinary dermatopathology (Table 11-1). Responses to injury will be illustrated by changes in the epidermis, dermis, adnexa, and panniculus.

Epidermis

Alterations in epidermal growth or differentiation

Basal cells, in their postmitotic state, migrate outward from the basal layer, eventually forming the cornified layers of the epidermis. In the normal epidermis, balance is established between the proliferation of the basal cells and the loss of differentiated cells from the surface, resulting in an epidermis of constant thickness. The orderly proliferation, differentiation, and cornification of epidermal cells are regulated by such factors as cytokines, vitamins, minerals such as zinc and copper, fatty acids, and hormones. The regulatory cytokines are produced by a variety of cell types (endothelial cells, leukocytes, fibroblasts, and other cell types, including keratinocytes). Keratinocytes, thereby, participate in a self-regulatory role; and inflammatory cells, among others, can influence keratinocyte growth and differentiation. The highly regulated process of epidermal proliferation, differentiation, keratinization, and desquamation is altered in some specific disease syndromes, such as primary idiopathic seborrhea of the cocker spaniel and schnauzer comedo syndrome, but can be caused by a variety of factors (i.e., inflammation, trauma, metabolic disorders, and nutritional imbalances). Mecha-

Table 11-1. Histopathologic diagnosis by use of lesion morphology (pattern)

Pattern	Brief features	Examples
Diseases of the epidermis		
I. Pustular diseases	Superficial epidermal pustules	Impetigo, pemphigus foliaceus
II. Bullous and vesicular diseases	Vesicles/clefts in deep epidermis or dermal-epidermal junction	Pemphigus vulgaris, lupus erythematosus, bullous pemphigoid
III. Necrotizing diseases	Individual keratinocyte necrosis or confluent necrosis	Burns, superficial necrolytic dermatopathy, erythema multiforme
IV. Spongiotic diseases	Intercellular edema → vesicles	Allergic contact dermatitis, eosinophilic plaque
V. Exudative and ulcerative diseases	Erosion or ulceration with cell migration → crusts	Miliary dermatitis, indolent ulcer
VI. Hyperplastic diseases	Proliferation of epidermis	Acral lick dermatitis, actinic dermatitis, acanthosis nigricans
VII. Hyperkeratotic diseases	Increase in epidermal and follicular keratin	Primary idiopathic seborrhea, ichthyosis, zinc-responsive dermatosis
Diseases of the dermis		
VIII. Perivascular diseases	Inflammation oriented around vessels	Hypersensitivity reactions, parasitic dermatosis
IX. Vascular diseases	Inflammation/degeneration of vessel walls	Immune-mediated vasculitis, septic vasculitis
X. Lichenoid (interface) diseases	Lichenoid or interface dermatitis	Mucocutaneous pyoderma, lupus erythematosus
XI. Infectious nodular and diffuse diseases	Macrophages and neutrophils in granulomas or diffuse	Actinomycosis, feline leprosy
XII. Noninfectious nodular and diffuse diseases	Macrophages and neutrophils in granulomas or diffuse	Foreign body reactions, histiocytosis, juvenile sterile granulomatous dermatitis and lymphadenitis
XIII. Nodular and diffuse diseases with eosinophils or plasma cells	Diffuse inflammation with eosinophils or plasma cells	Plasma cell pododermatitis, eosinophilic granuloma
XIV. Dysplastic/depositional diseases	Increased dermal substance or substance not normally found	Calcinosis cutis, calcinosis circumscripta, amyloidosis, mucinosis
Diseases of adnexal appendages		
XV. Pustular and nodular diseases without follicular disruption	Variable inflammation in and around follicles and adnexa	Superficial bacterial folliculitis, dermatophytosis, sebaceous adenitis
XVI. Pustular and nodular diseases with follicular disruption	Severe inflammation in and around follicles and adnexa with disruption of follicles	Folliculitis and furunculosis, acne, callus pyoderma
XVII. Atrophic diseases of follicles	Acquired hair cycle arrest with or without inflammation	Endocrine, telogen effluvium
XVIII. Dysplastic diseases of hair follicles	Abnormal growth or development	Color mutant alopecia, black hair follicle dysplasia
Diseases of the panniculus		
XIX. Diseases of the panniculus	Inflammation lobular/septal/diffuse with variable types of cells	Post–rabies vaccine alopecia, idiopathic sterile nodular panniculitis, feline pansteatitis

Information for this table was adapted with permission from Gross TL, Ihrke PJ, Walder EJ. Veterinary dermatopathology: A macroscopic and microscopic evaluation of canine and feline skin disease. St. Louis: Mosby–Year Book, 1992.

nisms that alter keratinocyte growth and differentiation vary with the disease syndromes and are often incompletely understood.

Hyperkeratosis is an increase in the thickness of the stratum corneum and occurs in two forms. In orthokeratotic hyperkeratosis (also referred to as hyperkeratosis), the cells are anuclear, and, in parakeratotic hyperkeratosis (also referred to as parakeratosis), the cells contain nuclei. Subtypes of hyperkeratosis include basket weave, compact, and lamellar. Both hyperkeratosis and parakeratosis are common, nonspecific responses to chronic stimuli (i.e., superficial trauma, inflammation), and occur specifically in certain diseases. Hyperkeratosis is a feature of ichthyosis, primary idiopathic seborrhea of the cocker spaniel (Fig. 11-

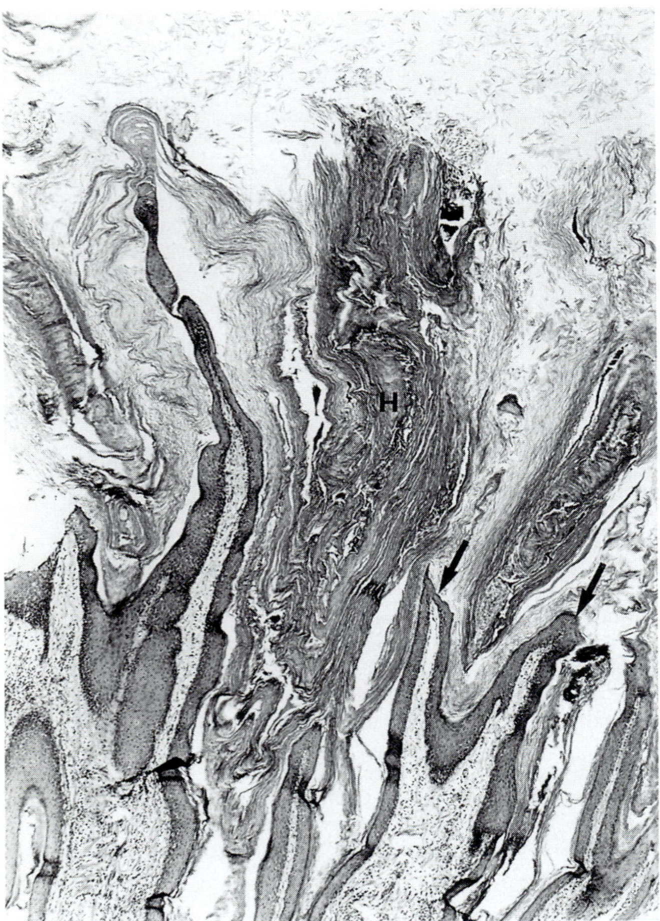

Fig. 11-4 Skin, haired; dog. Idiopathic seborrhea. Note the marked orthokeratotic hyperkeratosis (*H*). The keratin distends follicular ostia *(arrows),* creating a papillomatous appearance in the epidermis. H & E stain.

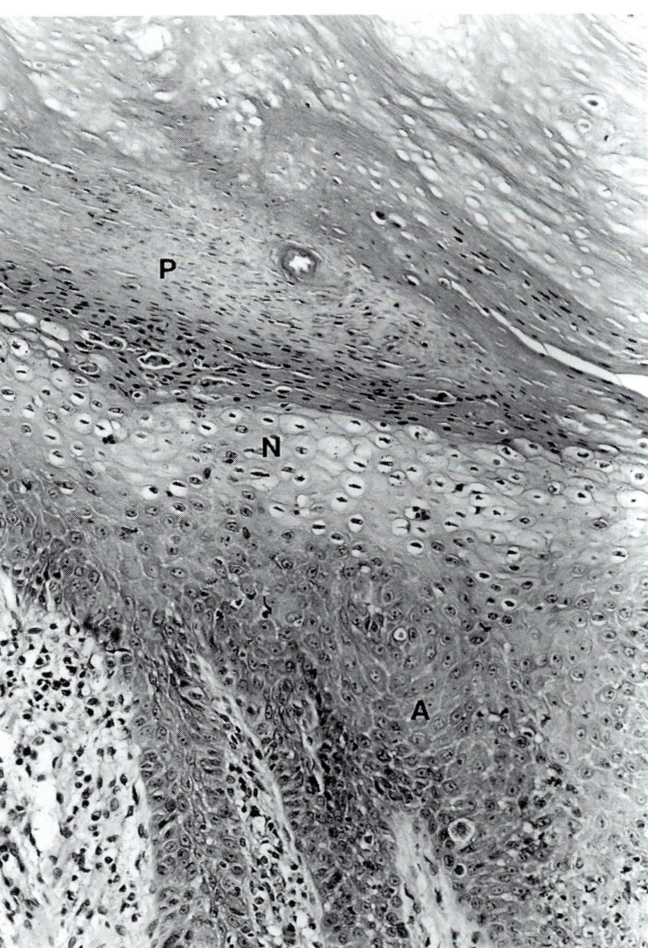

Fig. 11-5 Skin; dog. Superficial necrolytic dermatitis. Nuclear retention is present in the stratum corneum (parakeratotic hyperkeratosis [parakeratosis]) and a trilaminar pattern in the epidermis. Parakeratosis (*P*), edema/necrolysis (*N*), and acanthosis (*A*). H & E stain.

4), and vitamin A deficiency. Diffuse parakeratosis is a feature of zinc-responsive dermatosis and superficial necrolytic dermatopathy (hepatocutaneous syndrome) (Fig. 11-5). Hyperkeratosis and parakeratosis may be accompanied by alterations in the thickness of the granular cell layer. Generally, hyperkeratosis is associated with an increased thickness of the granular cell layer (hypergranulosis), and parakeratosis is associated with a decreased thickness of the granular cell layer (hypogranulosis).

Hyperplasia is an increase in the number of cells in the epidermis. The most significant hyperplasia is that of the stratum spinosum, called acanthosis. Hyperplasia is a response common to a variety of chronic stimuli and occurs in a variety of types, including psoriasiform, papillated, and pseudocarcinomatous (pseudoepitheliomatous) (Fig. 11-6) and in combination of types. In **psoriasiform hyperplasia,** regularly arranged epidermal projections extend downward into the dermis to interdigitate with dermal papillae. This type of hyperplasia is a feature of psoriasiform lichenoid dermatitis of the springer spaniel and porcine juvenile pustular psoriasiform dermatitis (pityriasis rosea). In **papillated epidermal hyperplasia,** the downward growth of the epidermis and fingerlike (papillary) projections to the exterior are increased. This hyperplasia is a feature of some papillomas, nevi, and calluses. **Pseudocarcinomatous hyperplasia** mimics some features of squamous cell carcinoma, such as increased mitotic figures and keratin pearls, but without invasion through the basement membrane and with differentiation of the epidermal cells. Pseudocarcinomatous hyperplasia is often seen in skin damaged by chronic actinic radiation prior to the development of squamous cell carcinoma or at the edges of chronic ulcers.

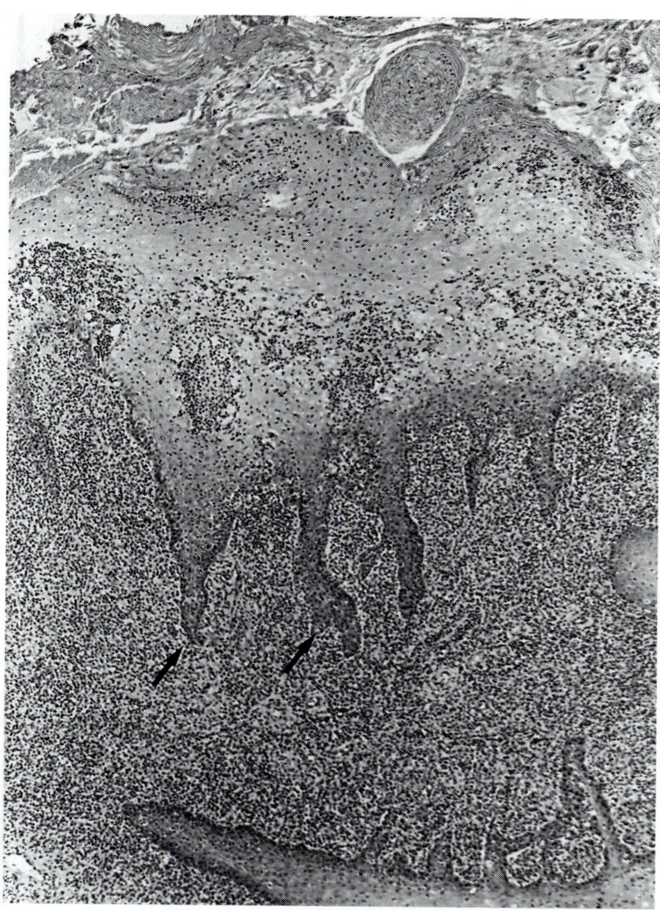

Fig. 11-6 Skin, lip; lamb. Contagious ecthyma. Epidermal hyperplasia, acanthosis, pseudoepitheliomatous hyperplasia *(arrows),* and inflammation are present. H & E stain.

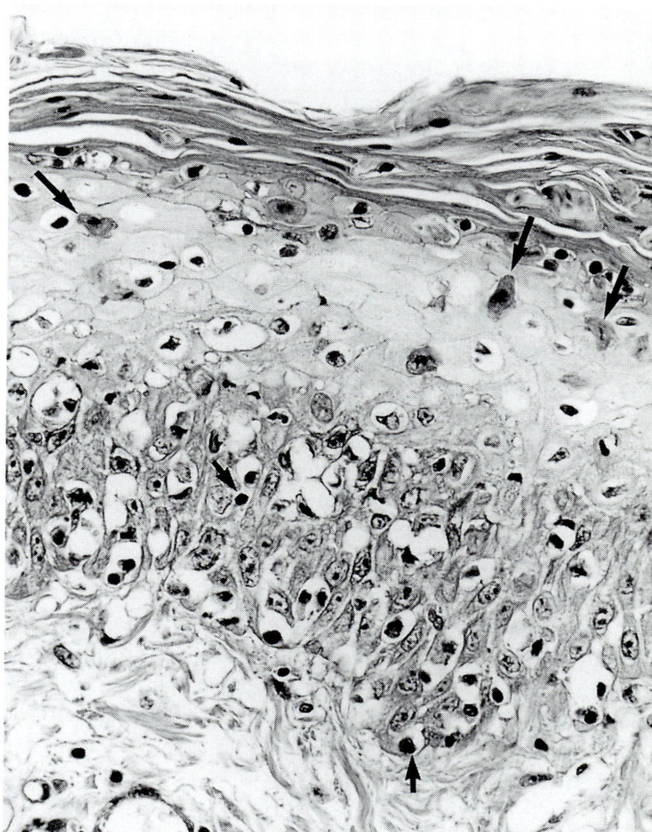

Fig. 11-7 Skin; dog. Erythema multiforme. Dyskeratotic (apoptotic) keratinocytes *(long arrows)* and lymphocytes *(short arrows)* are present in the epidermis. This histologic pattern is commonly seen in drug reactions. H & E stain.

Dyskeratosis is used to describe the morphologic features of premature or abnormal keratinization in the viable layers of the epidermis, i.e., the stratum spinosum. Dyskeratotic keratinocytes have brightly eosinophilic cytoplasm containing keratin filaments and a pyknotic nucleus. Dyskeratotic cells are shrunken and detached from adjacent keratinocytes. Dyskeratosis occurs in diseases with abnormal differentiation (parakeratosis), in neoplastic diseases (squamous cell carcinoma), and in immune killing of epidermal cells by lymphocytes or their products (erythema multiforme) (Fig. 11-7).

Apoptosis refers to programmed cell death. Apoptotic keratinocytes have morphologic features of dyskeratotic cells, such as brightly eosinophilic cytoplasm, a pyknotic nucleus with chromatin condensed along the margin, decreased size, and detachment from keratinocytes. Apoptotic cells are recognized and phagocytosed by adjacent keratinocytes. Phagocytosis before cellular disintegration prevents the development of an acute inflammatory response that would have been elicited by the liberated cellular constituents. Thus, the process of apoptosis is significantly different from necrosis. Apoptosis is seen with diseases such as lupus erythematosus and erythema multiforme (see Fig. 11-7) and in squamous cell carcinoma and basal cell neoplasms.

Necrosis refers to microscopically detectable death of epidermal cells in a living animal. The nuclei undergo pyknosis, karyorrhexis, or karyolysis; organelles swell; plasma membranes rupture; and cytoplasmic elements dispersed into the extracellular space initiate an acute inflammatory response by the liberation of complement activating factors, leukotrines or other arachidonate chemotaxins, or cytokines such as interleukin-1. Causes of epidermal necrosis include physical injury (lacerations, thermal burns), chemical injury (irritant contact dermatitis), and ischemic injury (vasculitis, thromboembolism).

Hypoplasia is a decrease in the number of cells in the epidermis, and **atrophy** is a decrease in the size of the cells within the epidermis. Hypoplasia and atrophy are uncommon and difficult to evaluate because haired skin in animals is normally quite thin. Hypoplasia and atrophy are most commonly and dramatically seen with hyperadrenocorticism in dogs and cats.

Alterations in epidermal cell adhesion

Edema may occur intercellularly or intracellularly. Intercellular edema is called spongiosis because, as the intercellular spaces widen with fluid, the epidermis develops a "spongy" appearance. Severe intercellular edema results in the formation of spongiotic vesicles and is common in inflammatory dermatoses. Intracellular edema, called hydropic, vacuolar, or ballooning degeneration, results in cellular swelling and, if severe, the swollen cells may burst, forming microvesicles enclosed by the cell walls of the ruptured cells. This type of epidermal damage is termed "reticular degeneration." Intracellular edema limited to the basal layer of the epidermis is termed **hydropic or vacuolar degeneration** and may result in the formation of intrabasilar vesicles. Hydropic degeneration is a significant lesion in lupus erythematosus, dermatomyositis, and drug eruptions. **Ballooning degeneration,** a form of intracellular edema in which swollen cells lose their intercellular attachments, is a feature of some viral diseases, particularly those caused by poxviruses.

Acantholysis, the loss of cohesion between epidermal cells, develops when antibodies form against protein components of desmosomes, as occurs in pemphigus foliaceus and pemphigus vulgaris. It also occurs secondary to damage to keratinocytes in vesicles formed in viral diseases and in epidermal pustular diseases. The microscopic lesions vary with the location of acantholysis. In pemphigus foliaceus, acantholysis occurs in the superficial epidermis, resulting in the formation of free-floating keratinocytes in superficial epidermal vesicles and pustules (Fig. 11-8). In pemphigus vulgaris, acantholysis occurs in the epidermis, just above the basal layer, resulting in the separation of the upper epidermis from the basal cells (often referred to as a row of tombstones) attached to the basal lamina (Fig. 11-9). Fluid accumulating between the separated layers forms a vesicle.

Vesicles (synonyms: blisters, bullae) are fluid-filled cavities (Fig. 11-10). Vesicles are generally 5 mm in diameter or smaller, whereas bullae are greater than 5 mm in diameter and develop in any layer of the epidermis or beneath the epidermis. Vesicles may form through acantholysis, epidermal or dermal edema, degeneration of basal cells, or other processes, such as frictional trauma and burns, that cause a lack of cohesion between the epidermal cells or between the epidermis and dermis. The location of vesicles or bullae is suggestive of certain diseases. Thus, intraepidermal vesicles occur in viral infections (see Fig. 11-10), suprabasilar vesicles in pemphigus vulgaris (see Fig. 11-9), intrabasilar vesicles in lupus erythematosus, and subepidermal vesicles in bullous pemphigoid.

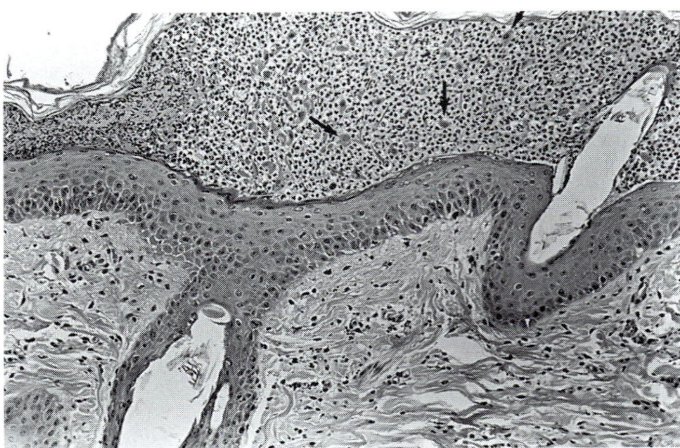

Fig. 11-8 Skin; horse. Pemphigus foliaceus. The subcorneal pustule contains acantholytic cells *(arrows)*. Clipping or scrubbing the surface of the pustule can lead to rupture and make the sample nondiagnostic. H & E stain.

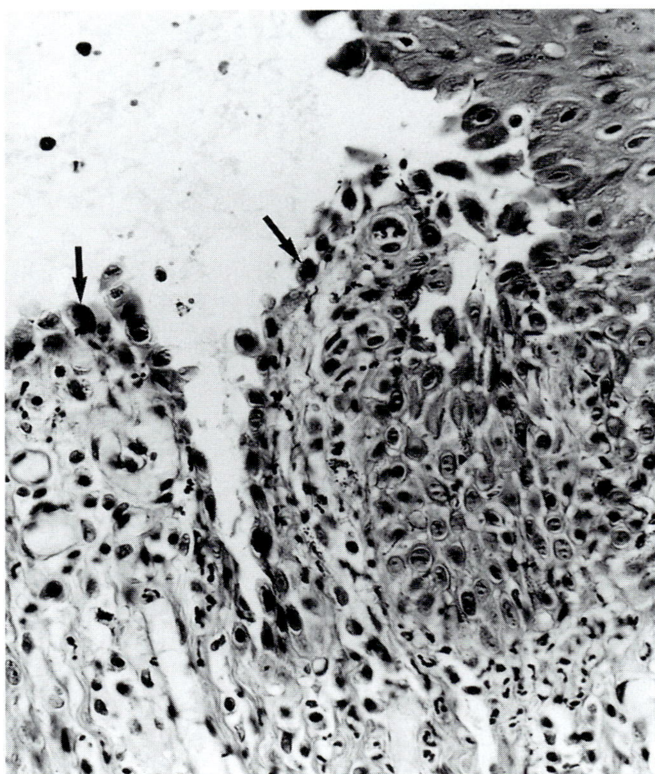

Fig. 11-9 Skin; dog. Pemphigus vulgaris. Suprabasilar clefting has left a row of basal cells *(arrows)* attached to the dermis. H & E stain.

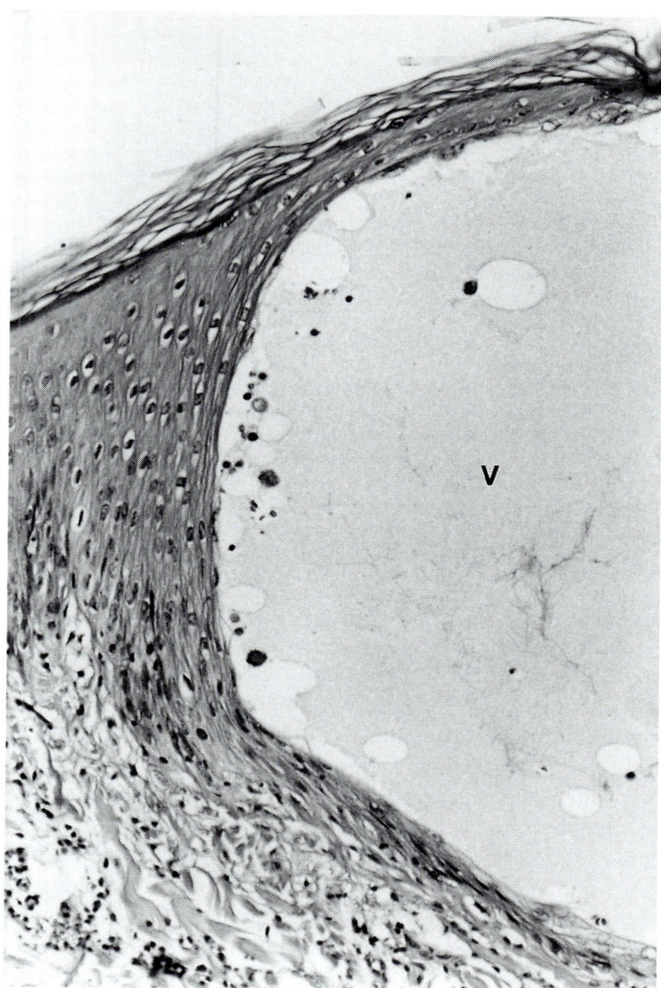

Fig. 11-10 Skin; chimpanzee. Herpesvirus infection (chickenpox). An intraepidermal vesicle (*V*) is present. H & E stain.

Inflammatory lesions of the epidermis

Exocytosis is the migration of erythrocytes or leukocytes into the epidermis. Exocytosis of leukocytes is common in inflammation and is usually accompanied by spongiosis (intercellular edema). Exocytosis of erythrocytes is associated with trauma, circulatory disturbances such as marked vasodilatation, and vasculitis.

Pustules (microabscesses) are vesicles filled with inflammatory cells (see Fig. 11-8) and vary with the types of contained inflammatory cells and location in the epidermis. The pustules of superficial bacterial infections generally contain degenerate neutrophils and coccoid bacteria and are often located beneath the stratum corneum. In ectoparasitic hypersensitivity, pemphigus foliaceus, and feline eosinophilic plaque, the pustules may be filled with eosinophils. The pustules of pemphigus foliaceus are subcorneal and contain acantholytic cells (see Fig. 11-8). Vesicles containing neoplastic lymphocytes are found in epidermotropic lymphoma.

Crusts, dried exudate on the epidermal surface, are indicative of a previous exudative process. Crusts are not specifically diagnostic but may hold the key to diagnosis in some diseases. For example, in dermatophilosis, the most diagnostic portion of the skin is the crust, which is multilaminated and contains the gram-positive, branching, and coccoid organisms, *Dermatophilus congolensis.* Similarly, crusts formed through aging of pustules in pemphigus foliaceus are multilaminated and, frequently, contain numerous acantholytic cells. Crusts may also contain hair shafts infected with spores and hyphae of dermatophytes.

Alterations in epidermal pigmentation

Pigmentary alterations include hyperpigmentation, hypopigmentation, and pigmentary incontinence. Melanin is produced by melanocytes of the stratum basale of the epidermis, the external root sheath and hair matrix of follicles, and, perivascularly, in the dermis. Melanogenesis takes place in membrane-bound organelles (melanosomes), using tyrosine as the substrate. Tyrosine is converted to dopa and dopaquinone by tyrosinase, a copper-containing enzyme. The two different forms of melanin are eumelanin (brown to black) and phaeomelanin (yellow and red). Melanosomes are transferred from the dendritic processes of the melanocyte to the adjacent keratinocytes by a process of endocytosis; the melanocyte and keratinocyte are termed the "epidermal melanin unit." Melanocytes have surface receptors for hormones, such as melanocyte-stimulating hormone, and these hormones regulate melanogenesis. Factors that influence melanogenesis are genes, ultraviolet light (most important in human beings), age, temperature, and inflammation. Melanogenesis is temperature dependent, which accounts for the darkly pigmented hair in the peripheral (cooler) parts of the body of Siamese cats. Inflammatory mediators may play a role in various ways, such as by influencing expression of receptors or by acting as mitogens. For instance, interleukin-1 affects the expression of receptors of melanocyte-stimulating hormone, and basic fibroblast growth factor is a mitogen for human melanocytes.

Hyperpigmentation results from increases in rate of production of melanosomes, in melanosome size, in maturation of melanosomes, or in numbers of melanocytes. Hyperpigmentation is common in chronic inflammatory diseases and in the endocrine dermatoses.

Hypopigmentation may be congenital or hereditary and develops due to a lack of melanocytes, failure of melanocytes to produce melanin, or failure of transfer of melanin to epidermal cells. Hypopigmentation may also be acquired via a loss of existing melanin or melanocytes (depigmentation). Because copper is a component of tyrosinase, production of melanin pigment is dependent on copper, and copper deficiency may result in reduced pigmentation. **Pigmentary incontinence** refers to the loss of melanin pigment from the basal layer of the epidermis due to damage to the

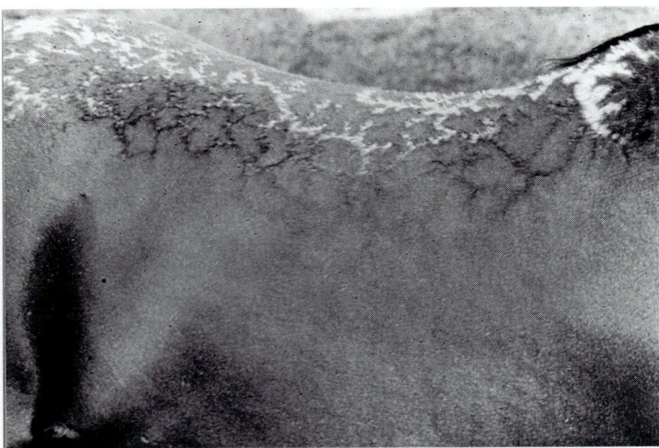

Fig. 11-11 Skin; horse. Leukotrichia (depigmentation of hair shafts). Leukotrichia is best visualized grossly. This horse has acquired leukotrichia in a reticulated pattern over the dorsum of the trunk. Histologically, the white hair shafts are devoid of melanin pigment. *Courtesy Dr. H. Power.*

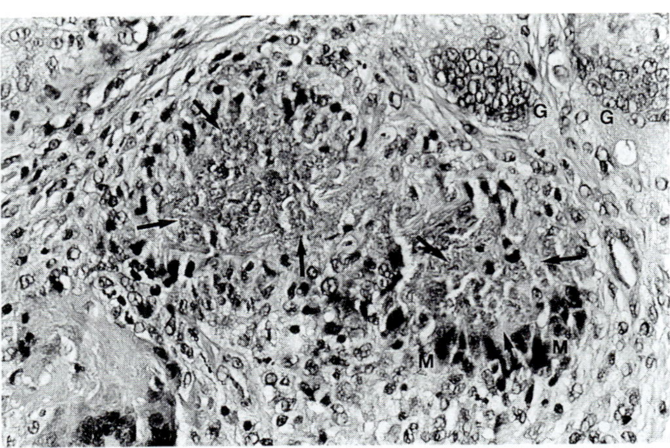

Fig. 11-12 Skin; cat. Eosinophilic granuloma. Fragmented collagen *(arrows)* bordered by a row of macrophages (*M*), some of which are multinucleated giant cells *(G),* and degranulated eosinophils. H & E stain.

cells of the basal layer and the accumulation of the pigment in macrophages in the upper dermis. Pigmentary incontinence may be a nonspecific lesion associated with inflammation; however, it is also seen with diseases that specifically damage the stratum basale, such as lupus erythematosus. Leukotrichia (Fig. 11-11) and leukoderma refer to decreased pigmentation of hair and skin, respectively.

Dermis

Alterations in growth or development

Atrophy, a decrease in the quantity of collagen fibrils and fibroblasts, results in a decrease in the thickness of the dermis. The principal causes of atrophy are catabolic diseases associated with protein degradation, such as hyperadrenocorticism in dogs and cats. In cats with hyperadrenocorticism, collagen loss is sufficient to increase fragility of the skin, which tears with normal handling.

Fibroplasia, an increase in the quantity of collagen, develops in response to various injuries, particularly ulceration. It consists of an increased number of fibroblasts and newly formed collagen fibrils that, in granulation tissue, are parallel to the surface of the skin and oriented perpendicular to proliferated vessels. Fibrosis refers to the gradual deposition and maturation of collagen to form a scar.

Collagen dysplasia is generally an inherited abnormality of collagen, resulting in decreased tensile strength and increased stretchability. The skin tears with minor trauma and heals by formation of scars. Microscopic features vary among the collagen dysplasia disorders, and, in some cases, the skin has no microscopic alterations. Collagen bundles may vary in size and shape and consist of tangled fibers with an abnormal organizational pattern.

Solar elastosis is caused by chronic exposure of the skin to the ultraviolet light rays of sunlight. In human beings, altered elastic tissue is the principal component of the ''elastotic material.'' The altered elastic tissue is chemically normal but structurally abnormal and considered newly formed as a result of altered function of fibroblasts rather than formed as a result of degenerative changes. Normally, elastic fibers and collagen fibers are eosinophilic in hematoxylin and eosin (H & E)–stained sections and, therefore, cannot be differentiated in such preparations. In solar-damaged skin, altered elastic fibers are basophilic in H & E-stained sections. Solar elastosis, most prominent in the horse, consists of increased numbers of thick, interwoven, basophilic fibers in the dermis in sun-damaged areas.

Degenerative disorders of the dermis

Collagen degeneration, characterized by increased granularity and staining intensity, develops in disorders associated with infiltrates of eosinophils (and subsequent eosinophil degranulation), such as reactions to insect bites, mast cell tumors, and eosinophilic granulomas (collagenolytic granulomas) (Fig. 11-12).

Collagen lysis, dissolution of collagen fibrils, develops subsequent to ischemia and in microbial and parasitic infections.

Disorders characterized by deposits in the dermis

Amyloid is a protein that may be deposited in the dermis either as a primary event of unknown cause or secondary to chronic infections, tissue destruction, or plasma cell neoplasms. Microscopically, amyloid consists of amorphous eosinophilic material.

Mucin, a normal component of the ground substance of the dermis, consists of protein bound to hyaluronic acid and may be deposited in increased quantity in focal areas or diffusely. Because hyaluronic acid has a great affinity for binding water, the skin in cases of **mucinosis** has a thick, puffy appearance. In cases of severe mucinosis, the skin may exude mucin (a stringy fluid material) when pricked with a needle. In histologic sections, much of the water is lost, and mucin appears as fine amphophilic granules or fibrils that replace dermal collagen. Examples of disorders with dermal mucin deposition include myxedema of hypothyroidism and mucinosis of the Chinese Shar Pei dog.

Calcium deposits in the dermis are secondary to alteration in dermal collagen (dystrophic calcification); develop in association with abnormal metabolism of calcium, phosphorus, and vitamin D (metastatic); or develop for unknown reasons (idiopathic). Calcification may involve individual or groups of collagen fibers, resulting in increased basophilia in stained sections and fragmentation of the fibers during sectioning. Calcium may also be deposited as amorphous nodular aggregates. Calcium deposits may be associated with a granulomatous inflammatory response.

Inflammatory disorders of the dermis

Dermatitis, inflammation of the dermis, follows the same sequences as in other tissues, including hyperemia, edema, and margination and immigration of leukocytes.

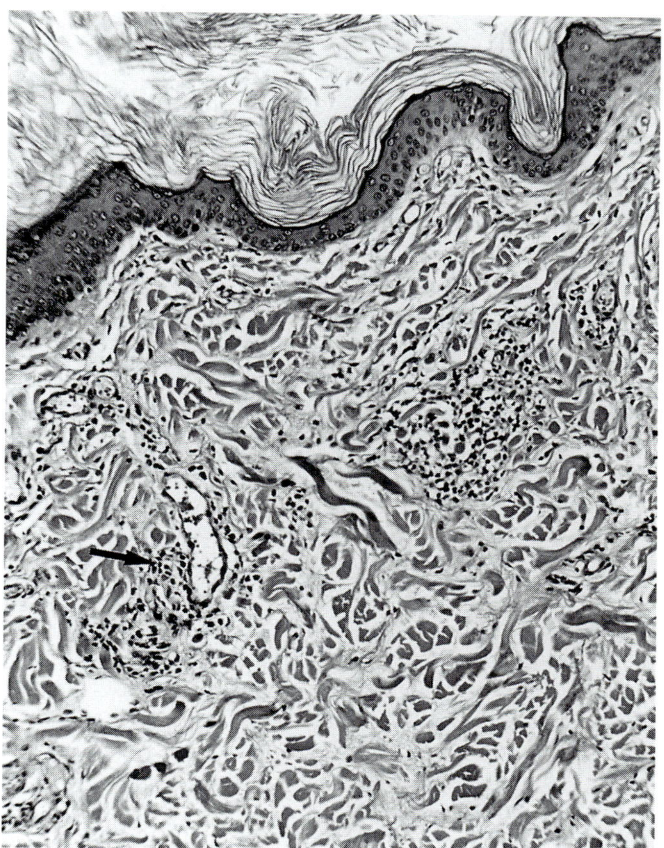

Fig. 11-13 Skin; dog. Perivascular inflammation. Vessels of superficial dermis are dilated and are bordered by leukocytes that have migrated through vessel walls into the surrounding perivascular dermis *(arrow)*. H & E stain.

The response is the same to many stimuli. However, the location and population of leukocytes can vary depending on cytokines, adhesion molecules, and other mediators. Thus, different patterns of cellular infiltrates are recognized such as perivascular (Fig. 11-13), lichenoid (interface), nodular, or diffuse. The types of cells present in the inflammatory infiltrate also vary. Perivascular and eosinophilic dermatitis is suggestive of hypersensitivity; lichenoid and lymphocytic dermatitis is suggestive of lupus erythematosus; and nodular and granulomatous dermatitis may be caused by infections with acid-fast bacteria and with fungi. Thus, patterns of inflammation and cellular composition of infiltrates are useful in microscopic diagnosis.

Adnexa

Adnexal structures include hair follicles and the associated glands. The follicles and glands tend to respond similarly to the same injury, and follicular epithelium responds with the changes described for the epidermis.

Alterations in growth and development of adnexa

Atrophy refers to gradual reduction (involution) in size and may be physiologic or pathologic. Physiologic atrophy is related to the normal cyclic changes of the hair follicle (see Anatomy and Histology of the Skin). Pathologic atrophy is greater than that expected for a given stage of the hair cycle, and causes include hormonal abnormalities, nutritional abnormalities, inadequacy of vascular supply, inflammation, and general state of health, including stressful events or systemic illness. Some types of pathologic atrophy can be reversed when the underlying cause is reversed. Pathologic atrophy associated with interference with blood supply (ischemic injury) can be severe enough to prevent regrowth of follicles or glandular adnexa, e.g., rabies vaccine–associated dermatitis due to injection of killed rabies vaccine into the subcutis, producing vasculitis. Destruction or total loss of the adnexa with scarring is due to damage to the germinal epithelium, as occurs in severe inflammation, chemical or thermal burns, and severe physical trauma.

Hypertrophy is an increase in the unit size of a structure or an individual cell. **Hyperplasia** is an increase in the number of cells in a structure. Enlargement of adnexa, a common response to injury, involves both hypertrophy and hyperplasia of cells and is observed in sebaceous and apocrine gland hyperplasia associated with chronic allergic dermatitis and follicular hypertrophy associated with acral lick dermatitis.

Follicular dysplasia refers to abnormal development, and several different and poorly characterized types of follicular dysplasia are described. Microscopic features vary and may include wavy distorted follicles (Fig. 11-14). The best understood forms of follicular dysplasia are color associated and include color mutant alopecia and black hair follicular dysplasia (see Fig. 11-14), where melanin pigment abnormalities serve as a marker for the dysplasia.

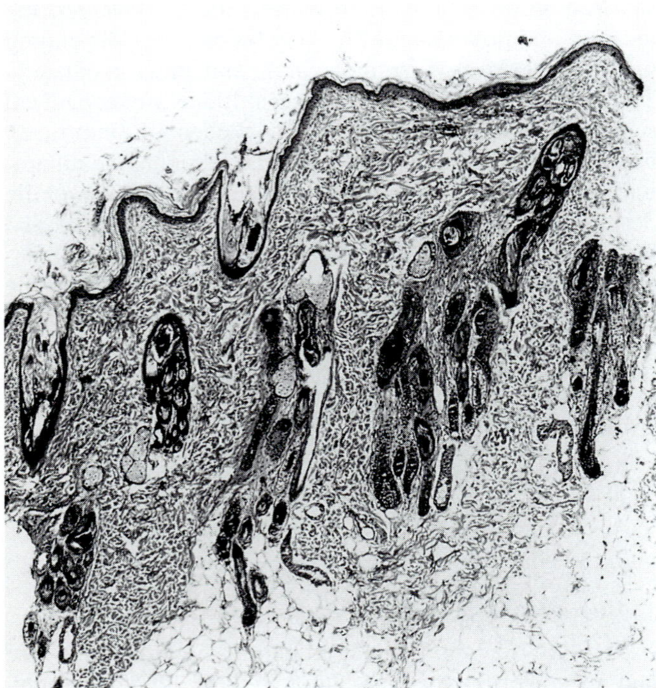

Fig. 11-14 Skin, haired; dog. Black hair follicular dysplasia. The follicles are irregular (wavy) and distorted. H & E stain.

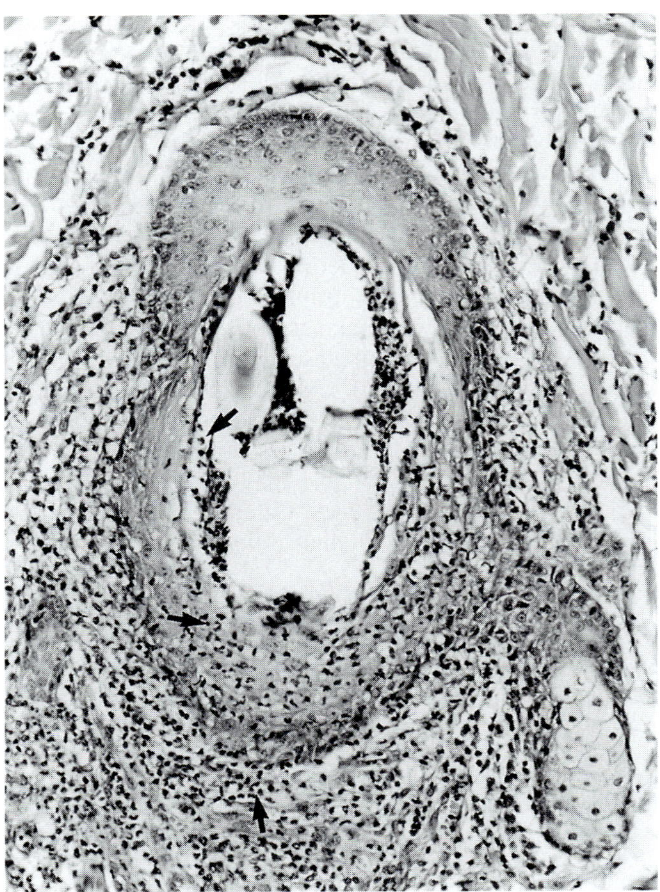

Fig. 11-15 Skin, haired; dog. Folliculitis. Neutrophils *(arrows)* are present in the lumen, wall, and perifollicular dermis. H & E stain.

Inflammatory disorders of the adnexa and panniculus

Perifolliculitis is inflammation surrounding the hair follicle. Inflammatory cells arrive via the perifollicular vessels and remain in perivascular sites. Perifolliculitis can be present at the same time as folliculitis. Perifolliculitis occurs as a specific lesion in alopecia areata, in which lymphocytes surround hair bulbs, causing the hair follicles to enter the resting stage of the cycle and the hair to shed.

Folliculitis is inflammation of a hair follicle, including the wall and often the lumen (Fig. 11-15). Mural folliculitis refers more strictly to inflammation of the follicular wall. Leukocytes migrate from the perifollicular vessels into the follicular wall and, often, subsequently the lumen. Superficial folliculitis predominantly involves the upper infundibulum, whereas deep folliculitis involves the entire infundibulum, isthmic (inferior) portion of the follicle, and the surrounding dermis. The inflammation may weaken the wall and predispose to follicular rupture (Fig. 11-16), resulting in **furunculosis** (perforating folliculitis). Released hair shafts, keratin, and sebum cause a foreign body–type response. Perifolliculitis, folliculitis, and furunculosis often follow in sequence. Specific causes include parasites *(Demodex, Pelodera),* bacteria (staphylococci), and dermatophytes *(Microsporum, Trichophyton).* Folliculitis and furunculosis also may follow reactions to drugs or insect bites (eosinophilic folliculitis) and develop as a secondary complication to pruritic dermatoses and to cornification and endocrine disorders. Follicular rupture as a complication to other dermatoses, such as cornification disorders, results because a plug of keratin at the follicular orifice causes accumulation of keratin, sebum, and sweat within the follicle to distend and weaken the follicular wall.

Sebaceous adenitis, inflammation of the sebaceous glands, may occur with folliculitis, demodicosis, uveodermatologic syndrome, or leishmaniasis. A specific inflammatory reaction targeting sebaceous glands occurs in dogs (Fig. 11-17) but is rarely seen in cats. Mild lesions are characterized by accumulations of lymphocytes around sebaceous ducts, but fully developed lesions consist of mixed populations of cells that have replaced sebaceous glands. Chronic lesions have total loss of sebaceous glands, scarring, and hyperkeratosis.

Hidradenitis, inflammation of apocrine glands, is seen in suppurative and granulomatous inflammations.

Panniculitis, inflammation of the subcutaneous adipose tissue, is the principal disorder of the panniculus and has a variety of causes, including infectious agents (bacteria, fungi), immune-mediated disorders (post–rabies vaccina-

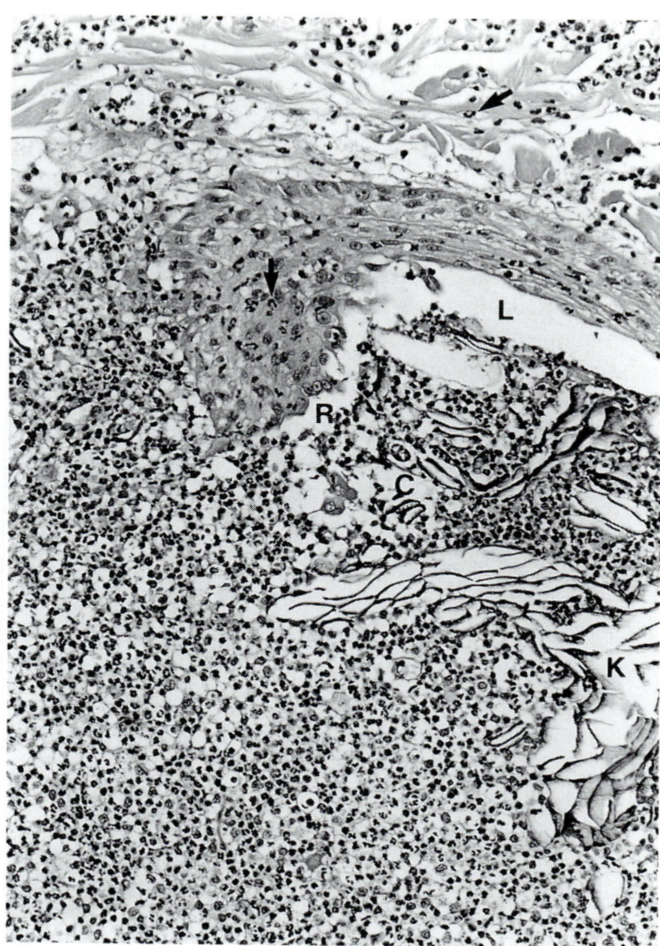

Fig. 11-16 Skin, haired; dog. Folliculitis and furunculosis. Note rupture (*R*) in the follicular wall, inflammatory cells (*C*) and keratin (*K*) in the follicular lumen (*L*), and neutrophils *(arrows)* in the follicular wall and perifollicular dermis. H & E stain.

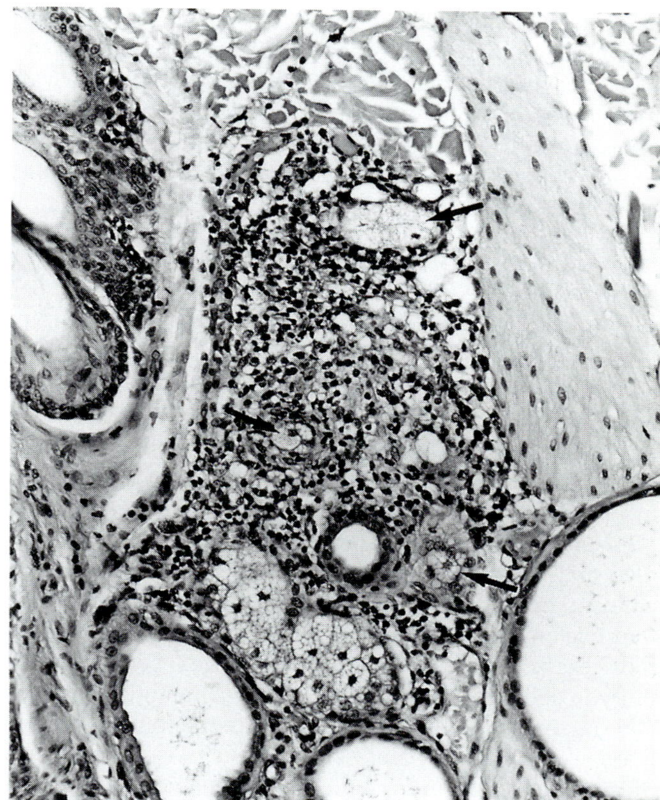

Fig. 11-17 Skin, haired; dog. Sebaceous adenitis. Inflammation is beginning to efface the sebaceous glands *(arrows)*. H & E stain.

tion alopecia, lupus erythematosus), physical injury (trauma, injection of irritant material, foreign bodies), nutritional disorders (vitamin E deficiency), and pancreatic disease. In some cases of panniculitis, an underlying cause is not known (idiopathic). Panniculitis may be primary or secondary to extension of inflammatory lesions in the contiguous dermis. Microscopically, lesions of a variety of inflammatory cell types may be concentrated in the fat lobules (lobular panniculitis) or in the interlobular septa (septal panniculitis) or involve both areas.

Pathologic Reactions of the Entire Cutaneous Unit

Responses of the skin to injury often involve multiple components; and lesions evolve through different stages, and some may resolve. Therefore, biopsy samples taken from multiple areas of a lesion often have different inflammatory stages involving multiple components creating different reaction patterns. The reactions of the various components of the skin can be illustrated by the example of a poxvirus infection. When a poxvirus invades the epidermis, the virus replicates in the cells of the stratum spinosum, causes cytoplasmic swelling (ballooning degeneration) and rupture (reticular degeneration) of some of the epidermal cells, and forms cytoplasmic viral inclusions in some cells. Ballooning and reticular degeneration result in the formation of a vesicle. Cellular constituents released from damaged epidermal cells are chemotactic for leukocytes. The chemotactic factors increase blood flow to the site of viral invasion by dilatation of vessels, cause margination of leukocytes along dermal vessel walls, increase vascular permeability (dermal edema), and cause migration of leukocytes out of the vessels into tissues. Initially, a perivascular dermatitis consists of lymphocytes and a variable number of neutrophils. Leukocytes in perivascular sites under the influence of inflammatory mediators from the epidermis migrate to the epidermis, followed by exocytosis and development of a pustule. Some poxviruses also cause epidermal hyperplasia by stimulating host-cell DNA synthesis, presumably by a viral gene product similar to epidermal growth factor, resulting in pseudoepitheliomatous hyperplasia (see Fig. 11-6). The pustule enlarges and eventually ruptures, releasing the exudate onto the skin surface; the exudate dries and forms crust (scab). In this way, multiple components of the skin participate in the development and resolution of the lesions and are responsible for the clinical stages of macule, papule, vesicle, pustule, crust, and scar.

BIOPSY TECHNIQUE

Biopsy Site Selection

Multiple cutaneous sites representative of the range of lesions should be selected for biopsy. Fully developed, nontreated primary lesions such as macules, papules, pustules, nodules, neoplasms, vesicles, and wheals are often the most useful for diagnosis. However, primary lesions may not be present, and secondary lesions (scales, crusts, ulcers, comedones, fissures, excoriations, lichenification, pigmentary abnormalities, and scars) then need to be sampled and evaluated. These secondary lesions may be diagnostic or contribute substantially to the diagnosis when multiple cutaneous sites are selected for biopsy. One of the most useful secondary lesions is the crust, because acantholytic cells from drying pustules in pemphigus foliaceus and organisms such as *Dermatophilus congolensis* or dermatophytes may be identified in crusts. Also, the margin of a chronic ulcer may represent a squamous cell carcinoma, or the scale at the edge of an epidermal collarette may represent a superficial, spreading pyoderma.

Biopsy Technique

Excisional biopsy samples (entire lesions) are recommended for large pustules or vesicles that may be damaged by use of a smaller punch biopsy instrument. Deeper excisional biopsy samples are generally necessary for diagnosis of lesions, such as panniculitis, that are deep to the skin. Digital amputation may be required, particularly in dogs, for the diagnosis of multifocal nail-bed lesions. Electrocautery should not be used for small biopsy samples, as the samples will be damaged and rendered nondiagnostic. Tissue forceps should grasp, if at all, only one nonaffected margin, preferably in the subcutis.

Biopsy Site Preparation

Generally, the skin at a punch biopsy site should not be surgically prepared because the procedure may remove the diagnostic portion of the sample (see Fig. 11-8). Gentle clipping of hair is acceptable. For an excisional biopsy of lesions deep to the epidermis, surgical preparation of the skin is acceptable.

Fixation

Punch biopsy specimens should be placed in 10 times the volume of 10% neutral buffered formalin (NBF). Thin excisional biopsy specimens should be gently attached to a flat object, such as a piece of tongue depressor, to avoid warping in the fixative. In cold climates during winter months, adding 1 part alcohol to 9 parts 10% NBF reduces the chance of freezing of the specimens during transport. For immunofluorescence evaluation, specimens should be placed in Michel's medium, which better preserves immunoglobulins and complement.

History

The diagnosis by a pathologist after histopathologic evaluation often requires knowledge of the gross features of the lesions. Therefore, it is essential to include with the biopsy samples the following information: age, breed, sex of the animal, location, gross appearance, duration of lesions, and the presence or absence of symmetry and pruritus. Clinical information—results of clinical laboratory evaluations, current medications, and response to therapy—should be included along with a list of clinical differential diagnoses.

CONGENITAL/HEREDITARY DISEASES

The terms ''congenital'' and ''hereditary'' are not synonymous. Congenital lesions develop in the fetus (in utero), are present at birth, and have a variety of causes. An example is hypotrichosis in the fetus, associated with maternal dietary iodine deficiency. Inherited conditions are transmitted genetically and are not always manifested phenotypically in utero or at birth. An example includes familial canine dermatomyositis, which may develop as early as 8 weeks of age.

Acanthosis Nigricans

Primary idiopathic acanthosis nigricans is considered a genodermatosis of young dachshund dogs. The disease is manifested by bilateral axillary hyperpigmentation, lichenification, and alopecia, which may involve large areas and include secondary seborrhea and pyoderma. Microscopically, the epidermis is thickened, principally by acanthosis. Hyperkeratosis and focal parakeratosis are accompanied by increased melanin pigment in the epidermis. The term ''acanthosis nigricans'' has also been used to encompass a variety of disorders which in the chronic form are manifested by axillary or more diffuse lichenification, alopecia, and hyperpigmentation.

Alopecia and Hypotrichosis

Alopecia or atrichia (absence of hair from skin where it is usually present) and hypotrichosis (less than the normal amount of hair) have been reported in most species of domestic animals. In some animals, the alopecia or hypotrichosis has been recognized as standard for the breed including the Mexican hairless dog, Sphinx cat, and Ulster pig. Degree, location, and age at onset of hairlessness vary. In some instances, the alopecia or hypotrichosis is not due to an absence or reduction of the number of hair follicles but to a failure of hair growth or failure to maintain hair within follicles, caused by an abnormality of the hair follicles (follicular dysplasia). Congenital alopecia has been associated with maternal iodine deficiency.

Collagen Dysplasia

Collagen dysplasia (cutis hyperelastica, dermatosparaxis, cutaneous asthenia) occurs in most domestic animals and comprises a clinically, genetically, and biochemically heterogeneous group of diseases. In each, the skin tears easily, is hyperextensible, and is loose, but the severity of these lesions varies among species. Specific enzyme defects of collagen synthesis or processing are the causes of some collagen dysplasia syndromes, and the cause of others has not been established. Grossly, cutaneous hyperextensibility and laxity (Fig. 11-18) are associated with numerous secondary scars. Microscopic features vary among the disorders of collagen dysplasia, and, in some cases, the skin is histologically normal. The histologic pattern is dysplastic; i.e., collagen bundles may vary in size and shape and have an abnormal organizational pattern. In some cases, electron microscopy or biochemical analysis is required to make a more definitive diagnosis.

Epidermolysis Bullosa (Red Foot Disease)

Epidermolysis bullosa refers to a group of mechanobullous diseases resulting in development of cutaneous blisters (bullae). The diseases vary in mode of inheritance, clinical manifestations, and anatomic location of the blisters. The diseases usually result in death of affected animals. Epidermolysis bullosa has been reported in some breeds of sheep, horses, cattle, and dogs. Lesions may be present at birth or develop shortly thereafter and are located where epithelial surfaces are traumatized such as oral mucosa, lips, and extremities, including the coronary band. Microscopic lesions are those of an epidermal vesicular disease in which vesicles form in different locations (subepidermal, epidermal-dermal junction, intraepidermal), depending on the specific disease. As healing occurs, the reepithelization causes more dorsal displacement of the vesicles, and, with secondary infection, the vesicles become pustules.

Epitheliogenesis Imperfecta (Aplasia Cutis)

Epitheliogenesis imperfecta results from the failure of the squamous epithelium and adnexa of skin and epithelium of oral mucosa to develop completely. The disease varies in severity and has been reported in most domestic species. It is inherited in some species, but inheritance is not proven in other species. Grossly, lesions consist of circumscribed variably sized areas in which the squamous epithelium is absent (Fig. 11-19). Without the protective covering of the squamous epithelium, the underlying tissue is easily traumatized and becomes infected, and bacteremia may develop.

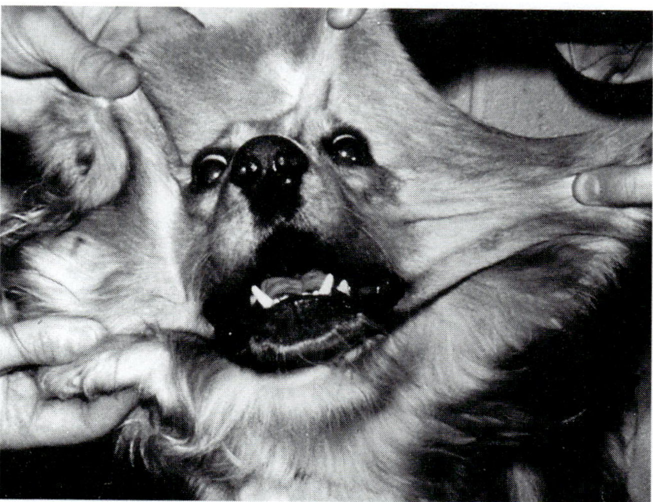

Fig. 11-18 Skin; dog. Collagen dysplasia. The skin is hyperextensible. *Courtesy Dr. B. Baker.*

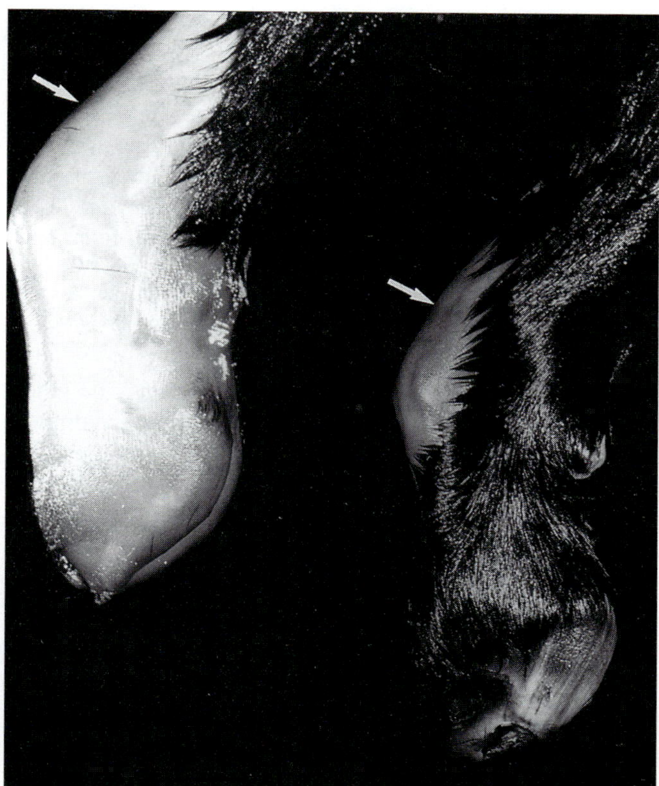

Fig. 11-19 Skin; calf. Epitheliogenesis imperfecta. Epidermis is absent multifocally over extremities *(arrows)*. *Courtesy Dr. M. D. McGavin.*

Hypertrichosis

Excessive growth of hair may be congenital or hereditary. Abnormally hairy fleece at birth develops subsequent to in utero infection of fine- and medium-wooled fetal lambs with the virus of Border disease. In addition to abnormal fleece, affected sheep have defective myelination of the brain and spinal cord, abnormalities of body conformation, poor growth, and reduced viability. Microscopically, primary follicles and wool fibers are enlarged, and the number of the secondary follicles and wool fibers is reduced. Hypertrichosis in lambs also has been associated with maternal hyperthermia.

Ichthyosis

Ichthyosis is an inherited cutaneous disease seen principally in dogs and cattle. The skin is thickened by marked hyperkeratosis and may crack into plates resembling fish scales, thus the origin of the name. The basic defect is increased adherence of keratinocytes, which prevents normal desquamation. In cattle, two forms of the disease have been described. One (ichthyosis fetalis) is lethal, and most calves are stillborn or die within days of birth. Grossly and microscopically, the skin is alopecic and covered by thick keratin with many fissures. In the second and less severe form (ichthyosis congenita), the skin is thickened and folded, with fissures and partial alopecia; more severe lesions occur on the limbs, abdomen, and muzzle. Microscopic lesions include a marked hyperkeratosis of the epidermis (lamellar hyperkeratosis), especially of the flexor areas and digital pads, alopecia, and lichenification. The skin is thickened by dry scales and keratin. In addition to the marked epidermal hyperkeratosis, hypergranulosis, keratinocyte vacuolation, and reticular degeneration are seen in skin of some affected animals.

Porcine Juvenile Pustular Psoriasiform Dermatitis (Pityriasis Rosea)

This disorder of suckling and young pigs may be inherited. Lesions are symmetric and develop on the abdomen, groin, and medial thigh, beginning as small papules covered by brown crusts. The lesions coalesce and spread and develop into umbilicated plaques with white centers and erythematous and scaly borders. Lesions resemble those of dermatophytosis but otherwise are of no significance. Microscopically, lesions are psoriasiform epidermal hyperplasia, parakeratosis, and epidermal pustules with superficial perivascular dermatitis.

Zinc-related Disorders

Lethal acrodermatitis is an autosomal recessive inherited disease in bullterrier dogs. Lesions generally begin between 6 and 10 weeks of age, and most afflicted dogs are dead by 15 months of age. Lesions begin between the digits and on foot pads, and progress to severe interdigital pyoderma, paronychia, and hyperkeratosis of foot pads. Lesions also develop on pinnae, muzzle, elbows, hocks, and, in some dogs, can become more generalized and consist of crusting, ulceration, and secondary pyoderma. Microscopically, the lesions consist of extensive diffuse orthokeratotic and parakeratotic hyperkeratosis and bacterial pustular dermatitis. Dogs do not respond to oral and parenteral zinc supplementation. An autosomal recessive inherited form of zinc deficiency has also been reported in young calves. The cutaneous lesions in the calves resolve with zinc supplementation.

ENVIRONMENTALLY RELATED DISEASES

Actinic Diseases

Sunlight comprises visible, ultraviolet (UV), and infrared light rays. The portion of the UV light most damaging to the skin is ultraviolet B (UVB) and is in the range of 290- to 320-nm wavelength. However, photodynamic chemicals, if present in the skin, can chemically react with longer wavelengths, creating cutaneous damage (photosensitization, phototoxicity). The amount of light reaching the skin is dependent on a variety of environmental and host factors such as ozone, smog, and cloud cover, which tend to absorb and scatter some of the UV rays. Altitude and latitude are also very important. The atmosphere at high altitude is thinner, with less oxygen and particulate matter to absorb and scatter UV rays. At higher latitudes, because of the angle of entry into the atmosphere, the path of sunlight through the ozone layer is longer than at lower latitudes, so more of the harmful UV light is absorbed by the ozone. The path of sunlight through the ozone layer is also one of the reasons the sunlight has more damaging UV rays in summer months and at midday. Host factors include quantity of hair, degree of pigmentation, and thickness of the stratum corneum. Therefore, solar damage is more prevalent at high altitude, low latitude parts of the world and in animals housed outside for long periods of time. Lesions generally develop in poorly haired or lightly pigmented sites.

Solar dermatosis and neoplasia

The damage to skin by UV light can be acute (sunburn) or chronic (solar dermatosis, neoplasia). An early transient erythema may be due to the heating effect of the light rays and, possibly, to photochemical changes. The later developing erythema is called ''sunburn erythema'' and is associated with warmth, tenderness, and swelling. The pathogenesis of sunburn erythema may involve diffusion of inflammatory mediators, such as cytokines, from radiation-damaged keratinocytes or from direct damage to endothelial cells by UV light. Pigmentation is increased in two stages: an immediate pigment darkening due to photooxidation of preexisting melanin and a longer term effect due to melanogenesis. UV light also depresses immune responses of the skin. Preneoplastic and neoplastic lesions are common chronic alterations in solar-damaged skin in domestic animals.

The mechanisms involved in development of solar lesions are multifactorial. Tissue damage occurs when UV light is absorbed, resulting in generation of reactive molecules—such as free radicals—which can damage nucleic acids and proteins. The damage may occur in nuclei, membranes, or organelles and may alter enzymes, cause mutations, or lead to neoplasms. One of the more influential alterations is the formation of thymidine dimers between pyrimidine bases of deoxyribonucleic acid (DNA). Before the cell undergoes mitosis, the damage can be easily and accurately repaired by an enzyme system that removes the damaged area and synthesizes a new strand of DNA. However, if the cell undergoes mitosis before the damage is repaired, a gap in the DNA strand is left at the location of the thymidine dimer. The gap is repaired by a postreplication repair method that is thought to be error-prone and may lead to mutations and the development of neoplasms. Factors that irritate the skin and increase the rate of cell division increase the number of cells repaired by the postreplication repair method, and, therefore, may enhance development of neoplasms. UV radiation may also alter immunologic reactivity by inducing suppressor T cells that favor growth of neoplastic cells.

Solar dermatitis

The lesions of sunburn occur in all domestic animals. In cats, gross lesions occur where there is little or no hair and little pigment—on external ear tips, eyelids, nose, and lips—and are most severe in white or multicolored cats. Dogs have lesions most commonly in nonpigmented, sparsely haired skin of ventral abdominal, inguinal, and perianal areas. Lightly pigmented younger pigs are more susceptible, and the pinnae and tip of the tail may slough if injury is severe. In lightly colored dairy goats, lesions may develop on the lateral aspects of the udder and teats. Grossly, lesions begin as erythema, scaling, and crusting. The skin becomes wrinkled and thickened, and squamous cell carcinomas may develop. Hemangiomas and/or hemangiosarcomas have developed in the nonpigmented conjunctiva of dogs and horses and in the skin of dogs and cats. The difference in type of neoplasm may be due in part to the thickness of the epithelium, which influences the depth of penetration of the UV rays.

Microscopically, in early UV-induced injury, the number of dyskeratotic cells scattered in the epidermis may be so numerous as to form a band of dyskeratotic cells along with intercellular edema, vacuolation of keratinocytes, and loss of granular cell layer. Within 72 hours, hyperkeratosis, parakeratosis, and acanthosis are present, along with dermal lesions of hyperemia, edema, perivascular mononuclear infiltrates, endothelial swelling, and hemorrhage. Hyperkeratosis, parakeratosis, and acanthosis may persist, and pseudoepitheliomatous hyperplasia and dermal fibrosis may develop. Actinic comedones may develop in some dogs. In some animals and in some anatomic locations, elastic tissue and collagen are damaged by solar radiation.

Photosensitization

Photosensitization occurs when long-wavelength UV or, less frequently, visible light is absorbed by a photodynamic chemical in the skin or by a complex of photodynamic molecule and a biologic substrate, which results in the activation of the photodynamic substance. Several mechanisms of tissue injury resulting from activation of the photodynamic substance have been proposed. For instance, furocoumarins (found in some plants) attach to the surface of the cell and, when activated, result in cell membrane damage and altered permeability. Porphyrins, on the other hand, become concentrated in lysosomes and, when activated, damage the lysosomal membrane, resulting in release of enzymes into the cytoplasm. The photodynamic substances activated by light of the appropriate wavelength generally cause membrane damage by producing oxygen radicals. Exposure to the photodynamic agent may be systemic (via the circulation) or by local application (direct contact).

Photosensitization can occur in several forms. The first, **primary** photosensitization, is often due to ingestion of preformed photodynamic substances contained in a variety of plants such as *Hypericum perforatum* and *Fagopyrum sagittatum* (buckwheat) or of fungal-contaminated plants. Administration of phenothiazine, tetracycline, thiazides, or sulfonamides also may cause primary photosensitization. Photosensitization may also develop due to **abnormal porphyrin metabolism.** These diseases usually are inherited due to an enzyme deficiency that results in abnormal synthesis of photodynamic agents, including uroporphyrin and coproporphyrin. Examples include bovine congenital porphyria and bovine erythropoietic (hematopoietic) protoporphyria. **Hepatogenous** (secondary) photosensitization is due to hepatic disease that impairs excretion of phylloerythrin, a product of chlorophyll metabolism. Hepatogenous photosensitization can occur secondary to inherited hepatic defects, biliary obstruction, or as a result of hepatic injury from ingestion of hepatotoxic plants (lantana) or fungal-contaminated plants (e.g., by the mycotoxin sporidesmin), exposure to chemicals (carbon tetrachloride), and infectious agents (diffuse inflammation in leptospirosis).

Grossly, in photosensitization, lesions are located in areas with little protection by pigment or dense hair or fleece and on parts of the body exposed to the sun, such as the blaze, muzzle, coronary band, cannon, and pastern in horses. In cattle, lesions occur in white areas and on the teats, udder, perineum, and muzzle. In sheep with heavy fleeces, lesions occur on the pinnae, eyelids, face, muzzle, and coronary band area, but, in shorn sheep, lesions may occur on the back. Sheep may have extensive edema of the head, resulting in the descriptions of "swelled head" and "facial eczema." Lesions initially include erythema and edema, followed by blisters, exudation, necrosis, and sloughing of necrotic tissues and keratitis in some animals. The microscopic lesions consist of subepidermal vesiculation with subsequent ulceration and secondary infection.

Photoenhanced dermatoses

Several immune-mediated cutaneous disorders aggravated by exposure to UV radiation include lupus erythematosus, dermatomyositis, and pemphigus erythematosus. Cytokines liberated from keratinocytes may play a role in photoenhancement. Photoactivated vasculitis in the white-haired extremities of horses is a poorly understood disorder associated with exposure to the sun. Lesions consist of well-demarcated erythematous, crusted lesions or hyperkeratotic plaques. Microscopically, mild vasculitis of the superficial dermal vessels and occasional thrombi are seen.

Chemical Injuries

Chemical injuries to the skin are due to local application and to systemic absorption. For a chemical to cause injury via local application, it must penetrate the hair and protective epidermal layers. Penetration is enhanced by physical damage to the stratum corneum, especially that caused by excessive moisture. Chemical injuries of the skin include contact irritant dermatitis; poisonings by such chemicals as arsenic, mercury, thallium, iodine, and organochlorines and organobromines; and poisonings by plants, fungal-contaminated plants, and plants containing selenium, mimosine, and tricothecenes.

Contact dermatitis

Of the two forms of contact dermatitis, one is immunologically mediated and the other is due to primary contact with irritant substances. Most cases of contact dermatitis are nonimmunologic and are due to direct contact with substances such as body or wound secretions; to the accidental exposure to irritants such as acids, alkalies, soaps, detergents, irritant plants; and to application of drugs. In dogs and cats, lesions of irritant contact dermatitis develop on the glabrous skin of the abdomen, axillae, flanks, interdigital spaces, perianal area, ventral tail, chest, legs, eyelids, and feet. Horses develop lesions on the muzzle, ventrum, lower limbs; where riding tack contacts the body; and on the perineum and caudal aspect of the rear legs. Grossly, erythemic patches and papules and, rarely, vesicles are the lesions, but self-inflicted trauma may lead to ulcers and crusts. Microscopically, lesions consist of spongiotic or hyperplastic dermatitis with superficial perivascular inflammation, except that corrosive substances (strong acids or alkalies) may cause epidermal necrosis.

Ergot

Ergot poisoning occurs when toxic alkaloids of the fungus, *Claviceps purpurea,* are ingested with the seed heads of grasses and grains. The toxic alkaloids include ergotamine, ergometrine, ergotoxine, and other chemicals, including histamine, acetylcholine, and tyramine. The alkaloids cause arterial and venous peripheral vasoconstriction and damage capillary endothelium, leading to thrombosis and tissue ischemia. Cold temperatures increase the severity of the lesions. The species most commonly poisoned are cattle fed contaminated grain and grazing pastures infected with the alkaloid-producing fungus. Lesions develop after about 1 week of consumption and begin as swelling and redness of extremities, particularly of the hind legs. Tips of pinnae and tail are affected with dry gangrene and may slough.

Fescue

Fescue poisoning due to excessive consumption of *Festuca arudinacea* develops after about 2 weeks of ingestion of the plant and consists of necrosis (dry gangrene) of distal extremities, with lesions identical with those of ergot poisoning.

Selenium

Selenium toxicity occurs worldwide, but, in certain regions, poisoning is more frequent; these include Nebraska, Wyoming, and the Dakotas in the United States and portions of Western Canada. Selenium poisoning develops after ingestion of plants that have accumulated toxic concentrations of selenium, but it can occur with overdosage of a selenium supplement. Some plants selectively accumulate selenium, regardless of soil selenium content. These selective accumulators (obligate accumulators, i.e., *Astragalus, Stanleya*) require selenium for growth, generally are not palatable, and are eaten only when other plant sources are unavailable. Many other plants, i.e., *Aster, Atriplex,* do not require selenium for growth but will accumulate toxic concentrations of selenium if grown in soil with high selenium concentrations (facultative accumulators). These facultative accumulator plants are commonly eaten by livestock and more often are the cause of poisoning. Selenium poisoning has been described in most domestic herbivores and, rarely, pigs, although susceptibility to selenium poisoning varies with species, dosage, diet, and other factors. In acute poisonings, signs relate to involvement of multiple organ systems. Herbivores with chronic selenium intoxication are emaciated, have poor quality hair coat, and have partial alopecia. Horses lose the long hair of the mane and tail, develop hoof deformities, and shed the hooves. The mechanism of action is not completely understood and is probably multifactorial. Replacement by selenium of sulfur in various molecules is a possible mechanism of toxicity.

Physical Causes

Acral lick dermatitis

Acral lick dermatitis (lick granuloma, neurodermatitis) is a relatively common psychogenic dermatitis usually of an extremity (acral = extremity) in dogs due to persistent licking and chewing (Fig. 11-20). Usually, a single lesion occurs on carpal, metacarpal, metatarsal, tibial, or radial areas. Grossly, lesions are circumscribed, hairless, and, sometimes, ulcerated. Microscopically, the hyperkeratosis is compact, and a marked hyperplasia involves the epidermal and follicular epithelium. The dermis is thickened by collagenous fibers oriented parallel with the hair follicles (vertical streaking) and contains perivascular and periadnexal plasma cell accumulations and hyperplastic sebaceous glands. A mild sensory polyneuropathy may be associated with lesion development.

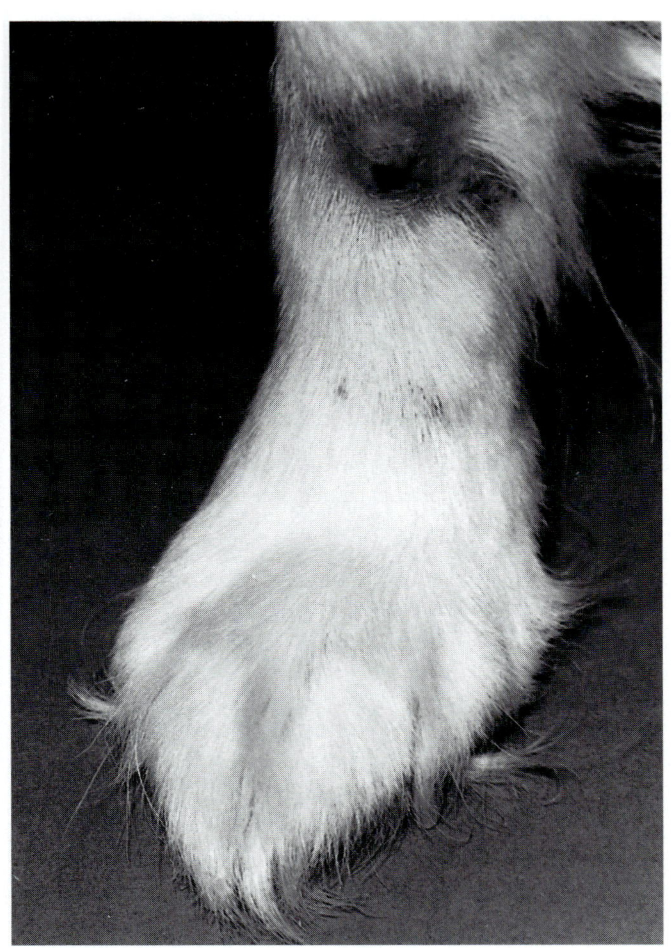

Fig. 11-20 Skin, leg; dog. Acral lick dermatitis. Area of alopecia with small dark ulcer is present.

Feline psychogenic alopecia

Psychogenic alopecia occurs in cats of the more emotional breeds and is multifactorial. A partial alopecia is due to broken hairs that develop after gentle, but persistent, licking. Linear or symmetric areas of alopecia are found along the dorsal midline or in the perineal, genital, caudomedial thigh, and abdominal areas. Microscopically, the skin is generally normal, but telogen follicles may be increased. Differential diagnoses include the rare endocrine alopecia and mild hypersensitivity disorders with associated persistent licking.

Callus

A callus is a raised, irregular, plaquelike area of cutaneous thickening that develops due to friction, usually over pressure points on bony prominences or on the sternum. Callosities can develop in all domestic animals but are particularly common in giant breed dogs and in pigs kept on concrete or other hard flooring without adequate bedding. Secondary folliculitis, furunculosis, and ulceration may develop. Microscopically, the epidermis and follicular epithelium are thickened by hyperkeratosis and acanthosis, and comedones and follicular cysts are present in some lesions. The follicular openings are widened by excessive keratin. Comedones and follicular cysts may rupture, releasing bacteria, keratin, and sebum, which will result in secondary pyoderma and a foreign body inflammatory response.

Injection site reactions

Injection of vaccines or therapeutic drugs into the subcutis can result in granulomatous nodules in the panniculus. These granulomas have central foreign and necrotic material bordered by macrophages and multinucleated giant cells and surrounded by a zone of granulation tissue, eosinophils, and perivascular lymphocytes that form lymphoid follicles in some lesions. In cats, fibrosarcomas have developed at some injection sites secondary to vaccination. In small breeds of dogs, especially poodles, injection of killed rabies vaccine has resulted in lymphoplasmacytic panniculitis and perivasculitis, mild vasculitis, and severe follicular atrophy (Fig. 11-21).

Intertrigo (skin fold dermatitis)

Intertrigo develops secondary to irritation and bacterial growth from skin friction and moisture of tears, saliva, cutaneous glandular secretions, and urine. Locations of intertrigo include the facial fold (common in brachycephalic breeds), lip fold (common in breeds with large lips such as Saint Bernard dogs), body fold, (common in the Shar Pei breed), vulvar fold (common in obese female dogs with a

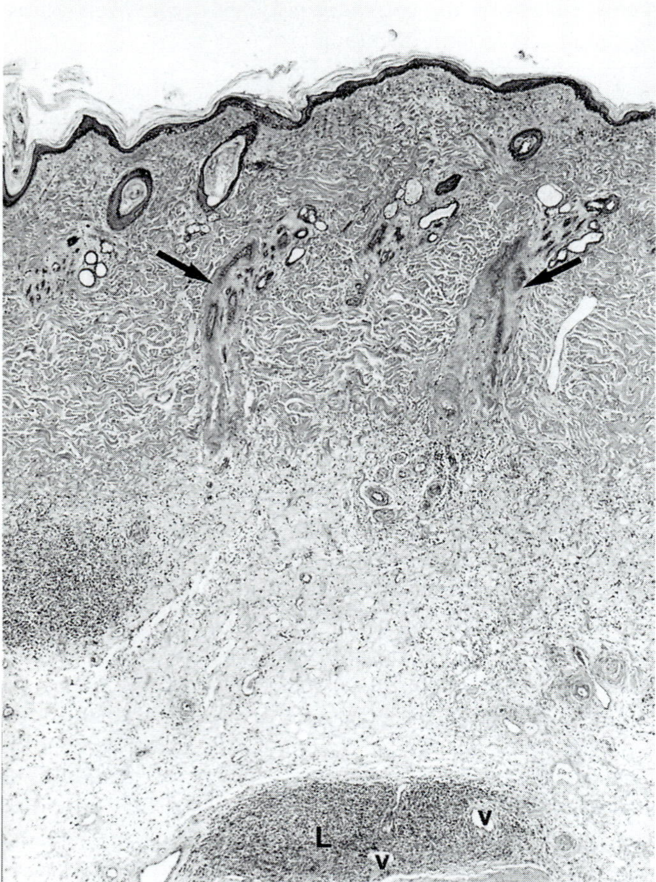

Fig. 11-21 Skin, haired; dog. Note injection site reaction with small, atrophic hair follicles *(arrows)* and lymphocytic perivasculitis *(L),* and vessels *(V)* H & E stain.

small vulva), and tail fold (common in dogs with corkscrew tails, such as English bulldogs) (Figs. 11-22 and 11-23). Intertrigo between the udder and medial thigh (udder-thigh dermatitis) develops principally in cows with a large, pendulous udder. Severe cases of udder-thigh dermatitis may have sloughing of the skin and subcutis.

Pyotraumatic dermatitis (acute moist dermatitis, ''hot spots'')

Pyotraumatic dermatitis, especially common in dogs, is secondary to irritation and is, principally, the result of self-inflicted trauma of biting or scratching because of pain and itching. Primary irritants include allergies, parasites, matted hair, and irritant chemicals. Dogs with long hair and dense undercoats are predisposed, and lesions develop more commonly in hot, humid weather. Grossly, the lesions are hairless, red, and moist; exude fluid; and have red and circumscribed edges. Microscopically, either superficial erosive to ulcerative exudative dermatitis or a deeper suppurative folliculitis (pyotraumatic folliculitis, deep pyoderma) is demonstrated. Biopsy is required to differentiate the more superficial pyotraumatic dermatitis from the pyoderma.

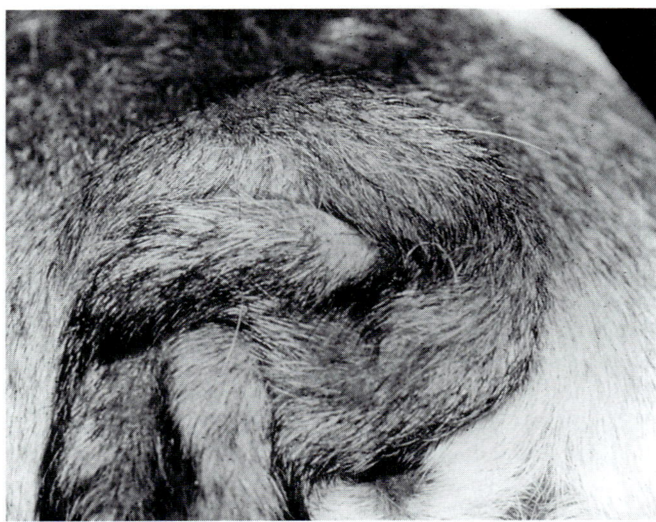

Fig. 11-22 Skin, tail; English bulldog. ''Screw tail.'' The skin is folded around the tail. *Courtesy Dr. A. Werner.*

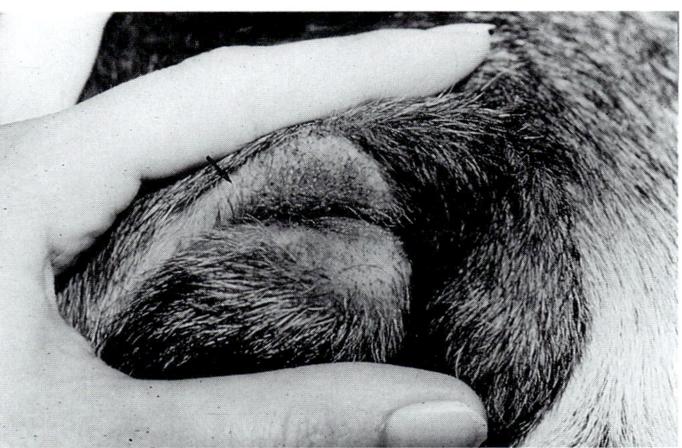

Fig. 11-23 Skin, tail; English bulldog. Intertriginous pyoderma. The lesion is present in the skin fold *(arrow)* of the dog depicted in Fig. 11-22. *Courtesy Dr. A. Werner.*

Radiation

Radiation injury may be due to electromagnetic (x-ray and gamma ray) or energetic particles (neutrons, protons, alpha particles, pi mesons, electrons, and heavy ions). Electromagnetic and particulate radiation cause damage by energy transfer. Radiosensitivity varies directly with the rate of cell division, and, therefore, dividing cells, especially the highly proliferative cells in the anagen hair matrix, are susceptible to radiation damage; and a sequela to cutaneous radiation is alopecia. Other sensitive cells include the germinal basal cells, melanocytes, and endothelial cells. Susceptibility of melanocytes to radiation injury is complex and dose dependent. At larger doses, melanocytes in the hair follicle are more susceptible than those in the epidermis, and those in telogen follicles are more susceptible than those in anagen follicles, with susceptibility related to the amount of cytoplasmic melanin pigment, a free-radical trap. Early cutaneous changes secondary to mild radiation damage include erythema that develops after 2 to 3 days. Depending on dosage and type of radiation, edema, epidermal blistering, erosion, and ulceration may develop between 2 and 6 weeks after exposure. Healing occurs with scarring and pigmentary changes (hyperpigmentation with smaller doses and hypopigmentation with larger doses that destroy melanocytes). Alopecia may be temporary or permanent, depending on the severity of the adnexal damage. Chronic changes, sometimes developing after a long latent period, include pigmentary alterations, scaling, alopecia, atrophy of epidermis and adnexal structures, vascular and elastic tissue degeneration, dermal and subcutaneous fibrosis, and ulceration. Squamous cell carcinomas may develop in some sites of severe radiation damage.

Temperature extremes

Extremes in temperature such as excessive and prolonged cold can cause injury by osmotic effects due to increased intracellular salt concentration, which develops when ice crystals form and dissolve, and by vascular injury. Slow chilling may produce vasoconstriction, some cellular damage, and secondary vasodilatation with the increased permeability followed by edema. Exposure to more severe and persistent cold causes vasoconstriction, increased blood viscosity, and tissue anoxia. Lesions due to cold temperatures are uncommon in well-nourished healthy animals but may develop in an animal recently moved from a warm to a cold climate and in neonates that are hypoglycemic or improperly dried. Lesions are located in the extremities such as the ear tips of cats, the scrotum of dogs and bulls, and ear tips, tail, and teats of cattle. Grossly, lesions consist of gangrene and sloughing of necrotic tissue.

Lesions due to excessive heat (local hyperthermia, burns) are variable and occur from exposure to liquids, flames, friction, electricity, and lightning. Burns are categorized as partial- or full-thickness lesions or first-, second-, and third-degree burns. Full-thickness burns have total destruction of the entire skin and dermal appendages; therefore, wounds must be repaired by grafting, scarring may develop, and the lesions are life threatening. Partial-thickness burns have preservation of some part of the epidermis or dermal appendages from which epithelial regeneration may develop. These lesions are less severe, lower temperatures are usually involved, and damage is due to accelerated cellular metabolism, inactivation of enzymes, and vessel injury. Grossly, lesions are those of erythema due to capillary dilatation, edema due to increased capillary permeability, and vesicle formation due to fluid accumulation at the dermal-epidermal junction (burn blister) (Fig. 11-24). Microscopically, partial-thickness burns have coagulation necrosis of the epidermis, subepidermal vesiculation due to accumulation of fluid from superficial capillaries, necrosis of superficial portions of follicles and adnexa, and degeneration of the subepidermal collagen. In more severe burns, the necrosis may extend to the panniculus. Due to coagulation of blood vessels, exudation may not develop; but cellular and vascular lesions, including vasculitis and thrombosis, will develop at the junction of viable and necrotic tissue. Secondary infection is manifested by accumulations of large numbers of neutrophils.

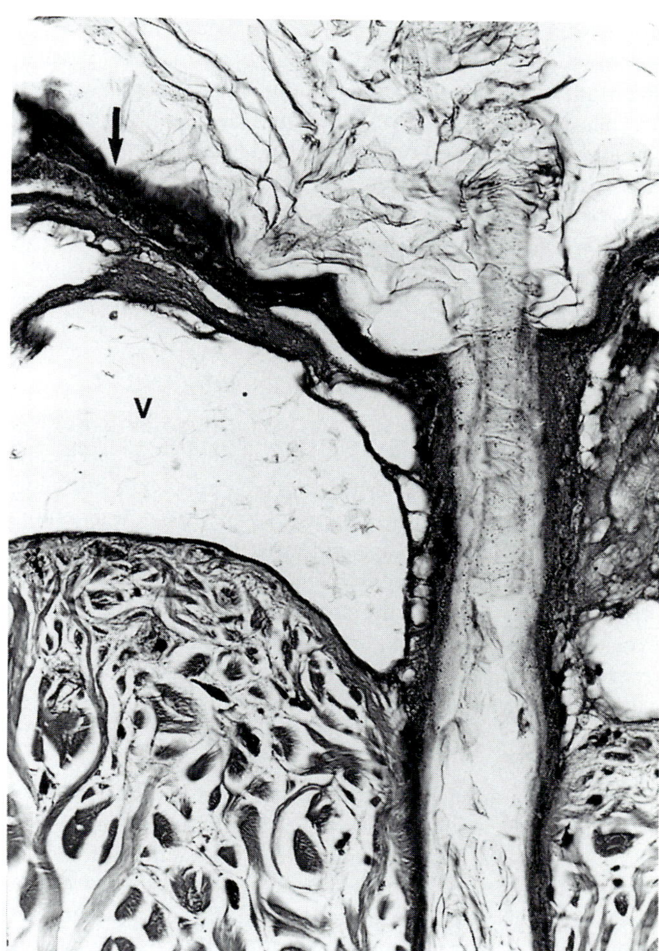

Fig. 11-24 Skin, haired; dog. Thermal burn. Necrosis of epidermis *(arrow)* and follicular epithelium are accompanied by subepidermal vesiculation (vesicle [*V*]). H & E stain.

Snakebites and spider bites

The families Elapidae (coral snake) and Viperidae (rattlesnake, water moccasin, and copperhead) contain the majority of the poisonous snakes in the United States. The genera *Latrodectus* (e.g., black widow) and *Loxosceles* (e.g., brown recluse) are the most common venomous spiders associated with cutaneous injury. Snakebites are most common on the extremities of large animals and cause swelling, erythema, and edema that may be followed by necrosis and sloughing of tissue and death of the animal. Spider bites are found on the face and legs, and the severity of lesions is dependent on the type of spider, with some bites becoming erythematous followed by necrosis and ulceration. Microscopic lesions of spider bites include an exudative, ulcerative dermatitis; dermal necrosis; neutrophilic and histiocytic infiltrates of the dermis and panniculus; and vasculopathy.

INFECTIOUS CAUSES OF SKIN DISEASE

Cutaneous infections develop when there is disruption of the defense mechanisms of the skin. Defense mechanisms include physical barriers such as hair coat, pigment, and stratum corneum and chemical barriers such as emulsion of lipids, electrolytes, proteins, vitamins, hormones, transferrin, immunoglobulins, and microbial flora. Predisposing factors to skin infections include friction, trauma, excessive moisture, dirt, matted hair, chemical irritants, freezing and burning, irradiation, inadequate diet, and parasitic infestation.

Poxviruses

Poxviruses are DNA epitheliotropic viruses that infect most domestic, wild, and laboratory animals and birds (Table 11-2). Dogs and cats are rarely infected with poxviruses, although infection with contagious ecthyma (parapoxvirus) has been reported in dogs and cutaneous infection caused by a poxvirus of the orthopoxvirus genus has been reported in cats in Europe. Poxviruses have major differences in the range of species they will infect, with some being species specific and others zoonotic. Many poxviruses of animals can cause skin lesions in human beings. Poxviral lesions develop secondary to viral invasion of epithelium, by ischemic necrosis due to vascular injury, and by stimulation of host cell DNA resulting in the formation of hyperplastic nodules or benign neoplasms. The severity of poxviral infection is variable, in part due to the localized or systemic nature of the infection and, in some instances, to secondary infections. Cutaneous poxviral sequential lesions consist of macule, papule, vesicle (variably severe), umbilicated pustule, crust, and scar. Sheep-pox and goatpox are the most pathogenic poxviruses; and infection causes significant mortality, especially in young animals, due to systemic disease, but these diseases do not occur in the United States or Canada.

Contagious ecthyma (contagious pustular dermatitis, orf, sore mouth)

This common localized infection of young sheep and goats is caused by a parapoxvirus with worldwide distribution. Less commonly, human beings, cattle, wild ungulates, and dogs are infected. Morbidity in lambs is usually great, and, although mortality is usually low, it can approach 15% in lambs. Lesions are initiated by abrasions from pasture grasses or forage, begin at the commissures of the mouth, and spread to the lips, oral mucosa, eyelids, and feet. Lambs may infect the teats of ewes, and the lesions may spread to the skin of the udder. Contagious ecthyma is of economic importance due to weight loss in lambs that are reluctant to eat because of oral and perioral lesions. Gross and microscopic lesions are consistent with the typical poxvirus lesions, except that the vesicle stage is very brief, the pustule stage is clinically prominent, and

Table 11-2. Poxviridae of domestic animals

Genus	Diseases	Species affected	Distribution
Parapoxvirus	Contagious pustular dermatitis	Sheep; goats; wild and captive ungulates; rarely, dogs	Cutaneous
	Papular stomatitis	Cattle	Cutaneous
	Pseudocowpox	Milking cows, zoonotic	Cutaneous
Orthopoxvirus	Cowpox	Some, such as cowpox and vaccinia, affect many species; others are more host specific	Cutaneous
	Vaccinia		Cutaneous
	Horsepox*		Cutaneous
	Equine papular dermatitis†		Cutaneous
Mulluscipox (tentative classification)	Mulluscum contagiosum	Horses	Cutaneous
Capripoxvirus	Sheep-pox	Most species specific	Systemic
	Goatpox		
	Lumpy skin disease	Cattle	Systemic
Suipoxvirus	Swine pox	Swine	Cutaneous
Unclassified poxvirus	Ulcerative dermatosis of sheep	Sheep	Cutaneous

*Horsepox may be due to human or cattle orthopoxviruses.
†Virus not fully characterized.

lesions are especially proliferative (see Fig. 11-6). Cytoplasmic inclusion bodies are only briefly detectable.

Herpesviruses

Herpesviruses are DNA viruses that are uncommonly associated with cutaneous lesions. Cutaneous lesions may develop in association with nondermatotropic herpesviruses such as infectious bovine rhinotracheitis (bovine herpesvirus-1) and equine coital exanthema (equine herpesvirus-3). Cutaneous lesions have rarely been reported in cats with feline herpesvirus-1 infection. Two dermatotropic herpesvirus infections with economic importance are bovine herpesvirus-2 and bovine herpesvirus-4. Herpesviruses may be latent, and lesions can recur at times of stress. Gross lesions consist of vesicles, ulcers, and crusts. Microscopic lesions in herpesvirus infections consist of the intraepidermal vesicle (see Fig. 11-10) associated with degeneration of epidermal cells and acantholysis. Degenerative changes include ballooning and reticular degeneration. Syncytial cells may be seen. Intranuclear inclusions develop but, because of rapidly developing necrosis, may not be found except at the margins of ulcers.

Bovine herpes mammillitis virus

Bovine herpesvirus-2, a dermatotropic virus (Allerton virus), may cause a more generalized disease (pseudo–lumpy skin disease) or, as seen in the United States, a localized infection (bovine herpes mammillitis). Localized infection occurs more commonly in lactating dairy cows, but may develop in beef cows, pregnant heifers, and suckling calves. Trauma is implicated in the pathogenesis, as normal skin is resistant to viral penetration. Bovine herpes mammillitis is of economic importance due to decreased milk production and secondary bacterial mastitis. Lesions develop on the teats and skin of the nearby udder or, occasionally, the perineum. Suckling calves may develop lesions on the muzzle.

Bovine herpes mammary pustular dermatitis

Bovine herpesvirus-4 causes a similar but milder disease than that caused by the localized form of bovine herpesvirus-2.

Other Viruses

Cutaneous lesions are seen with foot-and-mouth disease (picornavirus), vesicular stomatitis (rhabdovirus), swine vesicular disease (picornavirus), and vesicular exanthema (calicivirus). Some cats infected with either feline leukemia virus or feline immunodeficiency virus have skin lesions, probably due to immunosuppression produced by the viruses. A few cats with feline leukemia virus infection have developed cutaneous horns of the foot pads and dermatitis characterized by epidermal and follicular epithelial hyperplasia with epidermal giant cells, dyskeratosis, necrosis, and ulceration (Fig. 11-25). In immunoperoxidase-stained sections, the hyperplastic epidermis in cases with epidermal giant cells is strongly positive for feline leukemia virus. Rarely, feline calcivirus has been implicated as a cause of cutaneous lesions.

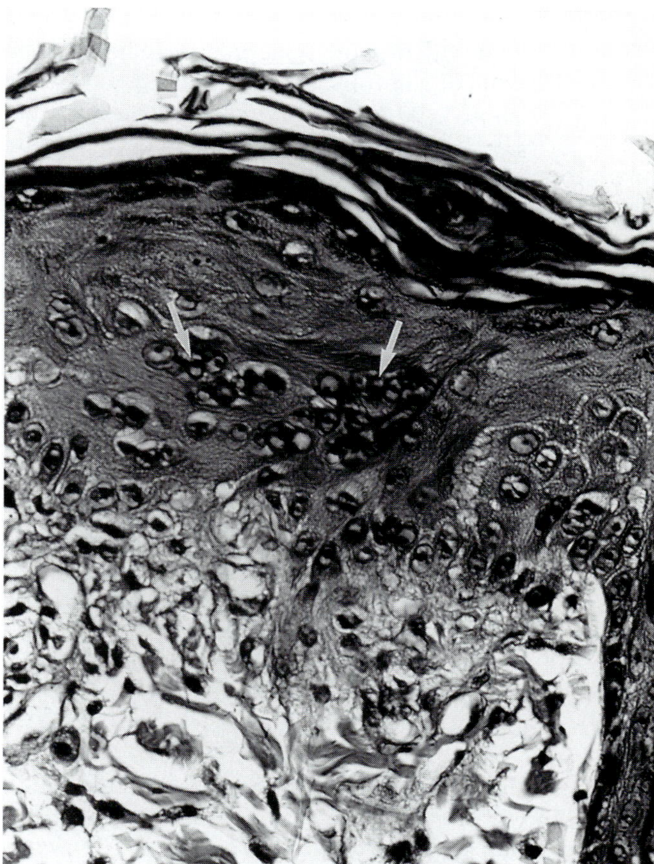

Fig. 11-25 Skin; cat. Cutaneous feline leukemia virus infection. Epidermal hyperplasia (acanthosis) and epidermal multinucleated giant cells *(arrows)* are present. H & E stain.

Rickettsial Infection

The most important rickettsial disease associated with cutaneous lesions is canine Rocky Mountain spotted fever. This disease, caused by *Rickettsia rickettsii,* is transmitted by ticks, and is observed during tick season in the Rocky Mountain region of the United States. In addition to systemic signs, affected dogs have cutaneous, ocular, genital, and oral erythema with petechiae, edema, necrosis, and ulceration due to vasculitis.

Bacterial Infections

Cutaneous bacterial infections are frequently referred to as **pyodermas** and are generally classified as superficial or deep. Pyodermas are among the most common lesions of the skin of dogs but are uncommon in cats and other domestic animals.

Superficial bacterial infections (superficial pyodermas)

These infections involve the epidermis, including the upper infundibulum of hair follicles, and usually heal without scarring; generally, the regional lymph nodes are not affected. Grossly, the lesions are erythema, alopecia, follicularly oriented papules and pustules, crusts, and epidermal collarettes (peripheral expanding rings of scaling). Microscopically, the patterns include intraepidermal pustular dermatitis and superficial suppurative folliculitis. Although bacteria are the cause of the lesions, they are not always microscopically demonstrable.

Superficial pustular dermatitis (impetigo)

This infection is observed in dogs, cats, piglets, cows, does, and ewes and is caused by coagulase-positive *Staphylococcus* sp. associated with such predisposing factors as cutaneous abrasions, viral infections, and poor nutrition. Older dogs with immunosuppression usually due to hyperadrenocorticism may develop a bullous impetigo. In cows, does, and ewes, lesions are predominantly on the udder. In kittens, the dorsum of the neck and shoulders are affected due to overzealous ''mouthing'' by the queen, and *Streptococcus* sp. and *Pasteurella* sp. are the more common bacterial isolates. Gross lesions consist of pustules that develop into crusts, principally (except in kittens) in nonhaired skin. The microscopic lesion is an interfollicular neutrophilic subcorneal pustule.

Dermatophilosis (streptothricosis) caused by *Dermatophilus congolensis,* is characterized by cutaneous lesions in cattle, sheep, and horses more often than dogs, cats, pigs, and goats. The bacterium is transmitted from carrier animals and is more common in tropic and subtropic countries and during wet weather. Lesions tend to develop more commonly on the dorsum of the back and distal extremities and after epidermal irritation from ectoparasites, trauma, or prolonged wetting of the skin, hair, or wool, which allows for the penetration of the damaged epidermis by the *Dermatophilus* ''zoospore.'' Proliferation of the bacterium in the outer root sheath of the hair follicle and superficial epidermis results in the development of gram-positive, filamentous branching organisms that are subdivided longitudinally and transversely (Fig. 11-26). These bacteria produce an acute inflammatory response in which neutrophils migrate from superficial vessels into the dermis and through the epidermis to form microabscesses. The inflammation inhibits further penetration of the bacterium. The epidermis regenerates, and the newly regenerated epidermis is reinvaded by residual bacterial organisms. Repeated cycles of bacterial growth, inflammation, and epidermal regeneration result in the formation of the multilaminated pustular crusts. Grossly, lesions consist of papules, pustules, and thick crusts, which may coalesce and mat the hair or wool (Fig. 11-27). The microscopic lesions are those of a hyperplastic superficial perivascular dermatitis

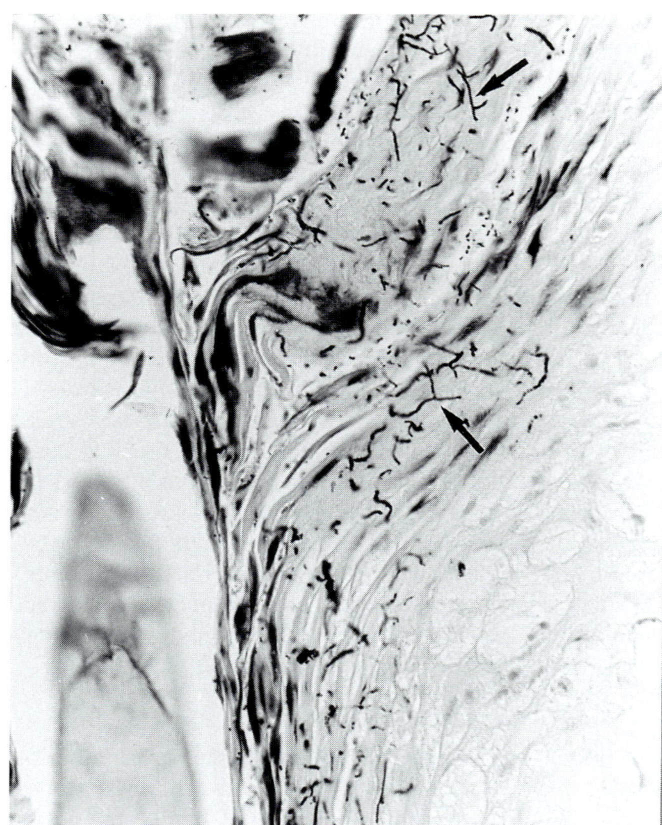

Fig. 11-26 Skin, haired; cow. *Dermatophilus* species infection. The stratum corneum contains filamentous bacteria *(arrows).* H & E stain.

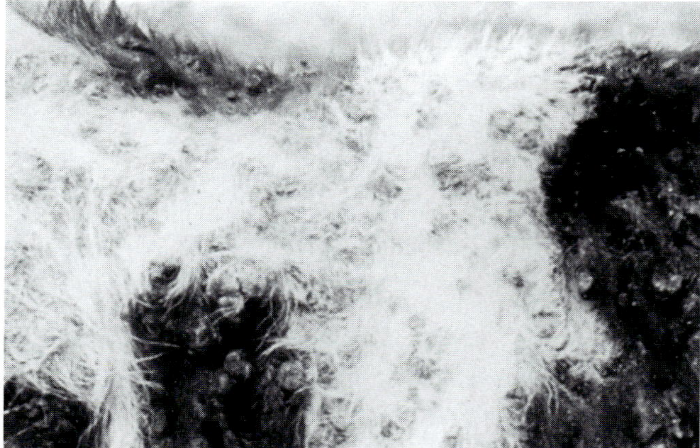

Fig. 11-27 Skin, haired; cow. *Dermatophilus* species infection. The hair is matted by a crust composed of dried exudate, keratin, and bacteria. *Courtesy Dr. F. Lozano-Alarcon.*

with multilaminated crusts of alternating layers of keratin and inflammatory cells.

Exudative epidermitis of pigs (greasy pig disease) caused by *Staphylococcus hyicus* is an acute, often fatal, dermatitis of neonatal piglets and a mild disease in older piglets. Predisposing factors include cutaneous lacerations, poor nutrition, and viral infections. In the course of the disease, a staphylococcal exotoxin called ''exfoliatin'' is produced, and the bacterial toxin binds to filaggrin in the keratohyalin granules of the stratum granulosum. This reaction may be responsible for the lesions of focal erosion of the stratum corneum, a brownish exudate, and a dermatitis that develops around the eyes, pinnae, snout, chin, and medial legs and spreads to the ventral thorax and abdomen. The lesions rapidly coalesce and become generalized, resulting in a greasy, malodorous exudate over a red underlying skin. If piglets survive, the exudate hardens and cracks, with the formation of fissures. Subacute disease develops gradually in older piglets, and lesions are generally localized to the skin of the face, pinnae, and periocular regions. Grossly, the epidermis is thickened with scaling. The early histopathologic lesion is subcorneal pustular dermatitis with extension to the hair follicle, resulting in superficial suppurative folliculitis. In the fully developed lesion, the epidermis is hyperplastic and has thick crusts of keratin, microabscesses, and cocci.

Other superficial pyodermas include ovine fleece rot (due to excessive moisture and *Pseudomonas*) and equine pastern folliculitis (grease heel), a secondary pyoderma of the caudal pastern and/or fetlock. Ovine fleece rot is important economically because it predisposes sheep to myiasis and reduces the value of affected wool.

Deep bacterial infections (deep pyodermas)

These infections are less common than superficial infections and develop most frequently in dogs. Deep bacterial infections involve the entire infundibulum, isthmic, or inferior portion of the hair follicles and the surrounding dermis and subcutis, often heal with scarring, and generally involve regional lymph nodes. These diseases are often secondary to immunosuppression, demodicosis (dogs), or disorders associated with follicular hyperkeratosis (chin acne, elbow callus). Deep pyodermas may originate as a sequela to superficial bacterial folliculitis. Grossly, the lesions include follicular crusted papules, pustules, alopecia, nodules, abscesses, ulcers, fistulas, and hemorrhagic bullae. Deep pyoderma in some dogs resembles pyotraumatic dermatitis. The microscopic patterns include pyogranulomatous folliculitis and furunculosis, nodular to diffuse dermatitis, and panniculitis. Draining sinuses may develop, often in association with a foreign body response to extruded follicular contents. Chronic lesions are associated with significant scarring and loss of adnexal structures. Bacterial organisms isolated include *Staphylococcus* sp., *Streptococcus* sp., *Corynebacterium pseudotuberculosis, Pasteurella* sp., *Proteus* sp., *Pseudomonas* sp., and *Escherichia coli. Staphylococcus intermedius* is the primary pathogen of canine skin.

Staphylococcal folliculitis and **furunculosis** develop most commonly in the dog (see Fig. 11-16), frequently affect the horse, goat, and sheep, but are uncommon in the cow, cat, and pig. In dogs, lesions are localized or generalized and develop on the muzzle, bridge of the nose, pressure points, interdigital areas, and chin. Deep pyoderma of adult German shepherd dogs of both sexes (German shepherd folliculitis, furunculosis, and cellulitis) is a unique deep pyoderma with an apparent genetic predisposition. Lesions are located on the dorsal lumbosacral, ventral abdominal, and thigh areas. Hypersensitivity to fleas or alterations in immune or neutrophil function have been proposed as predisposing causes, but most have been discounted. In horses, lesions develop most commonly in association with tack, especially around the saddle area or on the caudal aspect of the pastern or tail. In goats, the face, pinnae, distal limbs, and glabrous areas of the udder, ventral abdomen, medial thighs, and perineum are most commonly affected. In adult sheep, lesions develop on the face, limbs, and teats, whereas in lambs, the lips and perineum have lesions.

Subcutaneous abscesses are localized collections of purulent exudate located within the dermis and subcutis and are common in cats, due to the frequency of bacterial contamination of puncture wounds. The exudate may be surrounded by a collagenous wall and fibroblasts. Bacteria involved are frequently inhabitants of the mouth and include *Pasteurella multocida, Fusobacterium* sp., β-hemolytic streptococci, *Peptostreptococcus anaerobius,* and *Bacteroides* sp.

Bacterial granulomatous dermatitis is associated with bacteria that generally are saprophytes of low virulence. Grossly, lesions are diffuse or nodular and may ulcerate and drain to the skin surface via fistulas. Microscopically, collections of macrophages with or without multinucleated giant cells are present. Caseous necrosis and neutrophils are present in some lesions. Etiologic agents may be seen in the macrophages, exudate, or clear vacuolar spaces.

Mycobacterial organisms produce granulomatous to pyogranulomatous lesions in many species, including cattle, pigs, dogs, and cats. Cutaneous lesions are usually caused by *Mycobacterium lepraemurium* (feline leprosy) or the facultative mycobacterial organisms including *M. fortuitum, M. smegmatis, M. chelonei, M. phlei, M. xenopi,* and *M. thermoresistable* (atypical or anonymous mycobacterial infections). These facultative organisms are inhabitants of soil or water and contaminate wounds in several species. Cutaneous infections with *M. tuberculosis, M. bovis,* or *M. avium* are rare. Feline leprosy occurs in cats living along the Pacific coast of North America and de-

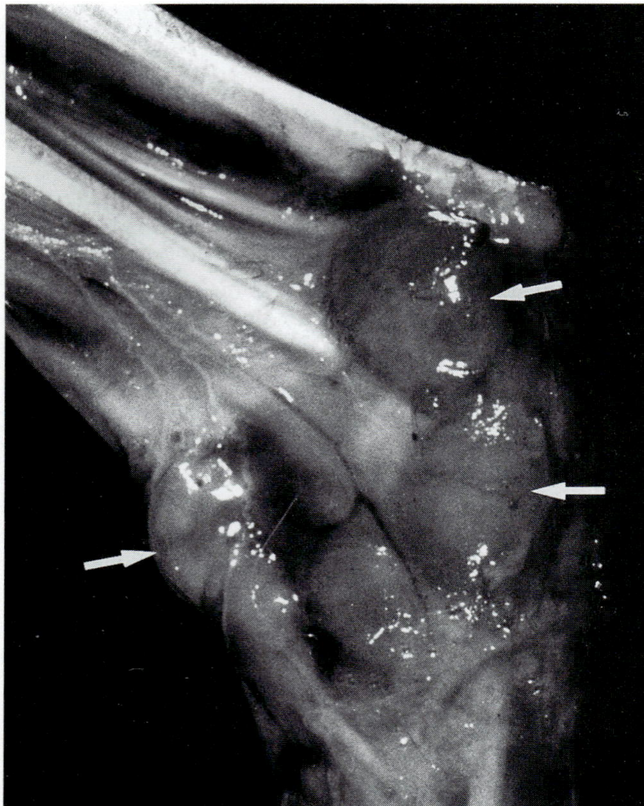

Fig. 11-28 Skin, leg; cat. Feline leprosy. Multiple nodules *(arrows)* consistent with the diagnosis of granulomatous dermatitis/panniculitis are present. (The epidermis and dermis have been removed.) *Courtesy Dr. C. Leathers.*

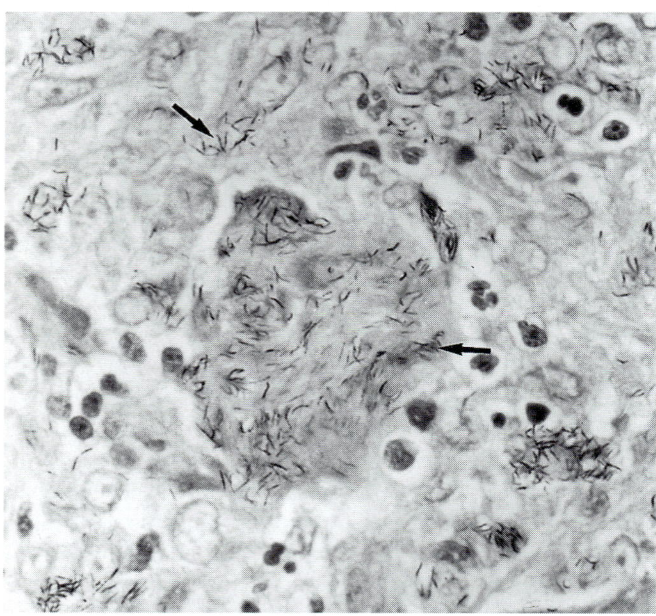

Fig. 11-29 Skin; cat. Feline leprosy. Macrophages contain numerous mycobacteria *(arrows).* Ziehl-Neelsen stain.

velops in cats without age, breed, or sex predilection. Lesions develop more commonly on the head, neck, and limbs but may occur anywhere (Figs. 11-28 and 11-29).

Botryomycosis is used as a diagnostic term for a granulomatous dermatitis caused by nonfilamentous bacteria (usually *Staphylococcus aureus*) when the bacteria form small, yellow "sulfur" granules. The granules consist centrally of bacterial colonies and peripherally of a homogeneous eosinophilic material often oriented in radiating club-shaped bodies about the bacterial colonies. The material, considered antigen-antibody complexes, is termed Splendore-Hoeppli material. Filamentous bacteria may form similar granules in tissue and can be differentiated from staphylococcal infections by Gram staining and culture. These organisms include various species of *Actinomyces, Actinobacillus,* and *Nocardia. N. asteroides* generally does not form granules, however. *Borrelia suilla* is a spirochete that causes ulcerative dermatitis (ulcerative granuloma, necrotic ulcer, porcine spirochetosis) in pigs that are kept under unsanitary conditions.

Digital infections of ruminants (bacterial pododermatitis)

Infections of the digits of cattle and sheep are usually mixed bacterial infections that are sometimes separated into two basic groups, **"contagious footrot"** and **"necrobacillosis of the foot,"** based on the contagious nature of the infection and the type of bacteria principally responsible for infection. Contagious footrot is caused principally by *Bacteroides nodosus* acting synergistically with *Fusobacterium necrophorum,* with other bacteria also frequently present. Necrobacillosis of the foot is caused principally by *F. necrophorum* with other bacteria, including *B. melaninogenicus* in cattle, also frequently present.

Contagious footrot has an initial colonization by a variety of microorganisms; and, if *B. nodosus* is present, footrot may be initiated, if predisposing factors such as moisture and trauma are present. *B. nodosus* elaborates proteases and growth-enhancing factors that aid bacterial penetration of the epidermis and encourages bacterial growth, especially of *F. necrophorum,* the bacterium responsible for most of the necrosis and inflammation. Contagious footrot in sheep occurs in virulent and benign forms; the virulent form is due to *Bacteroides* sp., which produces more proteolytic enzymes, allowing for more bacterial penetration of the epidermis. Early lesions are interdigital, affect both digits, and consist of red, moist, and swollen eroded skin. The inflammation spreads to the epidermal matrix of the hoof and results in separation of the horn by a malodorous exudate. The germinal epithelium is not destroyed, and regeneration is attempted, but the new horn is destroyed. In chronic infections, hooves may become long and misshapen. Benign footrot (scald) is mild, confined to interdigital skin, and may have slight separation of the horn of the heel; hoof overgrowth may occur. Footrot in cattle is similar to benign footrot in sheep.

Necrobacillosis of the foot of sheep includes ovine interdigital dermatitis and foot abscesses. Ovine interdigital dermatitis is an acute necrotizing dermatitis that clinically is similar to benign footrot. Ovine interdigital dermatitis is differentiated from footrot by the failure to demonstrate *B. nodosus* in smears or cultures of exudate. Foot abscesses include heel abscesses (infective bulbar necrosis) and toe abscesses (lamellar abscesses). Foot abscesses are more common in wet seasons and in heavy adult sheep. In addition to *F. necrophorum, Actinomyces pyogenes* may be isolated from the lesions.

Necrobacillosis (foul in the foot) of the bovine foot, an interdigital dermatitis and cellulitis, is caused by *F. necrophorum* and *B. melaninogenicus,* with trauma as a predisposing factor. Fissures with necrotic swollen edges are present in the interdigital space, and inflammation may extend into the joint spaces.

Systemic bacterial infections

Septicemic salmonellosis may cause cyanosis of the external ears and abdomen due to capillary dilatation and congestion. In addition, thrombosis may cause necrosis of distal extremities. Cutaneous lesions associated with erysipelas in pigs consist of rhomboidal, firm, raised, pink to dark purple areas (Fig. 11-30) and are due to vasculitis, thrombosis, and ischemia. Bacterial infections may also develop from direct extension of bacterial infections of deeper tissues, such as clostridial myositis and cellulitis. *Clostridium novyi* may also cause severe cellulitis, toxemia, and death in young rams with heads traumatized by butting during the breeding season. Spores in the soil gain entrance through cutaneous lacerations at the base of the horns, germinate, produce toxins, and result in cellulitis and toxemia. Swelling of the head and neck results in the common term "big head" or "swelled head." In horses, the purpura developing occasionally as a sequela to *Streptococcus equi* may be due to immune complex vasculitis.

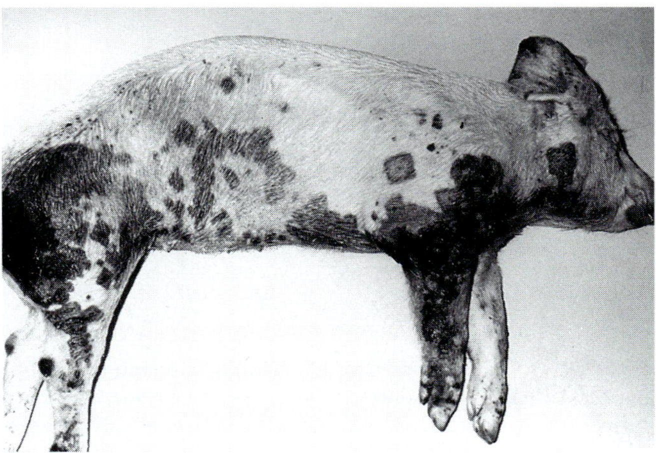

Fig. 11-30 Skin; pig. Erysipelas. Rhomboidal lesions are present in the skin. *Courtesy Dr. M.D. McGavin.*

Mycotic Infections

Mycotic infections have been classified into four basic categories: superficial, cutaneous, subcutaneous, and systemic. In general, mycotic infections tend to occur more commonly in animals with compromised resistance to infection, including those given broad-spectrum, long-term antibiotic therapy; those with debilitating diseases such as diabetes mellitus and neoplasia; and those undergoing therapy with immunosuppressive agents.

Superficial mycoses

Superficial mycoses are infections restricted to the stratum corneum or hair with minimal or no tissue reaction. Piedra, caused by *Trichosporon beigelii,* has minute swellings of the hair shaft.

Cutaneous mycoses

Cutaneous mycoses (considered as superficial mycoses by some authors) are infections of keratinized tissues, including hair, feathers, nails, and epidermis. The fungi are usually restricted to the keratinized layer, but tissue destruction and host response may be extensive. Infections in animals include dermatophytosis, cutaneous candidiasis, and malassezia dermatitis.

Dermatophytoses are fungal infections of the skin, hair, and nails of animals caused by taxonomically related fungi known as dermatophytes. Pathogenic genera include *Epidermophyton, Microsporum,* and *Trichophyton.* Dermatophytosis occurs worldwide, is the most important cutaneous (superficial) mycosis, and is common in human beings and animals, especially in cats. Dermatophytoses are more contagious than other fungal infections and are more common in hot, humid environments; young animals are more susceptible than adults. Animals kept in overcrowded, dirty, or damp areas and those with inadequate nutrition are also more susceptible. Species that more commonly infect domestic animals are included in genera *Microsporum* and *Trichophyton. Epidermophyton* is adapted to human beings (anthropophilic) and rarely infects animals. Zoophilic dermatophytes (e.g., *Microsporum canis*) are animal pathogens, and some, such as *Microsporum canis,* are so well adapted, especially in cats, that inapparent infections occur. Geophilic dermatophytes (e.g., *Microsporum gypseum*) occur in soil as saprophytes but, under favorable conditions, may infect human beings and animals.

Dermatophytes invade keratinized tissues (stratum corneum, hair shafts, and nails) by producing proteolytic enzymes, including "keratinase" and lipase, which help penetrate the surface lipid coat. The fungal hyphae invade the keratin, and the hyphae break up into chains of arthrospores. When the arthrospores are principally present on the outside of the hair, the invasion is referred to as "ectothrix." When the arthrospores are present inside the hair (rare in animals), the invasion is referred to as "endothrix." The products produced by the dermatophytes cause dermal irritation and damage to the epidermis. The fungal products and products released from damaged keratinocytes (cytokines) result in epidermal hyperplasia (hyperkeratosis, parakeratosis, acanthosis) and inflammation. Inflammatory cells arrive via the superficial vessels (superficial perivascular dermatitis) and, subsequently, migrate through the epidermal layers (exocytosis) to the invaded keratinized layers, forming intracorneal microabscesses. Exocytosis of inflammatory cells to follicular walls results in folliculitis and, if the follicular wall is destroyed, in furunculosis. Bacterial infection increases the severity of the folliculitis and furunculosis. Gross and microscopic lesions may be highly variable and range from an asymptomatic lesionless infection to a nodular eruptive lesion termed a "kerion" to a pseudomycetoma and to discolored, malformed, friable, broken or sloughed nails (onychomycosis). Gross lesions in haired skin are often circular or irregularly shaped, scaly to crusty patches of alopecia (Fig. 11-31) that may coalesce to involve large portions of the body. Areas of hair loss are due to broken hair shafts and loss of hairs from inflamed follicles. Follicular papules and pustules may be present. Fungi tend to die in areas of inflammation in the center of lesions and are viable peripherally, giving rise to the peripheral red ring and the term "ringworm." Microscopic patterns include perifolliculitis, folliculitis, or furunculosis as well as epidermal hyperplasia with intracorneal microabscesses. In many cases, septate hyphae or spores are present in the stratum corneum and keratin of hair follicles (Fig. 11-32).

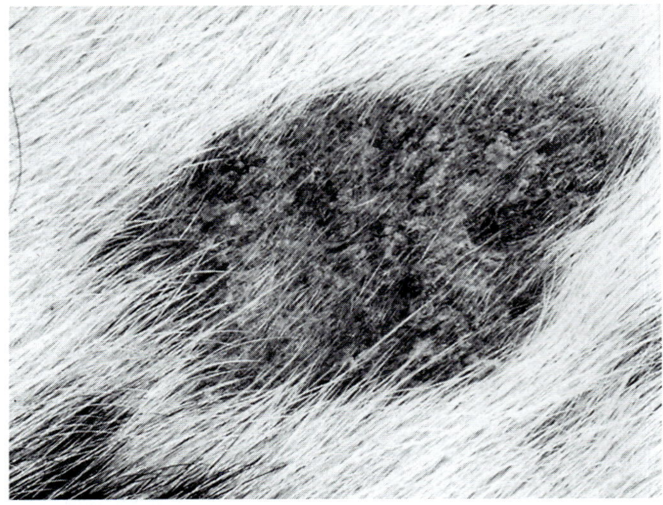

Fig. 11-31 Skin, haired; cow. Dermatophytosis. Note hairless encrusted area. *Courtesy Dr. H.D. Liggitt.*

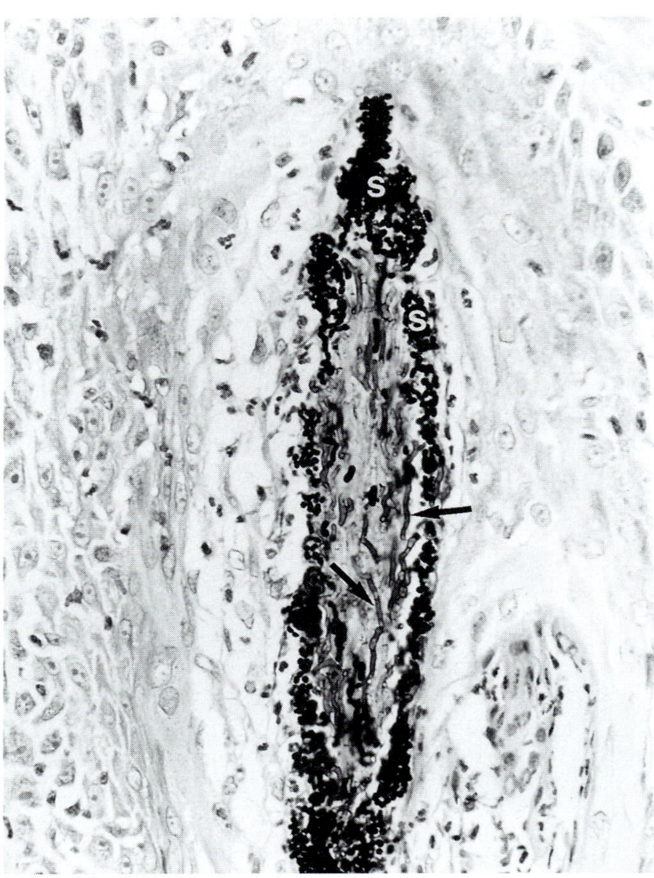

Fig. 11-32 Skin, haired, dog. Dermatophyte infection involving hair follicle. Note spores (*S*) along periphery and hyphae *(arrows)* within hair shaft. Gomori's methenamine-silver nitrate (GMS)–H & E counterstain.

Candidiasis is caused by *Candida* sp. that are normal inhabitants of the skin and gastrointestinal tract. Infection occurs when host resistance is compromised. Infections with *Candida* sp. are rare in domestic animals and tend to occur on mucous membranes and at mucocutaneous junctions. Exudative, papular, pustular to ulcerative dermatitis (cheilitis), stomatitis, and otitis externa may develop. Microscopically, spongiotic neutrophilic pustular inflammation with parakeratosis and ulceration are the lesions with organisms present in the superficial exudate.

Malassezia dermatitis is caused by *Malassezia pachydermatis (Pityrosporum canis),* a yeast isolated from normal external ear canal and skin. This yeast, which proliferates when the microclimate or host defenses are altered, may cause clinical disease. Lesions may be regional (interdigital, muzzle, otic, perianal) or more generalized. Grossly, the lesions are erythematous, often hyperpigmented, lichenified, alopecic, and scaly. Microscopic lesions consist of hyperkeratosis, focal parakeratosis, variable spongiotic pustular dermatitis, acanthosis, and the presence of *M. pachydermatis.* Because *Malassezia* organisms may be present in low number in animals without

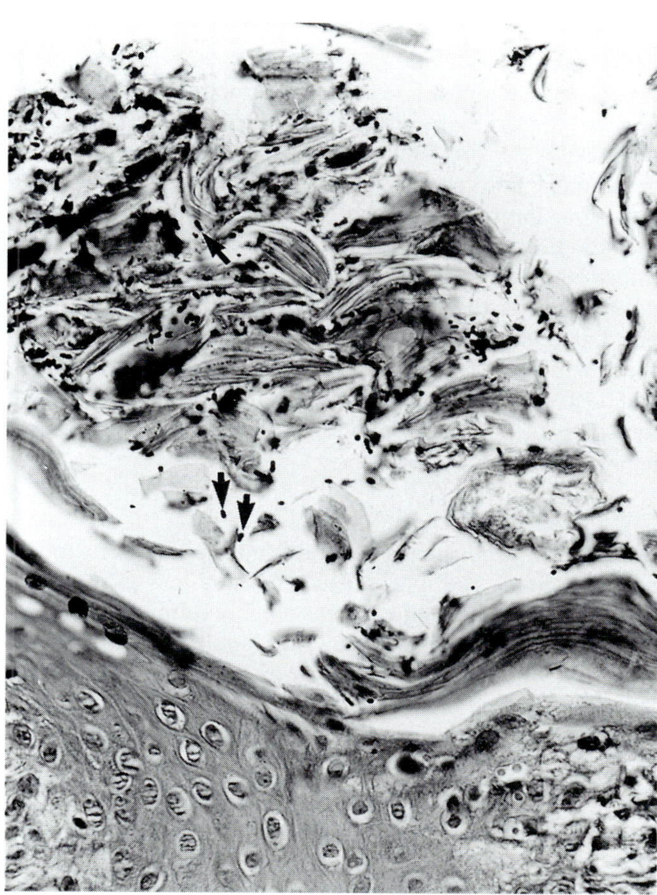

Fig. 11-33 Skin, haired; dog. *Malassezia*-associated dermatitis. Stratum corneum with numerous *M. pachydermatis* organisms. The *Malassezia* are bilobed (''peanut''-shaped [*arrows*]).

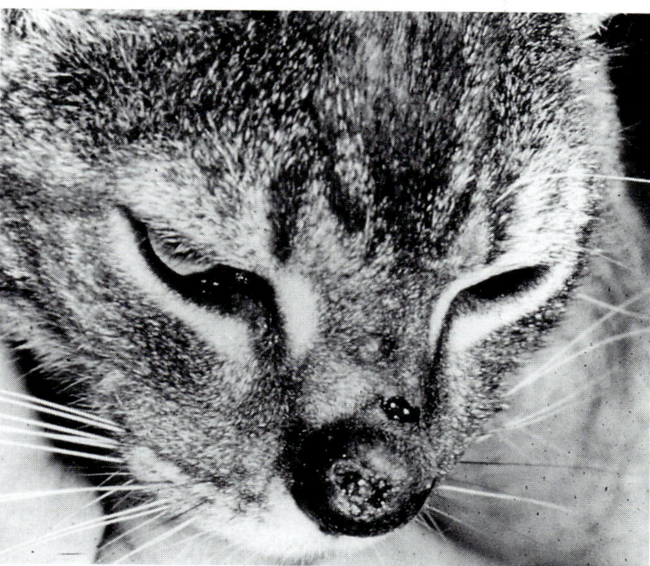

Fig. 11-34 Skin, nose; cat. Phaeohyphomycosis infection of nasal planum and dorsum of muzzle. Swelling and ulcerated areas are present. Exudate may drain from ulcerated areas. *Courtesy Dr. A. Werner.*

cutaneous lesions, identification of at least 3 to 5 yeasts per high-power field is considered necessary to implicate the yeast in lesion development (Fig. 11-33).

Subcutaneous mycoses

Subcutaneous mycoses are caused by fungi that invade cutaneous and subcutaneous tissues after their implantation via trauma. Some infections remain localized, but others spread to the lymph vessels. Diseases in this category include eumycotic mycetomas, subcutaneous phaeohyphomycosis, sporotrichosis, subcutaneous zygomycosis, and pythiosis. The gross appearance of subcutaneous mycoses and that of deep granulomatous infections caused by bacteria are similar; usually one or more nodular areas ulcerate and have draining fistulas (Fig. 11-34). Microscopically, the subcutaneous mycoses consist of nodular to coalescing, suppurative, pyogranulomatous or granulomatous inflammation.

Eumycotic mycetomas are rare tumorous enlargements of granulomatous inflammation in animals, occur chiefly in horses and dogs, and are caused by fungi. *Curvularia geniculata* is the more commonly isolated fungus in animals, and other fungal genera include *Madurella* and *Acremonium.* The exudate of mycetomas has granules that vary in size, shape, color, and texture. Microscopically, the hyphae are septate and branching and may be located within an acellular matrix.

Dermatophytic pseudomycetoma is a rare, deep, dermal and subcutaneous infection by *Microsporum canis* that develops predominantly in Persian cats, suggesting the possibility of a specific genetic deficit in natural or specific immunity in this breed. Gross lesions are similar to those of other subcutaneous mycoses. Microscopically, aggregates of fungal hyphae with irregular dilatations are found within the subfollicular dermis or subcutis, associated with a granulomatous inflammatory response. Hair shafts within adjacent follicles contain *Microsporum* hyphae and spores.

Phaeohyphomycosis is a mycotic infection caused by species of pigmented fungi (dematiaceous) of a variety of genera that have septate hyphae but no granules or sclerotic bodies. Genera include *Alternaria, Drechslera, Exophiala,* and *Phialophora.* Subcutaneous phaeohyphomycosis occurs in cats (see Fig. 11-34), cattle, horses, and, rarely, dogs.

Sporotrichosis, caused by *Sporothrix schenckii,* is an uncommon mycosis that may develop in cutaneous, cutaneous–lymph vessel, and disseminated forms in horses, mules, cattle, cats, and dogs. Cutaneous nodules ulcerate and fistulae may develop at the site of traumatic implantation and along lymph vessels, but visceral dissemination is uncommon. Organisms occur as ovoid to elongate (cigar-shaped) bodies and are often sparsely distributed and difficult to find, except they tend to be more numerous in cats. The exudate containing organisms is infectious to human beings, if introduced into cutaneous wounds.

Zygomycosis (phycomycosis, mucormycosis) is principally a disease of horses caused by *Basidiobolus haptosporus.* A similar disease in dogs and horses (pythiosis, oomycosis) is caused by *Pythium* sp. *(Hyphomyces destruens),* a funguslike member of the kingdom Protista, phylum Oomycetes. Zygomycosis and pythiosis occur in animals located in the warm, humid areas along the Gulf Coast. Cutaneous lesions occur on the head, limbs, and, usually, the ventral trunk. However, in dogs, the dorsolumbosacral region (presumably associated with flea bite dermatitis) is also affected. A unique gross feature is the presence of yellow, rough to jagged fragments of necrotic tissue and hyphae that can be dislodged from the granulomatous areas. Eosinophils are numerous in the lesions.

Because fungi may not be readily visible in H & E-stained sections, special stains such as Gomori's methenamine silver stain may be required to demonstrate the organisms microscopically, particularly the organisms of pythiosis. In many instances, fungal cultures are required to identify a specific agent.

Systemic mycoses

The lungs are almost invariably the primary site of infection in the systemic mycoses, but cutaneous and subcutaneous infections can occur as part of the disseminated disease or by direct implantation of fungi by trauma. Systemic mycoses include blastomycosis, coccidioidomycosis, cryptococcosis, and histoplasmosis. Infections with these fungi may occur in hosts with seemingly normal immune function. Grossly, one or more nodular areas may ulcerate and have draining fistulas. Histopathologically, the lesions are granulomas or pyogranulomas. Cryptococcosis may have a granulomatous response, but generally the inflammation is less severe than with the other fungi. The cryptococcal organisms have a mucinous capsule that does not stain with H & E. The capsules of the numerous organisms in a lesion give the tissues a "soap bubble" appearance. Cytology or microscopy is required for diagnosis, and, usually, the morphologic features of the organisms (including the mucicarmine-positive capsule) are sufficient for diagnosis.

Algal Infections

Protothecosis is a rare infection of animals caused by an achloric (colorless) alga of the genus *Prototheca.* Grossly, the lesions are nodular, and the microscopic pattern is nodular to diffuse granulomatous dermatitis and panniculitis. The organisms can be identified in tissues by means of Gomori's methenamine silver stain, by the immunoperoxidase reaction, or by culture.

Parasitic Infestations and Infections

Ectoparasites include mites and ticks (which have eight legs) and lice, fleas, and flies (which have six legs). The presence of these ectoparasites is called an infestation. Endoparasites causing cutaneous lesions include nematodes, trematodes, and protozoa, and their presence is called an infection. Parasites cause a number of untoward effects, including damage to hides and predisposition to secondary infection. Arthropod (jointed limbs) parasites also serve as vectors of bacterial, spirochetal, helminthic, rickettsial, protozoal, and viral infections. Cutaneous reaction to parasites varies with parasite number, location, feeding habits, and host immune response. The cutaneous reaction is often mediated in part by immune mechanisms (hypersensitivity).

Mites

Mite infestations cause serious cutaneous lesions in domestic animals and may cause economic loss in food animals. Sheep in the United States are free of mite infestation except for *Demodex* sp. and *Psorergates* sp. Cattle, however, can be infested with mites of *Sarcoptes, Psoroptes,* and *Chorioptes* genera, which are reportable diseases. Mite infestations can also cause serious cutaneous diseases in dogs, cats, and pigs. In *Sarcoptes scabiei* infestation, mites may be difficult to find, except for infestation of the external ears of pigs. *Demodex* sp. mites are normally inhabitants of hair follicles and sebaceous glands of all domestic species, and identification of large numbers of adult mites or an increased number of immature mites is required for diagnosis.

Demodicosis is caused by host-specific mites and, while uncommonly seen in cattle, goats, pigs, horses, sheep, and cats, it is a major problem in dogs. Most species of *Demodex* mites live in the lumina of hair follicles or sebaceous glands. Transmission from dams to offspring occurs during nursing. Canine demodicosis is caused by *D. canis* and occurs in two clinical forms, localized and generalized, both of which are more common in juvenile dogs.

Purebred dogs of many breeds are predisposed to infestation, suggesting an inherited basis for the disease related to a primary deficit in cell-mediated immunity. Secondary immunodeficiency due to T cell suppression is also associated with the disease in its complicated form. The secondary immunodeficiency improves as the demodicosis resolves. There are conflicting studies as to whether this immunodeficiency is due to the accompanying bacterial infection or to the mites. Demodicosis occurs in adult animals with underlying metabolic disorders (hypothyroidism, hyperadrenocorticism) or given therapeutic regimens (glucocorticoids or cytotoxic drugs) that may compromise the immune system. Idiopathic cases also occur.

Grossly, localized demodicosis consists of one or more scaly, erythematous, alopecic, macular areas on the face or forelegs (Fig. 11-35). The microscopic lesions are lymphoplasmacytic perifolliculitis (Fig. 11-36) with hyperkeratosis, sebaceous adenitis, focal mild degeneration of basal cells, pigmentary incontinence, and intraluminal mites in the upper third of the follicles. Generalized lesions consist of larger coalescing patches of erythema, alopecia, scales, and crusts. Microscopically, perifolliculitis and follicular hyperkeratosis may be associated with follicular plugging, bacterial proliferation, and bacterial neutrophilic folliculitis. The follicular plugging and mites may result in follicular rupture, a secondary foreign body furunculosis and, sometimes, cellulitis with lymphadenitis and septicemia.

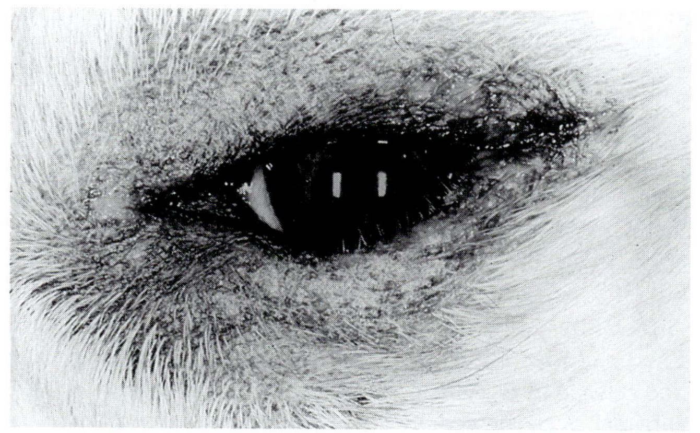

Fig. 11-35 Skin, periocular; dog. Localized demodicosis. Skin is alopecic, swollen, lichenified, and hyperpigmented.

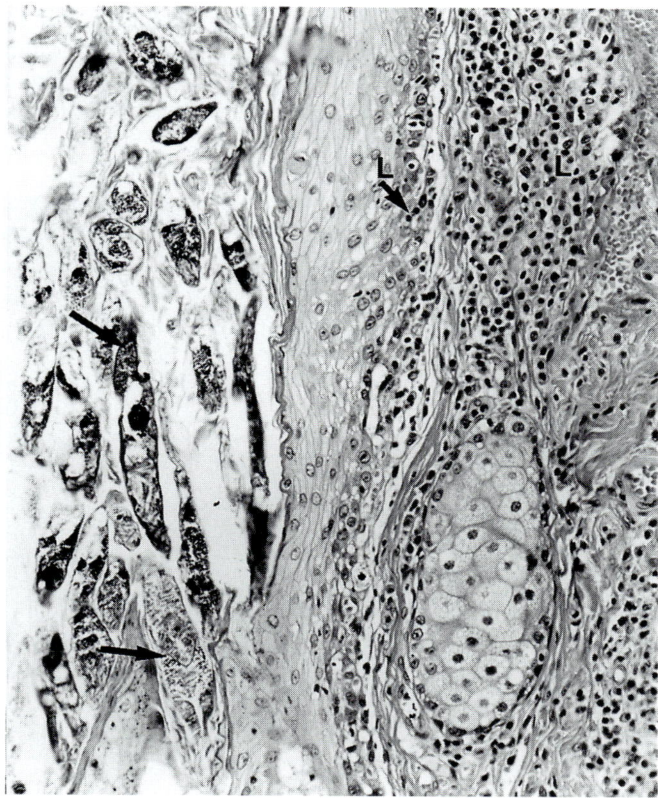

Fig. 11-36 Skin, haired; dog. Localized demodicosis. Lymphocytic perifolliculitis is present, (lymphocyte [*L*]) and elongated *Demodex canis* mites *(arrows)* are in the follicular lumen. H & E stain.

Scabies is caused by *Sarcoptes scabiei.* This highly contagious mite is the most important ectoparasite of pigs, is common in dogs, and is uncommon to rare in horses, cattle, sheep, goats, and cats. The mites burrow through the stratum corneum and cause intense pruritus due principally to hypersensitivity reactions, although irritation from secretions and excretions also plays a role. Lesions generally begin on the external ears, head, and neck and may become generalized. Gross lesions include erythematous macules, papules, crusts, and excoriations. Chronic lesions are scaly, lichenified, and hairless. Microscopically, the lesion is a hyperplastic, spongiotic, superficial perivascular dermatitis, with crusting and infiltration of eosinophils. Mite eggs or feces may be found in tunnels in the stratum corneum but are not commonly seen in tissue sections, due to small numbers of mites.

Notoedric mite infestation is a rare, but highly contagious, pruritic disease caused by *Notoedres cati.* The first lesion is an erythematous papular rash, followed by scales, crusts, and alopecia with lichenification when chronic. Lesions begin on the neck and pinnae and extend to the head, face, and paws and may become generalized. Microscopic lesions consist of epidermal hyperplasia, mild spongiosis, crusts, and superficial perivascular dermatitis with eosinophils.

Otodectic mite infestation caused by *Otodectes cynotis* occurs in the external ear canals of carnivores and, occasionally, may be present on other parts of the body. Hence, it is important to differentiate *Otodectes* from *Sarcoptes* and *Notoedres* mites.

Psoroptic mite infestation in sheep, cattle, horses, goats, rabbits, and other animals is caused by several species of host-specific mites. *Psoroptes cuniculi* infests the external ear canals of rabbits, horses, goats, and sheep. *Psoroptes equi* infests the base of the mane and tail and skin under the forelock of horses. *Psoroptes ovis* causes serious disease in cattle and sheep, producing parasitic lesions of thickened skin and dry scales and crusts that begin on the withers and spread because of persistent self-inflicted trauma. In sheep, psoroptic mite infestation is called "sheep scab." Lesions develop on the withers and sides. The wooled areas are chiefly involved with crusts that adhere to the matted fleece and, in time, expand and coalesce. Damage is due to self-inflicted trauma, resulting from the pruritus and from local irritation and hypersensitivity reactions. The microscopic lesion is a spongiotic, hyperplastic, or exudative superficial perivascular dermatitis with eosinophils.

Chorioptic mite infestation, caused by host-specific mites, develops in cattle, horses, goats, and, in some countries, sheep. Mites on the skin surface produce gross lesions, which are erythematous, papular, crusted, scaly, and hairless, and thickening of the skin on the lower hind limbs, scrotum, tail, perineum, udder, and thigh of cattle; lower limbs of horses; scrotum and lower hind limbs of sheep; and lower limbs, hindquarters, and abdomen of goats.

Cheyletiellosis, caused by infestation with *Cheyletiella* sp., occurs in dogs, cats, rabbits, wild animals, and human beings. In dogs and cats, lesions consist of hyperkeratosis manifested as dry, white, scaly dandruff along the back. Some infestations are asymptomatic, but, grossly, cats may have focal, multifocal, or generalized red papules or crusts. Microscopically, the lesion is a superficial perivascular dermatitis with eosinophils.

Psorergatic mite infestation caused by *Psorergates ovis* occurs in sheep in Australia, New Zealand, the United States, South Africa, and Argentina. The infestation produces lesions along the withers and sides of the body and is manifested by a pruritic dermatitis that may result in self-inflicted trauma.

Trombiculidiasis is infestation by harvest mites (chiggers). The larvae tunnel into the epidermis, inject saliva, and live on digested tissue fluids, producing an intensely pruritic dermatitis. Grossly, small, red papules or crusts contain several orange to red larvae and develop on parts of the skin in close contact with plants or the ground. The microscopic lesions are a hyperplastic, superficial perivascular dermatitis with eosinophils, mast cells, and intraepidermal mites.

Ticks

Ticks, both soft (argasid) and hard (ixodid), cause injury by loss of blood (producing anemia), by irritation due to bites, by hypersensitivity reactions, by acting as vectors of other diseases, by causing tick paralysis and toxicosis, and by predisposing to secondary bacterial disease and to myiasis. Local cutaneous reactions vary in severity with the tick and its secretions and the resistance of the host. Gross lesions consist of focal erosions, erythema, and crusted ulcers with alopecia and nodules in some individuals. Microscopic lesions include epidermal and dermal necrosis (triangular with the apex at the panniculus), and perivascular to diffuse inflammation at the margins of the necrotic area, with the exudate consisting of eosinophils, macrophages, and lymphocytes. Some lesions are granulomas (arthropod-bite granuloma) in which the inflammatory cells efface the tissue architecture and are interspersed among collagenous fibers and lymphoid follicles that form within the dermis. Cutaneous basophil hypersensitivity likely contributes to the reactions induced by tick bites.

Lice

Pediculosis, or infestation with lice, causes anemia, weakness, damage to hair and wool, and discomfort. Biting lice, feeding more on epithelial cellular debris and less on blood, cause less severe systemic signs. Pediculosis occurs more commonly in winter when temperatures are cooler, the wool or hair coat is longer, animals are congregated, and the plane of nutrition is lower. Infestations are relatively host specific, are spread by direct contact, and are relatively easy to control because the life cycle takes place entirely on the host. Pediculosis in swine is an economically important disease as the lice transmit *Eperythrozoon suis,* and the viruses of swinepox and African swine fever. Primary lesions caused by lice are few, and most are secondary to scratching. Gross lesions consist of papules, crusts, and secondary excoriations with lice and eggs visible in the lesions. Animals infested with sucking lice may be anemic.

Fleas

Flea infestation is principally a problem in dogs and cats. Fleas can cause severe skin irritation due to frequent biting and release of enzymes, anticoagulants, and histamine-like substances; hypersensitivity reactions to saliva; and secondary host-inflicted trauma from scratching and biting (Fig. 11-37). Severe infestations may cause blood loss (anemia), especially in puppies, kittens, or small, debilitated adults. Lesions occur over the dorsal lumbosacral region, caudomedial thighs, ventral abdomen, flanks, and, in cats, the neck area and consist of multiple red papules and secondary excoriations. *Ctenocephalides felis* is the most common flea causing infestation in dogs and cats and transmits the tapeworm *Dipylidium caninum.*

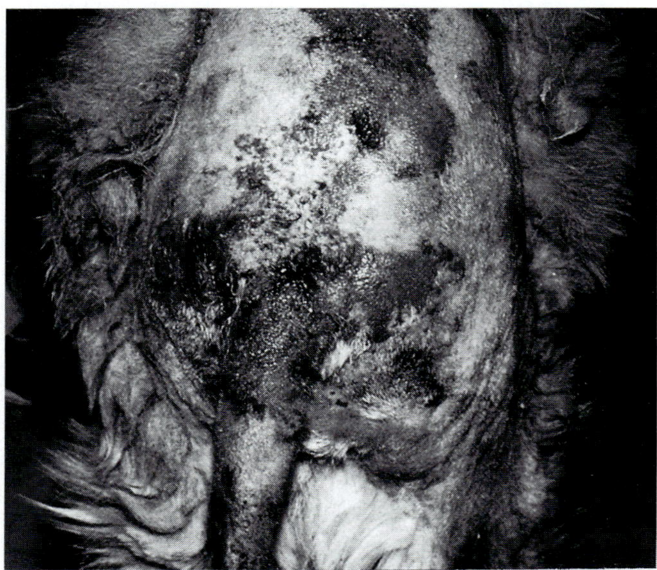

Fig. 11-37 Skin, haired; dog. Pyotraumatic dermatitis (acute moist dermatitis). Erosion, moist exudate, and crusting are present over rump of a dog with flea bite hypersensitivity (hair has been clipped). *Courtesy Dr. B. Baker.*

Flies

Cutaneous reactions to fly bites may be minor to severe and are due to bites by adult flies and to myiasis. Reactions to the bites of flies vary and include irritation, anemia, direct toxicity, and hypersensitivity. Biting flies include *Haematobia irritans* (horn fly), *Stomoxys calcitrans* (stablefly), and horse flies, deer flies, black flies, biting gnats, and mosquitoes. *Melophagus ovinus* (sheep ked) is another common ectoparasite that sucks blood. Lesions of biting flies are due to local irritation and include wheals and papules formed around a puncture wound that may bleed. Such lesions may persist with hair loss, scales, hemorrhagic crusts, erythema, and secondary excoriations due to self-inflicted trauma, especially if the animal is hypersensitive to the bites. Such hypersensitivity occurs with *Culicoides* sp. in horses (Queensland itch, sweet itch), and mosquitoes in cats (Fig. 11-38). Microscopic lesions include superficial perivascular dermatitis. Eosinophilic folliculitis, and furunculosis may also occur. Intraepidermal pustules filled with eosinophils and foci of necrosis (''nibble marks'') may be seen.

Myiasis is infestation of tissues by the larvae of dipterous flies (flies with two wings or winglike appendages) and is a disease of neglect occurring in moist areas of the body soiled by urine, feces, or bodily secretions. Flies are attracted by the malodor of such areas. Sheep are most commonly affected (ovine fleece rot). In myiasis due to blow flies (calliphorids) and flesh flies (sarcophagids), eggs are deposited on soiled hair or wool or in wounds. Grossly, matted hair or wool and multiple irregular holes or ulcers with an offensive odor are observed, and these areas may expand extensively due to the secretion of proteolytic enzymes by larvae. Death may occur and is due to septicemia or toxemia.

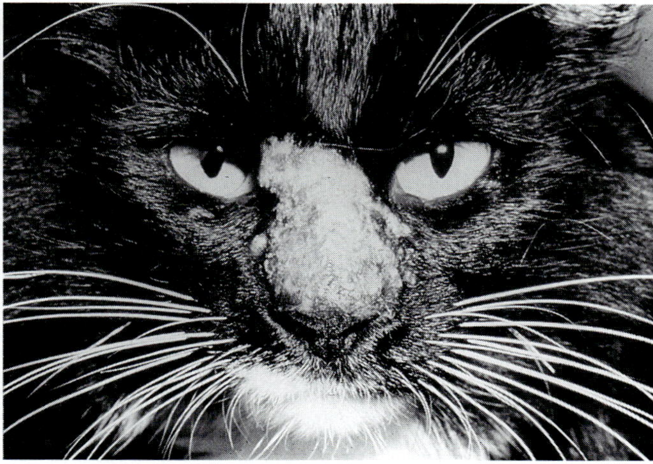

Fig. 11-38 Skin, face; cat. Mosquito bite hypersensitivity. Alopecia, depigmentation, and swelling are present in skin of the dorsum of muzzle. *Courtesy Dr. A. Werner.*

In **cuterebra myiasis,** *Cuterebra* sp. eggs are deposited on stones or vegetation, and young animals (rabbits, rodents, and, less often, cats and dogs) become infested by contact with the eggs. Nodules containing larvae are located in the subcutis and are associated with an opening in the skin for respiration by the larvae.

In **hypoderma myiasis,** larvae of *Hypoderma lineatum* and *H. bovis* penetrate the skin of the legs of cattle and, less frequently, horses and bison and migrate either through the esophagus or vertebral canal on their way to the subcutis of the back. The larvae become established in subcutaneous nodules similar to those of *Cuterebra* sp. (Fig. 11-39) with an opening for respiration. Microscopically, larvae are located in a cavity filled with fibrin and a few eosinophils and bordered by granulation tissue containing clusters of eosinophils.

Screwworm myiasis, caused by *Cochliomyia* sp. (*Callitroga* sp.) and *Chrysomyia* sp., is an important disease in domestic and wild animals. The disease occurs in Africa,

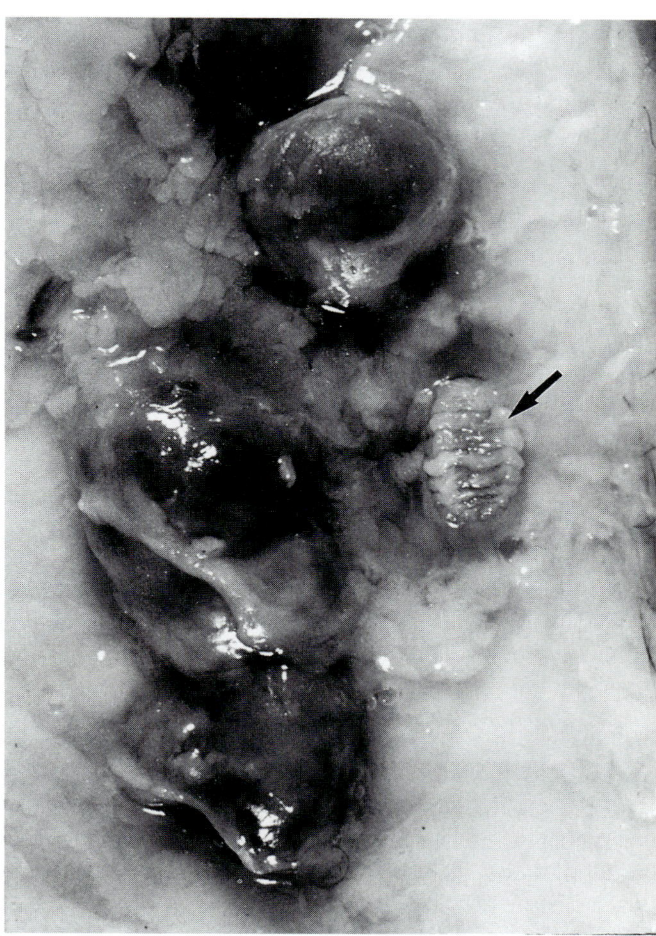

Fig. 11-39 Skin, subcutis; cow. *Hypoderma* species larva. Multiple nodules containing the larvae are present. One nodule is incised, exposing a larva *(arrow)*.

Asia, Central and South America, and Mexico, but has been eradicated in the United States and nearly so in Mexico. Screwworm flies deposit larvae in wounds or near mucocutaneous junctions of living animals; the larvae penetrate and liquefy tissue by secretion of proteolytic enzymes and feed on living tissues. Grossly, malodorous wounds contain larvae and shreds of tissue. Death may occur in untreated animals. When it is necessary to differentiate screwworm myiasis from cutaneous myiasis caused by other flies, larvae can be preserved in 70% alcohol and submitted for identification. Screwworm myiasis is a reportable disease in some countries, including the United States.

Helminths

Cutaneous infections with helminths are generally not life threatening but may be unsightly and irritating in companion animals and cause hide damage in food animals. Infections are due to migration of helminth larvae that, as adults, live in noncutaneous sites or by filarial infections (filarial dermatitis) in which adults or microfilaria spend some time in the skin or subcutis. Rarely, such adult helminths as *Dracunculus insignis* and *Anatrichosoma cutaneum* parasitize the skin.

Hookworm dermatitis is due to *Ancylostoma* or *Uncinaria* larvae. Red papules that coalesce into lichenified alopecic areas occur on the feet of dogs and, less frequently, on other areas in contact with an unsanitary environment contaminated by hookworm larvae. Foot pads may become soft, the keratinized portion may separate, and secondary bacterial dermatitis and paronychia may develop. Hyperplastic spongiotic perivascular dermatitis has eosinophils, serocellular crusts, and migration tracks as its principal lesions. Parasitologic evaluation of fresh tissue may provide larval identification.

Cutaneous habronemiasis (summer sores) occurs in horses and is caused by infection with the larvae of *Habronema* sp. or *Draschia* sp. deposited on the skin by houseflies or stableflies. Larval deposition and lesions occur on parts of the body where the skin is either traumatized (damaged), such as the legs, or moist and soft, such as the medial canthus of the eye and prepuce. Larvae are unable to penetrate normal skin, but the fly bites cause sufficient damage for larval penetration. Grossly, single or multiple, proliferative, ulcerated, red to brown tumorous masses have, on section, small, yellow to white gritty foci. The microscopic lesion is a nodular dermatitis with eosinophils, epithelioid macrophages, and, sometimes, multinucleated giant cells bordering larvae or necrotic debris. Granulation tissue infiltrated by neutrophils is prevalent along the ulcerated surface.

Other helminth parasites associated with cutaneous larval migration include *Pelodera, Necator, Strongyloides, Gnathostoma,* and *Bunostomum.* Schistosome cercariae, especially of birds, can cause similar lesions.

Onchocerciasis, a filarial dermatitis of cattle, buffalo, mules, donkeys, sheep, and goats, is principally a disease of horses which may develop severe Microfilaria, transmitted by intermediate hosts such as the Simuliidae (black flies, gnats) and Ceratopogonidae (biting midges), also may be present without significant dermal inflammation, and differences in lesion severity may reflect different degrees of hypersensitivity to microfilaria (living or dead). Adult parasites are located in nodules in connective tissue, and microfilaria are located in the dermis, particularly of the ventral midline. In equine onchocerciasis, lesions develop on the head, neck, medial forelimbs, ventral thorax, and abdomen. Gross lesions consist of patchy to diffuse alopecia, erythema, scaling, crusting, and pigmentary changes. Some horses have a characteristic, variably pigmented, circular area of dermatitis on the forehead. Keratitis, conjunctivitis, and uveitis are observed in some horses. Microscopic cutaneous lesions vary from none to a superficial and deep perivascular dermatitis with eosinophils, lymphocytes, and microfilariae.

Stephanofilariasis, a filarial dermatitis of cattle, buffalo, and goats, is transmitted by flies and caused by six species of parasites of the genus *Stephanofilaria.* Each species causes lesions in different body locations. *S. stilesi* occurs in cattle in the United States and causes ventral midline lesions that consist initially of circular patches with moist erect hairs, foci of epidermal hemorrhage, and serum exudation. Such foci expand and coalesce into a large area covered by crusts, which, upon healing, consist of thickened hairless plaques. Microscopic lesions are a superficial and deep perivascular dermatitis with eosinophils, adult parasites, and microfilaria along with epidermal hyperkeratosis, parakeratosis, acanthosis with spongiosis, eosinophilic microabscesses, and crust formation. Other causes of filarial dermatitis include *Elaeophora* sp., *Parafilaria* sp., *Suifilaria* sp., and, rarely, *Dirofilaria* sp. *P. bovicola* infection in cattle has increased in Europe; lesions consist of hemorrhagic nodules in the subcutis containing adult parasites. These may rupture and bleed.

Protozoa

In the United States, cutaneous protozoal infections may develop as part of systemic infections, principally with *Leishmania.* Leishmaniasis is caused by a variety of species of the protozoan parasite *Leishmania* of the family Trypanosomatidae. The disease, which can occur in cutaneous, mucocutaneous, or visceral forms, is rare in animals in the United States, except in endemic areas in Oklahoma and Texas. Sandflies serve as the vector for infection of animals; and dogs, cats, and rodents serve as reservoirs of infection for human beings. *Leishmania* organisms are found principally in monocytes and macrophages of the spleen, bone marrow, less often the liver, and rarely cells in peripheral blood. Cutaneous lesions in dogs consist of generalized alopecia with silvery white scales or more severe lesions that include nodules and ulcers. Lesions occur chiefly in areas where sandflies feed, e.g., around the muzzle, ears, and eyes. Microscopically, lesions include hyperkeratosis, parakeratosis, crusts, and granulomatous nodules in the dermis. Accumulations of macrophages, along with fewer lymphocytes and plasma cells, have a periadnexal pattern and may efface sebaceous glands. Organisms may be present in intracellular and extracellular locations.

IMMUNOLOGIC SKIN DISEASES

General

Immunologic diseases are classified as either hypersensitivity (allergic) or autoimmune. Hypersensitivity is a mild to severe reaction that develops in response to normally harmless foreign compounds, including antiserum, hormones, pollen, and insect venoms. Autoimmune diseases develop when antibodies or T cells are reactive against self-antigens rather than against foreign antigens. Ideally, at least three specific requirements should be met to classify a disease as ''autoimmune,'' but the requirements are seldom met in practice. These requirements are presence of an autoimmune-type reaction, evidence of primary tissue damage, and absence of another cause of the disease. ''Autoimmune disease,'' therefore, is a general term referring to a spectrum of diseases in which autoimmune mechanisms appear to participate in lesion production. Four basic immune reactions—types I, II, III, and IV—mediate the tissue damage in hypersensitivity and autoimmune diseases. Another reaction, cutaneous basophil hypersensitivity, is less well characterized, but may be operative in some hypersensitivity reactions, such as flea allergy in dogs. Most cutaneous hypersensitivity reactions are mediated either by type I or type IV reactions or by a combination of one or more of the four reactions. Autoimmune mechanisms tend to be mediated by type II or III reactions, although more than one mechanism may be involved. Hypersensitivity reactions are common in dogs and horses, less common in cats, and are uncommon in food animals. Autoimmune diseases with cutaneous manifestations are uncommon in domestic animals, accounting for 1% to 2% of dermatoses in most species. Of the cutaneous autoimmune disorders, pemphigus foliaceus is the most prevalent, followed in incidence by discoid and systemic lupus erythematosus. Dermatomyositis is widespread in the collie and Shetland sheepdog populations, but because dermatomyositis has only recently been described, prevalence of this disease in comparison with other immune-mediated diseases has not been determined. In domestic animals, certain breeds of dogs, horses, and cats seem to be predisposed to develop certain autoimmune diseases.

Mechanisms of Tissue Damage

Type I reactions

These inflammatory reactions are mediated by pharmacologically active substances released or formed de novo by mast cells and basophils following reaction between antigen and specific antibody (usually IgE) bound to receptors on the membrane of the mast cells or basophils. Released substances include histamine, serotonin, leukotrienes, prostaglandins, eosinophil chemotactic factor of anaphylaxis, and platelet-activating factor. Type I hypersensitivity can be systemic and/or local and, in the skin, may result in pruritic and circumscribed wheals with raised, erythematous borders. The reaction occurs in two phases, immediate (15 to 30 minutes) and late (6 to 12 hours), and is generally referred to as an immediate hypersensitivity reaction. The production of IgE is T cell dependent and genetically controlled, and therefore, inherited predispositions to type I hypersensitivity occur. Cutaneous type I hypersensitivity reactions include atopic dermatitis (most common), urticaria, angioedema, and hypersensitivity associated with bites of flies such as *Culicoides* sp., mites such as *Sarcoptes* sp., with gastrointestinal parasites, and with food. Traditionally, this type of reaction is characterized microscopically by capillary dilatation, edema, mast cell degranulation, and infiltrates of eosinophils.

Type II reactions

These cytotoxic reactions involve interaction of IgG or IgM with antigens bound on cellular membranes. Complement fixation frequently occurs, leading to cellular damage. Type II reactions involving the skin are caused by deposition of circulating antibody to protein components of desmosomes in intercellular areas or along the basement membrane of the epidermal-dermal junction and include such diseases as pemphigus (uncommon) and bullous pemphigoid (rare). The lesions vary with the location of the target antigen, and, in pemphigus and pemphigoid, vesicles develop either within the epidermis or subepidermally.

Type III reactions

These reactions, mediated by complement-fixing immune complexes, involve IgG or IgM immunoglobulins. When immune complexes deposit in tissues and fix complement, cytokines and other factors are generated that are chemotactic for neutrophils. Tissue damage results from lysosomal enzymes released from neutrophils, activation of complement and coagulation systems, platelet aggregation, and radical oxygen products. Immune complex vasculitis may be responsible for the purpura seen in infections with *Streptococcus equi.* Lesions of systemic lupus erythematosus are due to immune complex deposition. The lesions of familial canine dermatomyositis may be associated with immune complexes.

Type IV reactions

These reactions, termed ''delayed hypersensitivity reactions,'' take many hours to develop and are initiated by haptens, which bind to a carrier protein, usually epidermal. Langerhans' cells serve in antigen presentation. The reaction is mediated by sensitized T cells that, after contacting a specific antigen, release lymphokines (cytokines) and/or recruit other lymphocytes that are cytotoxic, but antibody and complement are not involved. Type IV hypersensitivity reactions are used in the diagnosis of diseases such as tuberculosis, histoplasmosis, and coccidioidomycosis. The skin reaction typically develops 24 to 48 hours after exposure to the specific antigen and consists of perivascular mononuclear cell accumulations.

Combination reactions

The strict categorization of hypersensitivity reactions is an oversimplification as the categories often overlap as do the lesions. Thus, hypersensitivity to fleas, ticks, *Staphylococcus* sp., hormones, and drugs is mediated by different combinations of types I, II, III, and IV reactions. The mechanisms are also interdependent. For instance, the production of IgE, which plays a significant role in type I reactions, is T cell dependent.

Hypersensitivity Reactions

Atopy

Atopy (atopic dermatitis, allergic inhalant dermatitis), an example of a type I hypersensitivity reaction, has the skin as the major target organ in dogs, cats, and horses, with the route of allergen exposure being predominantly respiratory, at least in dogs. Atopy is the second most common hypersensitivity dermatitis in dogs and accounts for 8% to 10% of skin disorders. In atopic dermatitis, T cells and cytokines interact to initiate lesions; for instance, type 2 T helper cells produce interleukin-4 (IL-4) and express interleukin-1 (IL-1) receptors. IL-4 enhances T-lymphocyte and mast cell multiplication. Interleukin-3 (IL-3) is synergistic, particularly in the facilitation of mast cell differentiation and development. IL-4 also stimulates B-lymphocytes to switch production from IgM to IgE. IgE activates mast cells. In dogs, IgE and subclasses of IgG are important in the allergic reaction. The predominant clinical sign of atopy is pruritus and, in dogs, is often manifested as face rubbing and foot licking. Clinical signs of feline atopy are varied and include those associated with facial pruritus, pruritic pinnae, generalized pruritus, miliary dermatitis, eosinophilic granuloma complex, and symmetric alopecia. Horses may have pruritus of the head, pinnae, ventrum, legs, and tailhead or recurrent urticaria. Skin lesions may not be seen, and those present are mostly the result of self-inflicted trauma. Dogs may have secondary pyoderma or seborrhea. Microscopically, the lesion is a hyperplastic superficial perivascular dermatitis with mixed populations of mast cells, nonmetachromatic mononuclear cells, and eosinophils. Some animals, particularly horses, have deep perivascular inflammation as well. Eosinophils are seen less frequently in dogs than in other species and are the predominant inflammatory cell in horses. Diagnosis of atopy is based on clinical signs, physical examination, intradermal skin testing, and the use of the radioallergosorbent test (RAST) and the enzyme-linked immunosorbent assay (ELISA) for elevated allergen-specific IgE.

Flea bite hypersensitivity

The most common hypersensitivity dermatitis in dogs and cats results from flea bites and involves type I and type IV reactions and cutaneous basophil hypersensitivity. Flea bite hypersensitivity is pruritic, and cutaneous lesions occur principally along the dorsal lumbosacral area (see Fig. 11-37), ventral abdomen, caudomedial aspects of the thighs, flanks, and, in cats, around the neck but may be generalized in highly sensitive animals (miliary dermatitis in cats). Secondary lesions are due to self-inflicted trauma. Grossly, there is a papular dermatitis with secondary excoriations. Some dogs with chronic disease have multiple firm, alopecic nodules (fibropruritic nodules) in the dorsal lumbosacral area. Microscopically, flea bite hypersensitivity is characterized by hyperplastic superficial perivascular dermatitis with edema, mast cells, basophils, lymphocytes, histiocytes, and eosinophils. Intraepithelial eosinophils may be seen. Fibropruritic nodules with a core of coarse, thick collagen bundles are covered by a hyperplastic epidermis.

Culicoides hypersensitivity

This is a common, worldwide pruritic dermatitis in horses, caused principally by type I and type IV hypersensitivity reactions to salivary antigens from bites of *Culicoides* sp. Signs and lesions may be seasonal or non seasonal depending on climate, usually develop in horses over 2 years of age, and arise in areas bitten by the species of *Culicoides* involved. Gross lesions consist of papules, crusts, alopecia, excoriations, and lichenification. Microscopic lesions include superficial and deep perivascular dermatitis with numerous eosinophils, epidermal hyperplasia with hyperkeratosis, and dermal fibrosis. Some horses will have eosinophilic folliculitis, intraepidermal pustules, and eosinophilic granulomas.

Allergic contact dermatitis

Allergic contact dermatitis, an example of a type IV hypersensitivity reaction, is due primarily to contact with chemicals such as aniline dyes in carpets, with plant resins, and, historically, with plastics in food dishes. The lesions are pruritic, resulting in self-inflicted trauma, are variable in severity, and are located in regions in contact with the antigen, typically, in glabrous areas unless the antigen is a liquid or aerosol. Grossly, erythema, papules with or without vesicles, and exudation develop into crusts. Chronic lesions are lichenified, hyperpigmented, and alopecic. Microscopic lesions include spongiotic superficial perivascular dermatitis with mononuclear cells, and, when chronic, epidermal hyperplasia. Some cases have many eosinophils, including eosinophilic epidermal pustules.

Hypersensitivity reactions to drugs

Hypersensitivity reactions to drugs are uncommon in dogs and cats, are rare in other domestic animals, and may result from any of the four types of hypersensitivity reactions. The drugs most commonly associated with hypersensitivity reactions include penicillins and trimethoprim-potentiated sulfonamides, but many drugs may cause a hypersensitivity reaction. Microscopic lesions are of several patterns and include perivascular dermatitis, lichenoid/interface dermatitis (see Fig. 11-7), vasculitis, vesiculopustular dermatitis, necrotizing dermatitis, panniculitis, or perforating folliculitis.

Autoimmune Reactions

Pemphigus

Pemphigus comprises a group of blistering diseases characterized by acantholysis associated with the binding of autoantibodies to desmosomal proteins and, subsequently, disruption of cell adhesion, resulting in the formation of vesicles. Acantholysis may result from a direct interruption of cell adhesion by binding of the autoantibody (also complement) to the antigen (an adhesion molecule) or indirectly by the synthesis of a plasminogen activator with subsequent activation of plasminogen and disruption of intercellular adhesion. **Pemphigus vulgaris** is rare and the most severe form of pemphigus, occurs in dogs and cats, and is characterized by vesicles or bullae, followed by erosions and ulcers in the oral cavity, at mucocutaneous junctions (nostrils, lips, eyelids, prepuce or vulva, anus, inner surface of pinna), and skin (axilla and groin). Microscopic lesions consist of suprabasilar vesiculation with a row of basal cells attached to the basement membrane (row of tombstones) (see Fig. 11-9) and a superficial perivascular dermatitis, sometimes with lichenoid infiltrates at the epidermal-dermal interface. **Pemphigus vegetans** occurs rarely in dogs, is predominantly truncal, and is a mild variant of pemphigus vulgaris; the lesions are vesicopustular dermatitis with epidermal hyperplasia, resulting in papillomatous formations. **Pemphigus foliaceus** is milder and occurs more commonly than pemphigus vulgaris in dogs, cats, horses, and goats. Lesions may be localized (muzzle, periocular, pinnae, foot pads, around nails) or generalized and consist of symmetric vesicular to pustular dermatitis with scales, crusts, alopecia, and superficial erosions (Figs. 11-40 and 11-41). Microscopically, subcorneal or intragranular pustules with acantholytic cells (see Fig. 11-8) and multilaminated crusts with acantholytic cells are observed. Crusts should be included in biopsy samples if pemphigus foliaceus is a differential diagnosis and if well-developed primary lesions are not present. The eosinophil is the predominant inflammatory cell in about one third of the canine and equine cases. **Pemphigus erythematosus** occurs in dogs and cats, is a mild variant of pemphigus foliaceus, and has lesions (including depigmentation and photodermatitis), usually limited to the face and external ears.

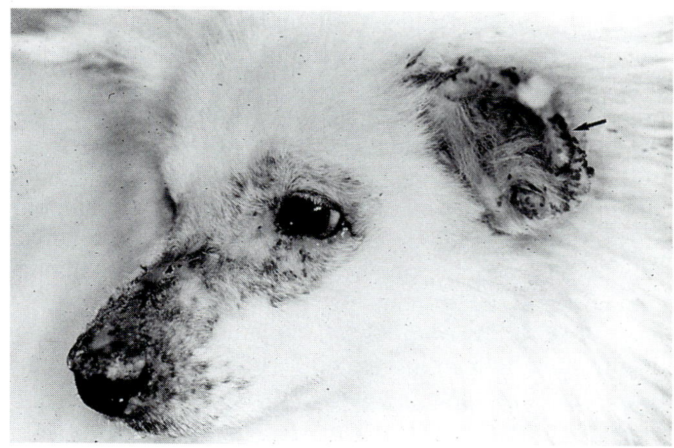

Fig. 11-40 Skin, face; dog. Pemphigus foliaceus. Alopecia, focal ulceration, crusting, and depigmentation are present on medial aspect of pinnae *(arrow),* periocular areas, and dorsum of muzzle, including the nasal planum (erythema is also present).

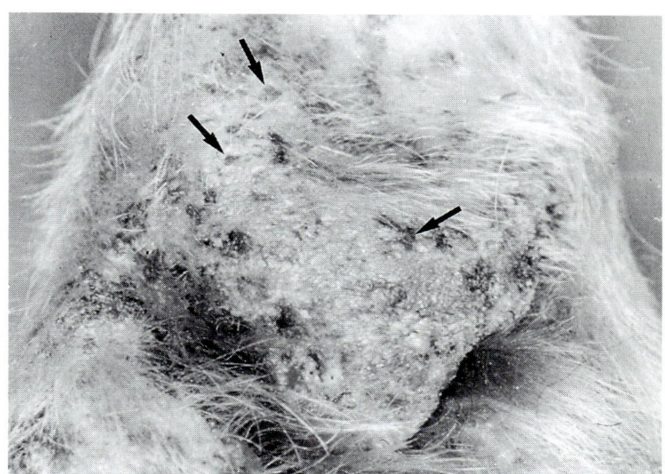

Fig. 11-41 Skin, foot pad; dog (same dog as in Fig. 11-40). Pemphigus foliaceus. Erosions *(arrows)* and depigmentation are present. Crusts are also a feature of this disease but are not present on this foot pad.

Bullous pemphigoid

Bullous pemphigoid is characterized by subepidermal vesicles and bullae associated with deposition of antibody in the basement membrane. In human beings, the antigen is considered to be a desmosomal plaque molecule, probably desmoplakin I. Vesiculobullous lesions result from activation of complement and leukocyte chemotaxis and activation; however, direct binding of antibody to hemidesmosomes may also occur, and immunoglobulins and/or complement may be demonstrated at the basement membrane. Grossly, bullous pemphigoid resembles pemphigus vulgaris and develops in dogs and horses; bullae are in the oral cavity, at mucocutaneous junctions, and in the axilla and groin. Microscopically, the subepidermal vesiculobullous lesions have basal cells lining the roof of the bullae and the basement membrane forming the floor. The bullae contain fibrin, neutrophils, or eosinophils. Acantholysis is not a feature, and dermal inflammation is minimal. Frequently, the bullae rupture and form ulcers, which stimulate a more severe inflammatory reaction.

Lupus erythematosus

Two forms of lupus erythematosus are recognized: systemic lupus erythematosus and discoid lupus erythematosus. Systemic lupus erythematosus (SLE) is a multiorgan disease of dogs, cats, and, rarely, horses. Factors involved in development include a genetic predisposition, viral infections, hormones, and UV light. SLE is a disease of immune dysregulation, which includes defective T cell suppressor function and cytokine dysregulation. The defective T cell suppression function could be due to anti–T cell antibodies or a primary suppressor T cell deficiency. B cell hyperactivity results in the formation of autoantibodies to a variety of cells and to nucleic acids. Immune complexes form by antigen-antibody binding and are deposited in a variety of tissues, including skin, and result in a type III hypersensitivity response. Cutaneous lesions may be localized or generalized; commonly involve the face, pinnae, oral mucosae, and distal extremities; and consist of erythema, depigmentation, alopecia, scaling, crusting, ulceration, and, sometimes, stomatitis or panniculitis. Microscopic lesions include a lymphohistiocytic interface dermatitis with basal cell degeneration, basement membrane thickening, vasculitis, and subepidermal vesicles.

Discoid lupus erythematosus is relatively common and is a mild variant of SLE with no involvement of other organs and a negative antinuclear antibody titer. Lesions—depigmentation, erythema, scaling, erosion, ulceration, and crusting—generally occur in the skin of the nasal planum, the dorsum of the muzzle, and, less commonly, the pinnae, lips, and periocular region and in the oral mucosae. Microscopically, a lichenoid interface dermatitis often has many lymphocytes, plasma cells, pigmentary incontinence, and basal cell degeneration.

Dermatomyositis

Dermatomyositis, an autosomal dominant disease of variable expressivity, is described in collies and Shetland sheepdogs (Fig. 11-42). Dermatomyositis occurs in puppies as young as 8 weeks of age, with lesions of a vesiculating dermatitis of face, lips, and external ears, and progresses to involve the distal extremities, especially over bony prominences and the tip of the tail. Myositis, and atrophy of muscles of mastication, distal extremities, and, sometimes, esophagus develop after the dermatitis. Ultrastructurally, endothelial cells in muscle contain inclusion bodies that resemble those produced by picorna-viruses (Fig. 11-43), and immune complexes seem to play a role in lesion development. Mild lesions heal without scarring, and moderate lesions heal with permanent foci of alopecia and hyperpigmentation. Moderately affected dogs have more of these lesions on the nose, periocular regions,

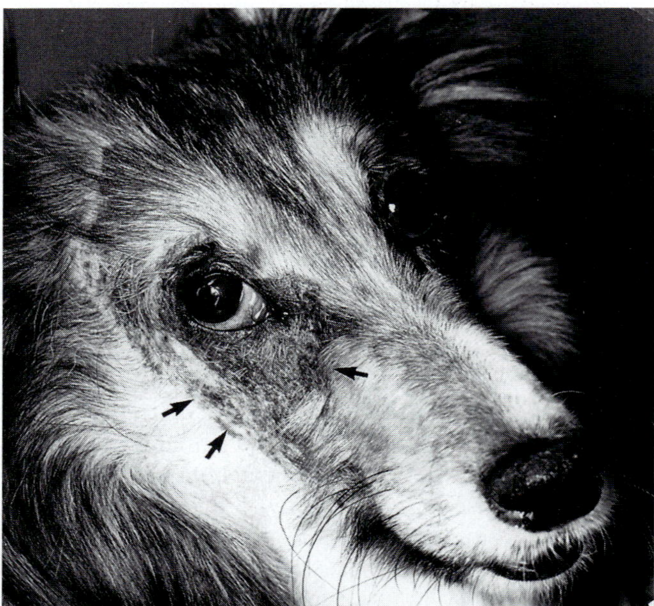

Fig. 11-42 Skin, face; dog. Dermatomyositis. Hair loss and hyperpigmentation are present in the skin around the eye and on the face *(arrows)*.

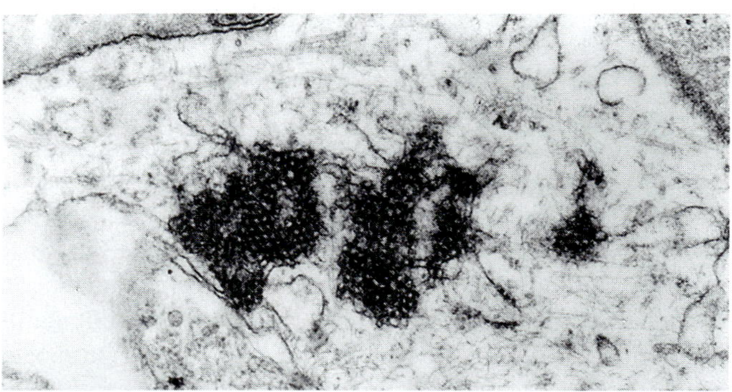

Fig. 11-43 Transmission electron micrograph. Muscle, endothelial cell; dog. Dermatomyositis. Viral-like inclusion consists of clusters of small, rounded bodies. Uranyl acetate–lead citrate stain.

distal extremities, and tip of the tail. Lesions in biopsy samples include interface dermatitis with basal cell degeneration of the epidermis and follicular wall, follicular atrophy, variable epidermal vesicles and pustules, and dermal scarring. Vasculitis is occasionally present. The anterior and most superficial portion of the temporalis muscle is the site of choice for biopsy to confirm the myositis.

Other uncommon to rare autoimmune or immune-mediated diseases with cutaneous lesions include cold agglutinin disease, cutaneous vasculitis, erythema multiforme, toxic epidermal necrolysis, linear IgA dermatosis, feline plasma cell pododermatitis, lichenoid dermatoses, alopecia areata, localized scleroderma, ulcerative dermatosis of the collie and Shetland sheepdog, and uveodermatologic syndrome (Vogt-Koyanagi-Harada (VKH)–like syndrome).

Diagnosis of autoimmune skin disorders

The diagnosis is based on distribution and appearance of gross and microscopic lesions. Other diagnostic tools include the demonstration of immunoglobulin (IgG, IgM, or IgA) and/or complement in intercellular areas (pemphigus vulgaris, pemphigus foliaceus, and erythematosus), at the basement membrane (pemphigus erythematosus, bullous pemphigoid, systemic lupus erythematosus, discoid lupus erythematosus, and linear IgA dermatosis), or in vessels (cutaneous vasculitis) and the results of clinical immunologic tests, such as antinuclear antibody titers and Coombs' test.

METABOLIC SKIN DISEASES

General

Cutaneous endocrine disorders are due to imbalances in hormones and generally are manifested as nonpruritic, bilaterally symmetric alopecia with the remaining hair coat dull and dry, easily epilated hair that fails to regrow after clipping, and pigmentary changes. These lesions are referred to as "endocrine alopecia." In disorders associated with alterations in sex hormones, the alopecia often begins in the perineal and genital areas and may extend cranially. However, it is not uncommon for a cutaneous endocrine disorder to have asymmetric alopecia and pigmentary changes along with secondary pyoderma or seborrhea. Microscopically, uncomplicated endocrine disorders of the skin consist of hyperkeratosis of superficial epidermis and of hair follicles; epidermal and follicular infundibular epithelial atrophy, hyperplasia, or normalcy; follicular dilatation; increased numbers of catagen and/or telogen hair follicles; empty hair follicles; and increased epidermal pigmentation. These changes may not be sufficiently specific to be diagnostic, and inflammation due to secondary seborrhea or pyoderma frequently complicates the diagnosis. Cutaneous endocrine disorders are more common in dogs than in cats, food animals, or horses.

Hypothyroidism

Deficiency of thyroid hormone is the most common endocrine disorder in dogs and is caused by idiopathic thyroid atrophy and lymphocytic thyroiditis. A variety of systemic and cutaneous signs and lesions result from thyroid hormone deficiency. Gross lesions consist of endocrine alopecia that develops, in most dogs, over the trunk and neck. Microscopically, in addition to the lesions associated with endocrine alopecia, dermal mucin is increased, resulting in dermal thickening (myxedema), and the epidermal and follicular infundibular epitheliae are acanthotic. Secondary pyoderma is a common complication.

Hyperadrenocorticism

Hyperadrenocorticism results in cutaneous lesions, principally in dogs and cats, due to excessive hormones derived from bilateral adrenal cortical hyperplasia secondary to a pituitary neoplasm, from a functional adrenal cortical neoplasm, or from the administration of exogenous glucocorticoids. In dogs, cutaneous lesions include endocrine alopecia, which generally spares the head and extremities, thinning of the skin, comedone formation, increased bruising, poor wound healing, and increased susceptibility to infection (Fig. 11-44). In some dogs, calcification involves the skin, particularly the dermis of the back, inguinal, and axillary regions (calcinosis cutis) (Fig. 11-45). In cats, the skin may tear with normal handling. Microscopically, the lesions of hyperadrenocorticism include epidermal, dermal, and follicular atrophy, comedones, and calcinosis cutis (dogs). Granulomatous inflammation and epidermal hyperplasia are commonly associated with the calcification.

Hyperestrogenism

Hyperestrogenism may develop in male and female dogs. In females, estrogen may be secreted by ovarian cysts

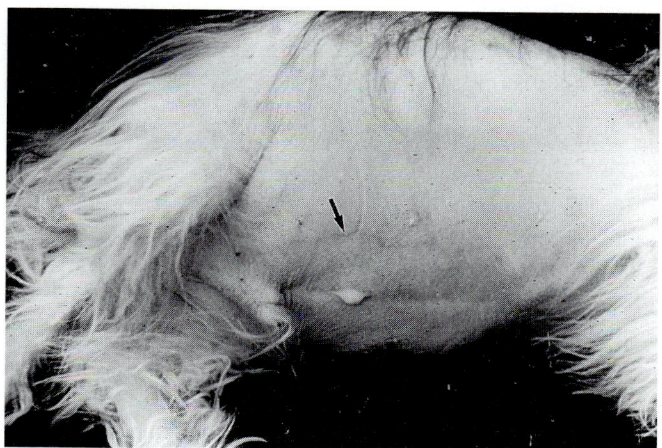

Fig. 11-44 Skin; dog. Hyperadrenocorticism. Truncal alopecia, distended abdomen, and thin skin are present. Vasculature is faintly visible *(arrow). Courtesy Dr. A. Mundell.*

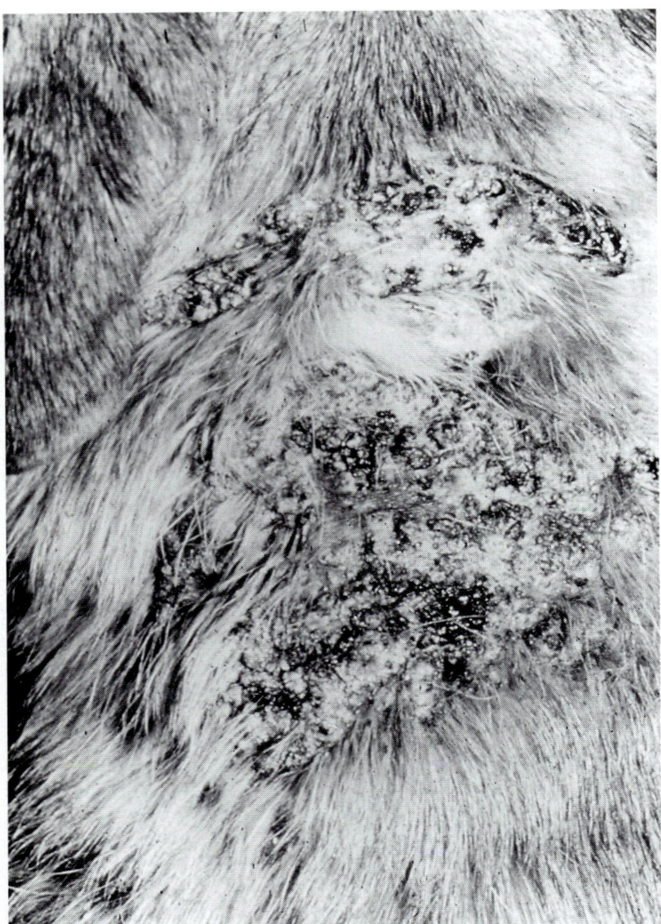

Fig. 11-45 Skin, dorsal neck; dog. Hyperadrenocorticism and calcinosis cutis. The skin is alopecic, thickened, and crusted. *Courtesy Dr. A. Mundell.*

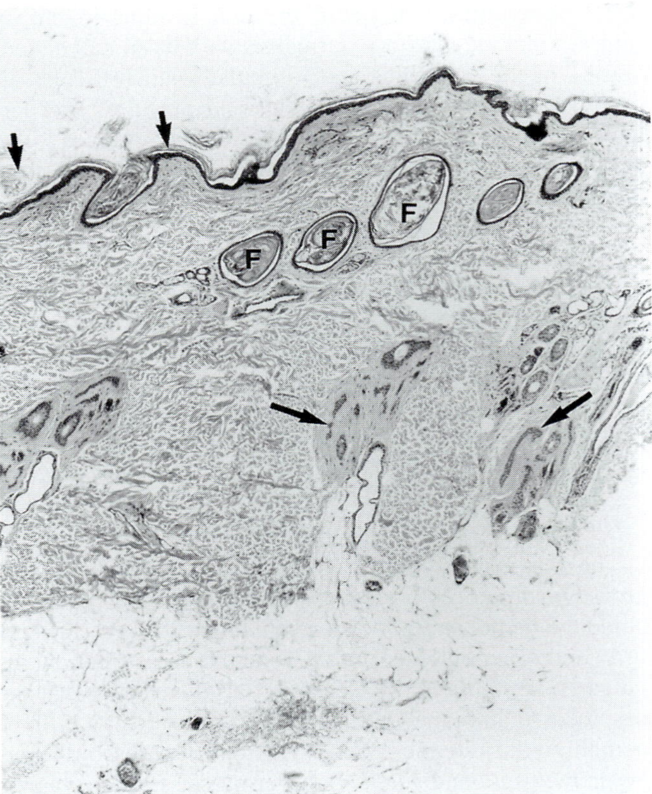

Fig. 11-46 Skin; dog. Hyperestrogenism. Male dog with latrogenic hyperestrogenism from diethylstilbestrol therapy. Note epidermal orthokeratotic hyperkeratosis *(small arrows),* follicles dilated with keratin *(F),* and small atrophic follicles *(large arrows).* H & E stain.

or, rarely, an ovarian neoplasm or be due to estrogen administration. In males, elevated serum concentrations of estrogen are usually derived from a functional testicular Sertoli cell tumor. Iatrogenic estrogen administration has also caused hyperestrogenism in male dogs (Fig. 11-46). In addition to endocrine alopecia, female dogs have an enlarged vulva and abnormalities of the estrus cycle. Male dogs may have gynecomastia, pendulous prepuce, or an enlarged prostate due to squamous metaplasia of the ducts. Microscopic lesions include, in addition to telogen follicles, hyperkeratosis and acanthosis of the epidermis and follicular infundibular epithelium.

"Castration-responsive Dermatosis" (Woolly Syndrome, Growth Hormone/Castration–responsive Dermatosis)

This syndrome, in which the hair coat is often fluffy and more woollike, develops mostly in intact male dogs of certain breeds. Symmetric alopecia develops over the perineum, thighs, ventral abdomen and thorax, and around the neck. Hyperpigmentation is sometimes present. Abnormalities in a number of hormones have been detected. In the Pomeranian dog, and possibly other breeds, partial deficiency of 21-hydroxylase enzyme results in disregulation of adrenal hormone synthesis and in hyperprogestinism and hyperandrogenism. Castration may provide a temporary response by removing testicular hormones. Microscopic alterations include increased numbers of catagen as well as telogen hair follicles and flame follicles (Fig. 11-47).

Hypersomatotropism

This syndrome, due to excess production of growth hormone, is rare in adult dogs and has cutaneous lesions of thick, folded skin over the head, neck, and extremities. Hypertrichosis may develop. Microscopic lesions consist of hyperplasia of the epidermis, dermal fibrosis, and mucinous degeneration of the dermis.

Hyposomatotropism

Deficiency of growth hormone in dogs less than 3 months of age is usually due to pituitary cysts that have destroyed the gland. Deficiencies of thyroidal, adrenal, and

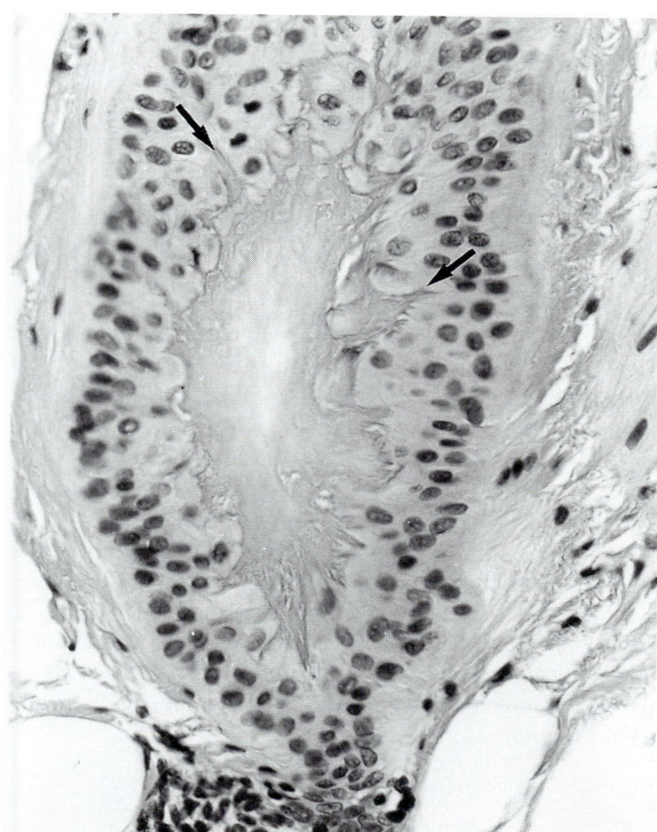

Fig. 11-47 Skin, haired; dog. Flame follicle. The hair follicle has excessive tricholemmal keratinization resembling the spikes *(arrows)* of a flame and consistent with a "flame follicle." H & E stain.

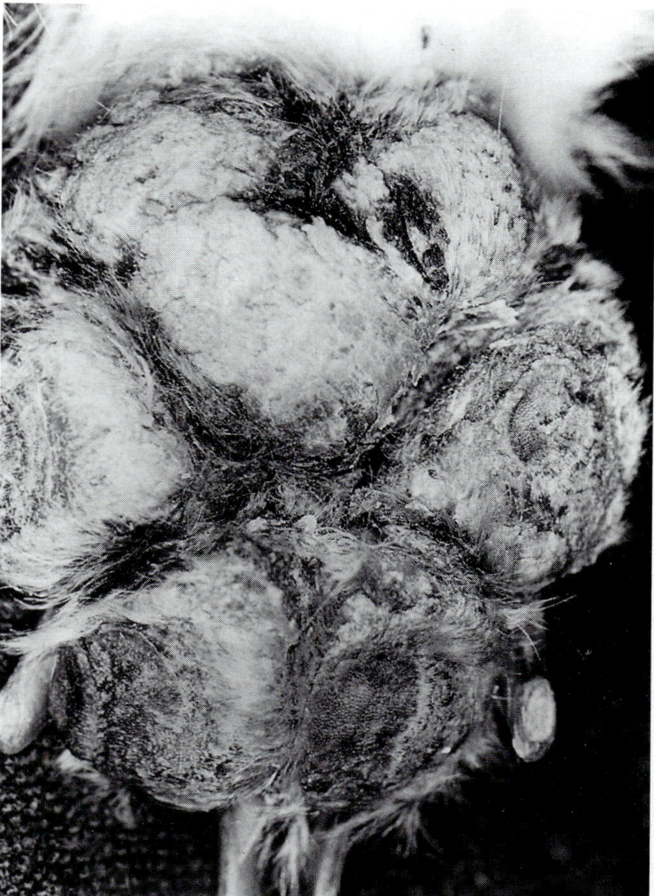

Fig. 11-48 Skin, foot pad; dog. Superficial necrolytic dermatitis. Crusting and fissuring are evident.

gonadal hormones are frequently accompanying problems. Pituitary deficiency results in failure to grow, retention of the puppy hair coat, and development of endocrine alopecia.

Superficial Necrolytic Dermatopathy (Diabetic Dermatopathy, Hepatocutaneous Syndrome)

This rare metabolic disorder develops in older dogs and is associated with diabetes mellitus, hepatic dysfunction, and pancreatic lesions rarely including glucagon-producing pancreatic islet cell tumor. Lesions of scaling, crusting, erythema, and alopecia develop on the face, distal extremities, genitalia, and foot pads with foot pad lesions consisting of crusting and fissuring or ulceration (Fig. 11-48). Microscopic lesions, when fully developed, are considered diagnostic and consist of a trilaminar thickening of the epidermis in which the outermost layer is parakeratotic, the intermediate epidermal layer is edematous (degenerate) and vacuolated, and the innermost layer is hyperplastic (see Fig. 11-5). Dermatophytes, probably a secondary infection, have been identified in the foot pads of some dogs with this syndrome.

NUTRITIONAL SKIN DISEASES

A variety of nutritional deficiencies result in similar cutaneous lesions. Inadequate diets may involve more than one dietary deficiency, as mineral and vitamin metabolism are sometimes interrelated (i.e., copper and molybdenum and vitamin E and dietary fatty acids). The lesions heal when the animal is fed a balanced diet. Deficiency diseases can develop through increased needs (pregnancy, neonatal growth, or cold weather) or through disease processes. Deficiencies affecting the skin include protein-calorie nutrition; fatty acid deficiency; hypovitaminosis A, C, and E; and deficiencies of riboflavin, pantothenic acid, biotin, niacin, iodine, cobalt, copper, and zinc.

Zinc Deficiency

Zinc deficiency occurs chiefly in pigs and dogs, is of less importance in ruminants, and results from diets containing high concentrations of phytic acid (binds zinc), low concentrations of zinc, high concentrations of calcium, or inherited absorptive or metabolic abnormalities. Zinc deficiency, although once common in pigs, occurs infrequently today because of dietary supplementation. The lesions are circumscribed, reddened papules and plaques, scales, and thick crusts and fissures along the ventral abdomen and medial thighs. Some pigs have generalized symmetric lesions, especially involving the lower limbs, periocular areas, pinnae, snout, scrotum, and tail. Microscopically, the lesions are parakeratosis, hypergranulosis, acanthosis, and pseudoepitheliomatous hyperplasia. Secondary bacterial invasion results in pustular dermatitis and folliculitis.

Canine zinc-responsive dermatosis

This dermatosis occurs in two forms. One form occurs principally in Siberian huskies and Alaskan malamutes, but other large breed dogs may be affected. Scaling and crusting develop in the skin around the mouth, chin, eyes, joints, scrotum, prepuce, or vulva (Fig. 11-49). Microscopically, the parakeratosis is diffuse and marked and extends into the hair follicles. The superficial perivascular dermatitis has eosinophils as the predominant cell type. The second form of zinc deficiency occurs in rapidly growing pups that have lesions of scaly plaques on the skin, foot pads, and planum nasale.

Zinc deficiency in ruminants

Zinc deficiency has been reported in cattle, sheep, and goats. Cutaneous lesions include alopecia, scaling, and crusting of the skin of the face, neck, distal extremities, and mucocutaneous junctions. Microscopically, the lesions consist of parakeratosis and, in some cases, hyperkeratosis.

Generic dog food dermatosis

Some dogs fed generic dog foods for 1 to 2 months develop bilaterally symmetric scaling and crusting involving the bridge of the nose, mucocutaneous junctions, pressure points, and distal extremities. Lesions include hyperpigmentation and lichenification, focal erosions, papules, pustules, and alopecia. Microscopically, the lesions are parakeratosis, dyskeratosis, and mixed cellular infiltrate in the dermis. The cause may be due partially to zinc deficiency, but multiple trace minerals, vitamins, or amino acids may be included.

Copper Deficiency

Copper is an essential component of tyrosinase, and deficient animals develop hair or wool depigmentation. Black sheep may develop bands of more lightly and darkly pigmented wool corresponding to variations in dietary intakes of copper. Cattle may develop a ''spectacle'' appearance due to depigmentation of hair around the eyes. The coat color also may change from black to reddish brown. In sheep, the wool becomes straight and is less desirable for commercial use due to imperfect oxidation of sulfhydryl groups in prekeratin, a process that requires copper.

Vitamin E Deficiency

Cats with vitamin E deficiency or fed diets with an excess of dietary fatty acids may develop steatitis. Grossly, the subcutaneous tissue contains firm, nodular, yellow to orange masses. Microscopic lesions include lobular to diffuse granulomatous panniculitis with macrophages and giant cells, fat necrosis, edema, infiltrates of neutrophils, and ceroid pigment.

Vitamin A Deficiency

Dogs with a vitamin A–responsive dermatosis have generalized scaling and microscopic lesions of marked follicular hyperkeratosis.

DISORDERS OF EPIDERMAL GROWTH OR DIFFERENTIATION

Seborrheic Disease Complex

Seborrhea is a chronic disease complex associated with abnormalities of cornification and/or function of sebaceous glands, increased quantities of free fatty acids and cholesterol, reduced quantities of diester waxes in surface lipids, and a change from nonpathogenic resident bacteria to pathogenic, coagulase-positive staphylococci. Seborrhea occurs most commonly in dogs and less commonly in

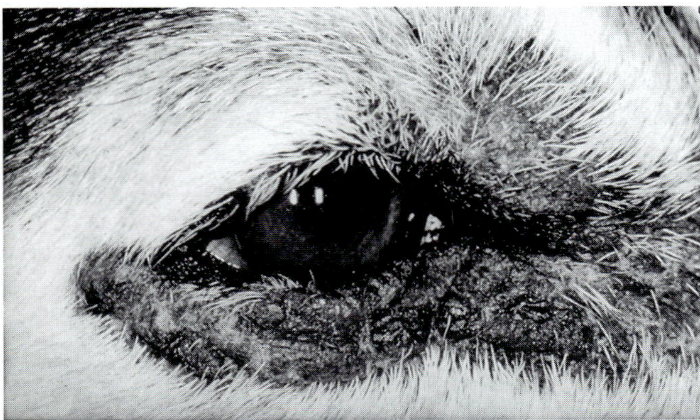

Fig. 11-49 Skin, periocular; Siberian husky dog. Zinc-responsive dermatitosis. Periocular skin is thickened, alopecic, pigmented, and covered by tightly adherent scale.

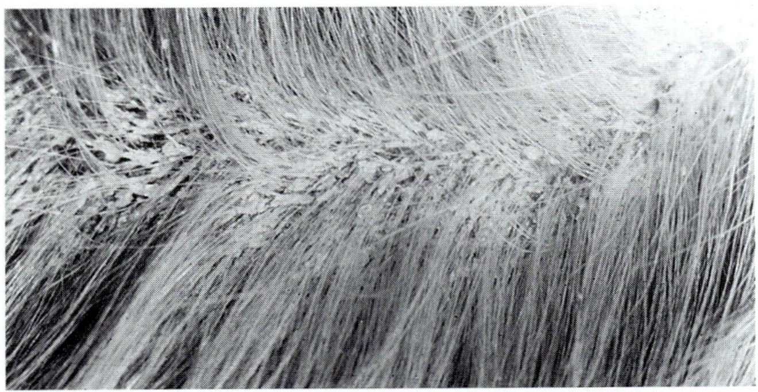

Fig. 11-50 Skin, haired; dog. Idiopathic seborrhea. Hair is parted to expose excessive scaling.

horses and cats. Clinically, seborrhea occurs either as a dry form (seborrhea sicca), with dry skin and white to gray scales (Fig. 11-50), or as a greasy form (seborrhea oleosa), with scaling and excessive brown to yellow lipids that adhere to the skin and hair.

Primary Idiopathic Seborrhea

This is a disorder of cornification with the epidermal turnover time reduced by about one third. Microscopic lesions include a papillary appearance to the epidermis due to disproportionate hyperkeratosis distending follicular ostia, parakeratosis at the edges of follicular ostia, and edematous, congested dermal papillae that support a spongiotic epidermis containing a few scattered leukocytes (see Fig. 11-4).

Secondary Seborrhea

Secondary seborrhea is common and develops in association with a variety of unrelated cutaneous disorders such as allergy, ectoparasitism, fungal infection, dietary deficiency, endocrine disease, and internal diseases. Microscopic changes include epidermal and follicular hyperkeratosis and/or parakeratosis and the lesions associated with the underlying disease.

Sebaceous Adenitis

Sebaceous adenitis occurs in a group of disorders with common lesions of inflammation of sebaceous glands, alopecia, and hyperkeratosis and a probable immune-mediated etiology. Sebaceous adenitis occurs most commonly in dogs, and lesions are diffuse in the longer haired breeds and multifocal, annular, and serpiginous in short-haired breeds. Microscopic lesions include inflammation of the sebaceous glands (see Fig. 11-17) and, in some cases, an extensive orthokeratotic hyperkeratosis. Chronic cases have no remaining sebaceous glands and a mild residual inflammation and fibrosis at the follicular isthmus.

DISORDERS OF PIGMENTATION

Hypopigmentation

Disorders associated with reduced pigment may be inherited or acquired, involve skin or hair, generalized or localized, and may be associated with other disease states or may be idiopathic. Terms used for these disorders include leukoderma and vitiligo for loss of pigment in the skin, leukotrichia for loss of pigment of the hair (see Fig. 11-11), hypopigmentation or incomplete albinism for generalized less-than-normal amount of pigment in the skin or hair, albinism for a hereditary lack of pigment, and dilution for reduced pigmentation. Examples of some of the disorders include Chediak-Higashi syndrome, color mutant (dilution) alopecia, the Maltese dilution of cats, leukoderma and/or leukotrichia of Doberman pincher and Rottweiler dogs, periocular leukotrichia in Siamese cats, and Arabian fading syndrome. Immune-mediated disorders associated with depigmentation include discoid lupus erythematosus and uveodermatologic syndrome (VKH-like disease).

Hyperpigmentation

Disorders associated with hyperpigmentation may result from inflammation or irritation, metabolic disorders, or pigmented neoplasms. A lentigo is a well circumscribed, macular to slightly raised plaque characterized by epidermal hyperplasia and hyperpigmentation.

DISORDERS CHARACTERIZED BY EOSINOPHIL INFILTRATES

Eosinophilic Plaques

These common lesions of the skin of cats, especially of the abdomen and medial thigh, are frequently associated with hypersensitivity reactions. Lesions consist of raised, variably sized, erythematous, pruritic, eroded to ulcerated plaques. Microscopically, epidermal lesions include acanthosis, variable spongiosis, erosion, and ulceration, accompanied by superficial and deep, perivascular to diffuse, predominantly eosinophilic dermatitis. Foci of collagen degeneration may be observed.

Eosinophilic Granulomas (Collagenolytic Granulomas)

Eosinophilic and granulomatous lesions with collagen degeneration (collagenolysis) occur in cats, dogs, and horses. The causes of these syndromes are poorly understood, but collagen degeneration may develop in any lesion with associated eosinophil degranulation, such as reactions to parasites or foreign bodies (including hair), or in mast cell tumors. Gross lesions include papules, nodules, plaques (sometimes linear), ulcers in the skin (Fig. 11-51), and nodular or ulcerated lesions in the oral mucosae of dogs and cats and foot pads of cats. Microscopically, nodular dermatitis (or stomatitis) consists of fragmented degenerate collagen fibers bordered by degranulated eosino-

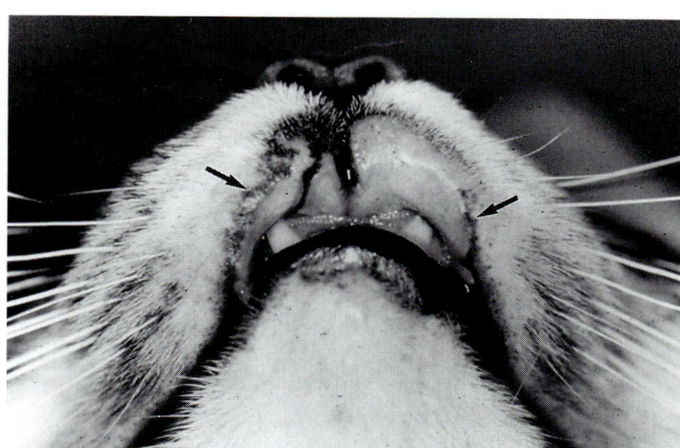

Fig. 11-51 Skin, lips; cat. Eosinophilic granulomas. Bilateral ulceration *(arrows)* of upper lip is present. One side is more affected.

phils and macrophages. Some indolent ulcers (rodent ulcers) on the upper lip of cats have areas of collagen degeneration and eosinophilic and granulomatous inflammation and are considered to be eosinophilic granulomas.

Eosinophilic Folliculitis and Furunculosis

Rarely, dogs, cats, cows, and horses develop folliculitis and furunculosis with infiltrates of eosinophils. Arthropod bites are the suspected cause. Lesion distribution varies among the species but may be multifocal in the horse.

STERILE GRANULOMATOUS DISORDERS

Juvenile Sterile Granulomatous Dermatitis and Lymphadenitis (Juvenile Pyoderma, Juvenile Cellulitis, Puppy Strangles)

This disorder of unknown cause occurs in pups less than 4 months of age (Figs. 11-52 and 11-53), with one or more of the pups of a litter having pustular and nodular dermatitis and edema of the face, ears, and mucocutaneous junctions. Microscopically, lesions are those of granulomatous or pyogranulomatous perifolliculitis, dermatitis, and panniculitis.

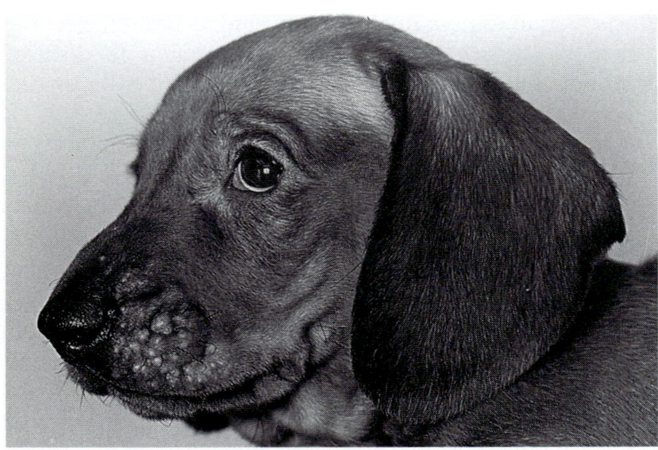

Fig. 11-52 Skin; dachshund puppy. Juvenile sterile granulomatous dermatitis and lymphadenitis (juvenile pyoderma). Pustular lesions of one day duration are present on muzzle. *Courtesy Dr. D. Prieur.*

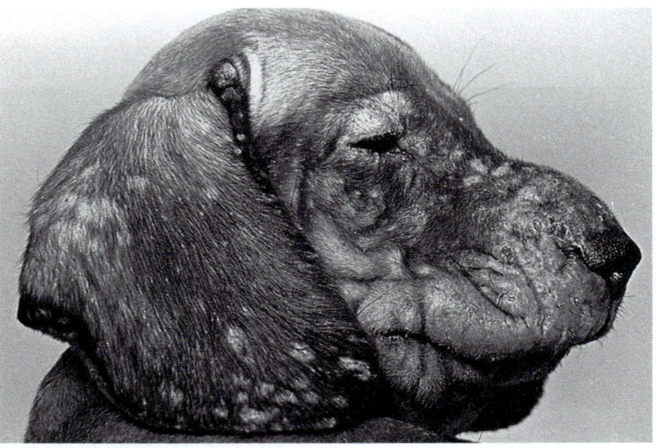

Fig. 11-53 Skin; dog (same as in Fig. 11-52). Juvenile sterile granulomatous dermatitis and lymphadenitis (juvenile pyoderma). The lesions, of 12 days duration, have progressed to include alopecia, edema, and crusting. *Courtesy Dr. D. Prieur.*

Other Sterile Granulomatous and Pyogranulomatous Disorders

These disorders develop in the skin of dogs and cats and include sterile granuloma and pyogranuloma syndrome, cutaneous xanthoma, cutaneous histiocytosis, systemic histiocytosis, malignant histiocytosis, and idiopathic nodular panniculitis. These lesions are characterized, grossly, by single or multifocal papules, plaques, or nodules and, microscopically, by discrete, coalescing, or, in some cases, diffuse accumulations of mixed populations of cells including, but not limited to, macrophages (histiocytes) and neutrophils. The lesions need to be differentiated from infectious granulomatous lesions and from neoplasms.

Equine Generalized Granulomatous Disease (Sarcoidosis)

This uncommon disorder of horses has cutaneous lesions and more widespread systemic involvement, resulting in anorexia and weight loss. Cutaneous lesions include generalized alopecia, scales, crusts, and, occasionally, nodules or tumorlike masses. Microscopic lesions are multifocal granulomas with multinucleated giant cells.

CUTANEOUS NEOPLASIA

The skin is a common site of neoplasms in most animals (Table 11-3), and the neoplasms are of ectodermal, mesodermal, and melanocytic origin. In female dogs, mammary gland neoplasms are the most common, and, in cats, mammary gland neoplasms are third in frequency to those of the skin and lymphoid tissues. Ectodermal neoplasms of the epidermis and adnexa tend to be benign, except for neoplasms of the apocrine glands, including sweat glands, glands of the anal sac, and mammary glands that include numerous carcinomas. Mesodermal neoplasms develop from fibrous tissue, muscle, adipose tissue, and vessels. More of the mesodermal neoplasms are malignant than the ectodermal neoplasms. Malignancy of melanocytic neoplasms depends in part on their location and size.

Benign neoplasms do not metastasize, do not invade the basement membrane, are circumscribed, grow by expansion, and are composed of well-differentiated cells that closely resemble the cells or tissue of origin. Malignant neoplasms often metastasize, invade basement membranes, and are composed of anaplastic cells with a high mitotic rate. Anaplastic cells are pleomorphic (vary in cell size and shape), have a large, vesicular nucleus with an increase in size and number of nucleoli, and have a decrease in number of normal organelles. Malignant cells develop surface alterations that allow invasion, implantation, and metastasis via blood or lymph vessels.

Text continued on p. 510.

Table 11-3. Selected cutaneous neoplastic and neoplastic-like lesions of domestic animals

Lesion	Cause	Species, age, breed, sex	Location	Gross pathology	Histopathology	Biologic behavior	Unique features
Cutaneous papilloma (wart) (verruca)	Often caused by papilloma virus	Common in horses, cattle Infrequent in dogs, goats, sheep Rare in cats Often young age Congenital in foals	Horse: about the nose, lips, inner aspect of ears (aural plaques) Any location, often the head	Flattened to papillary mass, single or multiple, on narrow or broad base Inverted variety occurs	Papillary projections of epithelium resting on collagen core Epithelium thickened by hyperkeratosis and acanthosis	Most benign and will regress Occasional transformation to squamous cell carcinoma	May regress May have viral inclusion bodies May have koilocytosis
Fibropapilloma	Bovine papillomavirus 2	Young bulls, cows	Glans penis of bulls Vulva and vagina of cows	Irregular mass attached to glans penis, less papillary than cutaneous papilloma	Proliferative epithelium with whorls and fascicles of fibroblasts and collagen	Look aggressive histologically and may recur after excision but do not metastasize	Location Viral cause
Cutaneous cysts Epidermal inclusion Follicular Dermoid Apocrine Ciliated	Inclusion (displaced epithelium/trauma) Follicular and apocrine (occluded follicles or ducts) Dermoid (genetic) Ciliated (developmental anomaly)	Any species, often dogs and cats	Anywhere on skin Dermoid: dorsal midline of Rhodesian ridgeback Ciliated: neck of cats	Cyst filled with soft, tan, greasy keratin and sebum (inclusion/follicular) and hair (dermoid) or clear fluid (apocrine and ciliated)	Cystic structure with wall comprised of epidermal or adnexal epithelium from which cysts arise Ciliated: from thyroglossal duct or respiratory epithelium	Nonneoplastic	Rupture and foreign body inflammation may develop
Cutaneous horn	Associated with benign or malignant epithelial tumors Cat: FeLV *Dermatophilus* associated	All domestic species	Any location Footpads of cats Areas of *Dermatophilus* infection in ruminants	Hard, conical, hornlike growth Greater height than diameter	Horn consists of laminations of compact keratin Base may be hyperplastic, neoplastic, or inflammatory lesion	Both neoplastic and nonneoplastic varieties Depends on nature of underlying lesion	Gross appearance
Hair follicle tumors Trichoepithelioma Trichofolliculoma Tricholemmoma Pilomatrixoma Trichoblastoma (hair follicle tumor of basal cells)	Genetic (breed predilections) May be multicentric in predisposed breeds	Dogs, occasionally cats Pilomatrixoma: Kerry blue terrier Trichoepithelioma: basset hound	Any location	Firm and discrete tumors Some cystic Some ulcerate Some mineralize	Variable, depending on tumor Resemble portion of follicle from which tumor arise	Benign behavior (some authors describe infiltrative and malignant trichoepithelioma)	May mineralize May result in foreign body response if cystic tumor ruptures

FeLV = feline leukemia virus.

Continued.

Table 11-3. Selected cutaneous neoplastic and neoplastic-like lesions of domestic animals—cont'd

Lesion	Cause	Species, age, breed, sex	Location	Gross pathology	Histopathology	Biologic behavior	Unique features
Intracutaneous cornifying epithelioma (infundibular keratinizing acanthoma)	Genetic (breed predilection)	Norwegian elkhound, may be multicentric	Often back and tail when multicentric	Dermal or subcutaneous mass, often with pore opening onto skin surface	Invaginated cyst with wall comprised of whorls and outward projections of stratified squamous epithelium	Benign	Resembles squamous cell carcinoma histologically
Squamous cell carcinoma (*in situ* carcinoma termed "Bowen's disease" in cats develops in haired skin, multicentrically)	Solar radiation Trauma Carcinogens Some unknown	All species, especially white cats, Hereford cattle, light-colored horses, white or partly colored dogs Less in pigs Adults to aged	Nonpigmented or lightly pigmented and sparsely haired skin Nail bed (dogs, cats) Penis/prepuce (horses)	Variable: nodular, proliferative, crusty, ulcerative Cutaneous horn may be present	Cords and islands of squamous cells Keratin pearls Dyskeratosis Intercellular bridges Basement membrane disrupted	May recur Metastasis to lymph nodes and beyond may develop Equine penis and feline nail bed carcinomas are more aggressive Solar-associated carcinomas are slow to metastasize	Keratin pearls, intercellular bridges Spindle-cell and pseudoglandular varieties occur
Benign basal cell tumor* (trichoblastoma synonym for canine and feline tumor of hair follicle origin) Basal cell carcinoma	Unknown	Benign basal cell tumor of epidermal origin (cats) Trichoblastoma (dogs and cats) Carcinoma (dogs and cats) Rare in other domestic animals	Often head, neck, and cranial trunk	All types: generally solitary firm nodules or plaques that are frequently ulcerated Carcinoma: may be multicentric	Benign feline: may have fusiform cells and melanin pigment Trichoblastoma: ribbon, trabecular, granular types Carcinoma: ragged margins, solid, clear cell, and keratinizing types	Benign feline type and trichoblastoma are benign Carcinoma locally aggressive with low potential for metastasis	Lack intercellular bridges May contain melanin pigment and can be confused with melanoma
Malignant pilomatrixoma (matrical carcinoma)	Unknown	Dogs	Any location Neck, thorax, tail	Generally deeper than basal cell carcinoma Large, lobulated, frequently ulcerated, poorly circumscribed Differentiates to parts of follicular wall	Not usually connected with epidermis Matrical keratinization (basal cells with abrupt transition to shadow cells)	Aggressive: all reported cases had metastasis to lymph nodes or lungs; recurrence also reported	Matrical keratinization May be difficult to differentiate from keratinizing basal cell carcinoma
Nail bed tumors Inclusion cyst Papilloma Keratoacanthoma Squamous cell carcinoma Melanoma	Unknown Trauma	Dogs; large breed, black-haired predisposed to multiple squamous cell carcinomas Cats	Nail bed May be multiple	Variable Swelling of nail bed Loss of nail Deformed nail	Depends on type of lesion/tumor	Malignant melanoma of dogs and squamous cell carcinoma of cats can be aggressive	Differentiate from pulmonary carcinoma in cat, which may metastasize to multiple digits
Apocrine adenoma Apocrine adenocarcinoma	Unknown	Older dogs and cats	Any location glands present Older female dogs: bilateral adeno-	Adenoma: small, slow growing, cystic, circumscribed	Benign: variable appearance, resemble glandular or ductal epithelium	Adenomas: benign Carcinomas: aggressive, may metastasize early	Carcinomas may resemble exudative dermatitis Anal sac carcino-

			carcinomas may develop from apocrine glands of anal sacs	Carcinoma: firm fibrous, infiltrative	Mixed type have myoepithelium, cartilage or bone Carcinomas of anal sac usually solid		mas are often associated with hypercalcemia
Sebaceous gland adenoma Sebaceous gland epithelioma Sebaceous gland carcinoma	Unknown	Adenoma common in adult dogs: cocker spaniel, poodle Less frequent in cats Rare in other animals	Head, neck, anywhere	Adenoma: gray-tan, greasy, lobulated, raised Epithelioma: discrete, firm, may ulcerate Carcinoma: often ulcerate	Adenoma: similar to sebaceous gland Epithelioma: more basal cells and mitoses Carcinoma: less fat in cells, less differentiated	Adenomas benign Epitheliomas may recur Carcinomas locally invasive; rarely metastasize	Eyelid meibomian gland tumors are similar Nodular hyperplastic lesions of sebaceous glands also very common
Perianal gland adenoma (circumanal or hepatoid gland) Carcinoma	Hormonal influence	Older dogs 90% male	Skin near anus, base of tail, prepuce, vulva, less elsewhere	One or more raised nodules often ulcerated, circumscribed, orangish-tan and greasy on cut surface	Adenomas resemble normal perianal glands; carcinomas are infiltrative, less differentiated, and have more mitoses	Most are adenomas which are benign In males, castration or estrogen therapy may cause regression of adenomas Carcinomas: low grade malignancy	Location Hormonal sensitivity
Canine cutaneous histiocytoma	Unknown	Dogs: more than half of tumors develop before 2 years of age Purebred dogs predisposed	Head, especially pinna, distal forelegs, and feet	Usually single Dome-shaped Circumscribed Often ulcerated	Sheets of large round cells (histiocytes) replace adnexa and collagen Frequent mitoses Later, necrosis and lymphocytic inflammation	Rapid growth followed by regression Rarely recur No metastasis	Young dogs Rapid growth Regression
Cutaneous histiocytosis	Unknown	Adult dogs Both sexes Variety of breeds	Face, neck, back, trunk	Multiple cutaneous and subcutaneous plaques and nodules	Histiocytic cells and variable mix of lymphocytes, plasma cells, neutrophils	Benign, but recurrent Nasal involvement may be present	Recurrent Steroid responsive May have nasal lesion
Systemic histiocytosis	Unknown Genetic	Bernese mountain dogs 2 to 8 years	Generalized, skin; especially scrotum, nasal planum, and eyelids	Multiple cutaneous nodules and lymph node enlargement, systemic involvement	Angiocentric, large histiocytic cells, fewer leukocytes, vasculitis	Remissions, relapses Prolonged course Systemic involvement Ultimately fatal	Multiple skin nodules and systemic lesions Breed
Cutaneous lymphoma Dermal form B cell type Epidermal form T cell type (mycosis fungoides)	Unknown	Dogs; less in cats and horses Age variable	Skin or oral mucous membranes Dermis or epidermis	Variable 4 basic forms: 1. Red scaly skin 2. Mucocutaneous ulceration/depigmentation 3. Single/multiple cutaneous masses 4. Infiltrative and ulcerative mucosae ± Systemic lesions	Dermal: sheets of lymphocytes in dermis (equine appear more inflammatory) Epidermal: lymphocytes in epidermis and adnexal epithelium	Ultimately fatal	Epidermal form may mimic dermatitis, autoimmune disease, or stomatitis

*Classification and terminology of benign basal cell tumors vary with authors. Differences appear largely related to epidermal versus follicular origin and, therefore, histologic appearance of the tumors. FIV = feline immunodeficiency virus; FeLV = feline leukemia virus; FeSV = feline sarcoma virus.

Continued.

Table 11-3. Selected cutaneous neoplastic and neoplastic-like lesions of domestic animals—cont'd

Lesion	Cause	Species, age, breed, sex	Location	Gross pathology	Histopathology	Biologic behavior	Unique features
Cutaneous plasmacytoma (extramedullary plasmacytoma)	Unknown	Dog; rarely, cat Aged adult Both sexes	Ear, lip, digit, and other mucocutaneous and cutaneous sites	Usually solitary, raised, reddish, discrete nodule	Densely cellular Single or multiple, variably sized nuclei Many mitoses Resemble plasma cells May have amyloid	Usually do not recur Subcutaneous or those with amyloid may be aggressive and recurrent Rare association with multiple myeloma	Cytoplasmic immunoglobulin present May have amyloid deposits
Mast cell tumor (mastocytoma)	Unknown Genetic influence Cats FIV associated?	Common tumor of dogs, especially boxers; less of other species Siamese cats have histiocytic variety Generally adults; less in neonates	Dog: often legs, trunk Feline: head	Solitary or multiple nodules Poorly circumscribed, edematous swellings May ulcerate early	Sheets of large round cells with bluish granular cytoplasm Not encapsulated Many eosinophils, in dogs especially Vasculitis Collagen degeneration	Canine: behavior may correspond to histologic grade May disseminate Feline: histiocytic may spontaneously regress Equine: generally benign	Metachromatic granules, eosinophils Other lesions: vasculitis, collagen degeneration, gastrointestinal ulceration Prolonged coagulation time
Melanoma Benign Malignant	Genetic factors Unknown	Common in dogs and pigs, and horses that fade to gray and white Less common in cattle and goats Uncommon to rare in cats, sheep	Dog: head, eyelids, legs, digits Horse: perineal skin and underside of root of tail Feline: head	Dog and cats: single Horse: multiple Macules to nodules Usually dark brown or black	Epithelioid to spindle-shaped cells containing variable quantity of pigment Nests of cells bordered by thin collagen septa Malignant melanomas are anaplastic and may be amelanotic	Canine: oral, mucocutaneous, subungual often malignant Haired skin often benign Gray horses: usually progressive and multicentric Location, size, mitotic index and cell morphology help predict behavior	Melanin pigment in cytoplasm Present in horses that fade to gray or white (storage disease?)
Fibroma Fibrosarcoma	Fibrosarcoma: FeLV and FeSV are associated in development of multiple sarcomas in young cats Vaccination in cats	Adult to aged All domestic animals Fibrosarcomas: mostly cats, less dogs, rare others	Head, legs, and sites of vaccination in cats	Circumscribed (fibroma) Firm to soft Resilient Gray-white	Whorls and interlacing bundles of fibroblasts and collagen	Fibromas benign Fibrosarcomas are infiltrative and often recur, but metastasis occurs uncommonly	In young cats: FeLV and FeSV have role in development of multiple sarcomas Vaccination is also a cause in cats
Equine sarcoid	Bovine papillomavirus has been identified in equine sarcoids and is probable cause	Most common skin tumor of horses Horse, donkey, mule	Skin of legs, trunk, and head	Types: Verrucous Fibroblastic Flat or occult	Fibroblastic proliferation with pseudoepitheliomatous hyperplasia	Locally invasive Frequently recur Do not metastasize	Autotransplantable Some regress

Canine hemangio-pericytoma	Unknown	Dogs Adult to aged More in females	Dermis and subcutis of extremities	Gray to pink Lobulated Firm and nodular or more gelatinous	Concentric laminations of spindle cells	Often recur Locally invasive Rarely metastasize	Concentric laminations of spindle cells around vessels
Myxoma Myxosarcoma	Unknown	Rare in domestic animals Adult to aged	Any location, often limbs	Poorly defined and infiltrative Soft and mucoid Gelatinous	Fusiform and stellate cells within mucinous matrix	Infiltrative, Recur frequently Myxosarcomas metastasize uncommonly	Some consider myxomas (sarcomas) to be a type of fibroma (sarcoma)
Nerve sheath tumors Neurofibroma Schwannoma Perineural fibroblastoma Neurilemmoma	Unknown	Cattle, dogs, less in others	Peripheral nervous system Cutaneous tumors are uncommon, more on head of cats and legs of dogs	Nodular Firm to gelatinous White-gray Associated with nerve	Bundles, whorls, and palisades of spindle cells	Dogs and cats: locally invasive, may recur Cattle: usually benign	Cells arranged in palisades Associated with nerve twigs
Lipoma Infiltrative lipoma Liposarcoma	Unknown	Lipoma: common in adult to aged dogs; less common in horse and cow; rare in cat, sheep, pig Infiltrative lipoma: adult dogs Liposarcoma: rare	Legs, thorax, abdomen	Lipoma: circumscribed, greasy, soft, white, and slightly translucent; floats in formalin Infiltrative lipoma: poorly delineated, soft enlargements of muscle or soft tissue Liposarcoma: firmer, nondiscrete, gray to white	Lipoma: mature fat cells Infiltrative lipoma: mature fat cells replacing normal muscle or collagen Liposarcoma: round to spindle-cell tumor, cellular, vacuolated cytoplasm	Lipomas: do not recur Infiltrative lipomas: locally invasive and recur but do not metastasize Liposarcomas: locally invasive, may recur, and rarely metastasize	Fatty tumor Float in formalin
Hemangioma Hemangiosarcoma	Unknown Trauma or solar radiation for some types	Adult to aged More in dogs; less in cats, horses, cattle, sheep, pigs Foals congenital hemangiomas	Hemangioma: dermis or subcutis Hemangiosarcoma: primary to skin or metastatic from visceral tumor Some more in white, poorly haired dermis, especially of dogs	Red, brown to black Circumscribed (hemangioma) Soft Ooze blood on cut surface Dermal may bleed	Interconnecting blood-containing channels lined by endothelium Hemangiosarcoma may resemble fibrosarcoma or have benign appearance (especially if metastatic)	Hemangiomas do not recur Hemangiosarcoma in white cat eartip and eyelid recur Metastatic potential is high in canine hemangiosarcomas	Thrombosis frequent in hemangioma Coagulation disorder may be associated with these tumors especially if tumors are large, malignant, or multifocal
Lymphangioma Lymphangiosarcoma	Some congenital	Uncommon to rare	Lymphatics associated with skin	Solid Cavernous Cystic May dissect along fascial planes	Interconnecting channels lined by endothelium without erythrocytes May be difficult to distinguish benign and malignant types	May be difficult to remove due to dissection along fascia	
Leiomyoma Leiomyosarcoma	Unknown	Very rare	Skin associated with arrector pili muscles or cutaneous blood vessels	Circumscribed Solitary Firm	Interlacing bundles of smooth muscle fibers tend to intersect at right angles Nuclei have blunt ends	Leiomyoma benign Leiomyosarcoma locally invasive	

Most cutaneous neoplasms are primary, as the skin is an uncommon to rare site for metastasis; however, the skin can be the site of secondary tumor growth. Examples include mammary gland neoplasms that invade into adjacent skin, feline pulmonary carcinomas that metastasize to multiple digits of multiple feet, and canine visceral hemangiosarcomas that may metastasize to the skin.

The causes of cutaneous neoplasms are generally unknown. However, trauma, solar radiation, x-radiation, and viruses have caused epidermal neoplasms. Hormones may play a role in the development of perianal gland and mammary gland neoplasms. Ovariohysterectomy before the first estrous cycle or after the first few estrous cycles can significantly reduce the number of mammary gland neoplasms. Perianal gland neoplasms tend to develop in intact male dogs and decrease in size after castration. Table 11-3 gives an abbreviated listing of the salient features of cutaneous neoplasms.

GLOSSARY

Acantholysis separation of keratinocytes.

Acanthosis thickening of the spinous cell layer (stratum spinosum).

Acral distal parts of the extremities.

Alopecia hair loss.

Anagen phase of hair cycle in which hair synthesis takes place.

Anaplasia lack of cellular differentiation and organization, a feature of neoplastic cells.

Apoptosis physiologic programmed cell death.

Atrophy reduction in size of a cell, tissue, organ, or part.

Blister (vesicle) localized collection of fluid usually in or beneath epidermis (< 0.5 cm).

Bulla large blister (> 0.5 cm).

Catagen transition phase of the hair cycle between growth and resting phases.

Comedo plug of keratin and dried sebum in a hair follicle.

Cornification production of stratum corneum by epidermal differentiation.

Crust material formed by drying of exudate or secretion on the surface.

Cytokines small-molecular-weight protein molecules (generally ≤ 30 kD) that are mediators of inflammation and mediators of growth.

Defluxion shedding of hair.

Dematiaceous naturally pigmented black or brown mycelium or conidium.

Dermatosis noninflammatory lesion of the skin.

Dermatophytosis infection of the keratin of the epidermis, hair, or nails with fungi of the genera *Microsporum, Epidermophyton,* or *Trichophyton.*

Dyskeratosis abnormal, premature, or imperfect keratinization.

Dysplasia abnormal development.

Effluvium shedding of hair.

Epidermolysis separation of the epidermis and dermis.

Eruption rapid development of skin lesion associated with redness.

Erosion loss of all or part of the epidermis.

Erythema redness of skin due to congestion of capillaries.

Excoriation superficial loss of epithelium due to physical trauma (scratching).

Exfoliation shedding of layers or scales.

Exudation escape of fluid, cells, or debris from blood vessels and deposition in or on other tissues.

Fissure cleft or groove.

Folliculitis inflammation of a hair follicle.

Furuncle circumscribed, painful nodule (accumulation of pus) in the dermis, associated with follicular rupture.

Genodermatosis genetically determined disorder of the skin.

Glabrous smooth; hairless.

Gynecomastia excessive development of mammary glands in the male.

Hydropic degeneration intracellular edema of basal epidermal cells.

Hyperhidrosis excessive sweating.

Hyperkeratosis histologic term for thickening of stratum corneum (keratin layer).

Hyperplasia increase in the number of normal cells.

Hypoplasia incomplete development.

Hypotrichosis less hair than normal.

Ichthyosis congenital skin disorder associated with marked hyperkeratosis.

Impetigo bacterial dermatitis characterized by pustules.

Indurated hardened.

Interface junctional zone between the epidermis and dermis, and inflammation at dermoepidermal junction with basal cell degeneration.

Intertrigo dermatitis that develops due to friction of skin on opposed surfaces.

Keratinocytes collectively, the cells of the epidermis that form keratin.

Keratosis excessive formation of keratin in localized areas.

Langerhans' cells antigen-presenting cells of the skin.

Lichenification thickening of skin with accentuation of skin creases.

Lichenoid two meanings, one clinical and one histopathologic. Histopathologic meaning of importance in veterinary medicine and refers to bandlike inflammation parallel to the epidermis, with or without basal cell degeneration.

Macule flat, circumscribed lesion of altered skin color.

Melanin dark, amorphous pigment consisting of dihydroxy indoxylic acid.

Melanophage macrophage containing ingested melanin.

Merkel cell neuroendocrine cell found in the stratum basale.

Mycelium mass of hyphae.

Myxedema nonpitting edema of the skin due to abnormal deposits of mucin.

Nevus circumscribed malformation of the skin consisting of excess of one or more of the normal components of the skin.

Panniculitis inflammation of subcutaneous adipose tissue.

Papule small, circumscribed, solid elevation of skin.

Parakeratosis retention of pyknotic nuclei in epidermal cells due to faulty or accelerated cornification.

Paronychia inflammation of skin around the nails.

Pemphigus cutaneous disease associated with blistering.

Phaeohyphomycosis mycotic disease caused by pigmented fungi (dematiaceous) of a variety of genera and species that do not form sclerotic bodies or granules.

Pigmentary incontinence melanin pigment released by previous injury to the basal layer cells and phagocytosed by dermal macrophages or located free in the dermis.

Plaque a flat-topped, solid elevation in the skin that occupies a relatively large surface area in comparison with its height.

Pruritus itching.

Pyoderma pyogenic or pus-producing bacterial infection of the skin.

Pustule small, circumscribed accumulation of pus within the epidermis.

Scale thin, platelike accumulation of keratin on the surface of skin.

Sebaceous pertaining to sebum.

Seborrhea nonspecific term for clinical signs of scaling, crusting, and greasiness; primary seborrhea is a more specific term applied to inherited cornification disorders.

Sebum secretion of sebaceous glands; thick, semifluid substance composed of fat and epithelial debris.

Spongiosis intercellular edema which, by widening of the intercellular space and stretching of the "intercellular bridges," creates a spongelike appearance to the epidermis.

Telogen resting phase of the hair cycle.

Ulcer loss of epidermis and at least superficial portion of dermis.

Urticaria vascular reaction in dermis consisting of transient wheals (hives).

Vesicle small blister within the epidermis or at or below the dermal-epidermal interface.

Vibrissa long, coarse hair located about the muzzle.

Vitiligo acquired disorder characterized by circumscribed areas of depigmentation in the skin.

Wheal smooth, circumscribed, slightly elevated area on skin caused by dermal edema.

Yeast unicellular budding fungus.

Acknowledgments

The author thanks Dr. Maron B. Calderwood Mays for chapter review; Dr. Emily J. Walder for review of neoplasia section; Dr. H. Denny Liggitt for photographic contributions; and Drs. Peter J. Ihrke, Anthony A. Stannard, Helen Power, Alexander Werner, and Alan C. Mundell for access to and discussion of clinical cases.

Suggested Readings

DeBoer DJ, ed. Advances in clinical dermatology. In: Veterinary Clinics North America (Small Animal Practice). Vol 20. Philadelphia: Saunders, 1990.

Goldschmidt MH, Shofer FS. Skin tumors of the dog and cat. New York: Pergamon, 1992.

Griffin CE, Kwochka, KW, MacDonald, JM. Current veterinary dermatology: The science and art of therapy. St. Louis: Mosby–Year Book, 1993.

Gross TL, Ihrke PJ, Walder EJ. Veterinary dermatopathology: A macroscopic and microscopic evaluation of canine and feline skin disease. St Louis: Mosby–Year Book, 1992.

Ihrke PJ, Mason IS, White SD. Advances in veterinary dermatology. Vol 2. New York: Pergamon, 1993.

Kunkle GA. Feline dermatology. Vet Clin North Am Small Anim Prac 1984; 14:1065-1087.

Muller GH, Kirk RW, Scott DW. Small animal dermatology. 4th ed. Philadelphia: Saunders, 1989.

Mullowney P, ed. Symposium on large animal dermatology. In: Veterinary Clinics North America (Large Animal Practice). Vol 6. Philadelphia: Saunders, 1984.

Scott DW. Large animal dermatology. Philadelphia: Saunders, 1988.

Stannard AA, Pulley LT. Tumors of the skin and soft tissues. In: Moulton JE, ed. Tumors in Domestic Animals. 3rd ed. Berkeley: University of California Press, 1990: 23-87.

Von Tscharner C, Halliwell REW. Advances in veterinary dermatology. Vol 1. Philadelphia: Bailliere Tindall, 1990.

Yager, JA, Scott DW. The skin and appendages. In Jubb KVF, Kennedy PC, Palmer N, eds. Pathology of Domestic Animals. 4th ed. New York: Academic, 1993: 531-738.

CHAPTER

12

Reproductive System: Female

HELEN M. ACLAND

DEVELOPMENTAL ANOMALIES OF THE FEMALE SYSTEM

The sex of an individual can be defined by several criteria—genetic, chromosomal, gonadal, ductal, and phenotypic. Normal mammalian chromosomal sex is XX for female and XY for male. The gene for the H-Y antigen was formerly proposed as the testis inducer but now appears not to be the essential element. On the Y chromosome, a gene (sex-determining region Y [SRY]) has been identified that may be the gene for the testis-determining factor (TDF). The differentiation of the gonad to a testis is dependent on the presence of this gene. In its absence, the indifferent embryonic gonad follows its default pathway and differentiates into an ovary. Gonadal sex is based on the histologic components of the gonad. Ductal sex is based on whether the elements are derived from the Müllerian (female) or the Wolffian (male) system. The appearance of the external genitalia is the criterion for phenotypic sex. There can be sexual ambiguity when the various definitions are in disagreement.

Abnormalities of Chromosomal Sex

Animals with abnormal chromosomal sex generally have underdeveloped rather than ambiguous organs. Examples are XXY males (Klinefelter's syndrome), XO females (Turner's syndrome), and XXX females.

Animals that are chimeras or mosaics for the sex chromosomes do have ambiguous reproductive organs. Chimeras and mosaics have two or more cell types, each with a different chromosomal constitution. The cells of a chimera come from a different source from one another, whereas the cells of a mosaic come from the same source. Several cases of canine chimeras have been described. The commonest chimera in domestic animals is the freemartin calf. This is the female of a set of male and female twins whose placental vascular anastomoses allow male hematopoietic cells to invade and colonize the female. Her gonad is small and can vary from an ovary with reduced number of or no germ cells, to an organ partially converted to a testis, or to an organ composed of structures resembling seminiferous tubules. The Müllerian duct derivatives vary from almost normal to cordlike structures, but there is never communication with the vagina (Fig. 12-1). The

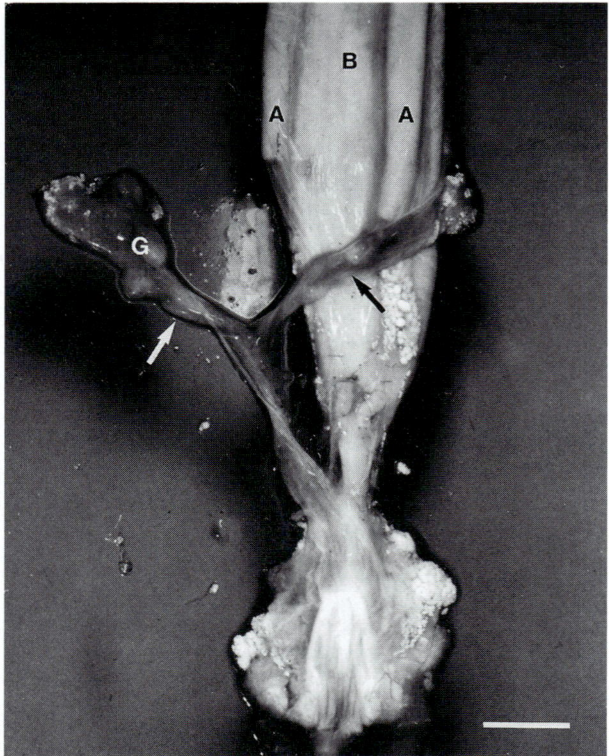

Fig. 12-1 Urogenital tract; freemartin, newborn calf. Compared with the normally sized urinary bladder (*B*) and umbilical arteries (*A*), the genital tract is very small. Seminal vesicles are present but not visible in this case because of the surrounding fat. (*G* = gonad; uterine horns = *arrows*). Bar = 2 cm.

source of Müllerian inhibitory factor seems to be the male twin's testes. Seminal vesicles are always present; other wolffian structures are present to varying degrees. Externally, the animal appears female, but the vestibule and vulva are hypoplastic and the clitoris is enlarged. The male twin is minimally affected.

Abnormalities of Gonadal Sex

Hermaphrodites have both ovarian and testicular tissue and can be further classified into three types: bilateral or unilateral, according to whether a combined organ, called an ovotestis, is present on one or both sides, and lateral, with a testis on one side and an ovary on the other. They have a genital tract that cannot be easily classed as male or female. True hermaphrodites are rare. In many cases, the mechanism for production of hermaphrodites is uninvestigated or unknown, but the pathogeneses of some are known—for instance, by means of chimera formation or by partial sex reversal when small amounts of testis determining factor (TDF) are expressed in an animal with XX chromosomes.

Animals in which the gonadal sex does not follow the chromosomal sex are labeled sex reversed. Examples are XX true hermaphrodites and XX males. In these animals, the TDF gene is present on an X chromosome or an autosome. Such partial or complete sex-reversal effects have been described in several species, including dogs, pigs and goats. From work in dogs, in which XX true hermaphrodites and XX males were found in the same family of cocker spaniels, it is likely that the two phenomena represent varying degrees of severity of the same defect. In cocker spaniel dogs, XX sex reversal is inherited as an autosomal recessive trait. The majority are XX true hermaphrodites, and 10% are XX males.

In goats, notably Saanans, the gene with the Y effect is close to the gene for polledness. The latter is a dominant gene. Goats heterozygous for polledness are hornless and have normal genitalia; goats homozygous for polledness are XY normal males, XX hermaphrodites, or pseudohermaphrodites with testes or ovotestes. The extreme variability in gonadal differentiation frequently seen among intersex goats could be explained by variability in the dose of sex-determining factor. Their external appearance ranges from normal male to female with an enlarged clitoris.

Abnormalities of Phenotypic Sex

Pseudohermaphrodites have the chromosomes and gonads of one sex and tubular organs modified toward those of the other sex. They are classified according to the type of gonadal tissue. Female pseudohermaphrodites are rare. In human beings, the adrenogenital syndrome is recognized. In this syndrome, cortisol precursors, which have accumulated as a result of adrenocorticotropic hormone (ACTH) production in response to low cortisol concentrations, are converted to androgen rather than cortisol, and the androgens masculinize the genitalia. The administration of sex steroid hormones during gestation or even shortly prior to conception carries the risk of masculinizing female fetuses.

Segmental aplasia of the Müllerian-derived duct system can have a wide variety of forms. The simplest is failure to make a proper connection with the urogenital sinus (Fig. 12-2), leaving in place a persistent hymen, the division between the two precursor elements. A perforated hymen often persists and is of no significance; but, if the completely imperforate hymeneal membrane persists, the vagina, cervix, and uterus fill with normal secretions, become atonic, and are subject to infections because of the potential microbial growth medium contained in the tract. More severe forms involve absence or rudimentary development of one or more segments of the vagina, cervix, uterine

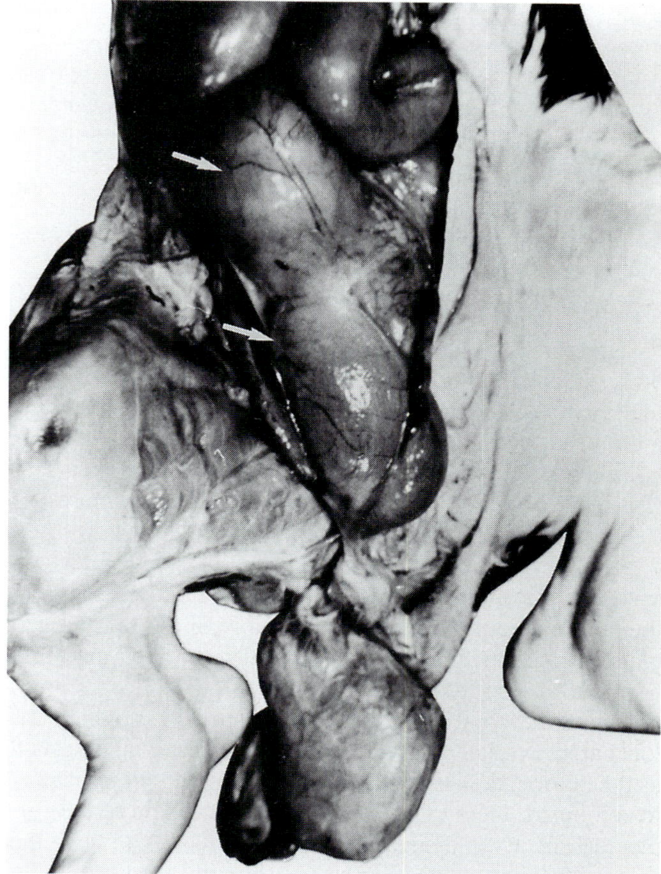

Fig. 12-2 Genital tract; calf. Developmental abnormalities (atresia) of the urogenital sinus and terminal alimentary tract. Obstruction of the outflow caudally has caused secretions to be retained and, thus, distended *(arrows)* the genital tract.

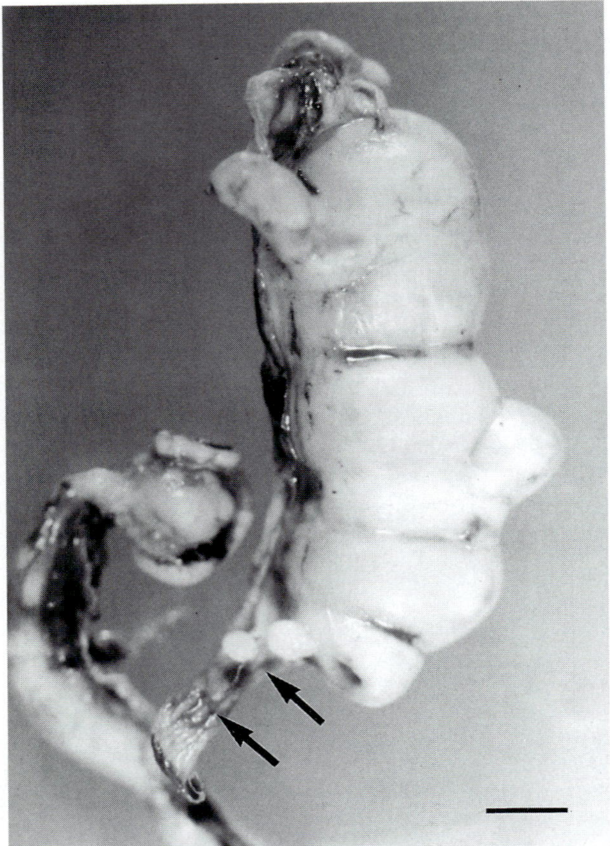

Fig. 12-3 Uterus, horn; cat. Segmental aplasia. Proximal to the region from which a segment is missing *(arrows)*, the horn is distended by secretions. Bar = 1 cm.

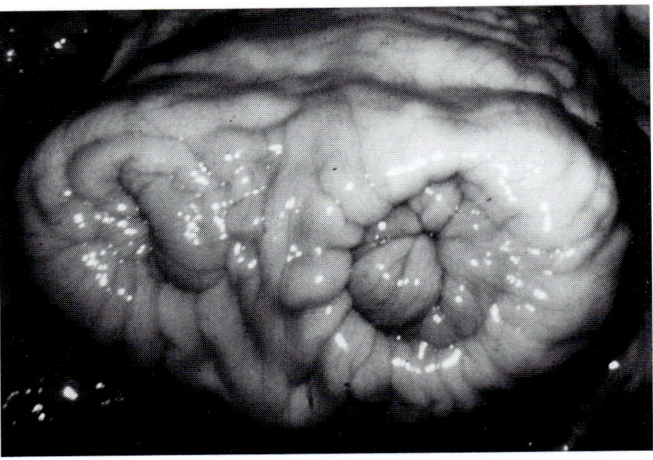

Fig. 12-4 Cervix; cow. Double cervices, side by side, caused by failure of normal fusion during development. *Courtesy Dr. R. Zemjanis.*

body, or uterine horns (Fig. 12-3). Generally, the ovaries, uterine tubes, and the most cranial parts of the uterine horns are present and normal, except for distention of the horns by secretion. Segmental aplasia of the Müllerian duct system most often occurs in Shorthorn cattle, in which it is associated with the recessive gene for white coat color.

An effect of segmental aplasia is that in species in which systemic transmission of $PGF_{2\alpha}$ from the endometrium to the corpus luteum is important, notably in the pig, prostaglandin can be synthesized in and released from the blind horn and have a lytic effect on the corpora lutea of pregnancy in the contralateral ovary. In species in which the local uteroovarian pathway is important for luteolysis, such as the bovine, the absence of a large segment of uterus may lead to insufficient $PGF_{2\alpha}$ for normal regression of the corpus luteum. Even a small segment of aplasia can have the same effect, by means of the tract cranial to the missing segment becoming distended with fluid and eventually losing ability to synthesize prostaglandin. In the dog and cat, the uterus does not play a role in regression of the corpus luteum.

Imperfect fusion of the paired Müllerian ducts is a common cause of anomalies. The normal sequence of fusion is that the two ducts unite first at the cloacal end to form the vagina and then the process moves cranially to form the cervix and, lastly, the uterine fundus. A double uterine fundus, called uterus didelphys, and double cervix are normal at an early stage of development. Malformations due to imperfect fusion are most common in and adjacent to the cervix. They range from a dorsoventral fibrous band in the cranial vagina together with a normal cervix; to failure of fusion of the caudal cervix, causing a bifurcation of the cervical canal; to complete duplication of the cervix and body of the uterus (Fig. 12-4).

VAGINA AND VULVA

Cysts in the vaginal wall of the cow arise from Gartner's ducts (Wolffian remnants) or Bartholin's glands. Stimuli for cyst formation are hyperestrogenism or inflammation. Gartner's ducts normally do not open into the vagina. When they become cystic, single or multiple cysts or a tortuous channel develops in the floor of the vagina, somewhere between the cervix and near the urethral opening (Fig. 12-5). Bartholin's glands become cystic when their openings into the lateral wall of the vagina or vagina-vulva junction become obstructed.

Tumefaction of the vulva is a normal phenomenon in animals in estrus. Overly large or persistent swelling is abnormal. These changes occur in hyperestrogenism, the most troublesome example of which is poisoning of swine by the mycotoxin zearalenone found in moldy corn. Other effects of the toxin are precocious mammary development, tenesmus leading to rectal prolapse, and the luteotropic activities of inducing anestrus or pseudopregnancy.

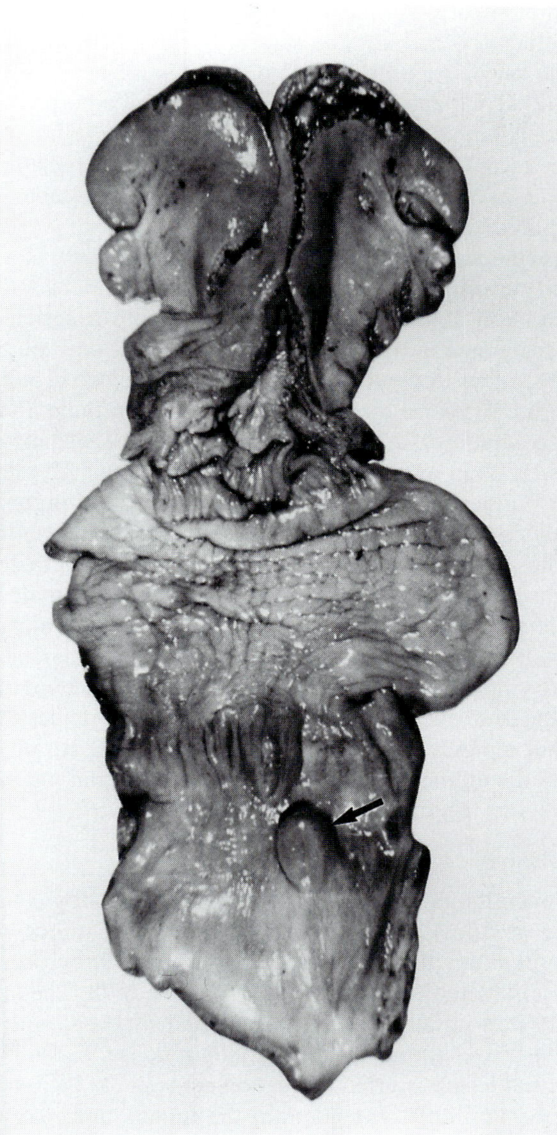

Fig. 12-5 Genital tract; cow. Cystic Gartner's duct. A unilateral cystic duct *(arrow)* is present on the floor of the vagina. Gartner's ducts, which are Wolffian remnants, are normally not visible and become apparent only when hyperplastic, inflamed, or obstructed.

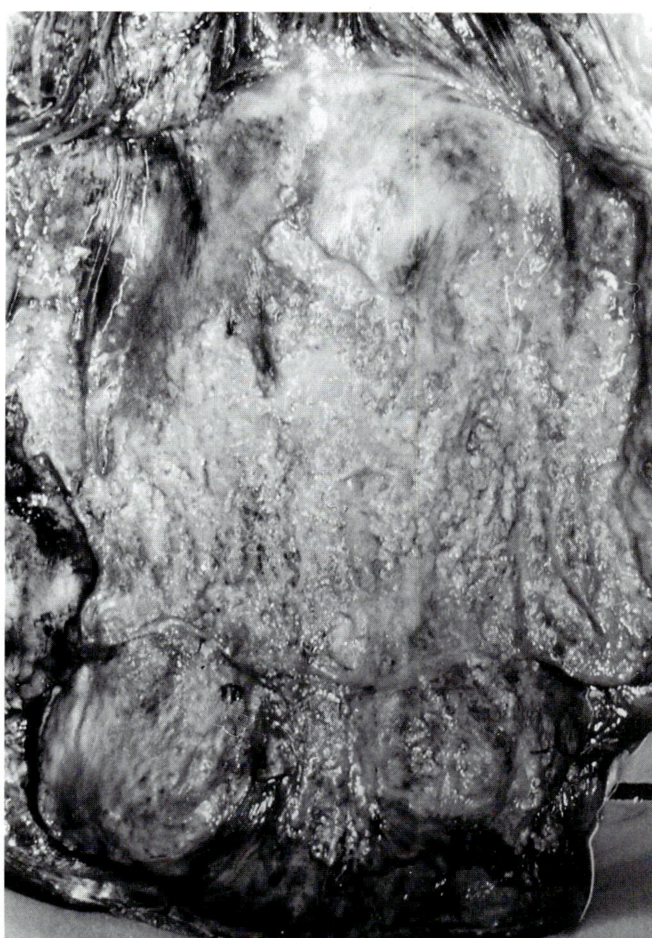

Fig. 12-6 Vagina; mare. The vaginal mucosa is thick, rough, and irregular because of severe, diffuse acute necrotizing vaginitis. Infection followed the trauma of dystocia and manual delivery of a foal.

Inflammation

The vagina and vulva are lined by stratified squamous epithelium that is fairly resistant to infection.

Postparturient vulvitis and vaginitis occur after there has been laceration or tearing during dystocia followed by infection (Fig. 12-6). Local trauma unrelated to parturition can progress similarly. Inflammation of the cervix and caudal vagina following dystocia is likely to have a much more serious outcome because of the possibility of local spread of infection to the peritoneal cavity.

Granular vulvitis of cattle is a disease in which the etiologic significance of *Mycoplasma* species and *Ureaplasma* species remains to be clarified. Granular vulvitis associated with *Ureaplasma* infection is characterized by a profuse, purulent vulvar discharge in the acute stage and a hyperemic vulvar mucosa in which 2 mm, raised granules are evident. The disease becomes chronic and resolves within 3 months. Reappearance of acute signs or reinfection is possible. In about 10% of affected cows, discrete, raised, white epithelial inclusion cysts, 2 to 5 mm in diameter, occur in rows or clusters on the dorsolateral wall of the vulva. Lowered fertility is explained by persistence of the organism in the uterus for up to 7 days following contamination from the vulvar lesions at coitus.

Infectious pustular vulvovaginitis of cattle is caused by a herpesvirus that is serologically indistinguishable from the virus of infectious bovine rhinotracheitis (IBR). The two diseases behave as separate entities, but their occurrence can overlap in a herd or in an individual. Vulvovaginitis is transmitted by coitus, artificial insemination, or close contact. Initially, hyperemia and edema of the vagina and vulva are followed by petechiae and slight nodularity of the mucosal surfaces over the normal 1 to 2 mm lymphoid nodules. Then, a rapidly coalescing, multifocal erosion and ulceration of the mucosa occurs over the lymphoid follicles. Microscopically, changes are present in the epithelium, the lamina propria, and the lymphoid follicles. The epithelium undergoes ballooning degeneration with intranuclear inclusions, necrosis, neutrophil infiltration, and desquamation, but without vesicle or pustule formation. The lamina propria becomes hyperemic and edematous and is infiltrated by inflammatory cells, mostly lymphocytes and plasma cells. The reaction of the lymphoid nodules is hyperplasia. Resolution is accomplished rapidly, leaving slightly thickened epithelium and hyperplastic lymphoid nodules. A similar set of lesions occurs on the penis of bulls. In the equine species, equine herpesvirus-3 (as distinct from equine herpesvirus-1, responsible for respiratory disease, nervous disease, and abortion) causes **coital exanthema,** which causes transient vesicles and erosions, morphologically similar to those of IBR, on the external genitalia of both mares and stallions (Fig. 12-7). **Infectious bovine cervicovaginitis,** or ''epivag,'' is a bovine disease seen in Africa and probably also caused by a herpesvirus. It is transmitted only by coitus. Lesions develop first in the anterior vagina, with intense congestion and a large amount of purulent exudate. Spread to the uterus, uterine tubes, and ovarian bursa follows.

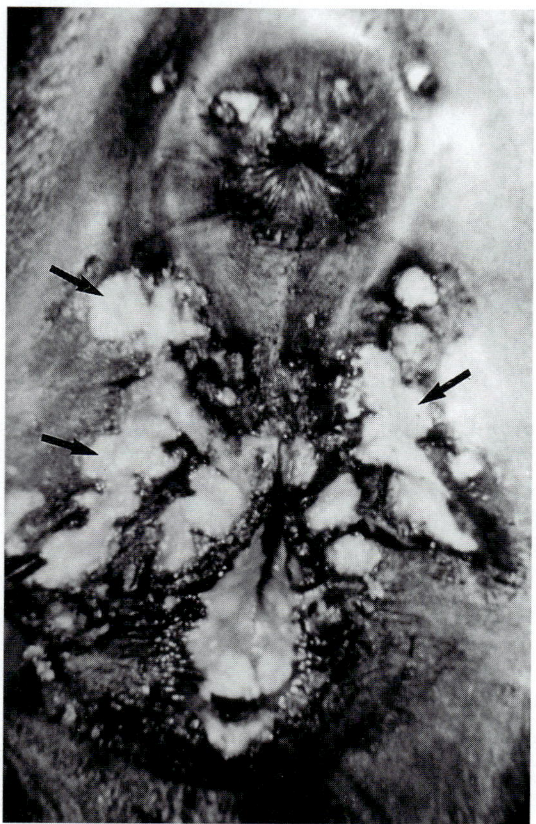

Fig. 12-7 Vulva; mare. Coital exanthema. Note the multiple circular ruptured vesicles *(arrows)*. *Courtesy Dr. L.J. Gleeson.*

Dourine, caused by *Trypanosoma equiperdum,* is a venereally transmitted disease of equidae that is enzootic in Africa, Asia, southeastern Europe, and South America. Organisms penetrate the intact genital mucosa and multiply locally, either in the lumen or in the wall, before becoming systemic. Trypanosomes can be observed in male and female genital discharges and in blood. The disease may involve the skin and nervous system as well as the genital tract. Variation is great in the virulence of the organism, resistance of the host, incubation period, persistence of the trypanosomes in the blood, length and severity of the clinical disease, and severity of the lesions. In the male and female genital tract, the acute lesion is edema, which can be extensive. With time, the edema becomes organized and firm. Lymphoid nodules of the genital tract are hyperplastic, and the overlying mucosa is ulcerated. Ulcers heal without repigmentation. In the wake of edema, atrophy involves the epithelial cells of the skin and genital mucosae, often with depigmentation.

Neoplasms

Transmissible venereal tumor (TVT) of the dog is transmitted at coitus and by the transfer of intact tumor cells. Both sexes are affected. TVT cells have 59 chromosomes, compared with the normal canine number of 78. The tumor begins as a nodule beneath the genital mucosa, with enlarging breaks through the overlying mucosa. In the bitch, the initial lesion is often in the dorsal vagina at its junction with the vestibule, extends into the lumen, and may protrude through the vulva as an ulcerated, friable mass. Microscopically, the tumor cells have poorly defined and lightly staining cytoplasm; are large and round or oval; and are uniform in size, with occasional large bizarre nuclei. The mitotic rate is high. Spontaneous regression is the rule, with multifocal necrosis, infiltration of lymphocytes, probable cell-mediated tumor cell lysis and decrease in number of tumor cells, and apparent transition of tumor cells to fibroblasts, with deposition of collagen. Metastases to other sites are few, although, in some parts of the world, metastases are relatively common. There is no explanation for the patchiness of the worldwide distribution of the disease.

Squamous cell carcinoma of the vulva occurs in the cow, ewe, and mare and in mature animals (Fig. 12-8). Solar radiation has been proposed as an etiologic factor. Ewes that have been subjected to the Mules' operation have a more exposed vulva and are more prone to develop squamous cell carcinoma. There is some correlation with ex-

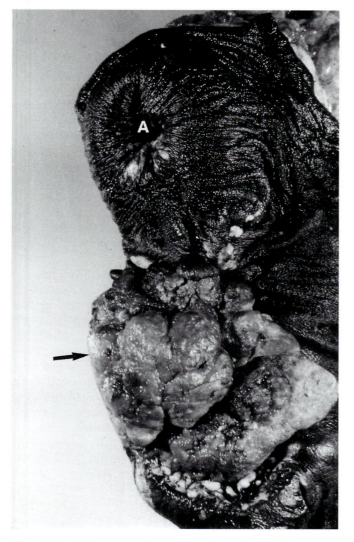

Fig. 12-8 Vulva; mare. Squamous cell carcinoma. The opening of the vagina is filled by neoplastic tissue *(arrow)*. (*A*, anus).

posure to sunlight and, at least in the cow, with lack of vulvar pigmentation. In the various species of animals affected, squamous cell carcinoma starts on the hairless skin of the vulva and has the same appearance and biologic behavior as squamous cell carcinoma at other sites. The neoplasm metastasizes late to the regional lymph nodes.

CERVIX

The cervix can participate in the range of abnormalities of the genital tract caused by failure of proper fusion of the paired elements of the Müllerian system. In cattle, some developmental abnormalities are peculiar to the cervix. These are hypertrophy or hypoplasia of the whole structure, aplasia of one or more of the five rugae, tortuosity or dilatation of the canal, or diverticulum formation.

Cervicitis is usually not seen alone but occurs with an overshadowing endometritis or vaginitis. This is true of specific infectious diseases, such as contagious equine metritis, and of nonspecific inflammations, such as postparturient metritis, cervicitis, and vaginitis. As an isolated lesion, inflammation of the cervix can be the result of traumatic artificial insemination. In the cow with acute cervicitis, the caudal rugae become edematous and prolapse into the vagina. Inflammatory exudate covers the mucosa and collects in the vagina. Cervical mucosa is relatively thin; the underlying fibromuscular tissue is relatively impervious to infection, and so most cases of cervicitis resolve readily. Those of traumatic origin are likely to involve deeper structures from the onset, and, with time, development of pericervical abscesses, fistulous tracts, stenosis with adhesions across the lumen in areas denuded of epithelium, or cysts filled with mucus retained because of disorganized healing can occur.

Neoplastic disease of the cervix of domestic animals is extremely rare.

UTERUS

Noninflammatory Abnormalities

Mechanical events can cause abnormal positions of the uterus. **Torsion** is of importance in pregnant animals, occurring mainly in the cow and, to a lesser extent, in the bitch (Fig. 12-9). Torsion can also occur when the uterus is enlarged by pyometra (accumulation of pus in the uterine lumen) or mucometra (accumulation of mucus in the uterine lumen). The mesovarium is a fixed point in both species, with the other fixed point influenced by the length of the horns and the presence and rigidity of the ligament between the horns. Rotation tends to occur about the cervix in the cow and the junction of the uterine horn and body in the bitch. The result of torsion is circulatory compromise; the veins, being thinner walled, are compressed and occluded before the arteries. The uterine wall and placenta become congested and edematous. The fetus dies and ei-

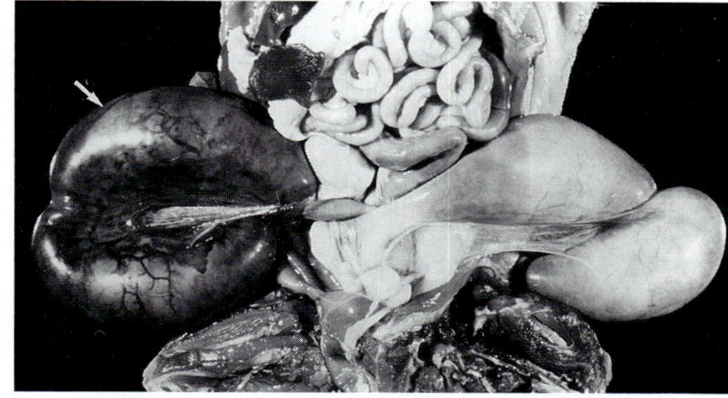

Fig. 12-9 Uterus; pregnant cat. Torsion. The affected *(right)* uterine horn *(arrow)* is purplish-black, whereas the normal horn is pink.

ther mummifies or putrefies, depending on whether the cervix allows organisms access or not. The uterine wall is friable and prone to rupture. Other situations in which rupture of the uterus occurs are in severe dystocia and during treatment by infusion. Rupture can be incomplete, involving just the mucosa, or complete. Torsion- and dystocia-related ruptures are likely to be in the caudal part of the uterus and are often fatal because of hemorrhage or infection. Ruptures that follow overvigorous infusion occur at the lesser curvature of a horn and dissect beneath the serosa and into the mesometrium, setting up a perimetritis.

Prolapse of the uterus is of some importance in the ewe, cow, and sow after parturition. Uterine inertia caused by such factors as prolonged dystocia, hypocalcemia, and ingestion of estrogenic plants is usually present. The structures involved can be restricted to the previously pregnant horn or may include the remainder of the uterus, the bladder, and even some intestine. Vascular compromise, shock, trauma, and sepsis follow.

Subinvolution of placental sites in the bitch causes a bloody vaginal discharge that lasts for weeks or months postpartum. Subinvoluted placental sites are about twice the size of normal sites at the same time after parturition. They are multiple segmental thickenings of the walls of the uterine horns interspersed with normal areas and are identifiable from the serosal surface (Fig. 12-10). The luminal surface of these thickened plaque areas is raised, rough, ragged, and gray to brown. The upper part of the plaques is composed of cellular debris, hematoma, thrombus, and regenerating endometrium. In the deeper part of the site, lesions include collagen deposition, hemorrhage, distention, and decreased density of endometrial glands. Trophoblast-like cells are abundant at the base of the collagen mass and, together with collagen, can invade the myometrium and, in some cases, even cause uterine perforation. Trophoblast-like cells are more numerous in subinvolution than in the normal placenta. In the normal placenta, trophoblast cells are found in the endometrium and around the small blood vessels of the myometrium, but they rapidly degenerate in the postpartum period. The retention of these cells may be the basis of the impairment of the involution process.

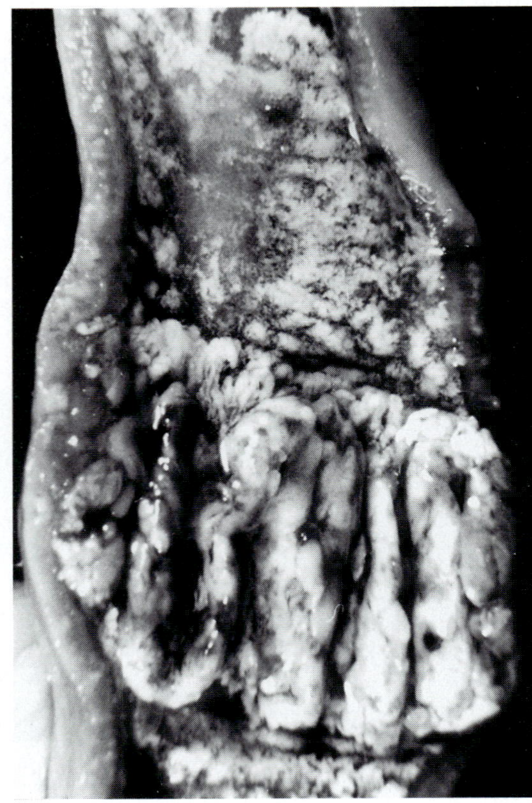

Fig. 12-10 Uterus; bitch. Subinvolution of placental site. Note the raised, rough plaque on the luminal surface of the uterus.

Endometrial atrophy can be due to loss of ovarian function secondary to hypopituitarism or, in some species, to old age or anestrus. The age effect is not seen in most domestic species. In the mare, an excellent example of diffuse endometrial atrophy occurs in anestrus. Much less commonly, equine endometrial atrophy is associated with the ovarian inactivity of debility and chromosomal aberrations. Some cases are of unknown cause. Focal rather than diffuse endometrial atrophy sometimes occurs in the mare, and the atrophic endometrium is thin and flat. In the mare, the longitudinal folds are not obvious, and, in the cow, the caruncles are flattened. The mare is the animal most studied histopathologically, because of the frequency with which uterine biopsies are taken. The endometrium of the anestrous mare has cuboidal surface and glandular epithelium and short, straight glands.

Endometrial hyperplasia is of importance in the ewe and bitch; occurs in the cow, cat, and sow; and is rare in the mare. In farm animals, the hormonal influence is prolonged hyperestrogenism. Ingested estrogenic pasture is the most likely source of hormone in the ewe. Cystic follicles, granulosa cell tumors, and phytoestrogens are associated in the cow, and the mycotoxin zearalenone is the cause in the sow. In the dog, the lesion occurs under the influence of progesterone but with priming by estrogen. Bitches may have a normal appearing corpus luteum and may be experiencing pseudopregnancy. In the cat, which is an induced ovulator, a strong association exists between the proliferative changes in the endometrium and prominent, active corpora lutea. However, the finding of endometrial hyperplasia in older queens, animals that often were not bred and without a corpus luteum, has led to the suggestion that the lesion is due to chronic stimulation of the endometrium by estrogen.

Simple endometrial hyperplasia may be overlooked or recognizable grossly by mild and patchy or diffuse thickening of the endometrium. After progression to the next stage, cystic endometrial hyperplasia, the lesion is more readily recognizable (Fig. 12-11). Cysts, about 1 cm in di-

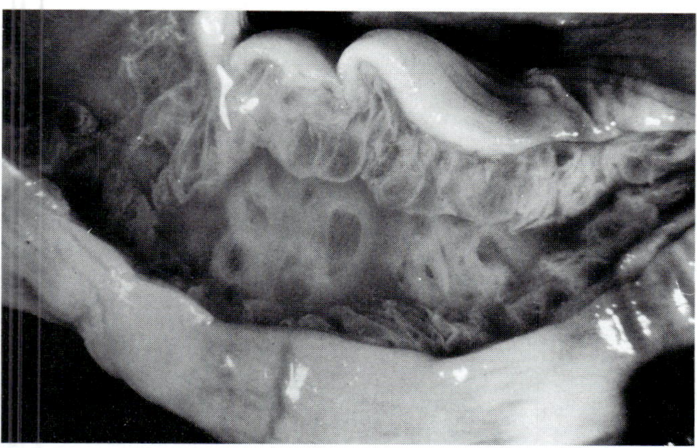

Fig. 12-11 Uterus; bitch. Cystic endometrial hyperplasia. The endometrium is diffusely thickened by numerous cysts. Progesterone is the dominant hormone.

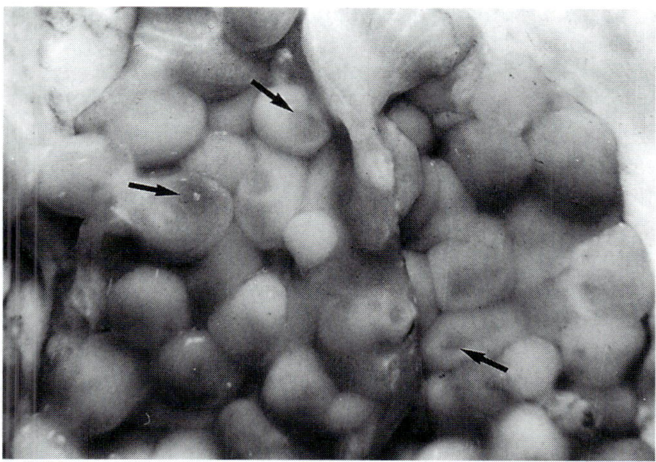

Fig. 12-12 Uterine body; ewe. Cystic endometrial hyperplasia. Cystic glands *(arrows)* are beside, beneath, and between the caruncles. Estrogen is the dominant hormone.

ameter in the ewe and up to 5 mm in diameter in the bitch, are filled with clear fluid. In the ewe, the cysts are both beside and beneath the caruncles (Fig. 12-12). Because of the prevailing influence of progesterone in the bitch and cat, infection can be superimposed, leading to cystic hyperplastic endometritis. Microscopically, the principal component of endometrial hyperplasia is an increase in the size and number of glands, with no increase in the stroma, except for edema. In the bitch and queen, the glandular epithelium is progestational, i.e., the cells are tall, hypertrophic, and hyperplastic, with clear cytoplasm. As glands become cystic and pressure of retained secretion increases, the epithelium becomes flattened. In all species, the cystic lesions are probably irreversible. Ewes with endometrial hyperplasia have reduced fertility, dystocia, and uterine prolapse due to uterine hypotonicity, and mammary development even when nonpregnant. Cysts may develop in the ovine cervix as well as the endometrium, and squamous metaplasia of the cervical epithelium can occur. Bitches and queens are likely to develop endometritis and then pyometra. Endometrial polyps, thought to arise from focal areas of endometrial hyperplasia, have been described in the dog and cat. Endometrial hyperplasia is not precancerous, as it can be in women.

Mucometra is the accumulation of mucus in the uterine lumen. The cause may be congenital or acquired obstruction of the outflow of mucus initially produced in normal amounts or the production of excessive amounts of mucus due to hyperestrogenism.

Adenomyosis and **endometriosis** are lesions of importance in primates, but adenomyosis, at least, is encountered occasionally in domestic animals, notably the queen, cow, and bitch, probably as a result of prolonged estrogen stimulation. Adenomyosis is the presence of nests of endometrium within the myometrium. The effect is negligible, or there may be diffuse, symmetric or focal, asymmetric enlargement of the uterus. Microscopically, endometrial glands or stroma or both have grown down from the basal endometrium well past the junction between endometrium and myometrium. Endometriosis is the presence of endometrial glands or stroma in locations outside the uterus. Sites most frequently involved are the ovary, the mesometrium, the peritoneum, and peritoneal surgical scars. The mechanism behind endometriosis is unknown; suggestions are metaplasia of coelomic epithelium, transformation of tissue rests, regurgitation of endometrium through the infundibulum of the oviduct at the time of menstruation, implantation at the time of uterine surgery, and dissemination by lymph or blood vessels.

Inflammation

Most uterine infections begin in the endometrium and are related to introduction of semen, pregnancy, parturition, or postpartum involution of the uterus. Resistance of the uterus to infection is influenced by humoral and cellular immune mechanisms, by the hormonal environment, and by physical factors.

Humoral and cellular immune mechanisms

Following infection, there is a rapid influx of fluid from the blood into the uterine wall and lumen. Recruitment of neutrophils from the blood occurs in response to chemotactic substances released by bacteria and to leukotriene B_4 from endometrium and leukocytes. Attracted neutrophils infiltrate the endometrium and enter the lumen, and contribute additional leukotriene B_4, creating more chemotactic stimulus. Neutrophils secrete substances that are toxic to gametes and embryos. Complement activation, directly by organisms by the alternate pathway or in the presence of specific antibody by the classical pathway, can lead to the elimination of organisms either by lysis following attack on their membranes or by enhanced phagocytosis following opsonization. Leakage of serum into the uterine lumen from the inflamed endometrium contributes to the antibody content of the uterine fluid. Opsonization of bacteria by antibodies, especially IgG, allows faster phagocytosis.

The role of immunoglobulins in protecting the female genital tract of domestic animals has been studied most often in the mare. IgG and IgA predominate in uterine secretions in the mare, and IgM has been detected. Immunoglobulins in the uterine lumen apparently are produced in the endometrium rather than coming from blood. Local immunity seems better developed in the equine than in other species. The influence of the estrus cycle on antibodies in the uterus is controversial, but most work suggests that concentrations of luminal immunoglobulins and immunoglobulin-containing cells in the endometrium are not influenced by the cycle. Demonstration of greater amounts of IgA and IgG in the uterine secretions of mares more susceptible to infection has led to the belief that immunoglobulins may play a minor role.

Locally produced IgA is neither directly bactericidal nor can it act as an opsonin or macrophage activator. It can, however, interfere with attachment of bacteria to mucosal surfaces and can activate complement via the alternate pathway. There is variation between species on the site in the tract where the concentration of IgA is greatest. It corresponds to the site of semen deposition (uterus in mares, vagina in cows).

Hormonal influences

In the normal estrus cycle, the cervix opens under the influence of estrogens, facilitating drainage. Infections are more easily overcome at estrus than at other stages of the cycle. Leukocytes are normally increased in the uterine wall at estrus. In different studies, leukocytic phagocytosis has been unchanged or increased under the influence of estrogen, but it is widely reported that neutrophil activity is suppressed under the influence of progesterone. In general, the uterus is more susceptible to infection when it is under the influence of progesterone. Progesterone reduces the migration of blood neutrophils and reduces phagocytosis and killing of bacteria by uterine neutrophils. The mechanism for action of sex hormones on neutrophils is unknown. Receptors for sex hormones have not been demonstrated on neutrophils. The nonpregnant uterus is highly resistant to infection.

Prostaglandins are normally produced by the endometrium, probably PGF in greater quantity by the epithelium and PGE in greater quantity by the stroma. In most species (excluding the dog, cat, and primates), prostaglandin is responsible for lysis of the corpus luteum. In acute inflammation, prostaglandin production by the endometrium is increased, via the release of arachidonic acid from the phospholipids of cell membranes, and lysis of the corpus luteum occurs earlier. When chronic inflammation progresses to a stage of loss of mucosal surface, production of prostaglandins is decreased and the corpus luteum persists.

The physical factor relating to infections that has received the most attention is conformation. In the mare, when a large proportion of the vulva is placed higher than the floor of the pelvic canal, there is a tendency for the vulva to become horizontal and to suck air and contaminants, including feces, into the vagina or even into the uterus. Urine, too, can pool in the vagina in mares with abnormal function of the muscles of the vestibule and vulva. The caudal parts of the tract become inflamed, while the more cranial parts become inflamed either at the onset from direct contact with environmental organisms or later from local spread of the inflammation. An additional physical factor influencing a female animal's ability to resist infection is the drainage allowed by the hormonally controlled normal relaxation and opening of the cervix and contraction of the myometrium during estrus.

Organisms that cause inflammation of the uterus can enter from the caudal parts of the tract (ascending infection) or can arrive in the blood. The former is the route for infections initiated at coitus and parturition, whereas the latter is the route for most of the specific infections that occur during pregnancy. A few specific uterine infectious agents do use the ascending route, especially in the mare, but ascending infections are more likely to be of a mixed flora. Organisms that cause placentitis, fetal infection, and abortion in most cases at the same time also cause inflammation of the maternal component of the placenta. In those species with a zonary or cotyledonary rather than a diffuse placenta, endometritis extends beyond the bounds of the part of the endometrium making close contact with the fetal part of the placenta. Postpartum metritis will occur to some degree even after a normal pregnancy and parturition, but it is especially common and more severe following an abnormal parturition (Fig. 12-13). Lochia is an excellent bacterial nutrient medium.

Endometritis is inflammation limited to the endometrium. Almost all uterine infections begin as endometritis. Mild acute endometritis may be unremarkable grossly. In more severe acute endometritis, the mucosa is swollen and has a rough surface, often with adherent shreds of fibrin and necrotic debris (Fig. 12-14). Microscopically, a few to many neutrophils are in the stroma and in the glands, and the surface changes range from desquamation of a few surface epithelial cells to extensive necrosis. Mild lesions may resolve completely or leave cystic glands and periglandular fibrosis (Fig. 12-15). The number of layers of periglandular fibroblasts and the number of fibrotic foci per field in an endometrial biopsy specimen are correlated directly with the ability of the equine uterus to carry a foal to term. In all species, severe acute endometritis often becomes chronic (Fig. 12-16), and the necrotic endometrium is replaced by granulation tissue and, ultimately, by fibrous scar

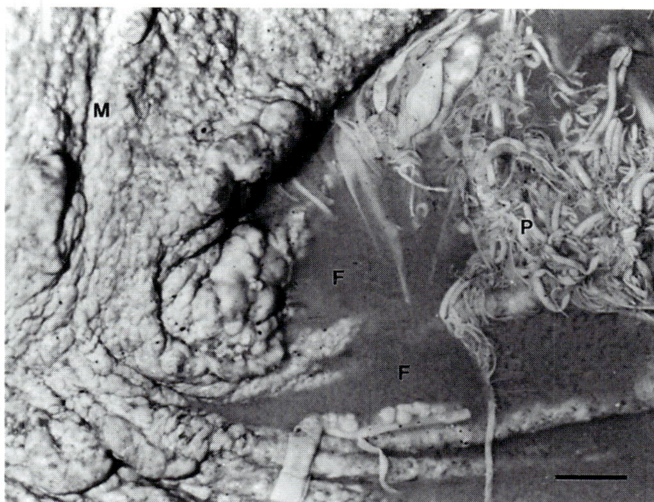

Fig. 12-13 Uterus; cow. Severe postcalving metritis. The mucosa (*M*) is coarsely nodular and is subacutely to chronically inflamed. Strings and shreds of disintegrating placenta (*P*) and brown fluid (*F*) are present in the lumen. Bar = 2 cm.

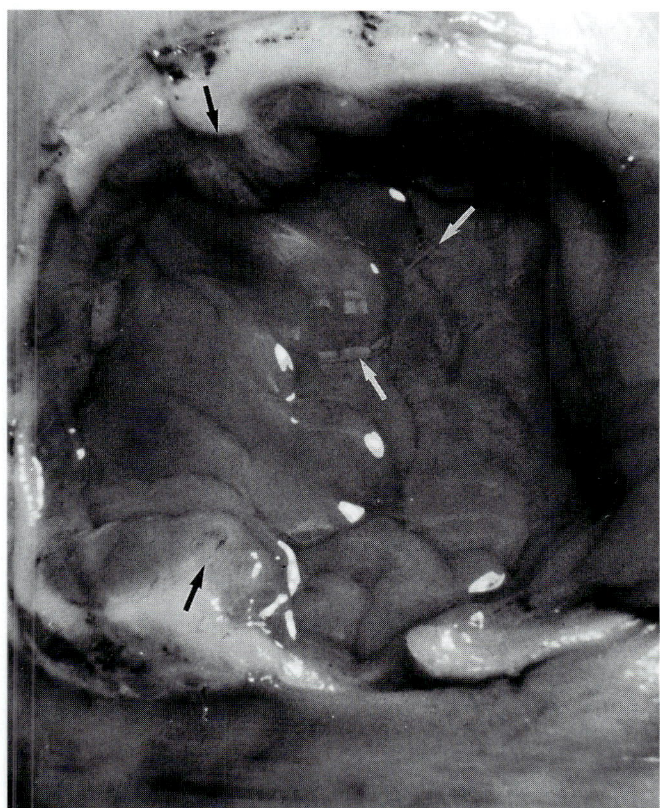

Fig. 12-14 Uterus; mare. Contagious equine metritis. In the acute stage, the endometrial folds are swollen because of edema, which is best seen at the cut edge *(black arrows).* The lumen contains increased mucus and strands of inflammatory debris *(white arrows).*

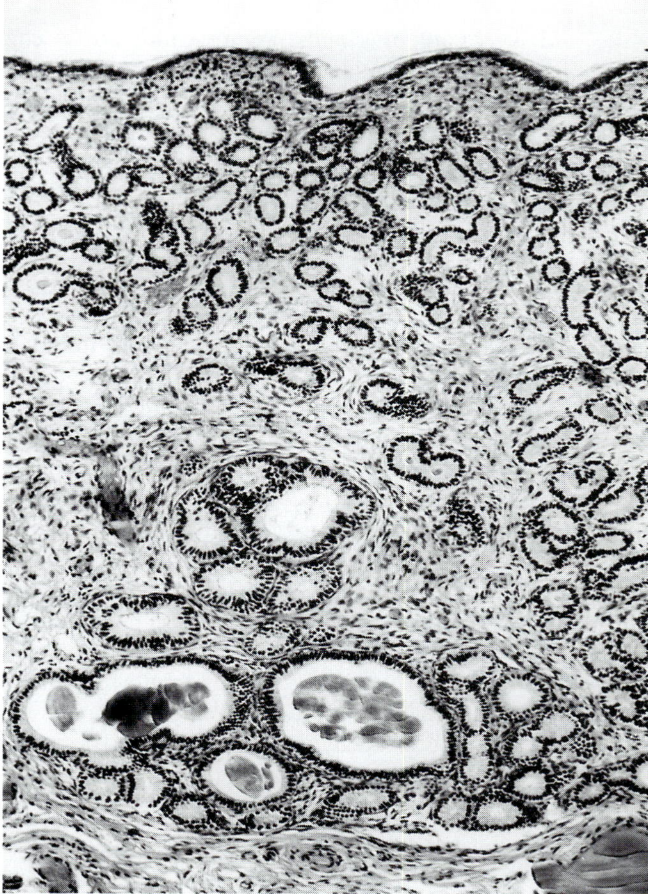

Fig. 12-15 Endometrium; mare. Mild fibrosis. Distended glandular lumina contain inspissated secretion. Nests of distended cross sections of glands are encircled by collagen and two or three layers of fibroblasts. Hematoxylin-eosin (H & E) stain.

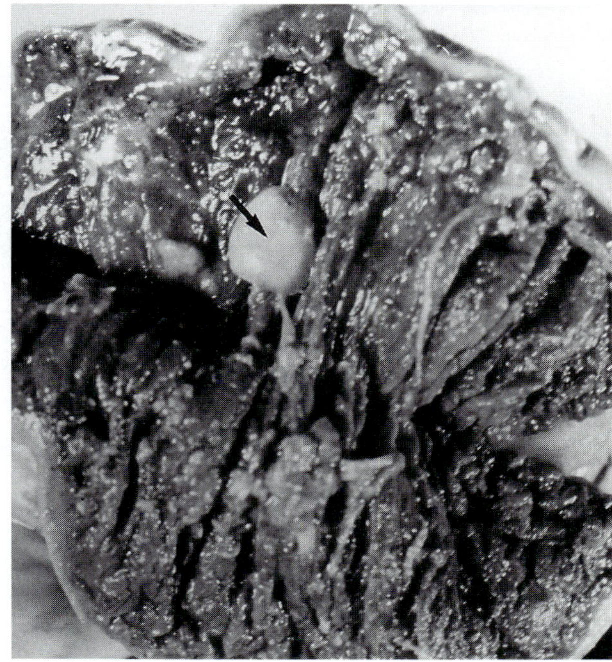

Fig. 12-16 Uterus; sow. Chronic staphylococcal endometritis. The endometrium is thickened and granular. Remnants of a macerated fetus, notably the cranium *(arrow),* are present.

tissue and is devoid of glands. Acute endometritis can cause synthesis of prostaglandin $F_{2\alpha}$ in large animals that have had 4 or 5 days of progesterone priming, leading to premature regression of the corpus luteum and shortening of the estrus cycle. The loss of endometrium in chronic inflammation can cause loss of ability to synthesize $PGF_{2\alpha}$, resulting in a persistent corpus luteum, especially in the mare and the cow.

Persistent endometritis is a problem in mares. Affected animals are unable to resolve the acute endometritis that usually follows mating. Defects in cellular and humoral defenses have been suggested. Neutrophils, the main phagocytic cells in the uterus, may be less able to migrate from the blood in susceptible mares than from the blood of resistant mares. Uterine neutrophils in susceptible mares may be less effective at phagocytosis. Uterine secretions may be deficient in promotion of neutrophil bactericidal activity, unrelated to generation of opsonizing complement components.

Metritis is inflammation of all layers of the uterine wall. In the acute stage, the serosa is dull, finely granular and has petechiae and fine adhering strands of fibrin. Microscopically, the subserosal tissue and muscle layer are edematous and infiltrated by inflammatory cells. Endometritis, as described above, is present.

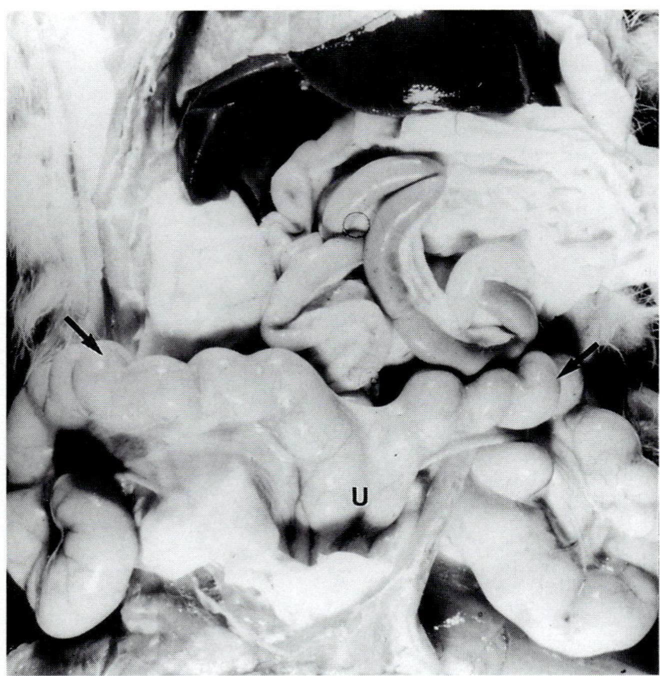

Fig. 12-17 Uterus; cat. Pyometra. Because the uterus (*U*) is greatly distended, it occupies a large proportion of the abdomen.

Pyometra may occur as a sequela to endometritis or metritis. It is an acute or chronic infection of the uterus, with accumulation of pus in the lumen in the presence of a closed cervix. The closing of the cervix is not always complete, allowing some discharge. In some instances, obstruction of the cervix is mechanical, but most cases involve functional obstruction of the cervix under the influence of progesterone from a retained corpus luteum. In the cow, the persistence of the corpus luteum is usually secondary to a pathologic process in the uterus, as no other lesions are present outside those of the genital tract. In the bitch and queen, most cases of pyometra occur as the result of bacterial infection secondary to endometrial hyperplasia, and most occur during pseudopregnancy. The color and consistency of the exudate vary with the type of bacterial infection. The uterus may be greatly distended (Fig. 12-17) but not necessarily uniformly. Necrotic, ulcerated, and hemorrhagic areas are present in the mucosa, as well as dry, white, thickened, finely cystic areas. The latter are due to hyperplasia, sometimes with squamous metaplasia. Lesions outside the genital tract, such as bone marrow depression, widespread extramedullary hematopoiesis, and immune complex glomerulopathy, are common.

Neoplasms

Leiomyomas occur in the bitch as multiple neoplasms, not only in the uterus but also in the cervix and vagina, often associated with other abnormalities, such as endometrial hyperplasia, ovarian follicular cysts, or mammary neoplasia. In other species, however, these neoplasms are rare, tend to be single, and lack any hormonal involvement. The neoplasms are discrete but not encapsulated, usually spherical with a wide range of sizes. Depending on size, they can be contained within the wall, project into the lumen, or project to the exterior. Some luminal neoplasms, especially those in the vagina, are pedunculated, creating the possibilities of their trauma and torsion. They are usually firm, pink or white, occasionally calcified or edematous. The color is related to the amount of fibrous tissue present along with the whorle smooth muscle cells; in some of the white neoplasms, smooth muscle is the predominant component.

Carcinoma of the endometrium is rare in domestic animals as a clinical problem, but it is well known as a lesion in the bovine uterus at slaughter. In the cow, starting in the depths of the endometrial glands of the horns more often than the body of the uterus, the neoplasm thickens the uterine wall without disturbing the overlying endometrium. A large amount of fibrous tissue is usually present, making the neoplasm firm and causing localized constriction bands visible from the exterior. The neoplasms can be small and annular or involve a large area of the uterine wall (Fig. 12-18). Microscopically, the neoplasm can readily be distinguished from normal endometrium by the epithelial cell

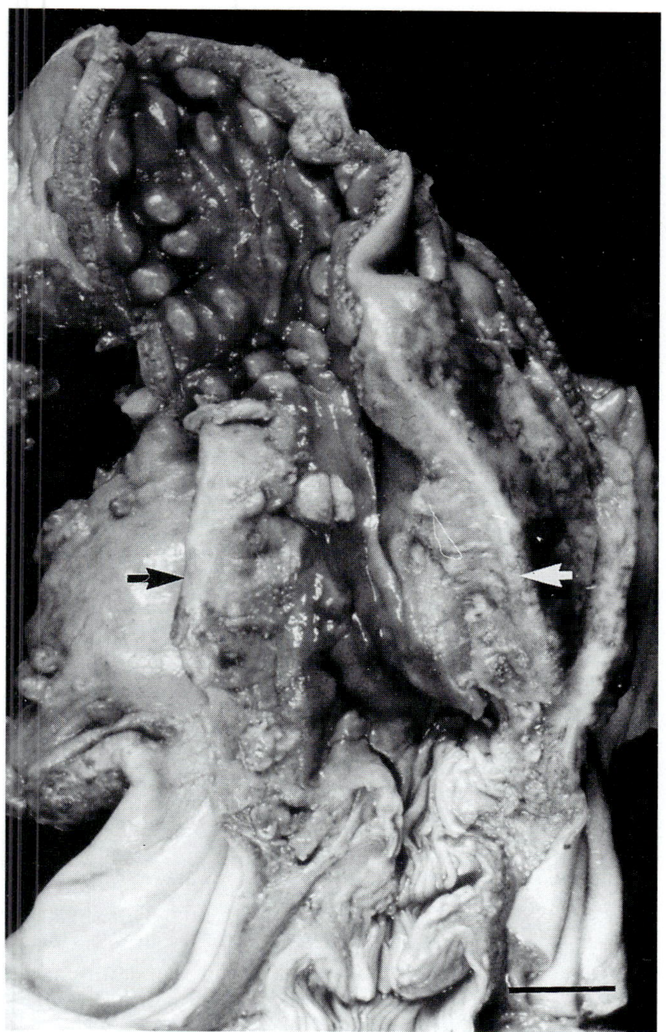

Fig. 12-18 Genital tract; cow. Endometrial carcinoma. The wall of the uterine body is thickened by the neoplasm and fibrous tissue *(arrows)*. Bar = 2 cm.

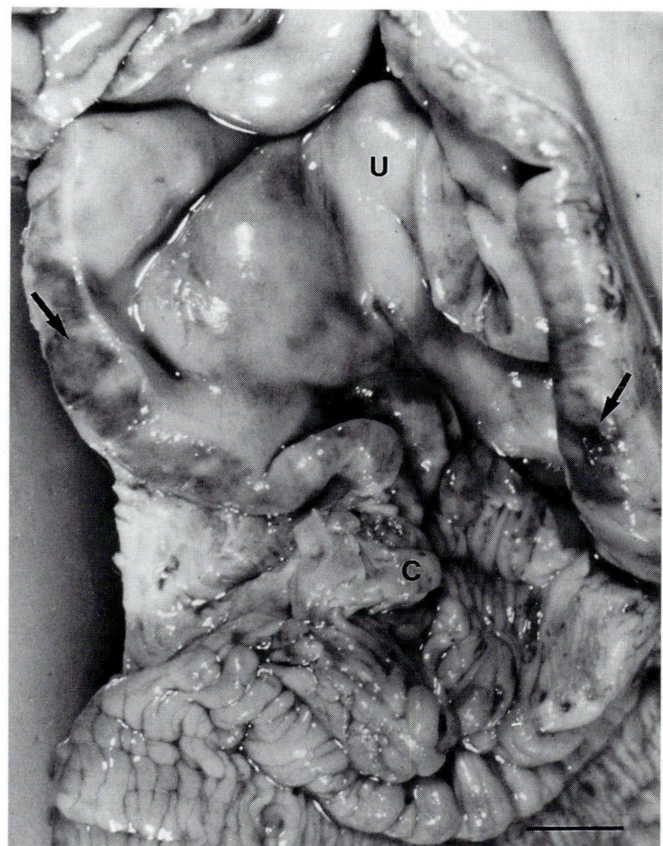

Fig. 12-19 Cervix (*C*) and uterine body (*U*); cow. Enzootic lymphosarcoma. The uterine wall is diffusely thickened by a light yellow neoplastic tissue with streaks of hemorrhage, best seen on cut surface *(arrows)*. Bar = 2 cm.

hypertrophy, pleomorphism, and cellular disarray. Metastases are found in the regional lymph nodes, lungs, and other organs.

Lymphosarcoma of the enzootic form in the cow caused by the bovine leukemia retrovirus commonly involves a tetrad of organs: namely, the heart, abomasum, lymph nodes, and uterus. In the uterus, as in other locations, the areas of infiltration can be focal, multifocal, or multifocally coalescing to becoming extensive (Fig. 12-19). Affected areas are light yellow, slightly friable, sometimes centrally necrotic plaques infiltrating or replacing part or the full thickness of the wall. It is not uncommon for the cervix and vagina to be involved as well as the uterus. In such cases, the vaginal lesions are multiple, small, often hemorrhagic nodules. An extensively involved uterus can support a pregnancy even to an advanced stage.

PLACENTA AND FETUS

Noninflammatory Disorders

Retention of fetal membranes for longer than normal after parturition is a common phenomenon and is prevalent in the cow. In the cow, membranes are considered retained if not shed by 12 hours postpartum. The cause is uncertain; infectious, nutritional, hormonal, circulatory, hereditary, and weather possibilities have been suggested. The membranes can act as a medium for exponential growth of bacteria from the environment, with the potential for the common, transient, mild postparturient metritis to become severe, even to the point of causing systemic disease. Normal shedding of the placenta involves maternal caruncles becoming smaller due to decreased blood supply in early uterine involution, degeneration of some maternal tissue, and autolysis of chorionic villi. There is no histologic difference prepartum between placentomes from cows that shed their placentas normally and those that retain them. In normal cows, a major decline in the number of binucleate giant cells in the placentomes occurs by 1 hour postpartum, whereas the same degree of reduction does not occur in cows that retain their membranes. Possibly these cells are concerned with the cell attachment at the fetomaternal interface, or possibly the necrosis of these cells liberates enzymes that destroy the ligands at the interface and allows separation.

Twinning is the most common noninfectious cause of abortion in the mare. Chorionic villi develop where there is contact between the endometrium and the chorion. In other areas, such as the contact area between chorion and endocervix and the contact area between the placentas of twins, chorionic villi do not develop and the chorion is smooth. The combined functional area of the chorions of both twins is only slightly larger than that for a normal singleton foal. Twin fetuses often have retarded growth. Aborted twin equine fetuses often appear to have died at different times. Death is thought to be due to placental insufficiency. In approximately 80% of cases, the available space in the uterus is divided evenly; both twins usually die and are aborted. However, in those cases in which there is great disparity in the apportioning of space, the favored twin has a chance of survival, while the other dies and mummifies.

In the mare, **endometrial fibrosis,** probably the result of a previous endometritis, reduces the area of the endometrium available for formation of the diffuse placenta. Although severely affected mares have no problem becoming pregnant, they do not carry the fetus to term because of the limitations of the placenta caused by endometrial fibrosis.

Premature placental separation in the mare has been described in two forms. One occurs around the time of parturition: the chorioallantois appears at the vulva with the cervical star intact, and tearing of the chorioallantois occurs across its body. The other type occurs some time before parturition, and the prematurely detached areas become brown and dehydrated. Another equine disease, albeit a rare one, in which fetal death and abortion occur as a result of placental insufficiency and fetal malnutrition, is **body pregnancy.** The fetus occupies the uterine body rather than the body and horns, and the placenta is underdeveloped in the horns.

Torsion of the umbilical cord is a cause of equine abortion. The cord is long and excessively twisted, and the twists are difficult to undo. For a twisted cord to qualify as being pathologic, there has to be a sign of vascular compromise such as edema and hemorrhage, with alternate dilatations and constrictions of the cord. There may be local distentions of the urachus (Fig. 12-20).

Adventitial placentation in ruminants, which is the formation of additional areas of fetal and maternal placental contact, is a response to inadequacy of the conventional placentomes and is most likely due to loss of caruncles as a result of endometritis (Fig. 12-21). Compensation may be achieved by enlargement of the existing functional maternal caruncles, followed by the establishment of additional areas of contact by simple villous interdigitation. These adventitious areas form initially adjacent to the placentomes but may expand to involve much of the surface.

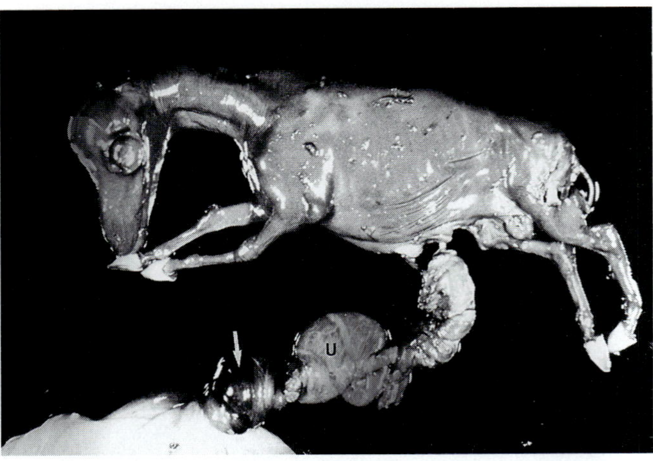

Fig. 12-20 Fetus; horse. Umbilical cord torsion. Fetal death and mummification. Early mummification is most easily recognized by the paucity of orbital contents. The vessels of the cord are congested in the twisted area *(arrow),* and the urachus (*U*) is ballooned on the fetal side of the twist.

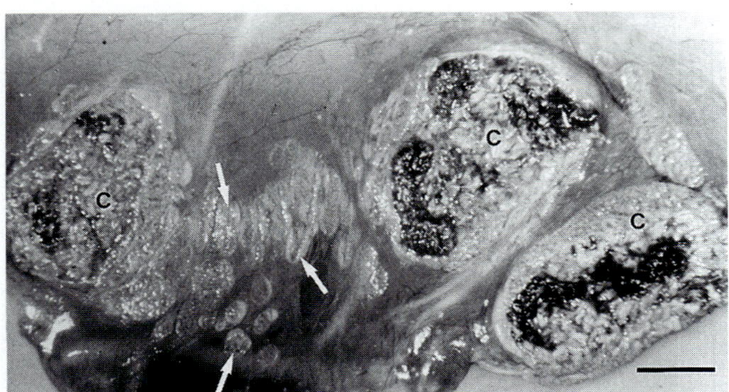

Fig. 12-21 Chorioallantois; cow. Adventitial placentation. Very severe inflammation and necrosis of cotyledons. Small adventitial cotyledons *(arrows)* are in between the major cotyledons (*C*). Bar = 2 cm. *Courtesy Dr. T.J. Van Winkle.*

Hydramnios and **hydrallantois** refer to the excessive accumulation of fluid in the amnionic and allantoic sacs, respectively. These lesions occur mostly in the bovine species, are fairly rare, and are not usually seen together. Amnionic fluid is viscid, resembling fetal saliva from which it is formed. Accumulation of excessive amnionic fluid occurs in association with certain fetal anomalies that involve the musculoskeletal system, especially abnormalities of the head. The implication is that serious nervous abnormalities impair the fetal drinking reflex. An association has been shown between fetal adrenal insufficiency and hydramnios. Allantoic fluid is formed from fetal urine, received through the urachus. In the cow, hydrallantois occurs in conjunction with adventitial placentation and in some twin pregnancies. Abortion or dystocia follows, with a dead and sometimes small anasarcous and ascitic fetus. The allantoic fluid composition changes from normal to one closely resembling maternal or fetal extracellular fluid. If membranes are retained after delivery of a fetus, fluid may continue to accumulate.

Embryonic and **fetal death** deprive the fetomaternal unit of whatever contribution the conceptus made to the continuation of pregnancy. Parturition or abortion in most large animal species is brought about by synthesis and release of $PGF_{2\alpha}$ from the endometrium, causing, in turn, regression of the corpus luteum and a decrease in progesterone production. In large animals, embryonic loss before expansion of placental membranes does not influence the time of return to estrus. If embryonic loss occurs after the membranes have expanded, the interval to the next estrus will be somewhat increased because the corpus luteum will have been programmed for prolongation of its life. The importance of the fetal component and the necessity of the presence of a corpus luteum for the entire pregnancy vary with species. For instance, the corpus luteum of the sow is needed throughout pregnancy, as progesterone production by the placenta is small; but, in the mare, the corpus luteum regresses halfway through pregnancy, and placental progesterone maintains pregnancy. Regardless of the source of hormones responsible for maintaining pregnancy in large animals, embryonic or fetal death is likely to permit the release of $PGF_{2\alpha}$ and expulsion of the embryo or fetus. The exact outcome is unpredictable, influenced by, among other things, species, stage of gestation, and number of fetuses involved. In the dog and cat, the life span of the corpus luteum is not very different in the pregnant and the nonpregnant animal. When embryonic or fetal death occurs in domestic carnivores, the demise of the corpus luteum is not a closely following consequence, and dead products of conception are retained until approximately the normal time of parturition.

The products of embryonic death have received relatively little study, because they were not available before decomposition has advanced, were resorbed, or were passed unnoticed. Probably in animals, as for human beings, many of the embryos that die have chromosomal abnormalities.

Mummification is one of the possible outcomes of fetal death. Rather than being expelled soon after death, the fetus is retained and progressively is dehydrated to become a firm, dry mass, colored brown or black by degraded hemoglobin and consisting of leathery skin enclosing the harder parts of the fetus (see Fig. 12-20). The cause of death can be infectious or noninfectious, but requisites for mummification are that organisms that promote lysis of dead tissue be absent and that the cervix be closed to prevent the entry of putrefactive organisms. The situations in which mummification most commonly occurs are in twin pregnancy in the mare and in parvovirus infection in the sow. In twin pregnancy in the mare, the mummified fetus and the longer surviving fetus are aborted together prior to term. In parvovirus infection in the sow, mummified fetuses are retained to be born at term along with live fetuses. In a singleton pregnancy, a mummified fetus can be expelled at any time or retained indefinitely.

Maceration of a dead fetus requires the presence of organisms in the uterus. These organisms can be the ones that caused the fetal death in the first place or putrefactive organisms that entered the uterus after the death of the fetus. Along with disintegration of the fetus, the uterus is also involved in the process, endometritis or pyometra will be present, depending on whether the cervix is open or not. If there is emphysema, such as caused by the invasion by clostridial organisms of a fetus dead because of dystocia, it is likely that maternal toxemia will be followed by death. Otherwise, both endometritis and pyometra tend to become severe and chronic, with voluminous pus. Fetal bones resist maceration (see Fig. 12-16), giving the added possibility that, if the uterus eventually regains some muscular tone, the bones will cause perforation.

Abortion in domestic animals is defined as expulsion of the fetus before development is sufficiently advanced to allow survival. An aborted fetus can be alive or dead at the time of abortion, but most are dead. **Stillbirth** is defined as the delivery of a dead fetus at a stage of development at which it should have been viable. Although these are useful terms, they do not give pathogenetic or diagnostic information. A particular intrauterine infection could cause a spectrum of effects from fetal mummification, abortion, or stillbirth to the birth of a live, but sick, fetus.

Fetal anomalies can take innumerable forms. Only those that have a direct influence on the reproductive process are mentioned here. First, some anomalies cause prolonged gestation because a fetal organ does not make its hormonal contribution to the birth process. One anomaly is aplasia or hypoplasia of the adrenal glands; another is displacement, dysgenesis, or absence of the pituitary gland. The classic example of a displaced pituitary gland causing prolonged gestation is in the fetal lambs from ewes that have ingested the plant *Veratrum californicum* on the fourteenth day of gestation. Absence of the pituitary gland occurs, probably as an inherited disease, in several breeds of cattle. It may occur alone or as part of anencephaly, another feature of which is a cyclopian malformation. Anencephaly is literally absence of a brain, but the term is used loosely to cover the far more common situation of absence of a forebrain, variable presence of a midbrain, and presence of a hind brain stem. The neurohypophysis is absent, as well as the adenohypophysis. The second large group of fetal anomalies that may interfere with the reproductive process is the type that causes mechanical problems in parturition. Examples are hydrocephalus, hydrops fetus, and arthrogryposis.

Inflammatory Disorders

Bacterial causes

Bacterial infections capable of causing inflammation of the placenta and fetus are numerous. Almost any organism causing septicemia can invade the uterus, but the following discussion concerns those organisms that have the placenta and fetus as a particular target. The route of invasion of the target organs for many animal species and many diseases is hematogenous, after the organisms have entered the dam through the digestive or genital tract. For some diseases, the method of spread can be either venereal or by ingestion. In the horse, most placental pathogens enter the pregnant uterus through the cervix. *Campylobacter fetus* var. *venerealis* can be a long-term inhabitant of the exterior of the bovine penis and the preputial cavity. It is transmitted venereally, can live for some time on the vaginal mucosa, but requires that the cow becomes pregnant in order to establish itself in the uterus. Embryonic or early fetal death are the most likely manifestations of campylobacteriosis, and often the only abnormality observed is irregular estrus cycles or return to estrus of an animal thought to be pregnant. Much less frequent is abortion at a later stage of pregnancy. Cows become immune to subsequent challenges by the organism. Gross and microscopic lesions in placentas are similar to those in brucellosis but less severe and with fewer organisms visible in the desquamated chorionic epithelial cells. Fetal lesions are nonspecific.

C. fetus in sheep is primarily an intestinal inhabitant, hence its designation as var. *intestinalis.* The organism is transmitted by ingestion rather than venereally, and the disease tends to occur in outbreaks, possibly with crows acting as vectors. The only important manifestation of its presence in sheep is involvement of the pregnant uterus during the septicemic phase. Infection of the pregnant uterus will result in late-term abortion or the birth of sick lambs. Immunity is gained after this episode. The placenta has an edematous intercotyledonary chorioallantois and friable, yellow cotyledons. The fetus may have no specific lesions, but about 25% of them have multiple yellow areas of hepatic necrosis up to 2 cm in diameter, with red, depressed centers. Microscopically, inflammatory infiltration of the chorioallantois occurs with a mixture of cells, many of which cannot be identified because of degeneration, but a large proportion are neutrophils. Inflammation is especially severe in the chorionic villi. Organisms are plentiful, as are the inflammatory cells. An additional feature diagnostically useful in *Campylobacter* infection is the presence of large, dense emboli of bacteria filling capillaries of the chorionic villi. The fetal liver has severe multifocal necrotizing inflammation, and, here too, the organisms are present in large numbers.

Brucella abortus in cattle gains access by ingestion of feed contaminated with the products of abortion. The initial lesion is a lymphadenitis, which becomes chronic. Bacteremic waves cause colonization of the spleen, lymph nodes, mammary glands, testes, accessory male glands, and synovial membranes. The organism is cleared from most organs, but some small nidus of infection usually persists. The pregnant uterus is particularly susceptible to infection, and the disease process becomes chronic, eventually clearing after abortion or parturition. Gross lesions in the placenta are edema of the intercotyledonary chorioallantois that has increased opacity and a leathery texture, light brown exudate on the chorionic surface, and variable extent of necrosis of the cotyledons. Such a placenta is grossly indistinguishable from the placenta of mycotic abortion or the rare case of campylobacteriosis with a late-term abortion. The fetus has nonspecific lesions of edema and fluid accumulation in body cavities and often has the more specific lesions of bronchopneumonia and pleuritis.

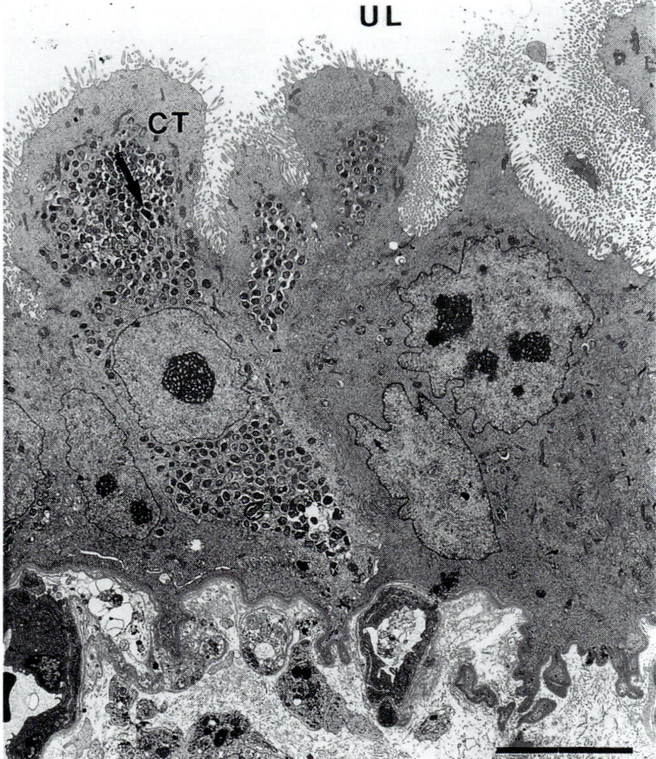

Fig. 12-22 Transmission electron micrograph. Chorioallantois; goat. *Brucella abortus* infection. In the nonplacentomal chorioallantois, the trophoblasts contain numerous *B. abortus* in dilated cisternae of the rough endoplasmic reticulum *(arrow)* and perinuclear envelope. A trophoblast (*CT*) is in the process of sloughing into the uterine lumen (*U*). Fetal capillaries *(fc)* and connective tissue are normal. *Courtesy Dr. T.D. Anderson.*

Microscopically, inflammation involves both the intercotyledonary chorion and the chorionic villi, and lesions are edema and infiltration of mononuclear cells and a few neutrophils. The striking feature is the presence of numerous coccobacilli within chorionic epithelial cells, many of which have sloughed to make up the considerable debris between maternal and fetal tissues. The sequence of events in ruminants infected with *B. abortus* appears to be release of organisms from the maternal circulation into the hematomas that normally occur at the tips of the maternal septa within the placentome, uptake of organisms by the erythrophagocytic trophoblasts at the base of the chorionic villi, replication in adjacent periplacentomal chorioallantoic trophoblasts (Fig. 12-22), trophoblast necrosis, chorioallantoic ulceration, and entry of organisms into the uterine lumen and chorionic villi, and, finally, hematogenous dissemination to fetal viscera. *B. abortus* appears to be taken up by endocytosis by erythrophagocytic trophoblasts, and then to replicate in the rough endoplasmic reticulum of the periplacentomal and interplacentomal trophoblasts, a unique mechanism of intracellular parasitism. Vasculitis in maternal and fetal tissues may be due to endotoxin released from the organisms. Most of the fetuses have some degree of pneumonia, even though the gross appearance can range from minimal to severe involvement. The pneumonia is chronic, either a bronchopneumonia with numerous mononuclear cells and some neutrophils in the exudate, or a fibrinous pneumonia. Microscopic granulomas that include multinucleate giant cells can be found in various organs, such as the liver, spleen, and lymph nodes.

B. canis infection is acquired by the dog either by ingestion or venereally. In both sexes, lymphadenitis involves, especially, the nodes of the head. Bacteremia is persistent. Epididymitis and testicular degeneration occur in male dogs, and females have placentitis and fetal endocarditis, pneumonia, and hepatitis. Microscopically, chorionic epithelial cells are packed with *Brucella* organisms. Common fetal lesions are bronchopneumonia, myocarditis, renal hemorrhage and subacute inflammation of the pelvic connective tissue, lymphadenitis, and hepatitis.

B. ovis infection in sheep is probably transmitted venereally, from a ram with epididymitis shedding large numbers of organisms in the semen. Placental lesions are essentially similar to those produced by *B. abortus* in cattle. Fetal lesions consist of nonspecific edema and fluid accumulation in the body cavities. Calcified plaques on the hooves have been noted, but there is some doubt as to their specificity. Microscopically, as with *Brucella* infections in other species, large numbers of coccobacilli are in chorionic epithelial cells. Bacteria are free in the chorionic mesenchyme, and vasculitis is present in the larger chorionic vessels. Pneumonia, lymphadenitis, interstitial nephritis, and a hypercellularity of portal tracts of the liver develop in the fetus. In younger fetuses, hyperplasia of monocyte-macrophage cells are found, as well as granulomatous inflammation; in older fetuses, the lymphoreticular response is indicated by well-formed nodules of macrophage-monocytes, lymphocytes, and plasma cells. *B. melitensis* infections in sheep and goats occur mainly in Mediterranean countries. Infection has a septicemic phase, with localization in the mammary gland and pregnant uterus. Goats suffer more severe febrile disease and more severe mastitis than do sheep.

B. suis infection in pigs causes a disease that is different in several respects from brucellosis in ruminants. The lesions are more widespread in the body, even having a predilection for bones and joints. Necrosis and caseation occur in many lesions. Pregnancy is not a prerequisite for endometritis in swine brucellosis. Miliary granulomas in the endometrium are mixed with multiple hyperplastic lymphoid nodules. Endometrial glands become distended by mucus and leukocytes, and surface epithelium partly sloughs or undergoes squamous metaplasia. Between placentas in the pregnant uterus, the mucopurulent exudate contains plentiful intracellular and free organisms. The chorioallantoic membranes have nonspecific edema and congestion.

Coxiella burnettii, the organism that causes Q fever in human beings, is sometimes responsible for abortion or the birth of dead or weak lambs or kids. Infection of goats is more common. Transmission of the organism is nonvenereal. The organism causes abortion in newly exposed animals, and repeat abortion is possible. The organism is shed in discharges at parturition and in the milk. In the affected goat, the placenta has a thick, leathery, yellow, discolored intercotyledonary chorioallantois with a moderate amount of surface exudate. Gross fetal lesions are nonspecific. Microscopically, the placental lesions of acute inflammatory infiltration are most severe in the intercotyledonary areas. Hypertrophic chorionic epithelial cells are packed with *Coxiella* organisms. Fetal lesions, if present, consist of peribronchiolar, renal medullary, and hepatic portal lymphoid accumulations.

Enzootic abortion of ewes is caused by a chlamydial organism. The disease has occurred as small outbreaks in several countries, producing late-term abortion in ewes and goats. Transmission is probably nonvenereal, and ewes seem to be immune after the first abortion. The affected placenta appears similar to the placenta infected by *Coxiella* or *Brucella.* Microscopically, the lesions are similar. Useful differentiating features are that in chlamydial abortion the cotyledons are more severely involved than the intercotyledonary areas; the organisms, even though they distend the chorionic cells, are difficult to visualize without the benefit of special stains; and there is no vasculitis. In the fetus, subacute inflammatory foci occur in several organs, especially the liver, lungs, and muscle.

Epizootic bovine abortion, also known as foothill abortion, occurs in California and adjacent states. It was thought for many years that the disease was caused by a chlamydial organism, but after it was found that normal bovine fetuses could harbor the same organism, attention shifted to a tick-transmitted virus. Now, it seems that the most likely cause is superinfection with a *Borrelia*-like spirochete. Abortion or the birth of weak calves occurs only in cows newly introduced into the territory of the tick *Ornithodorus coriaceus*. The fetal disease is a chronic one, and marked microscopic lesions develop 50 days after exposure of the dam to ticks. They are of sufficient specificity to make a diagnosis after 100 days. Lesions are ascites and an enlarged nodular liver (Fig. 12-23), lymph nodes, and spleen. Microscopic lesions center on the lymphoreticular system, with the development of severely hyperplastic lymph nodes and spleen and the transformation of the predominant lymphocyte from the small, darkly staining type to a larger cell with a less darkly staining nucleus. Lymphoid follicles are prominent, and large numbers of macrophages are present as well. The thymus is atrophic because of loss of cortical lymphocytes together with parenchymal and interstitial inflammation. Necrotic foci develop in several organs, especially the lymph nodes and spleen, and these foci frequently form pyogranulomas. Vasculitis, acute or subacute, occurs in any organ, and, if present, involves several organs. IgG and IgM are deposited in the vascular lesions.

Leptospirosis is another possible cause of abortion. Serologic evidence is that a high proportion of cattle and pigs are infected, but most animals do not have clinical signs. Several different serovars of leptospiral organisms are associated with abortion, especially serovar *hardjo* in cattle and *pomona* in swine. In adult animals, the organisms localize in the kidneys after the septicemic phase. Pregnant sows or cows may abort weeks after the septicemic phase, usually in the last trimester. Placental lesions are usually limited to edema. Fetal lesions often are mild and obscured by autolysis. A few fetuses are expelled near term in a relatively fresh state, and some of these have ascites, fibrinous peritonitis, nephritis, and necrotizing hepatitis. Leptospiral organisms can be demonstrated by silver stains in tubular lumina of fetal kidneys with or without morphologic changes.

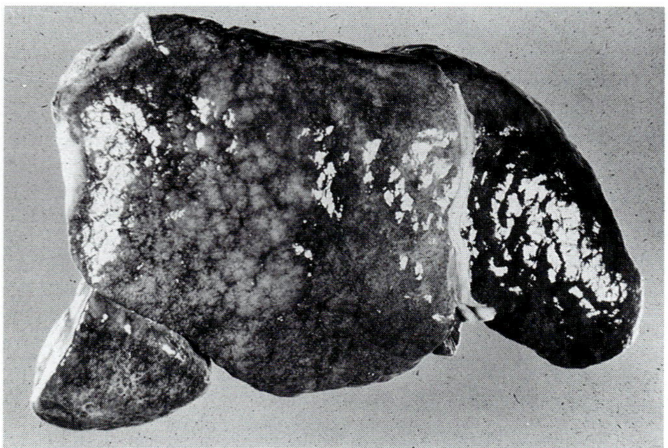

Fig. 12-23 Liver; aborted bovine fetus. Enzootic bovine abortion. Note the nodularity characteristic of the disease. *Courtesy Dr. P.C. Kennedy.*

Listeriosis is a cause of sporadic abortions in cattle, sheep, and goats and of outbreaks of abortion in sheep. Although it is possible for both the nervous disease and the reproductive disease caused by *Listeria monocytogenes* to occur in the same flock or herd, such a happening is a rarity. Listerial abortions occur in the last trimester of pregnancy, with or without maternal febrile disease due to septicemia or endometritis. The placenta can have severe diffuse necrotizing and suppurative inflammation of both the cotyledons and the intercotyledonary areas. The fetus may have an enlarged liver with numerous 1-mm yellow foci throughout. Microscopically, severe infiltration involves the mesenchyme of the villi and the upper intercotyledonary chorion; many of the inflammatory cells have degenerated beyond recognition, but some are neutrophils. Chorionic epithelium, especially in the areas between the villi, is packed with listerial organisms. Their identity is easy to ascertain because of their gram-positive staining. The acute, multifocal, necrotizing inflammatory lesions in the fetal liver are likewise packed with organisms, and other fetal organs will have similar microscopic lesions.

A variety of organisms that cause bacteremia in adult animals are capable of involving the placenta and fetus. Thus, in cattle, organisms such as *Salmonella* sp., *Pasteurella* sp., and *Haemophilus somnus* are potential causes of placentitis, fetal invasion, and abortion. In pigs, infection with various *Streptococcus* sp. may produce similar lesions.

Ureaplasmas can cause abortion in cattle. Focal or diffuse reddening of the amnion and chorioallantois may be accompanied by thickening and yellow discoloration of the amnion. Fibrosis, edema, inflammation, and necrosis of the amnion occur, together with focal inflammation and necrosis of the cotyledons and the intercotyledonary chorioallantois.

Various bacterial organisms can cause abortion in the mare. Hemolytic streptococci are the most frequently recovered from fetal organs, placentas, and uterine discharges. Other commonly encountered organisms are *E. coli, Pseudomonas, Klebsiella,* and *Staphylococcus.* Although some infections are hematogenous, the ascending route of infection, through the cervix, is the rule. Inflammation of the chorioallantois is most severe opposite the cervix, and forward extension of the involved area is greater ventrally than dorsally because of the help given by gravity. Affected parts of the placenta are edematous and brown, with a small amount of fibrinonecrotic exudate.

Gross fetal lesions may be only an enlarged liver and increased abdominal and thoracic fluid. Microscopically, in the areas with grossly visible lesions, a moderately severe subacute inflammation involves the stroma of the chorionic microcotyledons accompanied by sloughing of chorionic epithelium. Microscopic fetal lesions are usually equivocal, despite the ease with which bacteria can be recovered from many fetal organs. The prelude to abortion is either fetal death from septicemia or placental insufficiency from loss of functional area.

Fungal causes

Aspergillus and phycomycetes *(Absidia, Mortierella, Mucor, Rhizopus)* cause sporadic abortions in cattle and horses. In cattle, the organisms appear to arrive at the placenta hematogenously, because the placentomes are involved first and there is no selection of placentomes with regard to location. In the mare, as with bacterial placentitis, the fungi probably enter through the cervix, because the lesions in the chorioallantois are most severe in or even confined to the cervical area. In the affected bovine placenta, the cotyledons become enlarged, brown, and friable, and the intercotyledonary chorioallantois becomes leathery with a surface exudate (Fig. 12-24). The gross appearance of the placenta is, thus, similar to the classical descriptions of the placenta in bovine brucellosis. Affected areas of the equine chorioallantois are brown, initially swollen, and, later, shrunken and friable (Fig. 12-25). In both species, the amnion has thick white or yellow leathery areas. Small, white, raised plaques are present on the bovine fetal skin and, sometimes, involve the skin of fetal horses. Microscopically, inflammatory infiltration involves the allantoamnionic mesenchyme and chorionic mesenchyme, accompanied by sloughing of the chorionic epithelium. In the bovine species, the lesions are a vasculitis and fungal invasion of the larger vessels at the base of the cotyledons. In the fetal skin, the lesions include dermatitis and epidermal hyperkeratosis. Fungal hyphae, septate in the case of *Aspergillus* and nonseptate in the case of the phycomycetes, are plentiful in the lesions of the placenta and fetus. Fungi can be recovered from the fetal stomach, but fetal lesions usually do not extend beyond the fetal skin.

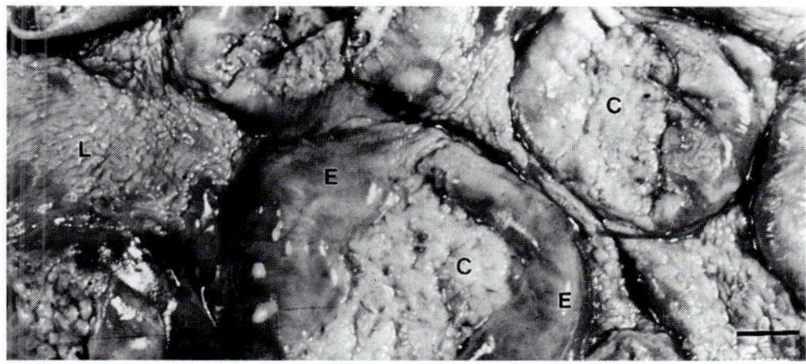

Fig. 12-24 Chorioallantois; cow. Mycotic placentitis. The intercotyledonary tissue is thickened and, in parts, is either leathery (*L*) or edematous (*E*). The cotyledons (*C*) are enlarged and friable and have surface inflammatory exudate. Bar = 1 cm.

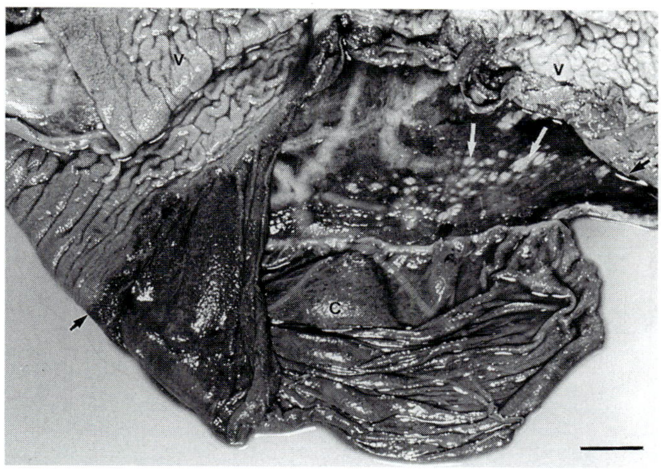

Fig. 12-25 Placenta, cervical area; mare. Mycotic abortion. The allantochorion (*C*) opposite to the cervix and adjacent uterus is torn, dehydrated, and friable and is clearly demarcated *(black arrows)* from the viable (*V*) allantochorion cranial to it. Note the fungal plaques *(white arrows)* on the allantoic surface. Bar = 1 cm.

Viral causes

Herpesviruses are well known as the cause of outbreaks of abortion in cattle, horses, and pigs. Abortions due to herpesvirus infection have also been described in goats and dogs (Table 12-1). Generally, applicable facts about the lesions in affected fetuses are that there is lymphoid necrosis, together with multiple, small foci of necrosis; mild acute inflammation; and intranuclear inclusion bodies in adjacent parenchymal cells in a wide range of organs, especially the liver, lungs, and adrenal glands (Fig. 12-26). Often the fetal liver is enlarged, and the focal lesions may be large enough to be visible as pinpoint white areas. Vascular lesions may be no more than endothelial swelling, but the effect can be pleural and peritoneal effusion and subcutaneous edema. Pulmonary involvement usually includes bronchiolar epithelial hyperplasia, with some necrosis and epithelial cell desquamation. Fibrinous bronchiolitis, grossly visible, is present in some fetuses, especially equine. The placenta may be edematous, but only in the pig has a specific lesion been observed. In that species, pseudorabies virus can cause mild inflammation of the chorion together with intranuclear inclusion bodies in chorionic epithelium.

Equine herpesvirus-1 (EHV-1) is now the name reserved for the abortogenic virus that formerly was called EHV-1

Table 12-1. Herpesviruses and fetal disease

Species	Virus	Disease in the fetus	Disease in the adult
Cattle	Infectious bovine rhinotracheitis	Fetus is usually autolyzed when expelled	Neonatal gastrointestinal ulceration Mastitis Infectious bovine rhinotracheitis Infectious pustular vulvovaginitis Encephalitis Respiratory disease—interstitial pneumonia
Horses	Equine herpesvirus-1 (also called equine rhinopneumonitis virus)	Multifocal inflammation and necrosis in liver, lungs, adrenal glands and lymphoid organs with intranuclear inclusions	Rhinopneumonitis Encephalomyelitis
Pigs	Pseudorabies virus (also called Aujeszky's disease virus)	Affected and unaffected litter members Inclusion bodies in chorionic epithelium	Dermatitis in pigs (rare) Encephalitis in cattle
Goats	Caprine herpesvirus	Little information available	Asymptomatic adults Enteritis in kids
Dogs	Canine herpesvirus	Multifocal inflammation and necrosis in any organ Newborn pups most susceptible	Not susceptible to disease after 2 weeks of age; inapparent infections common
Cats	Feline rhinotracheitis virus	Questionable cause of abortion	Upper respiratory disease, nonfatal

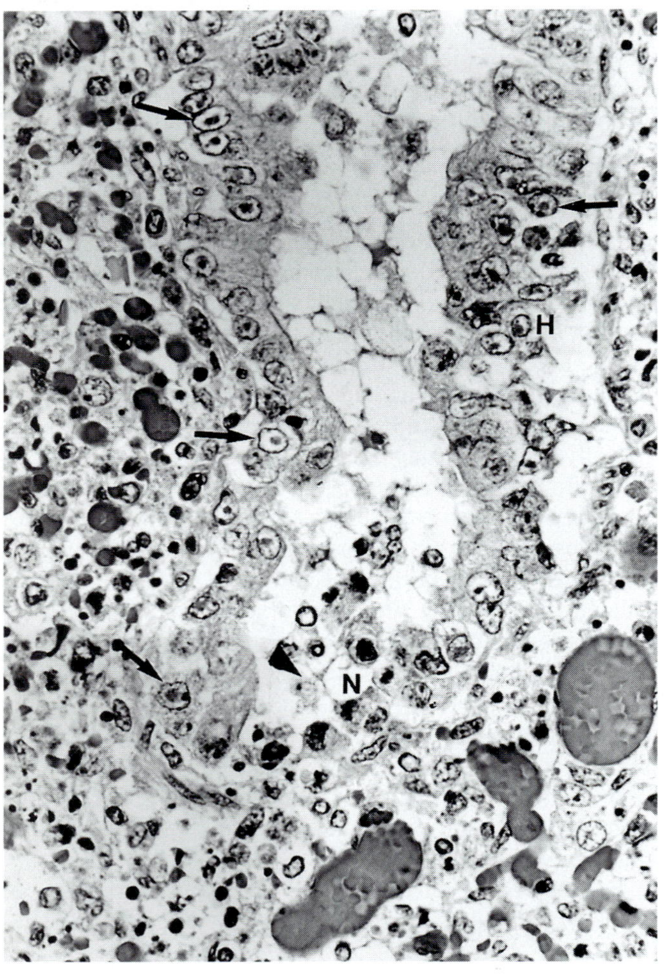

Fig. 12-26 Fetal lung; foal. Equine herpesvirus abortion. Bronchiolar epithelium is hyperplastic, and some necrotic epithelial cells have soughed into the lumen. Intranuclear inclusions are numerous *(arrows)*.

subtype 1. EHV-1 may be the most economically significant abortogenic animal herpesvirus. Viral infection of maternal uterine endothelial cells plays a major role in the pathogenesis of abortion. The lesions are multiple areas of thrombosis; perivascular infiltration by lymphocytes, neutrophils, and monocytes; perivascular edema; and subsequent avascular necrosis of endometrium. The fluid that escapes the damaged endometrium causes some separation of maternal and fetal elements of the placenta and can allow virus from maternal leucocytes and lysed endothelial cells to enter the fetus. Fetal endothelial cells are also targets for the virus, as well as the cells of a number of parenchymatous organs. In the cow, an affinity of herpesvirus for the endometrium has been demonstrated. After experimental intrauterine inoculation, infectious bovine rhinotracheitis virus produces an acute necrotizing endometritis in the uterine body or caudal parts of the uterine horns of the cow. Microscopically, the lesions vary in severity from mild focal lymphocytic endometritis to severe diffuse necrotizing metritis.

Flaviviruses in cattle, sheep, and pigs are capable of causing fetal death or malformation, depending on viral

Table 12-2. Pestiviruses and fetal disease

Species	Virus	Disease in the fetus	Disease in the adult
Cattle	Bovine virus diarrhea	Cerebellar hypoplasia Microphthalmia Retinal dysplasia	Bovine virus diarrhea
Sheep	Border disease	CNS myelin deficiency Decreased secondary hair follicles Skeletal immaturity	Caruncular angiopathy
Pigs	Hog cholera	One of the causes of congenital tremor syndrome	Hog cholera

strain, fetal age, and stage of development of the fetal immune system (Table 12-2). In the horse, equine viral arteritis virus causes abortion but, in the majority of cases, no fetal lesions. In this species, the mechanism is probably via fetal anoxia due to compression of uterine blood vessels by virus-induced myometritis, although a few cases of arteritis in the chorion and myocardium of aborted fetuses have been described.

Parvovirus in cats can cause congenital cerebellar hypoplasia. Feline panleukopenia virus causes selective necrosis of the rapidly dividing cells of the cerebellar extragranular layer. Porcine parvovirus is an important cause of embryonic and fetal loss, causing death and mummification of a proportion of affected litters. Swine fetuses infected before immunocompetence have widespread necrotizing lesions, together with inflammation and inclusion bodies, especially in the liver, lungs, kidneys and cerebellum. Damage to the fetal circulatory system leads to edema, hemorrhages, and the accumulation of serosanguinous fluid in body cavities.

Akabane virus and **Cache Valley virus** are bunyaviruses capable of causing fetal infection and abortion in sheep and other ruminants. The effect of the virus on the developing fetal central nervous system leads to a variety of lesions, such as hydranencephaly, microencephaly, cerebellar hypoplasia, and loss of spinal cord ventral horn neurons. Myositis and neurogenic muscle atrophy produce arthrogryposis (fixation of limb joints) and skeletal deformities, such as torticollis and scoliosis. In fetal lambs, developing hydranencephaly due to infection with bluetongue virus (an orbivirus) viral antigen can be found in immature neural cells associated with areas of necrosis in the subventricular zone of the cerebrum.

Protozoal causes

Toxoplasmosis caused by *Toxoplasma gondii* in sheep is an important cause of abortion. The organism has a cat-sheep life cycle, with contamination of sheep feed by cat feces and the ingestion of sheep fetal membranes by cats. Gross lesions in the fetal membranes are edema of the intercotyledonary chorioallantois and white, 1 to 2 mm foci in the cotyledons (Fig. 12-27). The fetus may have leucomalacia, believed to be a nonspecific effect of fetal anoxia secondary to placentitis. Microscopically, the cotyledonary lesions are distinctive because not only is there the inflammation common to many intrauterine infections, but there is also, at least in the stage before necrosis and sloughing, chorionic epithelial hypertrophy and hyperplasia, with rare groups of toxoplasmal organisms within chorionic epithelial cells.

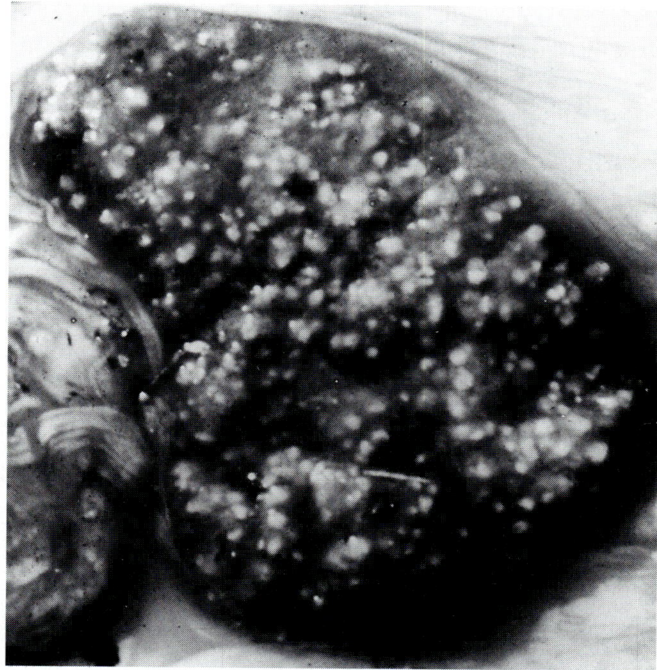

Fig. 12-27 Placenta; ewe. Placentitis and abortion due to *Toxoplasma gondii* infection. On the cotyledon are characteristic 1 to 2 mm white foci of inflammation, necrosis, and mineralization.

A protozoal organism resembling *Neospora caninum* has increasingly become frequently recognized as a cause of bovine abortion. Fetuses are of 3 to 9 months' gestation, with no gross lesions. In the brain, multiple foci of necrosis and gliosis are often adjacent to capillaries with hyperplastic endothelium. Protozoal organisms are in groups in these foci or are scattered more widely, sometimes in neural cells or endothelial cells. In the heart, the lesions are subacute multifocal inflammation of the epicardium, myocardium, and endocardium, with protozoal organisms present in myofibers or endothelial cells. Mononuclear portal hepatitis and multifocal hepatocellular necrosis with fibrin thrombi in sinusoids are common. Foci of mononuclear inflammatory cells can be present in a number of other organs, including the placenta.

Trichomoniasis, caused by *Tritrichomonas foetus* and transmitted by coitus in cattle, is another protozoal disease in which there may be abortion, mainly in the first half of pregnancy. Placentitis is mild, and no fetal lesion is observed, although the standard method of diagnosis is the demonstration of protozoa in the contents of the fetal stomach. Endometritis can be severe, and pyometra is a possible sequela.

UTERINE TUBES

Most lesions of the uterine tube are incidental or secondary to disorders elsewhere in the reproductive tract. In dogs and cats, it is considered that they are unlikely to affect reproductive performance. Lesions commonly encountered in small animals are duct remnants in the mesosalpinx. These are more often Wolffian (simple tubular structures lined by low columnar to cuboidal cells) than Müllerian (lined by a folded mucosa similar to the uterine tube mucosa).

Hydrosalpinx, distention of the uterine tube by clear fluid, is caused by mechanical or functional obstruction of the lumen. The obstruction can be at either end. The distention can be uniform or irregular and results in a thin wall and a tube increased in length and tortuosity. Extensive, multiloculated cysts form in the mucosa. The congenital type may be due to segmental aplasia of the uterine tube, present in freemartins, or, more likely, to segmental aplasia of the uterine horn. The acquired type is secondary to trauma or chronic inflammation; acute inflammation will cause pyosalpinx rather than hydrosalpinx. Trauma caused by manual interference with a corpus luteum in cattle may lead to the formation of an organizing hematoma about the uterine tube, causing obstruction from the peritoneal side. The same manipulation can force inflammatory exudate from the uterus into the tube, causing inflammation of the mucosa and obstruction of the lumen. Inflammatory exudate can be squeezed, manually or under the pressure of therapeutic uterine infusion, not only into the uterine tube but also into the ovarian bursa, where the ensuing inflammation can produce fibrous bands that compress the uterine tube. Hydrosalpinx or bacteriologically sterile pyosalpinx is one of the commonest causes of sterility in swine. It occurs almost exclusively in nulliparous animals and is almost always bilateral. The cause is unknown, but obstruction by embryonal rests of the Wolffian system has been proposed as a cause.

Salpingitis, in most cases, results from spread of infection from the uterus and is usually bilateral. Generally, it is not visible grossly, except perhaps for some hyperemia and thickening of the mucosa and the presence of a small amount of exudate in the lumen. Microscopically, the inflammation can vary from mild to severe and from acute to chronic (Fig. 12-28). Probably, even very mild inflammation interferes with fertility. Initially, loss of cilia and desquamation of epithelial cells occur at the tips of the mucosal folds. More severe salpingitis progresses to involve the remainder of the mucosa and, possibly, the muscle layer, with exudate in the lumen. With time, adhesions develop between the denuded areas, while adjacent mucosa becomes cystic, or the mucosa is replaced by granulation tissue.

Pyosalpinx has the same type of history as salpingitis. Grossly visible pus is present in loculi in the lumen follow-

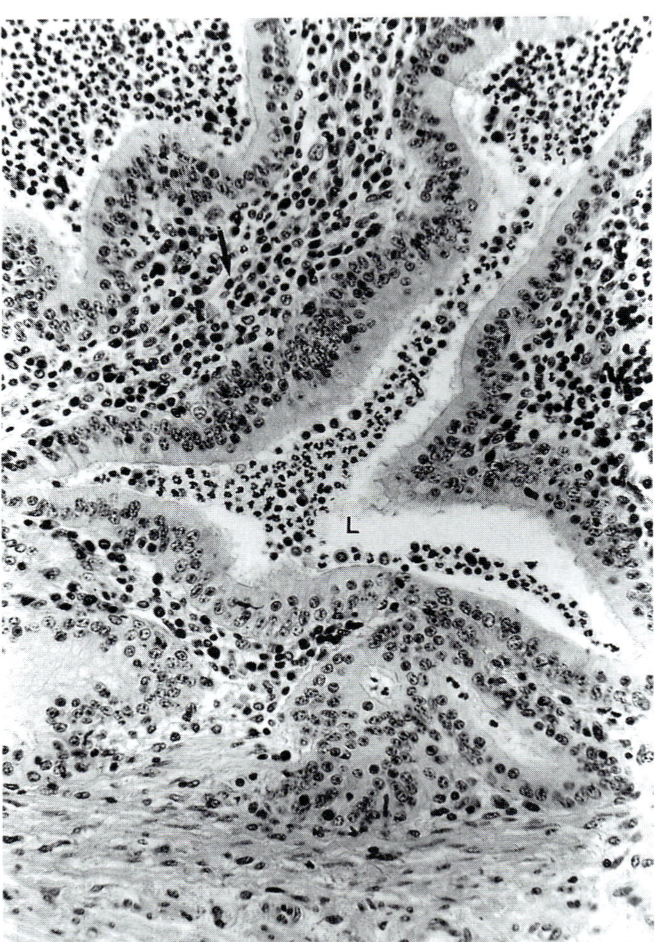

Fig. 12-28 Uterine tube; mare. Subacute salpingitis, contagious equine metritis. The lamina propria of the folds of the uterine tube is hypercellular and is infiltrated by inflammatory cells, mainly mononuclear *(arrow),* whereas the lumen (*L*) contains an inflammatory exudate that includes many neutrophils. H & E stain.

ing inflammation and obstruction. Microscopically, numerous neutrophils are present, along with other inflammatory cells, both within the tissues and in the mucosal cysts. Surviving epithelium may be scant; some of it undergoes squamous metaplasia.

OVARY

Developmental Anomalies

Occasionally, agenesis of one or both ovaries occurs. As part of the defect, tubular genitalia can be absent. In cases of bilateral agenesis, the tubular genitalia remain infantile. Another rare anomaly, duplication of an ovary, arises by two different mechanisms: by originating separately or by splitting from an already developing ovary. The latter type, an accessory ovary, is located close to the normally located organ and is usually connected to it.

Hypoplasia of the ovaries occurs in several species, but has been most studied in cattle. It is usually bilateral but nonsymmetric. The affected ovaries are small, usually without follicles but sometimes with cysts, and without surface scars from ovulation (Fig. 12-29). Microscopically, cortical stroma and ova are absent or poorly developed. Because the embryonic development of the female system happens passively, in the absence of testis-determining factor and not under the direction of gonadal hormone, it follows that ovarian hypoplasia does not lead to hypoplasia of the female genital tract. The tract, however, will remain infantile. Other causes of infantilism are malnutrition or some other form of debility. Infantilisms from the different causes are distinguishable from one another on morphologic grounds (by the presence of ovarian cortex) and on physiologic grounds (by response to gonadotropic hormones or the removal of the debilitating factor).

Hypoplasia with genetic or chromosomal abnormalities is reported. Swedish Highland cattle suffer ovarian hypoplasia from the effect of an autosomal recessive gene with incomplete penetrance. The defect is either unilateral or bilateral. There is a smaller-than-normal number of primordial follicles, a smaller-than-normal proportion of graafian follicles, and a tendency for luteinization to occur without ovulation. Cytogenetic abnormalities have been associated with ovarian hypoplasia. Examples are XXX chromosomes in the mare and cow and XO chromosomes in the mare. The latter type bears similarities to the XO disease in human females, called Turner's syndrome, in such features as small stature, lack of ovarian cyclic activity, and underdevelopment of the endometrium. The fetal gonad is normal, but the adult ovary contains no follicles.

Vascular hamartomas of the ovary are an incidental finding in the bovine, porcine, and equine species (Fig. 12-30). They form a dark red mass on the surface of the ovary and are composed of connective tissue and vascular channels lined by mature endothelial cells.

Cysts in the mesovarium adjacent to the ovary, called paraovarian cysts, arise from either the mesonephric or the paramesonephric duct. They can be up to several centi-

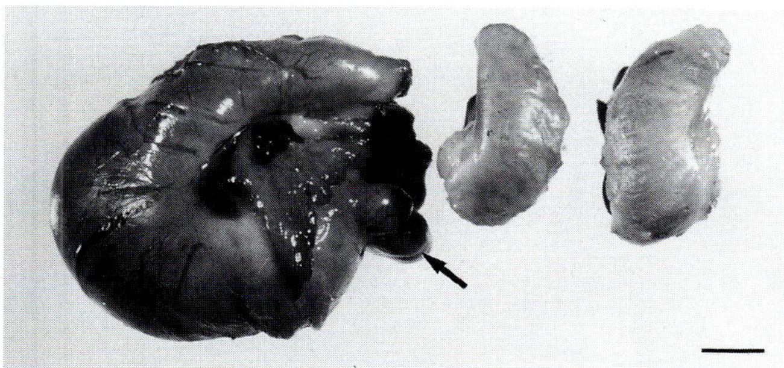

Fig. 12-29 Ovaries; two mares. Hypoplastic ovaries on the right, and normal ovary on left for comparison. Associated with the normal ovary are cysts *(arrow)* in the attached fimbriae of the uterine tube. Bar = 1 cm.

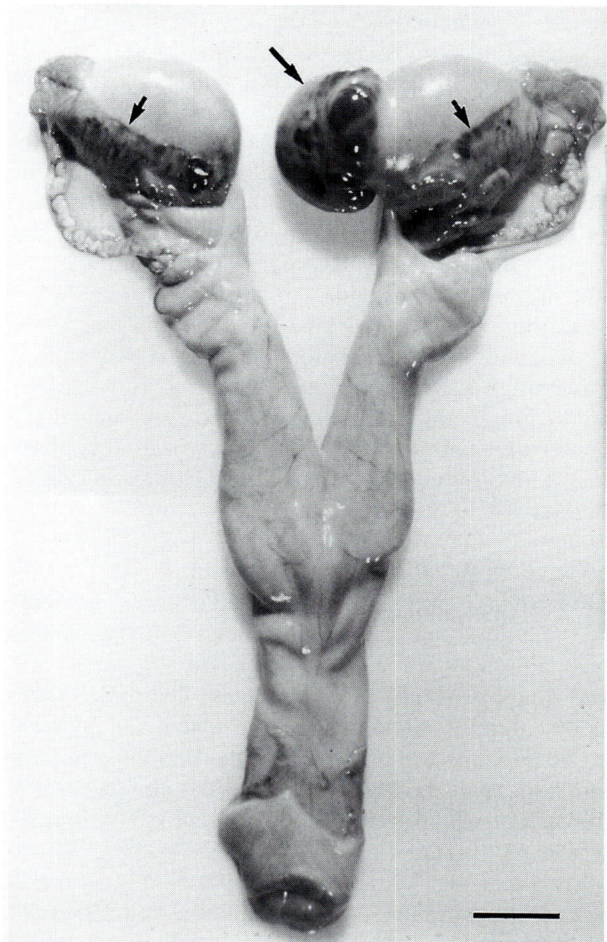

Fig. 12-30 Ovary, fetal foal. Vascular hamartoma *(long arrow)*. The margin between germinal epithelium and well-vascularized attachment zone is clearly demarcated *(short arrows)*. Bar = 2 cm.

meters in diameter. Those from the paramesonephric duct have less smooth muscle in their wall and are likely to be near the fimbriae of the oviduct. They occur most often in the mare. Cysts within the ovary are of three types: nongonadal stromal, gonadal stromal, and neoplastic. The latter two are described later. The nongonadal stromal cysts are not identical. One is a serous inclusion cyst, seen mostly in the bitch, and formed by a small area of surface lagging behind the rest in growth and losing continuity with the surface; the other is formed by cystic rete tubules, which can reach follicular size in the bitch and queen. Cystic rete ovarii is not as rare in the queen as had been thought. It expands into the ovarian stroma rather than into the mesovarium and is lined by ciliated columnar to flattened epithelium.

Acquired Ovarian Lesions

Oophoritis, inflammation of the ovary, is rare in domestic animals. Experimentally, infectious bovine rhinotracheitis virus induces necrotizing oophoritis in the postestrus cow, subsequent to viremia. Hemorrhages occur in the corpus luteum, and, in some cases, thick, cloudy, fibrinous fluid is in the follicles. Microscopically, the lesions in the corpus luteum vary from focal necrosis and infiltration of mononuclear cells to diffuse hemorrhage and necrosis. Most affected ovaries also have necrotic follicles and a diffuse mononuclear cell accumulation in the stroma.

Ovarian bursal adhesions are thin bands to large sheets of fibrous tissue crossing the space or binding together the walls of the ovarian bursa, a peritoneal pouch formed around the ovary by the broad ligament and the mesosalpinx. The lesion is often bilateral in cattle. It may be caused by ascending uterine infections resulting from complications of pregnancy, such as a retained placenta. Physical trauma from manipulations of the ovary is another possible cause. This lesion is common in beef heifers surveyed at slaughter.

Lesions Related to Cyclic Changes

Hemorrhage into follicles is sometimes present in calves; hemorrhage into cystic follicles happens occasionally in the bitch. Some hemorrhage, usually small, occurs at the time of ovulation in all species. The mare is an exception, normally shedding a large amount of blood into the cavity of the follicle, forming the **corpus hemorrhagicum.** Especially visible in the mare and cow, a focal area of serositis is set up at the point of ovulation. There is rapid progression through a fibrinous to a fibrous stage, forming an "ovulation tag." The manual expression of a persistent corpus luteum in the cow will sometimes be followed by severe hemorrhage. Organization of the blood clot can cause adhesions between the ovary and adjacent structures.

Atretic follicles are, in most cases, normal phenomena. In any estrus cycle, only one or a small number of follicles is destined to mature, while the others undergo atresia at various stages of maturation. A similar process occurs in seasonal anestrus and, in some species, in pregnancy. Follicular atresia is considered abnormal when it is part of any disease process that interferes with the release of, or the pituitary gland response to, gonadotropin-releasing hormone. Development of the follicle can be arrested at any stage, and this is followed, after an unknown amount of time, by degeneration. The ovum and zona pellucida undergo necrosis first; then, the granulosa cells become pyknotic, vacuolate, and desquamate. The follicle may persist in this form, a cyst with a thin partial lining of granulosa cells, or it may be invaded by macrophages, theca cells, and fibrous connective tissue to eventually become a small scar.

Cystic Graafian follicles are important in cows and sows. In dairy cows, the prolongation of the postpartum interval to first estrus is the main effect, as ovulation does not occur. Bovine cystic follicles are 2.5 cm or more in diameter and persist for 10 or more days without the formation of a corpus luteum (Fig. 12-31). They are probably due to an insufficiency of luteinizing hormone (LH), although the mechanism is not understood. An analysis of LH receptors,

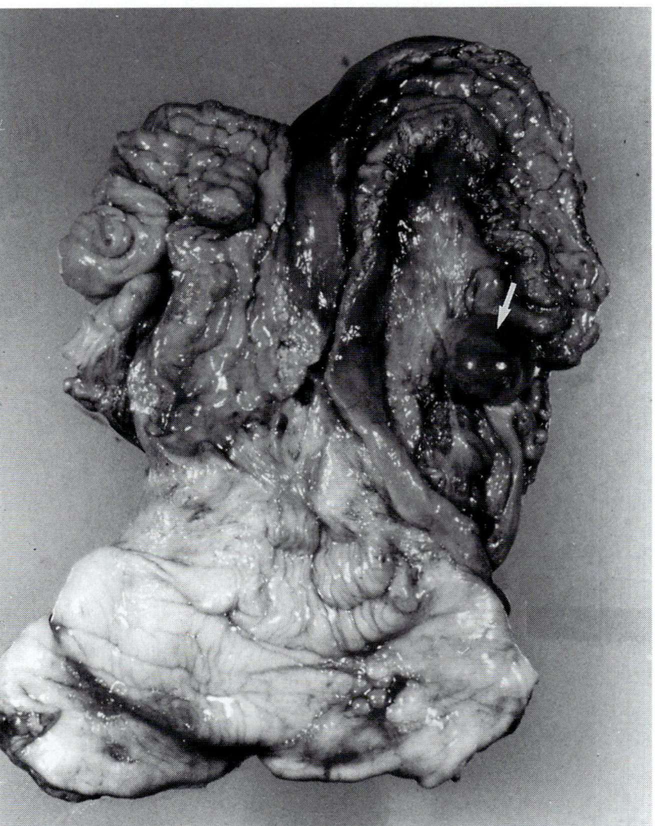

Fig. 12-31 Genital tract; cow. Cystic ovary. A large cyst *(arrow)* is present on one ovary.

especially an answer to the question of whether the full complement is acquired, would contribute to the understanding of cystic follicles. Cystic follicles were the most common genital lesion in a large slaughterhouse survey of beef heifers. There was an association with the use of melengestrol acetate, a compound resembling progesterone, used to inhibit estrus by suppressing LH release.

There is evidence of postpartum uterine infection causing cystic ovaries in dairy cows. To link the presence of cystic ovaries with the recovery of *E. coli* from the uterus and elevated concentrations of serum $PGF_{2\alpha}$ metabolites and cortisol, it has been proposed that bacterial endotoxins or prostaglandins produced because of damage by endotoxins stimulate the adrenal gland secretion of cortisol, which, in turn, suppresses preovulatory release of LH, resulting in development of cysts.

Follicular cysts in the cow may be single or multiple, may be unilateral or bilateral, and are usually thin-walled. Microscopically, the granulosa cell layer is thicker than normal or is degenerating, eventually becoming a flattened single cell layer, with no evidence of luteinization. The surrounding theca cell layer is thin, and the cells may become partially luteinized. Luteinization is more common when the granulosa cell layer is absent, and it is possible that only the theca interna cells become luteinized. Follicular cysts are capable of spontaneous regression; however, those that arise after the first postpartum ovulation are likely to be replaced by other follicles that become cystic. The remainder of the genital system may bear evidence of long-term estrogen stimulation.

Anovulatory luteinized cysts are thought to be caused by delayed or insufficient release of LH. The ovulation papilla is absent, because ovulation does not occur. The cystic cavity is lined by fibrous tissue, and an adjacent zone is composed of luteinized theca cells. Cystic follicles and luteinized cysts may be present in the same ovary. The degree of luteinization that must occur in a cystic follicle to justify its designation as a luteal cyst has not been defined.

Cystic corpus luteum has an uncertain pathogenesis. In cattle, it must be distinguished from an anovulatory luteinized cyst and from the small central cyst that can occur normally in a corpus luteum. Ovulation occurs, and a large irregular cyst develops. There is no interference with the length of the estrous cycle. It has been suggested that in swine, at least, the cysts found in ovaries are different degrees of the same aberration and that the morphologic form, whether it be an ovulated or unovulated follicle or a corpus luteum, is determined by the stage of the process at which the breakdown in the physiologic process occurs.

Supernumerary follicles are induced in the bovine ovary by drugs used to cause superovulation in preparation for embryo transfer. In these cows, it is not unusual for more than a dozen well-developed follicles or corpora lutea of the same age to be present (Fig. 12-32).

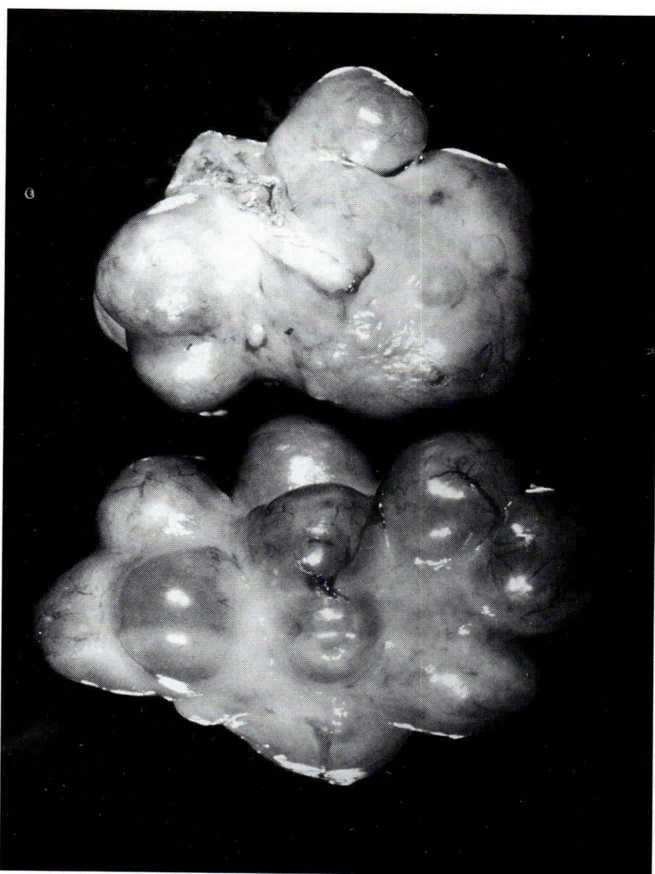

Fig. 12-32 Ovaries; cow. Numerous corpora lutea instead of the normal one or two. The cow had been treated with drugs that caused superovulation.

Neoplasms

Germ cell neoplasms

The ovum following fertilization differentiates to form embryonic and extraembryonic (placental or yolk sac) tissues. It would be expected that neoplasms arising from germ cells could be benign or malignant and undifferentiated or could differentiate along either embryonic or extraembryonic lines. In practice, in domestic animals, the great majority of neoplasms of germ cells are benign undifferentiated type (dysgerminoma) or benign with somatic differentiation (teratoma).

Dysgerminoma, a rare neoplasm composed of cells resembling primitive germ cells, has been described in the bitch, sow, and cow. The neoplasm is usually a solid lobulated mass with areas of hemorrhage and necrosis. It is analogous to seminoma in the male. Mitotic rate is high, but metastases are rare.

Ovarian **teratomas** are rare, usually well differentiated and benign. They arise from totipotential primordial germ cells and possess jumbled elements of at least two of the

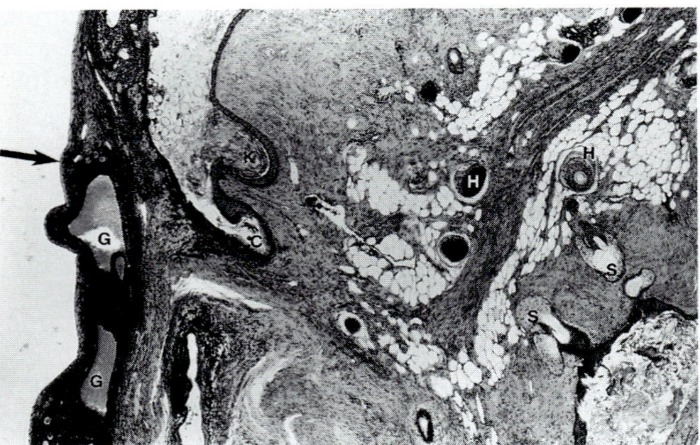

Fig. 12-33 Ovary; monkey. Teratoma. Note normal ovarian structures such as primordial follicles *(arrowhead),* and graafian follicles (*G*). Among the nonovarian elements are hair follicles (*H*), sebaceous glands (*S*), and keratinizing squamous epithelium (*K*) merging with columnar epithelium (*C*). *Courtesy Dr. T.G. Hodge.*

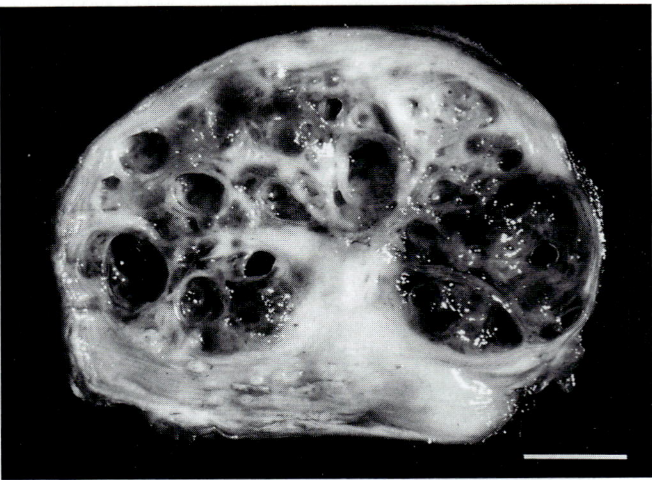

Fig. 12-34 Ovary; mare. Granulosa cell tumor. The ovary is greatly enlarged by multiple, fluid-filled cysts. The polycystic form is the most frequently encountered granulosa cell tumor. Bar = 1 cm. *Courtesy Dr. M.D. McGavin.*

three embryonic germ layers. Most teratomas are of the well-differentiated type, and many of these have a significant dermal component (Fig. 12-33). Malignant teratomas are even rarer, except in the dog.

Gonadal stromal neoplasms

Granulosa cell tumors are the most commonly found ovarian neoplasms in large animals. They are unilateral, smooth-surfaced, round and can be 20 to 30 cm in diameter. They can be solid, cystic, or polycystic (Fig. 12-34), with the fluid red-brown. Microscopically, the granulosa cells are not very different from normal granulosa cells and often are arranged as they would be in normal Graafian follicles, i.e., in single or multiple rows of round to columnar cells lining the fluid-filled spaces (Fig. 12-35). Sometimes, especially in cats, Call-Exner bodies are present in the fluid. These are rosettes of granulosa cells, some containing an eosinophilic body in the central space. In less differentiated areas, the neoplastic cells are arranged in sheets. The stroma can be sparse or plentiful; if the stroma predominates, the neoplasm is a **thecoma.** The cytoplasm of the thecoma cells may contain lipid droplets. Areas of luteinization in granulosa-theca cell neoplasms are not uncommon, but **luteomas,** neoplasms in which there is a uniform population of luteinized cells, are rare. Luteomas can probably develop from either granulosa or theca cells. Granulosa cell tumors are often malignant in the cat and sometimes in the bitch, but otherwise the sex cord stromal neoplasms are usually benign. Many stromal neoplasms produce steroids. The mare may have anestrus, nymphomania, or stallionlike behavior, whereas the bitch is likely to have prolonged estrus as well as lesions associated with

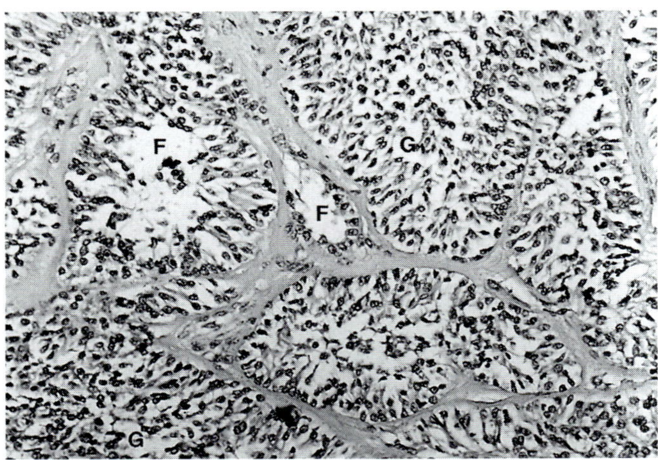

Fig. 12-35 Ovary; mare. Granulosa cell tumor. Granulosa cells are in large groups (*G*) without a central cavity as well as in structures resembling normal follicles (*F*). H & E stain.

progesterone production, namely, cystic endometrial hyperplasia and pyometra.

Surface neoplasms

The ovaries are covered by coelomic epithelium, the same layer of tissue that invaginates in early fetal life to form the lining of the genital tract. Neoplasms of the ovarian surface, thus, can resemble the several types of neoplasms of the endometrium. In practice, the serous type is the only important one in animals. Serous papillary cystadenoma and cystadenocarcinoma occur commonly in the

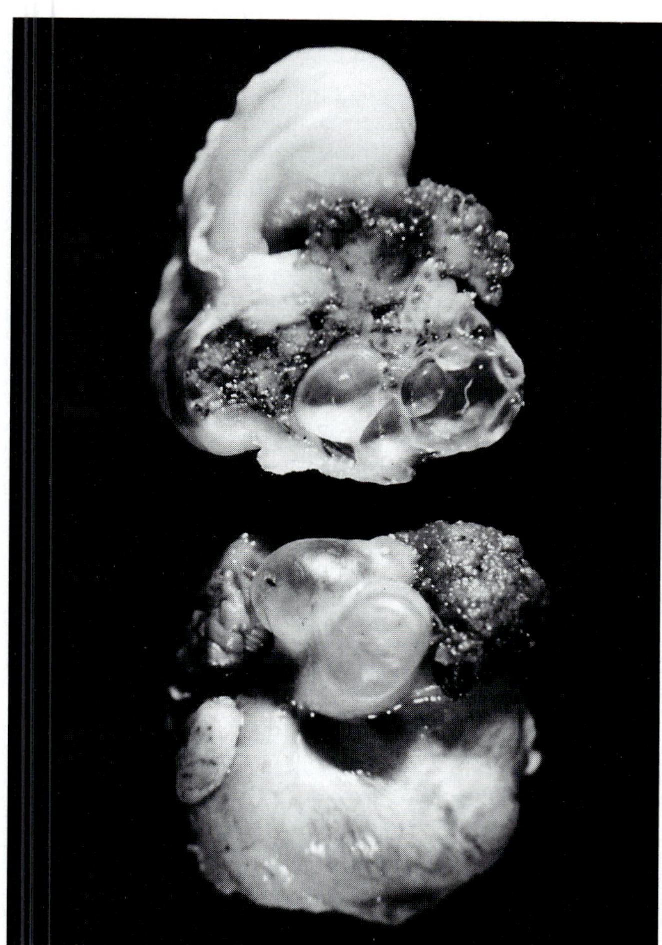

Fig. 12-36 Ovaries; bitch. Bilateral papillary cystadenocarcinoma. Large cysts and finely cystic tissue project from the surface of the ovaries.

bitch (Fig. 12-36). They originate from the epithelium of the surface or rest within the ovary or the rete ovarii. The neoplasms are frequently bilateral and shaggy-surfaced. Spread over the peritoneal surface occurs in the malignant forms. Ascites may result from obstruction of the diaphragmatic lymph vessels or from fluid secretion by the neoplasm.

MAMMARY GLAND

Inflammation

Mastitis in domestic animals is almost solely due to invasion by microorganisms. Bovine mastitis is a source of great economic loss. Because of increased vascular permeability, plasma components enter milk and ion balance is altered. The products of inflammation enter milk, altering its appearance. Alveolar epithelium damaged by inflammation or by pressure from adjacent inflammation secretes less milk.

The vast majority of organisms responsible for bovine mastitis are bacteria. These bacteria can be divided into those for which the mammary gland is the reservoir, such as *Streptococcus agalactiae, Staphylococcus aureus,* and *Mycoplasma* sp.; those for which the environment is the reservoir, into which group coliforms fall; and an overlap group, with organisms capable of persisting in either location, such as *Streptococcus uberis* and *S. dysgalactiae.* Cow-to-cow transmission is important for the mammary reservoir group, whereas contamination of the teat end by organisms from the environment is important for disease caused by the environmental group. The rates of new intramammary infections caused by environmental pathogens are greatest during the first and the last 2 weeks of a 60-day nonlactating period in dairy cows. These coliform infections and streptococcal infections from the environment that are established in the nonlactating period and are present at parturition cause clinical mastitis soon afterward.

Although hematogenous and percutaneous entry are possible, the usual route is via the teat canal (streak canal), the approximately 1-cm long, keratinized, stratified squamous epithelium-lined duct between the exterior and the teat sinus (teat cistern). Colonization of the lining of the teat canal may serve as a reservoir of bacteria for intramammary infection.

Non–Immune-mediated Defense Mechanisms in the Mammary Gland

The teat orifice and the teat canal offer mechanical resistance to the entry of organisms. Possibly the longer teat canal in cows protects against intramammary infection. The keratin of the teat canal may offer protection by adsorbing bacteria, desquamating when coated with bacteria, desiccating, and having bactericidal fatty acids. Infection and inflammation of the teat canal are rare.

The mammary gland has some intrinsic defense mechanisms that are not immune mediated. Regular milking out of the mammary gland probably is a natural defense mechanism, by virtue of the flushing of organisms and the products of inflammation. Lactoferrin, the major iron-binding protein of secretions, is a nonspecific natural protective factor in milk. The bulk of lactoferrin in milk is produced by mammary epithelial cells. It is increased in acute mastitis and in the involuting gland. The binding of iron withholds an essential nutrient from pathogenic bacteria, thus having a bacteriostatic effect. The lactoperoxidase-thiocyanate-H_2O_2 system temporarily inhibits some streptococci, coliforms, and *Staphylococcus aureus.* Lactoperoxidase is synthesized in mammary epithelium; thiocyanate is derived from certain green feeds, and H_2O_2 is produced by streptococci or comes from an exogenous source. Hypothiocyanite produced by the system damages the inner bacterial membrane. Lysozyme, synthesized locally or from blood, destroys bacteria by lysis of cell wall peptidoglycan. Of minor importance is complement activated by the alternate pathway in response to the presence of bacterial endotoxin.

Immune-mediated Defense Mechanisms in the Mammary Gland

Cellular mechanisms

The first elements bacteria encounter in the cellular defense system are cells of the lamina propria of the teat canal and the rosette of Furstenberg. The rosette is at the base of the teat cistern, immediately proximal to the junction between stratified squamous epithelium lining the teat canal and the one or two layers of cuboidal or columnar cell lining the teat cistern. The rosette area can be regarded as where the gland proper begins. The lamina propria of the teat canal and Furstenberg's rosette contain in their lining greater numbers of immunoglobulin-bearing leukocytes than parenchymal mammary tissue, in both uninfected and infected quarters. The number is greatest for Furstenberg's rosette in infected compared with uninfected quarters. In one study, the leukocytes were neutrophils and macrophages, not plasma cells, and the antibody was cytophilic or endocytosed. In another study, the subepithelial cells in Furstenberg's rosette were predominantly plasma cells and the major antibody produced was IgG_1.

In the mammary parenchyma, in both the alveoli and the interstitium, as well as in the lamina propria of the teat cistern, gland cistern, and interlobular and intralobular ducts, the macrophage is the resident cell involved in defense of the mammary gland against bacterial invasion. Macrophages are the most numerous cells in normal mammary secretions. Apparently at least 500,000 phagocytes per milliliter are needed for defense of the mammary gland against invading bacteria. In an uninfected bovine mammary gland, there are 50,000 to 200,000 neutrophils and macrophages per milliliter in milk, with macrophages predominating.

Upon stimulation by the presence of microorganisms, macrophages produce interleukin-1, which causes increased membrane phospholipase activity, with formation of arachidonic acid, which is a substrate for the production of prostaglandins and leukotrienes. Leukotriene B_4, produced by typical macrophages, is a powerful attractant of neutrophils. Whether the principle is followed by milk macrophages remains to be evaluated. Milk macrophages secrete less interleukin-1 than blood macrophages, a property common to macrophages from healthy and inflamed quarters of the mammary gland. Recruitment of neutrophils from the blood to an infection site is one of the first steps in an inflammatory response. Recruitment can be so rapid, that neutrophils are prominent even 2 hours after infection. Cell counts in milk average 700,000 per milliliter in subclinically infected quarters, and millions are common in clinical infections. Neutrophils are the principal effector cells in eliminating bacteria from the mammary gland. The principal method by which neutrophils kill bacteria is by phagocytosis after opsonization by antibody, with or without complement. A method of minor importance is lysis by antibody plus complement.

There is a cycling up and down every several days of the numbers of inflammatory cells (mostly neutrophils) in milk in experimental staphylococcal mastitis and an inverse cycling of the number of viable bacteria. As cell counts are at a peak, bactericidal activity per cell is most efficient, by as much as 10,000-fold, and phagocytosis is optimal. The frequency and periodicity of the cycle, as well as the amplitude of the cell and bacterial count, are independent for each infected quarter. The likely source of reinfection is those neutrophils that are inefficient at killing intracellular bacteria at the time of low cell count. As these cells undergo death and lysis, their protected bacteria are released to continue the cycle.

Although neutrophils recruited from the blood are so important in fighting infection in the mammary gland, they do not kill bacteria as well in milk as they do in blood. Some possible reasons are the absence of glucose (required for glycolysis by macrophages) in milk, decreased amounts of glycogen in neutrophils of milk, deficiency of opsonins and complement in milk, coating of the surface of neutrophils with casein, loss of neutrophil pseudopodia caused by ingestion of fat, and decrease of hydrolytic enzymes within neutrophils after ingestion of casein and fat.

In the first week after parturition, when neutrophils are likely to be most needed to deal with intramammary infections, bovine blood neutrophils already are defective before they pass into the mammary gland. They have significantly impaired chemokinesis and decreased superoxide anion production, antibody-dependent cell-mediated cytotoxicity, and ingestion of bacteria. The reason is probably some combination of the effects of stress, energy and protein demands of early lactation, and the hormonal fluxes of the stage of the reproductive cycle.

Interleukin-1 from macrophages also stimulates the immune system by activating T- and B-lymphocytes. The role of lymphocytes in defense of the mammary gland has not been established clearly, although they probably enhance phagocytosis through the production of specific opsonins. The stage of the reproductive cycle has an influence on lymphocytes. Bovine blood lymphocyte blastogenesis is markedly impaired in the first week after parturition. The proportion of T- and B-lymphocytes and macrophages in mammary gland secretion varies with the stage of lactation. In the postparturient period, the percentage of macrophages is greatest, and the proportion of T-lymphocytes is greatest in late lactation. The ratio of $CD4^+$:$CD8^+$ T-lymphocytes in mammary gland secretion is different from that in blood. Interleukin-2, one of the many T cell–derived cytokines, is present in smaller amounts in mammary secretions of the cow in the last week of gestation compared with 2 weeks prior to parturition, correlating with increased susceptibility to mastitis. The amount of TNF in mammary secretions increases toward the end of gestation. The increase is in concert with the increase in the number of macrophages, which are the source of TNF. The increased amount of TNF may contribute to the poor performance of mammary neutrophils in the postparturient period.

Humoral mechanisms

Antibody concentration in normal bovine milk is low, about 1 mg/ml. Most IgG is serum derived, and IgG_1 is selectively transferred into mammary secretion and is the major immunoglobulin class in milk. IgG_2 is both serum derived and locally produced. IgA and IgM are synthesized locally in the udder. Local production is by stimulation of subepithelial lymphocytes. Particulate antigens, such as bacteria, stimulate an antibody response in the mammary gland of the cow, whereas soluble antigens may not. In colostrum and in inflammation, antibody concentrations approach 50 mg/ml. Early in inflammation, IgG_1 and IgG_2 opsonize bacteria for enhanced phagocytosis by macrophages, but later the importance of IgG_2 as an opsonin increases as neutrophils enter the gland. IgM also functions as an opsonin. IgA does not opsonize but may prevent bacterial adherence to epithelium, inhibit bacterial multiplication, neutralize leucocyte-inhibiting bacterial toxins, and agglutinate bacteria.

Specific Pathogens in Mastitis

Streptococcus agalactiae was the most important pathogen for the bovine mammary gland in the days before the understanding of the importance of hygiene and before the availability of efficient antibacterial drugs. Resistance of cows to mastitis caused by this organism is subject to great individual variation; in general, resistance decreases with age. The mammary gland is the only organ affected by this organism, and *S. agalactiae* does not persist long in the environment. Once a cow is infected, however, the organism persists in the teat and gland cistern, with periodic waves of multiplication, increase in virulence, and tissue invasion. The initial response to invasion of streptococci is interstitial edema and influx of neutrophils into the interstitium and alveoli. The alveolar epithelium undergoes either brief hyperplasia or vacuolation and then desquamates. Macrophages are added to the cell population of invaded alveoli, and fibrosis rapidly obliterates the lumen of these alveoli. Edema, cellular infiltration, and fibrosis proceed around the alveoli invaded by streptococci and around adjacent alveoli, so that there is a pressure effect within the lobule and within adjacent lobules that causes stagnation of milk flow, thereby initiating premature involution of part of the gland. At the same time, the streptococci attack the ducts. After the acute phase, periductal fibrosis occurs, and granulation tissue replaces part of the normal cuboidal or columnar epithelium of smaller ducts, sometimes with the generation of polypous protrusions and the possible complete obstruction of milk flow. Restoration of epithelium can occur after cicatrization of the granulation tissue. The lobar ducts and sinuses, with their normally bistratified columnar epithelium, are similarly but less severely affected, often going through a phase of squamous metaplasia of the epithelium.

The gross appearance of the quarter with mastitis caused by *S. agalactiae* depends on the stage of the disease. Also, different stages are to be expected in different areas of a gland. Usually, more than one quarter is involved. In the acute stage, some hyperemia of the mucosa of the sinuses may be seen. Milk quality is altered, so that strands or floccules of debris are present or the milk is transformed into pus. The areas of parenchymal edema and cellular infiltration are gray and turgid. Groups of alveoli in which the secretion is retained because of obstruction of the duct by granulation tissue resemble small abscesses. Involuting and fibrotic parenchyma may be difficult to distinguish. Duct and sinus mucosae become granular and thickened because of underlying projecting areas of granulation tissue and surrounding fibrosis.

Isolates of *Staphylococcus aureus* from the bovine mammary gland range from apathogenic to highly pathogenic. Hemolysis and production of coagulase in culture are useful guides to pathogenicity. Extracellular products released during staphylococcal growth and the ability of the organisms to adhere to epithelial surfaces are important virulence factors. The severest form of staphylococcal mastitis is the gangrenous form (Fig. 12-37), usually occurring at the time of calving and affecting a variable amount of the udder. Stages of severe acute inflammation, with classical signs of heat, redness, swelling, and pain, progress to necrosis with coldness of the affected area, blue-black color, fluid exudation, and crepitation. Microscopically, in the first 48 hours after infection with *S. aureus,* infected tissue has more interalveolar stromal area, reduced alveolar luminal area, and more damaged and involuted alveolar epithelial area. Progressive swelling, vacuolar degeneration, and focal erosion and ulceration occur throughout the duct system and are most prominent near the junction of stratified squamous epithelium and columnar epithelium in the area of the rosette of Furstenberg. The organism attaches to epithelial cells, causes focal damage, and, later, can be seen on, within, and below ductal and alveolar epithelium. The

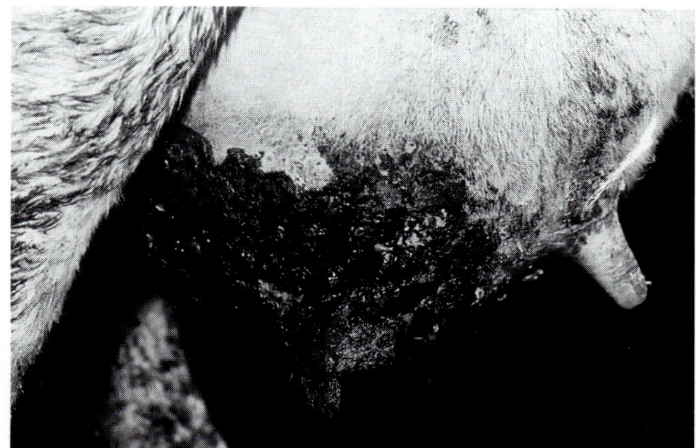

Fig. 12-37 Mammary gland; cow. Gangrenous mastitis. Acute staphylococcal or coliform mastitis has resulted in necrosis of the right hindquarter of the gland. Eventually, it will slough. *Courtesy Dr. M.D. McGavin.*

cellular response is rapid, with neutrophils initially in the subepithelial tissues of the distal parts of the duct system, then within the epithelium, and, later, in the secretory tissue.

Staphylococcal mastitis in the less acute form follows a course similar to that of the streptococcal disease. Initially, damage occurs to the epithelium of the cistern and larger ducts, and organisms move rapidly up the ducts to produce acute inflammation in groups of adjacent terminal alveoli. In chronically infected quarters, macrophages are the principal inflammatory cell type in the epithelial lining, lumens, and, especially, in the glandular interstitium. Lymphocytes also increase in number, but, sometimes, there is a lack of increase in plasma cells. This cytologic evidence suggests that mammary lymphocytes may become hyporesponsive to antigenic stimulation in quarters chronically infected with *S. aureus.* There is a suggestion that mammary lymphocyte function is compromised, from the observation of depressed blastogenesis in lymphocytes recovered from quarters infected with *S. aureus.* Plasma cells may be prevalent in the stroma of mammary glands with chronic *S. aureus* mastitis, and where there are more cells with IgA than IgG, and in IgA-containing cells. The prevalance increases as the disease progresses. It is unclear whether damaged alveoli redevelop secretory tissue or remaining healthy tissue undergoes compensatory hypertrophy or both.

Necrosis can be a prelude to abscess formation. Abscesses, scattered and often coalescing, range in size from microscopic to grossly visible. There is no evidence that the organisms pass through the alveolar epithelium into the interalveolar tissue before abscess formation. Sometimes, the staphylococci are surrounded by rosettes of immunoglobulin-containing club-shaped material. (The obsolete term botryomycosis was applied to such lesions.) An equally important and parallel set of events happening in the lobules not invaded by bacteria are the obstruction of milk flow by granulation tissue and the pressure from surrounding fibrosis, causing involution of those lobules. Disease caused by less pathogenic strains of staphylococci, such as nonhemolytic coagulase-negative strains, progresses less dramatically, not necessarily with obvious abscess formation, but has the same components of granulation tissue and fibrosis, causing obstruction and pressure, which, in turn, cause atrophy of adjacent lobules.

Coliform mastitis is caused after organisms from the environment contaminate the teat end. The most common organisms are *E. coli, Enterobacter aerogenes,* and *Klebsiella pneumoniae.* The coliform organisms probably exert their effect via endotoxin acting on the vasculature. In the acute disease, hyperemia, hemorrhage, and edema of the affected areas are found around ducts (Fig. 12-38), with fibrin thrombi in interstitial lymph vessels, and very little entry of inflammatory cells into alveoli (Fig. 12-39); but coliform organisms are numerous in the alveoli. The se-

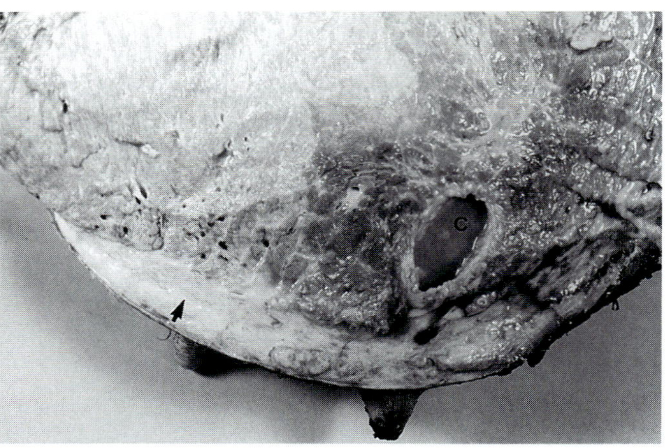

Fig. 12-38 Mammary gland, transverse section; cow. Severe acute coliform mastitis. Watery milk, flecked with fibrin, is in the gland cistern (*C*). Note the subcutaneous edema *(arrow). Courtesy Dr. M.D. McGavin.*

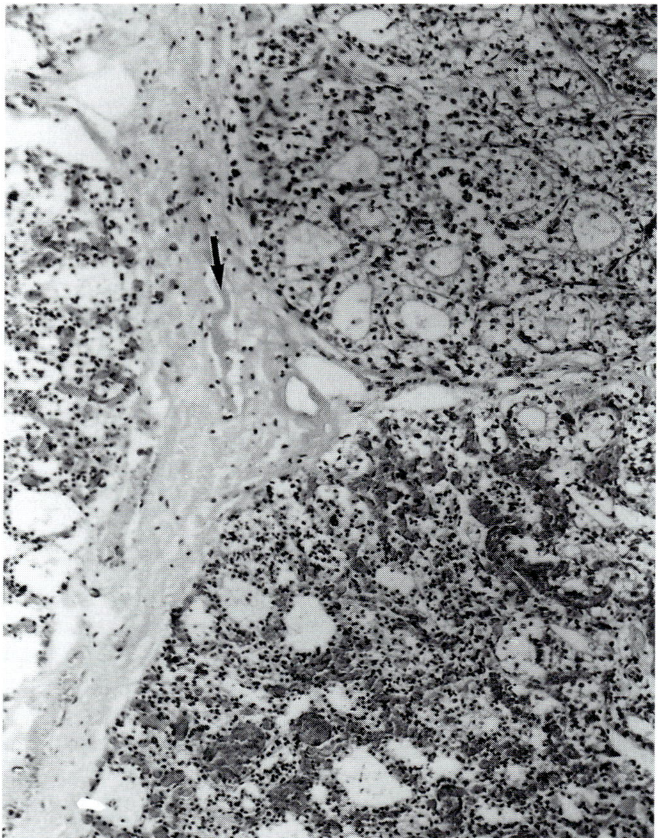

Fig. 12-39 Mammary gland; cow. Acute coliform mastitis. The connective tissue between adjacent hyperemic and nonhyperemic lobules is edematous. In the hyperemic lobules, there is much necrosis and sloughing of alveolar epithelium. A fibrinous thrombus is present in an interlobular lymphatic vessel. H & E stain.

verity of the disease in newly calved cows is attributed to a delay in the influx of neutrophils. However, the cow's response to endotoxin is influenced by the stage of the reproductive cycle. The nonlactating mammary gland responds much less to endotoxin than does the lactating gland in which phagocytosis of large numbers of organisms by secretory epithelium occurs.

Necrosis and sequestration of the necrotic tissue from viable tissue are the outcome of the acute disease if the animal survives. In cows in early lactation, the less severe coliform mastitis may go on to a chronic mastitis that has features of hyperplasia and disorganization and filiform processes of the epithelial cells of the teat and lactiferous sinuses.

Actinomyces pyogenes causes a disease in lactating, nonlactating, and even immature bovine udders, which is characterized by abscess formation in the large and small ducts. Fistulas can form at the base of the teat. In some glands, necrosis is extensive; whereas, in other glands, the result is diffuse fibrosis.

Mycoplasma mastitis in the cow occurs in herds in which the conventional forms of bacterial mastitis have been suppressed. Several mycoplasmas are capable of causing bovine mastitis, but *Mycoplasma bovis* is by far the most prevalent. The disease caused by *M. bovis* tends to involve the whole gland, with the production of a pronounced, purulent exudate in the early stages. Initially, the affected quarters are enlarged and firm, with light brown, nodular parenchyma. Abscesses up to 10 cm in diameter may form. Exudation of neutrophils into the lobular interstitium and alveoli is intense in the early stages. Early, vacuolation and degeneration of alveolar epithelium is followed by hyperplasia of alveolar and ductular epithelium, and, then, metaplasia to a relatively undifferentiated, multilayered lining. The exudate composition changes to include mononuclear cells. Lymphoid accumulations form in the lobular interstitium and around ducts. Focal erosions of duct epithelium are replaced by granulation tissue. Interstitial fibrosis and lobular atrophy occur in the late stages.

Granulomatous mastitis occurs naturally in some cases of bovine tuberculosis. It also occurs iatrogenically when contaminated therapeutic products are introduced through the teat canal of the cow.

Tuberculous mastitis exists in three forms—miliary, organ, and caseous—and all of them involve the ducts. In the cow, *Mycobacterium bovis* probably arrives at the mammary gland hematogenously. In most cases, it appears that the first lesions are in the alveoli, with later spread to the ducts, although progression in the opposite direction is evident in those few animals with minimal glandular involvement. Most cases are of the organ type, but a few are of the miliary type, which occurs when there has been massive release of organisms into a relatively naive organ, or of the caseous type, which occurs when the resistance of the organ is especially lowered. The miliary type is easy to recognize because of the very numerous, up to 1 cm, slightly yellow, often caseocalcareous nodules; and the caseous type is so named because of the large, irregular caseous areas bounded by zones of active granulomatous inflammation or fibrosis. The organ type of bovine tuberculosis, however, can be only slightly abnormal on gross appearance, even when the microscopic lesions are severe. The greater part of the organ can be involved, yet, on the cut surface, there is just an accentuation of lobulation, with a mild bulging of white or gray lobular parenchyma and distinct interlobular fibrous septa. Caseation is not prominent. Microscopically, the miliary type consists of classical tubercles, with central caseation surrounded by a zone of epithelioid macrophages and multinucleate giant cells, bounded by lymphocytes and fibrous tissue. In the more common organ type, the same cellular elements are present but with less orderliness. Milk quality is unaltered until very late in the course of the disease. Supramammary lymph nodes are usually involved, with a granulomatous lymphodenitis.

Iatrogenic granulomatous mastitis in the cow can be brought about when mastitis treatments introduced through the teat canal are contaminated with *Nocardia asteroides, Cryptococcus neoformans,* other *Mycobacterium* sp., or *Candida* sp. Nocardiosis can also be a spontaneous mastitis, from organisms resident in the soil. Features of the disease are systemic illness and the development of discharging sinuses from the mammary gland through the skin. An udder affected with cryptococcal mastitis has the same gray, gelatinous material that is typical of cryptococcal lesions elsewhere.

Mastitis in Nonbovine Species

Ovine progressive pneumonia virus is capable of causing mastitis in sheep. Clinical signs and gross lesions may be absent, but there is a diffuse interstitial accumulation of lymphocytes and focal degeneration of ductal epithelium. In more severe cases, the lesions are periductal lymphoid nodules with germinal centers and overlying epithelial hyperplasia, vacuolation, and focal necrosis. The mammary gland is a highly susceptible target organ of this nononcogenic retrovirus, possibly facilitating spread of the virus to other animals through the milk. Caprine arthritis-encephalitis virus, a closely related retrovirus found in goats, has been associated with diffuse and nodular infiltrates of lymphocytes and a few macrophages around ducts in the mammary gland. The virus can be recovered from the mammary gland of goats possessing antibody to the virus. In this disease too, involvement of the mammary gland is important from an epidemiologic standpoint.

Mycoplasma agalactiae causes mastitis in ewes and does, especially does, in Mediterranean countries. The disease is generalized, with localization to the joints and eyes as well as the mammary gland. Edema of the interstitium is the first mammary gland lesion, and, if the animal survives, interstitial fibrosis and glandular atrophy ensue.

Pasteurella haemolytica causes mastitis in lactating ewes, sometimes associated with rhinitis and pneumonia in their lambs. Usually only one of the two quarters is affected. There is an acute phase, with swelling of the gland and watery secretion, followed by blue discoloration due to necrosis. If the disease is not fatal at this stage, abscess formation and, then, sloughing will occur.

It is likely that coliform mastitis plays a part in the important clinical syndrome of mastitis-metritis-agalactia in sows. Some degree of visible mastitis is present in at least one gland in over 50% of affected animals, although metritis may not be a significant component. The lesions in the mammary gland have not received much descriptive attention, but it is likely that they are similar to those of acute coliform mastitis in the cow. The pathogenesis of the agalactia may be the suppression of prolactin production by the lipopolysaccharide of bacterial endotoxin, mediated at the level of the adenohypophysis or hypothalamus.

Mastitis is not common in dogs and cats, and, when it does occur, it is likely to be a sequela to minor lesions of the nipples or to be superimposed on mammary hyperplasia or neoplasia. The organisms most responsible are streptococci and staphylococci, which, in the acute phase, tend to cause suppurative and necrotizing inflammation, respectively.

Suggested Readings

Al-Bassam MA, Thomson RG, O'Donnel L. Involution abnormalities in the postpartum uterus of the bitch. Vet Pathol 1981; 18:208-218.

Allen GP, Bryans JT. Molecular epizootiology, pathogenesis, and prophylaxis of equine herpesvirus-1 infections. Prog Vet Microbiol Immunol 1986; 2:78-144.

Anderson JC. Progressive pathology of staphylococcal mastitis with a note on control, immunisation and therapy. Vet Rec 1982; 110:372-376.

Anderson TD, Cheville NF, Meador VP. Pathogenesis of placentitis in the goat inoculated with *Brucella abortus.* 11. Ultrastructural studies. Vet Pathol 1986; 23:227-239.

Anderson TD, Meador VP, Cheville NF. Pathogenesis of placentitis in the goat inoculated with *Brucella abortus.* 1. Gross and histologic lesions. Vet Pathol 1986; 23:219-226.

Barr BC, Anderson ML, Blanchard PC, Daft BM, Kinde H, Conrad PA. Bovine fetal encephalitis and myocarditis associated with protozoal infections. Vet Pathol 1990; 27:354-361.

Carmichael LE, Kenney RM. Canine abortion caused by *Brucella canis.* J Am Vet Med Assoc 1968;152:605-616.

Coignoul FL, Cheville NF. Pathology of maternal genital tract, placenta, and fetus in equine viral arteritis. Vet Pathol 1984; 21:333-340.

Cullor JS, Tyler JW, Smith BP. Disorders of the mammary gland. In: Smith B, ed. Large Animal Internal Medicine. St. Louis: Mosby, 1990: 1047-1067.

Cutlip RC, Lehmkuhl HD, Brogden KA, Bolin SR. Mastitis associated with ovine progressive pneumonia. Am J Vet Res 1985; 46:326-328.

Daley MJ, Oldham ER, Williams TJ, Coyle PA. Quantitative and qualitative properties of host polymorphonuclear cells during experimentally induced *Staphylococcus aureus* mastitis in cows. Am J Vet Res 1991; 52:474-479.

Edington N, Smyth B, Griffiths L. The role of endothelial cell infection in the endometrium, placenta and foetus of equid herpesvirus 1 (EHV-1) abortions. J Comp Pathol 1991; 104:379-387.

Frost AJ, Brooker BE. Hyperacute *Escherischia coli* mastitis of cattle in the immediate post-partum period. Aust Vet J 1986; 63:327-331.

Gelberg HB, McEntee K. Pathology of the canine and feline uterine tube. Vet Pathol 1986; 23:770-775.

Gudding R, McDonald JS, Cheville NF. Pathogenesis of *Staphylococcus aureus* mastitis: Bacteriologic, histologic, and ultrastructural pathologic findings. Am J Vet Res 1984; 45:2525-2531.

Hartley WG, Kater J. The pathology of toxoplasma infection in the pregnant ewe. Res Vet Sci 1963; 4:326-332.

Herenda D. An abattoir survey of reproductive organ abnormalities in beef heifers. Can Vet J 1987; 28:33-37.

Hill AW, Frost AJ. Progressive pathology of severe *Escherichia coli* mastitis in dairy cows. Res Vet Sci 1984; 37:179-187.

Jasper DE. The role of *Mycoplasma* in bovine mastitis. J Am Vet Med Assoc 1982; 181:158-162.

Kennedy PC, Casaro AP, Kimsey PB, Bon Durant RH, Bushnell RB, Mitchell GM. Epizootic bovine abortion: Histogenesis of the fetal lesion. Am J Vet Res 1983; 44:1040-1048.

Kennedy PC, Richards WPC. The pathology of abortion caused by the virus of infectious bovine rhinotracheitis. Pathol Vet 1964; 1:7-17.

Kennedy-Stoskopf S, Narayan O, Strandberg JD. The mammary gland as a target organ for infection with caprine arthritis-encephalitis virus. J Comp Pathol 1985; 95:609-617.

Kenney RM. Cyclic and pathologic changes of the mare endometrium as detected by biopsy, with a note on early embryonic death. J Am Vet Med Assoc 1978; 172:241-262.

Kesler DJ, Garverick HA. Ovarian cysts in dairy cattle: A review. J Anim Sci 1982; 55:1147-1159.

Lascelles AK. The immune system of the ruminant mammary gland and its role in the control of mastitis. J Dairy Sci 1979; 62:154-160.

Lawler DF, Evans RH, Reimers TJ, Colby ED, Monti KL. Histopathologic features, environmental factors, and serum estrogen, progesterone, and prolactin values associated with ovarian phase and inflammatory uterine disease in cats. Am J Vet Res 1991; 52:1747-1753.

Mahaffey LW, Adam NM. Abortions associated with mycotic lesions of the placenta in mares. J Am Vet Med Assoc 1964; 144:24-32.

Mattila T, Frost AJ. Induction by endotoxin of the inflammatory response in the lactating and dry bovine mammary gland. Res Vet Sci 1989; 46:238-240.

McEntee K, Nielsen SV. Tumors of the female genital tract. Bull World Health Organ 1976; 53:217-226.

Miller JM, Van Der Maaten MJ. Reproductive tract lesions in heifers after intrauterine inoculation with infectious bovine rhinotracheitis virus. Am J Vet Res 1984; 45:790-794.

Nickerson SC. Immune mechanisms of the bovine udder: An overview. J Am Vet Med Assoc 1985; 187:41-45.

Nickerson SC, Heald CW. Histopathologic response of the bovine mammary gland to experimentally induced *Staphylococcus aureus* infection. Am J Vet Res 1981; 42:1351-1355.

Nielsen SW, Misdorp W, McEntee K. Tumors of the ovary. Bull World Health Organ 1976; 53:203-215.

Osburn BI. The relation of fetal age to the character of lesions in fetal lambs infected with *Brucella ovis*. Pathol Vet 1968; 5:395-406.

Osebold JW, Osburn BI, Spezialetti R, Bushnell RB, Stott JL. Histopathologic changes in bovine fetuses after repeated reintroduction of a spirochete-like agent into pregnant heifers: Association with epizootic bovine abortion. Am J Vet Res 1987; 48:627-633.

Palmer NC, Kierstead M, Key DW, Williams JC, Peacock MG, Vellend H. Placentitis and abortion in goats and sheep in Ontario caused by *Coxiella burnetti*. Can Vet J 1983; 24:60-61.

Park YH, Fox LK, Hamilton MJ, Davis WC. Bovine mononuclear subpopulations in peripheral blood and mammary gland secretions during lactation. J Dairy Sci 1992; 75:998-1006.

Pattison IH. The progressive pathology of bacterial mastitis. Vet Res 1958; 70:114-117.

Politis I, McBride BW, Burton JH, Zhao X, Turner JD. Secretion of interleukin-1 by bovine milk macrophages. Am J Vet Res 1991; 52:858-862.

Potter K, Hancock DH, Gallina AM. Clinical and pathologic features of endometrial hyperplasia, pyometra and endometritis in cats: 79 cases (1980-1985). J Am Vet Med Assoc 1991; 198:1427-1431.

Ruhnke HL, Palmer NC, Doig PA, Miller RB. Bovine abortion and neonatal death associated with *Ureaplasma diversum*. Theriogenology 1984; 21:295-301.

Sandholm M, Vasenius H, Kivisto A-K. Pathogenesis of canine pyometra. J Am Vet Med Assoc 1975; 167:1006-1010.

Smith KL, Schanbacher FL. Lactoferrin as a factor of resistance to infection of the bovine mammary gland. J Am Vet Med Assoc 1977; 170:1224-1227.

Smith KL, Todhunter DA, Schoenberger PS. Environmental pathogens and intramammary infection during the dry period. J Dairy Sci 1985; 68:402-417.

Sordillo LM, Doymaz MZ, Oliver SP. Morphological study of chronic *Staphylococcus aureus* mastitis in the lactating bovine mammary gland. Res Vet Sci 1989; 47:247-252.

Van Der Maaten MJ, Miller JM. Ovarian lesions in heifers exposed to infectious bovine rhinotracheitis virus by non-genital routes on the day after breeding. Vet Microbiol 1984/85; 10:155-163.

Varner DD, Blanchard TL. An update on uterine defense mechanisms in the mare. J Equine Vet Sci 1990; 10:169-175.

Vermooten MI. Canine transmissible venereal tumor (TVT): A review. J S Afr Vet Assoc 1987; 58:147-150.

Watson ED. Uterine defence mechanisms in mares resistant and susceptible to persistent endometritis: A review. Equine Vet J 1988; 20:397-400.

Williams WF, Margolis MJ, Manspeaker J, Douglass LW, Davidson JP. Peripartum changes in the bovine placenta related to fetal membrane retention. Theriogenology 1987; 28:213-223.

CHAPTER

13

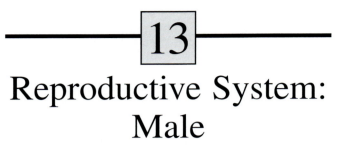

Reproductive System: Male

HELEN M. ACLAND

NORMAL MALE REPRODUCTIVE SYSTEM

The developing embryo has bipotential gonads, external genitalia, and a double set of ducts. The Müllerian or paramesonephric ducts are female precursors, arising by invagination of the celomic cavity; the Wolffian ducts are male precursors, arising from the duct of the primitive kidney, the mesonephros. Differentiation of female organs will occur by default. For a normal male system to develop, necessary ingredients are the presence of a Y chromosome acquired at fertilization and its gene for the testis-determining factor (TDF). The gene for testis determination has been mapped to the distal short arm of the Y chromosome and is highly conserved in mammals. It is expressed at the time and anatomic location of testis differentiation by somatic cells and not germ cells. The gene for H-Y antigen, a surface antigen on all male gonadal somatic cells and earlier thought to be the TDF, is on the long arm of the Y chromosome. After germ cells migrate from the yolk sac and the testis develops in genital ridge tissue, the organ produces two hormones. Sertoli cells secrete Müllerian inhibiting factor (MIF) for a limited time in embryonic development. The factor causes regression of the ipsilateral müllerian duct. Leydig cells secrete testosterone, which causes persistence and differentiation of the Wolffian duct system. After testosterone is converted to dihydrotestosterone by the enzyme 5α-reductase in the cells of the urogenital sinus, genital tubercle, and genital swellings, it induces the formation of the prostate and the closing of the urethral folds and the formation of the penis and scrotum. The production of testosterone is regulated by chorionic gonadotropin and luteinizing hormone (LH). The secretion of LH is under the control of a polypeptide hormone from the hypothalamus, the LH-releasing hormone (LHRH). Also under the control of LHRH is follicle-stimulating hormone (FSH), produced by the anterior pituitary. FSH regulates the activity of Sertoli cells and may, thus, influence MIF production. FSH-stimulated Sertoli cells produce a glycoprotein, androgen-binding protein, that fosters high testosterone concentration around the germ cells for the progression of spermatogenesis.

Descent of the testis into the scrotum is facilitated by the gubernaculum. It is a cord of mesenchymal tissue that attaches the developing testis and epididymis to the forming scrotal pouch. Part of the mechanism is the growth rate of the gubernaculum, which is slower than that of the surrounding pelvic structures. Also, the gubernaculum develops an enlargement just distal to the external inguinal ring, which allows traction to be exerted. The pulling is passive, as no contractile tissue is present in the gubernaculum. Subsequent regression of the gubernaculum aids in the migration of the testis. It seems that, although androgens play a role in descent of the testis, a nonandrogenic factor produced by the testis regulates the process and is needed for completeness of the process.

DEVELOPMENTAL ABNORMALITIES OF THE MALE SYSTEM: INTERSEXES

Abnormalities of Chromosomal Sex

Sex chromosomes can be abnormal in structure or number. Two examples of abnormal structure of the Y chromosome are deletion of the short arm and isochromosome formation (duplication of one arm and loss of the other). Affected animals have female phenotype and streak gonads. Duplication of one of the sex chromosomes in an animal with a Y chromosome (XYY or XXY) results in male external genitalia. Klinefelter's syndrome (XXY) is discussed under testicular hypoplasia. Chimeras, such as XX/XY, will have phenotypic sexual ambiguity.

Abnormalities of Gonadal Sex

Hermaphrodites have abnormal gonads, in possessing both testicular and ovarian tissue. There can be separate testis and ovary or one or both gonads can be mixed. The

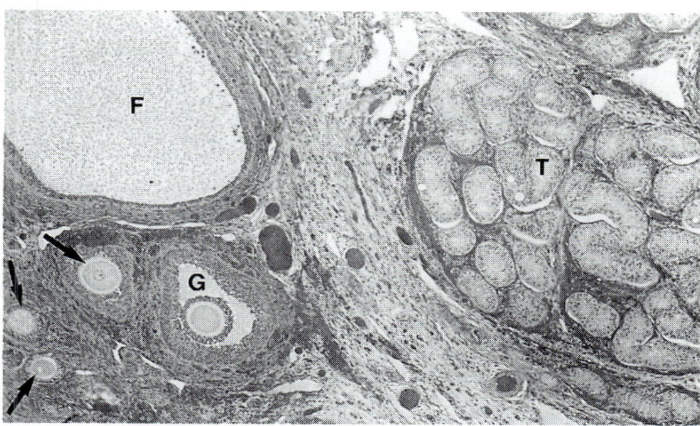

Fig. 13-1 Gonad; dog. Hermaphroditism. In this ovotestis, seminiferous tubules (*T*) are adjacent to a cluster of follicles. Two or more layers of nuclei of granulosa cells surround the oocyte in growing follicles *(arrows)*. The antrum of a small graafian follicle can be seen (*G*), as well as the cavity of a large follicle (*F*). Hematoxylin-eosin (H & E) stain. *Courtesy Dr. M.H. Goldschmidt.*

mixed organ is termed an ovotestis (Fig. 13-1). Most ovotestes have an end-to-end arrangement of ovarian and testicular tissue, with clear demarcation between the two. Each type of gonadal tissue is well developed and easily recognizable. Bilateral hermaphrodites have an ovotestis on each side, unilateral hermaphrodites have an ovotestis on one side, and lateral hermaphrodites have a testis on one side and an ovary on the other. The remainder of the genital tract in hermaphrodites is indeterminate. The basic mechanism for production of hermaphrodites is, in most cases, unknown. The majority have normal constituent of chromosomes, and more individuals are female than male. Cryptorchidism is a common feature in intersex disorders (both hermaphrodites and pseudohermaphrodites). The greater the ratio of testicular to ovarian tissue, the more likely an ovotestis will descend. A pure testis often lies in the scrotum, and an ovary is in its normal position. The ovary or the ovarian portion of an ovotestis is histologically normal, whereas the seminiferous tubules of a testis or ovotestis are abnormal because of a combination of cryptorchidism and the effect of estrogen produced by the ovarian tissue. Except for a few cases of scrotal testes, the tubules are filled with Sertoli cells, and spermatogonia are rare.

Sex reversal is the term used when the gonad is not the type corresponding to the XX or XY chromosomal makeup of the individual. XX males have been identified in several species and are discussed in Chapter 12. XY females are very rare, identified in mice and human beings, and suffer from a deletion or mutation of the testis-determining region of the Y chromosome. They have hypergonadotropic hypogonadism with absence of secondary sexual characteristics. The gonad is a streak of ovarian stroma.

Abnormalities of Phenotypic Sex

In male individuals with abnormalities of phenotypic sex, the chromosomal constitution is normal XY and the gonads are testes, but the development of the tract along male lines is slightly or greatly abnormal. Those with male/female ambiguity of the tract are termed **pseudohermaphrodites** (Fig. 13-2). Pseudohermaphrodites, in contrast to hermaphrodites, have only one type of gonadal tissue and are named male pseudohermaphrodites or female pseudohermaphrodites, according to the gonad present. In many cases, the mechanism of development is unknown. There is ample scope for gonadotropin deficiency or enzyme deficiencies to cause pseudohermaphroditism. Gonadotropin deficiency could be the reason for insufficient testosterone. It could be caused by deficient secretion or defective structure of LH or by abnormality or delayed appearance of the LH receptor on the Leydig cells. The synthesis of testosterone from cholesterol in the Leydig cells requires a series

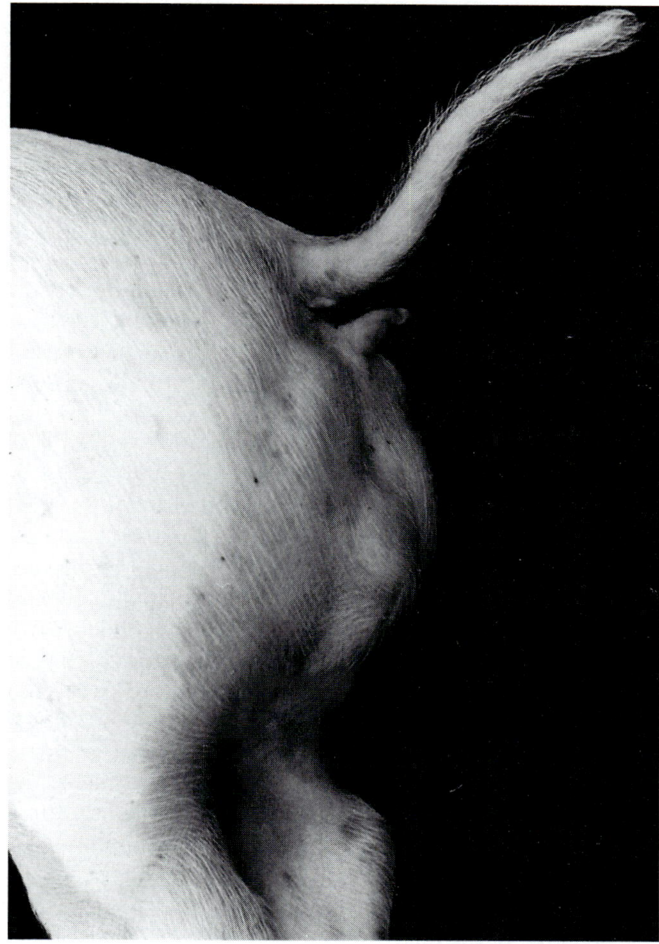

Fig. 13-2 External genitalia; pig. Pseudohermaphroditism. The external appearance is ambiguous, as the penis is short, is clitoris-like in length, but has a terminal urethral opening. Testes are in the scrotal sacs.

of enzymes, any one of which could be deficient. Three named male pseudohermaphrodite syndromes in which the pathogenesis is understood are persistent Müllerian duct syndrome, 5α-reductase deficiency, and androgen insensitivity.

Persistent Müllerian duct syndrome (PMDS) has been described in miniature Schnauzer dogs, with an autosomal recessive mode of inheritance, and in goats. Affected dogs have XY (or XXY) chromosomes, and, externally, are normal males with the common exception of unilateral or bilateral cryptorchidism. The testes, however, are attached to the cranial ends of uterine horns. When a testis has descended into the scrotum, the uterine horn passes through the inguinal ring. Vas deferens can be found microscopically within the myometrium. Cranial vagina and prostate gland are often present. MIF is present in the testes of normal male dogs up to 143 days of age. MIF is present in the testes of young affected dogs also and is bioactive. A reasonable hypothesis is that a mutation in the structural gene for the MIF receptor results in MIF resistance in PMDS-affected dogs. Dogs with unilateral or bilateral scrotal testes can be fertile. Sertoli cell tumor and pyometra are diseases to which PMDS-affected dogs are subject. Testicular abnormalities in PMDS, reduced spermatogenesis, and tubular sclerosis could be attributable to cryptorchidism.

Deficiency of 5α-reductase, inherited as an autosomal recessive trait in humans, has not yet been documented in animals but in all likelihood exists. The enzyme converts testosterone to dihydrotestosterone, which is required for the masculinization of the urogenital sinus, tubercle, and genital swellings. Without dihydrotestosterone, these structures passively become caudal vagina, vestibule, clitoris, and vulva, respectively. Internally, Wolffian structures develop. The testis is likely to be cryptorchid.

Androgen insensitivity, also called testicular feminization, is a rare X-linked, recessively inherited syndrome producing male pseudohermaphrodites. In domestic animals, it has been described in the equine, bovine, and feline species. Affected individuals are chromosomally male and have testes, often cryptorchid. The testes produce MIF, which has its effect. They also produce testosterone, but the stimulation of the Wolffian system is not achieved because of a qualitative or quantitative deficiency of cytosol receptors for the binding of androgen. External genitalia are female, but neither Müllerian nor Wolffian ductal system is present.

Embryonal and **fetal testicular regression syndromes** are described in men. There are five overlapping subtypes, related to absence of, or cessation of, testicular function at a particular stage of development. These are genotypic males in which testes may have never developed or may have developed but regressed in early, mid, or late gestation. The form of the duct system and external genitalia depends on the timing of regression of the testes. With absence of testes, the form is female. With regression of the testes very early, after some secretion of MIF but before much secretion of testosterone, neither duct system is present, and the external genitalia are female. Regression a little later will allow Wolffian duct derivatives and ambiguous external genitalia. With later still regression, the external genitalia are male, but the penis is small. With regression in late fetal life, the external genitalia are those of a normal male.

TESTIS

Developmental Abnormalities

Cryptorchidism is incomplete descent of the testis. In most mammalian species, the testis normally has descended into the scrotum by the time of birth. Cryptorchidism is more often unilateral than bilateral. The undescended testis can be anywhere along its path from caudal to the kidney to the scrotum, including just inside the inguinal ring and just outside the inguinal ring but not in the scrotal sac.

Cryptorchidism is the most common disorder of sexual development in the dog, occurring in as many as 13% of male dogs. It is likely that it has a genetic basis, and a reasonable working hypothesis is a sex-limited autosomal recessive mode of inheritance. It has been suggested that one gene might control internal testicular descent and organization of the epididymis and ductus deferens, and another gene controls external testicular descent. Pathogenetic mechanisms related to the gubernaculum are failure to develop, improper position, excessive growth, or failure to regress.

Many predisposing factors have been proposed for cryptorchidism, such as testicular hypoplasia, estrogen exposure during pregnancy, breech labor compromising blood supply to the testes, and delayed closing of the umbilicus, causing delayed ability to increase abdominal pressure. In the horse, there is a predominance of left unilateral cryptorchidism over right, explained by the relatively slower rate of descent of the left epididymis and testis, coupled with the consistent closure of internal ring at about the time of birth.

The gross appearance of the cryptorchid testis prior to puberty is normal. After puberty, the testis becomes progressively smaller and fibrotic. Atrophy is accompanied by interstitial collagen deposition, hyaline thickening of the tubular basement membranes, and atrophy of germinal epithelium, until only a few spermatogonia along with the Sertoli cells remain (Fig. 13-3). Interstitial cells appear relatively more numerous than they are in cases of descended testes. Epididymal differentiation is coordinated with testicular descent, and, consequently, it is retarded in some cases of cryptorchidism.

Cryptorchid testes are much more prone to neoplasia than normally placed ones, and the tendency is increased with the severity of retention. In the dog, Sertoli cell tumors

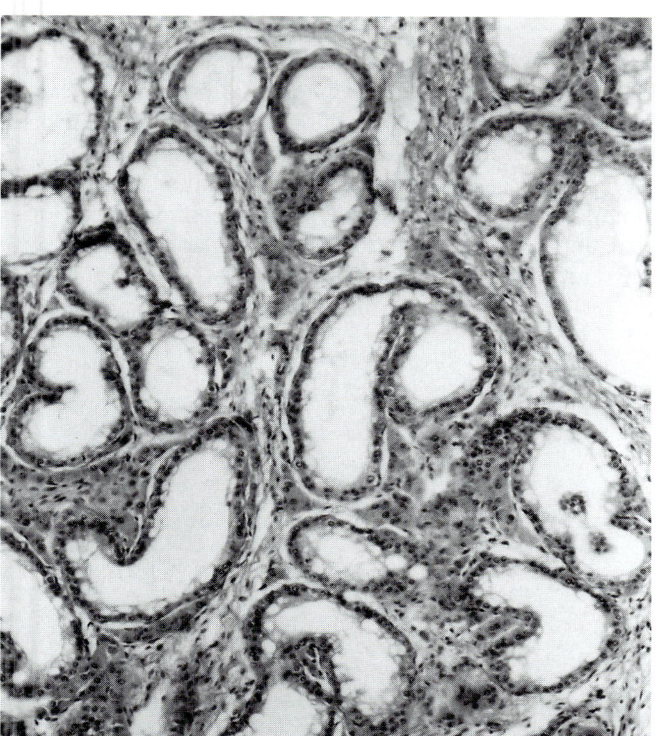

Fig. 13-3 Testis; horse. Cryptorchidism. Tubules are lined by Sertoli cells and a few spermatogonia. Note the numerous interstitial cells and moderate interstitial fibrosis. H & E stain.

are more likely in testes retained in the abdomen, while inguinal testes tend to develop seminomas. In men, undescended testes are prone to develop germ cell tumors (seminomas and teratomas). The contralateral testis is also at increased risk for development of neoplasms. A retained testis, enlarged by a neoplasm, is prone to torsion.

Hypoplasia of the testes is difficult to distinguish from testicular degeneration on morphologic grounds. Lesions of either testicular hypoplasia or degeneration can be seen on their own, with no apparent contributing or influencing factors, or can be seen associated with, secondary to, or as part of some other lesion. For testicular hypoplasia, examples of this second group of causally related factors include cryptorchidism, intersex development, poor general nutrition, zinc deficiency, specific genes in particular breeds of cattle, and endocrine and cytogenetic abnormalities. Endocrine disturbances capable of causing testicular hypoplasia are those related either to LH production by the pituitary gland, which in turn influences testosterone production by the interstitial cells, or to FSH production by the pituitary gland and its stimulation of the nurturing function of the Sertoli cells.

A whole range of cytogenetic abnormalities have been found, from translocations and mosiacs to nondisjunctions, causing polysomies of sex chromosomes. The best known example of the latter is the XXY karyotype of **Klinefelter's syndrome,** described in several species. In cats, the syndrome is recognized in male cats with the tricolor, tortoiseshell, or calico coat types. These cats can be XXY or XX/XXY or more complex chimeras or mosaics with two or more X chromosomes and one or more Y chromosomes. The gene for black and the gene for orange are carried one per X chromosome, so a normal male animal should not have both coat colors. In adult men with Klinefelter's syndrome, there can be a degree of eunuchoidism, and half the cases have gynecomastia. Their testes are usually only 1 cm in length and dark brown due to a predominance of Leydig cells. Before puberty, the microscopic abnormality is a decreased number of germ cells. At puberty, the tubules undergo irregular progressive sclerosis, becoming collagenous cords without the elastic fibers found in sclerotic, but previously normal, tubules. Leydig cells appear hyperplastic and clumped.

Hypoplasia of the testes often is not apparent until after puberty. Unilateral hypoplasia is more common than bilateral hypoplasia, but this could be a reflection of the relative ease of recognizing a size abnormality when the normal is available for ready comparison. Unilateral hypoplasia is difficult to explain when most of the causes would logically seem to act systemically and, therefore, produce the lesion bilaterally. The hypoplastic testis generally ranges in size from one quarter normal to near normal. Consistency of a hypoplastic testis is near to normal.

The severity of the hypoplasia can be graded histologically by the proportion of hypoplastic tubules scattered through the organ. Hypoplastic tubules have a small diameter, are lined by Sertoli cells and a few stem cells and spermatogonia, and have a thickened basement membrane surrounded by collagen deposits. Interstitial cells appear proportionally more numerous, but this is probably an illusion. In severe hypoplasia, most or all of the tubules are abnormal. The tubules are small in diameter, with uniform microscopic appearance, with only infrequent vacuolation of Sertoli cells and without a thickened basement membrane. In moderate hypoplasia, fewer tubules are small, and those of normal size have some differentiation of their seminiferous epithelium, a few reaching an advanced stage of development. Most, however, reach the stage of spermatocyte formation, and, then, the spermatocytes undergo degeneration, leaving a fenestrated tubular lining. The lumen of such tubules may contain cellular debris and multinucleate giant cells, formed when dividing cells fail to separate. Mild hypoplasia features only a few small tubules, lined mostly by Sertoli cells, whereas most of the tubules are active, many producing sperm. Multinucleate giant cells are present in the tubular lumina. Mild hypoplasia is difficult to distinguish from testicular degeneration. The number of hypoplastic tubules would not be expected to increase with age, as hypoplastic tubules do not arise after puberty.

Degeneration

Testicular degeneration is a relatively common lesion; the causes are many and often unknown. Degeneration can be unilateral or bilateral, depending on whether the cause is local or systemic. In young growing animals, the distinction between testicular degeneration and hypoplasia is often difficult to make on morphologic grounds. Both abnormalities are often present together, because hypoplastic testes are prone to degeneration. Inflammation, too, can be superimposed on degeneration when the cause is obstruction, leading to back pressure, rupture of seminiferous tubules, and spermatic granuloma formation. Recovery from degeneration is possible if the injurious agent is eliminated and damage is not too severe.

Specific causes of testicular degeneration are numerous. Locally acting factors include heat, obstruction of the flow of sperm, and vascular impairment. Fever or local heat from inflammation of the scrotal skin can injure the testis. Obstruction of sperm flow by developmental anomalies, local injury or inflammation of the epididymis, and vascular impairment from age-related mineralization of spermatic cord or testicular vessels, or from more dramatic vascular events such as Burdizzo castration or torsion of the spermatic cord, will cause testicular degeneration. Systemic factors include nutritional deficiency, hormonal aberrations, toxicities, and irradiation. Vitamin A and zinc deficiencies, and general malnutrition will cause testicular degeneration. Interference with gonadotropin-releasing hormones, LH and its control of androgen production by Leydig cells, or FSH and its effect on the production of androgen-binding protein by Sertoli cells will have a deleterious effect. Such interference could happen, for instance, by virtue of the presence of a space-occupying lesion in the pituitary gland or hypothalamus. Estrogen produced by Sertoli cell tumors induces testicular degeneration. Of the many toxins capable of causing testicular degeneration, most are toxic to the spermatogonia and dividing primary spermatocytes, but some are toxic to later stages, spermatocytes and spermatids, or even Sertoli cells. Some therapeutic drugs, such as amphotericin B, gentamicin, and chemotherapeutic compounds, cause testicular degeneration.

Initially, a degenerate testis will be swollen and softer than normal; progressive shrinkage follows. On the cut surface, the normal testis and the acutely degenerate testis bulge slightly. After the acute phase, the consistency becomes firmer, and small flecks or large areas of calcification are present. Locally acting agents are likely to produce local degeneration. Degeneration due to obstruction of efferent ducts is seen in the dorsal part of the testis. If the degeneration is due to ischemia after a vascular accident in the spermatic cord, small islands of parenchyma may survive by virtue of diffusion from vessels of the epididymis and tunica albuginea.

Microscopically, the appearance is similar to that of testicular hypoplasia; small seminiferous tubules with thickened basement membrane have decreased numbers of seminiferous epithelial cells, fenestrated tubular lining, intratubular giant cells, and interstitial fibrosis (Figs. 13-4 and 13-5). The degree of vacuolation of the lining is likely to be more severe in degeneration than in hypoplasia, reflecting the loss of germinal cells. A lesion helpful to distinguish between testicular hypoplasia and degeneration is that the basement membrane in degeneration is likely to have much more irregular outline because affected tubules

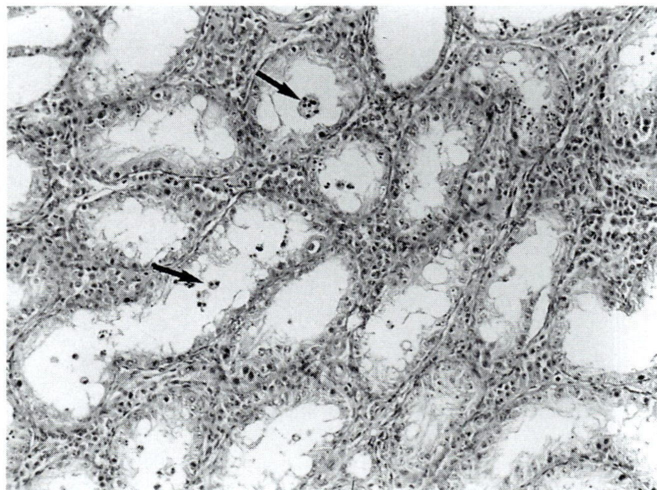

Fig. 13-4 Testis; horse. Testicular degeneration. Much of the epithelium lining the tubules has disappeared, and the remnants are vacuolated (fenestrated). Intratubular multinucleate giant cells have formed *(arrows)*. H & E stain.

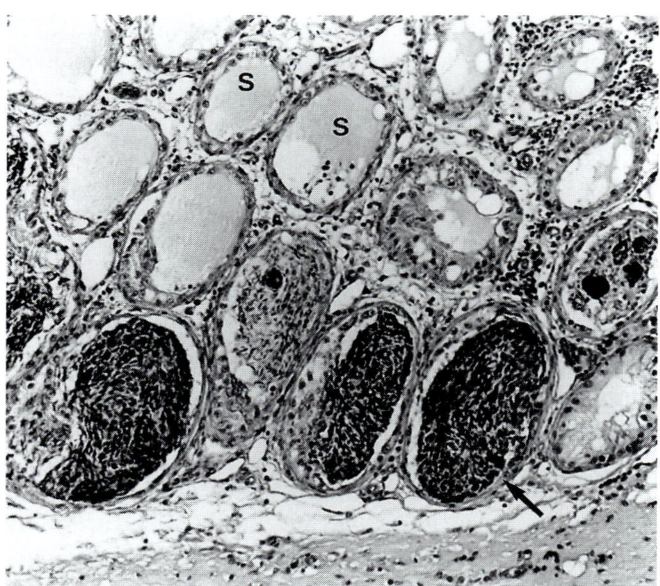

Fig. 13-5 Testis; ram. Testicular degeneration. Obstruction of seminiferous tubules has caused impaction of sperm *(arrow)*. Most tubules (*S*) are lined by Sertoli cells, and there are only remnants of seminiferous tubular epithelium. Tubular atrophy is mild. H & E stain.

had at some stage reached full size and then subsequently collapsed. At the end stage of testicular degeneration, Sertoli cells may be the only cells remaining. They also may disappear, leaving only the basement membrane. Calcification can involve intratubular cellular debris, tubular basement membranes, or the interstitium.

Inflammation

Sperm are sequestered within the seminiferous tubules, isolated from the general circulation by Sertoli cells, which completely line the basement membrane. The blood-testis barrier has two compartments: a basal compartment, containing spermatogonia and preleptotene spermatocytes, bounded by peritubular myoid cells and Sertoli cells below their tight junctions, and an adluminal compartment beyond the tight junctions between Sertoli cells, containing the later stages of spermatogenesis. Cell surface antigens undergo many remodelings during spermatogenesis, giving sperm surface antigens not present at the time in fetal life when immune self-recognition takes place. Yet, sperm are not normally recognized as foreign by the male animal. Sequestration is the mechanism most widely believed responsible. A second theory is that the barriers created by the numerous tight junctions of the Sertoli cells allow minute amounts of soluble sperm antigen into the host, and this soluble antigen activates suppressor lymphocytes involved in down-regulating cytotoxic immune responses. Lymphocytes have not been identified in the testicular interstitium. The absence of T-lymphocytes has been proposed as a mechanism that lessens the possibility of immune stimulation by sperm.

The formation of antisperm antibodies in men has been associated with major disruption of the blood-testis barrier. Surgical vasectomy is a common cause, but increases of sperm antibodies are known, with such injuries as vas obstruction, testicular trauma, malignancy, and infections. Disruption of the blood-testis barrier can allow the immune system to gain access to sperm. Antibody attached to sperm surface can interfere with sperm function. Antisperm antibodies have been identified in the seminal fluid or the serum of stallions with low sperm viability following trauma to the testis. If **autoimmune orchitis** occurs in domestic animals, it seems likely from experimental studies that the rete testis or efferent ducts are the sites at which the inflammatory process starts. When the disruption of the blood-testis barrier is so severe that sperm are outside their normal containment within the testis, epididymis, vas deferens, and urethra, a foreign body granulomatous reaction occurs.

Nonspecific orchitis, a mild, multifocal, subacute intertubular inflammation of unknown cause, is relatively common in bulls and stallions. There are no gross lesions. Microscopically, lymphocytic foci are present between tubules and around vessels. Other forms of orchitis, forms that produce grossly visible lesions, are much less common.

Intratubular orchitis probably arises by an ascending infection and starts as tubular inflammation that then spreads into the interstitium, as a mixture of the acute inflammation together with spermatic granulomas that form when sperm make contact with extratubular tissue. Intratubular orchitis appears grossly as poorly defined up to 1 cm, yellow foci that become firm and white as they become chronic. Initially, the affected tubules contain acute inflammatory cellular debris. The lining of the tubules is lost, but the tubular outlines are visible for some time. Spermatic granulomas and fibrosis later develop in the interstitium.

Necrotizing orchitis, the most severe form of orchitis, may begin as an intratubular disease, or it may arise hematogenously. The term implies that the affected areas are so severely inflamed and necrosis is so extensive that the original structures have disintegrated to form a caseous mass. In a few extremely severe cases, a fistula develops through the scrotum.

Granulomatous orchitis involves the formation of multiple, possibly coalescing, inflammatory nodules displacing and replacing parenchyma. Inflammation of the tunica vaginalis may accompany intratubular, necrotizing, or granulomatous orchitis. There may be an accompanying or even primary epididymitis.

Brucellosis in bulls is the most extensively studied orchitis in domestic animals. It is an intratubular orchitis that becomes necrotizing. Initially, the testis is swollen to the limited extent permitted by the tunica albuginea. Fibrinous exudate distends the cavity of the tunica vaginalis. Foci of necrosis in the testis expand and may coalesce, so that much of the testis is involved, becoming either liquefied or caseous. The surrounding tunicae and any surviving testis become densely fibrous.

Organisms that commonly cause orchitis are listed in Box 13-1.

Box 13-1 COMMON CAUSES OF INFECTIOUS ORCHITIS IN DOMESTIC ANIMALS

BULL
Brucella abortus
Bluetongue virus
Chlamydia psittaci
Actinomyces pyogenes
Lumpy skin disease virus
Mycobacterium tuberculosis
Nocardia asteroides

BUCK
Brucella melitensis

DOG
Brucella canis
Canine distemper virus
Escherichia coli
Proteus vulgaris
Pseudomonas pseudomallei

RAM
Brucella ovis
Corynebacterium ovis
Sheeppox virus

BOAR
Brucella suis
Pseudomonas pseudomallei

STALLION
Equine viral arteritis virus
Equine infectious anemia virus
Salmonella abortus equi
Strongylus edentatus

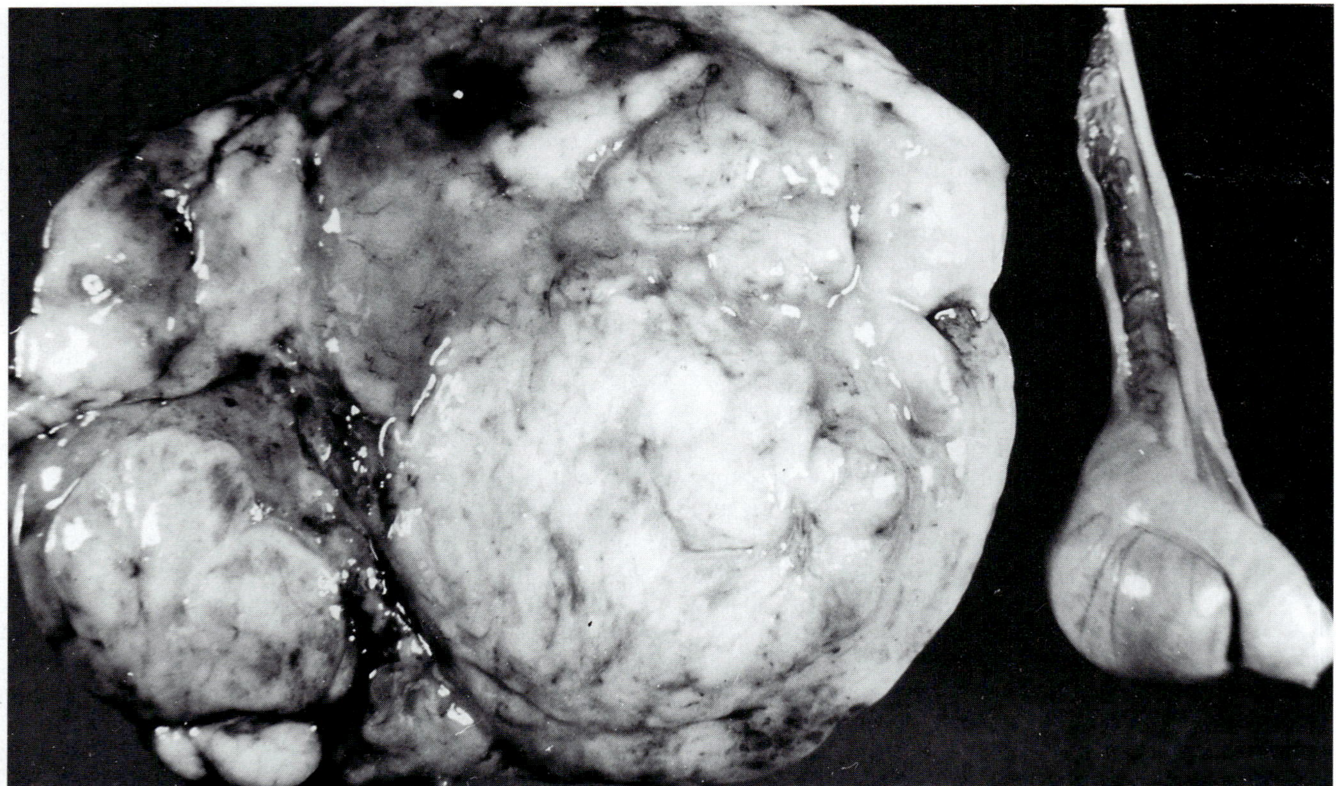

Fig. 13-6 Testis; dog. Seminoma. The tumor bulges from the cut surface, is discrete, and is divided by a few fibrous trabeculae.

Neoplasms

Testicular neoplasms are common in older dogs, occur in older bulls, and are rare in other species. They arise from germ cells or from gonodal stroma. Occasionally, neoplasms of testicular mesenchymal structures or metastatic neoplasms are found. The three common primary testicular neoplasms can occur singly or in combination. **Germ cell neoplasms** are seminoma, teratoma, and other rarer types.

Seminomas are the second most common canine testicular neoplasm, are the most common testicular neoplasm in the aged stallion, and are observed much less commonly in other species. They are more prevalent in cryptorchid testes than in descended testes. Arising from primitive seminiferous tubules, they do not produce hormones. Multicentric origins within the testis and local invasiveness are characteristic. The neoplasm is white or pink-gray, is firm and bulges when cut, and has fine fibrous trabeculae (Fig. 13-6). Seminomas, microscopically, can be found in an intratubular or diffuse arrangement of large, polyhedral, discretely demarcated cells with a large nucleus, variable nuclear size, and very little cytoplasm. Giant cells, with either a single or multiple nuclei, are sometimes present (Fig. 13-7). In immunocytochemically stained specimens from men, seminomas were negative for alpha-fetoprotein but were positive for human chorionic gonadotropin in the giant cells

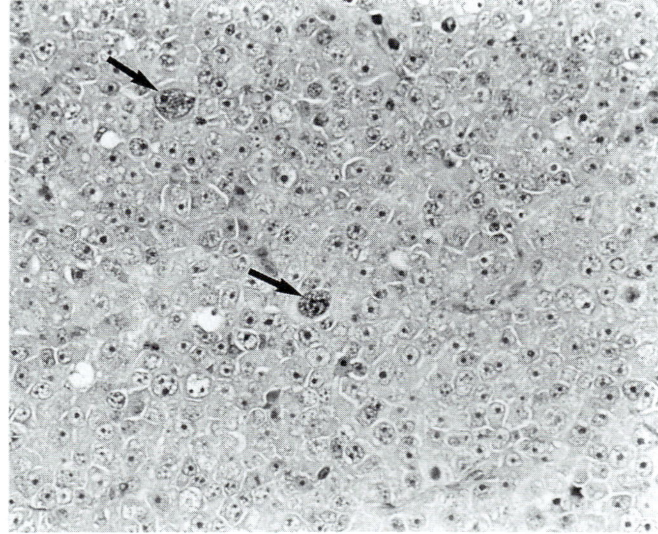

Fig. 13-7 Testis; dog. Seminoma. The tumor cells are large, polyhedral, discrete and their nuclei vary in size. A few giant cells *(arrows)* are present. H & E stain.

of chorionic origin but not in stromal giant cells. Lymphoid nodules are often present in seminomas. These neoplasms are seldom malignant. Pain from pressure created by the enlarging neoplastic mass may be the presenting sign.

Teratomas arise from totipotential primordial germ cells. These are uncommon but are best known in the horse, especially in the cryptorchid testis of the young horse. The tumor can be large, be cystic or polycystic, and can contain recognizable hair, mucus, bone, and teeth. Microscopically, derivatives of at least two of the three embryonic germ layers are present. A teratoma with well-differentiated organoid structures can be expected to be benign.

Other germ cell tumors are rare. Totipotential germ cells that become neoplastic are not restricted in their lines of differentiation. Germ cell tumors of the testis can be thought of as either seminomas or nonseminomas. Embryonal carcinomas are the stem type for the latter. In the array of derivatives of the embryonal carcinoma, there can be tumors of one histologic type or tumors of more than one histologic type, with differentiation into extraembryonic cell types (choriocarcinoma and yolk sac tumor) or embryonic cell types (ectoderm, mesoderm, endoderm, or teratoma). Immunohistochemical methods to demonstrate alpha-fetoprotein, human chorionic gonadotropin, and other germ cell tumor products are routinely used to classify germ cell tumors in human beings.

Gonadal stromal tumors are Leydig cell tumor, Sertoli cell tumor, and some other rare neoplasms.

Leydig cell tumor (interstitial cell tumor) is the most commonly found testicular neoplasm in the dog and bull. It is relatively rare in the stallion, with most cases found in undescended testes. It is readily identifiable grossly by its tan to orange color. The neoplasm is spherical and well demarcated (Fig. 13-8). The distinction between nodular

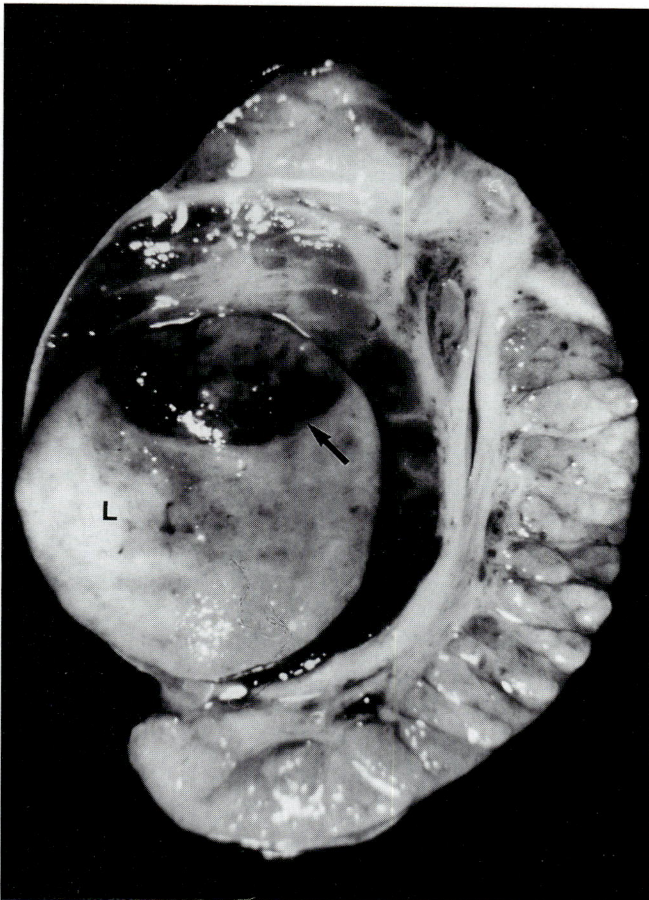

Fig. 13-8 Testis; dog. Leydig cell tumor (*L*). The tumor is distinctly demarcated and has an area of hemorrhage *(arrow)*.

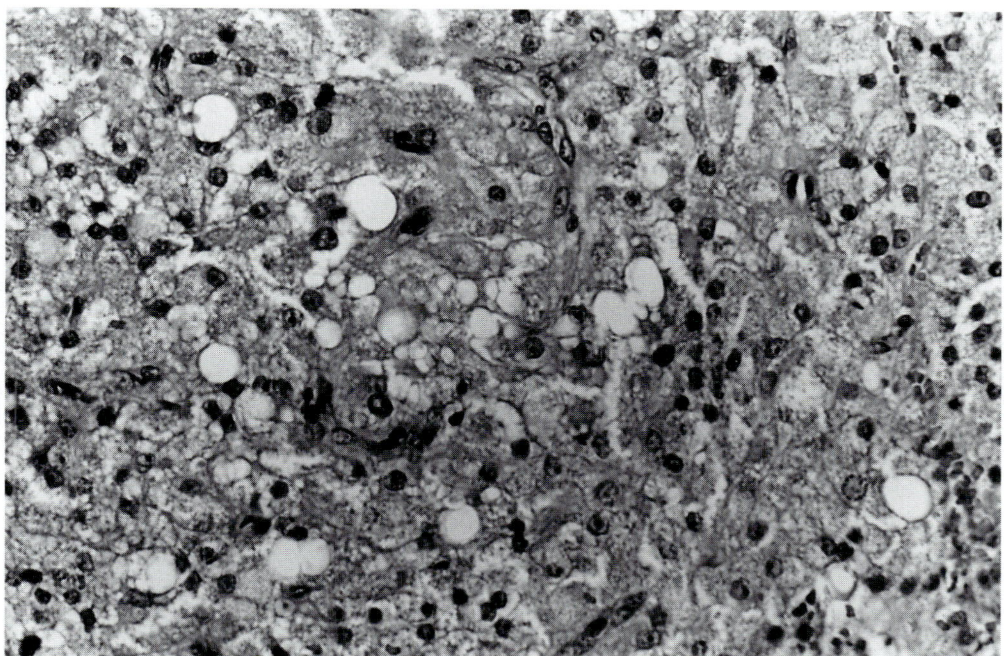

Fig. 13-9 Testis; dog. Leydig cell tumor. Tumor cells are in a sheet, and their cytoplasm is finely vacuolated, a characteristic of Leydig cells. H & E stain.

hyperplasia of Leydig cells and Leydig cell tumor is problematic. Whether the neoplasm produces hormones or not is unsettled. Microscopically, the bovine neoplasms have little cellular variation, but, in the dog, the cells can be large, round, and polyhedral or spindle shaped. The cells have plentiful cytoplasm that is often finely vacuolated and often brown. The cells are arranged in solid sheets or divided into small groups by fine fibrovascular trabeculae (Fig. 13-9). Although hemorrhage, necrosis, and cyst formation are common, Leydig cell tumors are noninvasive and are finely encapsulated.

Sertoli cell tumor is the third most common testicular neoplasm of the dog. It is rare in other species, but has been recorded in most. In the dog, more than 50% of Sertoli cell tumors are located in undescended testes. The neoplasm is firm, white, and is lobulated by fibrous bands (Fig. 13-10). It may cause enlargement of the affected testis, may invade the spermatic cord, and, occasionally, metastasizes to regional lymph node. Metastases beyond the regional lymph node have been reported but are rare. The neoplastic Sertoli cells may resemble normal Sertoli cells or may be more pleomorphic. They can have an intratubular or a more diffuse arrangement. The abundant amount of fibrous connective tissue present in Sertoli cell tumors is a feature that distinguishes them from the other two common types of testicular neoplasms. Neoplastic cells tend to palisade along the fibrous stroma (Fig. 13-11). In addition to the effects of pressure and local invasion, the other important consequence of the presence of Sertoli cell tumors is that about a third of them produce estrogen, which may have a feminizing effect, such as gynecomastia, on the host. A possibly life-threatening effect of estrogen secretion is myelotoxicity characterized by a nonregenerative

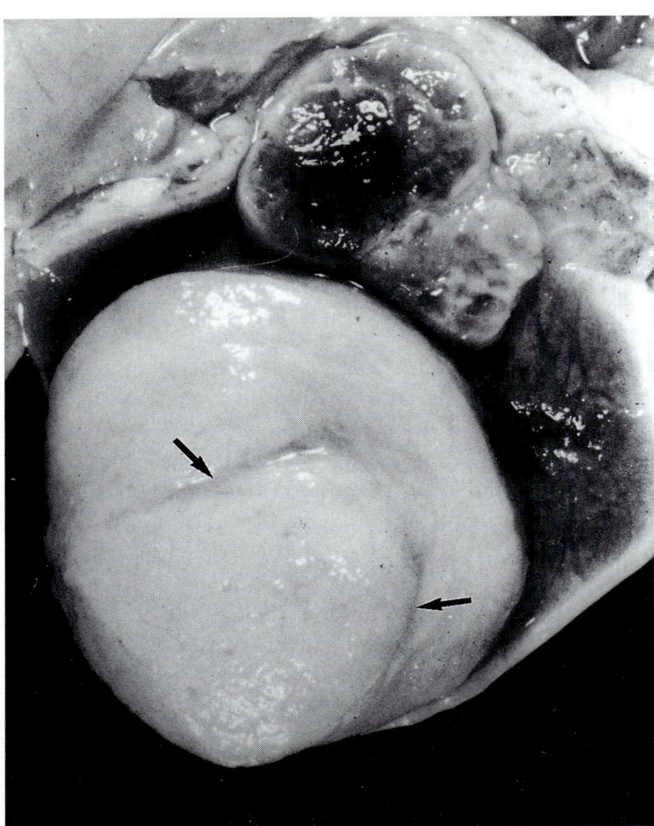

Fig. 13-10 Testis; dog. Sertoli cell tumor. Numerous white bands of fibrous tissue *(arrows)* dissect through the tumor.

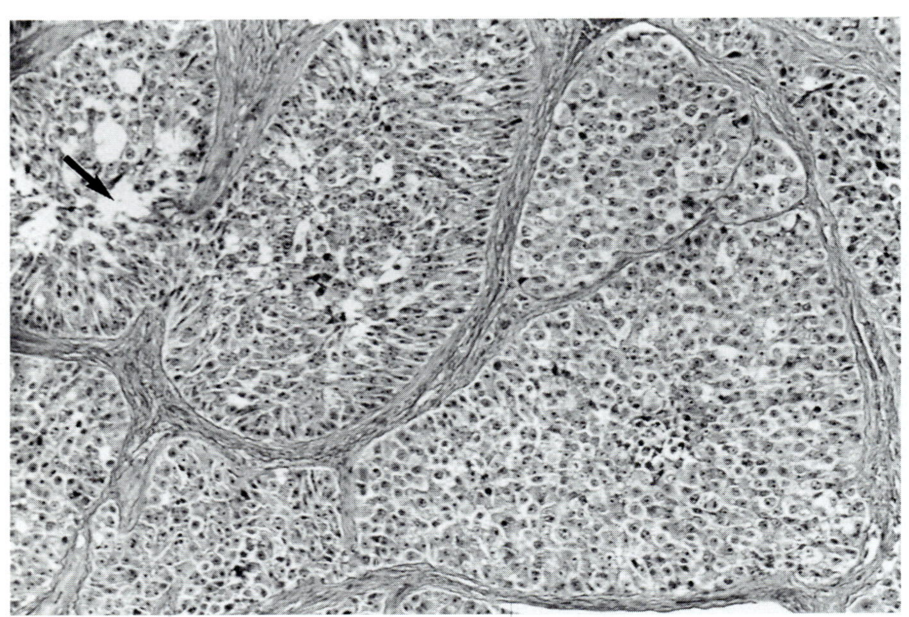

Fig. 13-11 Testis; dog. Sertoli cell tumor. Neoplastic Sertoli cells palisade along fibrous trabeculae and form solid tubules or tubules with a central space *(arrow)* or lumen. H & E stain.

anemia, granulocytopenia, and thrombocytopenia. Other effects of estrogen are induction of hypothyroidism and alopecia, hyperplasia and/or squamous metaplasia of the acini of the prostate, and adenomyosis of the epididymis. The amount of estrogen produced is generally proportional to the size of the neoplasm.

Other gonadal stromal neoplasms are rare and of somewhat uncertain origin. In addition to the above, granulosa cell tumor, mixed forms, and incompletely differentiated forms are recognized. Mixed cell tumors have been described recently in dogs. These occur in old dogs, with atrophy of the tumor-bearing testis, often in conjunction with cryptorchidism. There is an intimate intermingling of germ cells and Sertoli cells in tubular structures of various sizes. The germ cell component extends into the surrounding tissue. Staining for neuron-specific enolase and vimentin is useful to demonstrate the dual cell population.

SCROTUM

The scrotum is an outpouching of the perineum, composed of skin, tunica dartos, and scrotal fascia. It is fused with the parietal layer of the tunica vaginalis. The skin has a thin dermis, few hairs, and many sweat glands.

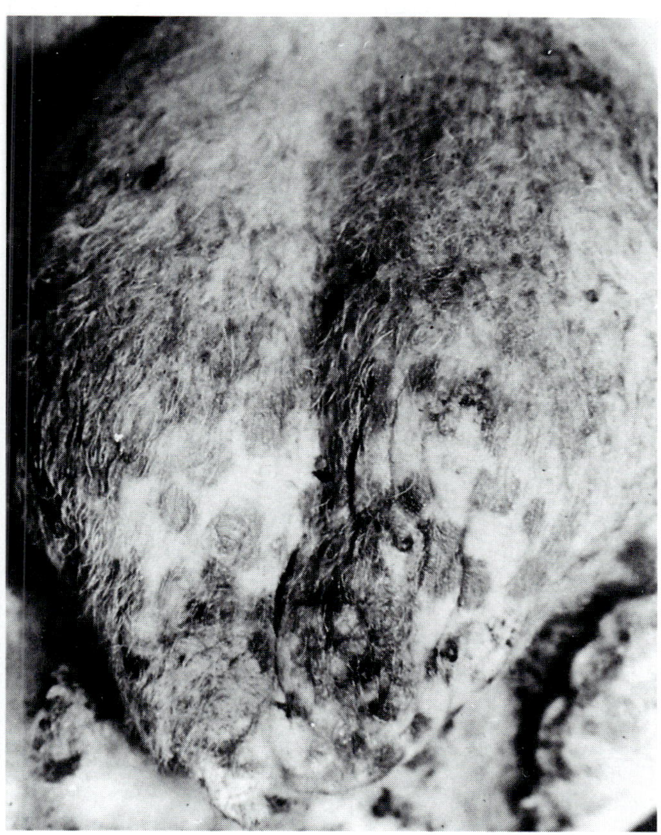

Fig. 13-12 Scrotum; ram. Dermatitis. The multiple coalescing areas of hyperkeratosis and inflammation are caused by the presence of *Chorioptes ovis* mites.

The fusion of the paired primordia of scrotal skin depends on hormones released from the gonad after it has differentiated into a testis. Disturbances in the formative stages may lead to various defects in the scrotum, such as failure of fusion, cleft formation, or bifurcation of the scrotum. Defects may be local, confined to the scrotum and penis, or part of a wider range of defects in an intersex animal.

Dermatitis of the scrotal skin is common. Often it is nonspecific, the result of trauma, frostbite, or exposure to environmental irritants. Some pathogens have the scrotum as a predilection site. These include *Dermatophilus congolensis* and *Besnoitia besnoiti* in the bull and *Chorioptes ovis* in the ram (Fig. 13-12). The heat generated in scrotal dermatitis may interfere with the thermoregulatory function of the scrotum, leading to testicular degeneration.

Neoplasms of any of the types that occur in the skin can occur in the skin of the scrotum, but are much less common here than elsewhere. Neoplasms occasionally encountered are mastocytomas and melanomas in the dog and papillomas in the boar. Vascular abnormalities, which may or may not be hemangiomas, occur on the scrotum of the dog and boar. The scrotal veins of bulls sometimes become varicose.

TUNICA VAGINALIS

The tunica vaginalis is the extension of the peritoneum that lines the scrotal sac as the parietal layer and covers the testis, epididymis, and spermatic cord as the visceral layer. The cavity between the two layers is continuous with the peritoneal cavity. The tunicae and the cavity, thus, are subject to all the diseases of the peritoneum and peritoneal cavity.

Inflammation of the tunica vaginalis as part of a systemic disease will have the characteristics of that disease. Inflammation of the tunica vaginalis without initial inflammation of the abdominal peritoneum can have a noninfectious, i.e., traumatic, or an infectious cause. The latter is likely to be an extension from orchitis or epididymitis. Especially well known causes are *Brucella ovis* and *Actinobacillus seminis* in rams and *Trypanosoma brucei* in several species. In general, traumatic inflammation of the tunica vaginalis is mild and focal, and inflammation with an infectious cause is severe and diffuse. Adhesions between the parietal and visceral tunica vaginalis, are fibrinous at first and, later, fibrous, and are common.

SPERMATIC CORD

Varicocele is the local dilatation of the spermatic vein in the pampiniform plexus. In the ram, associated subfertility has been proposed, with poor sperm motility, immature sperm in the semen, and testicular degeneration. The dilatation is great in the venous plexus near the inguinal ring and not involving the complex distal part. About half the cases are bilateral, and the unilateral cases are evenly divided between left and right. Thrombosis of affected vessels is the rule. Some degree of testicular atrophy appears to be associated with varicocele. Varicoceles can cause enlargement of the scrotum, even to the extent that it touches the ground.

Torsion of the spermatic cord can occur when the testis is undescended. Vascular occlusion may involve just the spermatic vein or the vein and artery, leading to infarction and necrosis of the testis.

Inflammation occurs after the contamination of a castration wound. Sometimes, the lesion is acute and necrotizing, but more often the chronic form, called scirrhous cord, is encountered. Great enlargement of the distal part of the cord is due to granulation tissue in which numerous small pockets of pus are scattered. Staphylococci are the organisms frequently recovered from the pus in the horse. The term ''botryomycosis'' has been used for these staphylococcal pyogranulomas. Radiating club-shaped bodies of Splendore-Hoeppli material are present around the central clusters of gram-positive bacteria.

MESONEPHRIC DUCT DERIVATIVES: EPIDIDYMIS, VAS DEFERENS, AMPULLA, SEMINAL VESICLE

The mesonephric duct forms the epididymis, vas deferens, ampulla, and seminal vesicle on each side. The seminal vesicle is an outpouching of the vas deferens. These latter two structures open in common or along side of each other into the prostatic urethra. The prostatic utricle or uterus masculinus is a Müllerian remnant located centrally between the two vasa deferentia. Male cats and dogs lack seminal vesicles.

Developmental Abnormalities

Improper linkage of derivatives of mesonephric tubules and duct

The testis is derived from gonadal cords that form between the gonadal ridge on the medial side of the mesonephros and remnants of mesonephric tubules. The rete testis and efferent ducts are derived from mesonephric tubules. Within the mesonephros, many mesonephric tubules enter the single mesonephric duct. It is from the within-mesonephros part of the duct that the epididymis is derived. The vas deferens, ampulla, and seminal vesicle are derived from the more caudal part of the mesonephric duct, outside the mesonephros. The developed testis has about 20 efferent ducts; the number varies with the species. Efferent ducts normally link in the head of the epididymis. Blind efferent ducts result when the connection to the epididymis is not made properly. They may be resorbed, persist, enlarge to form cysts, and/or rupture. Sperm that escape outside normal containment are reacted to as foreign bodies and incite an inflammatory response.

Unconnected with the lumen of the epididymal tubule or efferent ducts, remnants of tubules of the mesonephros can form **cysts** adjacent to the head of the epididymis (paradidymis externus) or within the head of the epididymis (paradidymis internus). Cysts, both connected and unconnected to the ductular system, are lined by ciliated columnar epithelium. They are clinically significant if they become large enough to cause stasis of sperm in adjacent structures, or if they rupture and liberate sperm into their surroundings. Of no clinical significance is the remnant left of the Müllerian duct, called the appendix testis, on the cranial surface of the testis near the head of the epididymis. Sometimes, this small nodule of tissue may appear cystic.

Segmental aplasia of mesonephric duct derivatives

Segmental aplasia of the epididymis, vas deferens, ampulla, or seminal vesicle can occur at any location but most commonly affects the epididymis alone and, less commonly, the epididymis and other structures. Segmental aplasia is reported mainly in the bull and most commonly in the body and tail of the epididymis. As expected, most cases are unilateral. Sperm become impacted because of obstruction; local dilatation or rupture of the structure occurs secondarily, allowing escape of sperm into surrounding tissues.

Spermatocele is a local distention of the epididymis that contains accumulated sperm. It can follow congenital or acquired (such as by vasectomy) occlusion of the lumen and often is followed by the escape of sperm into the connective tissue outside the duct through degeneration or rupture of the wall.

Immotile cilia syndrome, a rare disease identified in human beings, dogs, and rats, is caused by one or more of several defects in the axoneme of cilia all over the body and of the flagellum of spermatozoa. In dogs, a heterogeneity of ultrastructural abnormalities of microtubule doublets and their dynein arms or central microtubules is reported. The effect on the reproductive system is immotile or hypomotile sperm due to flagellar lesions, or oligospermia or azoospermia, presumably due to defective cilia in the epididymis and vas deferens. Because of defective cilia elsewhere, common associated lesions are rhinitis, bronchopneumonia, bronchiectasis, and hydrocephalus. Situs inversus also occurs, but the pathogenesis is unclear. Female infertility is related to defective function of cilia of the uterine tube. An autosomal recessive mode of inheritance is proposed.

Inflammation

Because the epididymis is only a single coiled tubule, any lesion along its length has the potential for causing obstruction of sperm movement. Epididymitis can be focal, multifocal or diffuse, unilateral or bilateral. It is most frequently encountered in unilateral, chronic, focal or multifocal form and, thus, can be recognized by comparing the size and shape of the abnormal organ with the normal one. In acute inflammation, the epididymis is soft and swollen;

in chronic inflammation, it is firm and swollen, because of the deposition of fibrous tissue, and likely to be nodular, because of distention of segments of the duct and the presence of spermatic granulomas and abscesses. Obstruction of the outflow of sperm is one of the causes of testicular degeneration. The testis is grossly atrophic. Local fibrinous or fibrous adhesions occur between the epididymis and the parietal tunica vaginalis lining the scrotal sac. If an abscess ruptures into the cavity of the tunica vaginalis, diffuse inflammation of the tunics may result, followed by adhesions across the cavity. In some cases, fistulae form through the scrotum.

Noninfectious causes of epididymitis include trauma and influx of urine along the vas deferens, as well as any lesion in which sperm escape from the lumen of the duct of the epididymis. Congenital and acquired obstructions account for most of the latter, but there is additional lesion, adenomyosis, that can be followed by escape of sperm. In adenomyosis, the epithelium of the duct invades the muscular layer, creating extensions of the lumen in which sperm may become entrapped. If these outpouchings rupture, sperm escape into the lamina propria. Sperm that have escaped their normal containment within the lumen of the excretory system incite a foreign body response (Fig. 13-13). An association has been observed between the occurrence of adenomyosis of the epididymis and the development of Sertoli cell tumor of the testis.

Microscopically, in epididymitis, the lumen contains a mixture of inflammatory cells, in which neutrophils are present and macrophages are prominent, together with desquamated epithelial cells, intact and fragmented sperm, and sperm within multinucleate giant cells. If the wall of the tubule is breached, inflammation spreads to the interstitium, where mononuclear cells become more numerous in the inflammatory exudate and collagen is deposited. There may be an accompanying hypertrophy of the smooth muscle layer of the wall of the epididymis, together with hyperplasia of the epithelium. The epithelial cells may proliferate irregularly, so that thick areas of epithelium appear to enclose thin areas, leading to "intraepithelial lumen" formation. Squamous metaplasia of the epithelium is a possible outcome in chronic epididymitis.

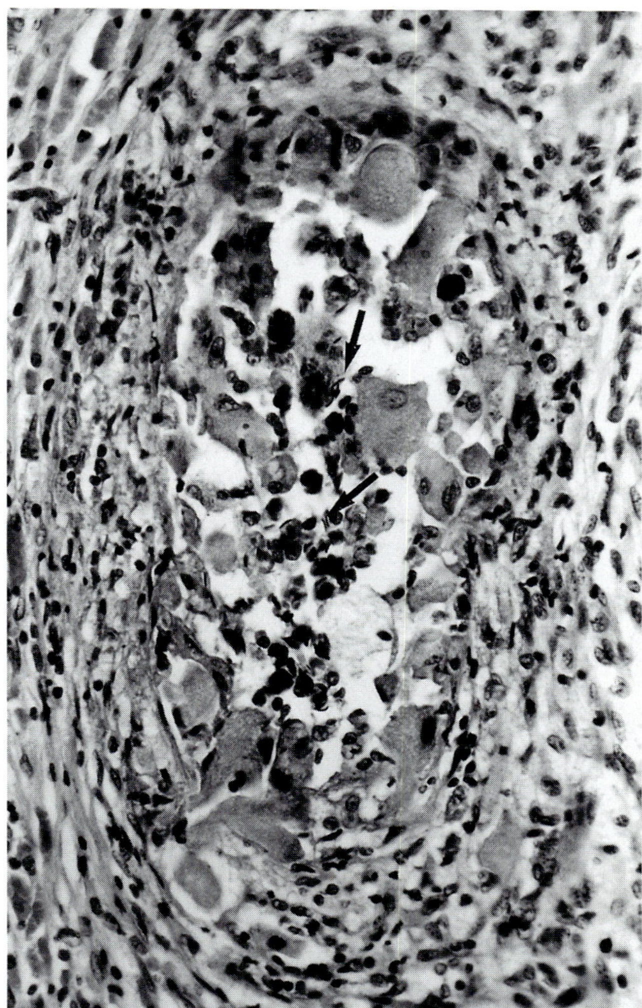

Fig. 13-13 Epididymis; ram. Spermatic granuloma. Sperm *(arrows)* that have escaped from the lumen of the ducts of the epididymis are surrounded by phagocytic cells, including multinucleate giant cells. H & E stain.

Infectious epididymitis is likely to be the result of the entry of organisms from the urinary tract rather than from hematogenous spread. *Brucella ovis* or *Actinobacillus seminis* infections in rams have epithelial hyperplasia and intraepithelial lumen formation as features of the early stages, with later progression to spermatic granuloma and abscess formation. Grossly, the abscesses are palpable in the tail of one or both epididymides. Testicular atrophy occurs secondarily. In *B. abortus* infection in bulls, epididymitis is accompanied by orchitis. Epididymitis occurs in mature dogs as a nonspecific infection (Fig. 13-14) or as part of a specific disease such as canine distemper. Intranuclear and intracytoplasmic inclusions can be found in the epithelial cells in distemper. *Brucella canis* infection causes epididymitis, testicular degeneration and atrophy, often unilateral, together with scrotal hyperemia and dermatitis and prostatitis.

Seminal vesiculitis is a significant problem in the bull, because fertility is reduced after the seminal vesicles contribute pus to the semen. Inflamed seminal vesicles are the most common source of inflammatory cells in bovine semen. The cause is most likely infectious, and various organisms, including viruses, protozoa, chlamydia, ureaplasma, mycoplasma, and other bacteria, have been investigated over the years. The seminal vesicles in bulls can be among the organs involved in *B. abortus* or *My-*

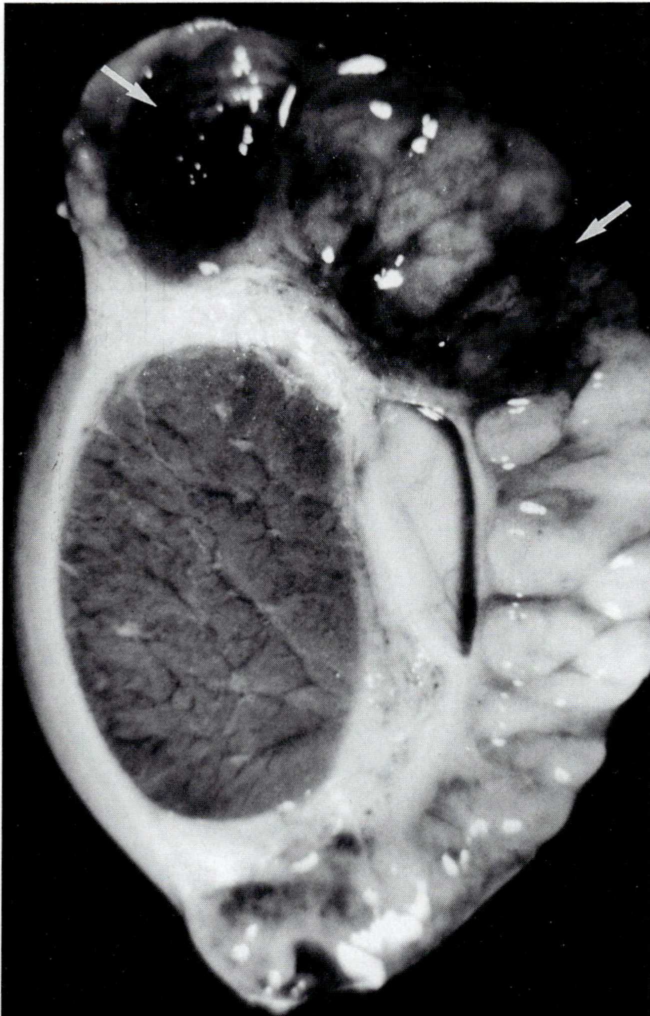

Fig. 13-14 Epididymis; dog. Epididymitis. Note the large area of hemorrhage and swelling of the head of the epididymis *(arrows).*

cobacterium bovis infections. In other species, seminal vesiculitis can be part of the range of lesions caused by *Pseudomonas pseudomallei,* by *B. abortus* in the boar, and by *B. melitensis* and *Actinobacillus seminis* in the ram. The pathogenesis too is uncertain. Ascending infection, descending infection, hematogenous spread, congenital malformation that prevents excretion of fluid and spermatozoa, and the reflux of spermatozoa or urine into the glands have all been proposed.

The common form of seminal vesiculitis is a chronic interstitial inflammation. In some cases, the gland is enlarged and has increased firmness with loss of lobulation. Collagen is deposited between the acini. A mixture of lymphocytes, plasma cells, macrophages, and a few neutrophils and eosinophils is present in the interstitium. The glands contain neutrophils, desquamated epithelial cells, and debris. Metaplasia of glandular epithelium to a stratified type is common. In some bulls, there is much epithelial disorganization and denuding.

PROSTATE

The prostate gland and the bulbourethral gland are derived from the urogenital sinus. Most domestic animals have both glands. The dog, however, has only a prostate gland. The central part of the prostate gland is of Müllerian origin. Both estrogens and androgens have tropic action on the prostate gland.

Prostatitis can be clinically significant if there is sepsis or the gland becomes large enough to cause urinary obstruction. In the dog, prostatitis can be found in old animals, often together with hyperplasia, or in young animals, without hyperplasia. Men with bacterial prostatitis have lowered zinc concentrations in prostatic fluid. Although increased concentrations of zinc in prostatic fluid are associated with antimicrobial properties in men and male dogs, resistance to infection and resolution of infection are not correlated with zinc concentrations in prostatic tissue in the dog. Prostatitis can usefully be divided into acute, chronic, abscessed, and specific *(Brucella canis)* forms. Organisms that can be isolated, *E. coli, Proteus vulgaris,* and others, invade from the urethra. The affected organ may be diffusely or focally involved, swollen, congested, and edematous (Fig. 13-15). The early histologic change is catarrhal inflammation of the acini, expanding later to involve the interstitium. The ensuing abscesses may persist or resolve to be replaced by fibrous scars. Also, in dogs, there is a more common, clinically insignificant chronic prostatitis of unknown cause. Prostatitis is part of the spectrum of lesions caused by *Brucella canis* in the dog, and the prostate may be the site of persistence of the organism. A subacute interstitial inflammation causes enlargement of some lobules and, later, fibrosis involves some lobules. Blastomycosis has granulomaloris prostatitis as one of the several organs involved.

Hyperplasia and **metaplasia** of the prostate are common only in the dog. Enlargement of the prostate is relatively common in old dogs, and the dog is the only animal species that spontaneously develops prostatic hyperplasia with age. Clinical consequences of prostatic hypertrophy are obstruction and infection of the urinary tract, hydronephrosis, and constipation. Enlargement of the prostate is hormone-related but the precise cause is unknown. Hypertrophy of the gland does not occur in castrated dogs. Removal of androgens by castration of affected dogs is therapeutic; administration of estrogens causes enlargement of the gland. Possibly, acinar hyperplasia is caused by androgen excess, and fibromuscular hyperplasia is caused by estrogen excess, but the contribution of these two elements to the enlargement of the gland can overlap considerably. Enlarge-

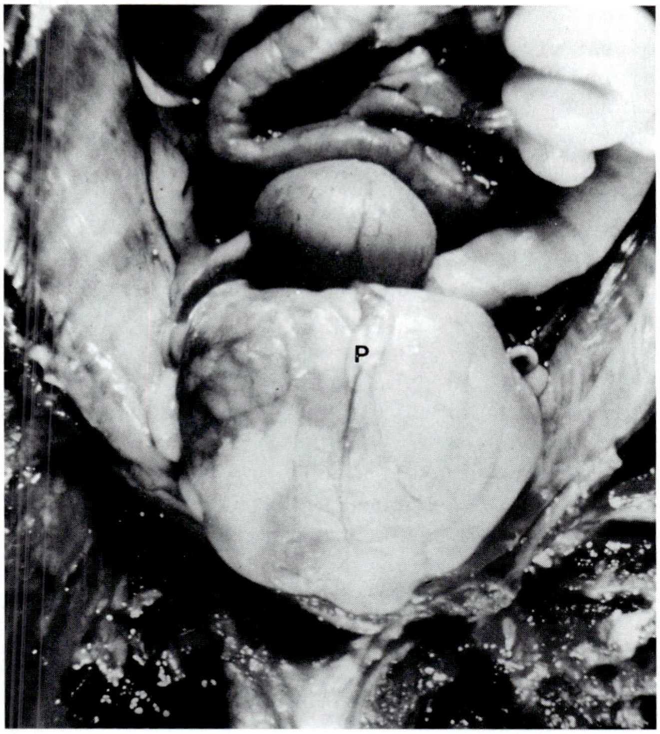

Fig. 13-15 Abdomen; dog. Prostatitis. The prostate (*P*) is enlarged.

ment of the gland may not be uniform. Large single cysts or multiple small cysts can develop.

Microscopically, hyperplasia of the interlobular and, to a lesser extent, the intralobular fibromuscular stroma occur together with hyperplasia of the acinar epithelium, often with the formation of papillae. Some acini are distended with fluid and lined by flattened epithelium. The presence of dilated cystic acini with attenuated epithelium is the basis for classifying prostatic hyperplasia as benign complex rather than benign glandular. In a study of the age-related changes in laboratory beagle dogs, complex benign prostatic hyperplasia was found in all animals over 6 years of age. Increases in size and weight of the prostate are primarily attributable to increases in interstitial tissues and to inflammation, with the inflammation being located primarily in the interstitial tissues. Increase in the glandular component is due to cystic dilatation not volume of glandular epithelium.

Estrogen-induced hypertrophy of the canine prostate, most often due to the presence of Sertoli cell tumor, has the added feature of squamous metaplasia of acinar epithelium, ducts, prostatic urethra, and uterus masculinus. Flattened keratinized squames are sloughed into the acini, and neutrophils and other inflammatory cells aggregate there too. Squamous metaplasia of the prostate in dogs is not preneoplastic. In castrated male sheep grazing clover pasture *(Trifolium subterraneum)* with a high estrogen content, hypertrophy, squamous metaplasia, and cyst formation occur in the accessory sex glands, especially the bulbourethral gland.

Adenocarcinoma of the prostate in the dog is the only prostatic neoplasm of any importance in domestic animals, and even it is rare. There seems to be an associated abnormal hormonal environment, as yet not well defined. Prostatic hyperplasia appears not to precede prostatic carcinoma, although the two lesions can be found together. The clinical signs of prostatic carcinoma are similar to those of prostatic hyperplasia, because of the enlargement of the organ, with the addition of cachexia and locomotory abnormalities caused by pressure and invasion of nearby structures, especially bones, by the neoplasm and its metastases. Grossly, the neoplasm is responsible for increased firmness, nonsymmetric enlargement, partial or complete loss of the median raphe, and cystic cavities in the prostate. The capsule may be ruptured by the outgrowing neoplasm, and often there is attachment to the floor of the pelvis.

Microscopically, prostatic tissue contains areas of hyperplasia and fibroplasia. Distinguishing between hyperplasia and neoplasia can sometimes be difficult; in hyperplasia, orientation of epithelial cells is regular against a basement membrane with little fibrosis and no invasion. Microscopically, prostatic adenocarcinomas can form acini, form undifferentiated sarcoma-like sheets, or invade the connective tissue as single cells. In men, it is recognized that the inner mass of the gland responds to estrogen stimulation and the outer mass to androgen stimulation. Hyperplasia most often occurs in the inner mass and neoplasia in the outer mass. In dogs, no specific region of the prostate has been associated with the development of hyperplasia or neoplasia.

PENIS AND PREPUCE

Developmental Abnormalities

The penis is subject to many abnormalities of size and form, such as congenital absence, hypoplasia, hyperplasia, duplication, directional deviations, and, in ruminants, absence of the sigmoid flexure and abnormal locations of retractor muscle insertions. These lesions are not common.

Hypoplasia of the penis and prepuce may simply be the result of extremely early castration. In intersex states, hypoplasia of these structures is part of a spectrum of abnormalities.

Persistent frenulum is a minor anatomic abnormality rather than a serious defect, but it can have an important deleterious effect in limiting the extent to which the penis can be protruded from the sheath (Fig. 13-16) and in causing the erect penis to be curved instead of straight. Persistent frenulum is of importance in bulls. Judging by the frequent occurrence of large flaps and tags of tissue on the ventral raphe of the penis, transitory persistence of the fren-

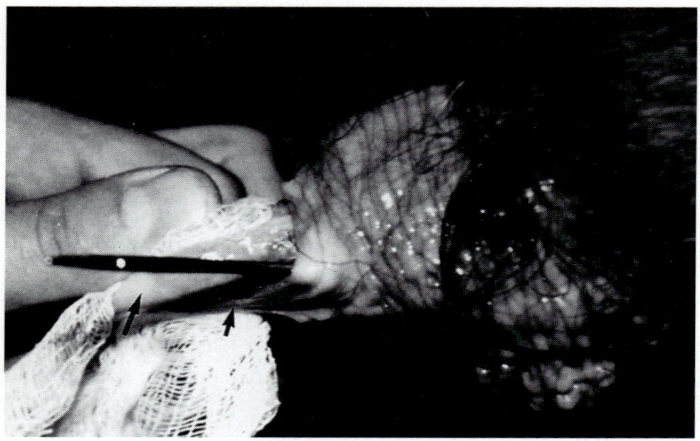

Fig. 13-16 Penis; bull. Persistent frenulum. The persistent frenulum *(short arrow)* permits only limited protrusion of the penis (*long arrow*). A probe has been inserted between the penis and the frenulum. *Courtesy Dr. E.A. Usenik.*

ulum is quite common. The raphe of the penis and sheath are remnants of the frenulum, a thin membrane, ventral to the penis, that normally ruptures, probably due to simple mechanical cause, at puberty. Persistent segments of frenulum are well vascularized, usually occur at the distal end of the penis, and can connect the penis to the sheath or the penis to itself.

Hypospadias and **epispadias** are malformations of the urethral canal that create abnormal openings of the urethra on the ventral surface of the penis (hypospadias) or on the dorsal surface (epispadias). Hypospadias can be regarded as a mild form of pseudohermaphroditism, with minimal ambiguity, as there is failure of proper closure of the urethral fold. In hypospadias, the urinary opening is ventral and proximal to the normal location, anywhere from the glans to the penile shaft, penoscrotal junction, or the perineum. Either hypospadias or epispadias may occur in animals with other malformations incompatible with survival, or they may occur alone. Their importance is in the potential for causing urinary obstruction and in interference with normal ejaculation.

Phimosis and **paraphimosis** are terms that in the human male refer, respectively, to inability to retract the prepuce over the penis because of too small a preputial opening and to the inability to replace the prepuce over the penis because of penile swelling. True congenital phimosis does not occur in animals because of the larger preputial cavity and opening. Inflammatory phimosis in animals occurs when inflammation causes swelling of the penis or prepuce so that the penis cannot be extruded from the sheath.

Inflammation

Inflammation of the glans penis is **balanitis;** inflammation of the prepuce is **posthitis.** Nonspecific inflammation of the penis and prepuce **(balanoposthitis)** can occur in a number of situations. A large and diverse microbial flora normally inhabits the preputial cavity. Inflammation occurs secondary to trauma, such as bite wounds in dogs and boars. Traumatic lesions occur in bulls of breeds with a pendulous sheath that can easily be torn by sticks or other sharp objects. Temporary protrusion of the penis from the sheath is common in these and other bulls; the everted preputial mucosa is subject to injury. In animals with phimosis, the initial problem is greatly exacerbated by urination into the preputial cavity, creating an environment for the overgrowth of organisms. Repeated protrusion of the penis into the normal preputial diverticulum of the boar, because of malformation or perverse behavior, likewise will predispose to local infection. Depending on the cause, balanoposthitis can take a wide range of forms, mild to severe, focal to diffuse, acute to chronic, possibly ulcerative, necrotizing, diphtheritic, catarrhal, or suppurative. Lymphoid nodules in the preputial lamina propria of the bull may be important in cell-mediated immunity in the preputial cavity.

Herpesviruses can cause balanoposthitis in several species. Infectious bovine rhinotracheitis virus causes a balanoposthitis in the bull. The disease progresses over the course of a few days from hyperemia and swelling to pustules and then 1 to 2 mm ulcers, especially on the glans penis. For a brief period in the pustule stage, intranuclear eosinophilic inclusion bodies are present in epithelial cells. Equine herpesvirus-3 causes equine coital exanthema, a disease in stallions and mares with a similarly short clinical course, but resulting in the formation of larger (15 mm) pustules with a predilection for the body rather than the glans of the penis. Canine herpesvirus in the dog causes inflammation at the base of the penis and the reflection of the prepuce but does not cause the formation of pustules or ulcers. Resolution of these lesions is rapid, leaving only hyperplastic mucosal lymphoid nodules and small areas of depigmented mucosa. In the bull, the herpesvirus persists in tissues in a latent state and is capable of becoming reactivated. It is not known whether the same phenomenon occurs in stallions and dogs.

Ovine ulcerative posthitis is caused by *Corynebacterium renale,* acting, when the urine has large amounts of urea, to produce ulceration of the prepuce near its orifice. Other factors, such as diet and season, play a role. Hormones seem to be involved, too, as the disease is mainly one of wethers, not rams. If the preputial orifice becomes blocked by swelling, the disease becomes much more severe, spreading beyond the initial small ulcer on the hairless skin of the prepuce to diffusely involve the mucosa, with ulceration of the glans penis and loss of the urethral process.

Other organisms are capable of causing balanoposthitis. These include *Strongyloides papillosus* in the bull, and the larvae of *Habronema* sp. in the horse. In equine habronemiasis, the gross lesion has the same elevated nodular bleeding surface as granulation tissue or a sarcoid. Microscopically, however, distinct tracts of larval migration are filled with debris and surrounded by an inflammatory exudate rich in eosinophils. The well-known bovine venereally transmitted diseases of **vibriosis** and **trichomoniasis** cause no lesions or minimal nonspecific lesions of the male external genitalia.

Neoplasms

The penis and prepuce may be involved in metastatic or multicentric neoplasms such as mastocytoma, melanoma, and lymphosarcoma. The following are the most important primary neoplasms of the penis and prepuce.

Transmissible venereal tumor of the dog is a neoplasm of uncertain histogenesis. In the male animal, it is found on the penis, more often on the caudal parts, and not often on the prepuce (Fig. 13-17). The neoplasm may be single or multiple, a few millimeters to 10 cm in diameter, with an inflamed, ulcerated, cauliflower-like surface. Microscopically, the neoplasm has the same appearance as it has in the bitch and is composed of sheets of neoplastic cells and minimal stroma. The neoplastic cells are large, uniform, with a large nucleus and nucleolus, indistinct cellular outlines, and numerous mitotic figures. Metastasis is not common. Regression and recovery are the rule. Virus particles have not been seen in neoplastic cells. Experimental transmissibility by intact cells, together with the repeatedly demonstrated constant karyotypic differences between normal dog cells and cells of the neoplasm, and the absence of host isoantigens on the neoplastic cells suggest that the neoplasm is a naturally occurring neoplasm of canine cells (allogeneic) that is transmitted from dog to dog by living cells rather than arising as the result of transformation of host cells.

Squamous cell carcinoma of the penis is of importance in the horse and, to a lesser extent, in the dog. In the horse, both stallions and geldings can have neoplasms, and the

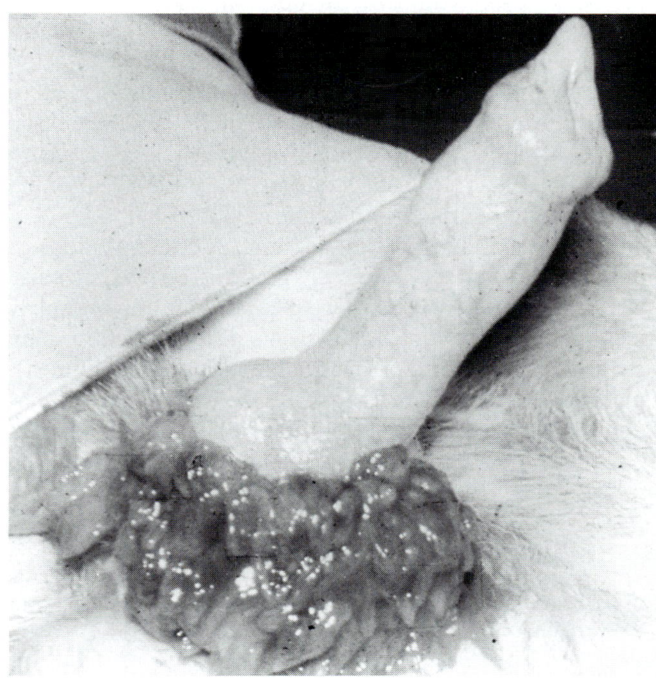

Fig. 13-17 Penis; dog. Transmissible venereal tumor. Soft, elongate tumor masses have formed in a cluster on the mucosa over the proximal end of the shaft of the penis. *Courtesy Dr. M.H. Goldschmidt.*

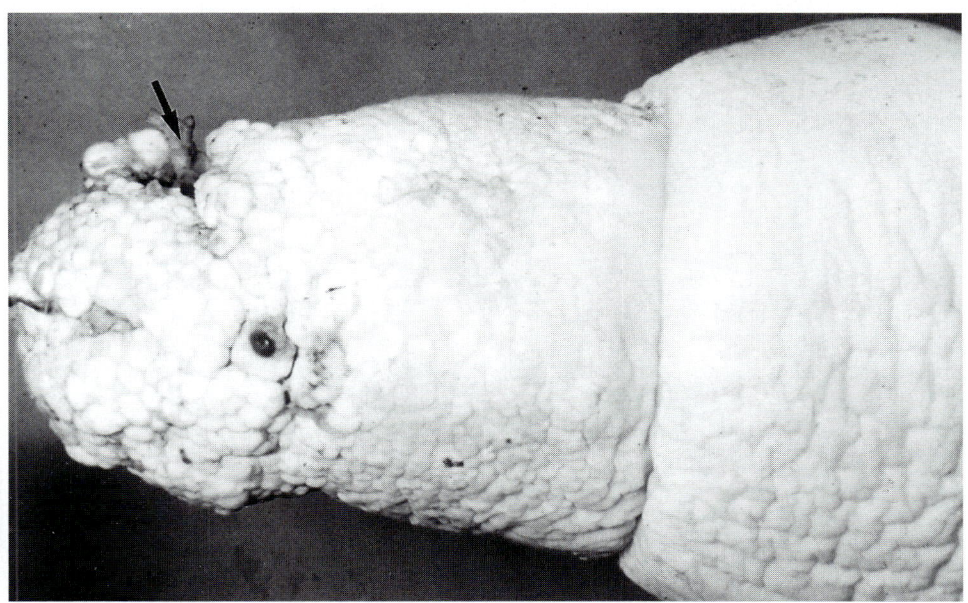

Fig. 13-18 Penis; horse. Squamous cell carcinoma. The carcinoma has invaded and has caused necrosis and subsequent ulceration of the glans penis *(arrow).*

common site is the glans penis. Rather than producing a proliferative mass, the neoplasm in this location in invasive, necrotic, and ulcerated (Fig. 13-18). Microscopically, the neoplasm is well differentiated, with well-developed keratin pearls. Metastases to the inguinal and iliac lymph nodes usually can be found. The sheath becomes edematous because of lymphatic obstruction, and the preputial cavity becomes distended by retained smegma, inflammatory debris, and urine.

Fibropapilloma of the glans penis of bulls occurs in younger animals. The age of the affected animals and the occasional observation of inclusion bodies suggest an infectious cause. The lesion consists of single or multiple warty growths, with a significant amount of fibrous core and a papilliferous epithelial covering. The proportions of epithelial and fibrous tissue vary greatly from case to case. There is often extensive surface ulceration following spontaneous necrosis or trauma. The size of the neoplasm may interfere with breeding or cause phimosis or paraphimosis. Other untoward possible sequelae are preputial hairs entangling the prolapsed penis and causing strangulation, and compression of the phimotic penis, causing rupture of the urethra.

Suggested Readings

Barsanti JA, Finco DR. Canine prostatic diseases. Vet Clin North Am Small Anim Pract 1986; 16:587-599.

Brown TR, Migeon CJ. Androgen receptors in normal and abnormal male sexual differentiation. Adv Exp Med Biol 1986; 196:227-255.

Edwards DF, Kennedy JR, Patton CS, Toal RL, Daniel GB, Lothrop CD. Familial immotile-cilia syndrome in English springer spaniel dogs. Am J Med Genet 1989; 33:290-298.

Ezzi A, Ladds PW, Hoffmann D, Foster RA, Briggs GD. Pathology of varicocele in the ram. Aust Vet J 1988; 65:11-15.

Gelberg HB, McEntee K. Equine testicular interstitial cell tumors. Vet Pathol 1987; 24:231-234.

Haas GG, Beer AE. Immunologic influences on reproductive biology: Sperm gametogenesis and maturation in the male and female genital tracts. Fertil Steril 1986; 46:753-766.

Humphrey JD, Ladds PW. Pathology of the bovine testis and epididymis. Vet Bull 1975; 45:787-795.

Leav I, Ling GV. Adenocarcinoma of the canine prostate. Cancer 1968; 22:1329-1345.

Lowseth LA, Gerlach RF, Gillett NA, Muggenburg BA. Age-related changes in the prostate and testes of the beagle dog. Vet Pathol 1990; 27:347-353.

Marshall LS, Oehlert ML, Haskins ME, Seldon JR, Patterson DF. Persistent mullerian duct syndrome in miniature schnauzers. J Am Vet Med Assoc 1982; 181:798-801.

McEntee K. Reproductive Pathology of Domestic Mammals. San Diego: Academic, 1990:224-384.

Meyers-Wallen VN, Donahoe PK, Ueno T, Manganaro TF, Patterson DF. Mullerian inhibiting substance is present in testes of dogs with persistent mullerian duct syndrome. Biol Reprod 1989; 41:881-888.

Meyers-Wallen VN, Patterson DF. Sexual differentiation and inherited disorders of sexual development in the dog. J Reprod Fert, Suppl 39 (1989), 57-64.

Meyers-Wallen VN, Wilson JD, Griffin JE, Fisher S, Moorhead PH, Goldschmidt MH, Haskins ME, Patterson DF. Testicular feminization in a cat. J Am Vet Med Assoc 1989; 195:631-634.

Paitnaik AK, Mostofi FK. A clinicopathologic, histologic, and immunohistochemical study of mixed germ cell-stromal tumors in the testis of 16 dogs. Vet Pathol 1993; 30:287-295.

Papa FO, Alvarenga MA, Lopes MD, Campos Filho EP. Infertility of autoimmune origin in a stallion. Equine Vet J 1990; 22:145-146.

Reif JR, Brody RS. The relationship between cryptorchidism and canine testicular neoplasia. J Am Vet Med Assoc 1969; 155:2005-2010.

Romagnoli SE. Canine cryptorchidism. Vet Clin North Am Small Anim Pract 1991; 21:533-545.

Zhang J, Ricketts SW, Tanner SJ. Antisperm antibodies in the semen of a stallion following testicular trauma. Equine Vet J 1990; 22:138-141.

CHAPTER

14

Pathology of the Eye and Ear

JAMES A. RENDER
WILLIAM W. CARLTON

GLOBE AND ADNEXA

The components of the eye (ocular apparatus) include the eyeball (globe), optic nerve, and accessory structures, including the eyelids, lacrimal apparatus, orbital fasciae, and oculomotor muscles. The eyeball has been defined as "a layer of neural light-sensitive tissue (the retina) held in place by surrounding coats which protect it (sclera) and nourish it (choroid) and served by an optical system of a lens of modified transparent epithelium behind a transparent anterior extension of the sclera (cornea), all of which combine to focus light on the retina." (Prince et al, 1960)

The eyeball is composed of three concentric tunics—fibrous, vascular, and nervous—and contains three refractive media—the aqueous humor, lens, and vitreous body. It is situated in the orbit, protected in front by the eyelids and conjunctiva and in the middle portion by the orbital ring. The orbit is a body fossa that separates the eyeball from the cranial cavity, surrounds and protects the globe, and provides pathways for nerves and blood vessels.

The tunicae of the eyeball consist of the fibrous, an external coat composed of an opaque posterior sclera and the transparent anterior cornea; the vascular (or uvea), lying internal to the fibrous tunic and composed of the iris, ciliary body, and choroid; and the nervous, composed of the retina, which is a thin delicate membrane representing an invaginated extension of the brain to which it is connected by the optic nerve.

The anterior and posterior poles are the central points of the anterior and posterior curvatures of the eyeball. The equator is an imaginary line drawn around the eyeball midway between the poles. Planes parallel to the equator are designated transverse, coronal, and frontal or radial planes. The meridional plane is a line drawn around the eyeball through the poles. Planes parallel to the meridional plane, but not passing through the poles, are called sagittal.

Ocular Embryology

The eyeball develops from several embryonic tissues, beginning with an envagination of the forebrain, the optic vesicle, connected to the forebrain by the optic stalk. The optic vesicle interacts with surface ectoderm and induces an invagination of the surface ectoderm to form the lens sac. The lens sac eventually develops into the lens vesicle, which pinches off from the surface ectoderm while the optic vesicle is invaginating to form the two-layered optic cup. The optic cup is incomplete due to a ventral optic fissure, which eventually closes. The developing lens is surrounded by a network of blood vessels (tunica vasculosa lentis) that connect with the hyaloid artery, a vessel extending from the posterior aspect of the lens to the optic disc. These embryonic vessels eventually regress. The surface ectoderm will give rise to the corneal epithelium, lens, ocular glands, conjunctiva, and skin of the eyelids. The neuroectoderm of the optic cup will form the epithelium of the iris and ciliary body and the retina. The mesenchymal tissue of the eyeball is presumed to be derived from mesencephalic neural crest cells. Interference with this development of the eye may result in anomalies that can involve some or all of these structures.

Anomalies of the Globe

Multiple anomalies of the globe and ocular adnexa are common in certain species, especially the dog, but are rare in most others. The severity of the anomalies varies greatly from the globe being absent (anophthalmia), through stages of congenital cystic globe, cyclopia, synophthalmia, and microphthalmia, to a normal-sized globe with missing portions of various layers (coloboma).

Congenital cystic globe, cyclopia, and synophthalmia

The congenitally cystic globe results when there is disruption of development of the evaginating optic vesicles.

In its extreme form, a variably pigmented optic vesicle is greatly distended and is frequently invested by choroidal and scleral tissues but does not have a lens, cornea, vitreous body, or anterior uvea. The developing globe is at risk of becoming cystic when each optic vesicle expands laterally to contact the lateral head ectoderm. In the area of contact, the neural retina is induced in the vesicle, and the lens ectoderm is induced in the surface ectoderm. When the vesicle fails to contact the surface ectoderm, these reciprocal interactions and all those flowing from them do not occur, resulting in the congenital cystic globe.

Cyclopia is a developmental anomaly characterized by the presence of a single median eye in a single median orbital fossa. Cyclopia is at one extreme of a spectrum of disorders; between cyclopia and the development of two normal lateral globes, any degree of either partial separation or fusion of the globes (synophthalmia) may occur. The nose either is absent or is present as a tubular appendage located above the orbit. Other anomalies associated with cyclopia and synophthalmia include hydrocephalus, lissencephaly, and absence of various structures of the brain and head.

Veratrum-*induced malformations*

Congenital malformations, varying in severity from cyclops to a slightly deformed upper jaw, occur in lambs born to ewes grazing certain alpine meadows in the western United States. Hydrocephalus, harelip, cleft palate, and displacement of the nose are associated anomalies. In severely malformed lambs, the cranium is domed; the cerebral hemispheres are fused into thin-walled, fluid-filled cysts; the olfactory bulbs are usually absent; and globes that are displaced centrally have only one optic nerve. Often, a proboscis-like protuberance, with either a fibrous or cartilaginous core, arises in the median plane dorsal to the eye. Anophthalmia is present in some lambs.

These anomalies are produced by the feeding of fresh green or dried *Veratrum californicum* to ewes from the 1st to the 15th day of gestation and in the lambs from ewes fed the plant only on gestation day 14. Ewes fed the plant on gestation day 11, 12, 13, 15, or 16 all have either normally developed fetuses or normally developed embryos that have died. The embryo at gestation day 14 is starting its early differentiation of the germ layers. Cyclopian-type deformities, identical to those in lambs, were produced in goats and calves by the feeding of *V. californicum* from the 14th day to 25th day of gestation. The teratogenic agents in *V. californicum* have been identified as steroidal alkaloids; three of these (jervine, cyclopamine, and cycloposine) are responsible for the cyclopian-type deformities.

Anophthalmia-microphthalmia

The clinical absence of a recognizable globe is called anophthalmia. Experimentally, some cases of clinical anophthalmia are degenerative in type, as optic rudiments are present early; but these degenerate, and animals are born with clinical anophthalmia. Complete absence of ocular tissue is uncommon; some rudiments usually can be recognized in the orbital tissue at microscopic examination.

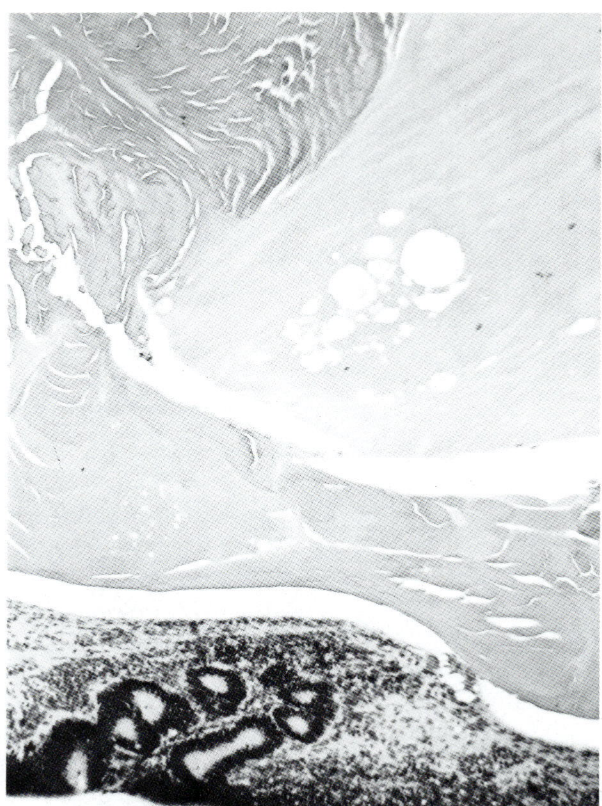

Fig. 14-1 Globe; canine. Microphthalmia. Multiple ocular anomalies include retinal detachment, retinal dysplasia, and cataract with retina adhered to lens. Hematoxylin-eosin (H & E) stain; ×63.

Microphthalmia, an abnormally small globe, has been described in all species and may be either unilateral or bilateral; the highest incidence has been described in pigs and dogs. Generally, microphthalmia is accompanied by other defects and anomalies of the ocular structures, and retinal detachment is a commonly associated defect. Detachment of the retina in the microphthalmic globe is apparently due to the difference in the growth rates of the inner and outer layers of the developing globe. Dysplastic changes also occur in the retina, including rosette formation, the presence of folds, and congenital detachment (Fig. 14-1).

Coloboma

A congenital absence of a portion of an ocular tissue is designated ''typical'' coloboma when located in the region of the fetal optic fissure and "atypical" when located elsewhere in the globe. Typical colobomas result from failure and/or aberrant closure of the fetal optic fissure and involve, most commonly, the choroid and retina but may involve the iris and ciliary body.

Collie ectasia syndrome (collie eye anomaly)

This inherited disease, described in the rough- and smooth-coated collie and Shetland sheepdog, has a worldwide distribution and is caused by defective mesodermal differentiation affecting posterior fibrous and vascular tunicae of the globe. The disease is characterized by several congenital defects involving the sclera, choroid, retina, and optic disc. The ocular lesions are always bilateral, although the severity of the lesions may vary in each globe. Abnormalities include choroidal hypoplasia, colobomas either in or adjacent to the optic disc, posterior scleral ectasia, retinal detachment, intraocular hemorrhage, microphthalmia, and central corneal opacity.

Globes that clinically have coloboma in the optic papilla microscopically have excavations of either the optic nerve or its sheath that often displace or distort the nerve. Deep in the colobomas, the body of the optic nerve contains aberrant neural tissue supported by a herniated scleral sheath. Colobomas of the optic nerve are lined by attenuated retina with the outer layers missing. Globes with posterior scleral ectasia clinically have orbital cysts in the region of the optic nerve. The posterior ectasia is supported by a greatly thinned sclera; the optic nerve is distorted and is replaced in part by an ectatic cavity lined partly by patches of proliferated unpigmented epithelium and partly by atrophic and disorganized retinal elements (Fig. 14-2).

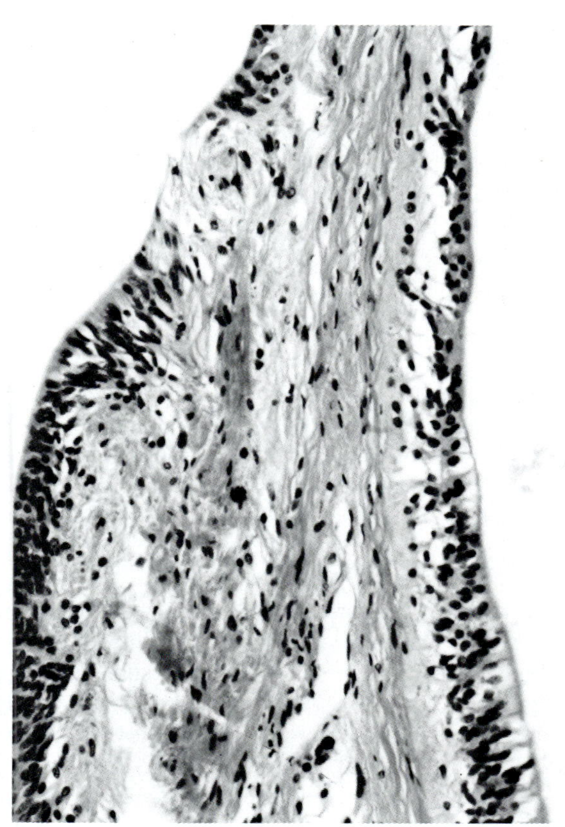

Fig. 14-2 Globe, optic nerve; canine. Collie ectasia syndrome. Ectatic spaces at optic nerve head are lined by dysplastic retinal tissue. H & E stain; ×160.

Bovine virus diarrhea

Ocular lesions, including microphthalmia, have been observed in calves born to cows infected during pregnancy with the virus of bovine diarrhea-mucosal disease. The microscopic ocular lesions include cataract, retinal atrophy, and optic neuritis. The retina may lose its normal layer organization. Gliosis can be severe in the optic nerve. In microphthalmic globes, the anterior chamber is shallow, the vitreous is filled with blood and aberrant tissue, and the lens is globular with the cortex cataractous and partially liquified. A cyclitic fibrovascular membrane forms in some globes from the posterior ciliary processes. The retina is dysplastic and may be sealed into the fibrovascular membrane that contains cartilage, bone, and bone marrow. Pigment may be present in all layers of the retina. The optic nerve is small and gliotic.

Ocular Inflammation

Inflammations of the globe are classified according to the character of the exudate (suppurative, nonsuppurative, granulomatous) and the extent of involvement of the ocular and periocular structures (endophthalmitis, panophthalmitis). Inflammatory processes in the globe are often difficult to classify because, in the early stages, the reaction may be suppurative and, later, it may be nonsuppurative. Panophthalmitis is an inflammation that is widespread in the globe and also involves the outer coat and Tenon's capsule. In endophthalmitis, the inflammation involves only the ocular cavities and their adjacent structures.

Suppurative inflammation

Panophthalmitis and endophthalmitis—fulminating, suppurative processes (Fig. 14-3)—cause variable degrees of destruction of the retina and uvea, abscess formation in the vitreous, and exudate in the anterior chamber. In panophthalmitis, extension of inflammation through the sclera produces tenonitis and orbital cellulitis.

Acute suppurative panophthalmitis and endophthalmitis are most often due to the introduction of bacteria by lacerated wounds, intraocular foreign bodies, extension of corneal infections through ulceration and perforation, surgical procedures, and septicemia with bacterial metastasis to the choroid and retina. Purulent and fibrinopurulent in-

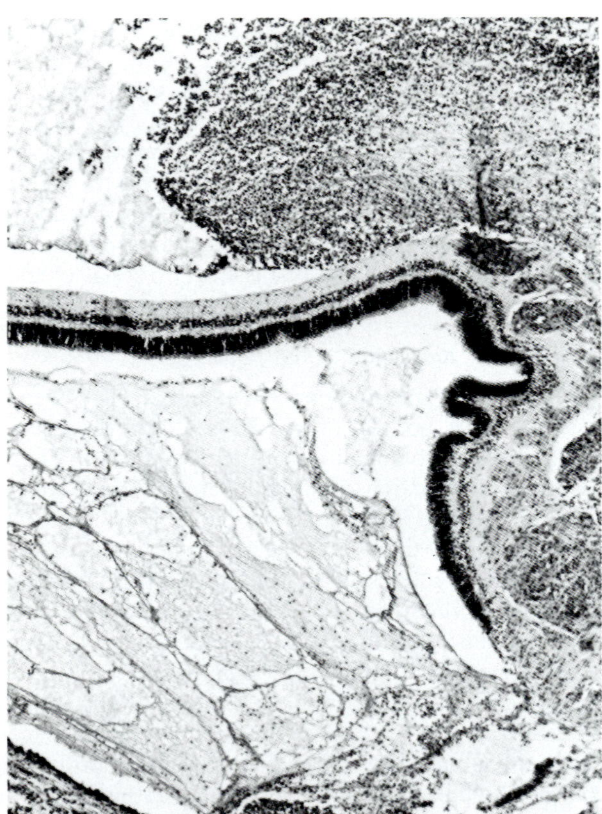

Fig. 14-3 Globe; equine. Suppurative endophthalmitis. The lesions include papillitis with exudate extending into the vitreous, retinal detachment, and a subretinal exudate. H & E stain; ×40.

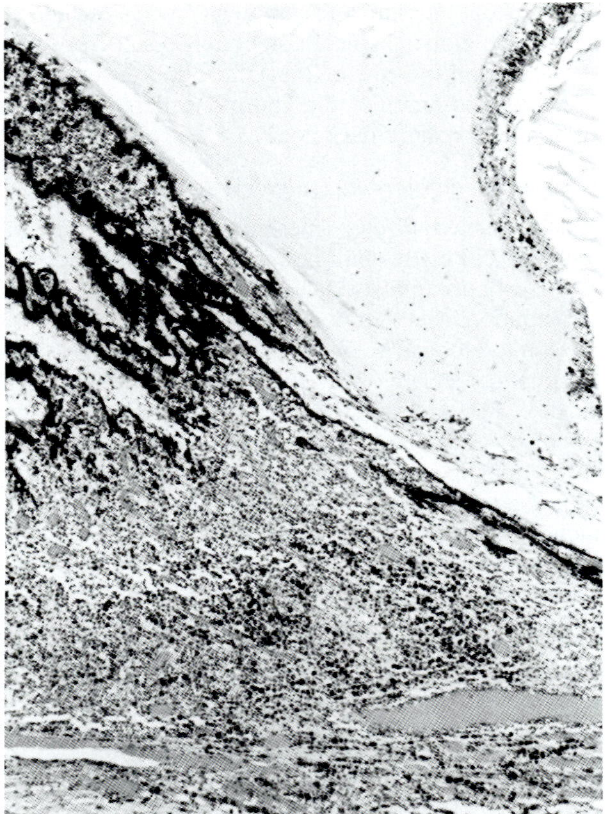

Fig. 14-4 Globe, ciliary body; canine. Nonsuppurative endophthalmitis. A diffuse mononuclear cellular exudate infiltrates base and processes of ciliary body, and a proteinaceous exudate fills the posterior chamber and subretinal space beneath a detached and atrophic retina. H & E stain; ×40.

fections of the globes of domestic animals are frequently hematogenous and may be associated with a necrotizing vasculitis. A variety of organisms may be responsible for suppurative panophthalmitis in animals, including coliform organisms, *Pseudomonas aeruginosa, Haemophilus somnus, Salmonella* spp., and *Streptococcus pneumoniae.*

Nonsuppurative inflammation

Surgical and other traumas that produce hemorrhages in the globe, foreign bodies, certain endogenous infections, and immune-mediated reactions often produce nonsuppurative ocular inflammation. The reaction is predominantly lymphocytic and plasmacytic. Microscopic features include much less tissue destruction and fewer infiltrating cells than are usual with suppurative inflammation. Mononuclear cells surround the vessels of the sclera, infiltrate the ciliary body (Fig. 14-4) and choroid diffusely, and form thick cuffs about retinal vessels (in species with retinal vessels). Mononuclear cells are present over the surface of the ciliary body and in the vitreous and are carried by the aqueous into the anterior chamber to form a layer on both surfaces of the iris. The aqueous becomes turbid with protein and floating cells, and these cells are deposited on the posterior surface of the cornea as keratic precipitates. The cornea may be spared if the changes are mild, but corneal edema and keratitis are to be expected if there is much exudation.

Granulomatous inflammation

Granulomatous inflammatory alterations of the globe and orbital tissues may follow trauma with introduction of foreign bodies, perforation of the lens and subsequent autosensitization to lenticular protein, posttraumatic endogenous fungal infections, microfilaria and larvae of parasites, and certain bacterial diseases, such as tuberculosis. The reaction is characterized by presence of epithelioid and giant cells, diffuse lymphocytic and plasma cell infiltrates, and some fibrosis. The reaction is often nodular, involving any portion of the globe but especially the iridal stroma, filtration area, ciliary body (Fig. 14-5), and choroid.

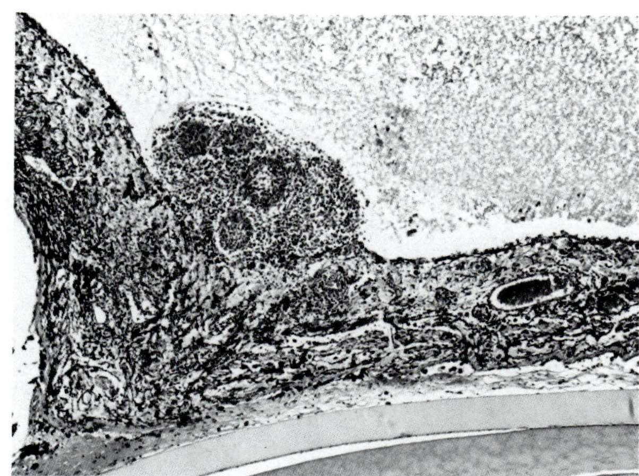

Fig. 14-5 Globe, iris; canine. Coccidioidomycosis. Granulomatous iritis with posterior synechia has nodules on the anterior face of iris, and proteinaceous exudate is in the anterior chamber. H & E stain; ×40.

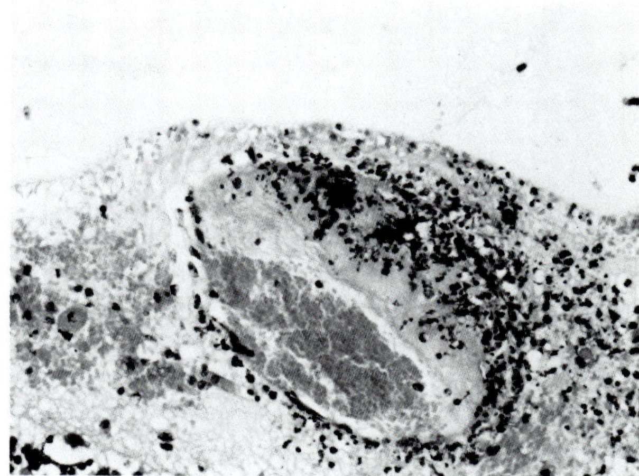

Fig. 14-6 Globe, retina; bovine. Thromboembolic encephalomyelitis. *Haemophilus somnus* infection results in vasculitis, thrombosis, and retinal hemorrhage and necrosis. H & E stain; ×250.

Complications of ocular inflammation

Complications of ocular inflammation include glaucoma, cataract, retinal detachment, atrophy of the uvea, and phthisis bulbi. Atrophy and phthisis refer to stages in the degeneration of injured or inflamed globes. Globes that have atrophy of internal structures without shrinkage are of normal size or slightly enlarged, and these result from chronic glaucoma. The internal architecture is well preserved, but atrophy diffusely involves the ocular tissues, especially the uvea and the retina, which may be detached. Some globes with internal atrophy are small and soft with scarred, small, flattened corneas. The anterior chamber may be absent, and both anterior and posterior synechiae are present. The lens is often cataractous, the internal architecture is relatively well preserved, but the retina is frequently detached by a cyclitic membrane.

Severely injured globes are disorganized and may be reduced to a shrunken, dense, white structure (**phthisis bulbi**). The cornea is shrunken, flattened, and opaque, and the sclera is markedly thickened. The contents of the globe are replaced by scar tissue, the retina is totally detached and atrophic, and osseous metaplasia may involve portions of the choroid.

Bacterial Causes of Ocular Disease

Many species of bacteria produce ocular disease when carried to the globe by the bloodstream and when introduced into the globe by traumatic penetrating wounds, by foreign bodies, and by surgery. The character, location, and severity of the ocular lesions vary, depending on the bacterial species (granulomatous with tuberculosis and suppurative with coliforms), the virulence of the organisms, the number of organisms in the inoculum, and whether the route of infection is hematogenous or traumatically introduced. Bacteria causing ocular disease include some of those that produce bacteremia and septicemia in domestic and laboratory animals. Focal choroiditis and cyclitis result from hematogenously introduced bacterial pathogens, as both ocular regions are especially sensitive and responsive to circulating bacteria and bacterial toxins. It is established that cases of bacterial meningitis, whether caused by streptococci, coliform organisms, or other bacteria, often have ocular lesions as well.

Diseases in which ocular inflammation have been described include colibacillosis in calves, pigs, and birds; streptococcosis in calves with meningitis and monkeys with either septicemia or meningitis; salmonellosis in pigs, calves, poults, and chicks; erysipelas in pigs; listeriosis in lambs and calves; brucellosis in dogs; tuberculosis in several species; and staphylococcosis in rats. *H. somnus,* the cause of bovine thromboembolic meningoencephalitis, produces ocular lesions centered about the vessels of the uvea and retina (Fig. 14-6).

Viral Causes of Ocular Disease

Bovine malignant catarrhal fever

Cattle with malignant catarrhal fever clinically have mucopurulent keratoconjunctivitis and corneal edema and ulceration. Microscopically, the panophthalmitis consists of mononuclear cellular infiltrations in the cornea, sclera, uveal tract, and retina and vasculitis of the uveal, scleral, and retinal vessels. Edema of the corneal stroma begins at the periphery and involves mainly the outer lamellae, accompanied by neutrophilic infiltration and intraepithelial edema with blister formation. The optic nerve seldom has lesions, although the meninges, adjacent extraocular mus-

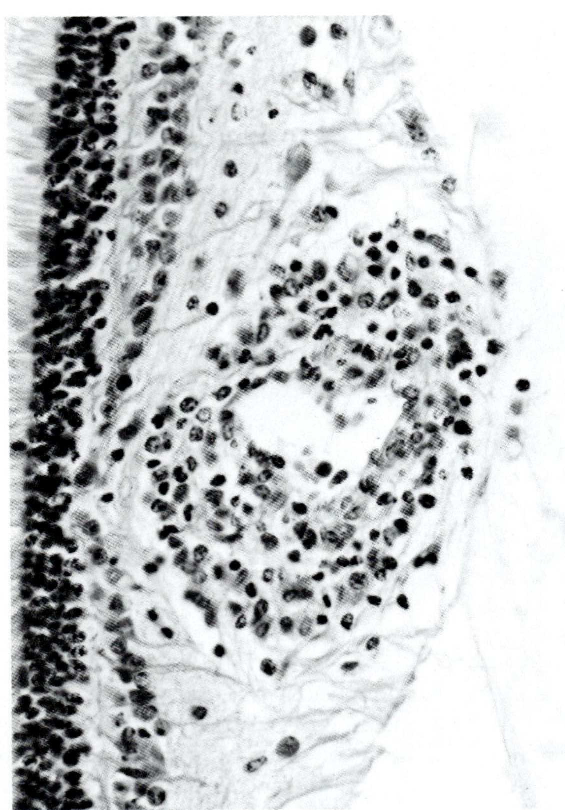

Fig. 14-7 Globe, retina; bovine. Malignant catarrhal fever. Retinitis characterized by mononuclear cells within and forming cuffs about retinal vessels. H & E stain; ×250. *Courtesy Dr. H.E. Whiteley.*

cles, and retina may have vessels infiltrated by inflammatory cells. Numerous retinal arteries and veins are cuffed by large mononuclear cells, varying from a single layer to massive cuffs that compress surrounding retinal tissue (Fig. 14-7). An acute iridiocyclitis is characterized by congestion, edema, and exudation of fibrin; mononuclear cells may be present along with synechia between either the iris and lens or iris and cornea.

Feline infectious peritonitis

Cats with infectious peritonitis may have unilateral or bilateral ocular lesions. Edema of the cornea is present in some cats, along with a mild aqueous flare and cells on the anterior surface of the iris. The irides maybe thickened and dull in appearance, and the retina may be detached. Cellular precipitates, which may occur on the face of the iris and adhere to the corneal endothelium, consist of necrotic macrophages, other mononuclear cells, and neutrophils. Focal, nonsuppurative to pyogranulomatous inflammation involves the iris, ciliary body, choroid, retina, optic nerve, and meninges of the optic nerve. The pyogranulomatous inflammation affects blood vessels, and the reaction is most intense in the uvea (Fig. 14-8). The choroidal blood vessels

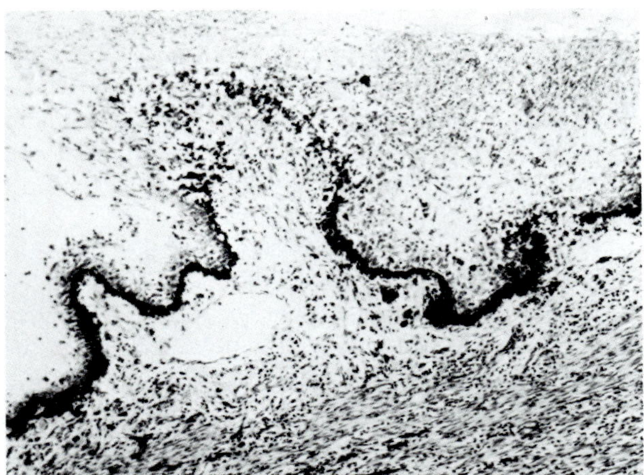

Fig. 14-8 Globe, ciliary body; feline. Feline infectious peritonitis. Uveal necrosis includes ciliary epithelium and is accompanied by exudate in posterior chamber about ciliary process. H & E stain; ×63.

exude cells and fluid; these collect in the subretinal space and cause retinal detachment.

Marek's disease

Ocular lesions are present in several tissues of the globes of chickens infected with the herpesvirus of Marek's disease. Proteinaceous exudate and inflammatory cells are present in the anterior and posterior chambers, and mononuclear inflammatory cells collect on the anterior face of the iris and about the pecten. Diffuse infiltrates or aggregates of lymphocytes and plasma cells are present in the iris and ciliary body. Cellular infiltrates may also occur in the choroid, retina, pecten, and optic nerve. The retina may become detached due to nodular accumulations of lymphoid cells in the choroid and subretinal space.

Parasitic Causes of Ocular Disease

Elaeophorosis in elk

Elaeophora schneideri is a relatively common parasite of deer and domestic sheep and is a cause of neuroophthalmic disease in elk. Elk are clinically blind due either to ocular or to brain lesions. The disease occurs predominantly in calves or yearlings of both sexes. Blind animals may have such signs as circling and ataxia and such gross lesions as necrosis of the muzzle and nostrils, dry gangrene of the ear tips, and abnormal growth of antlers. The larvae of *E. schneideri* are located predominantly in the arteries supplying the cephalic tissues from the ascending aorta and common brachiocephalic trunk, small leptomeningeal arteries supplying the brain, and the small arteries supplying the globe and optic nerve. Microfilariae are found chiefly in the small arteries, arterioles, and capillaries of the brain, globe, optic nerve, and skin of the head. Circulatory impairment follows lodgment of the parasite, and secondary ischemia results in lesions in the brain, globe, optic nerves, ears, muzzle, and other structures of the head region. In the globes, the lesions are bilateral and occur in the retina, choroid, and optic nerve and, early, consist of edema, focal degeneration, and necrosis, and, later, atrophy and sclerosis, primarily of the nontapetal region of the choroid and retina, and extend from the optic nerve head to the equator.

Onchocerciasis

In horses, microfilariae of *Onchocerca cervicalis* are found in the skin of the eyelids, with and without ocular lesions. In some acute cases, chemosis, conjunctivitis, keratitis, uveitis, and hypopyon are found. Chronic cases have follicular conjunctivitis, cataract, and uveitis with microfilariae in the cornea, anterior chamber, and other ocular tissues. Many globes with microfilariae have either no lesions or only perivascular cellular infiltrations.

Ocular larval migrans

Larval granulomatosis of the retina and choroid occurs in dogs due to larvae of *Toxocara* sp., especially *T. canis*. Ophthalmoscopic findings include elevated nodules in the fundus, retinal detachment, and retinal hemorrhages. The lesions are granulomas in the choroid and optic papilla. Those in the choroid extend into the subretinal space, resulting in retinal detachment and degeneration of the retina. Parasites are found within granulomas composed of mononuclear cells, fibroblasts, a few giant cells, and eosinophils. The lesions run the gamut from subacute to chronic inflammation, with fibrous connective tissue encapsulation, but are similar to the lesions seen in other organs of dogs with visceral larval migrans.

Ocular leishmaniasis

Ocular leishmaniasis *(Leishmania donovani)* is rare. The clinically detectable ocular lesions include pannus and exudate in the anterior chamber, over the iris, and in the vitreous. The microscopic lesions are those of marked bilateral nonsuppurative endophthalmitis with proliferation of fibrovascular tissue, cellular-proteinaceous exudate in anterior and posterior chambers, dense proteinaceous material and a few inflammatory cells in the vitreous, and infiltration of lymphocytes, plasma cells, and histiocytes into the uvea and cornea. Macrophages in several ocular tissues contain protozoal organisms.

Fungal Causes of Ocular Disease

Aspergillosis

Ocular infection with aspergilli (most commonly, *Aspergillus fumigatus*) is apparently most frequently encountered in birds, in which it occurs as part of systemic disease. It may also occur as a pure keratitis (Fig. 14-9), although intraocular structures become involved if the cornea is perforated. When part of a systemic infection, aspergillic fungi spread through the blood to lodge in the choroidal vessels

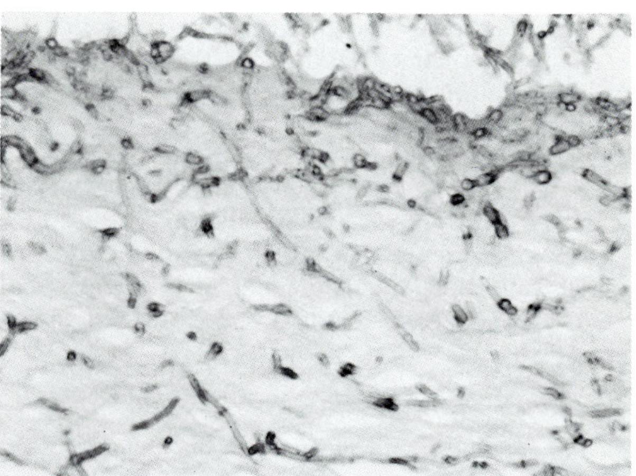

Fig. 14-9 Globe, cornea; avian. Aspergillosis. Fungal hyphae are in the corneal stroma and above the cornea. H & E stain; ×250.

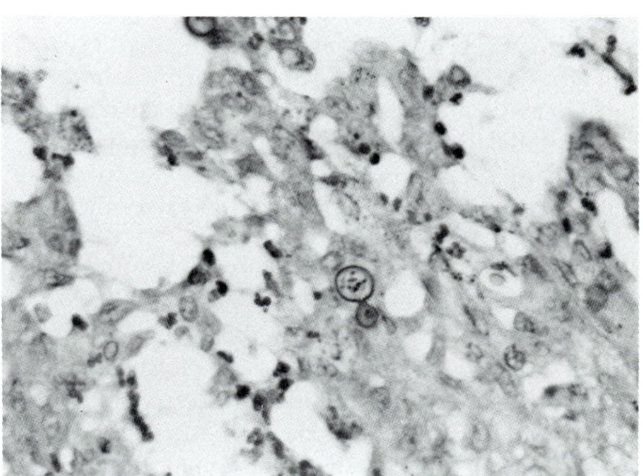

Fig. 14-10 Globe; canine. Blastomycosis. Budding blastospore of *Blastomyces dermatitidis* is in granulomatous exudate. H & E stain; ×400.

and, by extension, spread into the retina and vitreous, producing granulomatous endophthalmitis. Branching, septated fungal hyphae (3 to 6 μm in diameter) are present in several ocular structures. Organisms are demonstrated by such stains as periodic acid–Schiff (PAS) and Gomori methenamine-silver nitrate.

Blastomycosis

Ocular lesions due to infection with *Blastomyces dermatitidis* occur most often in dogs but are described in cats. Blindness, exophthalmos, scleritis, corneal edema, conjunctivitis, and purulent ocular discharge are present in affected dogs. The organisms spread to the globe through the bloodstream from either respiratory or cutaneous infections, resulting in either pyogranulomatous endophthalmitis or panophthalmitis. With involvement of the anterior uvea, exudate extends into the anterior and posterior chambers and into the vitreous. Exudate in the anterior chamber may lead to blockage of aqueous outflow and the development of glaucoma.

Lesions of the optic nerve consist of multiple granulomas containing fungal organisms. In most cases of ocular blastomycosis, lesions are found in other tissues. Fungal organisms are often numerous in areas of diffuse granulomatous inflammation and are budding, spherical bodies, are 8 to 15 μm in diameter, and have thick refractile walls (Fig. 14-10).

Coccidioidomycosis

Ocular infection with the fungus *Coccidioides immitis* has been rarely reported, although disseminated infection in dogs is common in endemic areas. The ocular lesions of a granulomatous endophthalmitis may involve the cornea (which may be opaque), ciliary body, iris, choroid, and retina. The lesions are nodular granulomas and contain spherules in all stages of development (Fig. 14-11). In some areas, especially about ruptured spherules, the inflammatory cellular reaction is mainly neutrophilic. Much exudate may be present in the anterior and posterior chambers and in the vitreal cavity. Exudate accumulating in the choroid causes detachment of the retina; extensive involvement of tissues of the filtration meshwork results in glaucoma.

Cryptococcosis

The incidence of intraocular infection with the fungus *Cryptococcus neoformans* appears to be fairly high in dogs and cats in endemic areas (Ohio and Mississippi River valleys). Involvement of the globe and, especially, the optic nerve may result from extension of infection from the meninges or by hematogenous spread, with trapping of the organisms in the choriocapillaris. The pathoanatomic alterations are bilateral and vary greatly from solid retinal and subretinal granulomas resulting in retinal detachment to honeycomb areas containing numerous cryptococcal organisms and little cellular exudate (Fig. 14-12), especially in immunosuppressed hosts.

Histoplasmosis

Ocular histoplasmosis in dogs and cats is usually a granulomatous endophthalmitis. Mononuclear cellular infiltrates in various ocular components include numerous macrophages containing spherical blastospores of *Histoplasma capsulatum.* The inflammatory process may extend from the choroid to the optic nerve head, the meninges about the optic nerve, and the outer retinal layers. The retina is separated from the retinal pigment epithelium by a proteinaceous exudate. The anterior chamber, filtration meshwork, and anterior uvea are filled with macrophages containing 2 to 4 μm, round, PAS-positive organisms.

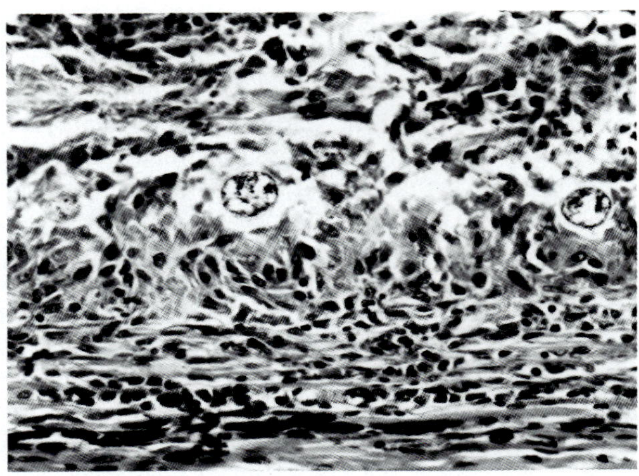

Fig. 14-11 Globe, choroid; canine. Coccidioidomycosis. Granulomatous choroiditis has spherule of *Coccidioides immitis.* H & E stain; ×250.

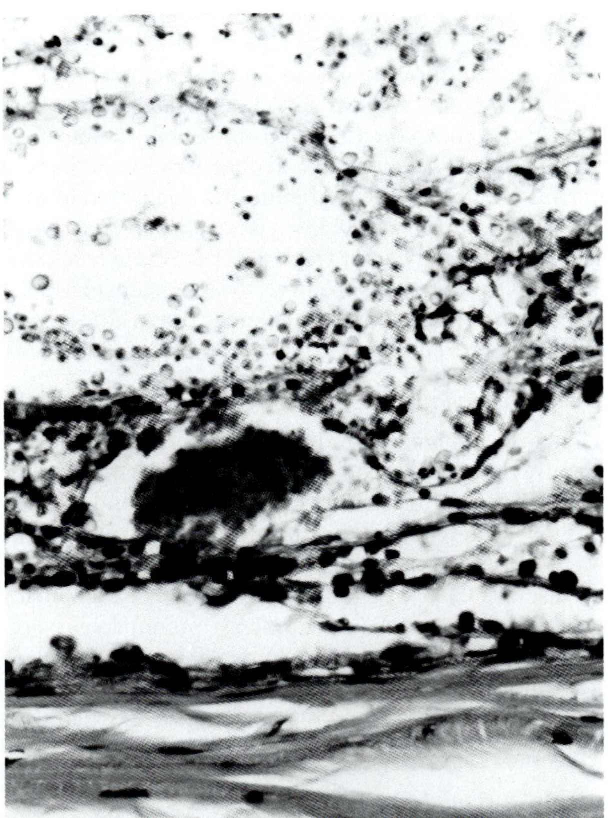

Fig. 14-12 Globe, choroid; canine. Cryptococcosis. Yeast forms of *Cryptococcus neoformans* are in the choroid, with little associated inflammatory reaction. H & E stain; ×250.

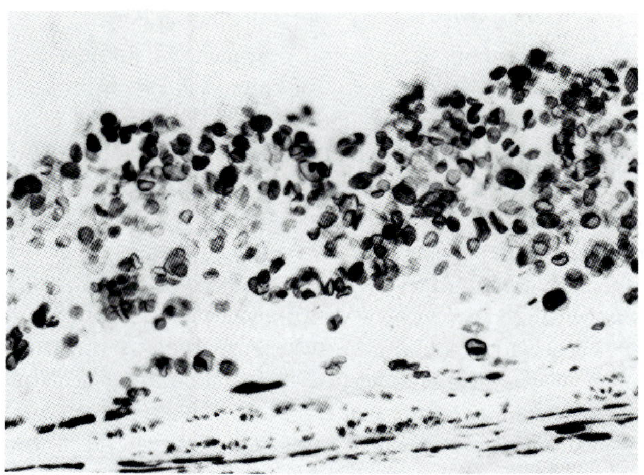

Fig. 14-13 Globe, choroid; canine. Protothecosis. Algal organisms of *Prototheca zopfii* are in the choroidal exudate. Gomori's methenamine silver (GMS) stain, ×250.

Algal Causes of Ocular Disease

Protothecosis

Prototheca species are microscopic, ovoid to globose, unicellular algal organisms with a hyaline, refractile, cellulose wall that surrounds granular cytoplasm. *Prototheca* species have been associated with lesions in several animal species and in a variety of tissues, but ocular lesions have been described only in dogs.

P. zopfii (in cases in which speciation was completed) has been the causative organism of canine protothecosis with ocular involvement. The globes can be severely damaged due to nonsuppurative endophthalmitis characterized by total retinal detachment, massive subretinal exudate teeming with algal organisms, and thickening of the choroid by exudate and organisms (Fig. 14-13). Posterior synechia, cataract, blood in the posterior chamber, iris bombé, retinitis, and optic neuritis with exudate and organisms in the connective tissue about the optic nerve are ocular alterations. Numerous organisms are present in the affected portions of the retina and in the subretinal exudate. The organisms appear round and oval and sometimes collapsed and crumpled. In size, they are 5 to 20 μm in diameter and have a thick, refractile cell wall in unstained smears. Multinucleate organisms are common.

CORNEA

Anomalies of the Cornea

Anomalies of the cornea include variation in size (**megalocornea, microcornea),** congenital opacities, congenital anterior synechiae, and dermoids. Megalocornea, in which the cornea is excessively large but otherwise normal, is rarely encountered in domestic animals. It must be distinguished from buphthalmos, in which there is a large cornea associated with an enlarged globe due to glaucoma. Microcornea is usually a part of microphthalmia but may occur alone. Congenital opacities of the cornea may be focal or diffuse and involve the superficial or deep stroma. Congenital opacities may result from a defect in development, e.g., Descemet's membrane usually is defective in the region of the opacity. Congenital anterior synechiae, consisting of isolated strands passing from the iris to the cornea, are common and are derived from the mesenchyme of the pupillary membrane, incompletely removed during development of the globe.

Dermoid

A dermoid is a congenital choristoma characterized as a piece of skin present on the cornea, conjunctiva, or both. The lesion has been described in several animal species but is probably most common in cattle. Dermoids are either unilateral or bilateral and are often located in the temporal region in dogs and are rare, superficial, and limbal in cats. Dermoids are congenital and are noticed either at birth or when the eyelids are opened. Because of irritation, their presence may be associated with a mucopurulent discharge and blepharospasm. Microscopically, dermoids have the structure of skin and may be cystic, pigmented, and with and without hairs.

Degenerations and Dystrophies

Keratoconjunctivitis sicca

This disease (dry eye, xerophthalmia), common in the dog but rare in other domestic animals, is a chronic disease of the cornea and conjunctiva due to inadequate tear production. Keratoconjunctivitis sicca may be primary, secondary, or of unknown cause. The primary type results from congenital lack of lacrimal secretion or in response to spontaneous senile atrophy of the lacrimal glands (inadequate production of aqueous layer). Secondary keratoconjunctivitis sicca follows canine distemper, traumatic damage to the lacrimal glands or to their nerve supply, occlusion of the lacrimal ducts due to chronic bacterial conjunctivitis, and toxic damage to lacrimal glands produced by certain drugs and may follow an immune-mediated inflammation.

The clinical signs vary greatly, depending on the severity of the reduction of tear production. Reduction in serous tear production results in decreased lubrication of the cornea and conjunctiva; these tissues become painful, resulting in blepharospasm and enophthalmos. With decreased tear formation, flushing of the surface of the cornea is inadequate, and a mucous residue accumulates and adheres to the conjunctiva. As the disease progresses, the residue becomes more tenacious and accumulates on the central cornea. The cornea becomes opaque, is ulcerated, and eventually becomes vascularized and pigmented. Corneal ulceration may extend to perforation.

Corneal alterations are degeneration, erosion, and thinning and ulceration of the corneal epithelium. The stroma contains vessels, and the epithelium undergoes epidermalization with development of rete pegs and keratinization in chronic cases. Pigment may be present in the stroma and in the epithelium in vascularized areas. Cellular infiltration is present in vascularized areas, and plasma cells and lymphocytes are abundant.

Corneal lipidosis

Fatty degeneration of the cornea occurs in adult dogs and often is associated with active or previous inflammation and with hyperlipoproteinemia resulting from thyroid atrophy, lymphocytic thyroiditis, and thyroidal carcinoma. Some cases in dogs are bilateral, unassociated with previous corneal disease or serum lipid abnormality, and qualify as a corneal dystrophy (such as observed in Siberian husky dogs). Pathoanatomic alterations are located in the superficial portion of the tunica propria and consist of deposits of neutral fats, fat-laden macrophages, and crystals of cholesterol. The fatty deposits may be accompanied by fibroblastic proliferation (Fig. 14-14).

Pigmentary keratitis

Corneal pigmentation is not common in domestic and laboratory animals and only melanosis is of significance. Melanosis may be either superficial or deep and is a common cause of blindness. The pigment may be accompanied in the outer layers of the substantia propria by vascularization and scarring. Superficial pigmentary keratitis in the dog is not a specific entity but is a manifestation of chronic keratitis. It is generally bilateral, often symmetric, and intimately related to corneal vascularization. Irritation of the cornea leads to vascularization accompanied by inward migration of limbal melanocytes. The first changes are small, discrete, dark brown or black plaques; these may coalesce so that the entire cornea is pigmented. Superficial pigmentary keratitis is present only in those corneas that have had superficial vascularization, but not all vascularized corneas are pigmented.

Pannus; degenerative pannus

In lesions characterized by corneal edema and inflammation, a fibrovascular tissue invades the cornea beneath the epithelium and is designated pannus. Masses of acellular and avascular hyaline material may accumulate in this

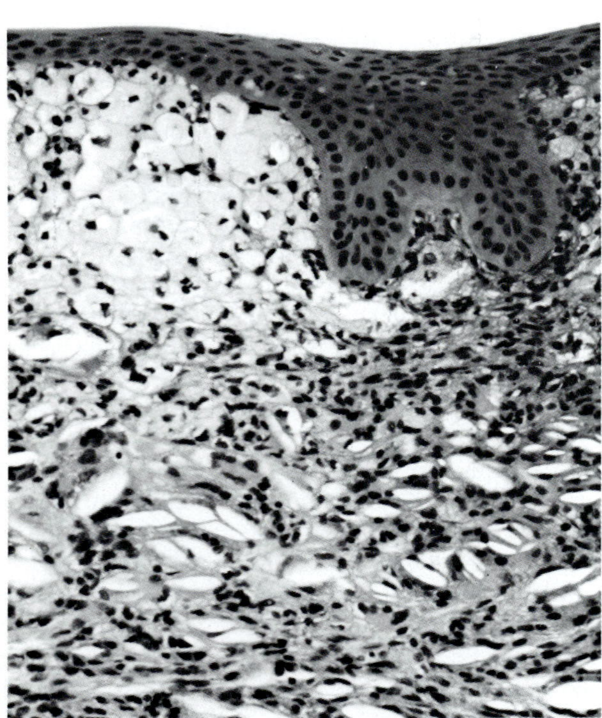

Fig. 14-14 Globe, cornea; canine. Lipid keratopathy. Granulomatous keratitis has lesions of cholesterol clefts and large foamy macrophages with associated epidermalization of corneal epithelium. H & E stain; ×160.

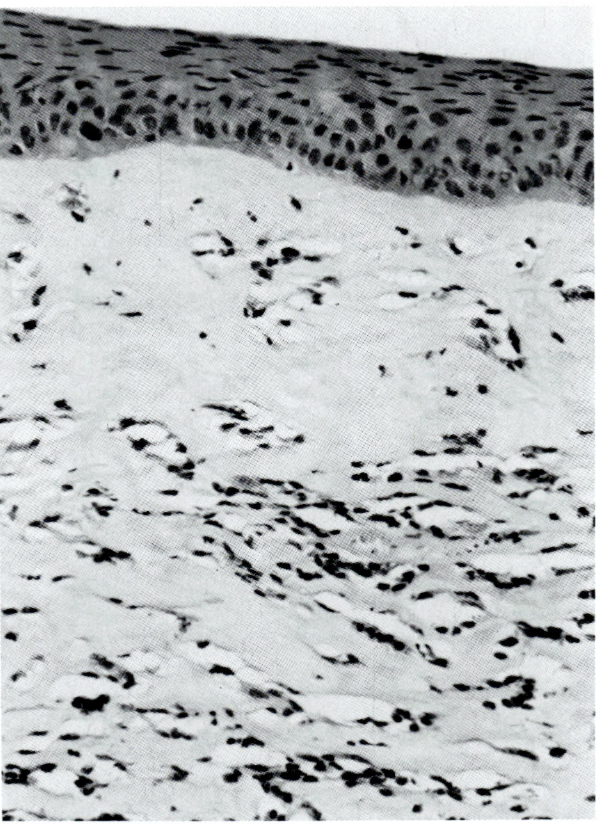

Fig. 14-15 Globe, cornea; equine. Degenerative pannus. Hyaline material separates vessels and a few inflammatory cells beneath a hyperplastic corneal epithelium. H & E stain; ×160.

area and replace fluid in bullae and vesicles. Eventually a thick, hyaline plaque elevates the epithelium (degenerative pannus). The degenerative pannus differs from the inflammatory pannus mainly by having much less lymphocytic and plasma cell infiltration and having the accumulated hyaline material (Fig. 14-15).

Band keratopathy

Band keratopathy (calcification of the cornea) as a clinical entity represents a degenerative process secondary to intraocular inflammation and hypercalcemia in hyperparathyroidism and vitamin D poisoning. It consists of deposition of calcium salts in the superficial layers of the cornea. It begins near the corneoscleral junction, gradually extends across the cornea in a horizontal plane, and merges centrally. Experimental corneal calcification may be produced by a combination of vitamin D treatment with various modes of corneal traumatization producing stromal edema.

Dystrophies

Corneal dystrophy denotes a primary, inherited, bilateral central corneal disorder unassociated either with a systemic disease or with preexisting corneal vascularization and inflammation. Few corneal diseases of animals qualify as corneal dystrophies, but cases include primary corneal lipidosis, edema, and crystalline deposits.

The opacity in the corneal dystrophy of Boston terrier and Chihuahua dogs is ascribed to edema. The corneas are blue-white without vascularization, pain, or conjunctival irritation. The opacity is bilateral, begins in the temporal quadrant, and extends to involve most of the corneal surface over 2 to 3 years. The cornea is thickened by edema, and epithelial bullae and epithelial erosions form secondarily to the chronic edema. Alterations include irregular thickenings of Descemet's membrane, occasional absence of endothelial cells, and a loss of compactness, decreased depth of staining, and reduced numbers of nuclei in the posterior portion of the corneal stroma. The number of endothelial cells is drastically reduced, and the typical hexagonal cellular outline is not discernable by scanning electron microscopy. The epithelial and stromal changes are considered secondary to fluid accumulation due to dysfunction of the endothelium.

Beagle dogs with corneal opacities characterized as a corneal dystrophy have ultrastructural lesions of the anterior corneal stroma; this zone is obscured by large numbers of stromal cells and by crystalline and vacuolar spaces containing cellular debris. The vacuoles within keratocytes are variable in size and are frequently empty; some vacuoles contain debris, dense material, and myelin bodies. Some keratocytes are degenerated, and others are necrotic. Crystal-shaped clefts are frequently associated with debris.

A progressive, apparently inherited corneal dystrophy in members of an inbred line of stump-tailed Manx cats had lesions of edema of the central and anterior half of the cornea. As edema becomes more severe, there is marked thickening, loss of staining of the corneal stroma, and development of a bullous keratopathy, with eventual breakdown of both corneal epithelium and stroma. The central superficial epithelium is thinned and squamous and often covers cystic areas. The basal cells are swollen, pale staining, and vacuolated. The endothelium appears structurally normal, but alterations are present in Descemet's membrane.

Inflammation of the Cornea (Keratitis)

The lack of vessels in the cornea modifies the early lesions of inflammation and the evolution of pathologic changes. Edema of the corneal epithelium and stroma accompanies corneal inflammation (Fig. 14-16). The fluid may arise by absorption of tears and from the aqueous due to damage to the corneal endothelium. Neutrophils migrate into areas of corneal injury, and the infiltration may be either superficial or deep. Following injury, macrophages from the limbal vessels and from transformed stromal cells appear at the injury site and phagocytose bacteria, dead neutrophils, and damaged corneal tissue. With healing, the

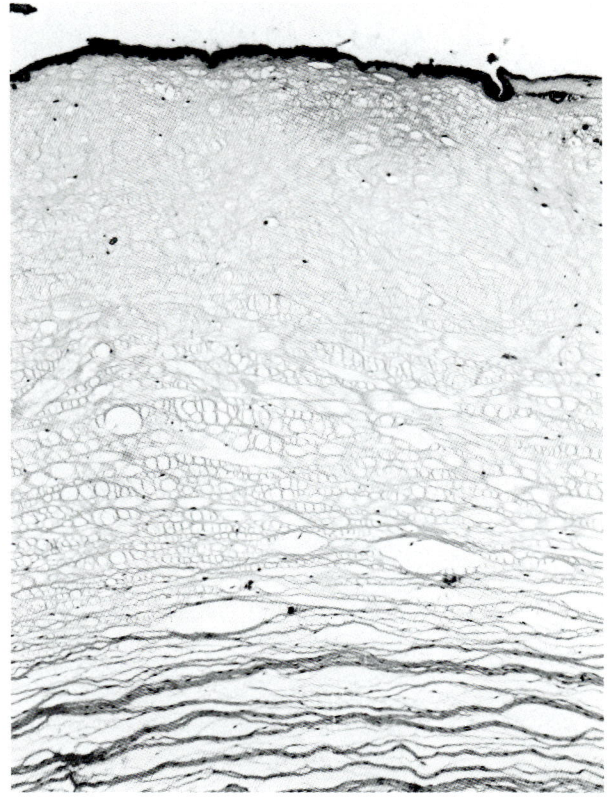

Fig. 14-16 Globe, cornea; porcine. Keratomalacia. The thickened edematous cornea is necrotic and has no viable keratocytes; corneal epithelium is missing, and the surface is covered by bacterial colonies. H & E stain; ×40.

inflammatory cellular exudate contains many lymphocytes and plasma cells. Keratitis is likely to be accompanied by pain, photophobia, blepharospasm, and lacrimation.

Nonulcerative corneal inflammation can be divided into epithelial, subepithelial, and deep stromal. Epithelial keratitis without ulceration is uncommon but may occur in certain viral diseases and as a prelude to stromal keratitis. The lesions may be punctate, discrete, and scattered over the central portion of the cornea. In areas of involvement, the epithelial cells are swollen and edematous. The corneal epithelium may be eroded but is not ulcerated.

Subepithelial keratitis is characterized by inflammatory cell infiltration into the stroma just beneath the epithelium and edema of the stromal, with splitting and degeneration of stromal fibers. Inflammatory cells are either neutrophils or lymphocytes, depending on cause and age of the lesion. Cellular infiltrates are at the margin of the cornea close to the epithelium. When there is vascularization, fibrosis, and cellular infiltration of the cornea, the lesion is a pannus. In chronic cases, the epithelium may be of the conjunctival type, with rete pegs, and it may be keratinized.

Stromal keratitis (Fig. 14-17) occurs when infections of the conjunctiva, sclera, and superficial cornea extend into the corneal stroma; it also occurs in certain systemic diseases. Inflammation may occur primarily in the cornea, develop by extension from the limbus, or spread from an uveitis and endophthalmitis.

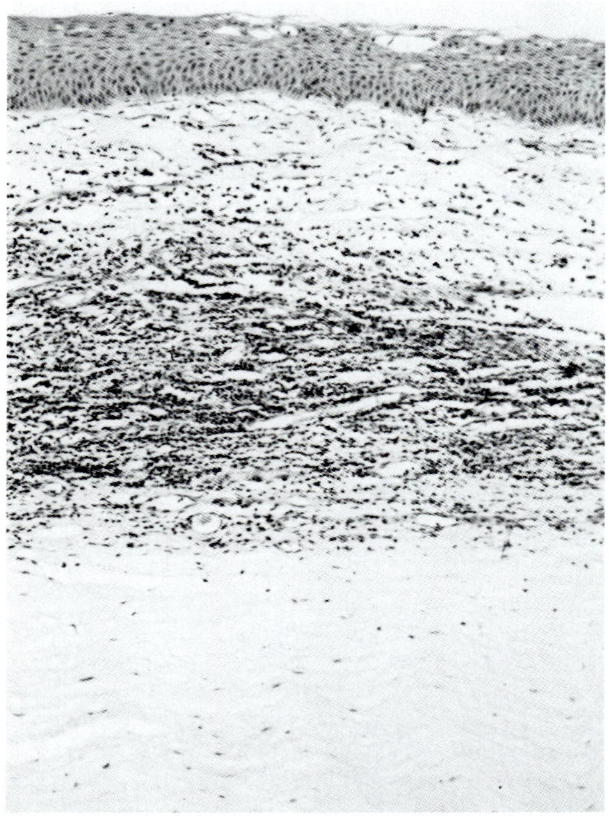

Fig. 14-17 Globe, cornea; equine. Keratitis. Dense cellular infiltrates along with vessels are present in the corneal stroma beneath a focally vacuolated corneal epithelium. H & E stain; ×63.

Corneal Vascularization

The cause of corneal vascularization remains unknown, but vascularization is associated with neutrophilic cellular infiltration. Thus, in models of corneal injury, corneal vascularization is a manifestation of the reparative phase of the inflammatory response. A conspicuous leukocytic infiltrate of the cornea from the limbal vessels precedes and accompanies the corneal vascularization in all models. The three phases include an early prevascular phase of leukocytic infiltration, a second phase with both blood vessels and leukocytes in the cornea, and a third phase in which blood vessels persist in the absence of leukocytes. The latent period preceding vascularization is directly related to the time of leukocytic infiltration. Vascularization is reduced but not completely prevented in the totally leukopenic animal. These results suggest that neutrophils augment neovascularization by the release of vasoproliferative factors.

Corneal Ulceration

Cornea ulceration (Fig. 14-18) may be due to bacterial, viral, and fungal infections. It may occur in cases of acute and chronic keratitis, suppurative ophthalmitis, trauma, and caustic damage. Most infectious ulcerative lesions of the cornea are due to bacteria, usually introduced into the tissues by trauma, because bacteria, with few exceptions, do not penetrate intact corneal epithelium. Bacterially induced corneal ulcers can result from infection by almost all virulent pyogenic organisms, but streptococci, staphy-

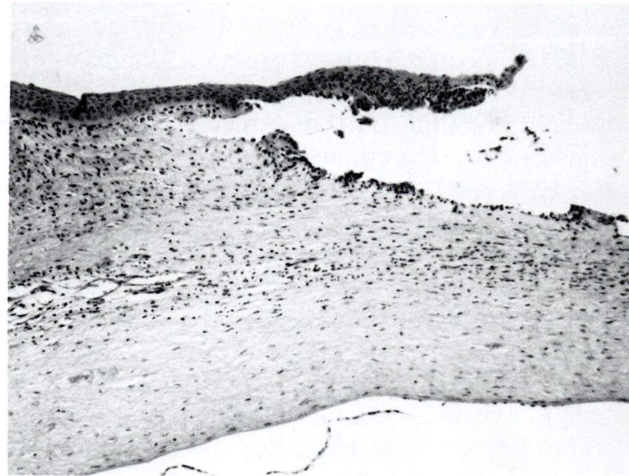

Fig. 14-18 Globe, cornea; bovine. Ulcerative keratitis. Portion of cornea is missing, the corneal epithelium is elevated (artifact), and the corneal stroma has vessels and cellular infiltrates.

lococci, coliform organisms, *Pseudomonas* species (equine), and *Moraxella bovis* (cattle) are perhaps the most frequently involved. Corneal ulceration produces clinical signs of blepharospasm, seromucoid ocular discharge, pain, and conjunctival hyperemia. The herpetic (dendritic) ulcer is a specific cornea ulcer of cats and is the direct result of viral invasion of the cornea. The ulcer is irregularly shaped and commonly accompanied by superficial conjunctivitis, chemosis, and blepharospasm. Fungally caused ulcers of the cornea most often follow injury and may develop as a complication of the treatment of a wound with antibiotics and corticosteroids for prolonged periods. Fungi most likely to be involved are members of the genera *Aspergillus* and *Mucor*. Other fungi causing corneal ulceration include *Candida albicans* and several species of the *Fusarium* genus.

Sequelae of Corneal Ulceration

Scars

These are common sequelae after corneal ulceration and result in opacification. Corneal opacities are classified according to the degree of density: nebula—faint, clouding; macula—definite gray opacity; and leukoma—dense, white opacity. Leukoma with a dark spot in the center due to attachment of pigmented uveal tissue is called leucoma adherens. Leukoma and adherent leukoma usually follow perforation of the cornea. Fibrosis and neovascularization of the corneal stroma are responsible for the corneal scarring.

Keratectasia

Bulging of a thinned, scarred cornea usually follows ulceration. Uveal tissue does not line the scar; thus, keratectasia is distinguishable from staphyloma and leukoma adherens, in which prolapse and incarceration of the iris occur in either a corneal ulcer or a perforating wound.

Descemetocele

Herniation of Descemet's membrane through the floor of a corneal defect may follow corneal ulceration. Descemet's membrane acts as a strong barrier to prevent loss of the anterior chamber. Microscopically, the membrane protrudes into the ulcer and, usually, is covered with a thin layer of fibrinous exudate, debris, and a few fibroblasts. The membrane usually is thinned, and the endothelium is missing in the thinned region.

Glaucoma and phthisis bulbi

These lesions may follow corneal ulceration, especially if the ulceration is followed by perforation, and, with extension of the inflammation, produce ophthalmitis. Whether glaucoma or phthisis follows ocular inflammation depends upon the severity of the alterations in the anterior and posterior segments of the globe.

Acquired Corneal Inflammations

Chronic superficial keratitis (inflammatory pannus; Uberreiter's disease)

This chronic progressive disease of the canine cornea has worldwide distribution, is most commonly seen in the German shepherd breed (over 80% in one survey), and is characterized by a chronic progressive inflammatory reaction, with formation of granulation tissue in the cornea and secondary deposition of melanin pigment. The cause of the disease is unknown. An immunologic mechanism (cellular hypersensitivity against corneal protein) has been proposed to account for its chronicity, and ultraviolet radiation could account for the greater incidence of the disease at higher altitudes. The disease has been observed in dogs of all ages but the greatest incidence is in 4- to 8-year-old dogs; there is no sex predilection.

The corneal lesions vary with the development of the disease. The initial stage is characterized by mononuclear cell infiltration of the subepithelial corneal stroma. The infiltrate consists mainly of plasma cells but includes lymphocytes, macrophages, and neutrophils. In the next stage, an extensive proliferation of blood vessels occurs within the superficial corneal stroma, accompanied by a massive, mixed inflammatory cell infiltrate composed predominantly of plasma cells. The corneal epithelium has degenerative, hyperplastic, and metaplastic changes, including cytoplasmic vacuolation, keratinization, and rete peg formation. Melanin pigment is present in both the corneal epithelial cells and the stroma. The next stage is characterized by a few foci of mononuclear inflammatory cells in the superficial stroma and fewer but larger blood vessels. The basement membrane of the corneal epithelium appears thickened and folded, but the epithelium appears nearly normal, with the exception of a variability in the number of cell layers. The quantity of pigment is increased in the corneal epithelium and stroma. The last stage has irregular foci of fibrous tissue, with few or no inflammatory cells and few vessels. Much melanin pigment is present, and the corneal epithelium varies in thickness.

Superficial indolent corneal ulcers

Superficial indolent (nonhealing) corneal ulcers are observed most frequently in the boxer dog but are seen in the Boston bull terrier and other breeds. The ulcers usually are eccentric, benign, and indolent, without any tendency to perforation. Ulceration usually affects both sexes and usually is unilateral but may be bilateral. Recurrence of ulceration may follow healing. Healing takes place by corneal vascularization, and the ulcers gradually fill with vascularized granulation tissue followed by reepithelization. The cause of the ulceration has not been established. The data thus far obtained suggest that the indolent corneal ulcer of the boxer dog may be associated with endocrine or senile disturbances or that the disease may be an epithelial dystrophy.

Feline chronic ulcerative keratitis with sequestrum

This distinct corneal disease—called corneal sequestrum, corneal mummification, focal corneal degeneration, and corneal nigrum—is characterized by chronicity and by the unilateral or bilateral formation of brown to black corneal plaques. The disease has been described in all breeds, in both sexes, and in young and old cats.

The cause of the disease has not been established. Exposure of the cornea to caustic chemicals, trauma, and infectious agents (as well as abnormal shape of the cornea and superficial corneal dystrophy) have been suggested, but not established, as causes.

The lesion is plaquelike, central or paracentral, well circumscribed, oval, and dark brown to black. It is accompanied by lacrimation, blepharospasm, corneal vascularization, corneal opacity, and corneal ulceration. The area of corneal dessication and necrosis may remain in place for an extended time.

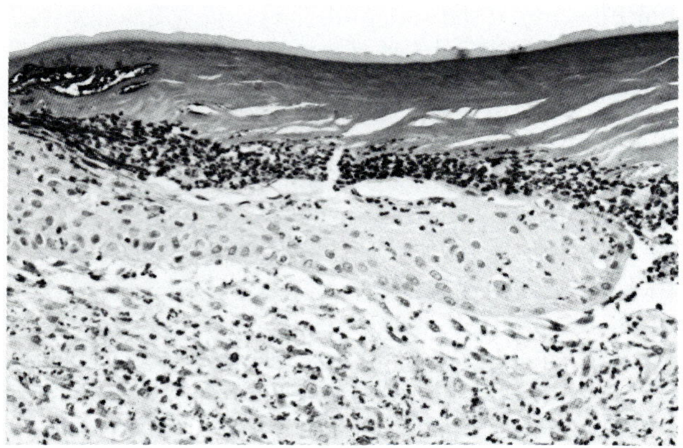

Fig. 14-19 Globe, cornea; feline. Feline chronic ulcerative keratitis. Dessicated pigmented corneal stroma overlays a zone of inflammatory exudate and hyperplastic corneal epithelium. H & E stain; ×160.

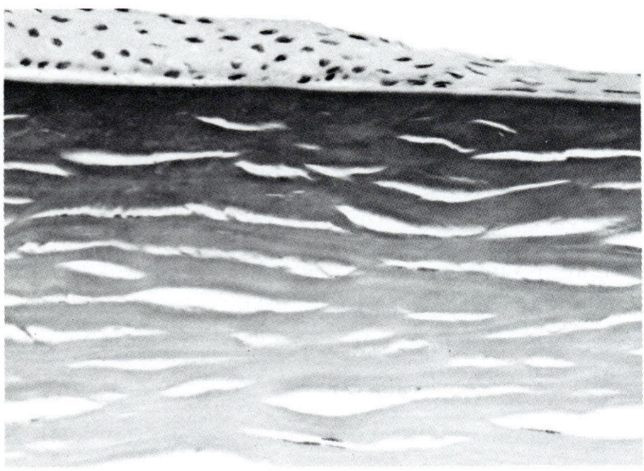

Fig. 14-20 Globe, cornea; feline. Feline chronic ulcerative keratitis. Sequestrum of pigmented necrotic tissue is acellular and avascular. H & E stain; ×63.

The principal alterations are those of a nonsuppurative ulcerative keratitis. The microscopic changes vary with the age of the lesion, and acute lesions have pigmentation and may have few cells. More typically, the corneal epithelium extends to the edge of the stromal lesions, which are heavily vascularized, with most of the blood vessels in the anterior corneal stroma (Fig. 14-19). The corneal stromal degeneration and necrosis extend to varying depths and can be extensive in some cats. The sequestrum is devoid of fibroblasts and inflammatory cells, except at its periphery and base (Fig. 14-20). Pigmentation of the sequestrum appears to be due to neither melanin nor hemosiderin but to dessication of the corneal stroma and pigment absorbed from tears.

Infectious keratoconjunctivitis of cattle (bovine pinkeye)

Infectious bovine keratoconjunctivitis is widely distributed among range, semirange, farm, and feedlot cattle on the North American continent and has been reported in all cattle-raising areas of the world. The disease is most prevalent among cattle during the summer, but epizootics have been described during the winter months. In tropic and subtropic areas, it is prevalent during all months of the year. The disease is considered highly contagious without regard to age, sex, or breed, but often young animals have the more severe form of the disease.

Transmission of infection can be by direct contact as well as by mechanical vectors, such as flies. The infectious organism, *Moraxella bovis,* is usually introduced into a herd by an infected animal, and up to 80% of cattle at risk may have the disease within 1 to 3 weeks. Predisposing factors include dust, sunlight, and various insects such as flies.

The clinical features are quite variable from herd to herd and between individuals within a herd. The acute phase is characterized by marked lacrimation, blepharospasm, conjunctivitis, vascular congestion, photophobia, and edematous swelling and hyperemia of the lower lid. The discharge from the eyes, initially watery, becomes purulent, and mats on the lashes and circumorbital hair. The eyelids are swollen, and the cornea becomes either partially or totally opaque and is covered by exudate. Opacity often begins in a spot just below the center of the cornea, and a shallow ulcer often starts in the same location. Keratitis is manifested by vesicles, flat spots, and ulcers, with and without accompanying corneal opacification. The chronic stage is characterized by extensive changes in the thickened, ulcerated cornea, and the keratitis is accompanied by an anterior uveitis and hypopyon. The ocular lesions can be quite variable and reflect the severity of the clinical disease. The earliest and mildest change is edema of the cornea with epithelial bullae formation. If central ulceration extends deep into the corneal stroma, the cornea may perforate with development of panophthalmitis and loss of sight.

Infectious bovine rhinotracheitis

This viral disease of cattle is manifested by various syndromes, including respiratory disease, pustular vulvovaginitis, and keratoconjunctivitis. In some field outbreaks, keratoconjunctivitis has been observed with and without respiratory signs and may be the only presenting sign. Ocular exudates (serous to mucopurulent), corneal opacity, and white plaques of the conjunctivae are common ocular lesions. The palpebral conjunctivae are intensely swollen and covered with fine petechiae. Lesions in naturally infected cattle include marked hyperplasia of lymph nodules in the conjunctiva and third eyelid. The propria of the eyelid contains variable numbers of mononuclear cells, endothelial cell hyperplasia, and capillaries filled with neutrophils. The epithelium over areas of lymphoid hyperplasia either is replaced by a fibrinonecrotic membrane or has vacuolar degeneration.

Keratoconjunctivitis in sheep

Contagious ovine keratoconjunctivitis (ovine pinkeye) is a common disease in sheep-raising countries, affecting a considerable proportion of flocks. It is considered highly contagious; is transmitted by contact with contaminated flies, dust, grass, seeds, and pasture plants; and usually spreads rapidly through a flock. Sheep of all ages are susceptible. The disease is not considered of major economic importance.

The cause of infectious ovine keratoconjunctivitis remains obscure, and, over the years, a number of organisms have been proposed either as the cause or as being associated with the disease. Mycoplasms have been recovered from affected sheep, and certain isolates have been considered the etiologic agent of ovine pinkeye.

The disease begins as a simple conjunctivitis, with the whole of the conjunctiva being reddened due to hyperemia, congestion, and petechiae. Excessive lacrimation is accompanied by photophobia. Keratitis often develops within a few days, and, later, blood vessels enter the cornea, producing either partial or complete corneal opacification. Ulceration of the cornea occurs in only a few cases, and, uncommonly, the cornea perforates with development of ophthalmitis. In the majority of sheep, the lesions are mild and, generally, there is no serious impairment of vision.

Keratoconjunctivitis in goats

Infectious keratoconjunctivitis (IKC) has been observed in goat herds in various parts of the world. The disease may occur either alone or as part of other ocular diseases. The etiology of some outbreaks of IKC in goats appears to be mycoplasmal organisms and, possibly, a species of *Acholeplasma.* The earliest signs are excess lacrimation and hyperemia of the palpebral conjunctiva. Other alterations in most affected goats include follicular conjunctivitis, corneal opacity with vascularization, ulceration, pannus, and iritis.

UVEA

Anomalies of the Uvea

Most congenital anomalies of the uvea are uncommon in domestic animals, and some are rare. Coloboma of the iris is not uncommon in the dog, and cases of persistent pupillary membrane are common in some breeds of dogs (basenji).

Aniridia

Complete absence of the iris is rare in all species. The iris, if deficient, is either rudimentary or incomplete and consists of a narrow rim of tissue. A rudimentary iris consists of underdeveloped ectodermal and mesodermal elements and is a feature of multiple ocular anomalies that occur in several breeds of dogs. Because aniridia is due to arrest in the differentiation of the anterior portion of the optic cup, associated abnormalities include cataract, microphthalmia, and corneal opacities.

Coloboma of the iris, ciliary body, and choroid

The absence of a sector of the iris produces variations in pupillary size and shape. Colobomas may be either unilateral or bilateral and may involve whole sections of the iris. The base of a typical coloboma is similar to the changes seen in aniridia, with the edge of the coloboma formed by rounded mesodermal stroma and by folded pigment epithelium. Coloboma of the ciliary body, an uncommon defect, may be associated with coloboma of the iris along the closure of the fetal fissure, with various remnants of mesodermal tissue in the defect. In coloboma of the choroid, the sclera is thin and ectatic, and the defect is covered by dysplastic retina.

Persistent pupillary membrane

The persistence of the vascular pupillary membrane is common in dogs and described in cattle, horses, cats, and nonhuman primates. Composed of nests of connective tissue cells in the anterior chamber, it is attached to the lesser iris circle; in the dog, it disappears by the age of 5 weeks. Strands of vascular connective tissue are present in the anterior chamber and may attach either to the lens or to the cornea. Attachment to the lens results in cataract, and attachment to the cornea may produce defects in Descemet's endothelium and membrane, thereby resulting in corneal opacities. Corneas with diffuse opacities have histologic changes in the corneal stroma; deeper regions are converted into laminated, hyaline material with only a few nuclei.

Heterochromia irides

Heterochromia irides has been described in cattle, swine, mouse, rabbit, cat, dog, and horse. In this lesion, differences in the coloration of the iris produce spots of color other than the basic color of the iris. The lesion occurs as a normal variant of iridal coloration and, in certain species, in association with white coat color (miniature swine), deafness, ocular anomalies, and systemic anomalies. The histologic changes include pigment anomalies, hypoplasia of the iridal stroma, reduction of iridal pigment, and clumping, irregular distribution, and partial absence of pigment in the iridal stroma. Pigment is reduced in other portions of the uveal tract as well.

Cysts of the iris and ciliary body

These occur on the posterior surface of the iris and the ciliary body. They result from separation of the two neuroectodermal layers. In dogs, iridal pigment cysts are not uncommon, may be bilateral, have been observed on the posterior surface of the iris in both young and old dogs, and represent either a congenital malformation or a senile change. Iridal cysts occur on both the anterior and posterior surfaces of the iris in horses. The cysts, in some cases, consist of heavily pigmented lining epithelium overlying a small amount of loose, vascularized, nonpigmented connective tissue. The cysts do not recur after removal.

Uveitis

The iris, ciliary body, and choroid alone and in various combinations are commonly involved in inflammatory processes. Inflammation may involve the anterior uvea (iritis, cyclitis, iridiocyclitis), the posterior uvea (choroiditis), or the entire uveal tract (panuveitis). The uveal tract may become involved by extension of inflammatory disease from the cornea, sclera, vitreous, retina, and optic nerve. These structures are almost always involved secondarily in uveal inflammation. Uveitis may be either suppurative or nonsuppurative, and the latter may be either granulomatous or nongranulomatous.

Suppurative uveitis

Pyogenic inflammation of the uvea follows accidental and surgical wounds, ulcerations of the cornea and sclera, and hematogenous spread of systemic bacterial infections. Purulent uveitis is a part of suppurative endophthalmitis. With purulent anterior uveitis, exudate in the anterior chamber (hypopyon) consists of neutrophils and fibrin. Exudate also fills the trabecular meshwork and is layered in the dependent portions of the posterior chamber, and leukocytes adhere to the posterior surface of the cornea. Vessels of the uvea are dilated and filled with leukocytes and fibrinous thrombi. The uveal stroma, especially of the ciliary processes, is edematous and infiltrated with neutrophils. In the choroid, the reaction begins in the inner vessel layer and, often, spreads to the retina.

Nonsuppurative uveitis

This inflammatory reaction is generally milder than purulent and granulomatous uveal inflammations. Diffuse and focal infiltrates of lymphocytes and monocytes are present in the uvea, with varying number of plasma cells and associated plasmacytoid cells and Russell's bodies. A fibrinous exudate may be present in the anterior and posterior chambers and the vitreal cavity. The choroidal inflammation is associated with perivascular cuffing of some retinal vessels by lymphocytes (species with retinal vessels). Idiopathic lymphocytic-plasmocytic anterior uveitis is a frequent cause of glaucoma in cats.

Granulomatous uveitis

Organisms causing tuberculosis, actinomycosis, coccidioidomycosis, blastomycosis, and cryptococcosis, and certain parasitic forms are found in uveal granulomas. The microscopic findings are similar in granulomatous uveitis, regardless of etiology. The vessels are dilated, keratic precipitates form on the corneal endothelium, and the aqueous humor contains a proteinaceous precipitate. Granulomatous inflammation occurs as small nodules and as diffuse involvement of the iris, ciliary body, and choroid accompanied by necrosis. The nodules consist of lymphocytes, plasma cells, epithelioid cells, and multinucleated giant cells. The epithelium of the iris and ciliary body and the retinal pigment epithelium atrophy in some areas, and, in other areas, these epithelia proliferate to form nodules.

Sequelae to uveal inflammation

Sequelae of uveal inflammation include posterior and anterior **synechiae.** Fibrinous adhesion of the iris to the lens is followed by fibrovascular organization; synechiae occur in all types of uveal inflammation. Peripheral anterior synechia forms as an adhesion either between the iris and the trabecular meshwork or between the iris and the cornea through the organization of particulate matter such as blood and inflammatory exudate. Inflammation may cause the corneal endothelium to proliferate around the false angle into the anterior surface of the iris with the production of Descemet's membrane. Blockage of the filtration meshwork by synechia can result in **glaucoma.**

Cyclitic membrane is a band of fibrovascular tissue that extends across the globe from one portion of the ciliary body along the posterior surface of the lens. Contraction of the cyclitic membrane results in partial detachment of the retina. Eventually, as the vitreous shrinks, the retina becomes totally detached. An **iris membrane** (Fig. 14-21) is a thin fibrovascular membrane on either the anterior or posterior surface of the iris. The membrane follows organization of an inflammatory exudate or blood and can result in **entropion uvea** or **ectropion uvea.** Preiridal fibrovascular membrane **(rubeosis iridis)** is a common lesion following uveitis and is also seen in globes with chronic glaucoma, intraocular neoplasms, and chronic retinal detachment. Neovascularization is present along the anterior face of the iris, beginning at the papillary margin and near the trabecular meshwork. The midportion of the iris also develops vessels.

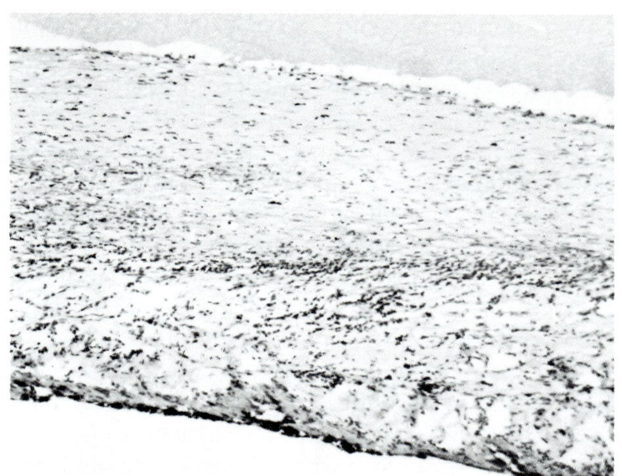

Fig. 14-21 Globe, iris; canine. Endophthalmitis, *Dirofilaria immitis.* Fibrovascular membrane lies on the anterior surface of the iris. H & E stain; ×63.

Atrophy and fibrosis of the uvea follow inflammation. Atrophy of ciliary processes leads to reduction of aqueous humor production and to development of lenticular degeneration and hypotony. Atrophy of the choroid may be diffuse or focal and may be accompanied by connective tissue and glial scars. Pigment epithelium of the retina may be heaped up at the edge of the scar. The scar in the choroid may contain hemosiderin, cholesterol, cartilage, and bone. Extensive scarring of the inner choroid is often associated with osseous metaplasia in cases of **phthisis bulbi. Detachment of the retina** follows choroiditis due to the formation of an exudate beneath the neural retina and, in cases of anterior uveitis, by the formation of a cyclitic membrane.

Acquired Uveal Inflammation

Equine recurrent uveitis

Equine recurrent uveitis (equine periodic ophthalmia), an inflammatory disease of the eyes of horses and mules, is the most common cause of blindness in these species and is characterized by recurring acute attacks of uveal inflammation alternating with quiescent periods of varying duration. One or both globes may be involved at quite unpredictable intervals. Acutely and early, the disease is primarily an iridiocyclitis, but, after several acute attacks, lesions are present in other ocular tissue, including the lens, retina, and vitreous, and these lesions eventually lead to impaired vision or blindness. Clinical features in the acute stage include conjunctival hyperemia, iridal discoloration, pupillary contraction, vascularization of the cornea, and exudate in the anterior chamber. The microscopic lesions include a neutrophilic exudate in the anterior chamber, within the iridic stroma, on the surface of the iris, in the posterior chamber, and over the lenticular capsule.

During the quiescent stage, the microscopic lesions are circumscribed lymphoid nodules in the iris and ciliary body. The vitreous humor contains lymphocytes, fibrin, and serum proteins, and a fibrinocellular exudate adheres to the lenticular capsule. Perivascular lymphocytic infiltrates are sometimes present in the optic papilla. After repeated attacks, exudative and degenerative changes are present in the retina, a serofibrinous exudate is between the layer of rods and cones and the retinal pigment epithelium, and the retina is focally detached.

After severe chronic uveitis, the globe is small, the cornea is more convex, and the sclera is thickened. Cataracts are common, as are posterior and anterior synechiae. The iris is torn and mottled, and the choroid is filled with thick-walled blood vessels. The ciliary processes are thickened and are covered and filled with an eosinophilic and PAS-positive exudate (Fig. 14-22). The retina commonly becomes detached due to subretinal exudates and is displaced forward, often into contact with the posterior surface of the lens. The retina becomes markedly degenerated and atrophied and may be represented by only a vestige of connective tissue. The optic nerve becomes atrophic and gliotic (Fig. 14-23).

Leptospirosis has been considered a cause of recurrent uveitis as *Leptospira interrogans* serovar *pomona* has been isolated from horses with acute recurrent uveitis. Also, horses with iridocyclitis have serum and aqueous antibod-

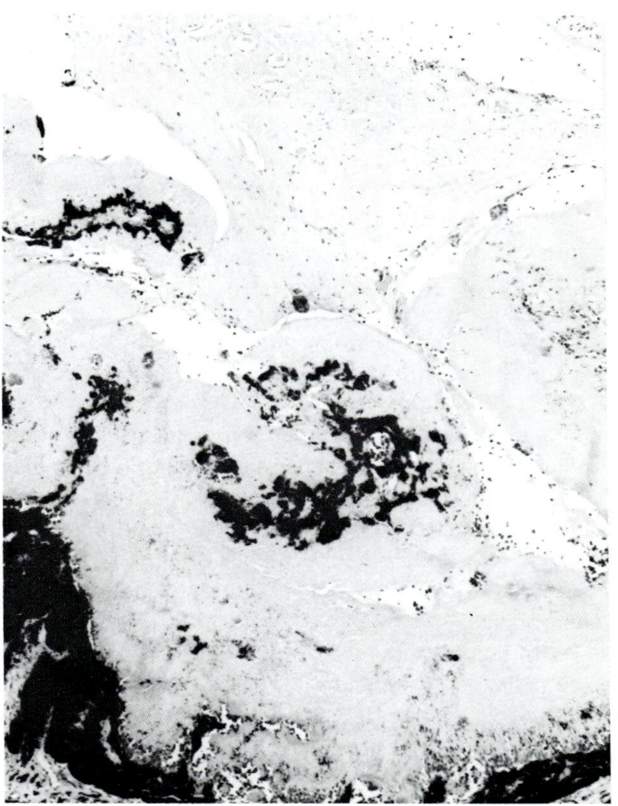

Fig. 14-22 Globe, ciliary processes; equine. Equine recurrent uveitis. A proteinaceous exudate covers and thickens the ciliary processes. H & E stain; ×40.

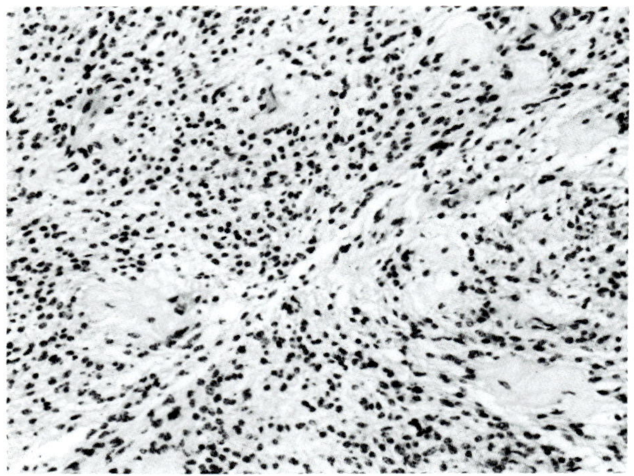

Fig. 14-23 Globe, optic nerve head; equine. Equine recurrent uveitis. Optic nerve head is atrophic and gliotic. H & E stain; ×160.

ies against *L. interrogans* serovar *pomona* and evidence of intraocular synthesis of antibody.

Lens-induced uveitis

Ocular inflammation due to leakage of lenticular proteins (phacolytic uveitis) is a mild lymphocytic-plasmacytic anterior uveitis. A severe uveitis (phacoclastic uveitis) follows release of lenticular material after extracapsular cataract extraction, trauma to the lens, and spontaneous rupture of the lenticular capsule. Presence of lenticular material within the globe does not always result in uveitis, but, in those cases that develop uveitis, the severity of the reaction varies with the amount of lenticular protein released within the globe. Clinical signs include keratic precipitates, posterior synechiae, secondary glaucoma, eyelid edema, chemosis, and corneal edema.

Lens-induced uveitis is apparently an immunologic disease. Antibodies to lenticular proteins are produced in animals sensitized with homologous lenticular protein. The crystallins can initiate a humoral immune response and produce an autoantigen-antibody reaction and, then, an inflammatory reaction. The lens-induced uveitis represents an autoimmune response to lenticular protein liberated through a ruptured capsule. Lens-induced uveitis is a zonal, granulomatous inflammation about lenticular material. Neutrophils surround lenticular material, and epithelioid and giant cells occur beyond the neutrophils. These cells may infiltrate into the lenticular cortex. Lymphocytes, plasma cells, and granulation tissue surround the epithelioid cells. The iris is usually encased in granulomatous inflammatory tissue.

Infectious canine hepatitis

Corneal opacity, usually unilateral, occurs sometimes during the convalescent stage of infectious canine hepatitis and after immunization for the disease. Opacification of the cornea is accompanied by moderate to severe iridocyclitis. Virus is detected by fluorescent antibody techniques in vascular endothelium of the iris and trabeculae, in macrophages, in the corneal endothelium, and in some cells of keratic precipitates.

The lesions in eyeballs with an opaque cornea are those of nonsuppurative uveitis with stromal keratitis of variable severity. The iridal and ciliary vessels are congested, and stromal edema involves the iris, ciliary body, and propria of the cornea (Fig. 14-24). Trabecular channels are filled with leukocytes. Predominantly, plasma cell infiltrates involve the iris. The cellular infiltrates are located mainly perivascularly and are most intense at the root. Lesions in the cornea consist of stromal edema and infiltration of inflammatory cells. In the corneal stroma, foci of necrotic inflammatory cells, mainly neutrophils, are present immediately anterior to Descemet's membrane. The endothelium of the cornea is either focally absent or the cells are swollen and distorted, especially in areas of keratic precipitates. The ocular lesions of canine hepatitis are considered manifestations of an Arthus-type hypersensitivity (type III).

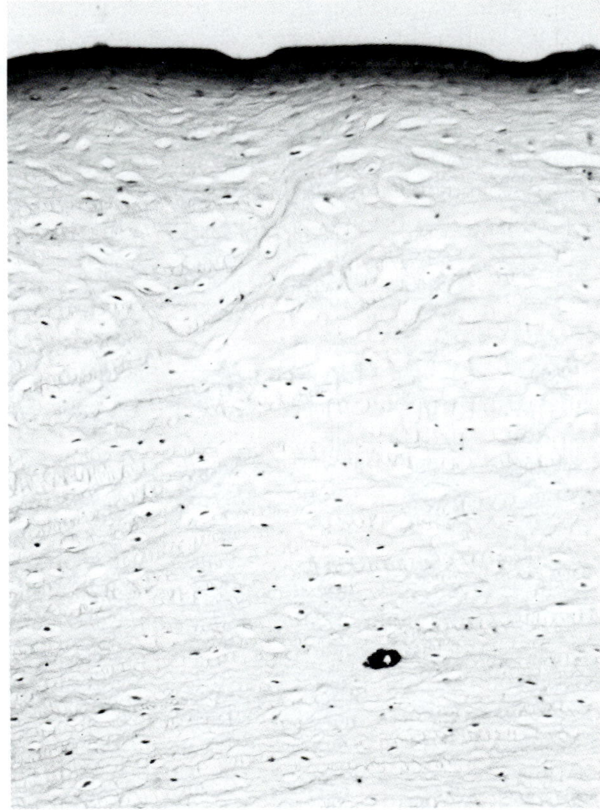

Fig. 14-24 Globe, cornea; canine. Canine viral hepatitis. The pale-staining corneal stroma is thickened by edema. H & E stain; ×63.

Canine granulomatous panuveitis and dermal depigmentation (Vogt-Koyanagi-Harada's syndrome)

Clinically, granulomatous uveitis accompanied by dermal depigmentation (nose and eyelids) in dogs has changes of episcleral congestion, corneal edema, iris injection, aqueous flare, keratitic precipitates, and a hypotonic globe. Some globes have a shallow anterior chamber, iris bombé, posterior synechia, and cataract. These globes are small and have retinal detachment, ocular hemorrhages, and a thickened anterior uvea. Uveal infiltrates, concentrated around vascular and neural emissaria, are composed of lymphocytes, plasma cells, epithelioid cells, and pigment-filled macrophages. Choroidal scarring is accompanied by thickening of the sclera and destruction of the retinal pigment epithelium and the overlying detached retina. Vitreal cavity contains blood and proteinaceous exudate in a liquified vitreous humor.

Avian encephalomyelitis

Chickens infected with the enterovirus *(Picornaviridae)* of avian encephalomyelitis have, in addition to lesions in the central nervous system (CNS), ocular alterations of lenticular cataract and nonsuppurative anterior uveitis. Blind chickens, with and without other signs of CNS dysfunction, have necrosis of lenticular epithelium, especially at the equator of the lens, with formation of clefts filled with protein-rich fluid and Morgagnian globules, and with proliferation of lenticular epithelium on both the anterior and posterior surfaces of the lens. The lenticular lesions accompany perivascular and stromal cellular infiltration of the anterior uvea. The infiltrates are composed mostly of lymphocytes with plasma cells and a few heterophils.

Injuries of the Uvea

Contusion of the iris may be followed by iridal tears, stromal atrophy, recession of the iris, and hemorrhage. Iridodialysis is characterized by separation of the iridal root from the ciliary body and may produce severe hemorrhage. Large hemorrhages usually clot, and, because reabsorption is slow, they produce inflammation, which results in adhesion between the iris, cornea, and lens. Extensive fibrosis may occur within the anterior and posterior chambers and on the anterior surface of the iris. Secondary glaucoma may follow severe contusion and usually is associated with massive anterior angle hemorrhage, which blocks the outflow of aqueous. Contusion of the ciliary body results in hemorrhages and exudation into the stroma as well as necrosis and rupture of the ciliary processes. Contusion of the choroid causes hemorrhage, detachment, tears, and inflammation.

Perforating injuries include mechanical and surgical lacerations and penetration by foreign bodies. Perforating wounds can lead to collapse of the anterior chamber and prolapse and incarceration of the iris. Perforating injuries of the limbus and anterior sclera produce severe damage to the ciliary body, with hemorrhage, detachment, and prolapse into the wound. Such injuries usually cause a marked endophthalmitis and may eventually lead to the sequelae of this lesion.

THE LENS

Anomalies of the Lens

In its development, the ectodermal lens is surrounded by vascular mesoderm, which provides its nutrition. Thus, abnormalities of the lens either may be associated with or result from anomalies of the surrounding tissues. Persistence of the posterior vascular tunic of the lens may be associated with a defective posterior capsule, invasion of the lens by fibrovascular tissue, and development of cataract.

The lens may be absent **(aphakia),** a rare anomaly associated with severe failure of ocular development; the globe is represented by a cyst with essentially no internal structure. In some severely microphthalmic globes, the lens is represented only by some small bits of tissue. False aphakia is more common, and the lens is represented by a wrinkled capsule containing some degenerated fibers.

In some cases of defective development, the lenticular capsule is thin, and it ruptures; the lens bulges, producing **lenticonus** or it may develop a spherical contour **(lentiglobus).** Eventually, with development of cataract and rupture of the capsule, degenerated lenticular substance is released into the vitreous and aqueous.

Cataract

The lesions of the lens are relatively few, and the most common and significant change is lenticular opacity, also known as cataract. Clinically, cataract signifies any opacity of the crystalline lens and its capsule. This change may be either congenital or acquired. Some congenital cataracts are inherited, and some are due to remnants of either the hyaloid vascular system or pupillary membranes. Congenital cataracts are often bilateral, multiple, and in a subcapsular location. Acquired cataracts are due to trauma, intraocular inflammation, glaucoma, and toxins. Topographically, cataracts can be either cortical or nuclear and involve the anterior or posterior poles of the lens and the dorsal or ventral equatorial regions of the lens.

The cortical lenticular fibers, when traumatized and subjected to toxic or adverse nutritional influences, may suffer rapid necrosis followed by liquefaction. Thus, the general morphologic changes in cataract are essentially the same, regardless of etiology. The fibers may lose fluid and shrink, and fluid collects in the resulting clefts and vacuoles (Fig. 14-25). Cell membranes disintegrate, vacuoles form and may coalesce, and, eventually, the fibers fragment into Morgagnian globules (Fig. 14-26). As the lenticular fragments disintegrate, protein is released, and the intercellular fluid becomes albuminous and stains pale pink (H & E section).

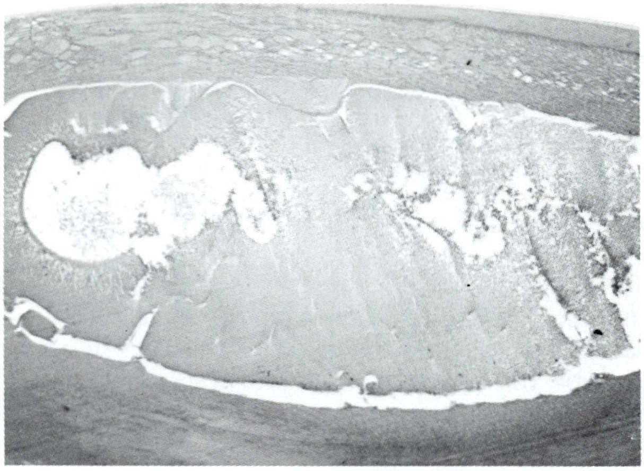

Fig. 14-25 Globe, lens; canine. Cataract. The lenticular fibers are necrotic and liquified, and the formed clefts are filled with finely granular proteinaceous material. H & E stain; ×63.

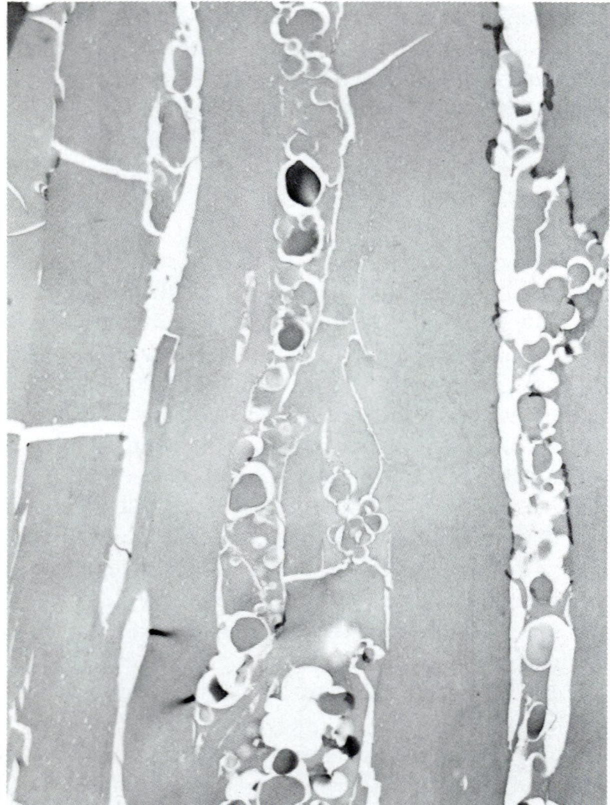

Fig. 14-26 Globe, lens; canine. Cataract. Globule formation (irregular, variably sized masses) from necrotic lenticular fibers. H & E stain; ×63.

The subcapsular epithelium reacts to injury by degeneration, necrosis, or proliferation. When stimulated by trauma and inflammation, the cells proliferate, resulting in opacity and anterior subcapsular cataract. The epithelium may become flattened and multilayered, and the lenticular cells appear like fibroblasts (Fig. 14-27).

Degeneration of the lenticular cells may be followed by proliferation of the capsular epithelium to form a continuous layer beneath the posterior capsule. With this change, the epithelial cells may become large, swollen, and vesicular, forming so-called bladder cells (Fig. 14-28). These represent abortive attempts to form lenticular fibers.

Primary cataracts with a heritable basis have been reported in a number of breeds of dogs. The mode of inheritance (autosomal recessive, autosomal dominant, polygenetic) varies, depending on the breed. In some cases, the cataract coexists with persisting pupillary membrane, retinal folds, microphthalmia, and hypotonia.

In cattle, cataracts have been reported as a primary entity and in association with other ocular anomalies. Bilateral congenital cataracts have been described in the Jersey, Holstein, and Hereford breeds, with a simple autosomal recessive inheritance in Jersey and Holstein breeds. In the Holstein, Jersey, and Shorthorn breeds, cataracts have occurred with other ocular anomalies, including lenticular luxation,

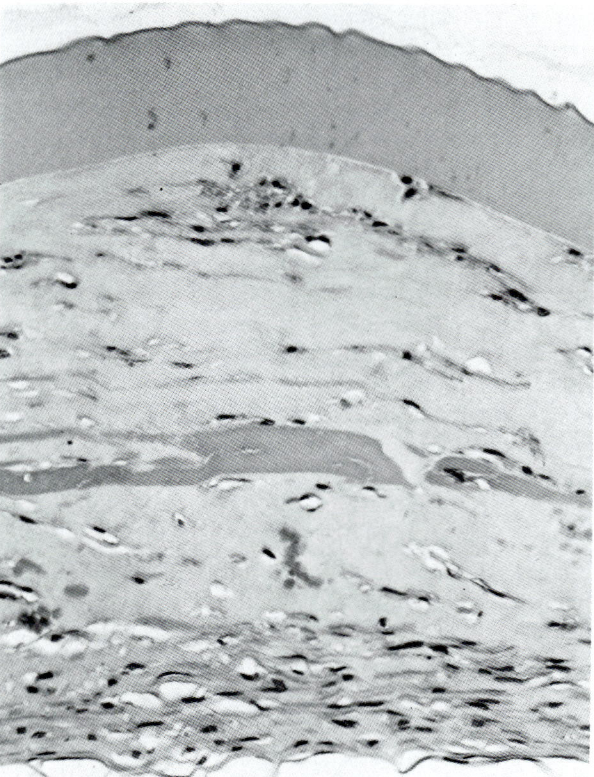

Fig. 14-27 Globe, lens; equine. Equine recurrent uveitis. Lenticular epithelium is hyperplastic and metaplastic, resembling fibrocytes. H & E stain; ×250.

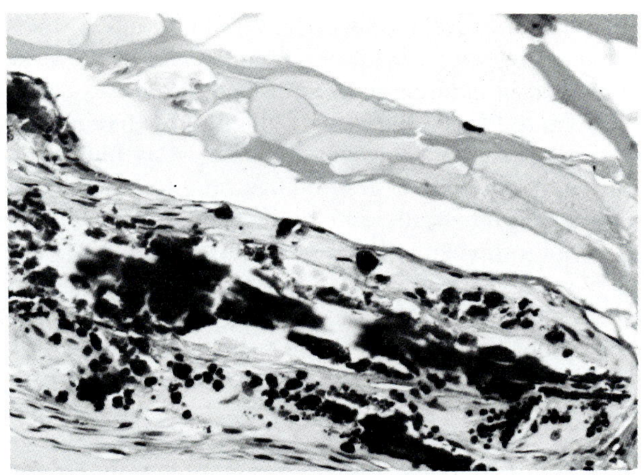

Fig. 14-28 Globe, lens; canine. Lenticular epithelium has proliferated along posterior lenticular capsule; some necrotic lenticular fibers are calcified, and some hyperplastic lenticular cells are swollen, finely granular, and have well-defined cellular membranes (''bladder cells''). H & E stain; ×160.

buphthalmia, microphthalmia, retinal detachment, and rupture of the lens. Congenital cataracts are not uncommon in foals and involve the nucleus, sutures, and cortex. Hereditary and congenital cataracts have been described in rats, rabbits, guinea pigs, bobwhite, quail, and mice. Several inherited cataracts in mice have been established as animal models.

Luxation of the Lens

Congenital dislocation of the lens occurs in dogs, calves, and horses as a part of multiple ocular anomalies. Acquired luxations are most common in dogs, and certain breeds such as Sealyham and wirehaired terriers are more susceptible. Primary lenticular luxation (spontaneous displacement as a result of rupture of the zonule, with no antecedent ocular disease) has been described in terrier breeds; the luxation has a high incidence, is sudden, and is often bilateral. Luxation in the Tibetan terrier has an autosomal recessive inheritance. In most cases, the dislocated lens passes forward into the anterior chamber and is likely to cause acute glaucoma. Enlargement of the globe can result in luxation due to stretching of the lenticular zonules as the globe enlarges. It may be impossible to determine if the lenticular luxation initiated the glaucoma or vice versa. Dogs with lenticular luxation and glaucoma have buphthalmic globes with corneal vascularization, corneal edema, and an aphakic crescent.

VITREOUS BODY

The vitreous (hyaloid) body is a transparent avascular gel filling the globe posterior to the lens. About 99% of its weight is water. It is a tenuous structure formed by a network of fine fibrous proteins permeated by the vitreous humor. It functions to retain the retina in position and prevents rapid spread of large molecules and cells while allowing small nutrient molecules to diffuse within it. The vitreous in human beings and nonhuman primates is attached to the optic disk, the retina, and the ciliary body; attachment is strongest along the peripheral retina, and the firmest attachment is anterior to the ora serrata in the region of the pars plana of the ciliary body. In domestic and laboratory animals, there is little or no attachment of the vitreous to the retina.

The vitreous body of mammals develops in three stages. A primitive vascular structure is first formed, then a nonvascular mass of vitreous develops, and, later, during embryonic growth, the tertiary vitreous constituting the zonule is formed. With formation of the lenticular capsule, the development of the primary vitreous ceases, and the secondary vitreous develops. In time, the hyaloid vessels atrophy, and the avascular vitreous humor continues to be formed by the retinal Müller cells and, possibly, by hyalocytes.

Anomalies of the Vitreous Body

Persistence of primary vitreous

Either complete or partial persistence of the hyaloid vascular system may occur in postnatal life. The hyaloid artery may contain blood or appear as a fine thread of fibrous and glial elements extending from the optic nerve head to near the lens. Only the posterior portion may persist attached to the optic disc, and, if patent, it forms a vascular loop extending into the vitreous **(Bergmeister's papilla).** Hyaloid remnants without clinical disease are especially common in the ox.

Persistent hyperplastic primary vitreous (PHPV)

This uncommon lesion in domestic animals has been described in dogs, especially the Doberman pinscher. It consists of the fibrovascular tunic of the lens and the hyaloid vascular system. The pathologic features of PHPV include

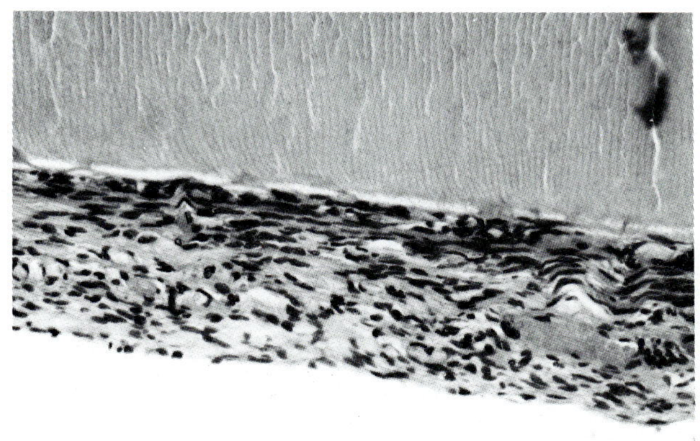

Fig. 14-29 Globe, lens; canine. Persistent hyperplastic primary vitreous. A fibrovascular membrane extends along the posterior surface of the lens. H & E stain; ×160.

pigmented fibrous dots or fibrous plaques located retrolentally on the posterior capsule of the lens with some plaques extending halfway to the equator. Microscopically, the plaques consist of fibrous connective tissue (Fig. 14-29) with melanin pigment and may contain cartilage, bone, and adipose tissue. The fibrous tissue is more dense on the surface facing the vitreous. In some cases, the fibrous tissue extends into defects of the lens, and the fibrous tissue contains collections of lenticular epithelial cells. Posterior lenticonus is present in some affected dogs, along with components of the hyaloid-tunica vasculosa lentis system, retinal rosettes, Bergmeister papilla, and persistent pupillary membrane.

Reactions of the Vitreous Body

The pathologic reactions of the vitreous are largely passive and, usually, are characterized by liquefaction and opacification. Its avascularity and relative acellularity account for its susceptibility to infection. Liquefaction is the most common degenerative change of the vitreous. A number of causes are possible, but the most important in domestic animals are endophthalmitis and panophthalmitis.

In the early stages of iridiocyclitis, chorioretinitis, and papillitis, the entire vitreous may become opaque due to its being flooded with a protein-rich fluid (**plasmoid vitreous**) and inflammatory cells. The vitreous is often displaced anteriorly, and the subvitreal space contains varying amounts of proteinaceous and cellular exudate. Early, acute inflammation of the vitreous (hyalitis) is usually purulent, but, later, mononuclear cells become numerous, and fibroblastic proliferation occurs. Fibroblastic cells may form a wall about abscesses and may diffusely invade the vitreous.

Asteroid hyalosis

Asteroid hyalosis is the occurrence of spherical or disk-shaped white bodies (Fig. 14-30) in the vitreous, which either appears normal or may be liquified. Asteroid bodies are roughly spherical, usually stain weakly with H & E, and appear crystalline with polarized light; they stain for lipids (oil red O, Sudan black B); and they give a positive reaction for acid polysaccharides with alcian blue and colloidal iron methods. These bodies consist chiefly of calcium-containing lipids and stain positively with alizarin red in microincinerated sections.

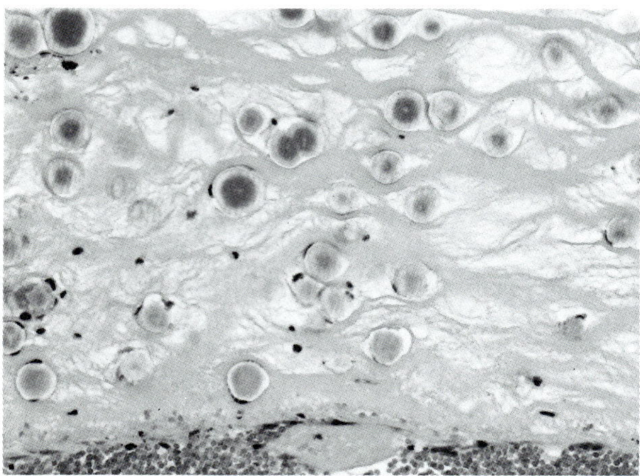

Fig. 14-30 Globe, vitreous; canine. Asteroid hyalosis. Spherical crystalline bodies (calcium-lipid) in liquified vitreous. H & E stain; ×160.

RETINA

The retina is composed of the retinal pigment epithelium and the sensory retina, both derived from neuroepithelium. The tissues of the retina arise from the optic vesicle: the pigment layer arises from the outer wall of the optic cup, and the sensory layer is derived from the inner wall. The retinal pigment epithelium, a single layer of rectangular cells, normally is nonpigmented over the tapetum, but, over most of the fundus, the cells contain pigment granules. The sensory retina, a delicate transparent layer, is firmly attached only at the optic disc and anteriorly at the ora ciliaris retinae. Otherwise, it is held against the retinal pigment epithelium by the turgid vitreous body. The sensory retina is composed of nine layers, from outward to inward these are the following:

1. Layers of rods and cones
2. External limiting membrane
3. Outer nuclear layer
4. Outer plexiform layer
5. Inner nuclear layer
6. Inner plexiform layer
7. Ganglion cell layer
8. Optic nerve fiber layer
9. Internal limiting membrane

In the dog, the main retinal vessels are in the ganglion cell and outer optic fiber layers; they do not protrude above the general level of the inner limiting membrane. Such protruding vessels occur in bovine animals (Fig. 14-31), sheep, and pigs.

Anomalies of the Retina

Retinal dysplasia

Retinal dysplasia has been described in most species, but especially in several breeds of dogs. It is characterized microscopically by a series of straight branching tubes that represent abortive elements to form the rod and cone layer, external limiting membrane, and outer nuclear layer and by the formation of rosettes (Fig. 14-32). A rosette is formed mainly of cells of the outer nuclear layer, with a mixture of cells from the inner nuclear layer arranged radially around a lumen lined by the external limiting membrane. The limbs of the rods and cones are usually absent; the lumen of the rosette may be round, oval, or flattened. Dysgenesis of the retina may include the ganglion cells and be accompanied by extensive gliosis. Other abnormalities may occur in common with retinal dysplasia, especially in dogs, and these include microphthalmia, cataract, persis-

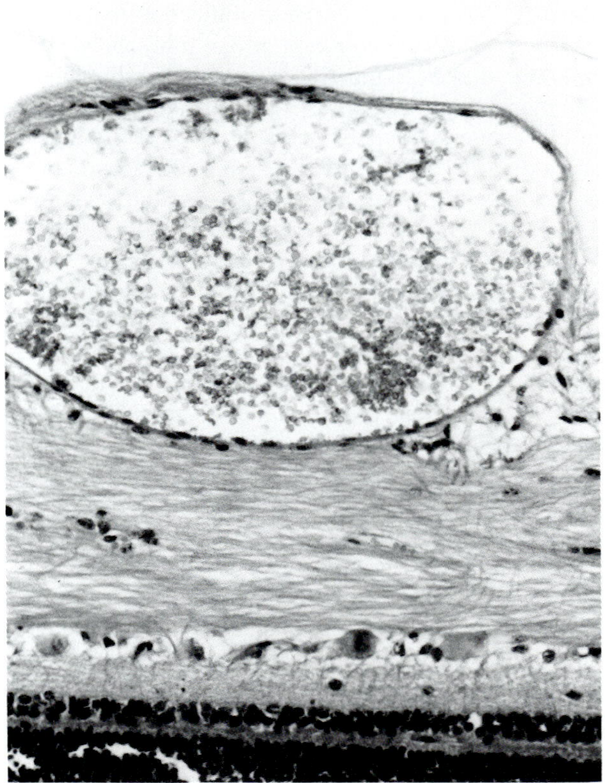

Fig. 14-31 Globe, retina; bovine. Normal animal. Retinal vessels in calf normally protrude above surface of the retina. H & E stain; ×63.

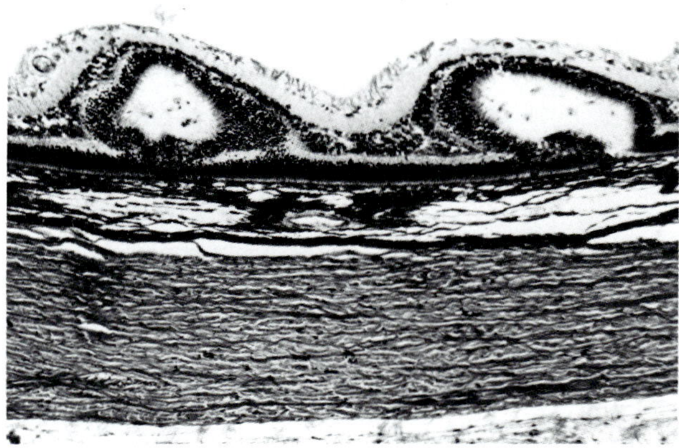

Fig. 14-32 Globe, retina; bovine. Retinal dysplasia. Rosettes present in retina have central, irregular to oval cavity. H & E stain; ×250.

tence of the primary vitreous, and coloboma of the uveal tract and optic nerve.

Lambs born of ewes given bluetongue virus vaccine during the first half of gestation have developmental anomalies of the brain and globe. The ocular lesions are retinal dysplasia, retinitis with perivascular cuffs of mononuclear inflammatory cells, and necrosis of the retina.

Hereditary Retinal Atrophy: Dog

The hereditary retinal degenerations in the dog, termed progressive retinal atrophy (PRA), have been subdivided into generalized and central forms. Generalized PRA includes several recessively inherited retinal dysplasias and degenerations that differ in functional and structural features. The disease has been described in many breeds and in mongrel dogs. It seems likely that any dog, whether either purebred or mongrel, can be affected with PRA.

The syndromes of PRA include rod dysplasia in the Norwegian elkhound, rod-cone dysplasia in Irish setter and collie breeds, cone dysplasia in the Alaskan malamute, and rod-cone degeneration in the miniature poodle. In these breeds, PRA is inherited as a simple autosomal recessive trait.

Rod dysplasia of Norwegian elkhound

In this progressive retinal disease, the rods are involved early and never reach functional maturity before degeneration. Young dogs (6 months) have impaired vision in dim light, and, by 3 to 5 years of age, affected dogs are both day and night blind. Ophthalmoscopic changes are detected at about 5 months of age when the tapetal retina has a tan to brown discoloration with a swirling granular appearance. In time, tapetal hyperreflectivity is most marked in the posterior pole just above the optic nerve head. Vascular thinning becomes prominent after 2 years of age, and the end result is an avascular retina.

No retinal lesions are seen by light microscopy in the globes of dogs 6 months of age, but, in those of dogs 2 years of age, the outer layers of the retina are thinned due to loss of the outer limbs of the rods and cones and by club-shaped deformation of the inner segments. Both the outer nuclear layer and the outer plexiform layer are thinned. Older dogs have complete retinal disorganization, gliosis, and pigment cell migration.

Rod-cone dysplasia of Irish setter

In this progressive retinal atrophy, onset of night blindness occurs early, and affected dogs invariably become blind. The rods and cones never attain functional maturity before degeneration, and the disease represents a development defect (dysplasia) rather than a premature degeneration (abiotrophy).

The outer segments of both rods and cones throughout the retina are abnormal by 24 days of age, and the deviation from normal is greatest in the central portion of the retina and in the rods. The outer segments are disorganized, fewer in number, and shorter and have reduced number of lamellae. The outer nuclear layer contains pyknotic rod nuclei. The retinal pigment epithelium contains few phagosomal inclusions. In the 14-week-old pup, some rod nuclei are pyknotic, and the internuclear space is greatly expanded by cytoplasmic processes of Müller cells. Outer segment material of both rods and cones is scant and disorganized. The outer plexiform layer is thinned. There is never any buildup of outer segment material.

The rod-cone dysplasia of the Irish setter has been associated with a defect in cyclic guanosine monophosphate (cGMP) metabolism. There appears to be deficiency in cGMP phosphodiesterase, which causes an accumulation of cGMP within the photoreceptor cells. The content of cGMP is 10 times greater in the retinas of affected dogs than in those of normal dogs.

Rod-cone dysplasia of collie

The disease in the collie dog is similar to that found in the Irish setter breed and is usually seen within the first year of life. It is inherited as an autosomal recessive trait by present evidence and is inherited independent of the collie eye anomaly. Clinically, the dogs are night blind by 6 weeks of age and are nearly totally blind by 1 year of age. The central tapetal fundus has a granular appearance at about 14 to 16 weeks of age. Affected dogs have a markedly deficient electroretinographic (ERG) response.

Lesions are present in the photoreceptor cells and retinal pigment epithelium (RPE). The RPE is thickened early (9 to 25 days), and outer segments of the rods and cones are nearly absent, with the space between the RPE and sensory retina filled with cellular debris. Degenerative changes are also present in the plexiform and inner nuclear layers. Affected collies have greater amounts of cGMP in the retina.

Progressive retinal (rod-cone) degeneration of miniature and toy poodles

This familial, bilateral, and progressive retinal degeneration is characterized initially by night blindness, followed by deterioration of day vision. Results of ERG studies indicate that the rods and cones attain functional maturity prior to degeneration. It is seen in both sexes and in all coat colors. Ophthalmoscopic observations include attenuation of retinal vasculature, hyperreflectivity of the tapetal area, and optic atrophy. Cataracts are common.

Lesions occur in the outer retinal layers, are most severe at the periphery, and consist of loss of the layer of rods and cones and reduction in width of the outer nuclear and outer plexiform layers. As the disease progresses, the retina loses layer organization and becomes reduced in width.

Cone dysplasia of Alaskan malamute and miniature poodle

Afflicted dogs are without ophthalmoscopic abnormalities, but day blindness is apparent in most affected dogs by 8 to 10 weeks of age. Night vision is not impaired. The disease was relatively common at one time but nearly has been eliminated from the Alaskan malamute breed.

The microscopic and ultrastructural features are the presence of degenerated cones in young dogs (6 months) and absence of cones in mature (4 years) hemeralopic dogs. In affected dogs, the rods and the inner retinal layers are normal. Results of ultrastructural studies indicate that the cones develop normally but degenerate with age. In the 2-year-old dog, few cones remain, and those present have no outer segments and short inner segments. Large bundles of filaments are present in the perinuclear zone of surviving cones. The outer segments slowly disappear, and the inner segments subsequently degenerate. Eventually, the cone nuclei are lost.

Central progressive retinal atrophy (pigment epithelial dystrophy)

Central progressive retinal atrophy is a specific pigment epithelial dystrophy and is uncommon in dogs of North America. The pigment epithelial cells become hypertrophied and hyperplastic, and these changes cause a secondary retinal degeneration. The disease is recognized in many breeds of dogs, and almost any breed can be affected.

Early ophthalmoscopic abnormalities are small, irregular, pigmented foci in the tapetal region near the area centralis; the tapetal fundus becomes increasingly spotted by clumps of pigment that vary in size, shape, and number. In late stages of the disease, the pigment foci disappear and the retina is atrophic.

The early change is hypertrophy of individual retinal pigment epithelial cells with accumulation of a light-brown granular material. The photoreceptor outer segments are shortened and bent. With time, large areas of the pigment epithelium consist of a monolayer of hypertrophied cells containing light-brown, granular, autofluorescent pigment. Retinal atrophy follows, with focal loss of photoreceptor and outer nuclear layers associated with multicellular nests of hypertrophied retinal pigment epithelial cells, some of which contain drusenlike bodies joined to the basement membrane. Gross retinal atrophy follows, with accompanying gliosis, aggregates of hypertrophied pigment epithelial cells, and migration of pigment-bearing cells into the retina.

Senile Retinal Degeneration

Changes in the globes of senile dogs include the common cystic degeneration of the peripheral retina (Fig. 14-33) and retinal breaks. Retinal breaks may be complete without retinal detachment and include holes, ruptured peripheral retinal cysts, holes associated with abnormal vitreous strands, and breaks associated with choroidal colobomas. The most common type of defect is the atrophic hole; these globes contain large patches of chorioretinal atrophy and areas of retinal thinning to the point of hole

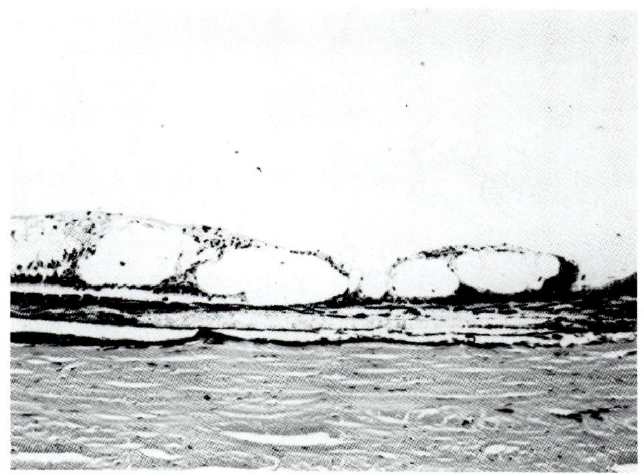

Fig. 14-33 Globe, retina; canine. Aged dog. Cystoid degeneration of peripheral retina consists of multiple variably sized cysts with replacement of retina. H & E stain; ×63.

formation. Holes may coalesce and spread, giving rise to retinoschisis.

Inflammatory Retinal Degeneration

Degeneration followed by atrophy can involve the retina of various species due to inflammatory changes produced by several infectious agents, including certain bacteria, viruses, fungi, and parasites.

Canine distemper

Retinal atrophy in the dog can follow infection with the virus of canine distemper. The lesions include degenerative changes in the retinal ganglion cells, perivascular cuffing, and the presence of eosinophilic intranuclear inclusion bodies. Chorioretinal damage in canine distemper may be of several types, including a peracute generalized retinitis (congestion, edema, perivascular cuffing) occurring during the initial stages of the acute encephalitis, a chronic generalized retinopathy in dogs with delayed onset of neurologic sequelae, a dystrophy of the cells of the pigment epithelium with or without evidence of other damage to the retina, and scattered foci of advanced degeneration with atrophy and sclerosis of the retina. The principal changes occur in the inner layers of the retina, are those of retinitis, and may be accompanied by optic neuritis with myelin destruction and astrocytic gliosis. In some dogs with distemper, lesions include swelling of the retinal pigment epithelial cells over the tapetal fundus, migration of retinal pigment cells into the retina, compression atrophy of the outer limbs of the rods and cones, and focal detachment of the sensory retina.

Pseudorabies

Ocular lesions occur in some swine infected with the herpesvirus of pseudorabies. The ocular lesions include perineuritis of the optic nerve, optic neuritis with perivascular lymphocytic cuffs, degeneration of ganglion cells, and focal retinal gliosis.

Toxoplasmosis

The clinical signs in affected animals have included those of anterior uveitis (aqueous flare, keratic precipitates, hyphema) and retinochoroiditis (retinal hemorrhage and detachment). Microscopic lesions in affected globes include multifocal necrosis of the retina with little inflammatory reaction (mainly plasma cells), retinitis with mononuclear cellular cuffs about retinal vessels, papillitis with gliosis and cuffed vessels, and nonsuppurative uveitis. Toxoplasmal organisms are usually found within active ocular lesions.

Toxic Retinal Degeneration

Progressive retinal degeneration (bright blindness) of sheep

This characteristic blindness has been observed for decades in hill flocks in the Yorkshire moors of northern England, has been observed in Scotland, and probably occurs in Wales. The disease is confined to those flocks grazing bracken fern *(Pteris aguilina).* The incidence is greatest in 3- to 4-year-old animals, and the disease is seldom seen in ewes less than 2 years of age. Clinically, affected sheep become permanently blind, adopt an alert attitude, and have bilaterally dilated pupils.

Lesions are bilateral and confined to the retina, and the early lesions are present in the layer of rods and cones, outer nuclear layer, and inner nuclear layer. With loss of the outer layers, the pigment epithelium abuts directly onto the thinned inner nuclear layer. Early cases have fragmentation and swelling of the outer segments of the rods and cones, and these structures also occur as a fine granular material internal to the pigment epithelium. The lesions develop earliest and are most severe in the central region.

Nutritional Retinal Degeneration

Feline nutritional retinal degeneration (taurine deficiency)

Retinal degeneration in cats fed a semipurified diet with casein as the protein source is progressive, begins with the layer of rods and cones, and, in time, involves other retinal layers. The retinal degeneration is associated with a selective decrease in plasmal and retinal taurine concentrations. Methionine and cysteine (taurine precursors) are present at concentrations comparable with those of controls, and supplementation of the taurine-free casein diet with either methionine or cysteine does not prevent the retinal degeneration. The cat converts only a limited amount of cysteine to taurine, apparently because the enzyme required for this synthesis is limiting in activity.

Early alterations in the retina include degeneration of the photoreceptors cells in the area centralis and, later, of the photoreceptors in the peripheral retina. The most extensive loss of photoreceptors occurs where the concentration of ganglion cells is greatest. In areas of minimal disruption, the outer segments are shortened and fragmented. Some areas have loss of both inner and outer segments and either thinning or absence of the outer nuclear layer, accompanied by a widened profile of the inner nuclear layer. The pigment epithelium appears unaltered, but a severe disorganization of the lattice arrangement of tapetal rods occurs in cats fed a taurine-deficient diet.

Diabetic Retinal Degeneration

Only a few cases of diabetic retinopathy have been described, and these were in dogs. The retina of diabetic dogs contains several saccular capillary microaneurysms and exudates typical of those observed in human diabetic retinopathy. Also, a generalized loss of pericytes and pericyte ghosts are present. Some aneurysms are hyalinized, and others have the classic endothelial proliferation within the aneurysmal wall. Oversized capillaries occur singly or in groups and tend to be diffusely hypercellular, whereas most of the remaining capillaries are either acellular or deficient in pericytes. Subcapsular cortical cataract with degeneration of the lenticular fibers and vacuole formation are additional ocular lesions. The subcapsular epithelium is focally proliferated, but no glycogen vacuoles are present in the pigmented epithelium of the iris as seen in human patients.

Retinal Degeneration by Visible Light

The retina of various species can be damaged by light, both fluorescent and incandescent illumination, that is not intense enough to burn or cause thermal injury. Several types of lasers are capable of producing retinal damage, and damage can be produced in the retina of monkeys and dogs exposed to the light of the indirect ophthalmoscope.

The extent of damage to the retina is modified by such variables as wavelength of light, intensity of the source, duration of exposure, body temperature, age, and photoperiodicity. The wavelengths most efficient in producing retinal damage are those most efficient in bleaching rhodopsin; the order of damage from most to least is blue, green, white, and red.

Damage to the retina increases with increasing light intensity; it also increases with increasing duration of exposure at lower intensity. The rate of degeneration is directly related to the intensity of the illumination. The extent of degeneration and the involvement of the pigment epithelium are greater with greater intensity illuminants. The rate and extent of retinal damage can be increased by raising the body temperature of the animal during the duration of exposure to the light. Temperature can also alter the tissue affected; thus, raising the body temperature can increase the likelihood of destroying the retinal pigment epithelium with a given intensity of illumination. Age influences the severity of light damage, as susceptibility to light damage is increased in older animals.

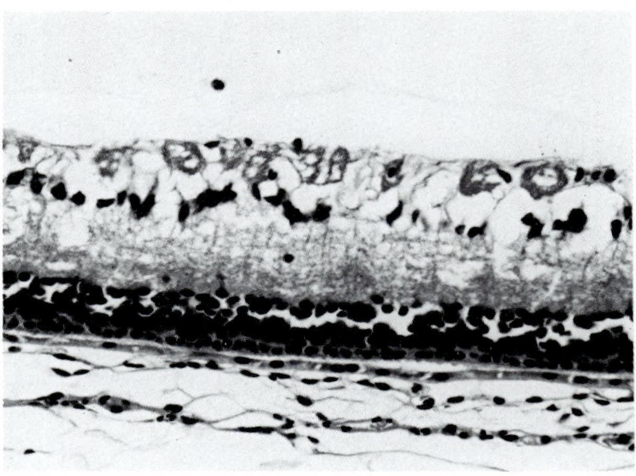

Fig. 14-34 Globe, retina; murine. Light retinopathy. Atrophy involves the outer retinal layers (loss of layer of rods and cones and much of outer nuclear layer) in a rat exposed to continuous light for several weeks. H & E stain; ×250.

Continuous light produces early effects on the outer segments of the photoreceptor cells. Microscopically, the segments develop a stratified appearance, separate from the retinal pigment epithelium, and, later, become fragmented and are removed by phagocytes. The nuclei become pyknotic, and eventually the photoreceptor cell and the outer plexiform layers are lost (Fig. 14-34). With lower intensity illumination, the retinal pigment epithelium is not damaged.

Retinal Detachment

The retina is firmly attached only at the optic nerve head and at the ora ciliaris retinae. The potential space between the retina and the retinal pigment epithelium is a vestige of the central cavity of the optic vesicle. Accumulation of fluid, exudate, blood, or neoplastic cells within this potential space constitutes detachment of the retina. Retinal detachment (or nonattachment) is part of congenital ocular anomalies of the collie ectasia syndrome and retinal dysplasia in other breeds and is also part of microphthalmia. The consequence of detachment is degeneration and necrosis of the retina; degenerative changes occur in the outer segments of the photoreceptor cells within 2 to 6 weeks of detachment. The rods and cones rapidly atrophy and disappear. Pseudorosettes then form by a folding of the outer retinal layers. Atrophy of the retina is slow but progressive, affecting the several layers in turn; it ultimately extends to the optic fiber layer, which becomes edematous and develops cystoid spaces (Fig. 14-35). The retinal pigment epithelium tends to proliferate (Fig. 14-36).

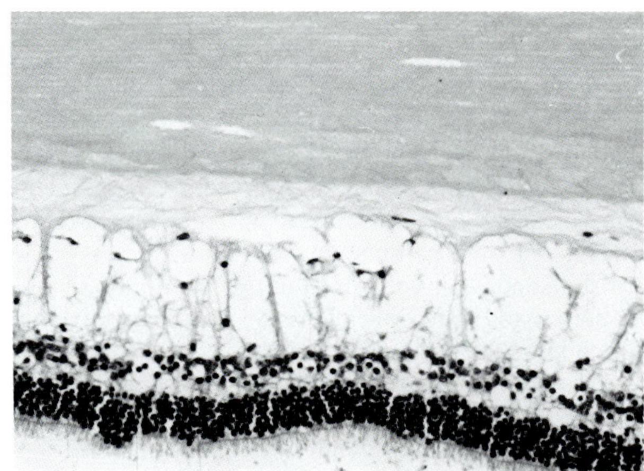

Fig. 14-35 Globe, retina; canine. Retinal detachment. Detached retina lies in contact with posterior lenticular capsule and has microcystoid degeneration of the inner layers. H & E stain; ×160.

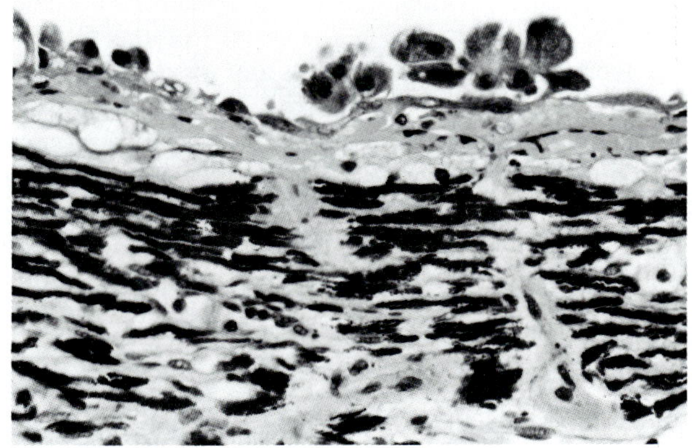

Fig. 14-36 Globe, choroid and retinal pigment epithelium; canine. Retinal detachment. Hypertrophy and hyperplasia of retinal pigment epithelium occur when the retina is detached. H & E stain; ×250.

OPTIC NERVE

The optic nerve consists of the axons of the ganglion cells of the retina and is a white fiber tract of the CNS, extending from the eyeball to the optic chiasma. It consists of ocular, orbital, and intracranial portions. In most species, the optic fibers within the globe are unmyelinated and take on a myelin sheath as they leave the globe at the lamina cribrosa. In the dog and the rabbit, myelinated fibers occur within the optic disc. Also, there is variation in the entrance of the vessels that supply the retina, in the density of the lamina cribrosa, and the amount of connective tissue within the nerve. The nerves vary in size and the angle at which they leave the globe. Primates have a functional central retinal artery and vein; other species normally do not have a central artery, but vessels enter the nerve at the sclera. The lamina cribrosa is very dense and prominent in horses, cows, and dogs and essentially is nonexistent in rabbits and rodents.

In cross section, the axis cylinders of the nerve fibers appear as small, faintly stained eosinophilic dots surrounded by clear halos—the myelin sheath. The normal nerve is rather pale with a somewhat spongy appearance microscopically. Glial cells are neither normally large nor numerous, and the nerve appears hypocellular. In diseases of the optic nerve, myelin may be lost and collagenous tissue increased. The nerve is then less spongy, more compact, and more eosinophilic because the nerve tissue contains increased numbers of glial and mesenchymal cells. Marked pigmentation of the nerve head is observed in many animal globes and should not be considered abnormal when melanin pigmentation is the only change. An aging change present in the optic nerve of dogs is increased connective tissue, especially about blood vessels.

Anomalies of the Optic Nerve

Aplasia

Aplasia of the optic nerve is rare in animals. In true cases, the optic disc, optic nerve, and optic tracts are absent. The optic nerves are represented by thin and fragile cottonlike strands that extend from the globe to the brain with no recognizable chiasma. Ganglion cells are not present in a retina that contains rosettes in its central and peripheral portions.

Hypoplasia

Hypoplasia of the optic nerve is a rarely reported lesion and has been found as an isolated defect in several species. It can result from failure of development of the ganglion cell layer and absence of a corresponding number of optic nerve fibers. The extent of the reduction in size of the nerve varies from a severe form, in which only a thin filament remains, to mildly affected nerves that only are reduced in diameter as compared with those of controls. The optic chiasms and optic tracts are hypoplastic.

Coloboma of the optic nerve

This lesion may occur alone, but it is often associated with microphthalmia, mainly in dogs, in which it is part of the collie eye anomaly syndrome. Colobomas of the optic papilla have been described in incompletely albino cattle, in cats, in collie and basenji dogs, and as an inherited syndrome in Charolais cattle. Excavation of the optic papilla often extends into the nerve and may communicate with cavities in the choroid and sclera. True optic colobomas are confined to the optic disc and nerve. The anomaly may involve the lamina cribrosa and may produce an ectasia of the sclera. Coloboma of the optic nerve is often accompanied by dysplasia of the adjacent retina. In the colobomatous cavities, the retina and the choroid are extremely thin, and hypertrophy and hyperplasia affect the retinal pigment epithelium.

Papilledema

Papilledema (disc edema) is edema with swelling of the nerve head from any cause. Lesions that alter the pressure gradient so that flow of tissue fluid is outward (from optic nerve into the globe) result in papilledema. Such diverse lesions as space-occupying intracranial lesions, increased venous pressure, meningitis, and orbital neoplasms all tend to increase pressure posterior to the lamina cribrosa and produce papilledema. The microscopic changes of papilledema are similar, regardless of cause. The vessels of the papilla may be congested, and the nerve head is pale-staining and swollen (Fig. 14-37). It protrudes against the vitreous and bulges laterally, and swelling of the nerve head may cause buckling of the retina. Some proteinaceous exudate may occur between the retina and the pigment epithelium. Papilledema, if present for an extended period, results in degenerative changes and the development of irregular varicosities and cytoid bodies in the optic nerve head. In chronic papilledema, the optic nerve head is atrophic and gliotic.

Inflammation

Optic neuritis is the involvement of any part of the optic nerve by inflammatory, vascular, or degenerative disease. The term papillitis is used when the nerve head is involved, and the term neuroretinitis is used when there are associated alterations in the retina. Lesions of the optic papilla are rarely primary in animals but are almost always secondary to lesions in the globe, optic nerve, and brain. Optic papillitis is part of retinitis and ophthalmitis and is characterized by edema, perivascular cuffing, and gliosis. Topographically, optic neuritis can be subdivided into perineuritis—leptomeningitis of the optic nerve; periaxial optic neuritis—extension of meningial inflammation along the pial septa into the parenchyma of the optic nerve; axial neuritis—selective involvement of the inner portions of the optic nerve; and transverse neuritis—severe and extensive destruction of the optic nerve.

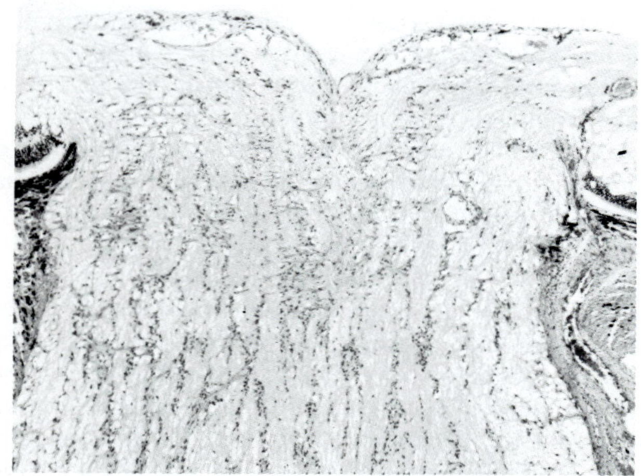

Fig. 14-37 Globe, optic nerve; canine. Papilledema. Optic nerve head is pale-staining, is swollen, and protrudes into vitreous (rafoxanide toxicity). H & E stain; ×40. *Courtesy Dr. R. Brown.*

The optic meninges and meningial spaces are continuous with those of the brain, and perineuritis is an expected complication of primary (especially bacterial) cerebral leptomeningitis. It results from an extension of inflammation along the meninges of the optic nerve, or it may develop as a direct extension of localized inflammation in the sinuses, orbital space, or globe.

Degeneration

The optic nerve is a special white-matter tract of the CNS, is composed of the axons of the ganglion cells of the retina, and reacts to injury differently than do peripheral nerves. Because the optic nerve is part of the CNS, the nerve fibers have no Schwann cells and little or no capacity for regeneration. Glial, meningeal, and connective tissue components of the optic nerve respond to injury by proliferation. Optic nerve degeneration may be ascending when lesions affect the ganglion cells of the retina and nerve fiber layers. The process may be either focal or general in the nerve, depending on the extent of the lesions in the retina.

Secondary optic nerve degeneration

These lesions in the optic nerves are due to either inflammation or vascular disease near the globe. Although optic atrophy may be of unknown cause, it often can be related to retinal degeneration, inflammation, prolonged papilledema, glaucoma, or inflammatory and destructive lesions of the optic nerves and tracts. A pronounced reaction of glial and mesenchymal tissues of the optic nerve head may obscure the essential degenerative features.

Rafoxanide neuropathy is caused by a halogenated salicylanilide with fasciolicidal activity. The drug produces brain and ocular lesions in dogs and sheep. Papilledema and increased cerebrospinal fluid (CSF) pressure are accompanied, in the dog, by spongy degeneration of the white matter of the corpus callosum, fornix, and periventricular areas of the brain, and the periphery of the optic chiasma and optic nerves. Lesions in sheep include status spongiosus of varying severity in the CNS with predilection for such areas as the periventricular area of the lateral ventricles, optic tracts, lateral geniculate bodies, and optic fasciculi. In the retina, necrotic nerve cells are present in the ganglion cell layer. The blindness in the sheep and dog could be due to the lesions in the retina and optic nerves and to status spongiosus lesions in the brain.

Retrobulbar optic neuropathy (male fern toxicity) was observed in calves grazing a paddock containing rhizomes of male fern *(Dryopteris [Aspidinum] felix mas; D. austriaca).* These plants contain a complex mixture of phloroglucin derivatives. Fundic lesions are hemorrhages on and near the optic disc associated with papilledema in the acute stage. In the chronic stage, the optic disc is sunken and has a light gray color. The blood vessels of the disc and retina are thin and irregular. The optic nerve is swollen and increased in size. Degenerative changes are vacuolation (Fig. 14-38) and destruction of fibers, with development of lacunae containing gitter cells and debris. The number of axons and the amount of myelin are markedly reduced. In some areas, the destruction of nerve fibers is nearly total, and these areas have abundant gitter cells. There is no regeneration.

Optic neuropathy occurs in calves fed vitamin A–deficient diets. These calves are blind and have alterations of edema of the optic papilla, engorged and distorted retinal vessels, constriction of the optic nerve, and elevated CSF pressure. Blindness in calves can vary in severity from a reversible night blindness to the irreversible blindness of retinal degeneration and optic nerve necrosis and atrophy.

Calves deficient in vitamin A have gross changes in the bones of the skull. These bones are increased in thickness and reduced in density. The size of the optic foramen is reduced due to encroaching bone. Early, the nerves are swollen and contain red-brown zones of hemorrhage. The optic nerve in the region of the constriction is necrotic and atrophic. In older lesions, the necrotic segment is sharply contracted from the normal nerve proximal and distal to the constriction. An advanced lesion is composed of an atrophic segment of white fibrous tissue within a constricted optic canal.

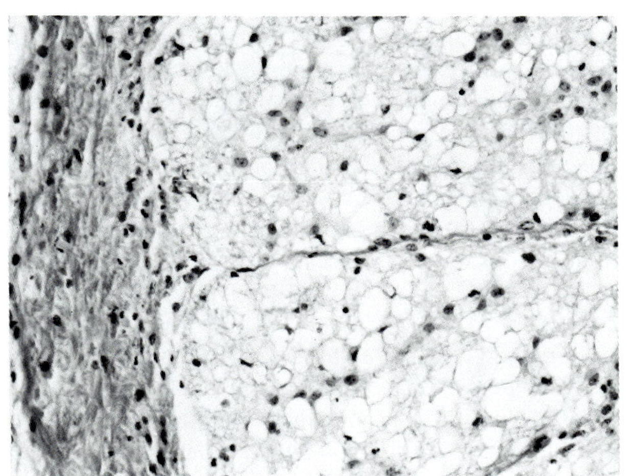

Fig. 14-38 Globe, optic nerve; bovine. Male fern optic neuropathy. Spongy degeneration (edema, demyelination, vacuolation) involves the peripheral portion of the optic nerve. H & E stain; ×160. *Courtesy Dr. D.R. Lucas.*

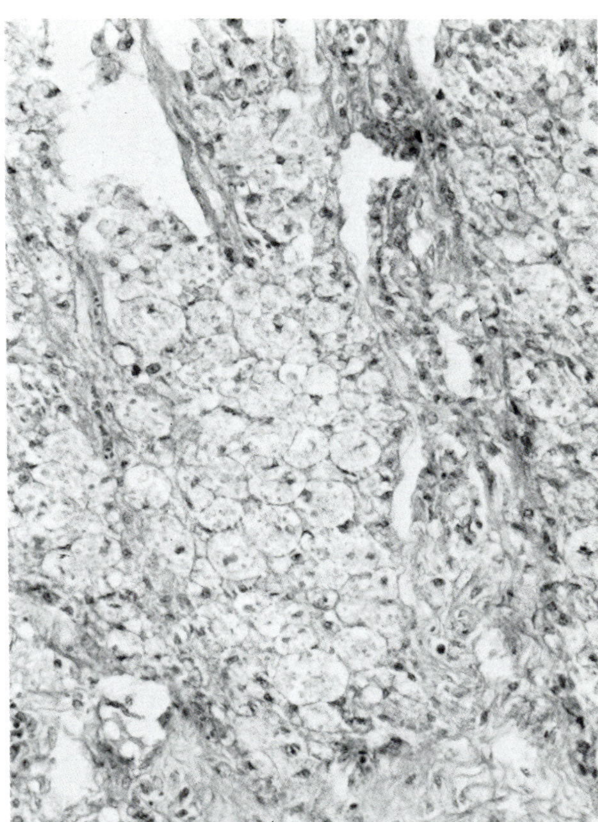

Fig. 14-39 Globe, optic nerve; bovine. Vitamin A deficiency. Necrosis of optic nerve is accompanied by replacement with large foamy macrophages (''gitter cells''). H & E stain; ×160. *Courtesy Dr. S. Nielsen.*

Microscopically, areas of necrosis and gitter cell accumulation are present in the region of greatest constriction (Fig. 14-39). Fragmented axons are numerous in some nerves and are absent in the most chronic lesions. Older lesions have thickened leptomeningeal septums and extensive astrocytic gliosis in the adjacent viable nerve.

Proliferative Optic Neuropathy

The clinical appearance of this lesion in horses varies from a whitish-gray, oval, elevated structure to a round, protuberant, whitish mass at the optic disc. The lesion usually is unilateral, and visual disturbances are not detected.

The thinly encapsulated mass is composed of large, plump, round to ovoid cells with small, dense, eccentrically placed nuclei and palely eosinophilic, foamy to vacuolated cytoplasm (Fig. 14-40). Foamy cells are present in the optic nerve, both at the level of the lamina cribrosa and deeper

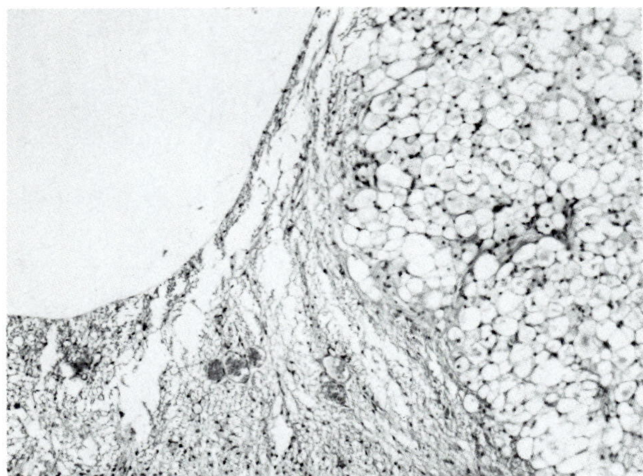

Fig. 14-40 Globe, optic nerve head; equine. Proliferative optic neuropathy. Circumscribed lesion is composed of sheet of large cells with vacuolated cytoplasm. H & E stain; ×63.

in the nerve. A portion of the nerve posterior to the mass may be demyelinated.

Storage Diseases

The storage diseases reported in animals have ocular lesions, and many different cells of the globe and optic nerve, especially neurons of the retina, accumulate materials within lysosomes due to enzyme deficiency and faulty degradation.

Gangliosidosis

Gangliosidosis with retinal lesions has been described in the dog, cat, and calf. Corneal opacities occur due to polysaccharide accumulation within the corneal endothelium and in stromal fibroblasts. Retinal ganglion cells and amacrine cells have swollen, foamy, granular, and PAS-positive cytoplasm (Fig. 14-41). Ultrastructurally, membranous cytoplasmic inclusions are present in neurons of the retina, brain, and ganglia. Axon degeneration is present in the optic nerve.

Mannosidosis

Ocular lesions have been described in animals with α- and β-mannosidosis. Nubian goats affected with β-mannosidosis have small palpebral fissures, a paucity of myelin in the optic nerves, and the presence of numerous, nonstaining spherical intracytoplasmic vacuoles in retinal ganglion cells, ciliary epithelium, retinal pigment epithelium, keratocytes, corneal endothelial cells, other retinal cells, and ocular mesenchymal cells. Similar lesions, except for vacuolation of the retinal pigment epithelium, have been observed in Salers cattle. Vacuolated retinal cells have been described in cattle with α-mannosidosis.

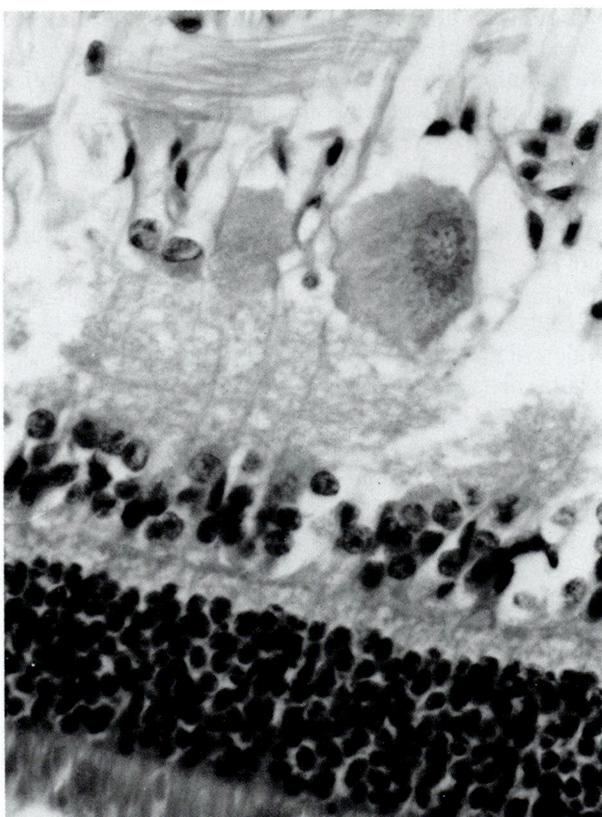

Fig. 14-41 Globe, retina; bovine. GMI Gangliosidosis. Retinal ganglion cells are enlarged, are swollen, and have granular cytoplasm. H & E stain; ×400. *Courtesy Dr. B. Sheahan.*

Mucopolysaccharidoses

These storage diseases are characterized by biochemical derangements in metabolism of glycosaminoglycans. Ocular lesions have been described in cats affected with mucopolysaccharidosis I and IV (MPS I and MPS IV). In cats with MPS I, intracytoplasmic vacuolation is observed in connective tissue cells of the cornea, conjunctiva, sclera, choroid, iris, and ciliary body; in the epithelium of the iris and ciliary body; and in the retinal pigment epithelium. The ocular lesions observed in cats with MPS IV are similar.

GLAUCOMA

Glaucoma is a sustained increase in intraocular pressure and the changes produced in various ocular structures. The increased pressure is almost always due to tissue changes that reduce the outflow of aqueous, and many different causes and processes may be responsible. Thus, glaucoma results from a complex of ocular diseases, all having in common the elevation of intraocular pressure as a result of obstruction to aqueous outflow in the region of the anterior chamber angle and trabecular meshwork. The most important aspects of the pathology of glaucoma are the various changes induced in the intraocular tissues by the continued elevated intraocular pressure.

When the block in aqueous outflow is a complication of an ocular disease, the glaucoma is called secondary. If the elevation of pressure occurs without prior ocular disease, the glaucoma is classified as primary. Glaucoma appearing at or shortly after birth as a consequence of some developmental error is called congenital glaucoma. Some cases of congenital glaucoma in animals may be secondary to ophthalmitis arising from an intrauterine bacterial infection.

Primary Glaucoma

Primary glaucoma, including both closed- and open-angle types, has been described in several breeds of dogs. In dogs with clinical evidence of glaucoma, the filtration angles are compressed with loss of trabecular meshwork, and the iris root is displaced forward into apposition with the cornea and is accompanied by collapse of the scleral venous plexus. Extensive anterior synechiae, scleral stretching, and collapse of ciliary cleft and trabecular meshwork are other ocular lesions found in glaucomatous globes.

In cases of primary glaucoma in the basset hound dog, the filtration angles are anomalous, and the root of the iris is pulled forward over the trabecular meshwork by a band of tissue that merges into the posterior corneal surface. This type of glaucoma is due to mesodermal dysgenesis of the filtration angle.

Light-induced Avian Glaucoma

In domestic chicks reared from hatching under continuous light, the developing glaucoma has such features as elevated intraocular pressure, impaired outflow facility, globe enlargement, increase globe weight, retinal damage, and, eventually, blindness. The retina is detached, and peripheral anterior synechiae may form prior to rupture of the globe. With time, the ocular chambers are fibrosed and contain foci of metaplastic bone. The development of glaucoma in light-exposed chicks is apparently not a simple angle-closure type because iridectomy neither prevents nor alters the course of the development of the glaucoma.

Secondary Glaucoma

Most cases of glaucoma in animals are of the secondary type and are complications of a large number of intraocular diseases, including inflammatory, traumatic, neoplastic, and degenerative lesions. Most cases are unilateral and occur in the globe with causative lesions. Most cases of filtration-angle obstruction result from acute or chronic inflammation directly, and many are due to the presence of preiridal fibrovascular membranes (Fig. 14-42). Glaucoma usually develops in animals with a neoplasm of the anterior segment. Intraocular neoplasms may produce peripheral anterior synechiae by displacing the iris forward against the trabecular meshwork, and neoplasms of the iris and ciliary body, whether primary or metastatic, may invade and obstruct the filtration angle.

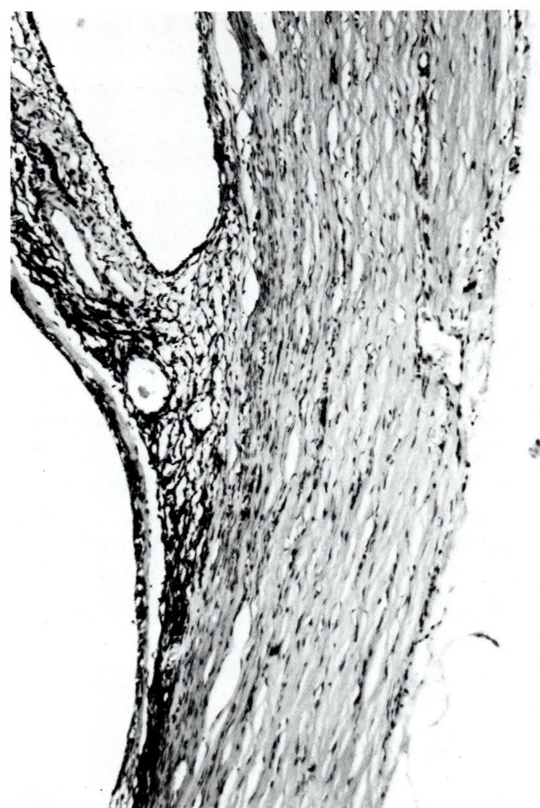

Fig. 14-42 Globe, filtration area; canine. Secondary glaucoma. The filtration angle is open, and the trabecular meshwork is obliterated and fibrosed with base of iris pulled forward. H & E stain; ×160.

Secondary angle-closure glaucoma can be caused by pupillary block, which obstructs the flow of aqueous between the posterior and anterior chambers. Annular adhesions, because of organization of inflammatory exudate, develop between the lens and the pupillary part of iris in certain cases of iritis; and, if complete, the pressure increase in the posterior chamber pushes the iris forward, producing iris bombé. If iris bombé is chronic, peripheral anterior synechia forms at the site of contact between the iris and trabecular meshwork. Adhesions may form due to iridal swelling and exudates in the filtration angle. As the intraocular pressure increases, the root of the iris is displaced forward to further decrease the width of the filtration angle.

A dislocated lens may cause pupillary blockage and angle closure. Extreme pupillary block occurs when the lens is dislocated into the anterior chamber with the iris pressed against the posterior surface of the lens. It is not always possible in the late stages of glaucoma to distinguish primary from secondary forms.

Ocular Effects of Glaucoma

In chronic cases of glaucoma, most of the tissues of the globe are altered. The globe is enlarged, its tunics are thinned, the uvea is atrophied (Fig. 14-43), and the iris is displaced forward. Globe enlargement is usual in the dog and cat but is uncommon in other domestic animals, which have a thicker sclera. Important damage occurs at the optic disc, which gradually becomes excavated (Fig. 14-44).

Changes in the retina include atrophy of the nerve fiber and ganglion cell layers (Fig. 14-45), which may progress to complete absence of these tissues. The nontapetal retina is usually more severely affected than the tapetal retina. Some secondary gliosis may occur, but the outer neuronal layers are usually without lesions until late in the disease. The iris stroma becomes atrophic and fibrotic, and the ciliary body and ciliary processes also become atrophic, hyalinized, and fibrotic. The choroid may be thinned, and the vessels are sclerosed.

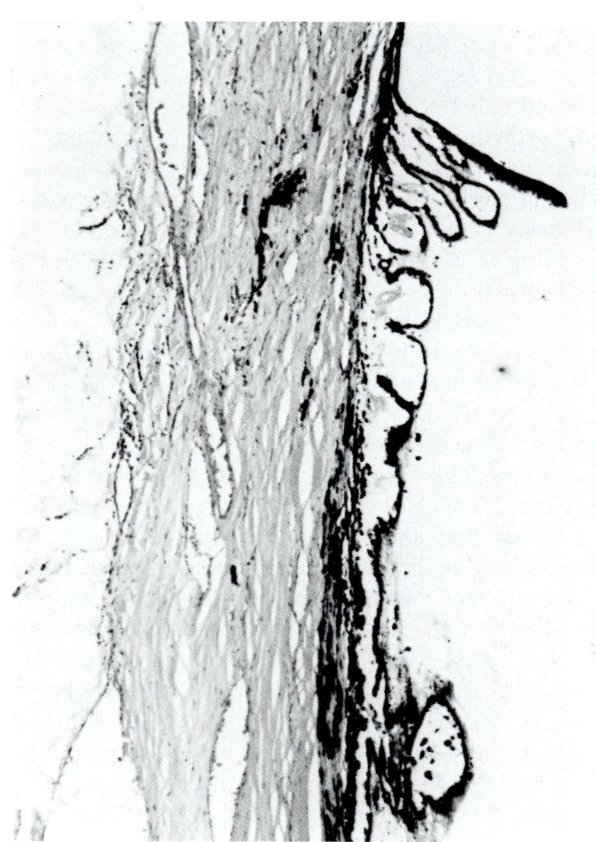

Fig. 14-43 Globe, ciliary body; canine. Secondary glaucoma. The ciliary body and ciliary processes are severely atrophic. H & E stain; ×40.

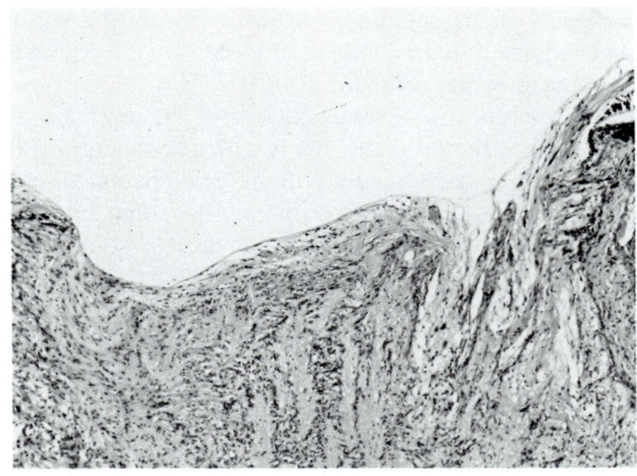

Fig. 14-44 Globe, optic nerve; canine. Secondary glaucoma. The optic nerve head is atrophic and "cupped," with nerve head displaced below level of choroid. H & E stain; ×40.

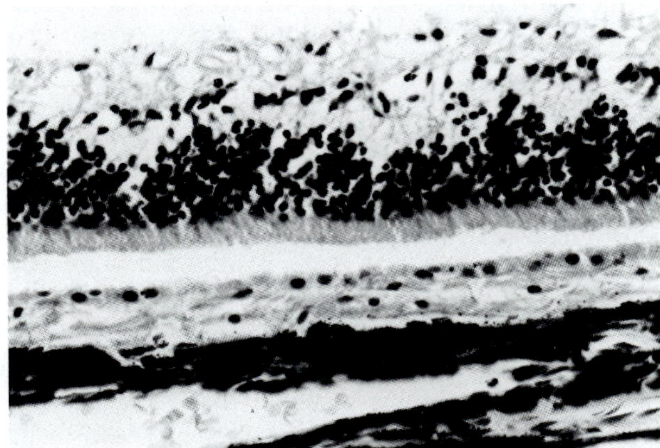

Fig. 14-45 Globe, retina; canine. Secondary glaucoma. The inner layers of the retina are atrophied with only single row of nuclei remaining of inner nuclear layer. Outer nuclear layer and layer of rods and cones appear unaffected. H & E stain; ×250.

CONJUNCTIVA

Conjunctivitis

Bacterial conjunctivitis is common, especially in dogs and cattle. Species of several genera of bacteria are responsible for conjunctivitis in domestic and laboratory animals. These organisms include staphylococci, streptococci, *Pseudomonas aeruginosa, E. coli,* and *Moraxella bovis.* The conjunctiva is very sensitive to bacterial infection, and some organisms—including those of tularemia,

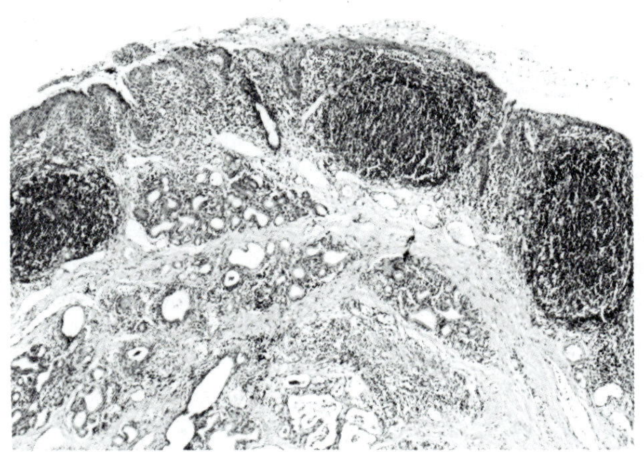

Fig. 14-46 Eyelid, conjunctiva; canine. Follicular conjunctivitis. The lymphoid tissue is hyperplastic with follicle formation. H & E stain; ×40.

listeriosis, and brucellosis—penetrate the intact conjunctiva. The clinical signs of acute infective conjunctivitis are much the same, regardless of cause. Epiphora, at first serous, later becomes either mucoid or mucopurulent, and the ocular discharge is accompanied by a congested, swollen, edematous, and chemotic conjunctiva.

The microscopic alterations in the conjunctiva are very similar in many cases of acute infective conjunctivitis. Edema, hyperemia, cellular degeneration, and necrosis are accompanied by neutrophilic infiltration of the epithelium and underlying stroma. Numbers of plasma cells and lymphocytes vary, depending on the age of the lesion and the inciting organism. The epithelium of the conjunctiva is not keratinized normally but readily becomes keratinized when chronically irritated. Also, the goblet cells and the small lymphoid aggregates normally present in the conjunctival propria undergo hyperplasia. Lymphoid hyperplasia can proceed to produce rather large follicles and increased numbers of follicles **(follicular conjunctivitis)** (Fig. 14-46). Clinically, the conjunctiva has a roughened, cobblestone appearance.

Chlamydia (feline pneumonitis; *Chlamydia psittaci*) and mycoplasma may act in concert to produce conjunctivitis in cats. Lesions may be unilateral or bilateral, and clinical signs are lacrimation, conjunctival edema, and catarrhal, purulent exudate. The conjunctiva is chemotic, smooth, shiny, and gray-pink. Small lymphoid nodules form in the third eyelid. Feline mycoplasmal conjunctivitis follows some stress and either as a sequela to or in conjunction with viral respiratory disease. In severe cases, a pseudomembrane forms on the membrana nictitans. Mycoplasma are coccoid to coccobacillary and occur in clusters either on or near the surface of the epithelial cells. The subepithelial tissue is infiltrated by a mixture of inflammatory cells, and the epithelium is focally eroded. A mycoplasma-like organism may produce a follicular conjunctivitis in swine.

Feline infectious conjunctivitis

Ocular lesions in cats infected with feline herpesvirus occur in kittens 2 to 4 weeks of age and consist of conjunctivitis, keratitis, corneal ulceration, and perforation of the globe. Acute feline herpesvirus conjunctivitis is characterized by blepharospasm, slight epiphora, and mild conjunctival vascular injection. The ocular discharge soon becomes profuse and seromucoid; chemosis involves the conjunctiva of the globe and membrana nictitans. Histopathologic alterations include a pseudodiphtheritic membrane, ulcerative keratitis, and lesions of keratoconjunctivitis sicca.

EPISCLERA

The episclera is the well-vascularized connective tissue between the bulbar conjunctiva and the sclera. Few lesions involve this structure.

Nodular Episcleritis (Nodular Granulomatous Episclerokeratitis)

Nodular episcleritis (nodular fasciitis, fibrous histiocytoma) is a benign nodular lesion of connective tissue. It is rare in animals but has been described in the dog. Firm, nodular growths involve the conjunctiva, sclera, membrana nictitans, and corneal stroma. The masses are composed of interlacing bundles of fibrous connective tissue, numerous capillaries, and a mixture of histiocytes and fibroblasts with a sprinkling of inflammatory cells, mostly lymphocytes and plasma cells (Fig. 14-47).

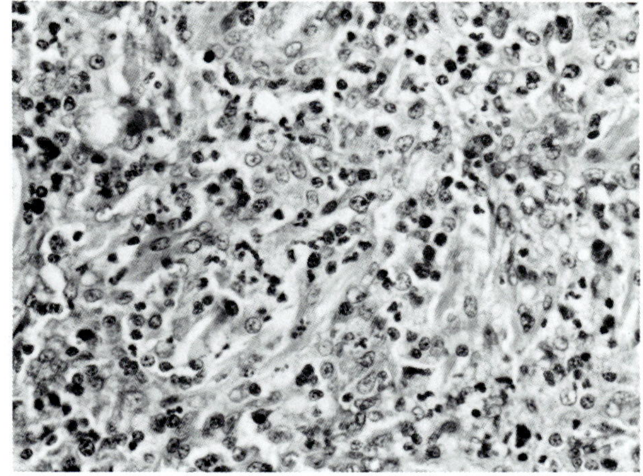

Fig. 14-47 Eyelid; canine. Nodular fasciitis. Mass is composed of fibroblasts and histiocytes with sprinkling of mononuclear inflammatory cells (lymphocytes and plasma cells). H & E stain; ×250.

EYELIDS

The disease processes that affect the skin of the eyelids include many that involve the skin in other locations. Afflictions peculiar to the skin of the eyelids include trichiasis, districhiasis, entropion, and ectropion. These lesions, if not corrected, will result in conjunctivitis and keratitis. Other lesions include epidermoid and dermoid cysts and cysts of the membrana nictitans. Inflammation of the gland of the membrana nictitans and hyperplasia of lymphoid follicles are lesions that enlarge the third eyelid and cause it to protrude.

Inflammation

Inflammatory lesions include blepharitis, hordeolum, internal hordeolum, and chalazion. In blepharitis, the reactions of the skin of the eyelids include hyperemia, edema, and serous exudation. Fluid accumulates among epithelial cells, producing vesicles and degeneration. In more severe infections, necrosis, ulceration, and intense leukocytic infiltration occur. **Hordeolum** is a folliculitis due to pyogenic infection of the perifollicular tissue. Abscess formation in the follicle or glands of a cilium of the eyelid is a complication of bacterial blepharitis; after localization, the abscess breaks into the skin to produce a cellulitis. Pyogenic infection of meibomian (tarsal) glands, **internal hordeolum,** results in occlusion of the duct and abscess formation. Swelling, redness, and evidence of pain are observed as the focal lesion develops into an abscess. Chronic inflammation of meibomian or Zeis glands **(chalazion)** generally is granulomatous due to the chronic irritation produced by the released sebaceous material. The center of the granulomatous inflammatory lesion may liquify and, if encapsulated, a cyst is formed. Rupture of the cyst through the eyelid produces a mass of granulomatous tissue. The essential feature is that granulomas and abscesses form around sebum released from damaged sebaceous glands. Giant cells, macrophages, lymphocytes, and plasma cells are part of the granulomatous inflammation (Fig. 14-48).

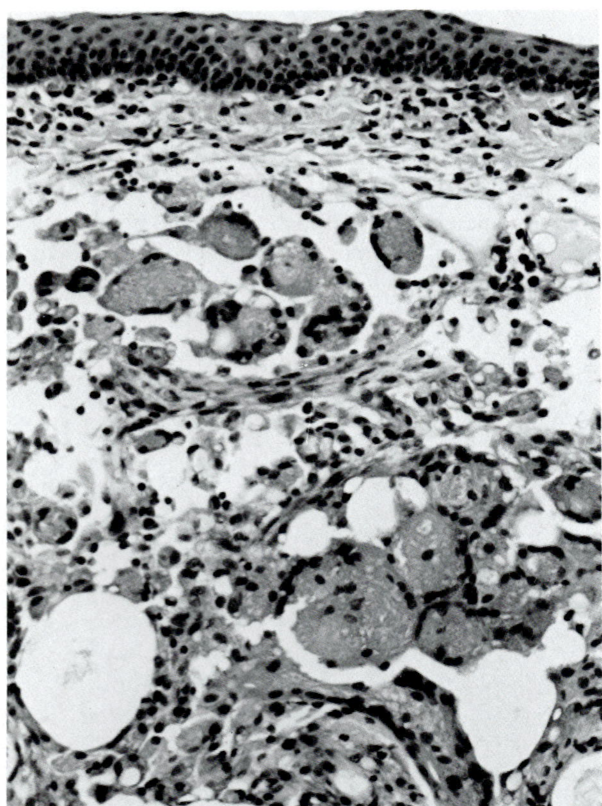

Fig. 14-48 Eyelid, meibomian glands; canine. Chalazion. Granulomatous inflammation with giant cells with foamy cytoplasm due to sebum released from necrotic meibomian glands. H & E stain; ×160.

LACRIMAL APPARATUS

Inflammation of the lacrimal gland (dacryoadenitis) can be primary or secondary due to the spread of disease processes from the conjunctiva and from the orbit, in cases of orbital cellulitis. When inflammation is acute and diffuse, the sequela may be an abscess that may rupture. Inflammation of the lacrimal gland may also accompany chronic granulomatous panophthalmitis and orbital cellulitis, especially in dogs.

Sialodacryoadenitis of Rats

Sialodacryoadenitis is a coronavirus infection that is highly contagious, is nonfatal, and spreads easily and rapidly among susceptible rats by contact, aerosol, and fomite. Sucklings and weanling rats are most susceptible. This common disease of rats involves the salivary glands, the intraorbital and harderian lacrimal glands, cervical lymph nodes, thymus, eyes, and, sometimes, the lungs. The acute disease in sucklings, when well developed, is distinctive, as the neck becomes thickened by the enlarged submaxillary salivary glands and surrounding edema to produce a "mumpslike" appearance. Grossly, gelatinous edema involves the intermandibular space and the submaxillary glands are swollen. In some rats, only the harderian gland is involved, and the disease is sometimes indicated by "red tears" (chromodacryorrhea) due to secretion of porphyrin by the harderian gland. Usually, mortality is low, and the disease, if mild, might go undetected in affected rats. Keratoconjunctivitis has been associated with some natural outbreaks, and affected rats have photophobia, lacrimation, corneal opacity, corneal ulcers, pannus, hypopyon, and hyphema.

Lesions in salivary and lacrimal glands are an acute inflammatory process and necrosis of the ducts and acini. Lobules are widely separated by edema and an exudate composed of a varying mixture of neutrophils, lymphocytes, and histiocytes. The parenchyma may be difficult to recognize owing to the massive cellular infiltration and to degeneration and necrosis of the acinar epithelium. With repair, the epithelium of the ducts is converted into stratified epithelium that occludes some lumina. Squamous metaplasia subsides within about a month postinfection, and the cytoarchitecture is restored. Nasopharyngeal lesions include multifocal necrosis of respiratory epithelium with edema of the lamina propria. Nasal meatuses contain an exudate of necrotic cellular debris. Mild tracheitis with focal necrosis may be present.

ORBIT

Space-occupying lesions of the orbit result in deviation or protrusion of the eyeball **(exophthalmos).** Exophthalmos may be slight; if severe, there is prolapse of the globe. Causes of exophthalmos include retrobulbar abscess, salivary gland cysts, orbital parasites, sinus neoplasms, myositis, foreign bodies, and retrobulbar neoplasms such as lymphosarcoma. Retrobulbar abscess is a common entity in the dog, and affected dogs have fever, anorexia, and dysphagia as well as exophthalmos. The exophthalmos seen in cases of canine masticatory eosinophilic myositis is due to swelling of the temporal muscles, with an associated increase in pressure on the retrobulbar fat. Exophthalmos, if prolonged, can result in exposure keratitis and excessive drying of the cornea.

Orbital inflammation, called cellulitis, is acute and is characterized by congestion and edema but is not common in domestic animals. Orbital inflammation that extends either to or from inflammation of the eyelids and conjunctivae is usually bacterial in origin. Orbital cellulitis can be caused by parasites and fungi, penetrating foreign bodies, and spread of infection from paranasal sinuses, infected teeth, and suppurative or granulomatous panophthalmitis through the sclera. Most orbital inflammation is suppurative.

NEOPLASMS OF THE GLOBE AND OCULAR ADNEXA

Neoplasms of the Eyelids

Neoplasms of the eyelids are those that occur in the skin generally and arise from epithelial, mesenchymal, and melanogenic cells. Eyelid neoplasms are found in all domestic animals but are uncommon to rare in all but cattle and dogs. Sebaceous gland neoplasms (arising commonly from meibomian glands) are most numerous in dogs, and squamous cell carcinoma is most frequent in cattle. Melanogenic neoplasms and squamous cell papilloma also occur with a fairly high frequency in the eyelids of dogs.

Mesenchymal neoplasms of the eyelids may arise from a variety of cell types including fibroblasts, mast cells, histiocytes, and endothelial cells. None of the mesenchymal neoplasms are common in the eyelids.

Conjunctival and Corneal Neoplasms

Epithelial neoplasms of the conjunctiva and cornea include squamous cell papilloma and squamous cell carcinoma. Squamous cell papillomas occur at the limbus and on the caruncle and the lid margin of cattle, horses, and dogs; they are most frequent in cattle. These neoplasms occur as either soft or hard, pedunculated or sessile, gray-red or pigmented masses. Microscopically, the squamous papilloma of the conjunctiva resembles those found in the skin of the eyelid and is composed of fronds consisting of proliferated squamous prickle cells about a connective tissue core. The prickle cells may undergo keratinization. Squamous cell carcinomas of the conjunctiva have been described in most domestic animals but are uncommon in all except cattle and horses. In horses, the neoplasms involve the cornea and conjunctiva, with the primary sites being the medial and lateral limbi and membrana nictitans. The neoplasms vary in size and present as ulcerated pink to white, irregular masses. Histologic features are those of this neoplasm in other locations.

Bovine ocular squamous cell carcinoma

Neoplasms of the globe or circumocular structures have been described in several breeds of cattle, including beef types from several continents and countries. In North America, ocular squamous cell carcinoma is of economic importance only in the Hereford breed. The incidence in cattle is greatest in those geographic areas with longest hours of sunlight per year and ultraviolet radiation. The lesions have a marked predilection for the medial and lateral aspects of the globe, portions not generally covered by the eyelids. This indicates that exposure to sunlight is a factor in the development of the lesions.

Breed contribution to susceptibility is related to the degree of pigmentation of the bulbar conjunctiva. The genetic basis of susceptibility is an indirect one, depending on the degree of pigmentation. Lesions develop when pigment is lacking from some area of the corneoscleral junction, regardless of the pigment status of the lids and the surrounding area.

The incidence of benign and carcinomatous lesions is greatest on the eyeball and least frequent on the nictitating membrane. The corneoscleral junction is the most common site; about 75% are either at the limbus or on the cornea proper, and lesions tend to be located along the line of the palpebral fissure.

The lesions are plaque, squamous cell papilloma, early squamous cell carcinoma, and invasive squamous cell carcinoma. Plaque and squamous cell papilloma represent early stages. Most of the lesions are squamous cell carcinomas (Fig. 14-49).

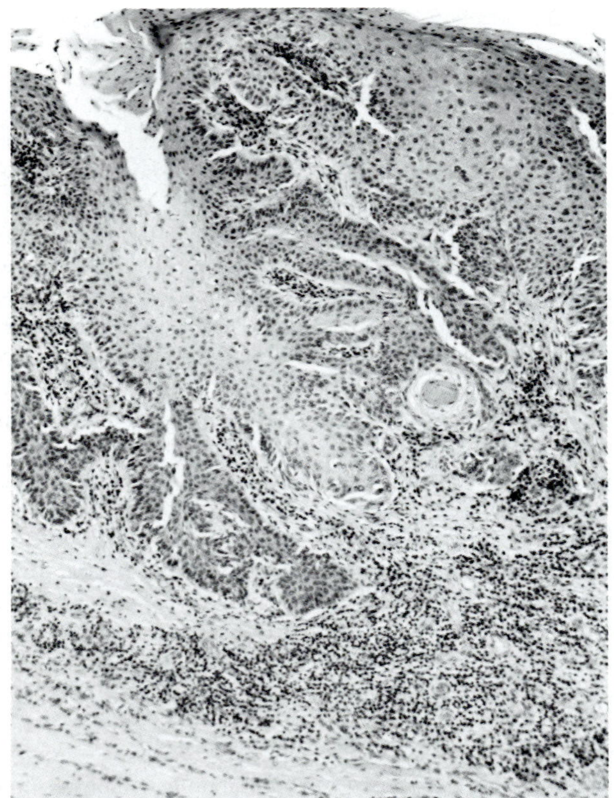

Fig. 14-49 Globe, cornea; bovine. Squamous cell carcinoma. Infiltrating cords of neoplastic squamous cells are accompanied by an inflammatory cell infiltrate in the corneal stroma. H & E stain; ×63.

Vascular lesions

Hemangiomatous lesions occur in the perilimbal conjunctiva in dogs, and most are located at the lateral limbus. Most lesions begin as small hemorrhages in foci of vascular ectasia with single or multiple, small, well-circumscribed, blood-filled spaces and are considered hematocysts. Larger lesions composed of variably sized, endothelial, blood-containing spaces are considered hemangiomas. The cells vary in size and shape, are occasionally multinucleated, and contain ovoid, vesicular nuclei with multiple nucleoli.

Angiokeratoma

These lesions are discrete superficial ectasias consisting of dilated and engorged small blood vessels with reactive hyperplasia of the overlying epithelium. These lesions have been described in the conjunctiva of the dog, appearing as a smooth red mass on the nictitating membrane and as a black mass of the bulbar conjunctiva. Microscopically, large vascular channels are covered by a hyperplastic epithelium.

Lacrimal Gland Neoplasms

Neoplasms of the lacrimal glands, including the gland of third eyelid of animals, are rare and are either adenomas or adenocarcinomas. Mixed neoplasms (epithelial and myoepithelial components) are extremely rare in animals. The adenoma and adenocarcinoma cause exophthalmos and deviation of the globe. The adenomas are composed of tubular profiles of closely packed cuboidal epithelium. The adenocarcinoma has features of histologic and cellular anaplasia (Fig. 14-50).

Harderian gland neoplasms

The harderian gland is present in most laboratory animals with a third eyelid (except the dog). The gland lies within the orbit, medial to the eyeball; and, in rats and

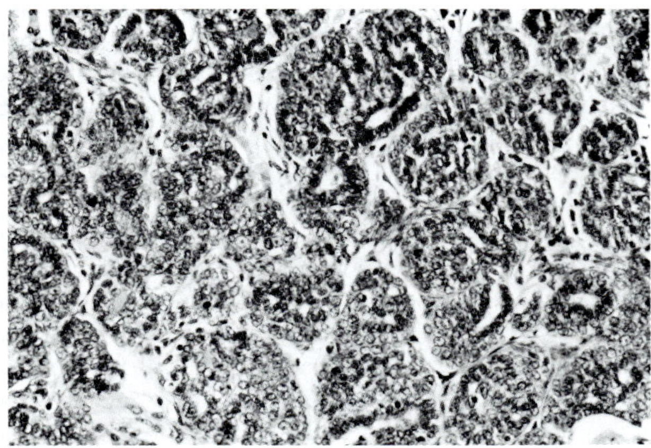

Fig. 14-50 Membrana nictitans, lacrimal gland; canine. Adenocarcinoma. Neoplastic epithelial cells from nests of closely packed cuboidal cells, forming tubular profiles. H & E stain; ×160.

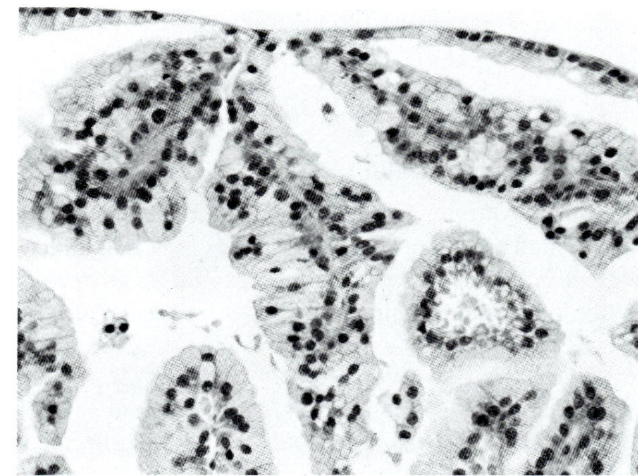

Fig. 14-51 Harderian gland; mouse. Adenoma. Trabeculae of adenoma are composed of large columnar cells with vacuolated cytoplasm and uniform basally located nuclei. H & E stain; ×250.

mice, it has a horseshoe shape and partially encircles the optic nerve. This tubuloalveolar gland, divided into lobes and lobules, has alveoli lined by columnar epithelial cells with round, pale-staining, basally located nuclei. Spontaneous neoplasms, usually adenomas, occur in mice and hamsters but are rare in rats. These neoplasms cause protrusion of the globe, are usually papillary, and may be cystic. The cells of the neoplasms resemble those of the normal gland and have foamy cytoplasm and basally located nuclei (Fig. 14-51). These neoplasms are readily produced by certain chemical carcinogens in mice and rats.

Neuroectodermal Neoplasms

The neuroepithelial intraocular neoplasms are classified morphologically into adenoma and adenocarcinoma if they arise from mature neuroepithelium and into retinoblastoma, medulloepithelioma, and teratoid medulloepithelioma if they arise from the primitive medullary epithelium. Primary pigmented neoplasms have been reported in most animal species. Retinoblastoma is an extremely rare neoplasm in domestic and laboratory animals.

Medulloepithelioma and teratoid medulloepithelioma

The medulloepithelioma contains poorly differentiated neural tissue that may resemble embryonic retina. It is composed of single and multilayer columnar epithelium that forms festoons and lines glandlike structures, cysts, and tubes. Some areas resemble retinoblastoma, with areas of necrosis and the presence of ill-defined rosettes (Fig. 14-52). In teratoid medulloepithelioma, areas of neuroglia and foci of cartilage occur, as well as ganglion cells, striated muscle, and tissue resembling neurophil. The teratoid medulloepithelioma imitates and probably arises from either the embryonic neuroepithelium of the optic cup during organogenesis or from rests of such tissue during neonatal life.

Adenoma and adenocarcinoma

Adenoma and adenocarcinoma of the iridociliary epithelium are uncommon in animals. Most cases have been observed in the dog and cat. Clinical signs are extremely variable, depending on location, size, and duration. Scleral injection, interstitial keratitis, iris bombé, hyphema, retinal detachment, corneal edema, and glaucoma are described in cases of ocular neoplasia.

Grossly, the mass may be solid, be white or pink, and occupy variable amounts of the intraocular space. Small neoplasms of the uvea displace the lens, and large ones fill much of the intraocular space. Variable amounts of blood and protein coagulum are present in the ocular chambers. Displacement of the iris anteriorly can result in peripheral anterior synechia. Severe involvement of the anterior uvea can result in hypotony and a phthisical globe.

Microscopically, the neoplasms are composed of cuboidal to columnar cells with round to ovoid vesicular nuclei and moderate amounts of cytoplasm arranged in papillary, tubular, glandular, and rosette-like formations (Fig. 14-53). Cells about the lumina of tubular formations and pseudorosettes may have fine processes that extend to a thin membrane or to a blood vessel. Mitotic figures may be either numerous or rare. In some areas, cells in palisade formation are lined up along thin stromal trabeculae in single parallel rows forming closed acinar units. In other areas, the rows of cells are separated by groups of tubular and pseudorosette structures. Adenocarcinoma has features of cellular and histologic anaplasia (Fig. 14-54). Metastasis of adenocarcinoma arising from iridociliary epithelium is rare, but the neoplasm may penetrate the globe and invade the orbit.

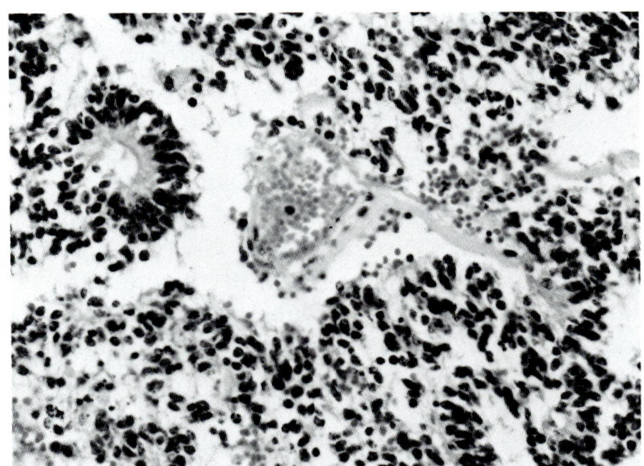

Fig. 14-52 Globe, anterior uvea; canine. Medulloepithelioma. Neoplasm composed of bands of undifferentiated epithelial cells with some ill-defined rosettes. H & E stain; ×250.

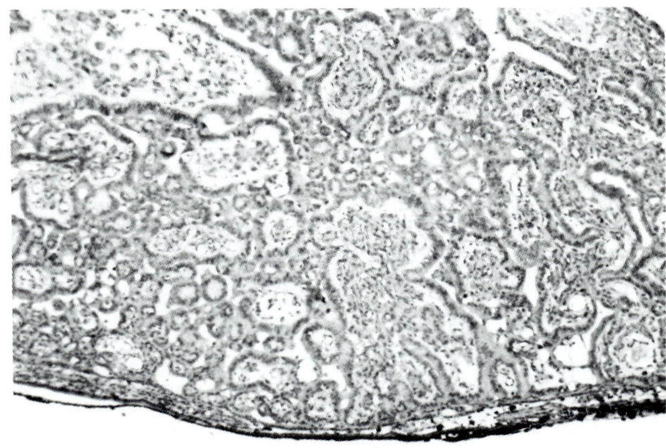

Fig. 14-53 Globe, anterior uvea; canine. Adenoma. Neoplasm composed of glandular and papillary formations of closely packed cuboidal epithelium. H & E stain; ×63.

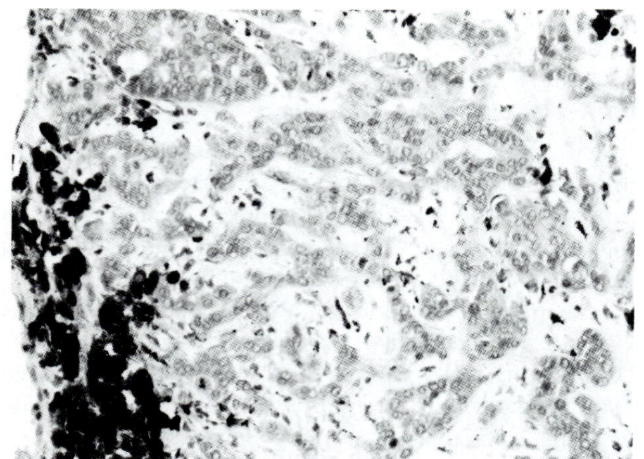

Fig. 14-54 Globe, anterior uvea; canine. Adenocarcinoma. Neoplasm composed of interconnecting trabeculae and variably sized nests. H & E stain; ×160.

Mesenchymal Neoplasms of Globe

Primary mesenchymal neoplasms of the globe are extremely rare, and few cases have been reported. These include cases of hemangioma, leiomyoma, leiomyosarcoma, and chondrosarcoma.

Feline trauma-associated sarcomas

Sarcomas, spindle cell and osteosarcoma, have been observed in the globes of cats years after trauma to the globe. The affected globes may be normal, bulging, or phthisical and firm and irregular in shape. Microscopically, the sarcomas extensively involve the globe, line the inner aspect, and extend into the optic nerve. The most extensive area of involvement is the choroid, with infiltration of the retina and stroma of the ciliary body. The neoplasms are composed of anaplastic spindle cells (Fig. 14-55) with deposits of osteoid. The osteoid is surrounded by well-differentiated cells and is considered metaplastic.

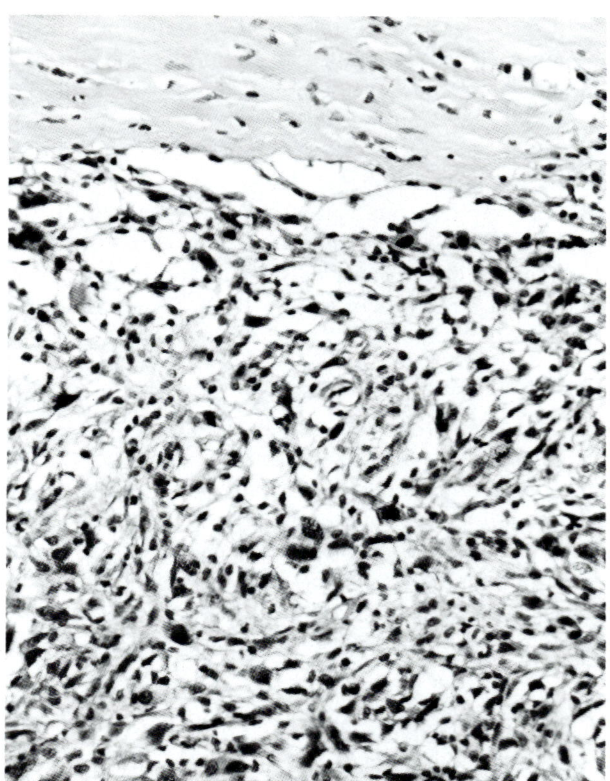

Fig. 14-55 Globe, anterior uvea; feline. Trauma-associated sarcoma. Neoplasm is composed of anaplastic, mesenchymal, spindle-shaped cells that filled the anterior chamber and invaded the cornea. H & E stain; ×160.

Melanogenic Neoplasms

Melanogenic neoplasms (both benign and malignant forms) involving the conjunctiva and skin of the eyelids are frequent only in the dog. In the eyelids, the neoplasms are frequently dome-shaped or sessile enlargements that may be either amelanotic or dark brown to black. Microscopically, sheets, bundles, and nests of spindle and/or epithelioid cells may contain abundant or scant melanin pigment. Melanophages occur in varying numbers in most melanomas. These cells are larger than the neoplastic cells and contain coarser melanin granules. Melanomas may be mainly cellular or mainly fibrous. In the fibrous type, melanocytes are grouped in irregular bundles and mixed with fibroblasts. Amelanotic fibrous melanomas resemble fibrosarcoma, and the amelanotic cellular type can be confused with undifferentiated carcinoma.

Epibulbar (limbal) melanomas

These neoplasms arise in the sclera and subconjunctival tissue at the limbus and appear as raised, firm, outward bulging, pigmented masses at the corneal-scleral junction. The broad-based masses are firmly attached to the sclera and may invade the cornea. Microscopically, the neoplasms have two cell types in varying proportions. One cell type is a small, lightly pigmented spindle cell, and the second cell type is a large, round, pigment-laden cell (Fig. 14-56). The spindle cells are of A type, with plump, oval nuclei with moderate amounts of heterochromatin. The pigment-laden cells are filled with dispersed, mature melanin granules and have round to oval vesicular nuclei and prominent nucleoli. These large cells differ from the epithelioid cells of ocular neoplasms in that they lack the features of nuclear and cytoplasmic anaplasia. Multinucleate cells are common. The epibulbar melanomas are considered benign; they grow slowly and appear not to metastasize.

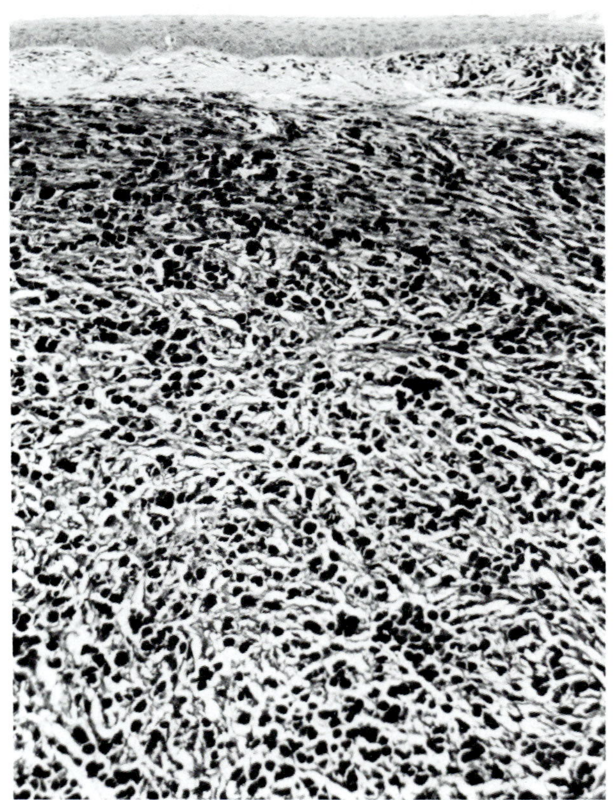

Fig. 14-56 Globe, bulbar conjunctiva; canine. Epibulbar melanoma. Neoplasm composed of pigment-filled spindle and round cells. H & E stain; ×63.

Uveal melanomas

These are the most common primary intraocular neoplasms in domestic animals, but few cases of intraocular melanoma have been recorded in animals except for the dog and cat. Nearly all the animal cases have involved the anterior uvea, but a few **choroidal melanomas** have been recorded in the dog. The usual clinical sign is the presence of a pigmented mass in the anterior uvea that is observable in the iris. Secondary glaucoma resulting from obstruction of the filtration angle often follows the initial observation of the neoplasm. Other signs produced by intraocular melanomas include an irregular pupil loss of pupillary space, filling of the anterior chamber and drainage angle, increased iridial pigmentation, and thickening and/or folding of the iris. Gross features may vary widely, depending on the origin of the neoplasm, its malignancy, the extent of invasion of adjacent structures, and the pigment content of the neoplasm.

Intraocular melanomas in the dog include anterior uveal melanomas and choroidal melanomas. Choroidal melanomas are raised, darkly pigmented masses of the choroid with irregular margins arising usually adjacent to the optic nerve. The neoplasms are composed of large polygonal cells with abundant melanin pigment. These neoplasms do not metastasize but may infiltrate along the optic meninges.

Anterior uveal melanomas are composed of epithelioid to spindle-shaped cells. The benign melanomas are composed predominantly of large round cells with abundant melanin pigment. Neoplasms considered malignant are less numerous than benign ones and have pleomorphic cells and mitotic figures; metastasis occurs but is infrequent.

Uveal melanomas in cats are present in the anterior uvea, beginning along the anterior margin of the iris; with progression, the neoplasm involves much of the iris leaf and spreads to the ciliary body, filtration meshwork, and adjacent sclera. Uveal melanomas are malignant much more commonly in the cat than in the dog, regardless of cell type, which may be epithelioid, spindle-shaped, or mixed type.

Orbital Neoplasms

Oribital and retrobulbar neoplasms arise from mesenchymal and epithelial tissues of the globe and orbit and by direct extension from adjacent tissues and from the nasal cavity and sinuses. Hematogenous spread of neoplasms to the orbit may occur, but the hematogenous route to the orbit appears to be rare except for lymphosarcoma.

Orbital neoplasms produce similar clinical signs, regardless of neoplasm type. The clinical sign most indicative of an orbital neoplasm is unilateral exophthalmos, but other signs associated with orbital neoplasms include swelling around the globe, prominent and/or hypertrophied third eyelid, exposure keratitis, deviation of the globe, dilated or eccentric pupil, and elevation of the retina from its medial attachment.

Metastatic Intraocular Neoplasms

Secondary intraocular neoplasms may arrive at the interior of the globe by extension of an orbital or adnexal neoplasm or hematogenously in cases of disseminated neoplasia. The hematogenous route accounts for most of the reported cases. Secondary intraocular neoplasms may be of epithelial, mesenchymal, or melanogenic origin, and secondary mesenchymal neoplasms are the most common. None of the metastatic intraocular neoplasms are at all common; most can be considered rare, but, of those, lymphosarcoma, especially in the dog, has been reported most often.

Except for neoplasms of the mammary gland, only a few case reports of epithelial neoplasms metastatic to the globe have been reported, and most of these have been in the dog. Epithelial neoplasms metastatic (or extending) to the globe have included those arising in the nasal epithelium, epidermis, sweat gland, conjunctiva, thyroid gland, testes, pancreas, kidneys, urinary bladder, uterus, and mammary glands.

Neoplasms arising from mesenchymal tissues represent

the majority of metastatic intraocular neoplasms in the dog and cat due to the prevalence of intraocular metastasis of lymphosarcoma.

Lymphosarcoma

Most cases of ocular lymphosarcoma are bilateral. Clinical signs include a variety of changes in the conjunctiva and cornea as well as iritis, leukemic retinopathy, intraocular hemorrhage, glaucoma, and hydrophthalmus. An intraocular neoplasm should be suspected in cases of unilateral glaucoma. Although all segments of the globe can be invaded by neoplastic lymphoid cells, the anterior uvea is the primary site of metastasis. If only a few cells are present in the globe, they are generally found in the anterior ciliary body and root of the iris. When ocular infiltration is extensive, the anterior uvea is most severely involved and the choroid less so.

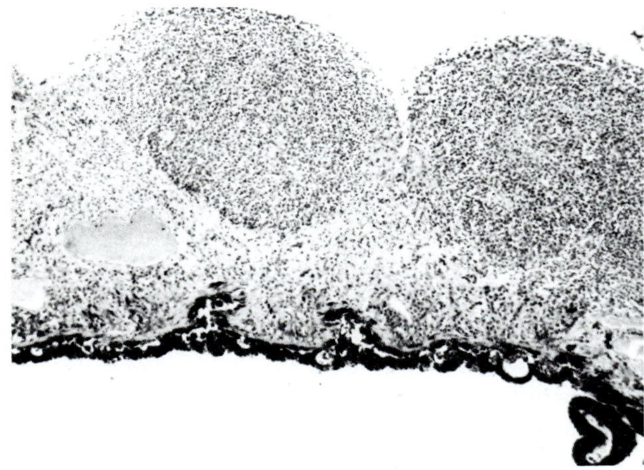

Fig. 14-57 Globe, iris; canine. Lymphosarcoma. Iris has multiple nodules and diffuse infiltrate of neoplastic lymphoid cells. H & E stain; ×63.

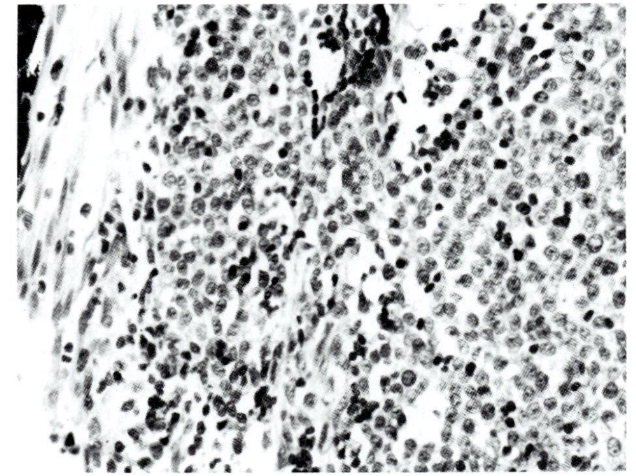

Fig. 14-58 Globe, iris; canine. Lymphosarcoma. Nodule composed of sheets of lymphoid cells. H & E stain; ×250.

In the anterior uvea, the neoplastic cells are present in the interstitial tissue and appear fairly evenly distributed when the infiltration is extensive. In less extensive infiltration, the neoplastic lymphoid cells are often perivascular, occurring as collars or clumps of cells around smaller vessels. Neoplastic cells often form a thin layer on the anterior surface of the iris and are often free in the filtration angle and meshwork. Neoplastic cells often form large nodular masses that either distort or replace the anterior uvea (Figs. 14-57 and 14-58).

COLLECTION AND PREPARATION OF OCULAR TISSUES

The structures of the eyeball, especially the retina, undergo autolysis rapidly after death or removal from an animal. Thus, the globe must be removed quickly and gently and placed in fixative. Because the most commonly used fixative, 10% neutral buffered formalin (NBF), does not penetrate rapidly, fixation time can be reduced and fixation enhanced by the injection of a small amount of 10% NBF into the vitreal cavity (0.3 to 0.5 ml for a canine globe) using a 25- to 27-guage needle. Injection of the solution is done slowly and continued until the globe is firm. The globe, cleaned of all tissues, is then submerged in fixative with 10:1 to 20:1 fixative/globe ratio. Eviserated globes should be examined microscopically to exclude presence of an intraocular neoplasm.

EAR

The ear is a sensory organ composed anatomically of the external ear, middle ear, and the inner ear (labyrinth). The labyrinth is divided into two anatomic and functional divisions: the cochlea for hearing and the vestibular system for equilibrium. Sensory information from these two structures is transmitted to the brain via the eighth cranial nerve and then through the central auditory pathway. Any portion of the ear may be involved in disease. To identify and describe lesions, one must have an appreciation of otic embryology, normal macroscopic and microscopic anatomy, and terminology.

External Ear

The external ear is composed of the auricle (pinna) and the external auditory meatus, which ends medially at the tympanic membrane. All these structures may be easily examined grossly. The pinna is composed of a flat sheet of cartilage covered by skin. The external auditory meatus is supported laterally by cartilage and medially by bone and is lined by epidermis containing sebaceous glands, as well as sudoriferous and modified sweat glands (ceruminous glands). Rodents do not have ceruminous glands, but rats have lobulated sebaceous glands (Zymbal's glands) ventral to the base of the external ear. The tympanic membrane is formed by epithelium of the external auditory meatus, connective tissue, and mucosa of the tympanic membrane.

Alterations of the external ear include congenital anomalies, necrosis, and lesions due to trauma, generalized or regional dermatologic diseases, infections, and neoplasia.

Congenital anomalies

At birth, the pinna may be normal or abnormally large (macrotia) or abnormally small (microtia). An absence of the pinna (anotia) is an inherited defect in sheep and may occur with other deformities in the dog. Extra pinnae (polyotia) may be the result of a recessive mutation in the cat. Deafness may result from an absence of the external auditory meatus (atresia) or failure of the meatal plug to be shed (persistent meatal plug), which occurs in the dog between 14 to 17 days after birth. Nubian goats affected with β-mannosidosis are born with abnormally shaped pinnae.

Ear-tip necrosis and fissures

Necrosis of the tip of the pinna may be due to frostbite (pigs, calves), ergot poisoning (cattle), septicemia (pigs), and trauma. Trauma may result from scratching, rubbing, or head-shaking; these are clinical signs associated with inflammation of the external ear (otitis externa). Fissures may develop on the distal edge of canine pinnae as the result of trauma.

Auricular hematoma

Auricular hematomas may result from an intrachondral fracture of the pinnal cartilage. They present as fluctuant, blood-filled swellings on the concave surface of the canine pinna near the apex and, with maturation, are replaced by granulation tissue. Contraction of granulation tissue can result in distortion of the pinna. Auricular hematomas are the result of violent head-shaking and scratching; an immune-mediated reaction has been suggested as a possible contributing factor.

Dermatologic diseases

The external ear may be involved in either generalized or regional dermatologic diseases. Regional diseases include idiopathic pinnal alopecia in Siamese cats, feline solar dermatitis, marginal seborrhea, and equine aural plaques. **Feline solar dermatitis** is a chronic actinic disorder of the margin of the pinna characterized by erythema, acanthosis, scaling, epithelial necrosis, ulceration, and superficial perivascular dermatitis with basophilic degeneration of superficial dermal collagen. The disease may progress through epithelial hyperplasia, dysplasia, and carcinoma in situ to invasive squamous cell carcinoma. **Marginal seborrhea** is characterized by numerous, small, greasy nodules of orthokeratotic and/or parakeratotic hyperkeratosis of the pinnae of dogs. In severe cases, the lesions include inflammation, necrosis, ulceration, and pinnal deformity. **Equine aural plaques** are solitary or multiple, raised, flat-surfaced, nonpigmented, scaly to crusty lesions of the inner aspects of the pinnae caused by infection with a papilloma virus. The lesions consist of epithelial hyperplasia and hypertrophy. The enlarged cells have clear cytoplasm and keratohyaline-like granules in the stratum spinosum and granulosum.

Table 14-1. Mites and ticks affecting the external ears of animals

Name	Type	Host
Amblyomma spp.	s, t	Dog, horse, ruminants
Boophilus spp.	s, t	Cattle, other ruminants, horse
Demodex canis	s, m	Dog
Dermacentor nitens	s, t	Horse, ruminants
Haemaphysalis leporis-palustris	s, t	Rabbit
Ixodes cati	s, m	Cat
Otobius megnini	e, t	Dog, cat, horse, ruminants, swine, others
Otodectes cynotis	e, m	Cat, dog
Psoroptes cuniculi	e, m	Rabbit, sheep, goat, white-tailed deer, horse
Rallietia auris	e, m	Cattle
Rhipicephalus spp.	s, t	Dog, horse, ruminants, others
Sarcoptes scabiei	s, m	Dog, pig

s, skin; e, ear; m, mite; t, tick.

Parasitic otitis externa

A variety of parasites can infest the external ear (Table 14-1). Otoacariasis is a common problem and may be due to either ear or skin mites. Transmission of mites among animals readily occurs. The otitis externa resulting from parasitic infestations may have an allergic basis. A parasitic otitis externa in the dog may be due to the spinose ear tick, *Otobius megnini,* but many genera of ticks have a predilection for the external ear (Table 14-1). Since pinnae have less pelage, they are sites of sandfly bites that may result in auricular nodules due to *Leishmania* infections.

Mycotic otitis externa

Dermatomycosis of the external ear (otomycosis) is caused by fungi of the genera *Microsporum, Candida, Trichophyton, Aspergillus,* and *Peyronellaea. Malassezia pachydermatis (Pityrosporum canis)* is frequently cultured from ears of dogs and cats with (Fig. 14-59) and without externa media, so the importance of its role as a pathogen is uncertain.

Bacterial otitis externa

Bacterial otitis externa has been frequently reported in dogs, cats, and pigs, and mycoplasmas have been isolated from the external ears of goats. In the dog and cat, *Staphylococcus intermedius, S. aureus,* β-hemolytic *Streptococcus* species, *Proteus* species, *Pseudomonas* species, and *E. coli* may colonize and infect the external ear. *Actinomyces*

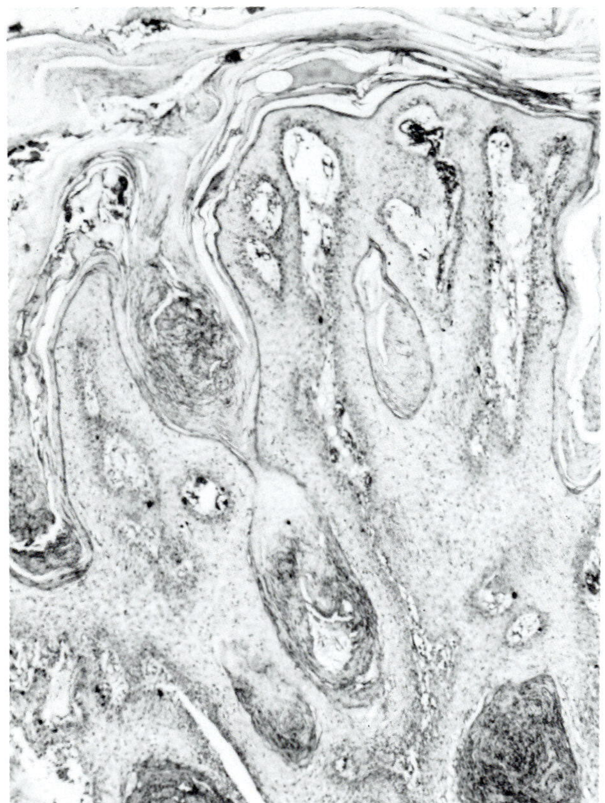

Fig. 14-59 Ear, pinna; canine. Otitis externa. Epidermal hyperplasia and hyperkeratosis due to infection with *Malassezia pachydermatitis.* H & E stain; ×40.

bovis produces granulomatous inflammation in the perichondral subcutis of the external ears of swine, resulting in a thick and indurated auricle.

Noninfectious otitis externa

Noninfectious causes of otitis externa include foreign bodies and hormonal imbalances. The awns of certain grasses, especially foxtail grass in the western United States, may become embedded foreign bodies in the tissue of the external ear. Hypothyroidism, ovarian imbalances, and Sertoli cell tumors have been associated with ceruminous otitis externa.

Lesions of otitis externa

The gross and light microscopic lesions of otitis externa are similar to those of skin diseases but generally nonspecific. The external auditory meatus may contain tenacious, dry, brown cerumen that microscopically may contain serum, leukocytes, and epithelial debris. If the cause is parasitic, ova and parasites at various life stages may be present within the exudate and/or within the epidermis. Chronic lesions may include epidermal hyperplasia with acanthosis, parakeratosis, perifolliculitis, folliculitis, and either glandular atrophy or ectasia. Scabs often occur from epidermal burrowing of mites, and ulceration is associated with infection by *Pseudomonas* species. The meatus may become narrowed due to the inflammatory changes, and the inflammation may spread through the tympanic membrane to the middle ear.

Neoplasms of the external ear

Neoplasms of the external ear originate from the auricular skin, auricular cartilage, and the ceruminous glands. Squamous cell carcinoma occurs in the pinnae of white cats exposed to sunlight for prolonged periods. Other reported neoplasms of the external ear include canine histocytoma, basal cell epithelioma, plasmacytoma, equine sarcoid, chondroma, and chondrosarcoma. Adenomas and adenocarcinomas of ceruminous glands occur in old cats and dogs as nodular and pedunculated masses, usually less than 2 cm in diameter, that protrude into the external auditory meatus. The majority of the neoplasms in dogs are benign, whereas many ceruminous gland neoplasms in cats are malignant. Adenomas are composed of cuboidal epithelium arranged in well-differentiated tubules and acini containing eosinophilic to golden-brown pigment. Malignancy is based on anaplasia and invasiveness (Fig. 14-60). Metastasis to regional lymph nodes occurs occasionally.

Middle Ear

The middle ear develops from a lateral extension of the first pharyngeal pouch, which connects with the first pharyngeal cleft to form the tubotympanic recess. This widens to become a cavity within the temporal bone and communicates with the nasopharynx via the eustachian (auditory) tube. In the horse, a portion of the auditory tube develops into a diverticulum, the guttural pouch. The middle ear is lined, usually by a two-layered, ciliated or nonciliated, secretory or nonsecretory mucosa containing goblet cells, a mucosa that resembles modified respiratory mu-

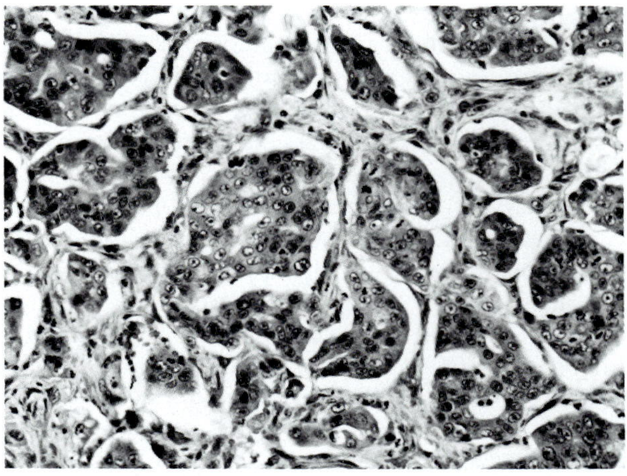

Fig. 14-60 Ear, pinna; feline. Ceruminous gland adenocarcinoma. Neoplasm is composed of pleomorphic epithelial cells arranged in clusters of tubuloacini. H & E stain; ×250.

cosa. This mucosa also forms the inner layer of the tympanic membrane, a structure that is in contact with the manubrium of the malleus, one of the three tympanic ossicles. The malleus articulates with the incus that articulates with the stapes. The footplate of the stapes articulates with the membrane of the vestibular (oval) window of the cochlea. Collectively, the middle ear, through the ossicles, communicates sound-induced vibrations of the tympanic membrane to the inner ear.

Gross examination of the middle ear

Gross examination of the middle ear includes examination of the tympanic bullae and the guttural pouches in the horse. The external wall of the bullae should be thin and smooth; irregular and thickened bullae occur with chronic bacterial infections of the middle ear, especially in cattle. Structures within the bullae include the tympanic septum in cats; bony septa and air spaces in pigs and cattle; the cochlear promontary, ossicles, and the tympanic membrane in all domestic and laboratory animals. The guttural pouch may be examined by viewing the caudal aspect of the head after it has been removed at necropsy.

Otitis media

The principal alteration involving the middle ear is inflammation (otitis media), although the middle ear may be the site of metastatic and primary neoplasms. Otitis media is usually due to bacterial infection (Table 14-2). In dogs, infections are due to *Candida* species, *Aspergillus* species, and *Malassezia pachydermatis.* Routes of infection may occur via the auditory tube, especially in pigs and cattle, and from an otitis externa with inflammation of the tympanic membrane (myringitis), especially in dogs and cats. Otitis media has been associated with eustachitis in pigs. Otitis media due to *Pasteurella* species has been associated with pneumonia in lambs and cattle. A possible sequela to otitis media is an otitis interna that may lead to meningoencephalitis; a pharyngitis could follow otitis media and develop into pneumonia. Cholesteatomas may form in rabbits and guinea pigs.

Table 14-2. Bacteria causing otitis media in animals

Name	Host
Actinomyces pyogenes	Pig, calf, sheep
Corynebacterium pseudotuberculosis	Cattle
Coryneform group E	Swine
Escherichia coli	Dog
Mycoplasma pulmonis	Rat, mouse
Pasteurella haemolytica	Lamb, cattle
Pasteurella multocida	Rabbit, cat, cattle, swine
Proteus mirabilis	Dog, gorilla
Pseudomonas aeruginosa	Pig, mouse
Staphylococcus spp.	Dog
Streptococcus spp.	Pig, dog

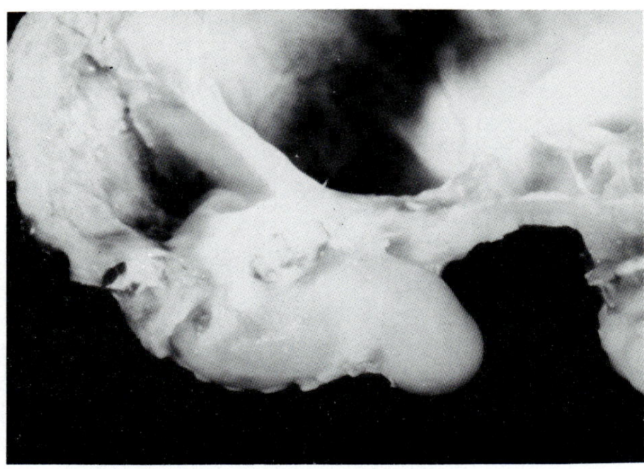

Fig. 14-61 Ear, middle ear; feline. Nasopharyngeal polyp. The polyp is located within the opened tympanic bulla, auditory tube, and nasopharynx.

Nasopharyngeal polyps

In cats, a response to inflammation is the formation of nasopharyngeal polyps from the mucosa of the tympanic cavity (Fig. 14-61), middle ear, and auditory tube. The polypoid masses may fill the tympanic cavity, extend through the auditory tube into the nasopharynx, and recur after excision. The masses are composed of well-vascularized, fibrous to myxomatous connective tissue diffusely infiltrated by lymphocytes and covered by nonciliated or ciliated columnar or squamous epithelium. The masses may contain mucous glands and lymphoid nodules. Polyps present in the nasopharynx may be ulcerated and superficially infiltrated by neutrophils.

β-mannosidosis

This storage disease has been observed in Nubian goat kids and Salers calves, and deafness was reported in affected goats. The cavity of the middle ear is narrowed in Nubian goats affected with β-mannosidosis, and numerous coalescing mucosal folds are present. Epithelial and connective tissue cells of the middle and inner ear contain intractyoplasmic vacuoles. The cells include hair cells, other cells of the organ of Corti, and histiocytes. Salers calves had a similar distribution of cellular vacuolation.

Eustachitis

Eustachitis, inflammation of the auditory tube, is common, can occur in association with otitis media in swine, and usually involves the guttural pouches of horses. Alterations of the auditory tube include empyema, tympany in young horses, foreign bodies, abscesses, and, rarely, neoplasms. In mycotic eustachitis of the guttural pouches, a fibronecrotic inflammation can extend to and cause rupture of the adjacent internal carotid artery. Empyema is the accumulation of a suppurative exudate occurring as a sequela to an upper respiratory infection. The causative agent is usually *Streptococcus* species in horses, although *Pasteurella multocida* and *Actinomyces pyogenes* can be causes in swine. Alterations present in chronic eustachitis include mucosal swelling and formation of granulation tissue.

Inner Ear

The inner ear (labyrinth) consists of membranous channels (membranous labyrinth) lining cavities within the petrous temporal bone (bony labyrinth). Portions of the membranous labyrinth are separated from the bony labyrinth by a fluid (perilymph). The body labyrinth is divided into three parts: the cochlea, semicircular canals, and the vestibule. The cochlea and semicircular canals each contain a portion of the membranous labyrinth of similar shape, with the cochlea containing the cochlear duct. The vestibule contains the endolymphatic duct, the utricle, and the saccule of the membranous labyrinth.

The sensory organ of hearing is the organ of Corti, a portion of the cochlear duct. It is supported by the basilar membrane and consists of external hair cells, internal hair cells, and supportive cells. The hair cells are stimulated by movement of the stereocilia, which extend into the overlying gelatinous tectorial membrane. Hair cells then stimulate the nerve endings of bipolar neurons that have their cell bodies in the ganglion (cochlear or spiral) in the central bony core of the cochlea (modiolus). Axons of these neurons constitute the auditory portion of the eighth cranial nerve.

The sensory end-organs of the vestibular system include the maculae within the utricle and saccule and the cristae ampullares within the ampullae of the semicircular canals. The maculae contain a gelatinous mass with calcareous bodies (otoliths or otoconia) that are affected by gravity during accelerated motion. The cristae ampullares contain a gelatinous mass (cupula) that moves during shifts in the position of the head. On stimulation, impulses are transmitted through the bipolar neurons with cell bodies located in the vestibular (Scarpa's) ganglion of the vestibular nerve.

Dysplasia and degeneration of the cochlear duct

Dysplasia and degeneration of the cochlear duct result in deafness that may be detected by examination of auditory brain stem–evoked potentials. The causes of deafness include hereditary, toxic, acoustic, senile, inflammatory, and neoplastic lesions. Hereditary deafness due to dysplasia of the cochlear duct has been reported in a variety of animals, including white cats, white (Hedlund) mink, Dalmatians and other breeds of dog (Fig. 14-62), Japanese dancing (shaker) mice, waltzing guinea pigs, and others. Ototoxic compounds causing degeneration of the cochlear duct include aminoglycoside antibiotics, loop diuretics, salicylates and other analgesics, and several other compounds. Regardless of the cause, the lesions of the cochlear duct may include loss of inner and/or outer hair cells, loss of supporting cells, vacuolation of hair cells, collapse of Reissner's membrane, distortion of the tectorial membrane, and general atrophy of the organ of Corti. Inflammation of the inner ear (otitis interna, labyrinthitis) and metastatic neoplasia, such as lymphosarcoma, result in destruction and loss of the cochlear duct, along with destruction of the structures of the vestibular labyrinth. The inflammation may be severe and extensive and may cause an osteomyelitis and a vestibulocochlear neuritis. Infections may be due to viral, bacterial, fungal, or algal agents.

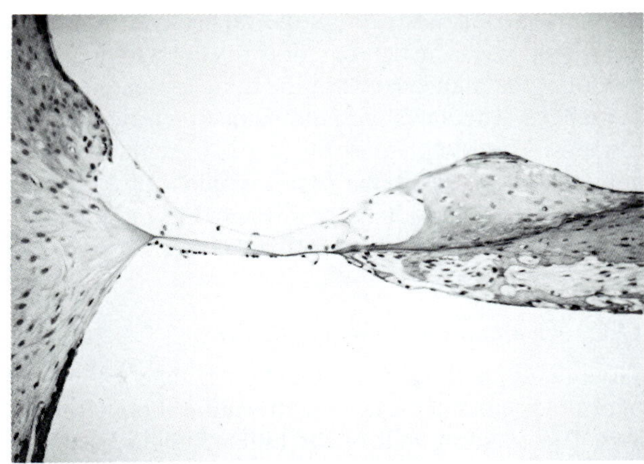

Fig. 14-62 Ear, inner ear, cochlear duct; canine. Dysplasia of organ of Corti. Organ of Corti and tectorial membrane are underdeveloped with collapse of Reissner's membrane. H & E stain; ×400. *Courtesy Dr. D.J. Zappia.*

Vestibular disorders

Congenital vestibular disorders have been reported in dogs and cats and have been associated with a "screw-neck syndrome" in pastel mink. This syndrome, due to a reduction in the number of or to the absence of otoliths, can be prevented by a dietary supplement of manganese. Vitamin A deficiency in guinea pigs may result in progressive metaplastic changes of the macular epithelium and loss of hair cells. Vestibular dysfunction in the cat has been caused by infiltrative squamous cell carcinoma extending to the inner ear from a primary location in the middle ear.

Neoplasms of the middle and inner ears

Neoplasms are rarely found in the tissues of the middle and inner ears of domestic animals. The described cases have been principally in older animals and have included squamous cell carcinoma in the middle and inner ears of domestic cats and adenoma of the respiratory epithelium of the middle ear of dogs. The adenomas fill the tympanic cavity and are solid or papillary and are composed of small tubular formations of cuboidal to columnar ciliated epithelial cells.

Suggested Readings

Adcock JL, Hibter CP. Vascular and neuro-ophthalmic pathlogy of elaeophorosis in elk. Pathol Vet 1969; 6:185-213.

Aguirre G. Hereditary retinal diseases in small animals. Vet Clin North Am 1973; 3:515-528.

Aguirre G, Carmichael L, Bistner S. Corneal endothelium in viral induced anterior uveitis. Ultrastructural changes following canine adenovirus type-1 infection. Arch Ophthalmol 1975; 93:219-224.

Aguirre GD, Laties A. Pigment epithelial dystrophy in the dog. Exp Eye Res 1976; 23:247-256.

Binns W, Shupe JL, Keeler RF, James LF. Chronologic evaluation of teratogenicity in sheep fed *Veratrum californicum.* J Am Vet Med Assoc 1965; 147:839-842.

Branis M, Burda H. Inner ear structures in the deaf and normally hearing Dalmatian dog. J Comp Pathol 1985; 95:295-299.

Brightman, II AH. Keratoconjunctivitis sicca. J Am Vet Med Assoc 1980; 176:710-711.

Brown TT, Bistner SI, DeLahunta A, Scott FW, McEntee K. Pathogenetic studies of infection of the bovine fetus with bovine viral diarrhea virus. II. Ocular lesions. Vet Pathol 1975; 12:394-404.

Bussanich MN, Rootman J, Dolman CL. Granulomatous panuveitis and dermal depigmentation in dogs. J Am Anim Hosp Assoc 1982; 18:131-138.

Carlton WW. A case of blastomycosis in a dog with pulmonary, cutaneous and ocular lesions. J Am Anim Hosp Assoc 1974; 10:586-590.

Carlton WW, Austin L. Ocular protothecosis in a dog. Pathol Vet 1973; 10:274-280.

Carlton WW, Feeney DA, Zimmermann JL. Disseminated cryptococcosis with ocular involvement in a dog. J Am Anim Hosp Assoc 1976; 12:53-59.

Delack JB. Hereditary deafness in the white cat. Compend Cont Educ Pract Vet 1984; 6:609-619.

Dubielzig RR. Ocular sarcoma following trauma in three cats. J Am Vet Med Assoc 1984; 184:578-581.

Gelatt KN, Das ND. Animal models for inherited cataracts: A review. Curr Eye Res 1984; 3:765-778.

Gelatt KN, Peiffer RL, Stevens J. Chronic ulcerative keratitis and sequestrum in the domestic cat. J Am Anim Hosp Assoc 1973; 9:204-213.

Halliwell RE, Brim TA, Hines MJ, Wolf D, White FH. Studies on equine recurrent uveitis. II: The role of infection with *Leptospira interrogans* serovar *pomona.* Curr Eye Res 1985; 4:1033-1040.

Hayes KC, Nielsen SW, Eaton HD. Pathogenesis of the optic nerve lesion in vitamin A–deficient calves. Arch Ophthalmol 1968; 80:777-781.

Jubb KV, Saunders LZ, Coates HV. The intraocular lesions of canine distemper. J Comp Pathol 1957; 61:21-29.

Lanum J. The damaging effects of light on the retina. Empirical findings, theoretical and practical implications (Review). Survey Ophthalmol 1978; 22:221-249.

Leipold HW, Huston K. Congenital syndrome of anophthalmia-microphthalmia with associated defects in cattle. Pathol Vet 1968; 5:407-418.

Martin CL. Conjunctivitis: Differential diagnosis and treatment. Vet Clin North Am 1973; 3:367-383.

Martin CL, Dice PF. Corneal endothelial dystrophy in the dog. J Am Anim Hosp Assoc 1982; 18:327-336.

Martin CL, Wyman M. Primary glaucoma in the dog. Vet Clin North Am 1978; 8:257-286.

Monlux AW, Anderson WA, Davis CL. The diagnosis of squamous cell carcinoma of the eye (cancer eye) in cattle. Am J Vet Res 1957; 18:5-33.

Murray JA, Blakemore WF, Barnett KC. Ocular lesions in cats with GMI gangliosidosis with visceral involvement. J Small Anim Pract 1977; 18:1-10.

Patz A, Maumenee AE. Studies on diabetic retinopathy. I. Retinopathy in a dog with spontaneous diabetes mellitus. Am J Ophthalmol 1962; 54:532-541.

Percy DH. Feline histoplasmosis with ocular involvement. Vet Pathol 1981; 18:163-169.

Prince JH, Diesem CD, Eglitis I, Ruskell GL. Anatomy and Histology of the Eye and Orbit in Domestic Animals, Springfield, Ill.: Charles C Thomas, 1960:13.

Roberts SR. Color dilution and hereditary defects in collie dogs. Am J Ophthalmol 1967; 63:1762-1775.

Rubin LF, Saunders LZ. Intraocular larva migrans in dogs. Pathol Vet 1965; 2:566-573.

Ryan AM, Diters RW. Clinical and pathologic features of canine ocular melanomas. J Am Vet Med Assoc 1984; 184:60-67.

Saunders LZ. The histopathology of hereditary congenital deafness in white mink. Pathol Vet 1965; 2:256-263.

Saunders LZ, Barron CN. Intraocular tumors in animals. IV. Lymphosarcoma. Brit Vet J 1964; 126:25-35.

Schmidt GM, Krehbiel JD, Coley SC, Leid RW. Equine ocular onchocerciasis: Histopathologic study. Am J Vet Res 1982; 43:1371-1375.

Schmidt SY, Berson EL, Hayes KC. Retinal degeneration in cats fed casein. I. Taurine deficiency. Invest Ophthalmol 1976; 15:47-52.

Shively JN, Whiteman CE. Ocular lesions in disseminated coccidioidomycosis. Pathol Vet 1970; 7:1-6.

Slatter DH, Lavach JD, Severin GA, Young S. Ubereiter's syndrome (chronic superficial keratitis) in dogs in the Rocky Mountain area: A study of 463 cases. J Small Anim Pract 1977; 18:757-772.

van der Linde-Sipman JS, Stades FC, de Wolff-Rouendaal D. Persistent hyperplastic tunica vasculosa lentis and persistent hyperplastic primary vitreous in the Doberman pinscher: Pathological aspects. J Am Anim Hosp Assoc 1983; 19:791-802.

Watson WA, Terlecki S, Patterson DSP, Sweasey D, Herbert CN, Done JT. Experimentally produced progressive retinal degeneration (bright blindness) in sheep. Brit Vet J 1972; 128:457-469.

Whiteley HE, Young S, Liggitt HD, DeMartini JC. Ocular lesions of bovine malignant catarrhal fever. Vet Pathol 1985; 22:219-225.

Wilcock BP. The eye and ear. In: Jubb KVF, Kennedy PC, Palmer N, eds. Pathology of Domestic Animals. Vol 1. 4th ed. New York: Academic, 1993:441-530.

Index

NOTE: *f* following a page number denotes a figure.

B

C

E

F

G

H

I

N

O

P

Q

R

U

V